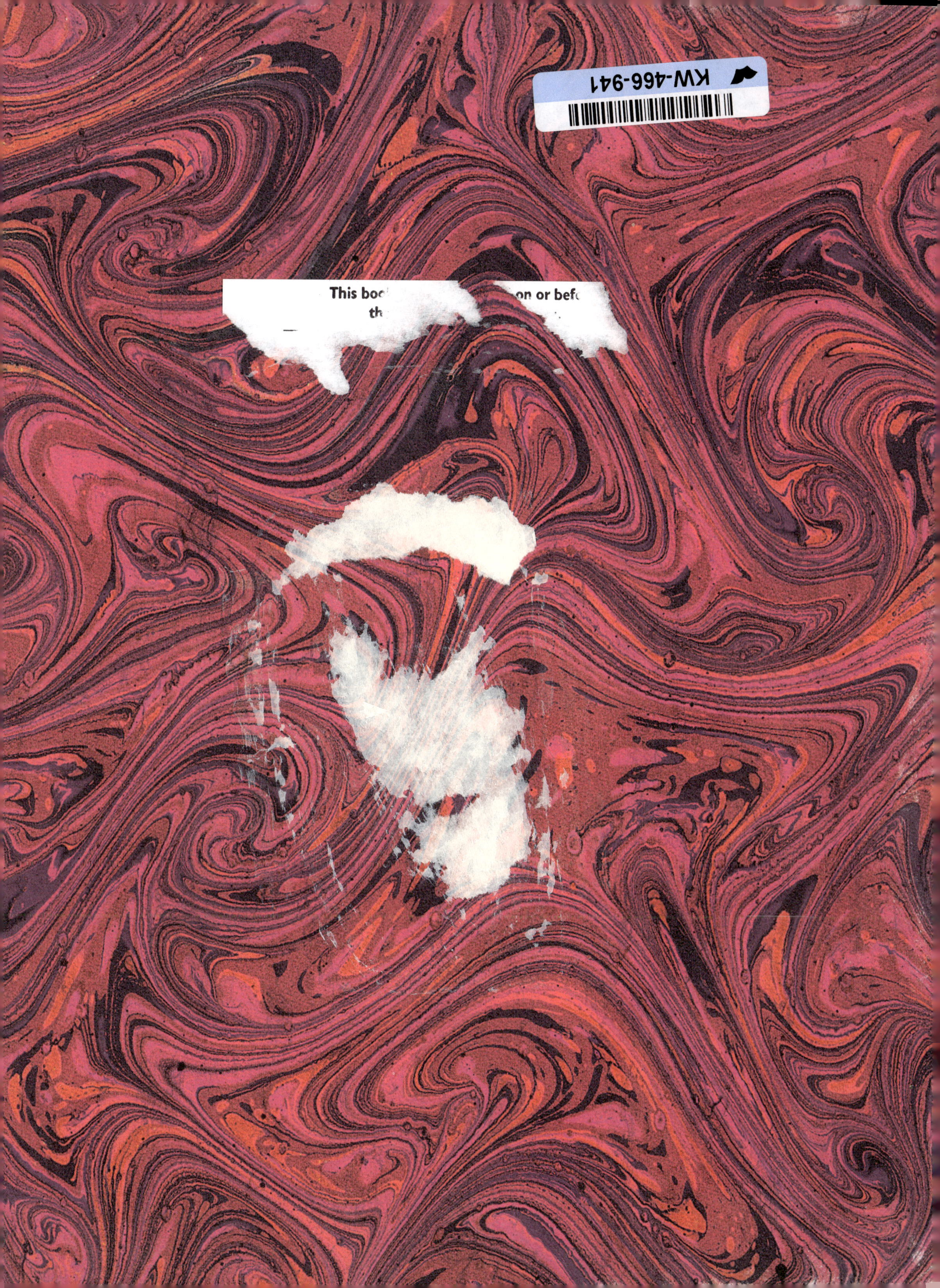
KW-466-941

The Retina Atlas

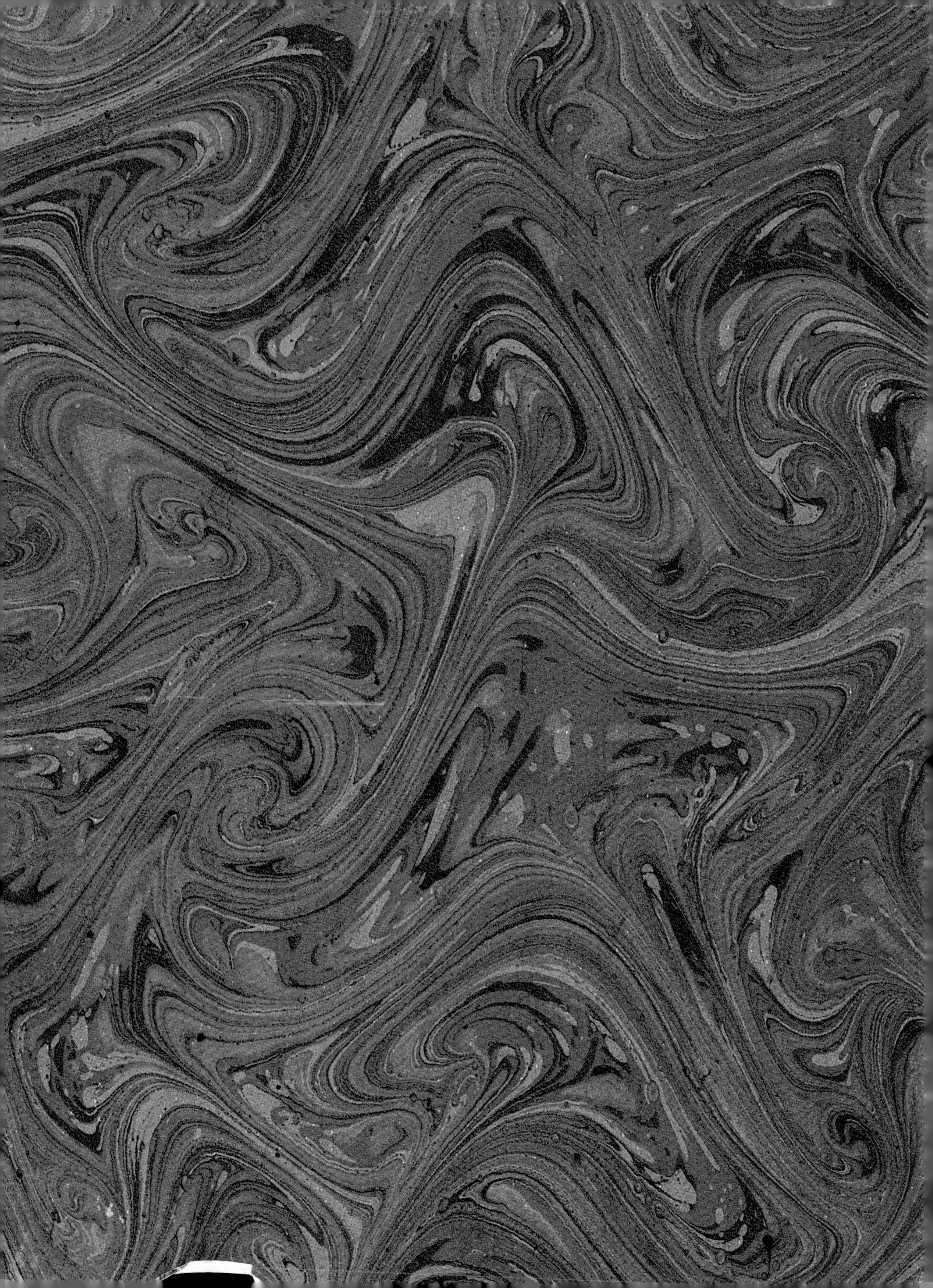

The Retina Atlas

Lawrence A. Yannuzzi, M.D.
Vice Chairman and Director of Retinal Services
Manhattan Eye, Ear, and Throat Hospital
Professor of Clinical Ophthalmology
Columbia University Medical School
New York, New York

David R. Guyer, M.D.
Director of Residency Training
Manhattan Eye, Ear, and Throat Hospital
Clinical Associate Professor of Ophthalmology
Cornell University Medical Center
New York, New York

W. Richard Green, M.D.
Professor of Ophthalmology and Pathology
International Order of Odd Fellows Professor
of Ophthalmology
Johns Hopkins University School of Medicine
Baltimore, Maryland

with 1693 *illustrations*

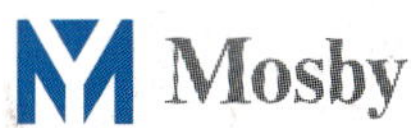

St. Louis Baltimore Boston
Carlsbad Chicago Naples New York Philadelphia Portland
London Madrid Mexico City Singapore Sydney Tokyo Toronto Wiesbaden

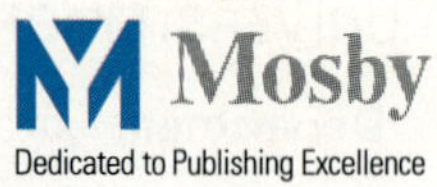

A Times Mirror
Company

Editor: Laurel Craven
Developmental Editor: Dana Battaglia
Project Manager: Linda Clarke
Production: Deborah Ann Cicirello
Interior Design: Sheilah Barrett
Cover Design: Nancy McDonald
Electronic Production Coordinator: Christine H. Poullain
Manufacturing Manager: Theresa Fuchs
Medical Illustrator: Kimberly M. Battista

Additional credit information can be found at the end of the text.

Printed in Spain
Composition by Mosby Electronic Production, Philadelphia
Printing/binding by Grafos S.A.

Mosby–Year Book, Inc.
11830 Westline Industrial Drive
St. Louis, MO 63416

Library of Congress Cataloging-in-Publication Data

Yannuzzi, Lawrence A., 1937-
The retina atlas / Lawrence A. Yannuzzi, David R. Guyer, William R. Green ; with illustrations by Kimberly M. Battista, medical illustrator.
p. cm.
Includes bibliographical references and index.
ISBN 0-8151-3432-0
1. Retina—Diseases—Atlases. I. Guyer, David R. II. Green, William Richard. III. Title.
[DNLM: 1. Retinal Diseases—atlases. WW 17 Y23r 1995]
RE551.Y36 1995
617.7'3'0222—dc20
DNLM/DLC
for Library of Congress 94-31577
CIP

95 96 97 98 99 / 9 8 7 6 5 4 3 2 1

To the memory of a dear friend,
LuEsther T. Mertz,
with admiration, gratitude, and love

L.A.Y.

To my parents
for their constant and incredible support,
love, and encouragement

D.R.G.

To Janet, Parke, and Gordon

W.R.G.

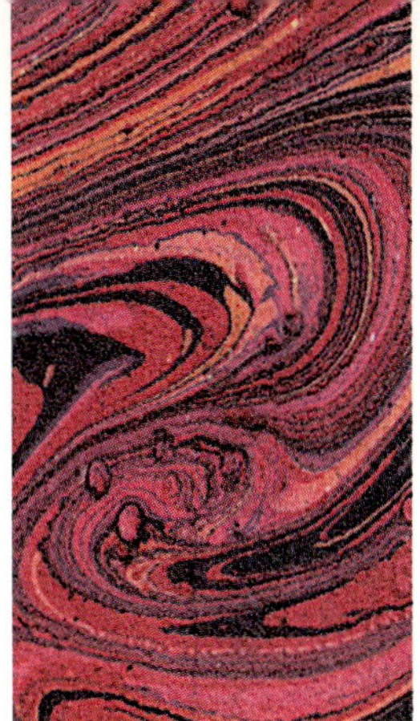

Foreword

"Often," wrote Carlyle, "I have found a portrait superior in real instruction to half a dozen biographies." So begins the foreword written by William Holland Wilmer for his own *Atlas Fundus Oculi,* published in 1934 by the MacMillan Company in New York. This book, with glorious hand painted fundus images created by Annette Burgess at the Wilmer Eye Institute, was the most influential color atlas of its type and era. Dr. Wilmer noted that "it is impossible to reproduce perfectly by artificial means the beauty and the brilliancy of the ever-changeful, living fundus designed by the greatest of all artists—Nature." In Dr. Wilmer's time, fundus photography was a newly emerging technique, and he was convinced that "it cannot take the place of reproductions in color by the brush." Of course, technology advances, and new diagnostic procedures, such as angiography of the fundus, are invented. In the current volume, the authors have amassed, much as a curator would, wonderfully illustrative fundus photos, angiograms, and histopathologic photomicrographs. They constitute a remarkable compendium of dramatic and educational photographs of diseased human fundi. Yes, phenocopies and genocopies exist, mimicking each other, because living tissues, including the retina and choroid, often have limited ways of responding to different pathologic insults. Suprisingly, however, the retina and choroid have such a diversity of response patterns that precise diagnosis is often possible by simple ophthalmoscopic inspection. Dr. Wilmer would be delighted with the advance of ophthalmoscopic and photographic skills in the years since he so laboriously compiled his remarkable atlas, and I believe he would be particularly stimulated by progress made possible by angiography and histopathology.

More than most other physicians, ophthalmologists are required to be adept at pattern recognition. This skill is particularly desirable for retinal specialists, because expert clinicians should be able to identify disease patterns (and often specific etiologies) on the basis of characteristic and sometimes pathognomonic appearances in the fundus. Disease categories, such as congenital, inherited, traumatic, toxic senescent, infectious, and others, can often be accurately identified ophthalmoscopically. Moreover, in the case of an infectious disease, for example, careful ophthalmoscopy is often sufficient to differentiate among various etiologies, including bacteria, viruses, fungi, and even protozoa. Similar diagnostic specificity applies to almost all of the other major disease categories also. The unique ability of a retinal specialist to visualize living internal structures of the body through noninvasive means provides unparalleled diagnostic and therapeutic potential, along with enormous professional and emotional gratification for the physician.

In Dr. Wilmer's day, the color plates of the fundi went through complex printing, often with 8 to 16 impressions for each final version in offset lithography. Personal inspection of Mrs. Burgess' original illustrations in the collection of the Wilmer Institute reveals that the publisher did a remarkably faithful job in reproducing her magnificent and lifelike paintings. Because today's printing processes are vastly superior to older ones, the illustrations in the current volume are, as one would anticipate, more accurate and instructive, and, as one would also expect, the precision of diagnosis has markedly improved over the last six decades.

This volume represents a labor of love by expert ophthalmologists and clinical scientists. Their efforts will be rewarded by the gratitude of clinicians and patients and by the incalculable pleasure their photographs bring to both the casual and the discerning reader.

Morton F. Goldberg, M.D.
Director
The Wilmer Eye Institute
Baltimore, Maryland

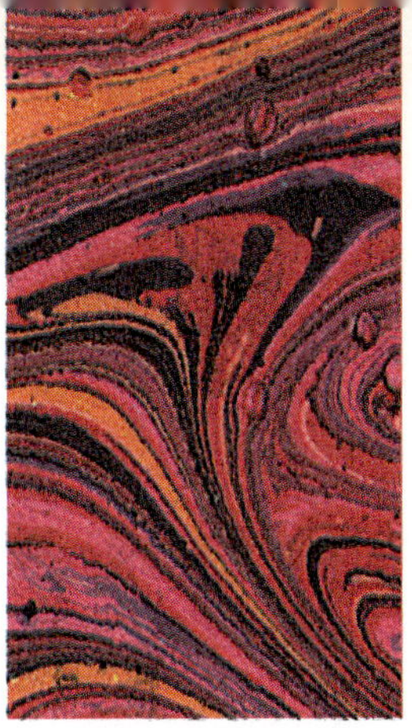

Preface

The Retina Atlas is devoted to medical retinal diseases. The medical retinal specialty finds its origins in the classic 1967 description of "The Pathogenesis of Disciform Detachment of the Neuroepithiums," by Dr. J. Donald Gass, which was published initially as a supplemental issue of the American Journal of Ophthalmology. Prior to this milestone in the field, specialists in "retina" were essentially "bucklers"—individuals trained to excel in indirect ophthalmoscopy in order to find "breaks" to reattach the retina.

Armed with a new diagnostic adjunct (fluorescein angiography), inspired by Gass's brilliant and original work along a broad chorioretinal front, and catalyzed by the potential for new forms of treatment (most notably laser photocoagulation), a new breed of retinal specialists began to emerge in the beginning of the 1970s.

Coincidental with and consequential to evolutionary changes in ophthalmologic subspecialization was the proliferation of a number of superb medical retina texts and atlases by a score of academicians. Although many important literary contributions on the retina preceded this period, a few notable contributions from distinguished international figures who emerged at this time set the trend for future developments in the medical retinal specialty. These individuals included Dr. Koichi Shimizu (Japan), who wrote "Atlas of Fluorescein Fundus Angiography" in 1968 (with Dr. Shin-ichi Shikano), "Microangiopathy of the Ocular Fundus" in 1973, and "Fluorescein Angiography" in 1974; Dr. Achim Wessing (Germany), who wrote "Fluorescein Angiography of the Retina" in 1969; Dr. Emanuel Rosen (England), who wrote "Fluorescence Photography of the Eye" in 1969; and Dr. J. Donald Gass (United States), who wrote "Stereoscopic Atlas of Macular Diseases" in 1969. At the same time a coincidental and unexpected development—the advent of medical lasers—was to have a major impact on the specialty. This monumental advance resulted originally from the pioneering work by Dr. Gerd Meyer-Schwekerath on *Licht Koagulation* in 1969, then subsequently from the introduction of the "Argon laser delivery system through a slit-lamp biomicroscope for applications in ophthalmology" by Dr. Lloyd Aiello, Dr. Francis L'Esperance, Dr. Arnall Patz, and Dr. H. Christian Zweng. This innovative technology justified medical retinal pursuits simply because of the potential for treatment of chorioretinal diseases.

The first medical retinal specialists were soon to be joined and eventually supplanted by an elite corps of academic clinicians who were exquisitely trained in the meticulous, diagnostic, and therapeutic methodologies of the discipline and skilled in critical and factual analysis of their observations. The other texts and atlases that would also serve as primers in the 1970s for future medical retinal specialists were *Arlie House Symposium on the Treatment of Diabetic Retinopathy*, edited by Dr. Morton Goldberg and Dr. Stuart Fine in 1968; a text, *Laser Photocoagulation and Retinal Angiography,* by Dr. H. Christian Zweng, Dr. Hunter L. Little, and Dr. Robert R. Peabody in 1969; *Stereo Atlas on the Differential of Intraocular Tumors* by J. Donald Gass in 1970; *The Retinal Circulation* by Dr. George Wise, Dr. Colin Dollery, and Dr. Paul Henkind in 1971; a text and atlas called *Hereditary Dystrophy of the Posterior Pole* by Dr. August Deutmen in 1971; a text and atlas entitled *Hereditary Retinal and Choroidal Diseases* by Dr. Alex Krill in 1972; *A Stereoscopic Atlas on Ocular Photocoagulation* by Dr. Francis L'Esperance in 1975; a text and atlas called *Interpretation of Fundus Fluorescein Angiography* by Dr. Howard Schatz, Dr. Tom Burton, Dr. Lawrence Yannuzzi, and Dr. Maurice Rabb in 1978; *The Macula: A Comprehensive Text and Atlas*, edited by Dr. Lawrence Yannuzzi, Dr. Kurt Gitter, and Dr. Howard Schatz in 1979; and a series of texts, slides, and atlases on diabetic retinopathy and other retinal vascular diseases (1971 through 1983) from the Wilmer Eye Institute, principally authored by Dr. Stuart Fine, Dr. David Orth, and Dr. Arnall Patz.

Collectively, these publications formed a literary chronicle of the early history of the medical retina specialty; their scholarly text and beautiful illustrations documented technological improvements in imaging of the fundus, newly identifed and better defined chorioretinal entities, and established treatment strategies. As knowledge accumulated, many other texts and atlases followed; these were written by new authors who elucidated the multiple, tortuous ways in which the medical retina specialty evolved. These textbooks provided a practical, current, comprehensive, and authoritative account of the field, embellished with succinct and unique concepts in design. Within collaborative formats, these individuals and others performed research to establish incontrovertible forms of treatment based on fundus imaging as a guide for laser treatment, beginning with diabetic retinopathy and branch retinal vein occlusion and extending more recently to neovascularized maculopathies. The National Institutes of Health played a key role in supporting such research by virtue of collaborative trials such as the Diabetic Retinopathy Study and the Macula Photocoagulation Study, which defined and legitimized laser treatment concepts that were eventually described in the ophthalmic literature.

So, why another medical retinal text? The rationale for our book's existence originated in the independent, but ultimately conjugate opinions of three sources: the publisher, a few colleagues, and the authors. First, there was recognition of an apparent, particular need which had not been filled. Previous textbooks on the retina, like any other published product in any other discipline, were generally limited in their mode of presentation and level of comprehensiveness by several factors, a predominant one being cost containment. Mosby–Year Book, Inc., was in 1994 preeminent in the ophthalmic publishing field in the area of retina, by virtue of two very prestigious and successful texts; the new edition of *Stereo Atlas of Macular Diseases,* by Dr. J. Donald Gass, and *Retina,* a three-volume multiauthored text edited principally by Dr. Stephen Ryan. Limitations in size and publishing costs restricted the use of color illustrations in Gass's book to attached stereo slides which required a viewer. Likewise, the use of color in the Ryan series was limited because of the sheer size and complexity of the three volume work.

At the suggestion of colleagues, the publisher approached Lawrence A. Yannuzzi and David. R Guyer in early 1994 with a proposal: the opportunity to publish a comparatively large, color atlas on medical retinal diseases; essentially a companion to the Ryan text. In spite of several elegant and sophisticated imaging systems commonly available and generally developed within the field, there was an assumption that no clinical picture was as dynamically instructive and as asthetically pleasing to ophthalmologists as color illustrations. If it is true that physicians are attracted to the field of ophthalmology because of an interest in visual images, retinal specialists must have an inherent passion for the same experiences. In what other internal medical specialty can clinicians witness a disease entity, its natural progression, and its response to treatment so vividly?

Although angiography and other forms of imaging are diagnostic adjuncts of tremendous clinical value, there is no substitute for the physician-in-training as well as the experienced specialist to see, and recognize or diagnose, a manifestation or disease "as is" in the clinical setting in full, natural color.

We agreed that there was a need for a single volume in which every consequential medical retinal disease could be presented in color—or, if you will, *in vivo*, since no such text was available or known to be in preparation. We were convinced that a text of this sort could best serve as a contemporary compendium for the study of medical retinal diseases if strengthened by the addition of clinicopathological correlations. This decision to expand the concept of the atlas was predicated on the belief that the greatest reward for readers would be the recognition of a clinical manifestation or entity and the acquisition of greater insight on the pathophysiologic mechanisms of diseases of the ocular fundus.

Enter Dr. W. Richard Green, undeniably the world's most knowledgeable and prestigious ocular pathologist in the area of retinal disease. As a tireless educator who has never learned to say "no" to an invitation to teach or to any academic challenge, particularly one with reasonable promise to provide yet another documentation of his legendary work, he joined the team of authors quite willingly and enthusiastically.

Given the rationale for the text, the next phase was to conceive a useful design that would best serve professionals in the field of eye care, ranging from physicians-in-training to medical retinal specialists, and including general ophthalmologists without particular expertise in the area of retina. The chapters were set-up to correspond to the Ryan text, which was also to provide definitive text, relevant references, and an exhaustive bibliography. However, the plan was to expand the text's usefulness so that it could largely stand alone to provide the field of ophthalmology with a timely and pertinent source of information. The urge to include stereo photography, while compelling, was abandoned simply because of its impracticality. The inclusion of every conceivable case was also deemed impossible on the basis of traditional limitations in publishing. Some newer concepts in layout and production were devised in an attempt to facilitate the presentation of the material in a "reader friendly" and instructional format. These included multicolored schematic line drawings and group photo identification.

The authors began their search for illustrations by rummaging through a retinal attic to harvest a trunk's worth of cases from classic illustrations of common findings (for necessary clinical knowledge and for general enhancement of pattern recognition) and certain unusual or rare manifestations and typical variations on clinical themes—even a few that have not been previously reported in the ophthalmic literature. Despite nearly 30 years of collecting slides, there were still conspicuous absences for a comprehensive text. There is no better way to fill such voids than to call on colleagues and friends—good friends—who uniformly fulfilled our expectations by promptly combing through their files to provide us with examples of missing, pertinent material. So, our gracious thanks to many, particularly Dr. Norman Byer, Dr. Ronald Carr, Dr. Lee Jampol, Dr. Irene Maumenee, Dr. William Mieler, Dr. Jerry Shields, Dr. Stuart Fine, Dr. Kurt Gitter, and Dr. Mike Trese.

There are also some cases in the text that we purposely recruited from certain sources or individuals, specifically to provide accurate or standardized representations of entities which they described in the literature or classified with currently accepted definitions. For example, the standardized diabetic retinopathy photographs for Diabetic-2000's classifications, the clinical definitions for the Retinopathy of Prematurity Study Group, and the descriptive terms recommended by the Macular Photocoagulation Study Group for neovascularized age-related macular degeneration were provided by these groups, not by us. Similarly, an example of North Carolina Dystrophy was provided by Dr. Kent Small, who extensively described this maculopathy, not by us. Dr. Norm Byer provided us with a representative series of his own, classical peripheral retinal photographs. The list continues.

The penalty for trying to be comprehensive and instructive solely with color illustrations and within the confines of a publishing schedule predictably led to a compromise in the quality of some of the slides. Although we worked closely with the publisher to ensure quality in the graphic reproductions, there were still some photographs for which the authors—not the publishers must take the blame. Some photographs, selected for their unique features, were not of the best quality, nor were they "originals"; instead they were "copies" or even "copies of copies." This resulted in accentuation of contrast and annoying colormetric imbalances that were technically unavoidable. Furthermore, we simply could not find perfect examples of every important disorder. For these limitations and flaws, we apologize to the readers. If general acceptance of the text dictates a future edition; that is if the book establishes a tradition of excellence, an attempt to remedy these deficiencies is pledged.

So, we thank the publishers (particularly Linda Clarke and Laurel Craven) for their encouragement and assistance; our office and research staffs for technical and editorial work; the Macula Foundation, Inc. (particularly Lisa Meyer and Joan Daly) for its support; our librarian, Dede Silverstone, for her research assistance; William Comstock, for his typing assistance; our colleagues and friends for their inspiration and contributions; and above all, our families for their understanding and love. Thanks to them, we hope that *The Retina Atlas* will find a meaningful and valued place in the *libraries of ophthalmologists, today and in the future.*

Lawrence A. Yannuzzi, M.D.

David R. Guyer, M.D.

W. Richard Green, M.D.

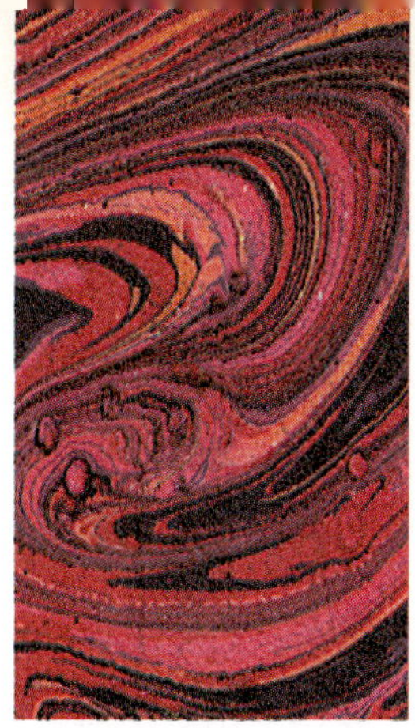

How to Use This Atlas

This atlas follows the chapter order of Stephen Ryan's textbook, *Retina.* Although this order was not necessarily the most logical for an atlas, we have preserved the order so that the two textbooks can more easily be used together. Only chapters describing clinical disorders were included; those sections on basic science material and treatment modalities were not included in this atlas. Thus, the reader can use the atlas to better illustrate the material in Ryan's *Retina* or can use *Retina* to provide detailed information on a topic seen in the atlas. The atlas's purpose is to photographically highlight the various retinal disorders. No attempt was made to provide detailed narrative about the various conditions. These factual details are easily found in the accompanying chapter in *Retina.* In addition, the atlas's purpose is to highlight macular disorders; surgical and peripheral retinal conditions are discussed only briefly.

In general, we have tried to illustrate basic findings of each disorder in the beginning of each chapter and then present more esoteric and rarer cases at the end of the chapter.

A color scheme has been introduced to make this atlas easier to use. Blue or green borders around photographs indicate that these photographs are from the same patient. Red borders indicate a clinicopathologic correlation.

We hope that you will find this atlas not only informative, but "user friendly."

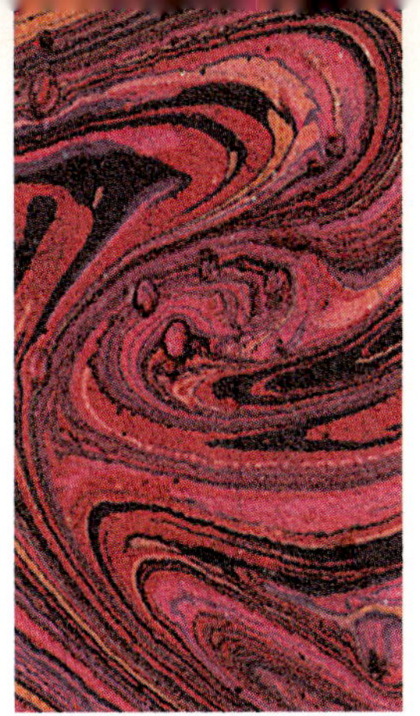

Contents

Part VII Retinal Vascular Diseases

Part VIII Inflammatory Diseases

Part IX Other Diseases

Part X Optic Nerve Diseases

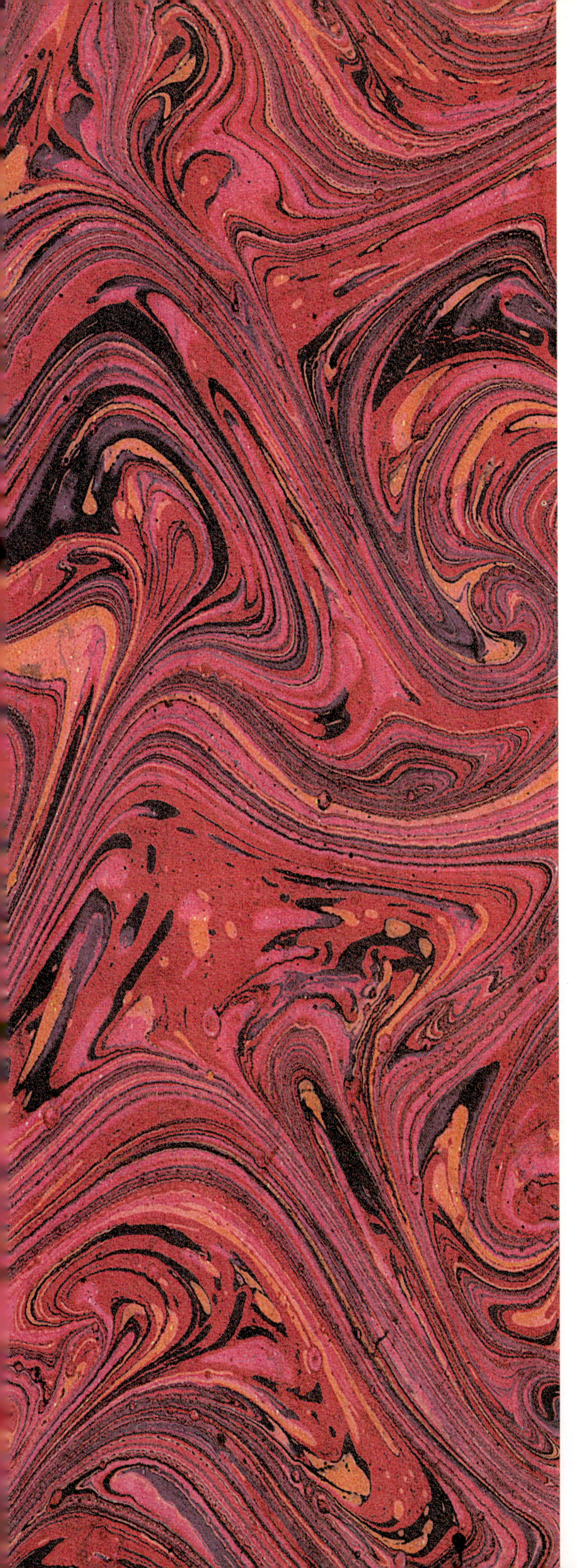

Part I

Retinal Degenerations and Dystrophies

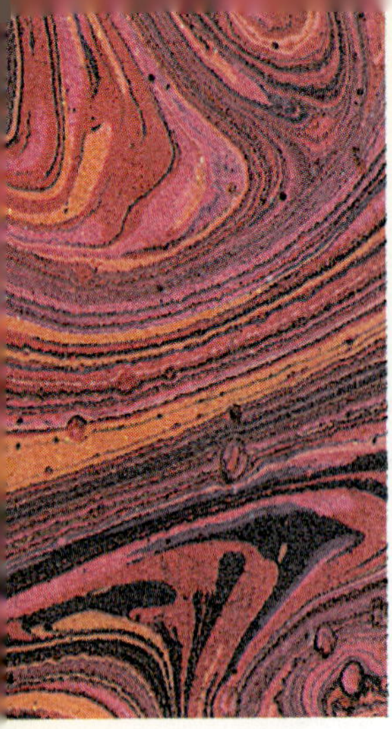

Chapter 1

Retinitis Pigmentosa and Allied Disorders

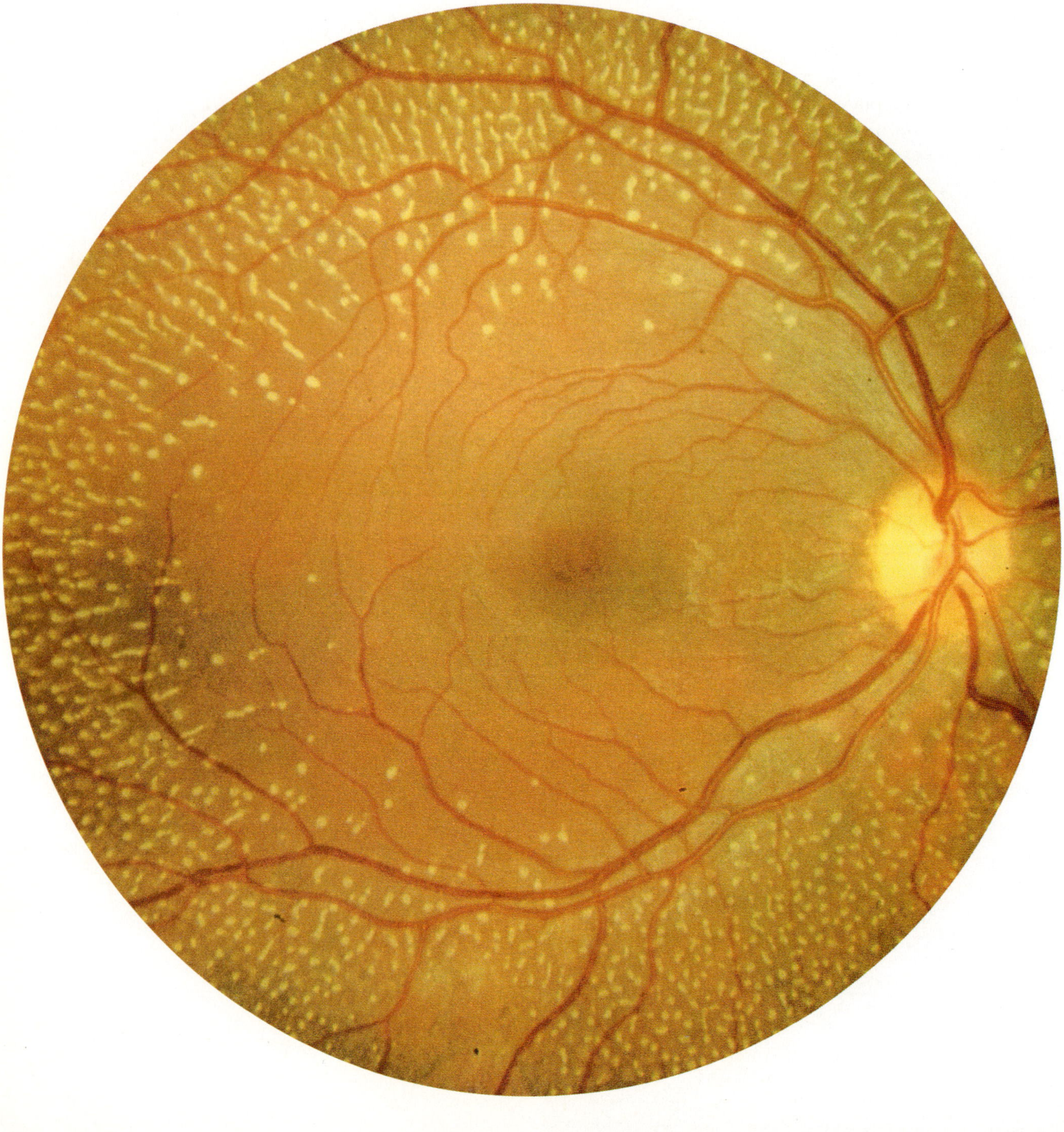

Retinitis pigmentosa is the most common hereditary retinal dystrophy. The condition has various inheritance patterns, which include an autosomal dominant pattern (10%–24%), an autosomal recessive pattern (13%–69%); and an X-linked recessive pattern (5%–21%). The condition may also be sporadic. Affected patients often note difficulty with night and/or peripheral vision early in life. The classic retinal findings include midperipheral paravenular bone spicules, attenuated arterioles, and a waxy pallor of the optic disc. Other findings may include retinal pigment epithelium mottling and atrophy, cystoid macular edema, epiretinal membranes, optic nerve drusen, a Coats'-like response, and posterior subcapsular cataracts. In addition, these patients may have vitreous changes, including veils, condensations, detachment, and pigmented cells.

Various systemic diseases may be associated with a pigmentary retinopathy. Usher's syndrome is an autosomal recessive condition consisting of retinitis pigmentosa and deafness. Vestibulocerebellar ataxia and a pigmented retinopathy occur with Hallgren's syndrome. Laurence-Moon and Bardet-Biedl syndromes are autosomal recessive disorders that consist of retinitis pigmentosa, mental retardation, and hypogenitalism. Patients with Bardet-Biedl syndrome may also demonstrate polydactyly and/or obesity; in patients with Laurence-Moon syndrome, hemiparesis may be noted. Some investigators lump these syndromes into one condition. Bassen-Kornzweig disease (abetalipoproteinemia or hereditary acanthocytosis) is an autosomal recessive syndrome consisting of ataxia, fat intolerance due to internal malabsorption, and defective erythrocytes (acanthocytosis). Treatment with vitamin A may be effective. Kearns-Sayre syndrome is an autosomal dominant disorder consisting of progressive external ophthalmoplegia, pigmentary retinopathy, cardiac arrhythmias, and heart block. Patients with this condition demonstrate ragged red fibers on muscle biopsy; the disease is of mitochondrial origin. Pseudoretinitis pigmentosa may be associated with syphilis, drug toxicity, trauma, pigmented paravenous chorioretinal atrophy, and chorioretinitis.

1–1

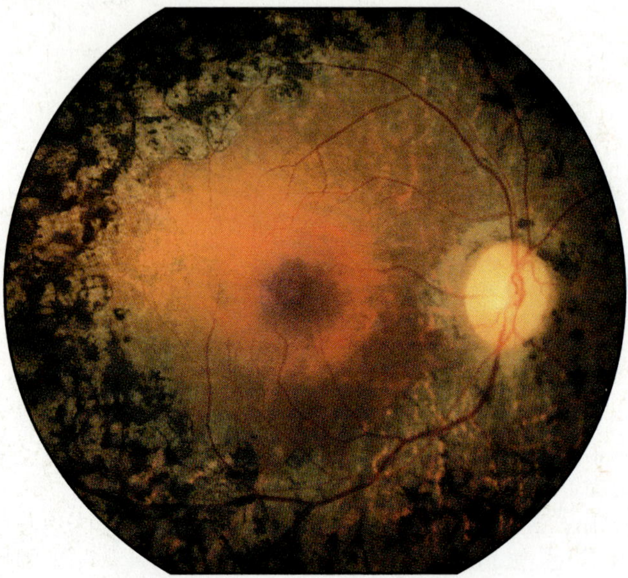

1–1 This patient illustrates the classic clinical features of retinitis pigmentosa. Note the bone spicules, epiretinal membrane, attenuated retinal vessels, and the waxy pallor of the optic disc.

1–1, *Courtesy of Mark Croswell.*

1–2

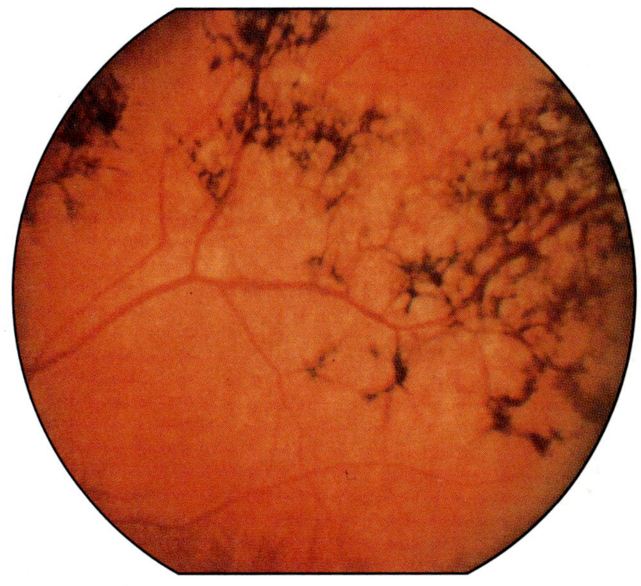

1–3

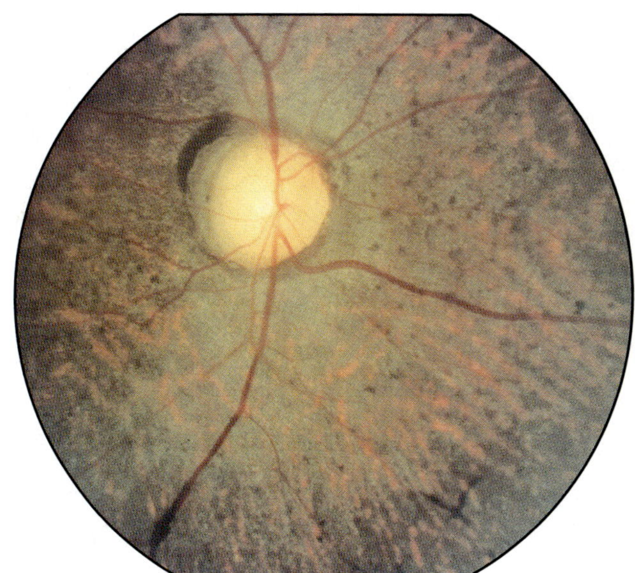

1–4

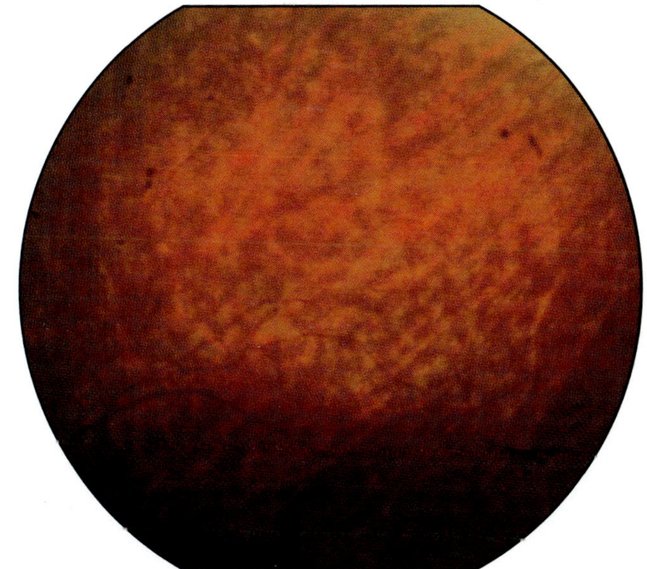

1–5

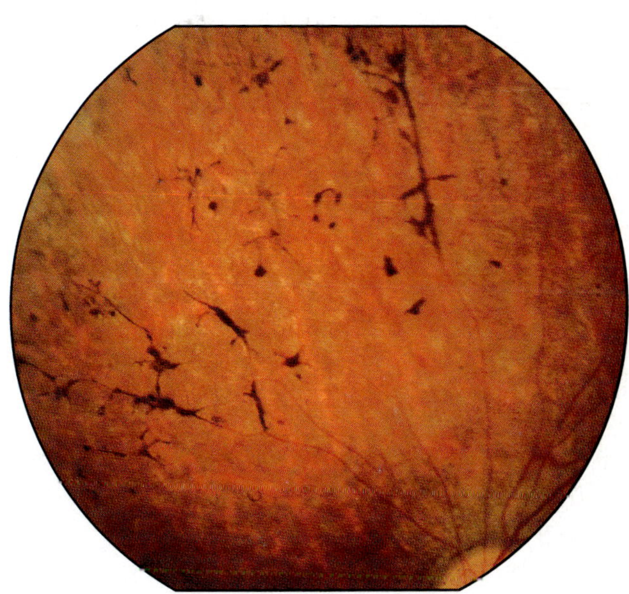

1–2 Bone spicules are noted in the midperiphery in this patient with retinitis pigmentosa.

1–3 Waxy optic disc pallor, attenuated retinal vessels, atrophic retinal pigment epithelium, and bone spicules are demonstrated in this patient.

1–4 Atrophic retinal pigment epithelial changes in the midperiphery may be an early sign in patients with retinitis pigmentosa.

1–5 Classic bone spicules noted in retinitis pigmentosa may be seen within atrophic areas. Attenuated retinal vessels can also be appreciated.

1–6

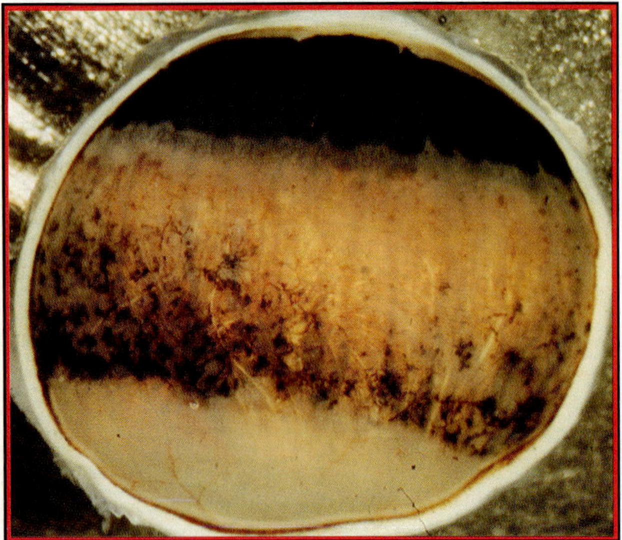

1–7

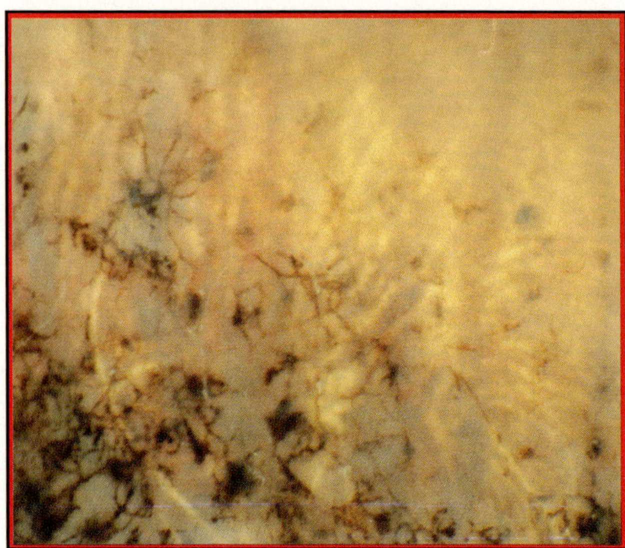

1–8

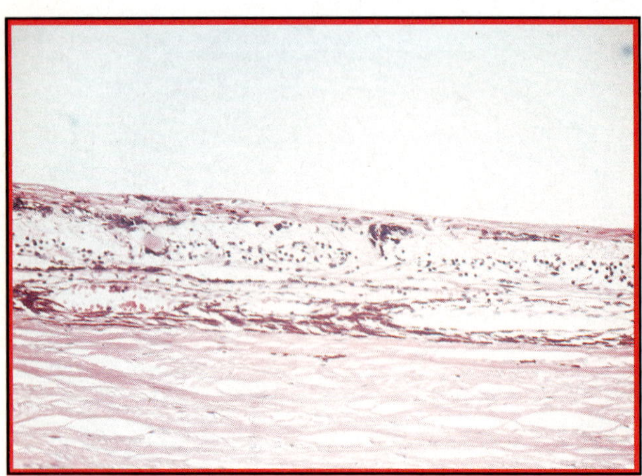

1–6 This patient has retinitis pigmentosa and drusen of the optic nerve head. The first photograph shows the gross pathologic findings of bone spicules.

1–7 Higher magnification reveals the bone spicule pattern.

1–8 Atrophy of the photoreceptor cell layer with hyperplasia and migration of the retinal pigment epithelium into the retina in a perivascular pattern accounts for the bone-spicule appearance.

1–9

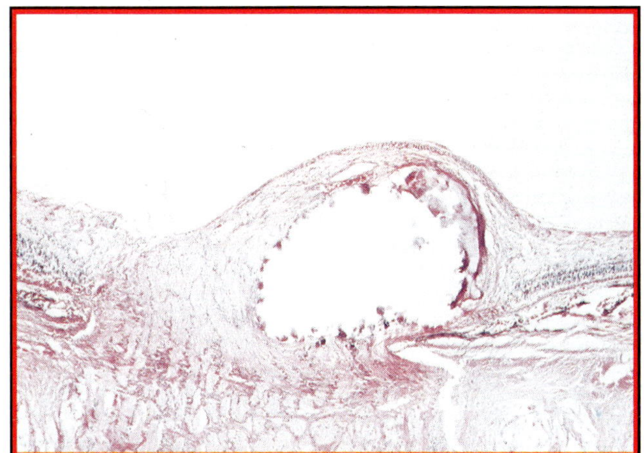

1–10

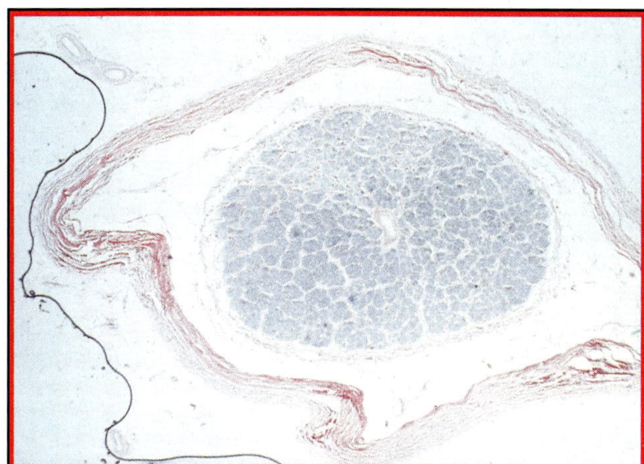

1–11

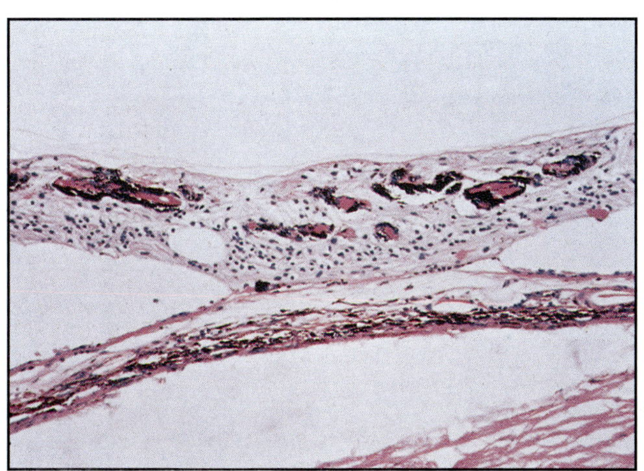

1–9 and 1–10 A 1.25- × 1.0-mm acellular druse of the optic nerve head (1–9) is associated with a sector area of optic atrophy (1–10).

1–11 Another histopathologic case shows photoreceptor atrophy with retinal pigment epithelium hyperplasia and migration into the retina in a perivascular distribution.

1–12 COATS'-LIKE RESPONSE IN RP

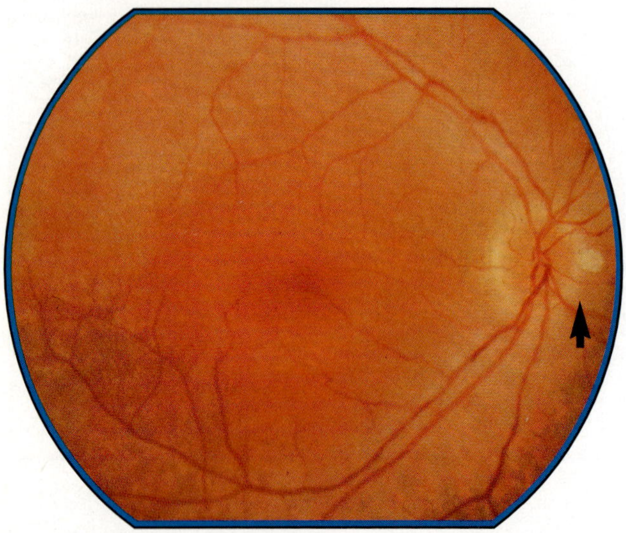

1–13 **1–14**

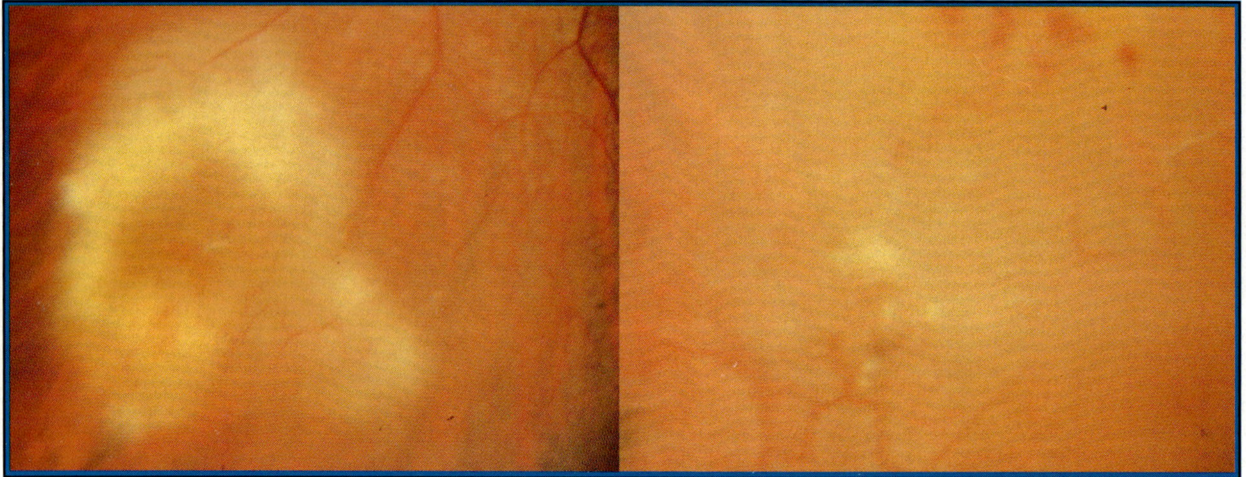

1–12 This patient illustrates the Coats'-like response that occurs in some patients with retinitis pigmentosa. Atrophic areas of retinal pigment epithelium can be seen in the surrounding temporal and infratemporal macula. An astrocytoma of the optic disc is also present *(arrowhead)*.

1–13 and 1–14 Peripheral views of this patient demonstrate the Coats'-like variant of the disease with telangiectasia and marked exudation.

1–12, 1–13, *and* ***1–14,*** *Courtesy of Dr. Stuart L. Fine.*

1–15 ANGIOMA WITH RP

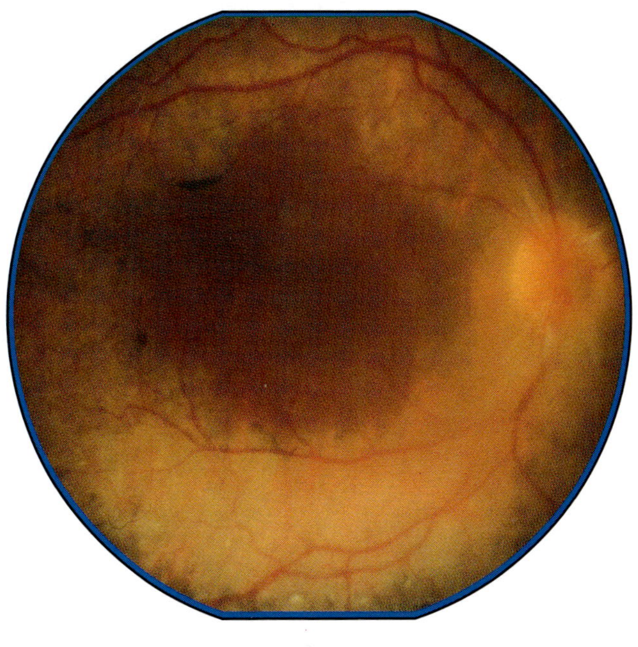

1–16

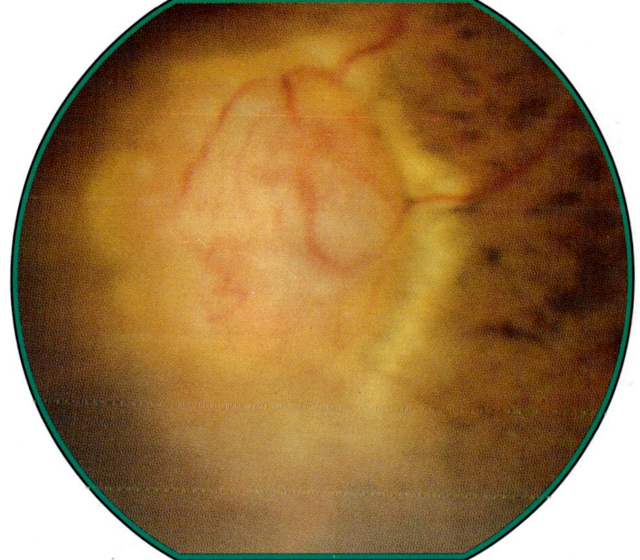

1–17

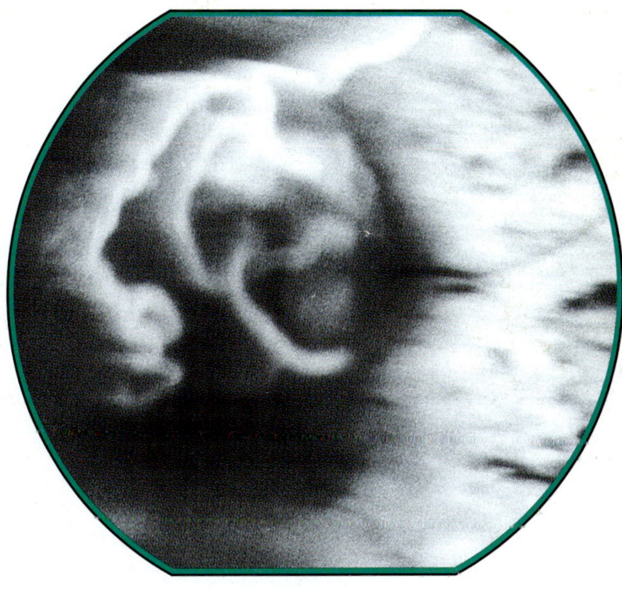

1–15 through 1–17 These Coats'-like findings can range from the telangiectatic-like changes as noted in the last patient to angiomatous-like changes, as seen in this patient. An angiomatous-like lesion is noted in the periphery in this patient with retinitis pigmentosa (1–15, 1–16, and 1–17). Note the classic posterior pole findings of retinitis pigmentosa (1–15). An angiomatous lesion with surrounding lipid exudation is demonstrated in the periphery (1–16). Note the bone-spicule changes next to the lesion. Fluorescein angiography reveals the vascular filling pattern of the tumor (1–17).

1–18 CYSTOID MACULAR EDEMA WITH RP

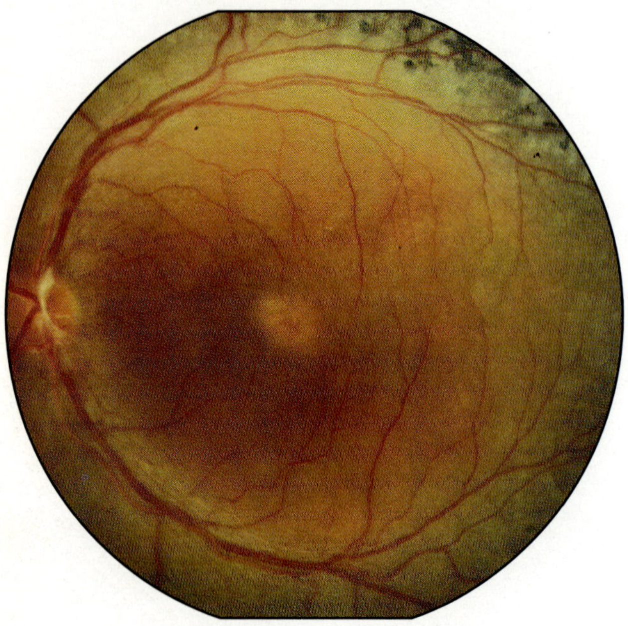

1–19 **1–20**

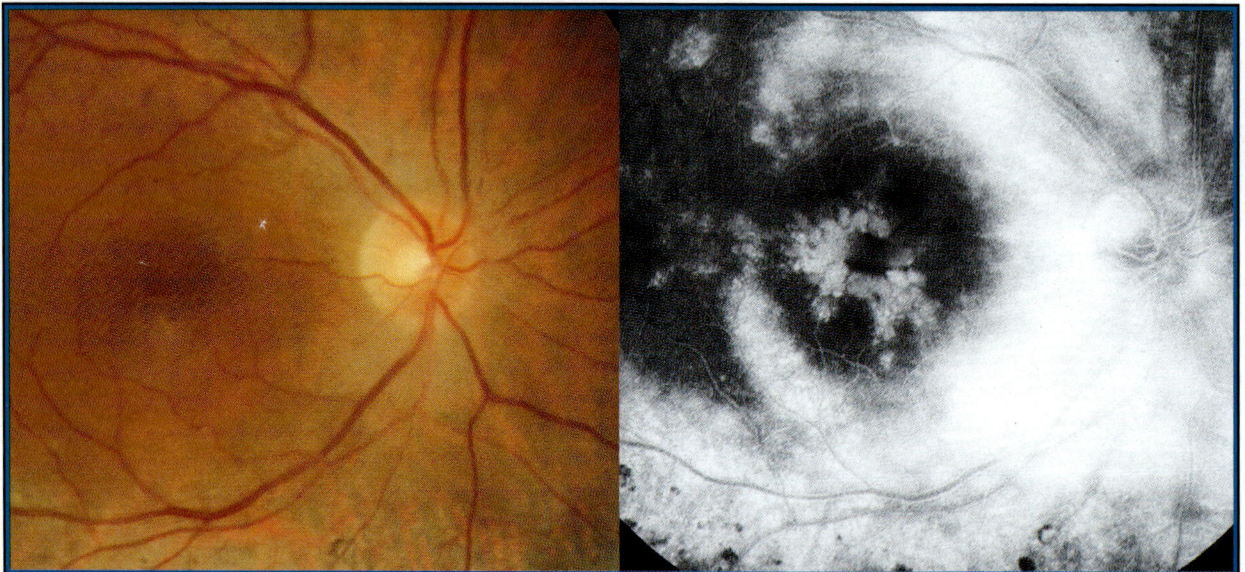

1–18 Cystoid macular edema is another feature that can be seen in patients with retinitis pigmentosa. Note the cystic lesion.

1–19 and 1–20 Cystoid macular edema (1–19) reveals a classic petalloid-like pattern on fluorescein angiography (1–20).

1–21 MACULAR HOLE WITH RP

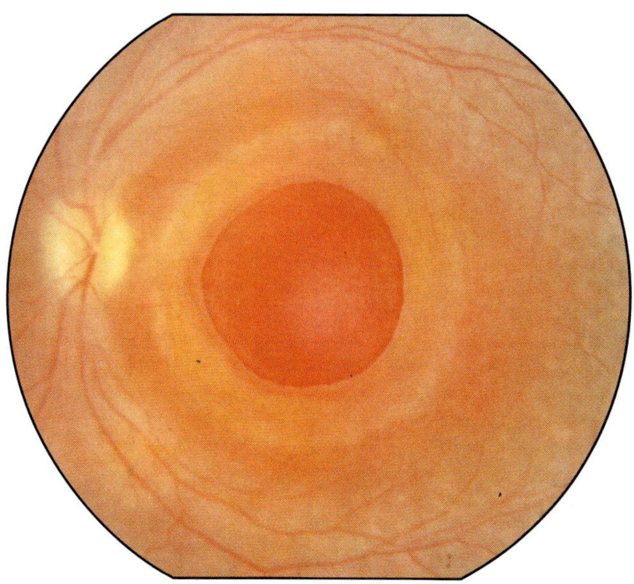

1–22 BARDET-BIEDL SYNDROME

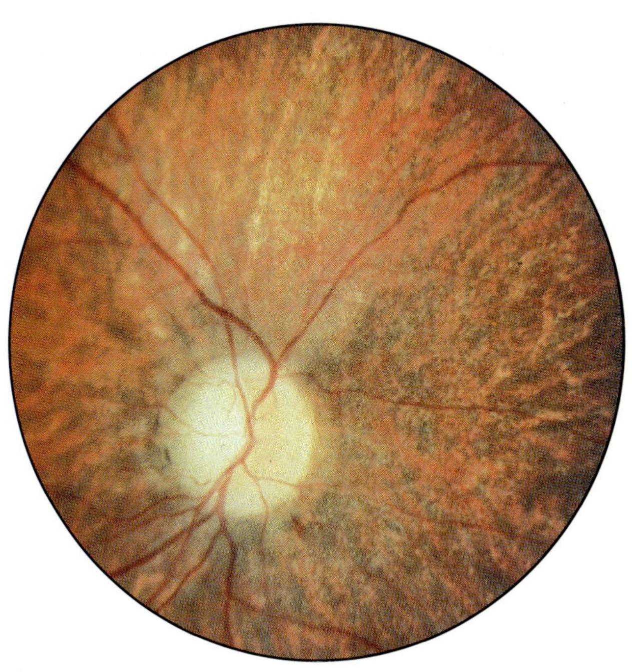

1–23 LAURENCE-MOON SYNDROME

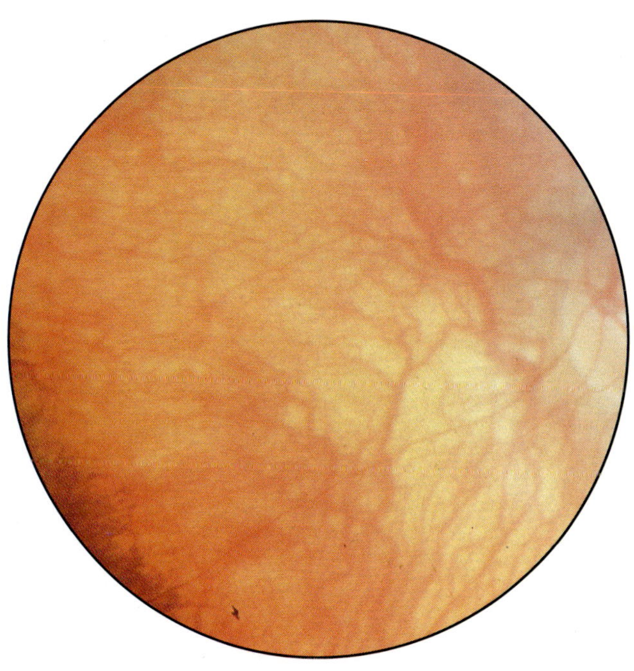

1–21 This patient with retinitis pigmentosa developed a large macular hole, which may or may not be related to the generalized retinal disease.

1–22 Patients with the Bardet-Biedl syndrome demonstrate a pigmentary retinal dystrophy, obesity, mental retardation, hypogenitalism, polydactyly and syndactyly. Ophthalmologic features usually are similar to those of retinitis pigmentosa. In this patient with the Bardet-Biedel syndrome, note the optic atrophy with sheathed vessels and an atrophic pigmentary retinopathy.

1–23 The Laurence-Moon syndrome has characteristics similar to the Bardet-Biedl syndrome. However, polydactyly and obesity are not noted. In addition, patients with the Laurence-Moon syndrome often develop hemiparesis. Ophthalmologic examination may reveal extensive chorioretinal atrophy, as seen in this patient. In more severe cases, the atrophy may resemble choroideremia.

1–22, *From Ryan, SJ: Retina, ed 2, St Louis, 1994, Mosby–Year Book. Courtesy of Bateman, Lang, and Maumenee.* ***1–23,*** *Courtesy of Dr. Irene Maumenee.*

1–24 ALAGILLE'S SYNDROME

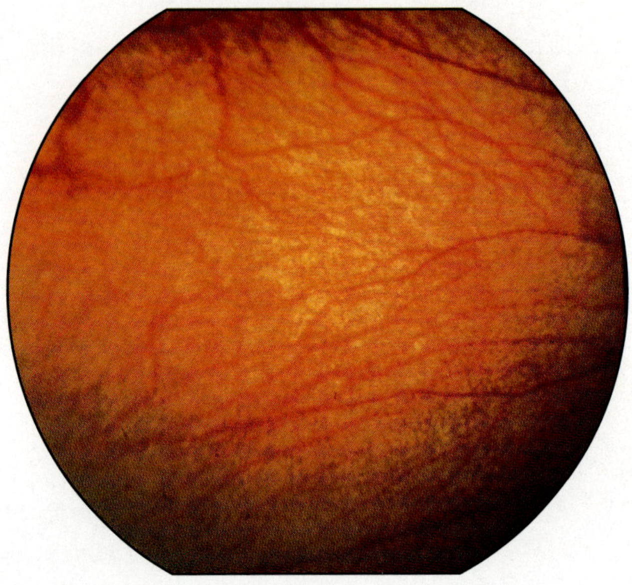

1–24 Alagille's syndrome, or arteriohepatic dysplasia, is characterized by intrahepatic cholestasis with neonatal jaundice, itching, and failure to thrive. Various ocular manifestations include posterior embryotoxon, Axenfeld's anomaly, and a peripheral pigmentary retinopathy. An atrophic pigmentary retinopathy characteristic of this syndrome is demonstrated in this patient

1–24, *Courtesy of Dr. Irene Maumenee.*

1–25 KEARNS-SAYRE SYNDROME

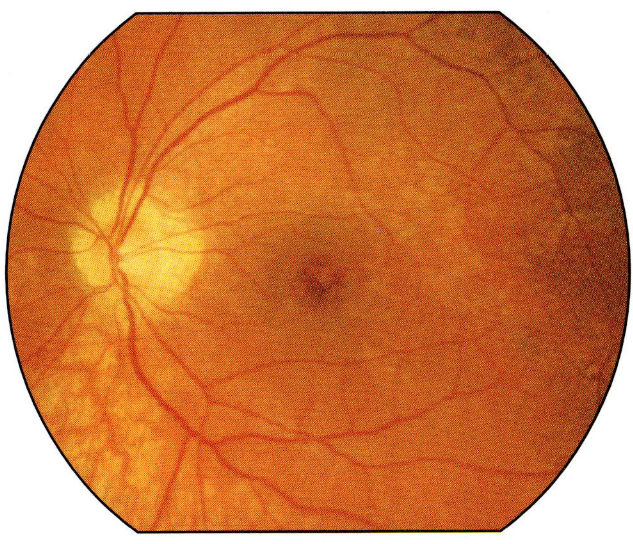

1–26

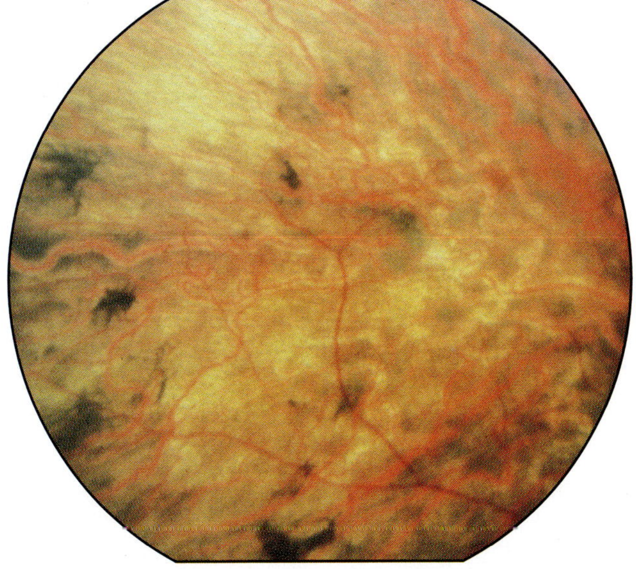

1–27

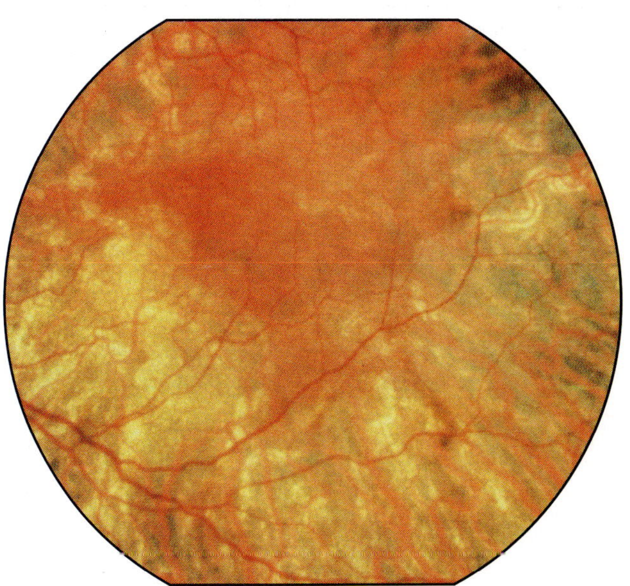

1–25 Pigmentary retinopathy, external ophthalmoplegia with ptosis, and heart block may be noted in patients with the Kearns-Sayre syndrome, which is an autosomal dominant condition. Other characteristics of this syndrome include deafness and hypogonadism. This condition is due to a mitochondrial abnormality and has been termed a "ragged" red fiber myopathy. A widespread salt-and-pepper retinopathy may occur. Pigmentary changes of the peripapillary area are common. The optic disc and retinal vasculature are usually normal. This patient demonstrates pigment mottling in the posterior pole. Also notice the depigmentation in the peripapillary region, especially inferiorly.

1–26 and 1-27 A retinitis pigmentosa–like picture can occasionally be observed (1–26) or more hypopigmented atrophic areas may be noted (1–27).

1–25, *Courtesy of Dr. William Mieler.* ***1–26*** *and* ***1–27,*** *Courtesy of Dr. Irene Maumenee.*

1–28 BASSEN–KORNZWEIG SYNDROME

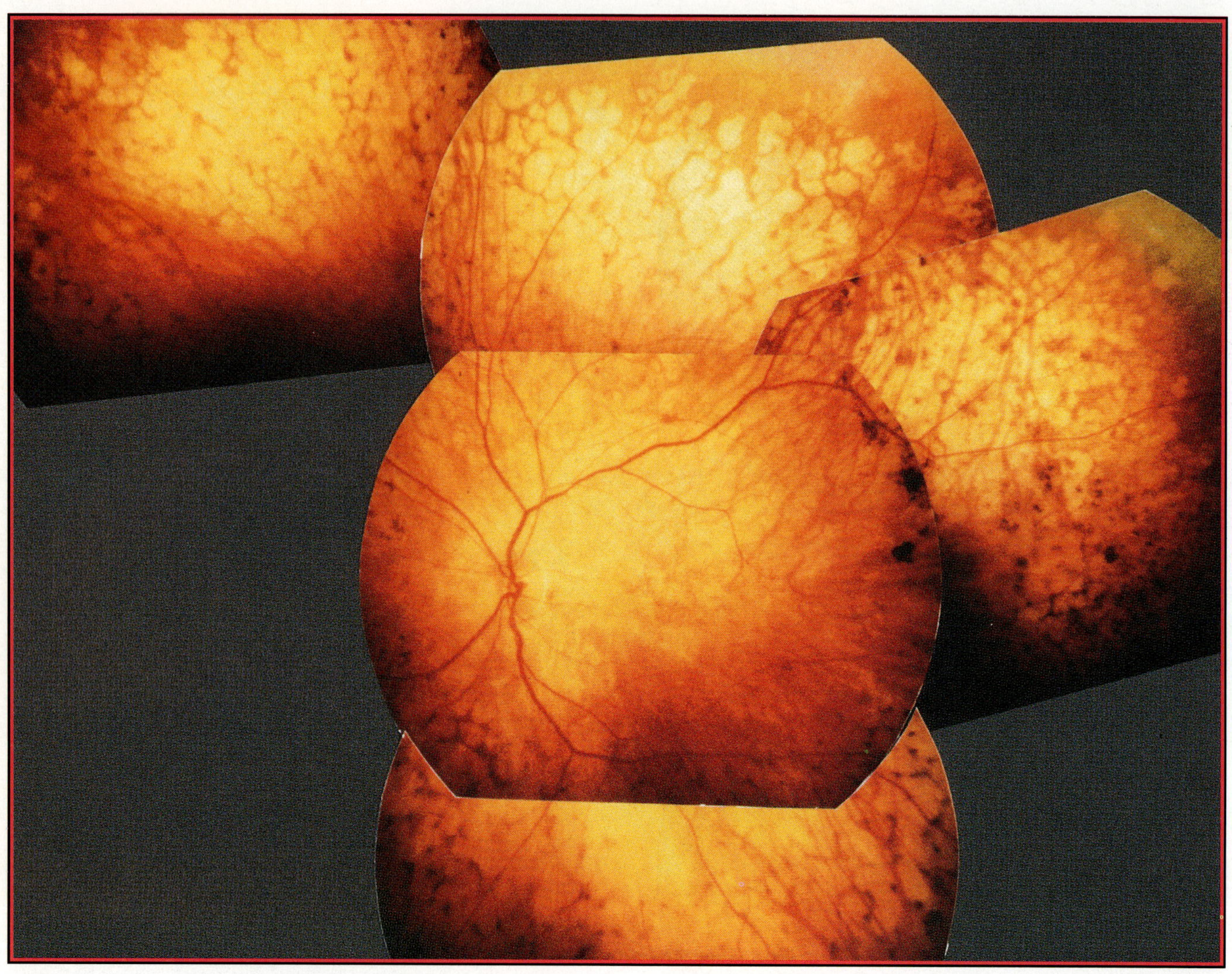

1–29

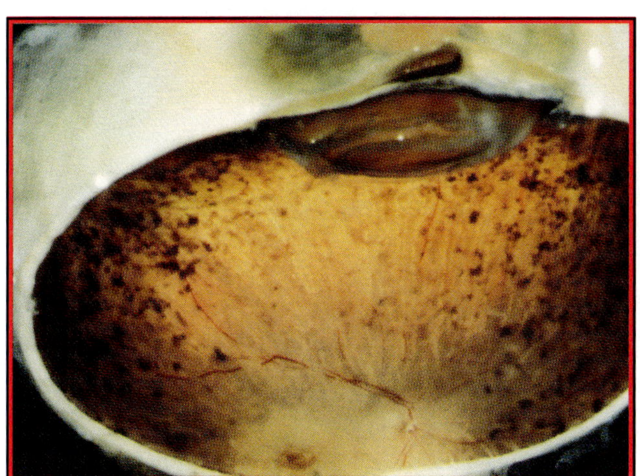

1–30

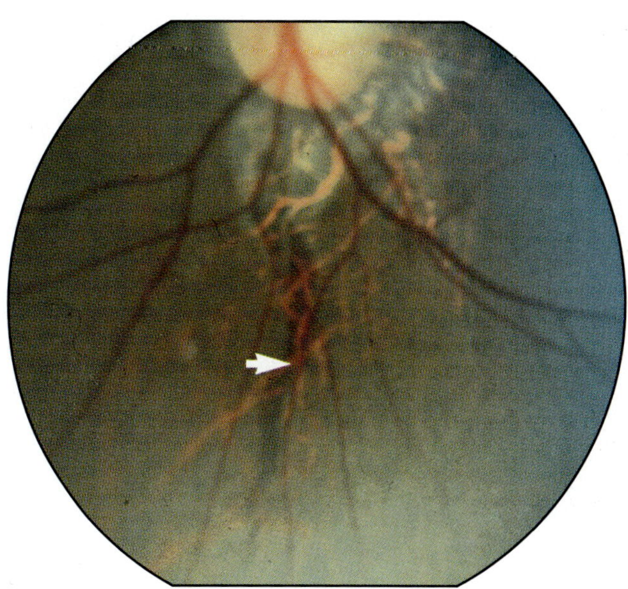

1–28 through 1–30 Patients with the Bassen-Kornzweig syndrome demonstrate a pigmentary retinopathy associated with night blindness and cerebellar ataxia. Affected patients often have celiac syndrome with acanthocytosis. The liver and retina are deprived of vitamin A. Abetalipoproteinemia is common. These patients usually develop a pigmentary retinopathy with a waxy pallor of the optic disc, attenuation of the retinal vessels, and retinal pigment epithelial atrophic changes. The montage illustrates such a patient with a generalized atrophic and pigmentary retinopathy (1–28). Histopathologic evaluation reveals bone spicules (1–29). This patient also has abetalipoproteinemia (1–30). Note the attenuation of the retinal vessels. This patient also has angioid streaks *(arrowhead)*.

1–28 *and* ***1–29,*** *Courtesy of Dr. A. Rodriguez.*

1–30, *Courtesy of Dr. Irene Maumenee.*

1–31 and 1–32 HALLERVORDEN–SPATZ SYNDROME

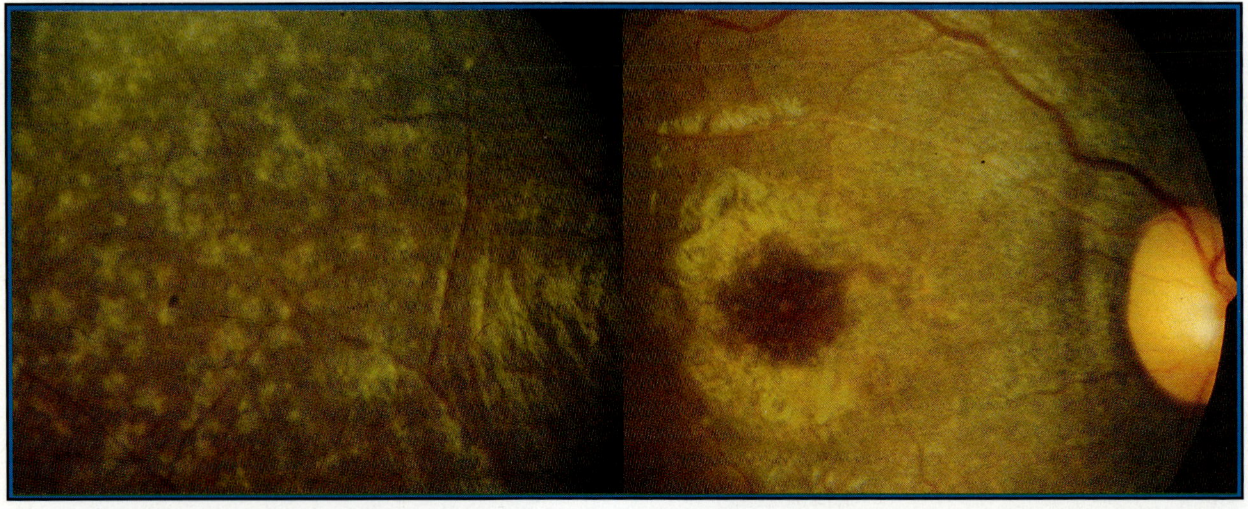

1–33

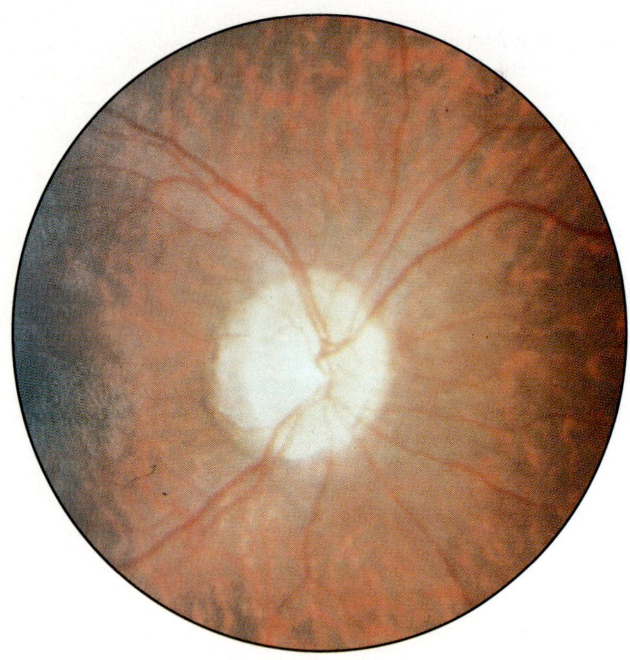

1–31 to 1–33 Hallervorden-Spatz syndrome is an autosomal recessive neural degenerative disorder. Extrapyramidal motor signs, dementia, dysarthria, and rigidity may occur. Associated acanthocytosis has been demonstrated. Approximately one-quarter of patients with this condition have a retinal degeneration and may experience a more rapid course with death occurring in late childhood. The retinal degeneration may consist of retinal flecks (1–31), a bull's eye maculopathy (1–32), retinal pigment epithelium mottling, and a retinitis pigmentosa–like pattern. In this patient with Hallervorden-Spatz syndrome, acanthocytosis, and a pigmentary retinopathy, note that the midperipheral areas of the retina have various yellow-white flecks of varying size and shape located deep to the retinal vessels (1–31). The bull's eye appearance of the macular region reveals an incomplete annulus of atrophy surrounding a hyperpigmented central macula (1–32). Deep to the retinal vessels, an annular deposition of yellowish material is noted. A second patient with this syndrome demonstrates a pigmentary retinopathy, optic atrophy, and attenuated retinal vessels (1–33).

1–31 *and* ***1–32,*** *From Luckenbach, MW, Green, WR, Miller, NR, Moser, HW, Clark, AW, Tennekoon G: Ocular clinicopathologic correlation of Hallervorden-Spatz syndrome with acanthocytosis and pigmentary retinopathy. Am J Ophthalmol 95:360–382 ,1983.*

1–34 USHER'S SYNDROME

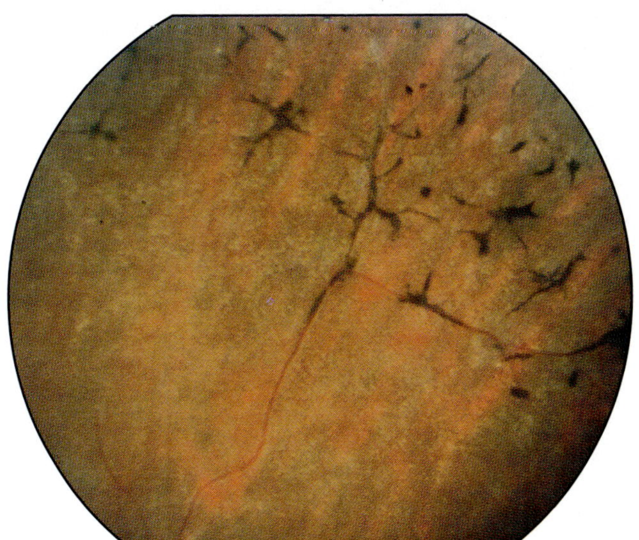

1–35 PSEUDORETINITIS PIGMENTOSA

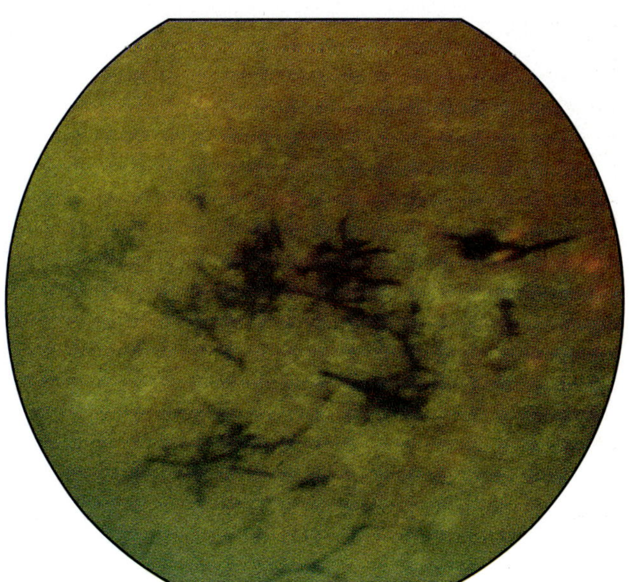

1–34 Patients with Usher's syndrome may demonstrate a retinitis pigmentosa–like picture associated with deafness

1–35 Pseudoretinitis pigmentosa may be associated with syphilis, trauma, ocular inflammation, and previous retinal detachment.

1–34, *Courtesy of Dr. Irene Maumenee.*

1–36 PIGMENTED PARAVENOUS CHORIORETINAL ATROPHY

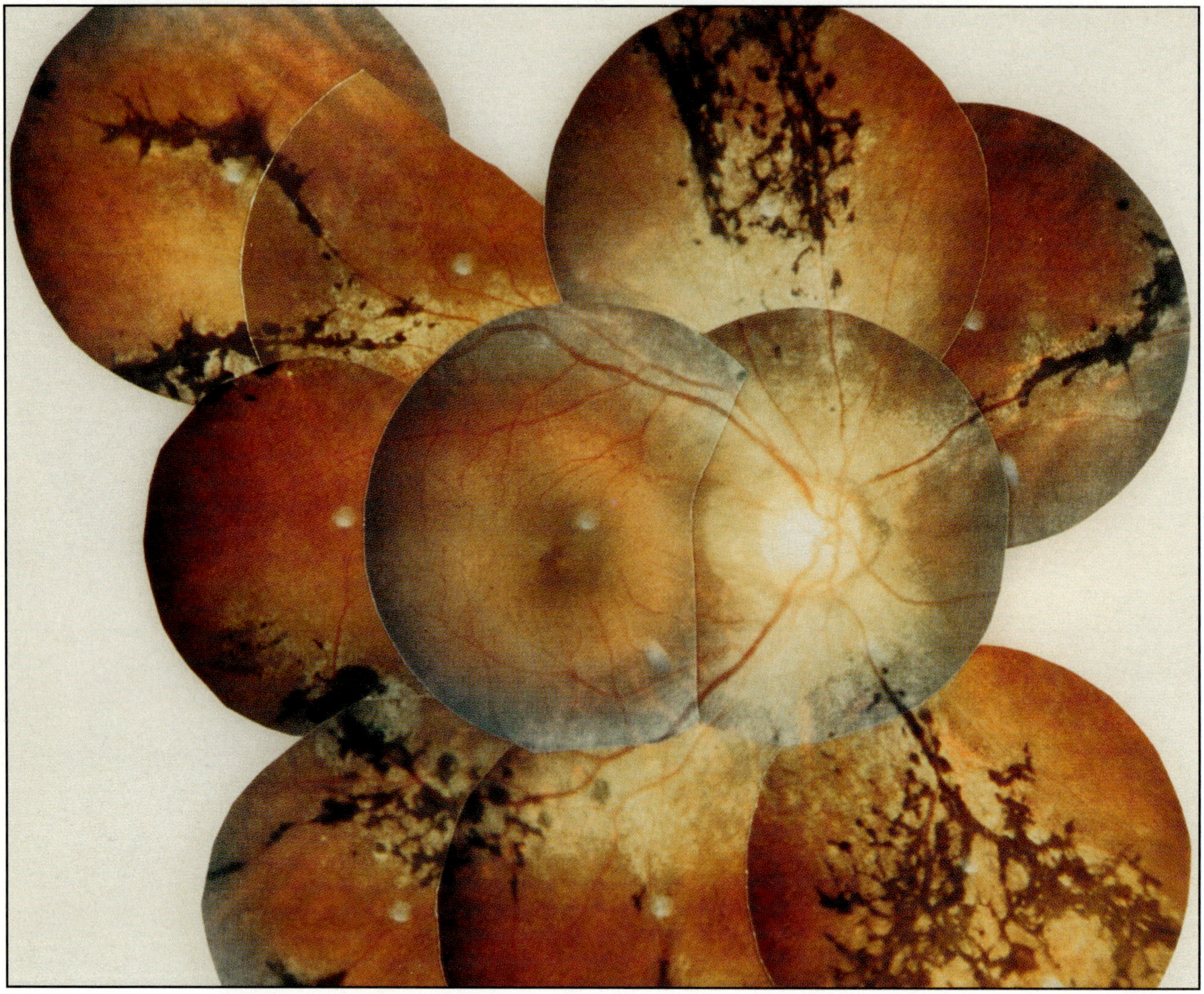

1–37

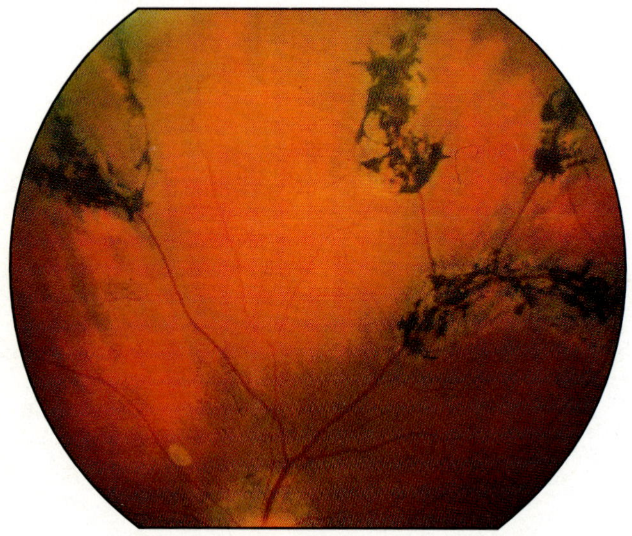

1–36 and 1–37 Pigmented paravenous chorioretinal atrophy is a sporadic pigmentary retinopathy in which the changes are in the distribution of the retinal veins. This condition may be caused by an infectious or inflammatory mechanism. This composite shows the widespread extent of pigmented paravenous chorioretinal atrophy throughout the fundus (1–36). Note how the hyperpigmented lesions follow the venules (1–37). This condition may be distinguished from retinitis pigmentosa by the venular distribution of the pigmented changes. The recognition of this disorder is important, as it has a more benign prognosis than retinitis pigmentosa.

***1–36** and **1–37,** Courtesy of Dr. Kent Small. From Arch Ophthalmol 109:1408–1410, 1991.*

1–38

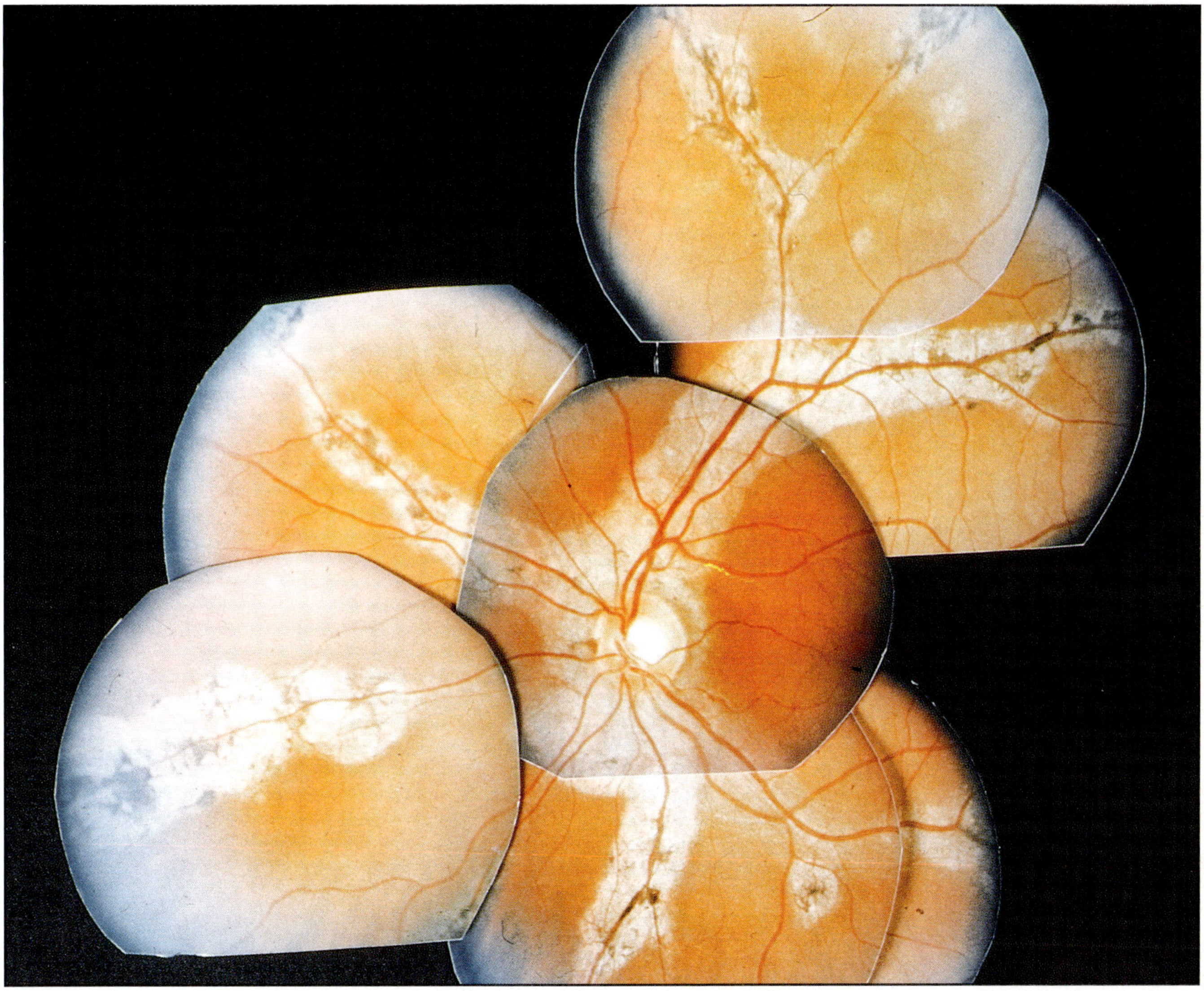

1–38 and 1–39 These paravenous changes may also be hypopigmented.

1–39

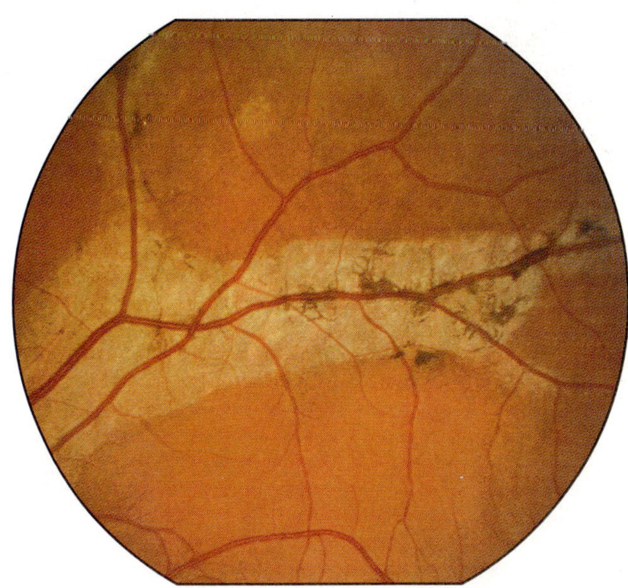

1–40 FUNDUS ALBIPUNCTATUS

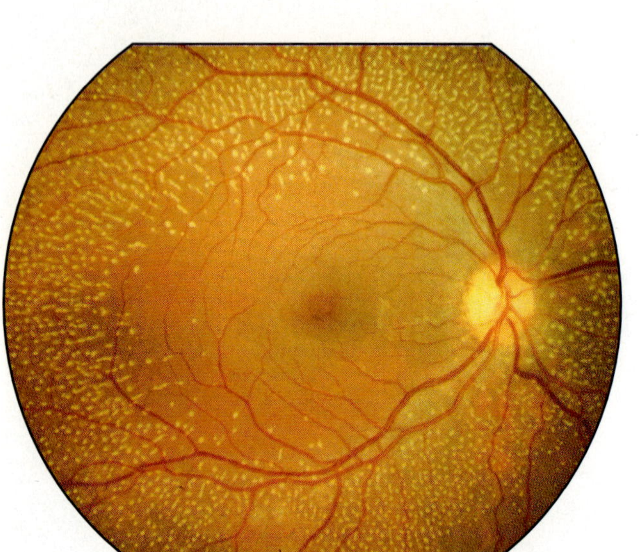

1–41

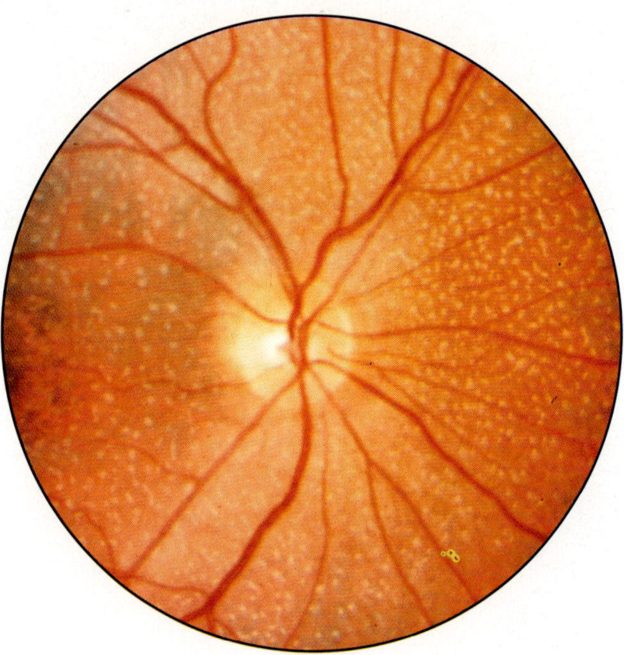

1–42

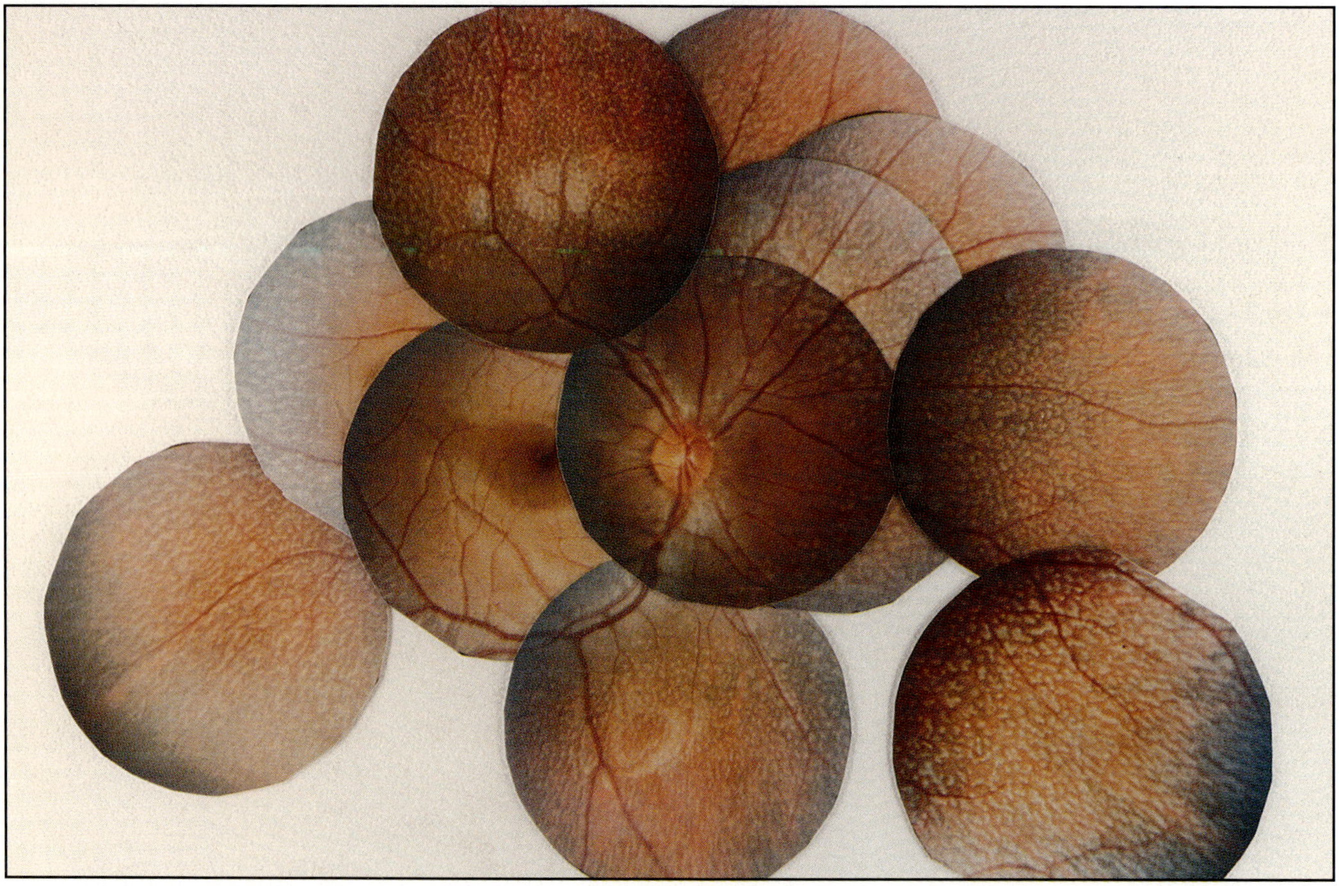

1–43 RETINITIS PUNCTATA ALBESCENS

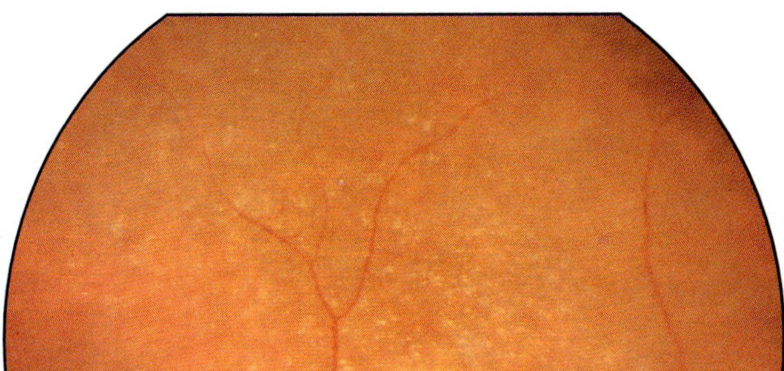

1–44 LEBER'S CONGENITAL AMAUROSIS

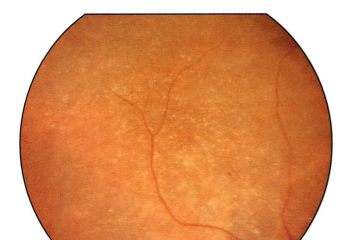

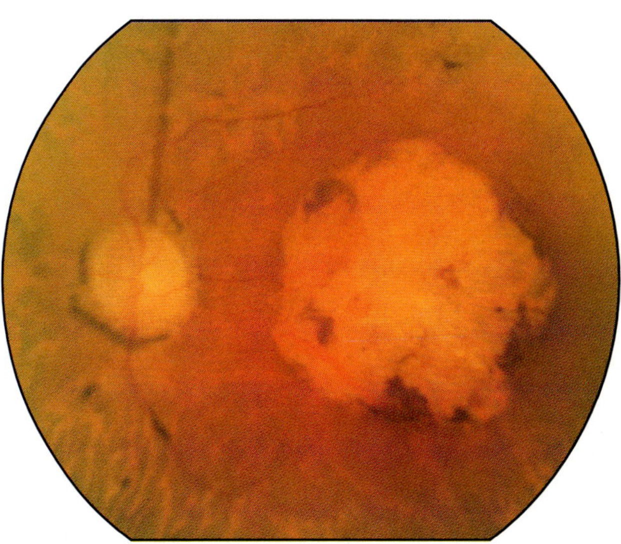

1–40 and 1–41 These patients with fundus albipunctatus demonstrate the characteristic whitish-yellow spots seen in this condition. Affected patients complain of night blindness and are noted to have small whitish spots deep in the retina. However, these changes are usually stationary.

1–42 This montage illustrates diffuse fundus lesions that involve more of the retina than is usually seen with fundus albipunctatus. Fundus albipunctatus shows the unusual electrophysiologic feature of an abnormally slow regeneration of the visual pigments with a long dark-adaptation period.

1–43 Retinitis punctata albescens has a clinical picture similar to fundus albipunctatus but is progressive in nature. These two similar conditions can be differentiated based upon electrophysiology studies. The electroretinogram is severely depressed or absent in retinitis punctata albescens.

1–44 Leber's congenital amaurosis is a group of autosomal recessive disorders characterized by severe vision loss in infancy. Findings may include nystagmus. A spectrum ranging from a normal retina to retinal pigment epithelium changes or a more severe retinal degeneration may be noted.

1–40, *Courtesy of Dr. Sheila Margolis.* ***1–41,*** *Courtesy of Drs. Sheila Margolis, Ron Carr, and I. Siegel.* ***1–42,*** *Courtesy of Dr. Sheila Margolis.* ***1–41*** *and* ***1–42,*** *From Margolis, S, Siegel, IM, Ripps, H: Variable expressivity in fundus albipunctatis. Ophthalmology, 94:1416–1422, 1987.*

Suggested Readings

Berson, EL: Retinitis pigmentosa and allied disease: applications of electroretinographic testing, Int Ophthalmol 4:7–22, 1981

Berson, EL, Rosner, B, Sandberg, MA, Weigel-DiFranco, C, and Dryja, TP: Ocular findings in patients with autosomal dominant retinitis pigmentosa and rhodopsin, proline-347-leucine, Am J Ophthalmol 111:614–623, 1991

Birch, DG, Anderson, JL, and Abdi, H: Natural history of rod loss in retinitis pigmentosa (abstract), Invest Ophthalmol Vis Sci 33(ARVO Suppl 4):1395, 1992

Bird, AC, and Blach, RK: X-linked recessive fundus dystrophies and their carrier states, Trans Ophthalmol Soc UK 90:127–138, 1970

Boughman, JA, and Fishman, GA: A genetic analysis of RP, Br J Ophthalmol 67:449–454, 1983

Breageat, P, and Amalric, P: Postmeningoencephalitis bilateral paravenous chorioretinal degeneration. In Henkind, P, Shimizu, K, Blodi, FC, Polack, FM, and Veronneau-Troutman, S, eds: Acta: XXIV International Congress of Ophthalmology, vol 1, Philadelphia, 1983, JB Lippincott, pp 454–457

Byrne, E, Marzuki, S, Sattayasai, N, Dennett, X, and Trounce, I: Mitochondrial studies in Kearns-Sayre syndrome: normal respiratory chain function with absence of a mitochondrial translation product, Neurology 37:1530–1534, 1987

Carr, RE: Abetalipoproteinemia and the eye, Birth Defects 12:385–399, 1976

Carr, RE, and Heckenlively, JR: Hereditary pigmentary degenerations of the retina. In Duane, TD, and Jaeger, EA, eds: Clinical ophthalmology, vol 3, Philadlephia, 1987, JB Lippincott, pp 1–28

Chew, E, Deutman, A, Pinckers, A, and Aan de Kerk, A: Yellowish flecks in Leber's congenital amaurosis, Br J Ophthalmol 68:727–731, 1984

Ellis, DS, and Heckenlively, JR: Retinitis punctata albescens: fundus appearance and functional abnormalities, Retina 3:27–31, 1983

Fishman, GA, Alexander, KR, and Anderson, RJ: Autosomal dominant retinitis pigmentosa: a method of classification, Arch Ophthalmol 103:366–374, 1985

Fishman, GA, Fishman, M, and Maggiano, J: Macular lesions associated with retinitis pigmentosa, Arch Ophthalmol 95:798–803, 1977

Heckenlively, JR: X-linked recessive retinitis pigmentosa (X-linked pigmentary retinopathies). In Heckenlively, JR, ed: Retinitis pigmentosa, Philadelphia, 1988, JB Lippincott, pp 162–187.

Heckenlively, JR, Martin, DA, and Rosales, TO: Telangiectasia and optic atrophy in cone-rod degenerations, Arch Ophthalmol 99:1983–1991, 1981.

Illingworth, DR, Connor, WE, and Miller, RG: Abetalipoproteinemia: report of two cases and review of therapy, Arch Neurol 37:659–662, 1980

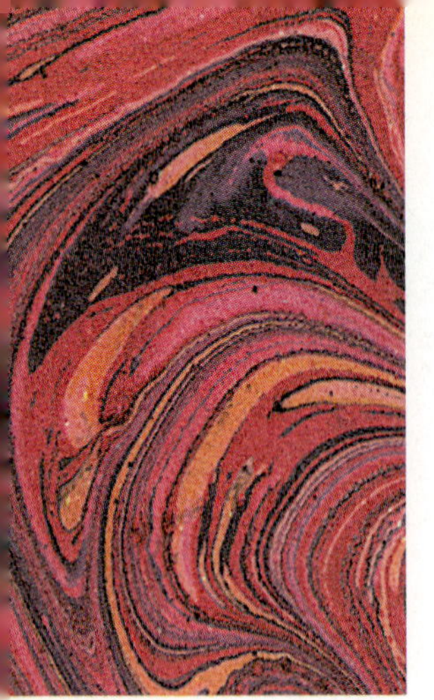

Chapter 2

Congenital and Hereditary Chorioretinal Disorders

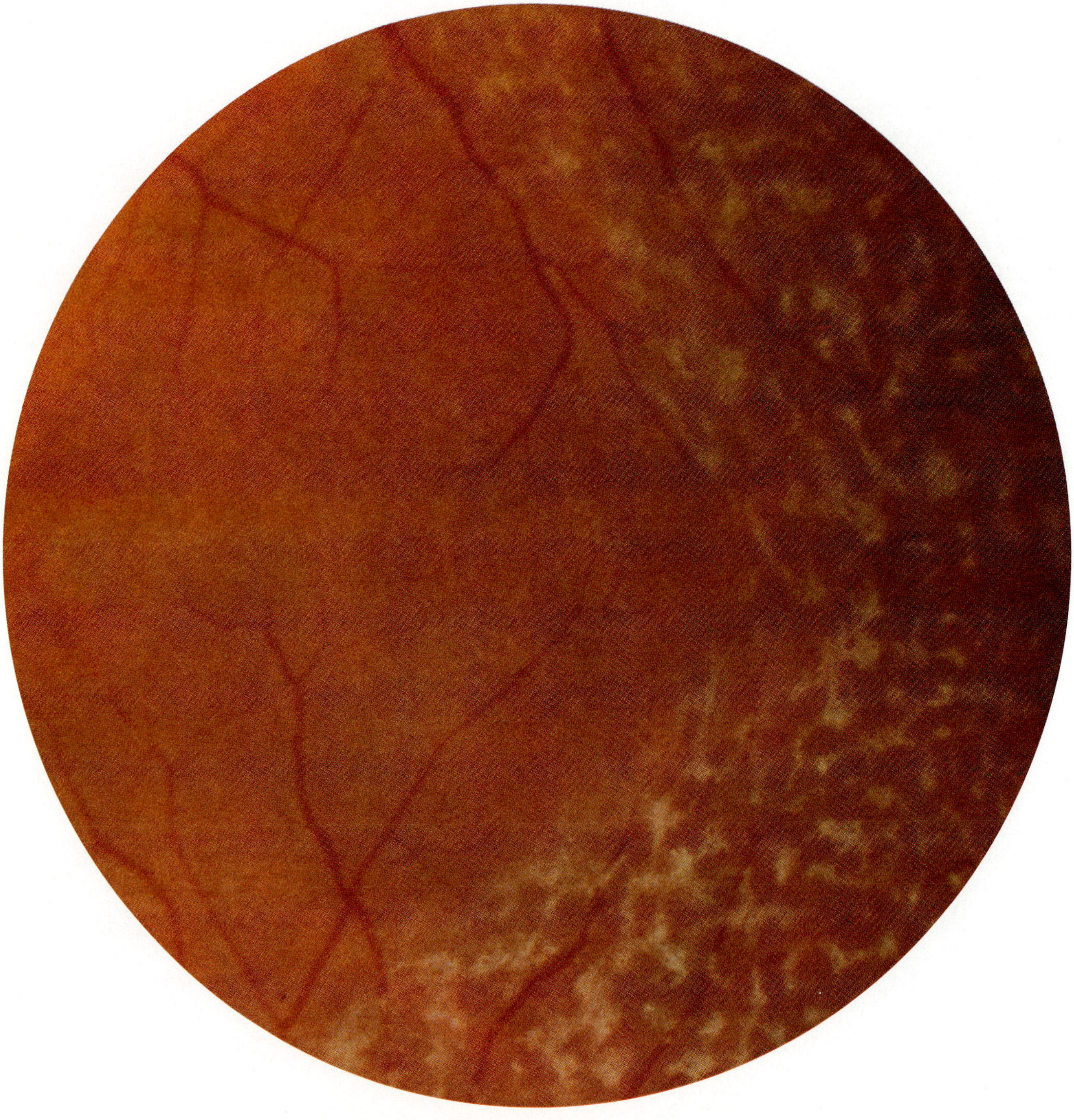

Various congenital and hereditary disorders may affect the choroid and/or retina. The congenital disorders include aberrant retinal veins, cilioretinal arteries, congenital arteriovenous shunts, myelinated nerve fibers, colobomas, and fistulas.

Numerous hereditary conditions can also affect the choroid and/or retina. These diseases include storage diseases, choroideremia, gyrate atrophy, Alport's disease, Cockayne's syndrome, and olivopontocerebellar atrophy. Other dystrophies that may affect the choroid and retina include central areolar choroidal dystrophy, peripapillary choroidal dystrophy, Bietti's crystalline dystrophy, rod monochromatism, cone dystrophy, and Oguchi's disease. Albinism is another hereditary condition that may commonly affect the eye. Rare hereditary disorders such as the Aicardi syndrome may also affect other organ systems.

2–1 CONGENITAL DISORDERS

2–2

2–3

2–4

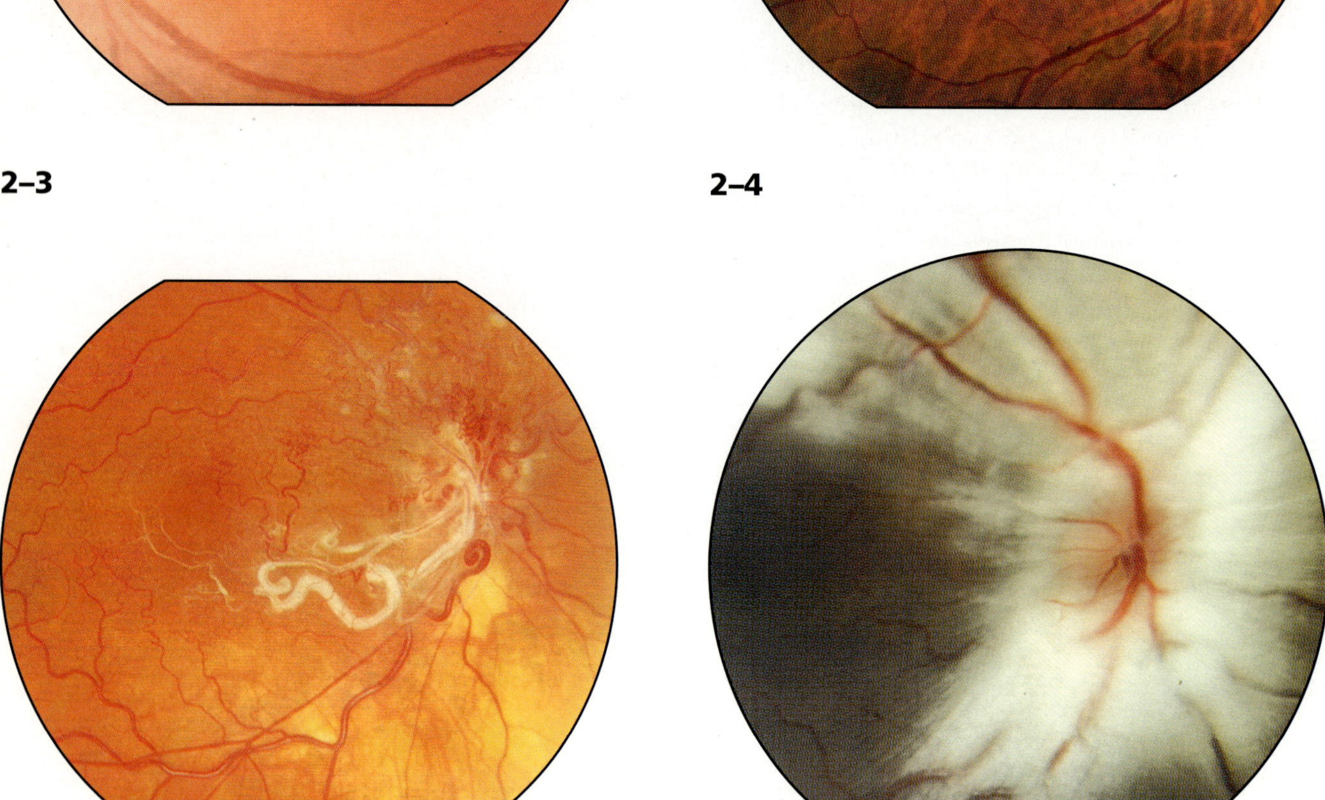

2–1 and 2–2 Various congenital abnormalities may involve the choroid and/or retina. An aberrant retinal vein may occur in the macular region (2–1) or a cilioretinal artery may traverse the fovea (2–2).

2–3 This patient has a congenital arteriovenous shunt that developed a retinal vein occlusion with sclerosis of the vessels.

2–4 Extensive myelinated nerve fibers are present around the optic disc in this patient.

***2–1** and **2–2,** Courtesy of Terry George. **2–3,** Courtesy of Dr. Dennis Han.*

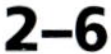

2–5 COLOBOMAS

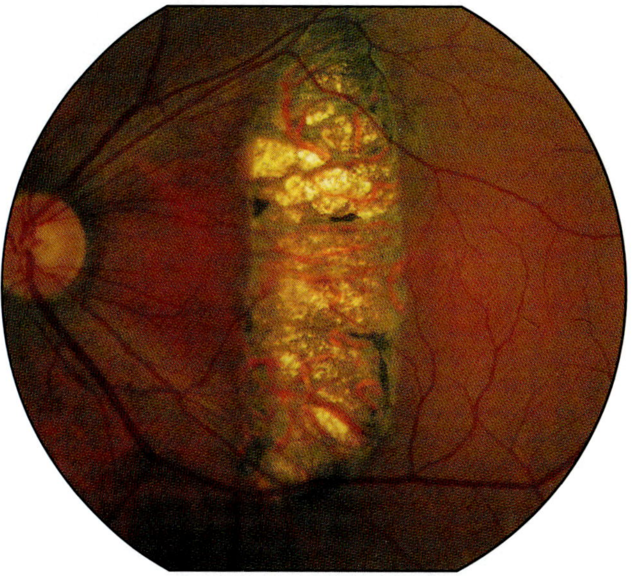

2–6

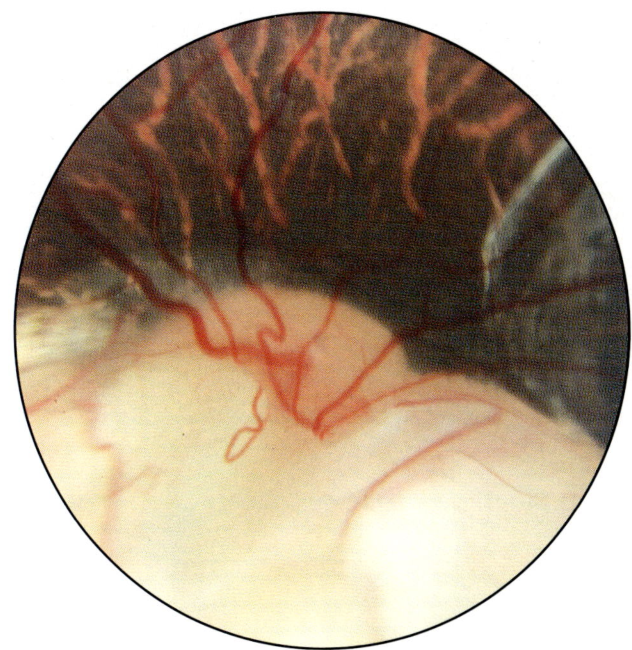

2–7

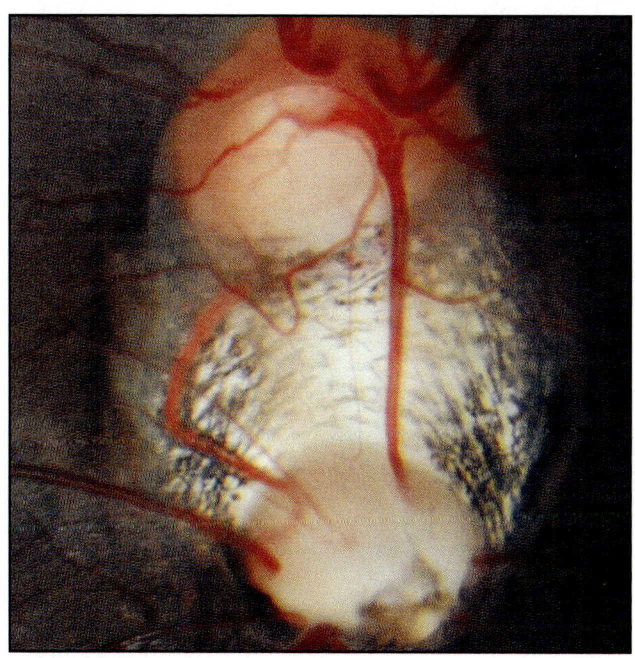

2–5 and 2–6 Macular (2–5) or combined optic disc and choroidal (2–6) colobomas may occur.

2–7 This combined optic disc and choroidal coloboma is associated with a retrobulbar fistula that simulates a double optic nerve.

2–8 COLOBOMA

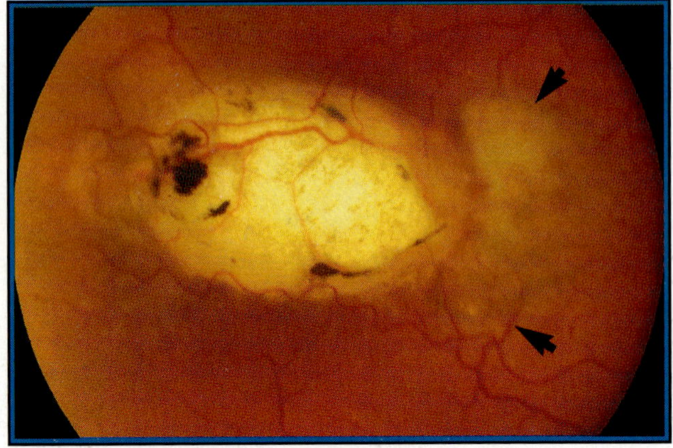

2–9

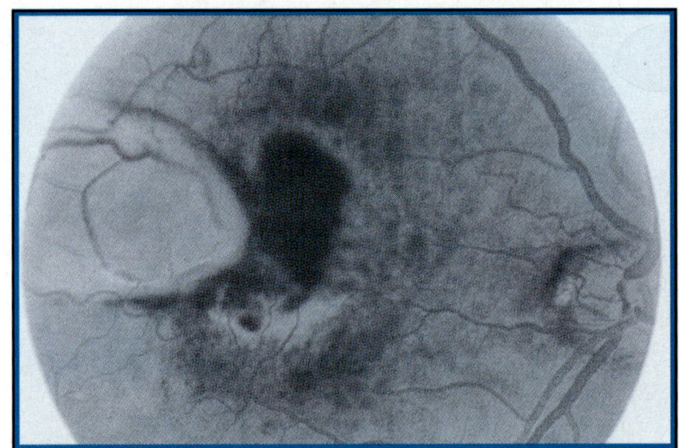

2–10 MORNING GLORY SYNDROME

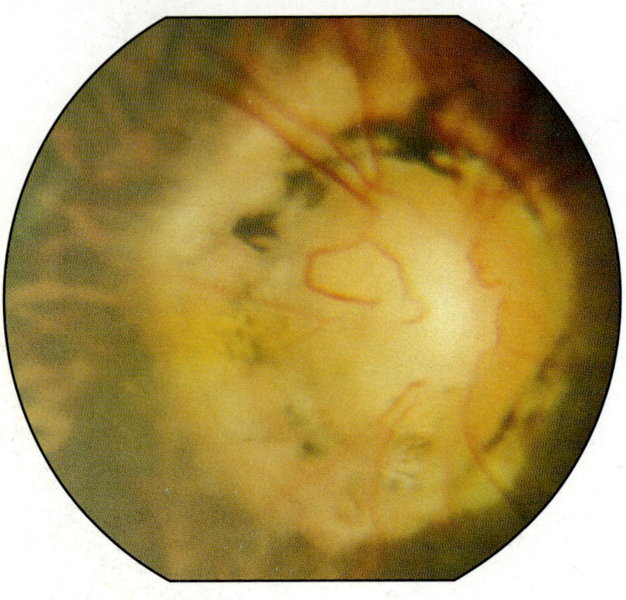

2–11

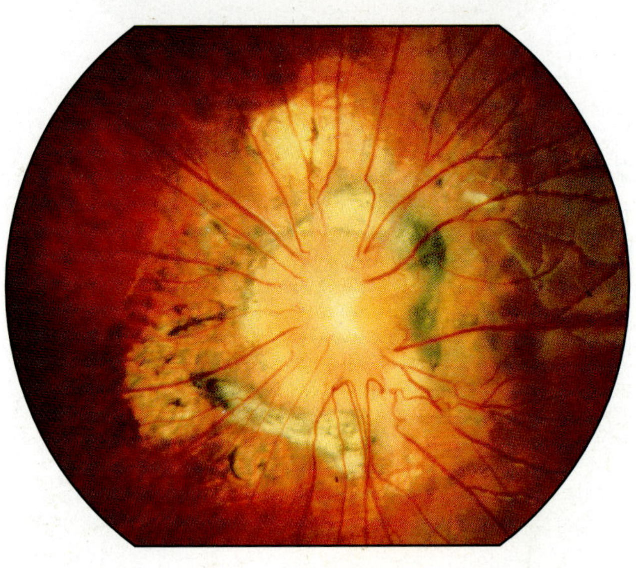

2–8 and 2–9 Colobomas may rarely be associated with choroidal neovascularization *(arrowheads)* as illustrated in this patient.

2–10 and 2–11 The morning glory syndrome is a developmental abnormality of the optic disc. Extensive central excavation of the optic nerve head is noted in affected patients. A complete staphyloma can be observed. Retinal detachments may sometimes occur with this syndrome.

Hereditary Disorders: Storage Diseases

2–12 MUCOPOLYSACCHARIDOSIS TYPE II (HUNTER'S SYNDROME)

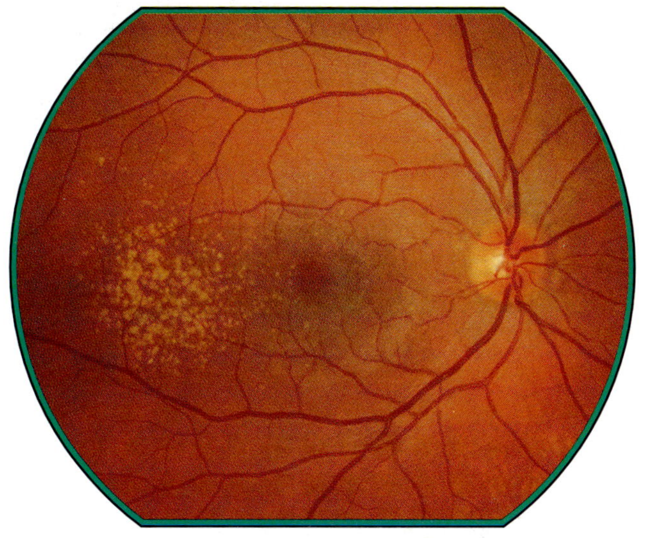

2–13

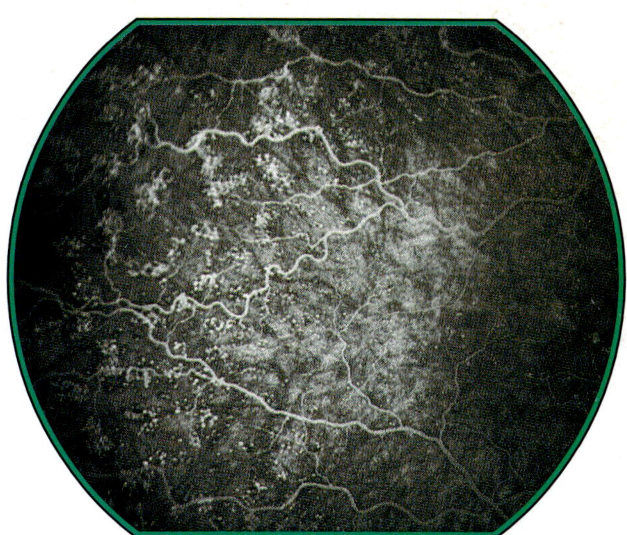

2–14

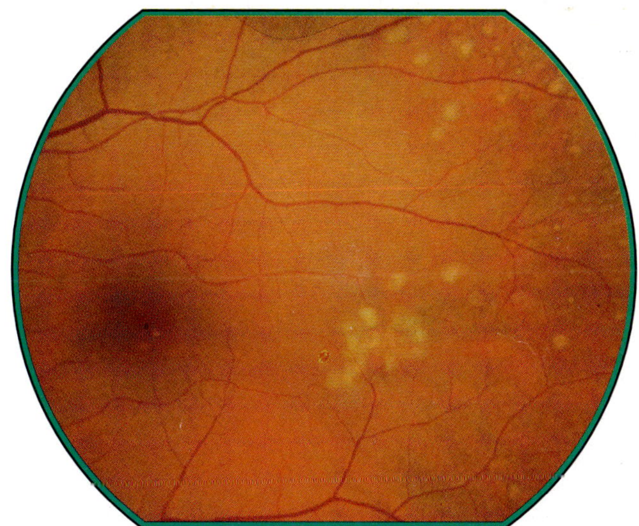

2–15

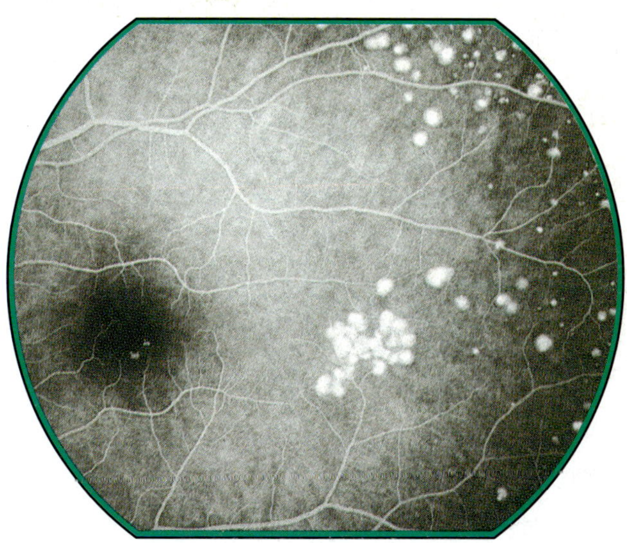

2–12 through 2–15 Storage diseases may be associated with a pigmentary retinopathy. Affected patients with mucopolysaccharidosis type II (Hunter's syndrome) show drusenoid-like lesions in the macula and the periphery, which stain on fluorescein angiography. In some patients, the lesions are larger and nummular-like.

***2–12** through **2–15**, Courtesy of Dr. William Mieler.*

2–16 MUCOPOLYSACCHARIDOSIS IIIA (SANFILIPPO SYNDROME)

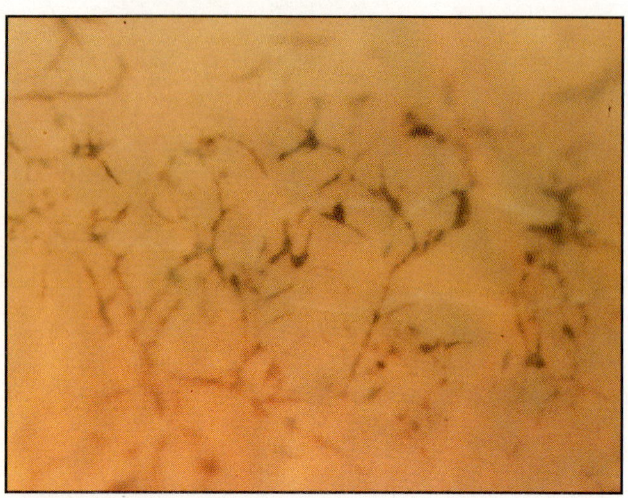

2–17 CEROID LIPOFUSCINOSIS (BATTEN-VOGT SYNDROME)

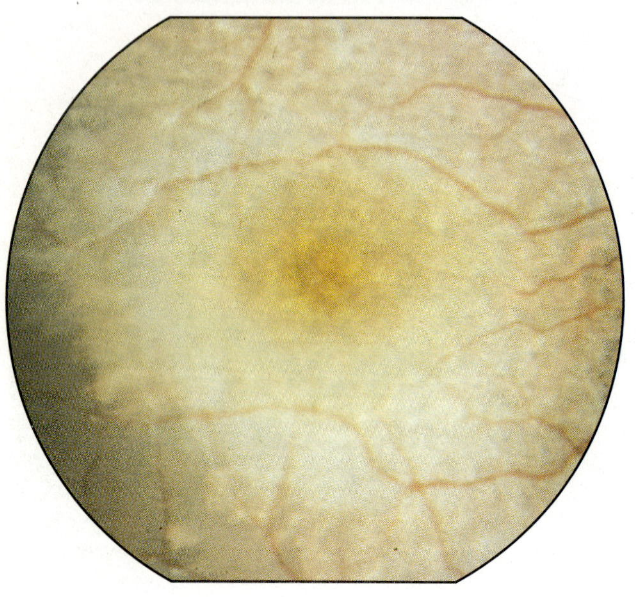

2–18 CEROID LIPOFUSCINOSIS (HAGBERG–SANTAVUORI SYNDROME)

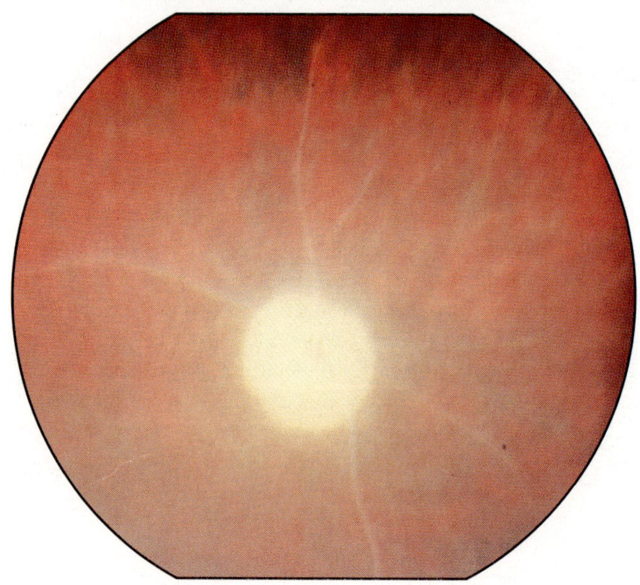

2–16 Patients with mucopolysaccharidosis IIIA or Sanfilippo's syndrome may demonstrate a retinitis pigmentosa–like appearance due to hyperplasia of the retinal pigment epithelium. Migration into the retina occurs in a perivascular distribution. Optic atrophy also may be present. Retinal vascular attenuation and sheathing is present but masked by the pigmentary changes.

2–17 Ceroid lipofuscinosis (Batten-Vogt syndrome) findings may include a diffuse atrophic area with patchy parafoveal pigmentary disturbances or a bull's eye configuration.

2–18 Hagberg-Santavuori syndrome is an infantile type of neuronal ceroid lipofuscinoses. Affected patients demonstrate mental and motor regression, ataxia, and hypotonia. This patient has the ocular findings of vascular sheathing, retinal degeneration, and optic atrophy known to be associated with this disease.

***2–16,** From Spencer, W: Ophthalmic pathology: an atlas and a textbook, ed 3, vol 2, Philadelphia, 1985, WB Saunders. **2–17,** Courtesy of Dr. Irene Maumenee. **2–18,** From Ryan, SJ: Retina, ed 2, St Louis, 1994, Mosby–Year Book. Courtesy of Bateman, Lang, and Maumenee.*

2–19 SPHINGOMYELIN LIPIDOSIS (NIEMANN-PICK DISEASE)

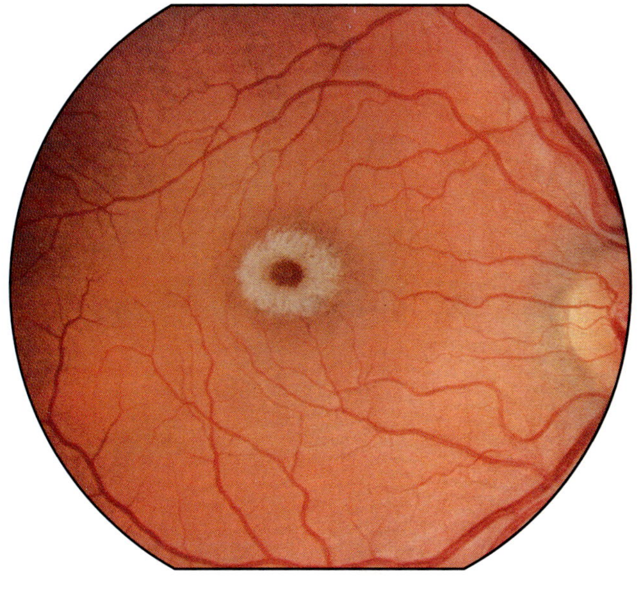

2–20

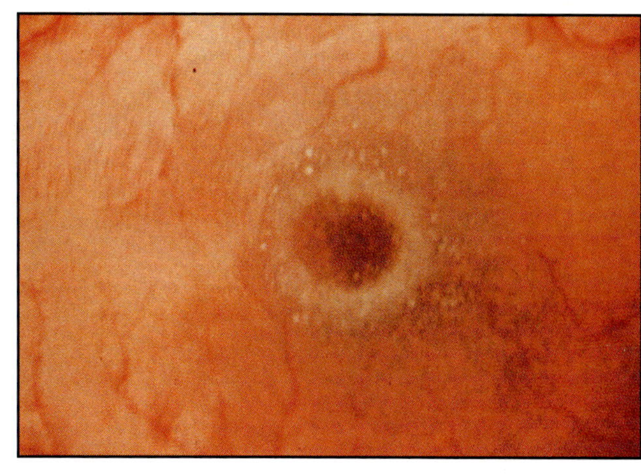

2–21

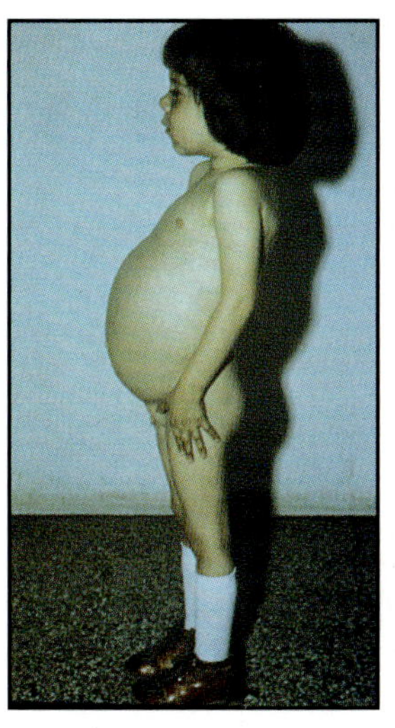

2–22

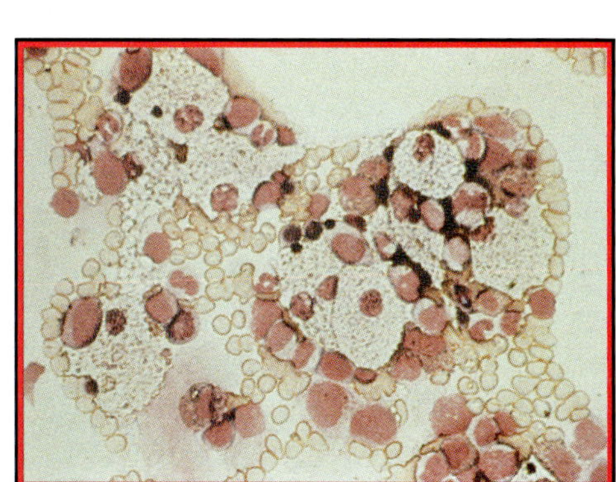

2–23

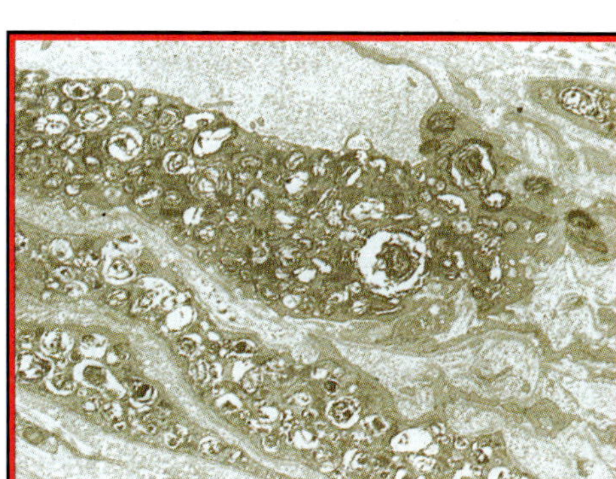

2–19 and 2–20 An enzyme deficiency that causes storage of sphingomyelin and cholesterol is responsible for Niemann-Pick disease (sphingomyelin lipidosis). A macular halo is classically observed. In this patient (2–20) the deposits are multifocal, as well as inside and outside the ring. This finding may be associated with normal vision.

2–21 Sphingomyelin and cholesterol are also accumulated in the abdomen, causing a characteristic appearance in these patients.

2–22 and 2–23 Light microscopy (2–22) and electron microscopy (2–23) reveal lipid accumulations.

2–19, *Courtesy of Dr. John Matthews. Reprinted from Matthews, JD, Weiter, JJ, and Kolodny, EH: Macular halos associated with Niemann-Pick type B disease, Ophthalmology 93:933–937, 1986.* ***2–20,*** *From Ryan, SJ: Retina, ed 2, St Louis, 1994, Mosby–Year Book.* ***2–20*** *through* ***2–23,*** *Courtesy of Dr. Irene Maumenee.*

2–24A GANGLIOSIDOSIS TYPE I (TAY-SACHS DISEASE)

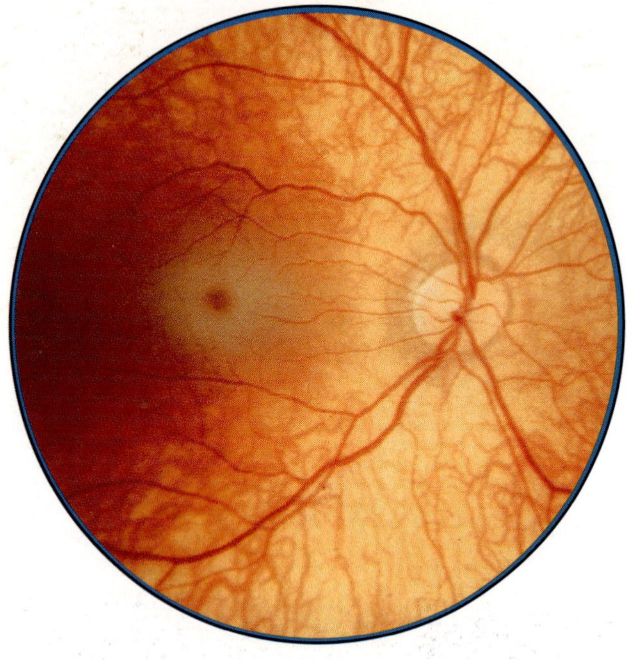

2–24B

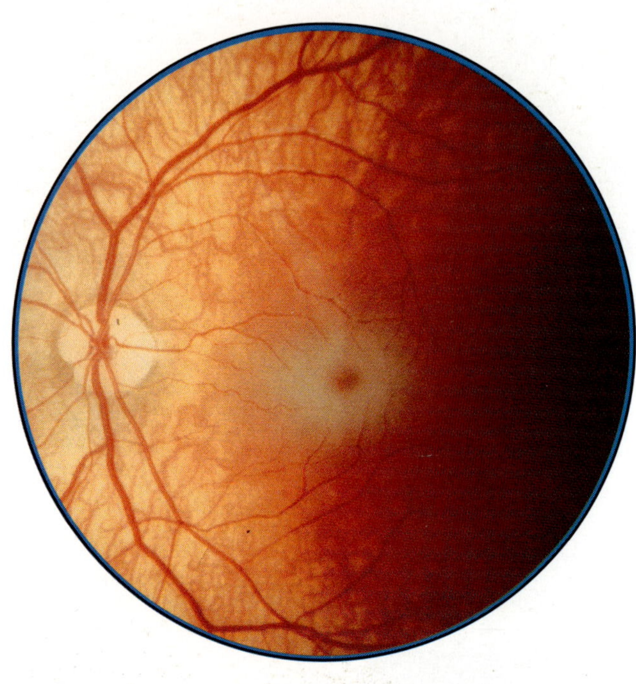

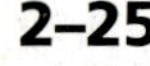

2–25

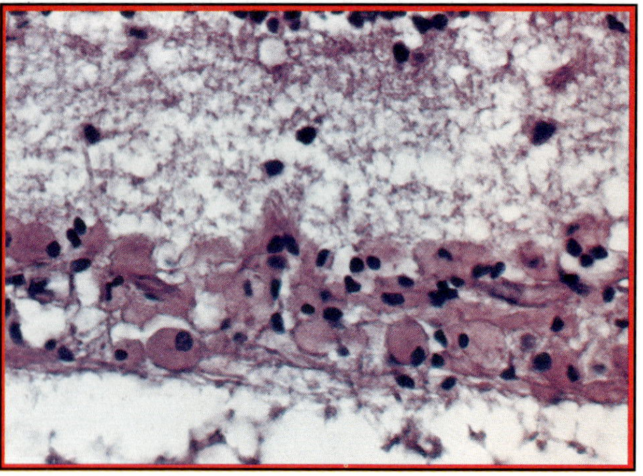

2–26

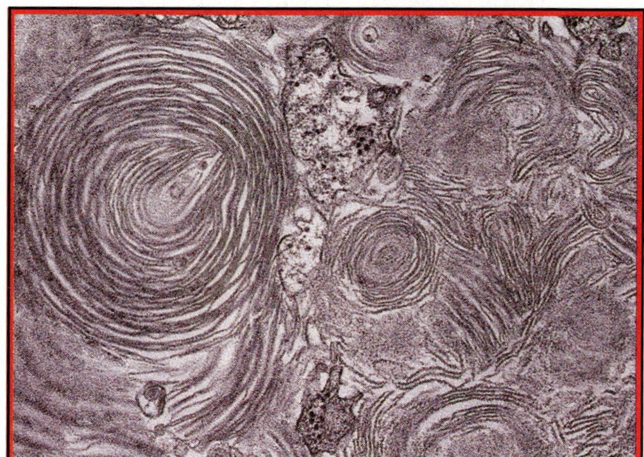

2–24 Patients with Tay-Sachs disease may have cherry-red spots. Tay-Sachs disease, or gangliosidosis type I, is caused by a deficiency of hexosaminidase A.

2–25 Note the appearance of distended ganglion cells of the retina from a patient with Tay-Sachs disease.

2–26 The material that accumulates in Tay-Sachs disease appears multimembranous.

__2–24__ and __2–25__, Courtesy of Dr. Albert Aandekerk. __2–26__, From Spencer, W: Ophthalmic pathology: an atlas and a textbook, ed 3, Philadelphia, 1985, WB Saunders.

2–27 SIALIDOSIS

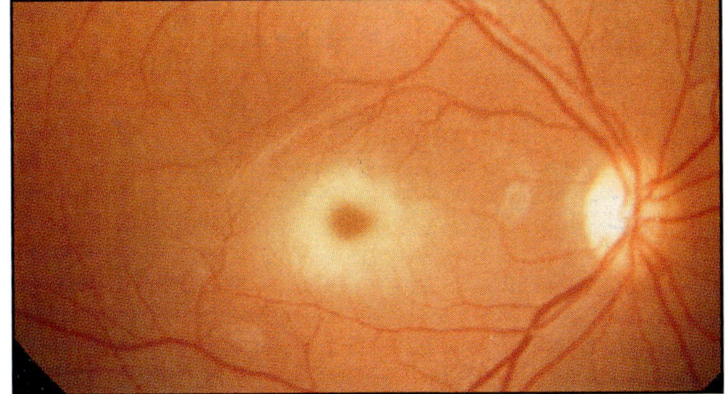

2–28

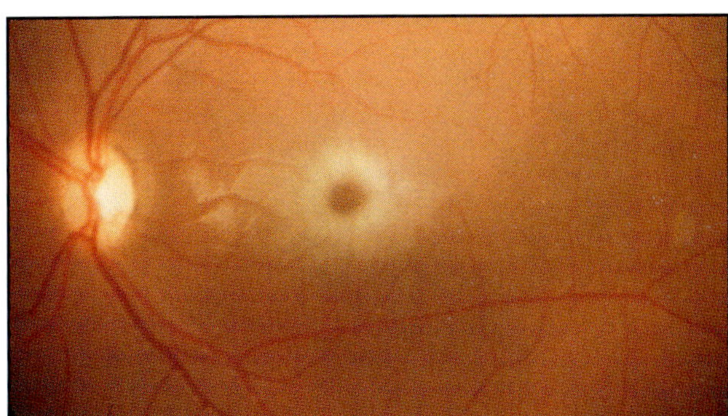

2–29 GAUCHER'S DISEASE

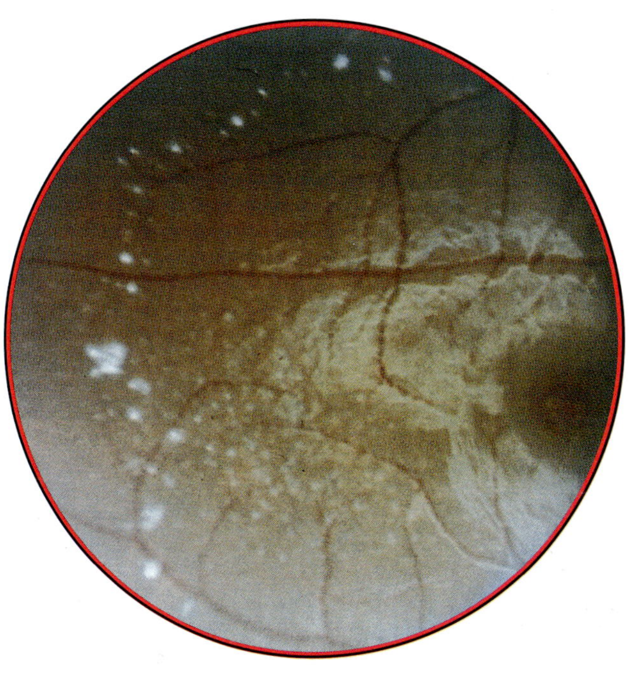

2–30

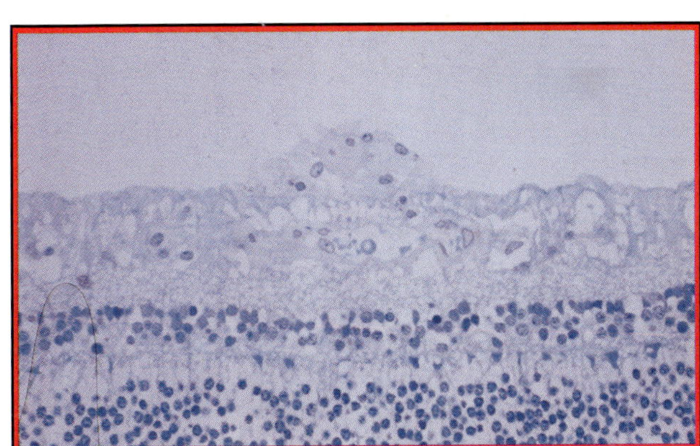

2–27 and 2–28 Cherry red spots may also be seen with sialidosis type II (mucolipidosis) as in this case, or with Landing's disease (gangliosidosis), Farber's disease (disseminated lipogranulomatosis), or metachromatic leukodystrophy.

2–29 This patient with juvenile Gaucher's disease shows discrete deposits in a semicircular pattern temporal to the macula.

2–30 The deposits are clusters of Gaucher's cells within and on the retina.

***2–27** and **2–28,** Courtesy of Dr. Stefanos Kokolakis. **2–29** and **2–30,** From Ueno, SS, Kamitani, T et al: Clinical and histopathologic studies of a case with juvenile form of Gaucher's disease, Jpn J Ophthalmol 21:98–108, 1977.*

2–31 **FABRY'S DISEASE**

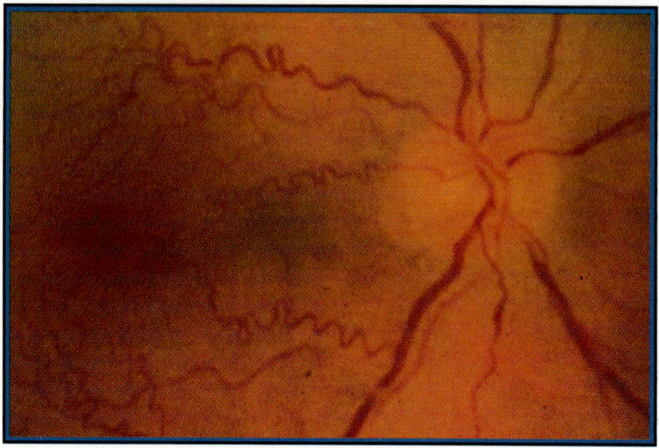

2–32

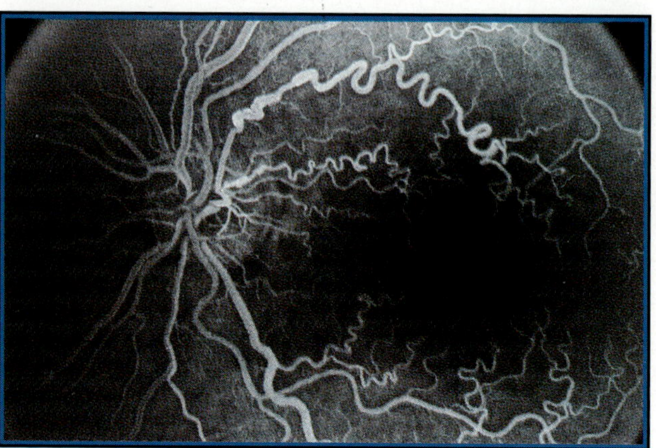

2–33 **MULTIPLE SULFATASE DEFICIENCY**

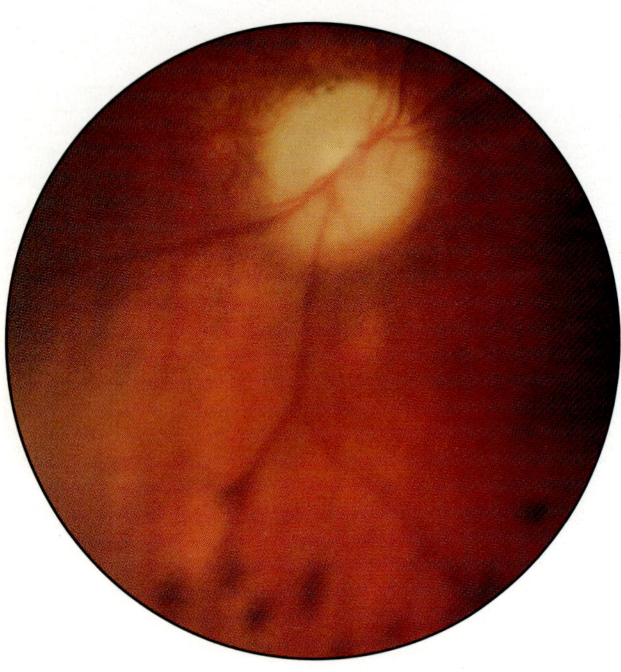

2–31 and 2–32 Fabry's disease is an X-linked disease in which there is a sphingolipid storage abnormality. The disease is due to a defective alpha-galactosidase A. Verticillate corneal epithelial opacities may be noted due to ceramide trihexoside deposition. The conjunctiva may show tortuosity. The retina also may show tortuous-like vessels, as in this bilateral case. The fluorescein study shows normal flow and accentuates the tortuosity. The vessels do not stain.

2–33 Multiple sulfatase deficiency is an autosomal recessive condition due to sulfatase enzyme deficiencies. Systemic findings include psychomotor retardation, organomegaly, and ichthyosis. This 11-year-old boy has multiple sulfatase deficiency. Note the optic atrophy and retinal dystrophy.

2–31 *and* ***2–32,*** *Courtesy of Dr. Tom Weingeist.* ***2–33,*** *From Ryan, SJ: Retina, ed 2, St Louis, 1994, Mosby–Year Book. Courtesy of Bateman, Lang, and Maumenee.*

2–34 CYSTINOSIS

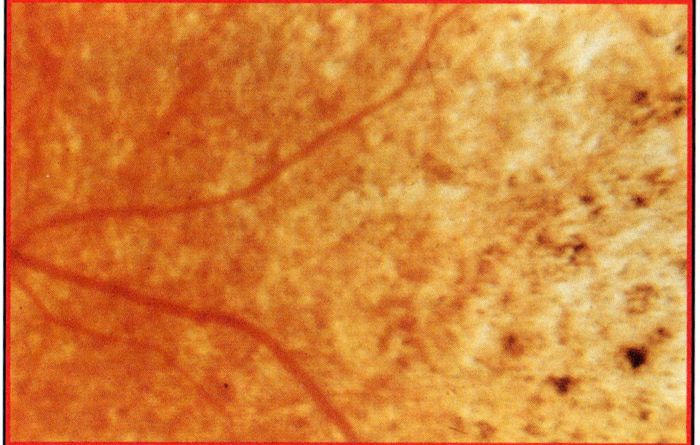

2–35

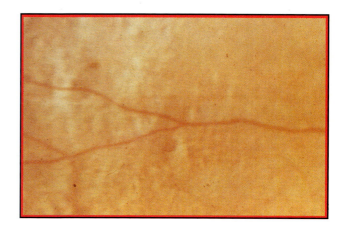

2–36

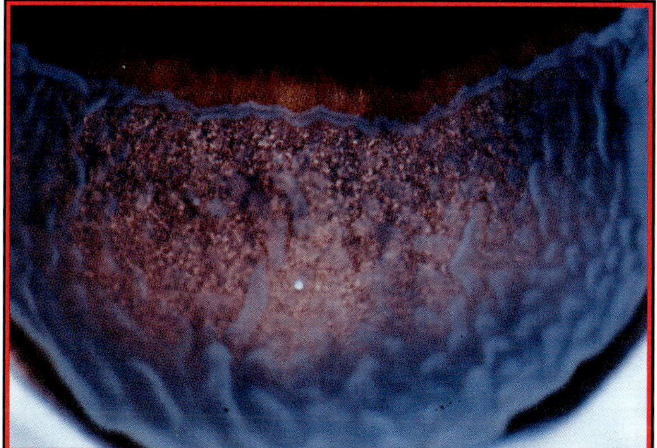

2–37

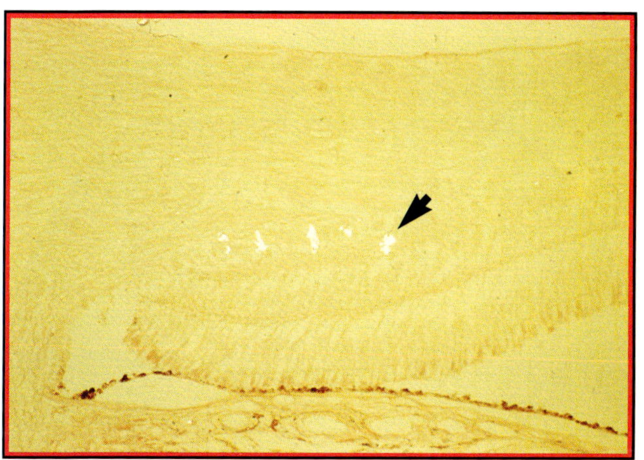

2–34 and 2–35 Cystinosis is an inborn error of metabolism that results in accumulation of intracellular cystine. Several forms of this autosomal recessive disease exist. In the infantile or early onset form of the disease, nephropathy is demonstrated. Usually renal failure occurs during the teenage years. Affected patients note photophobia. Cystine crystals may be noted in the cornea, conjunctiva, and iris. In the peripheral retina areas of pigmentary changes are noted.

2–36 Gross examination reveals the pigmentary changes of the peripheral retina seen in these patients.

2–37 Accumulation of cystine crystals is noted in the retina *(arrowhead).*

***2–34** through **2–37,** Courtesy of Dr. V. G. Wong.*

2–38 CHOROIDEREMIA

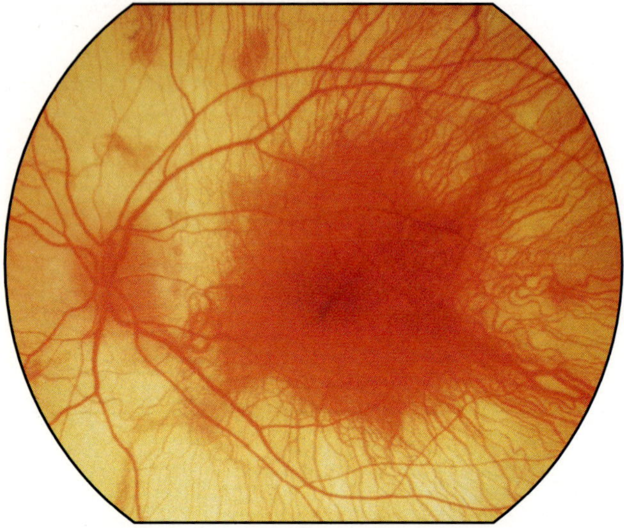

2–39

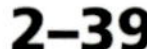

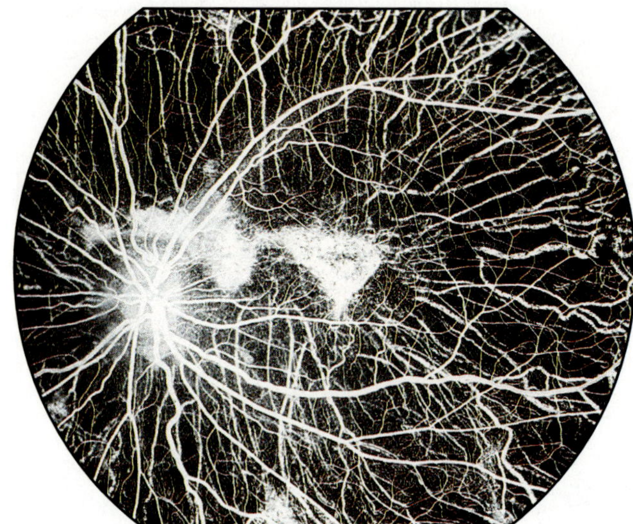

2–40

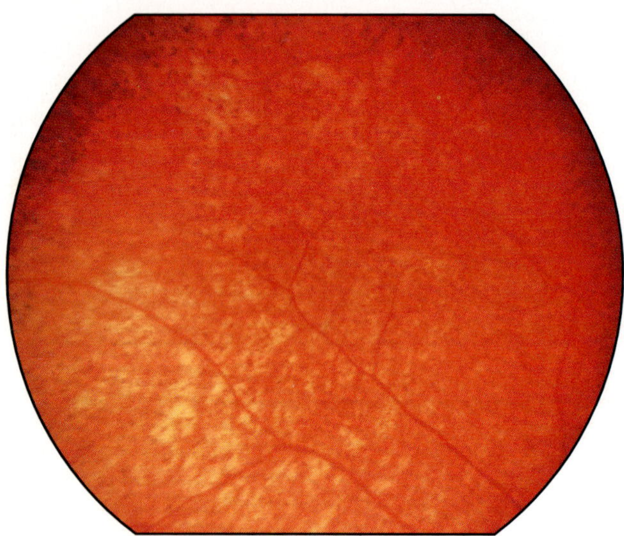

Choroideremia is a sex-linked generalized chorioretinal disorder. Males note difficulties with night vision and peripheral vision early in life. Later in life, visual acuity may be affected. The choroidal and retinal pigment epithelium atrophy begin in the midperiphery and then progress both anteriorly and posteriorly. A small macular area may eventually be the only normal tissue noted. Later, optic disc atrophy and retinal vessel attenuation often occur.

2–38 This patient illustrates the extensive chorioretinal atrophy with macular sparing noted in such patients.

2–39 The preserved central macula of another patient demonstrates a stellate appearance. Note that the fluorescein angiogram shows extensive atrophy and allows visualization of the underlying choroidal vessels.

2–40 This patient with early choroideremia has midperipheral atrophy with pigmentary granularity.

2–40, *Courtesy of Dr. Irene Maumenee.*

2–41

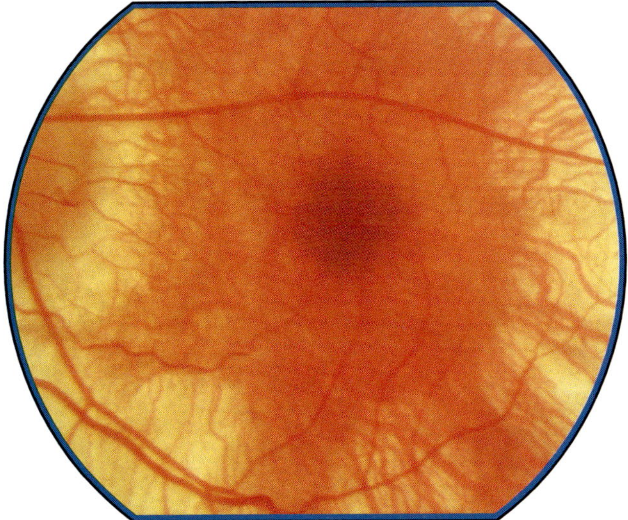

2–42

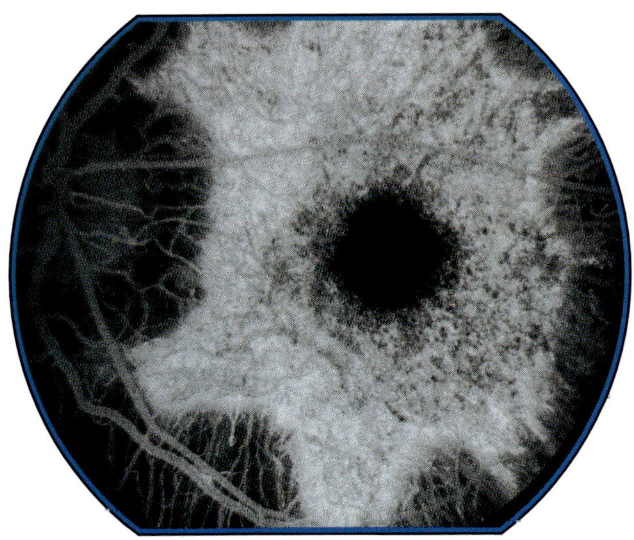

2–41 Another patient with choroideremia also reveals areas of atrophy in the posterior pole that does not involve the macula.

2–42 Note the "skip" areas of atrophy, which are hypofluorescent on the fluorescein study.

2–41 *and* ***2–42,*** *Courtesy of Dr. Jim Tiedeman.*

2–43 CHOROIDEREMIA

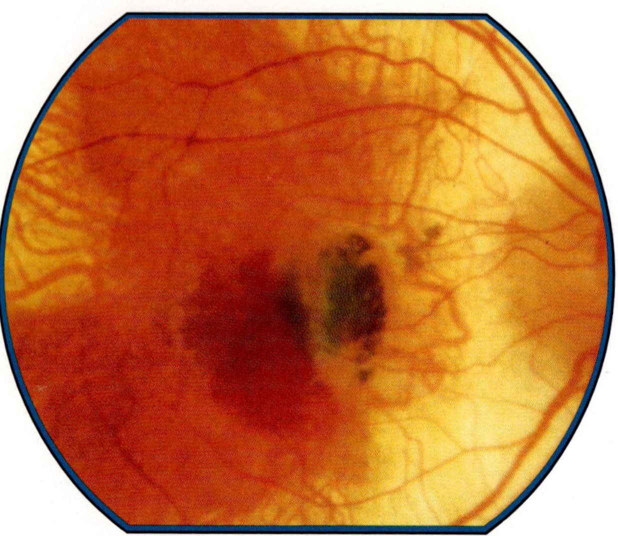

2–44

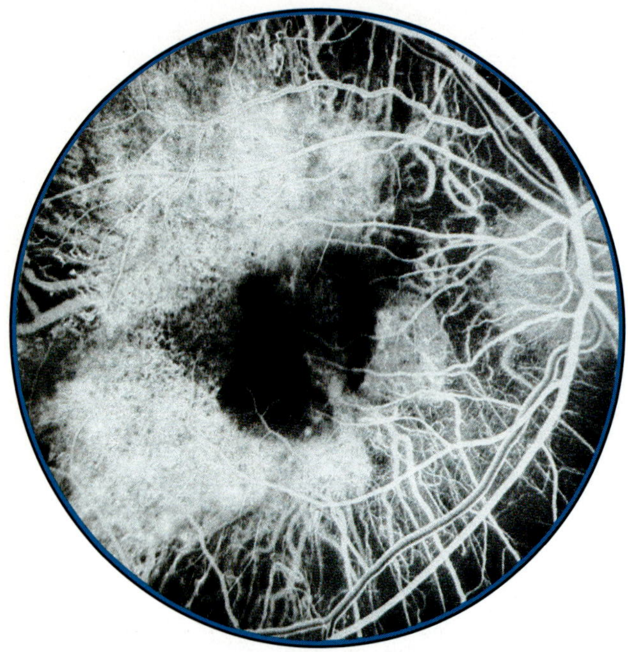

2–43 and 2–44 The next patient illustrates that choroidal neovascularization can be associated with choroideremia. This patient has subretinal hemorrhage secondary to choroidal neovascularization. The accompanying fluorescein angiogram reveals blockage secondary to the subretinal hemorrhage, as well as hyperfluorescence consistent with neovascularization (2–44). These vessels originate where the choriocapillaris is still intact.

2–43 *and* ***2–44,*** *Courtesy of Dr. Jim Tiedeman.*

2–45

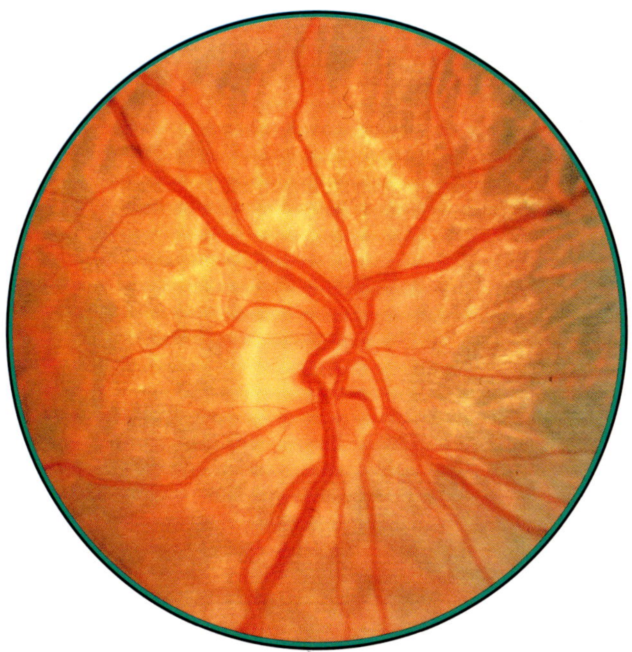

2–46

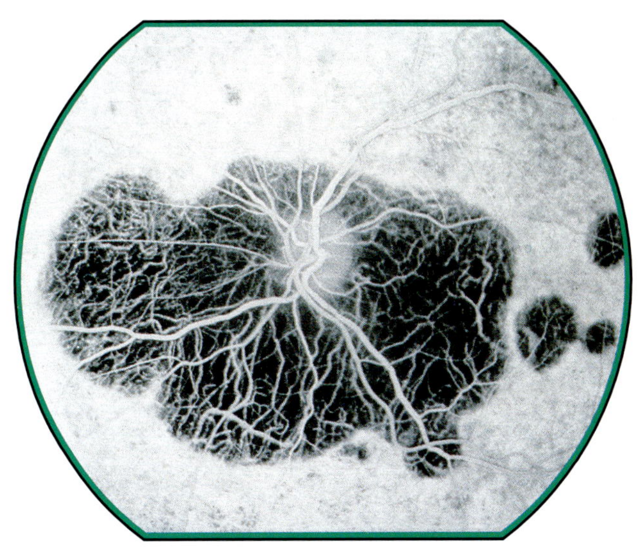

2–47

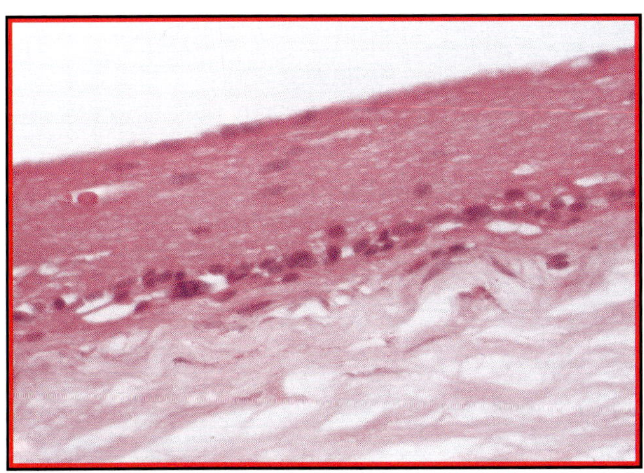

2–45 Carriers of choroideremia may show retinal pigment epithelial changes with normal visual function. This 55-year-old female is a carrier of choroideremia. She has one son and two nephews with the disorder. Note the chorioretinal atrophy around the optic disc. Visual acuity was 20/20.

2–46 Note the peripapillary atrophy and "skip" lesions evident on the fluorescein study.

2–47 Histopathologic examination of an eye from a patient with choroideremia reveals a loss of the choroid, retinal pigment epithelium, and outer retinal layers.

***2–45** and **2–46,** Courtesy of Dr. Ron Carr.*

2–48 GYRATE ATROPHY

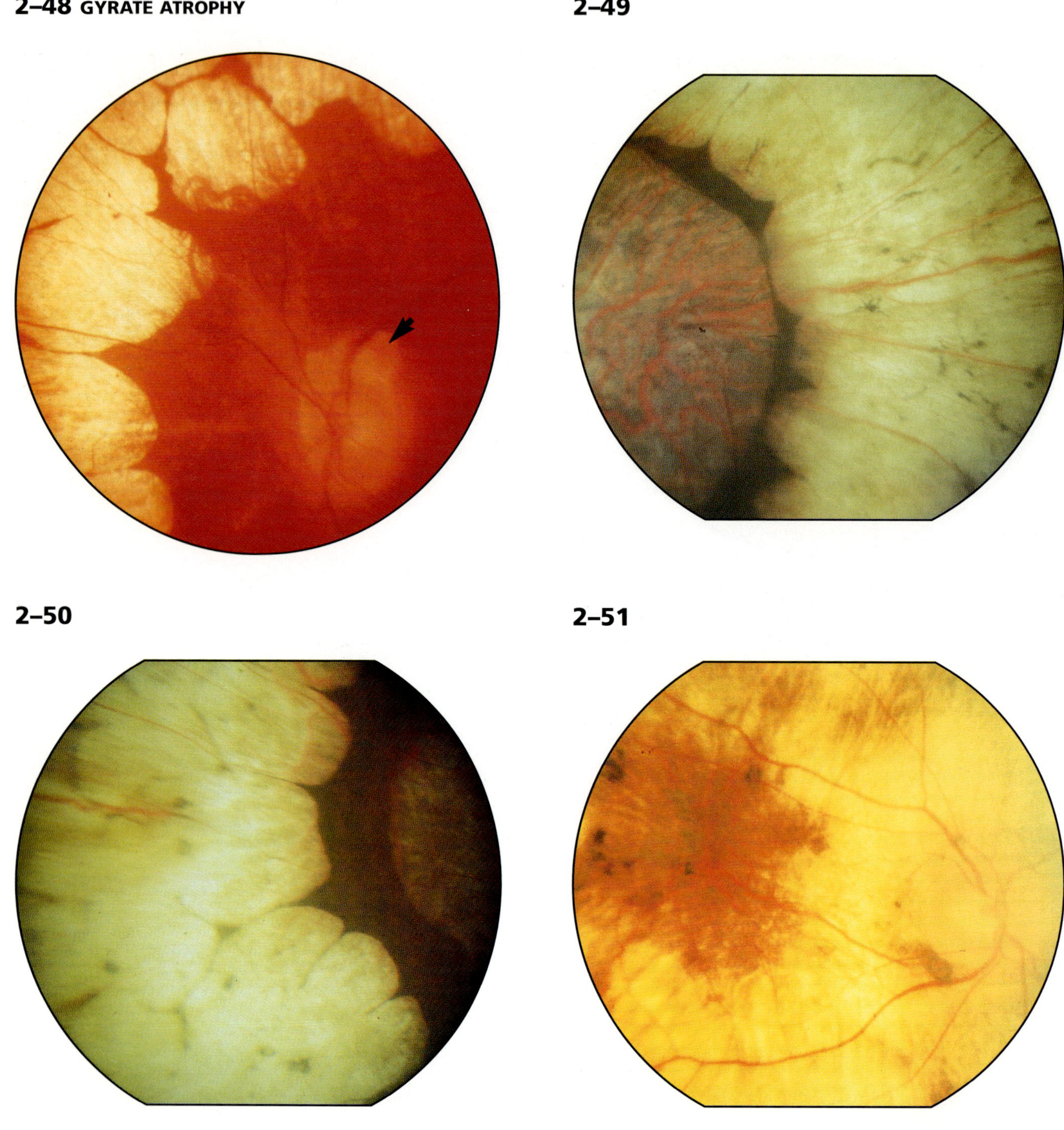

2–49

2–50

2–51

Gyrate atrophy or ornithine aminotransferase deficiency is a rare autosomal recessive condition, which is also a progressive generalized chorioretinal disorder. Laboratory evaluation may confirm the diagnosis. Patients with gyrate atrophy usually have high myopia and a characteristic chorioretinal atrophy with well-delineated scalloped-like borders. Like choroideremia, these lesions start in the midperiphery and then extend in each direction. Loss of night vision occurs early in life. Visual acuity and peripheral field changes are noted over time. Results of pyridoxine supplementation and dietary restrictions upon the progression of the dystrophy are controversial.

2–52

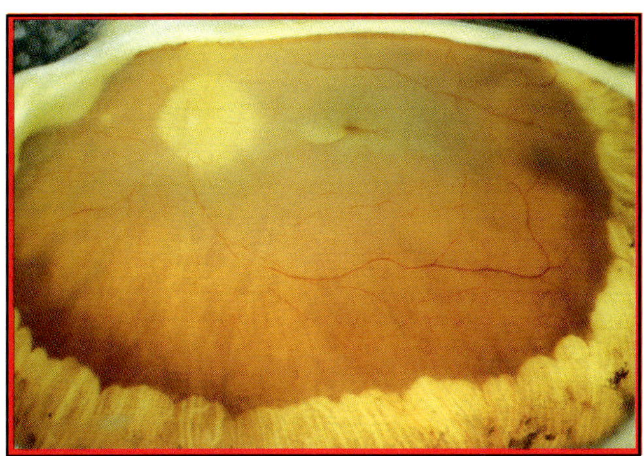

2–53

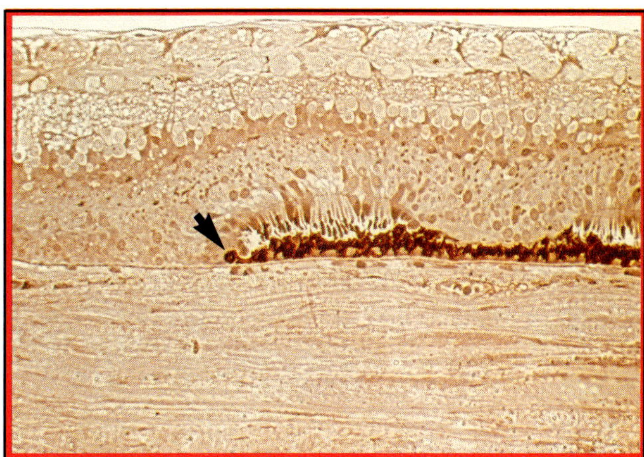

2–54

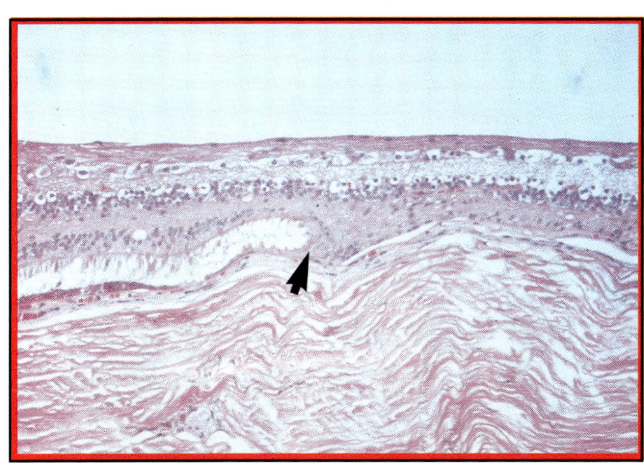

2–48 through 2–50 The scalloped geographic atrophic areas in these patients are characteristic of gyrate atrophy. Note the preservation of some bands of retinal and retinal pigment epithelial tissue between atrophic areas. Optic disc drusen can be seen in 2–48 *(arrowhead)*.

2–51 Note that the progression of the atrophy extends into the macular region in this patient and resembles choroideremia. Laboratory evaluation is essential in determining the diagnosis.

2–52 through 2–54 Gross (2–52) and microscopic (2–53 and 2–54) appearance of an eye with gyrate atrophy reveals sharply circumscribed areas of atrophy with scalloped margins. Note the junction between unaffected and affected areas on the phase-contrast and light microscopy photographs *(arrowheads)*. There is an absence of the choroid and outer retinal layers in the affected areas.

2–48, *Courtesy of Terry George.* ***2–49*** *through* ***2–51,*** *Courtesy of Dr. Irene Maumenee.* ***2–52*** *through* ***2–54,*** *From Wilson, DJ, Weleber, RG, Green, WR: Ocular clinicopathologic study of gyrate atrophy, Am J Ophthalmol 111:24–33, 1991.*

2–55 ALPORT'S DISEASE

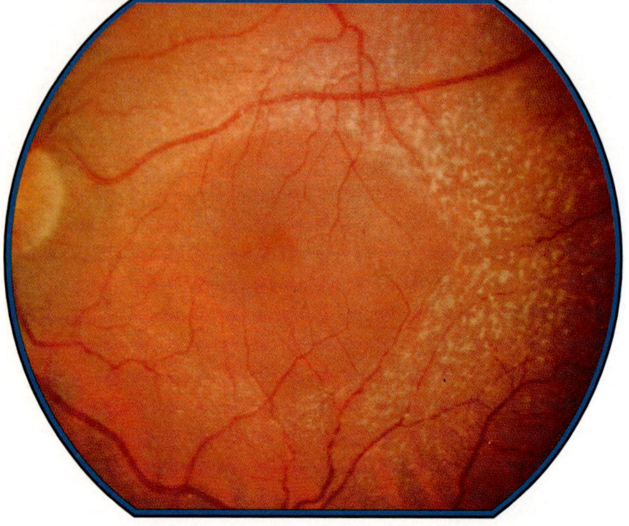

2–56

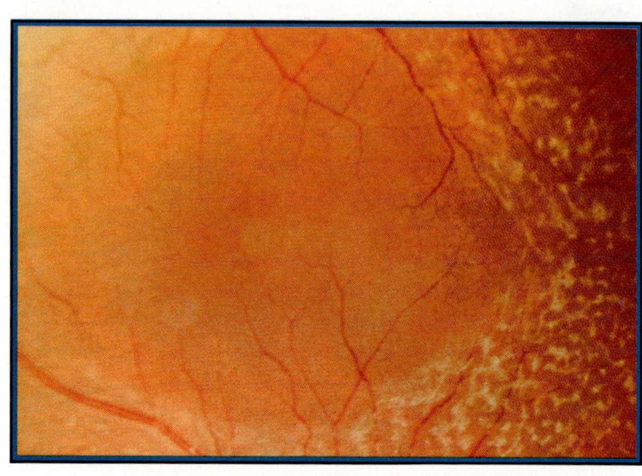

2–57

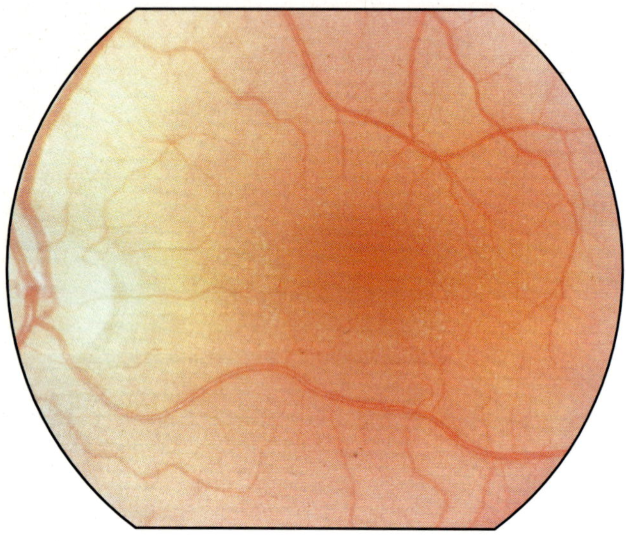

2–58 COCKAYNE'S SYNDROME

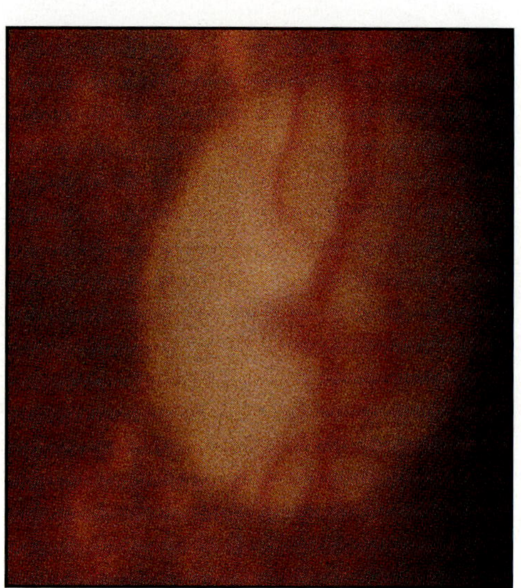

Alport's Disease

2–55 and 2–56 Alport's disease is a hereditary condition consisting of neurosensory deafness and nephritis. Anterior lenticonus may occur. An advanced case of Alport's disease shows crystalline deposits in a lacy configuration.

2–57 An early case shows the deposits in the inner retina.

Cockayne's Syndrome

2–58 Cockayne's syndrome is a progressive autosomal recessive condition. Systemic findings include gastrointestinal abnormalities, short stature, decreased hearing, photosensitivity, and mental retardation. Ocular findings include cataracts, miosis, keratopathy, and a pigmentary retinal dystrophy with bone spicules. Optic atrophy and vascular attenuation may also occur. This 9-year-old female with Cockayne's syndrome shows retinal degeneration and optic atrophy.

***2–55** and **2–56,** Courtesy of Dr. Scott Sneed. **2–57,** Courtesy of Dr. Irene Maumenee. **2–58,** From Ryan, SJ: Retina, ed 2, St Louis, 1994, Mosby–Year Book. Courtesy of Bateman, Lang, and Maumenee.*

2–59 OLIVOPONTOCEREBELLAR ATROPHY

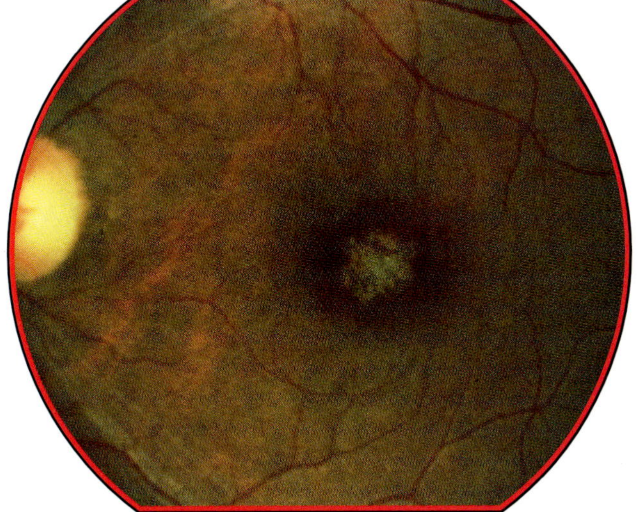

2–60

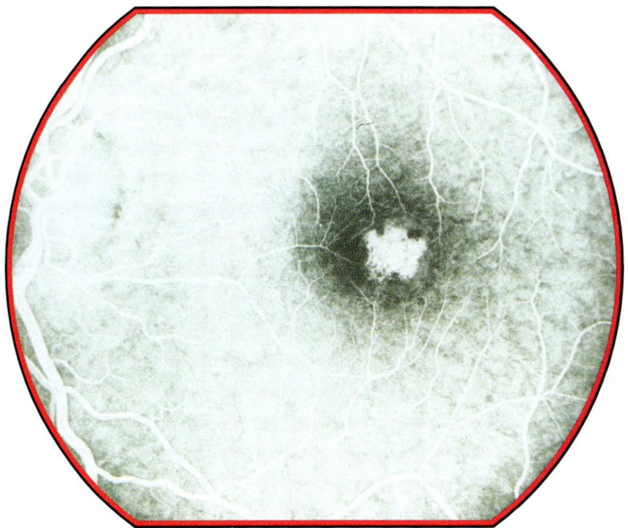

2–61

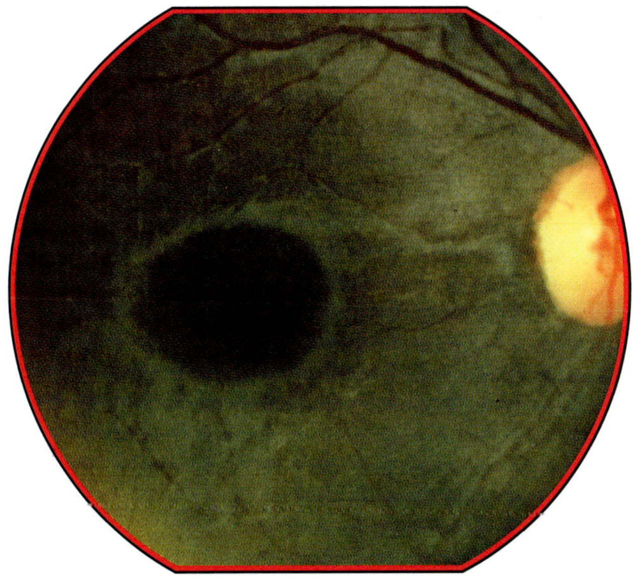

2–62

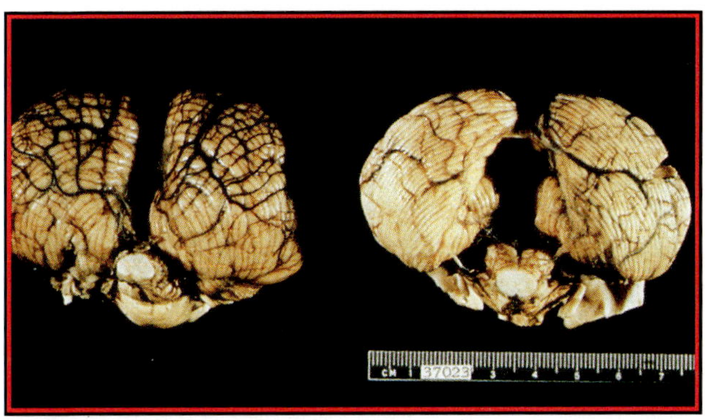

2–63

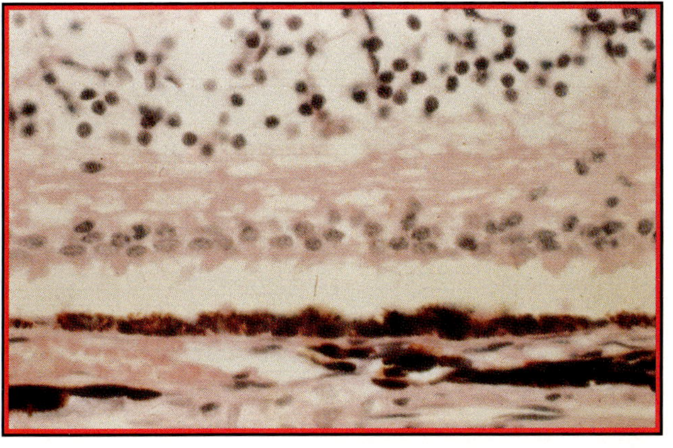

Olivopontocerebellar Atrophy

2–59 and 2–60 Olivopontocerebellar atrophy type III is an autosomal dominant disease associated with a retinal dystrophy. In this condition, cerebellar ataxia occurs with an associated atrophic, granular, or bull's eye type of maculopathy.

2–61 A polymorphic macular sheen is noted early. Late in the disease, a bull's eye appearance can be seen as atrophy evolves in the perifoveal region. The optic disc is atrophic.

2–62 Cerebellar degeneration also occurs.

2–63 Histopathologic examination reveals that the retinal pigment epithelium is relatively intact. Total loss of the outer segments is noted with near total loss of the inner segments and a reduction in the outer nuclear layer. These changes suggest that the primary defect is in the photoreceptor cells.

***2–59** through **2–62**, Courtesy of Dr. Irene Maumenee.*

Hereditary Choroidal Diseases

2–64 CENTRAL AREOLAR CHOROIDAL DYSTROPHY

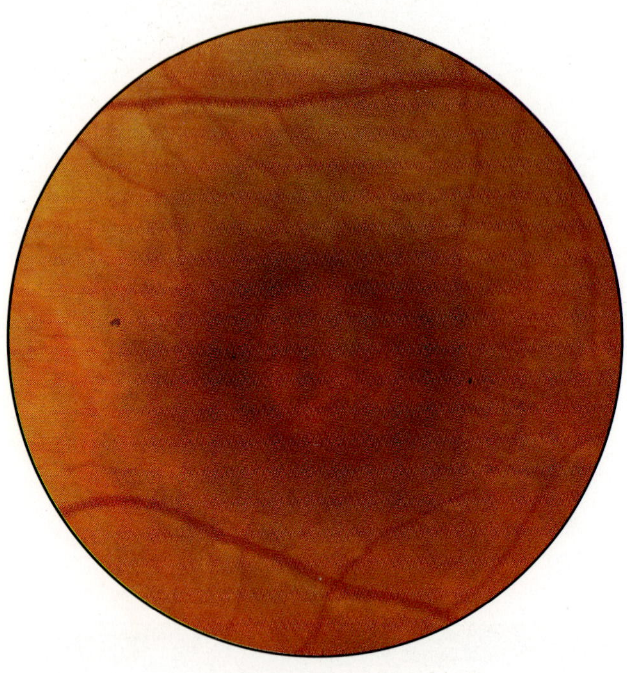

2–65

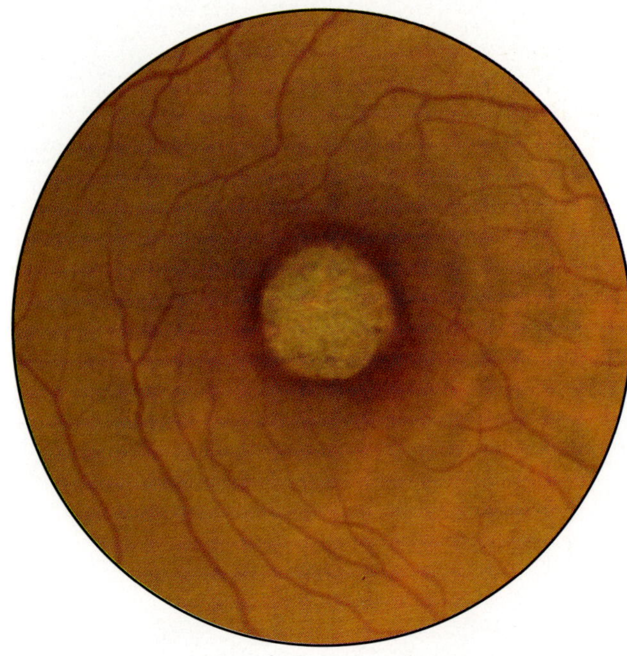

2–66

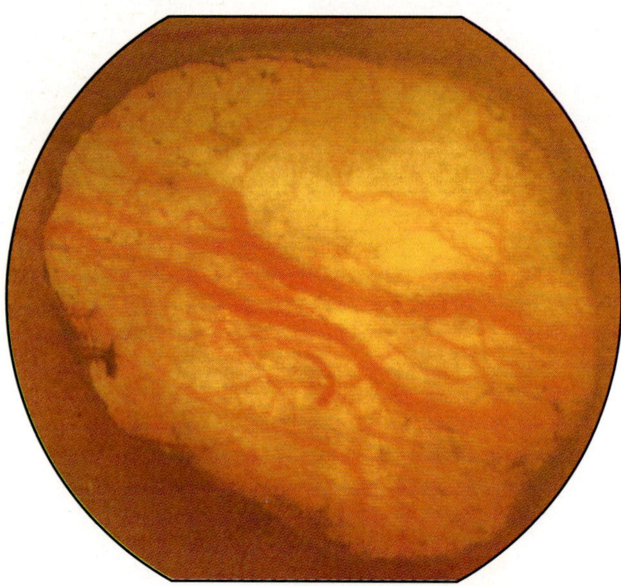

2–64 and 2–65 The macular region is initially affected in central areolar choroidal dystrophy, which is an autosomal dominant disorder. In the early stages of this condition, a mild atrophic change (2–64) occurs and later more advanced atrophy is noted (2–65).

2–66 Even later in the disorder, there is an extensive loss of the retina and choroid in a parafoveal distribution. The remaining choroidal vessels are seen overlying the sclera.

***2–64** and **2–65,** From Ryan, SJ: Retina, ed 2, St Louis, Mosby–Year Book. Courtesy of Drs. Ron Carr and Ken Noble. **2–66,** Courtesy of Drs. Ron Carr and Ken Noble.*

2–67 PERIPAPILLARY CHOROIDAL DYSTROPHY

2–68

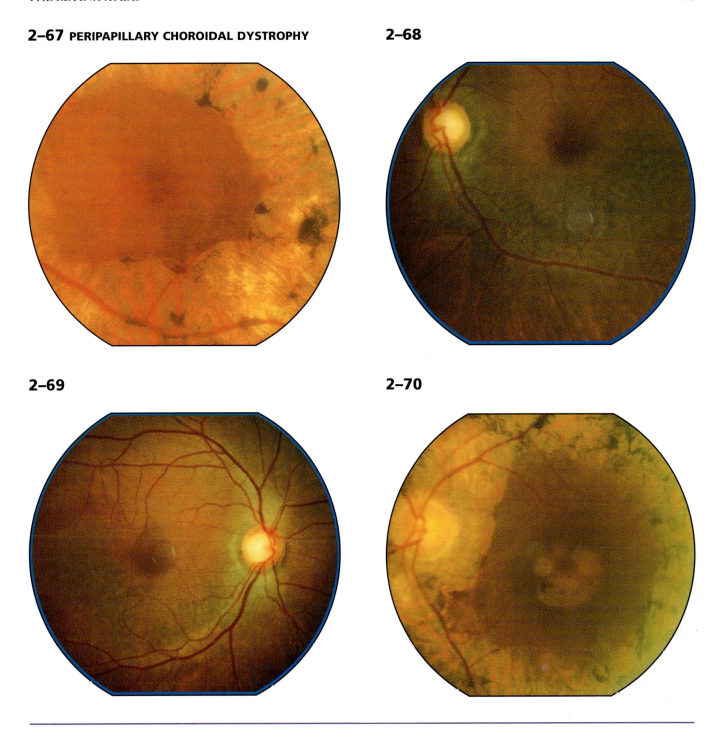

2–69

2–70

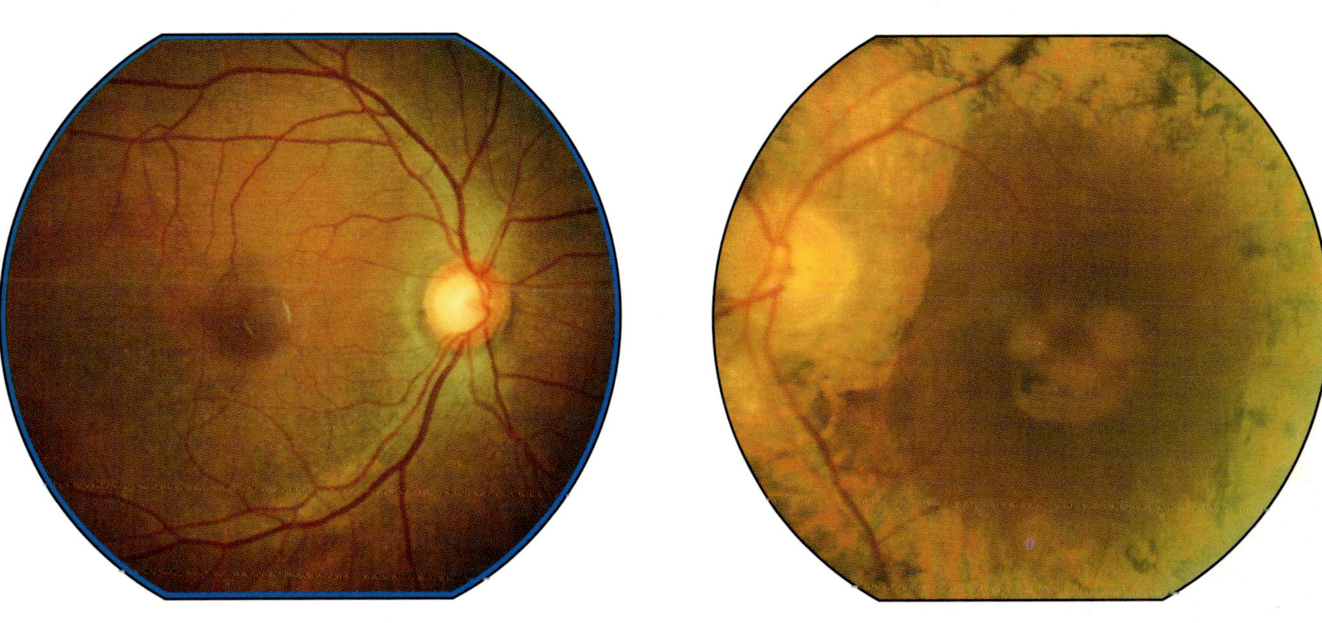

2–67 This autosomal dominant disorder is extremely rare. Unlike central areolar choroidal dystrophy, which remains localized in the macula, peripapillary or pericentral choroidal dystrophy initially involves the peripapillary area and radiates along the vascular arcade sparing the macula.

2–68 and 2–69 A more subtle case shows peripapillary atrophy that radiates along the vascular arcade and spares the macula.

2–70 Later, the macula may become involved.

2–67 *and* ***2–70,*** *Courtesy of Drs. Ron Carr and Ken Noble.* ***2–68*** *and* ***2–69,*** *Courtesy of Dr. Dan Rosberger.*

2–71 BIETTI'S CRYSTALLINE DYSTROPHY

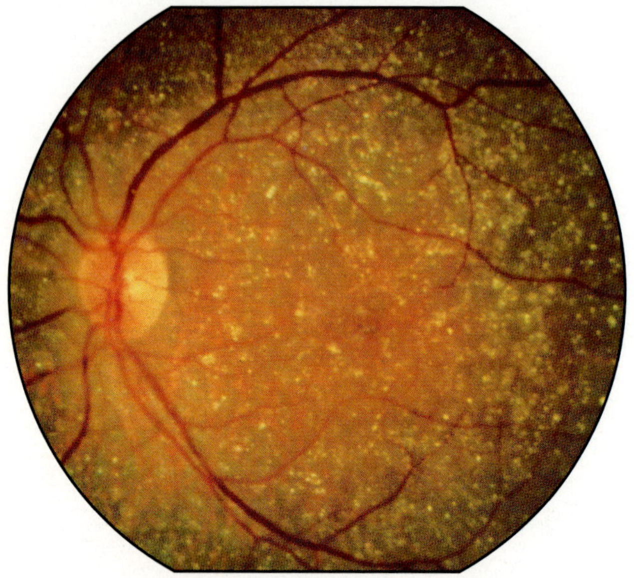

2–72

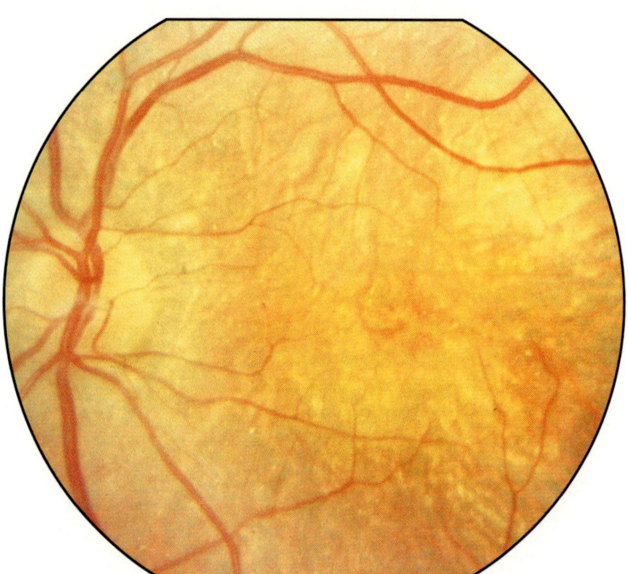

2–73 ROD MONOCHROMATISM

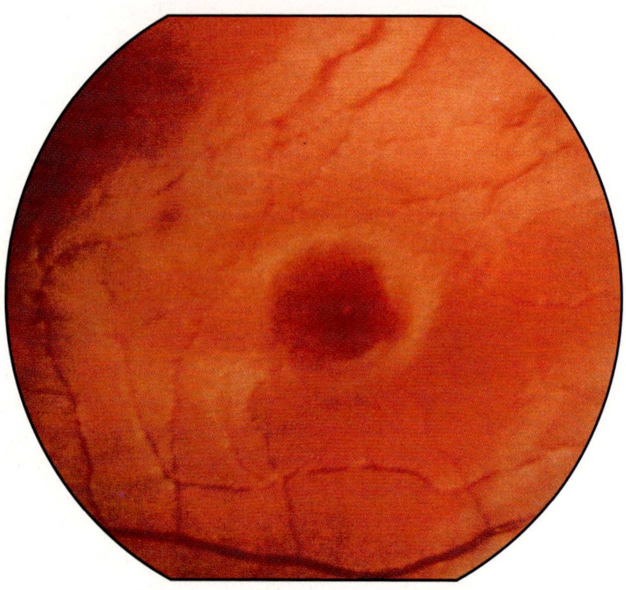

Bietti's Crystalline Dystrophy

2–71 This rare autosomal recessive disorder consists of marginal corneal crystals associated with a crystalline retinopathy. Choroidal and retinal pigment epithelium (RPE) atrophy also occur. Crystalline deposition is noted in this patient.

2–72 In a more advanced case, zones of atrophy are found throughout the fundus. Crystalline deposits in this stage are now less apparent in the atrophic areas.

Rod Monochromatism

2–73 Rod monochromatism is a congenital absence of cones. Vision is poor at birth, and nystagmus often is noted. Electroretinogram (ERG) studies reveal an absent cone ERG with a normal rod ERG. The fundus often is normal in these patients. Nonspecific RPE changes or a bull's eye pattern may occur.

2–71, *Courtesy of Dr. Carmen Puliafito.* **2–72,** *Courtesy of Dr. Irene Maumenee.*

2–74 CONE DYSTROPHY **2–75**

2–76 **2–77**

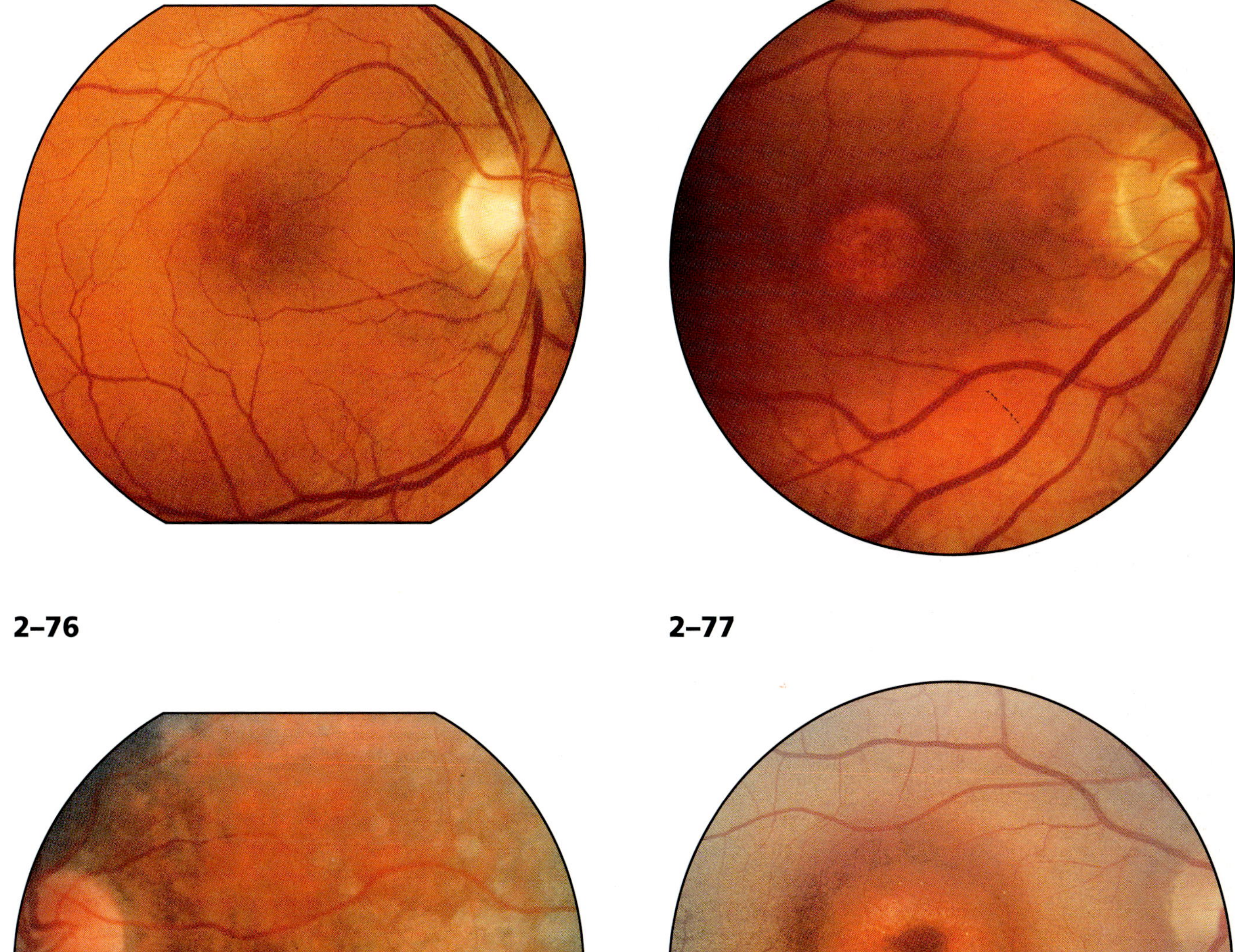

Cone Dystrophy

2–74 through 2–76 Progressive cone dystrophy may be inherited in several genetic modes or occur sporadically. The macula may vary from minimal pigmentary changes in the perifoveal regions (2–74), to a more pronounced, discrete perifoveal disturbance (2–75), or to more widespread atrophic and pigmentary retinopathy (2–76).

2–77 The macula may have a bull's eye pattern. However, more commonly, nonspecific pigmentary changes are noted.

***2–74** through **2–77,** Courtesy of Drs. Ron Carr and Ken Noble.*

2–78 OGUCHI'S DISEASE

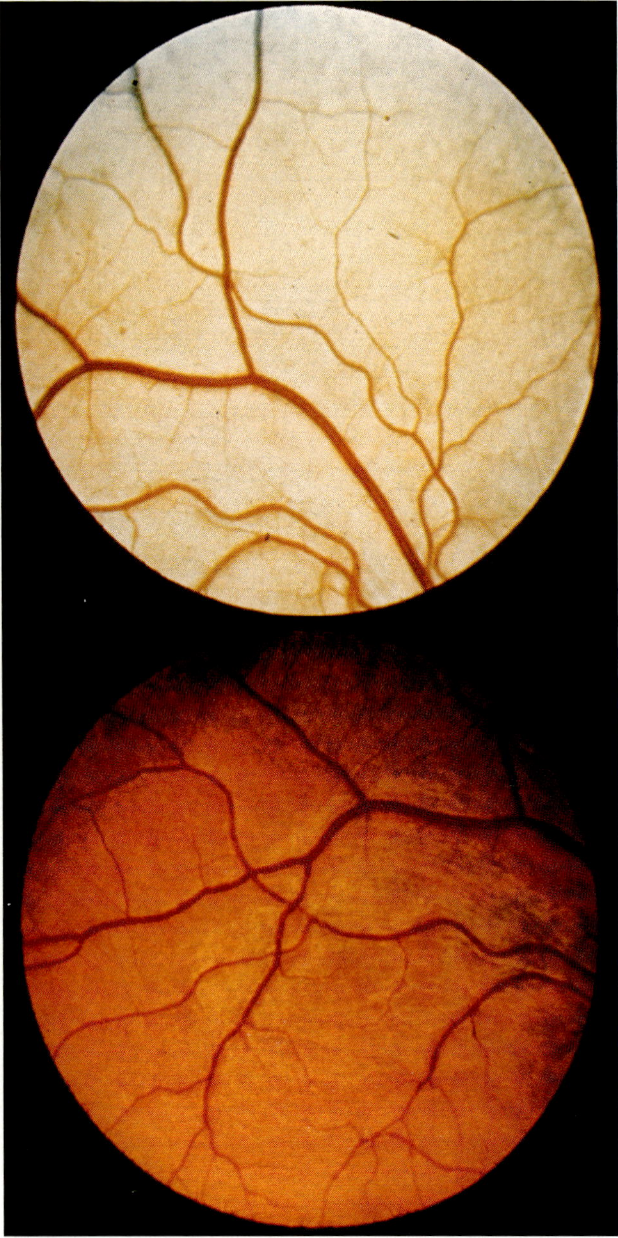

2–79

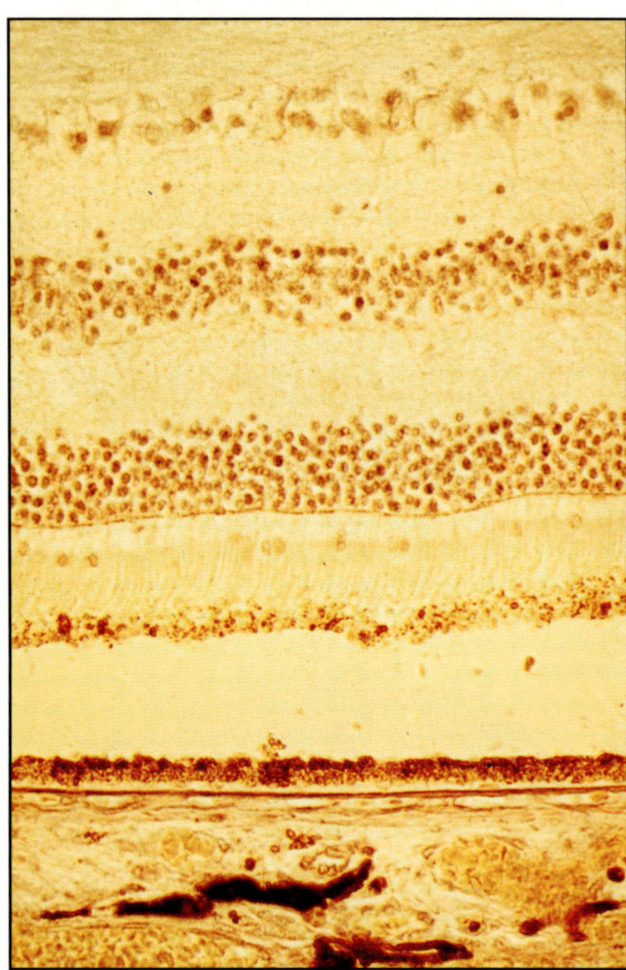

Patients with Oguchi's disease, an autosomal recessive condition, have difficulty with night vision and dark-adaptation abnormalities. This disorder is a type of congenital stationary night blindness.

2–78 The characteristic ophthalmologic features of Oguchi's disease include a peculiar grayish-white discoloration of the retina with a change from dark to light adaptation, which is termed Mizuo's phenomenon. This case demonstrates Mizuo's phenomenon in a patient with Oguchi's disease.

2–79 Histopathologic examination of a patient with Oguchi's disease reveals that the retina is normal except for the accumulation of pigment between the photoreceptors and the retinal pigment epithelium. There is also migration of the photoreceptor cell nuclei into the inner segment area.

2–78 *and* ***2–79,*** *Courtesy of Dr. Jeffrey Shakin.*

2–80 ALBINISM

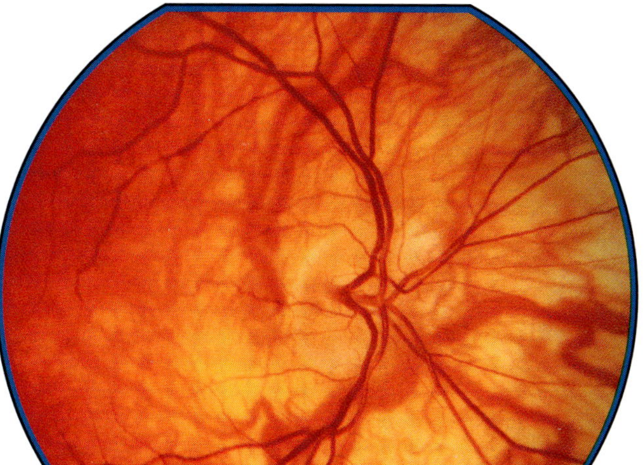

2–81

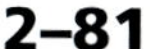

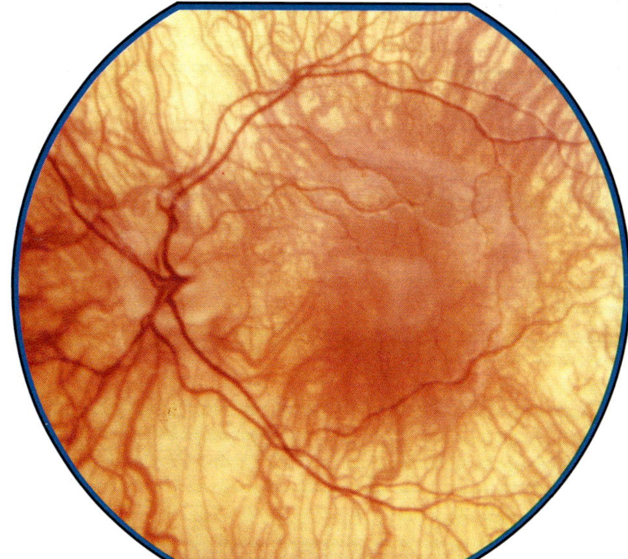

2–82

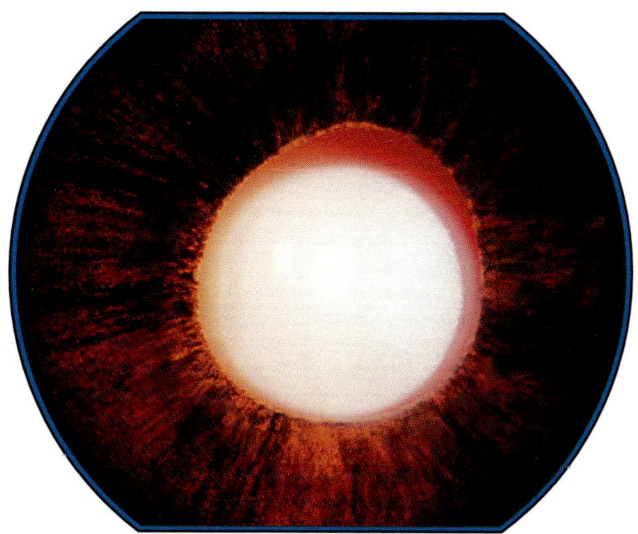

2–80 and 2–81 Oculocutaneous albinism occurs by autosomal recessive inheritance, whereas ocular albinism is usually transmitted by X-linked or autosomal recessive inheritance. These patients with albinism demonstrate the hypopigmented fundus characteristic of this disorder. Note the enhanced visualization of the underlying choroid. The fovea is often indistinct, and foveal hypoplasia may occur.

2–82 Transillumination of the iris is often noted.

***2–80** through **2–82,** Courtesy of Dr. Jeffrey Shakin.*

2–83 ALBINISM

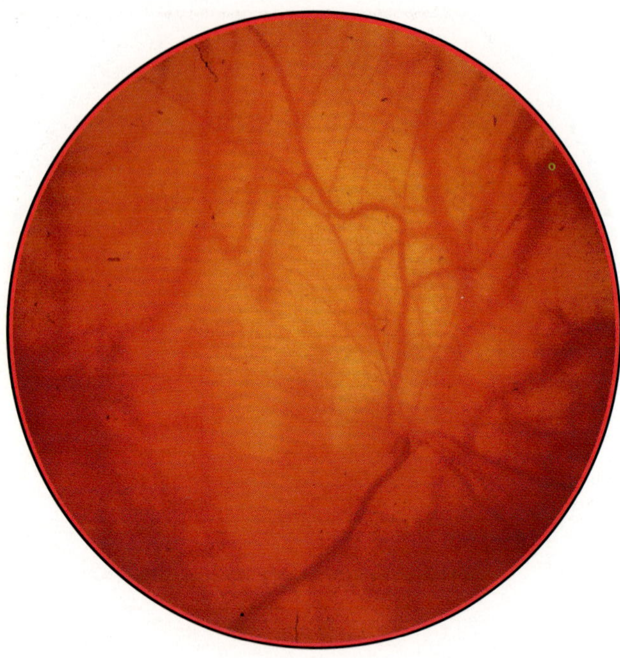

2–84

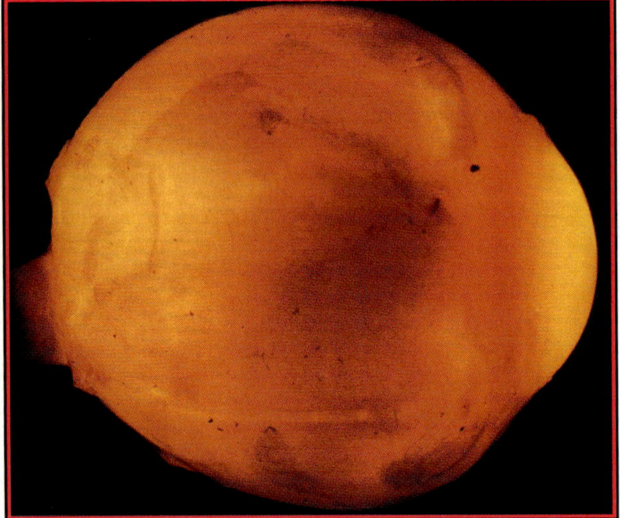

2–85

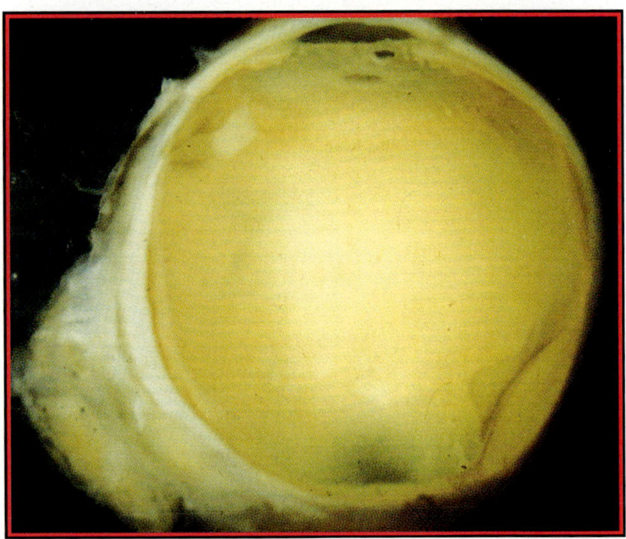

2–83 through 2–85 This clinicopathologic correlation of a patient with oculocutaneous albinism reveals total absence of melanin pigment as seen by fundus photography (2–83), transillumination (2–84) and gross examination (2–85).

2–83 *through* ***2–85,*** *Courtesy of Dr. Jeffrey Shakin.*

(Case continued on next page.)

2–86

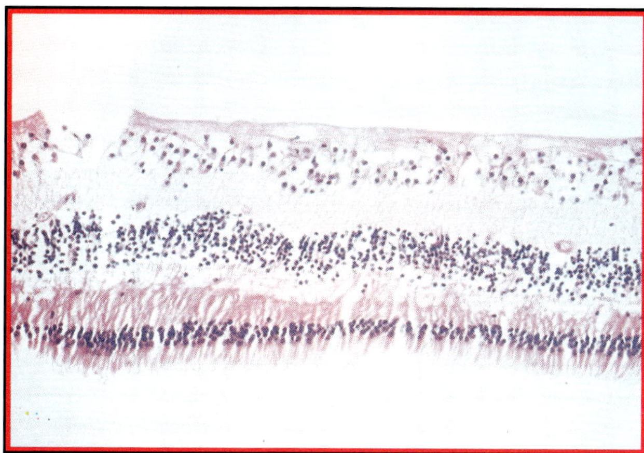

2–87

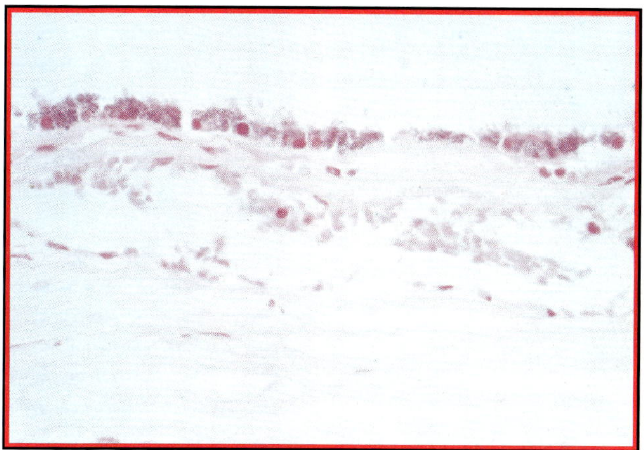

2–88

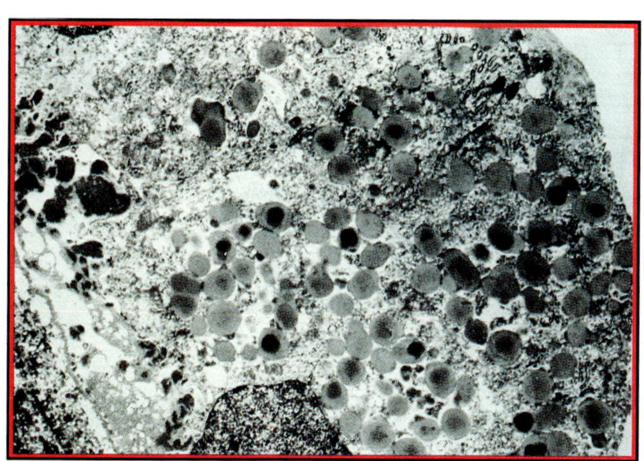

2–86 Histopathologic serial sectioning through the center of the macula shows a lack of foveal differentiation.

2–87 and 2–88 Some pigmentation in the retinal pigment epithelium is due to the accumulation of lipofuscin.

2–86 *through* ***2–88,*** *Courtesy of Dr. Jeffrey Shakin.*

2–89 CARRIERS OF ALBINISM

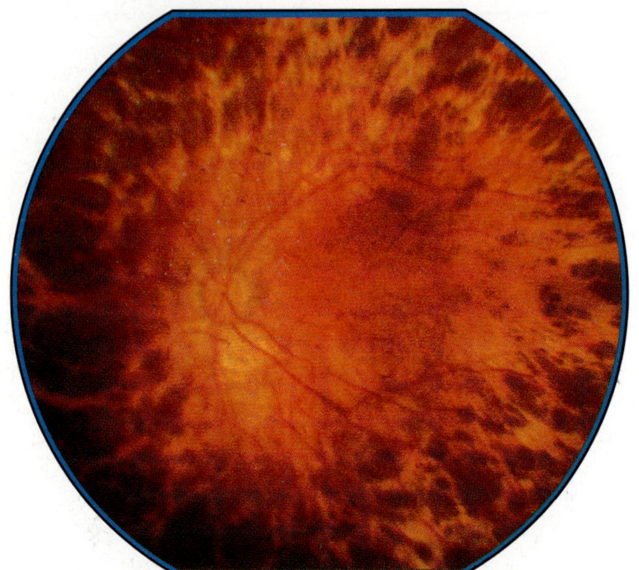

2–90

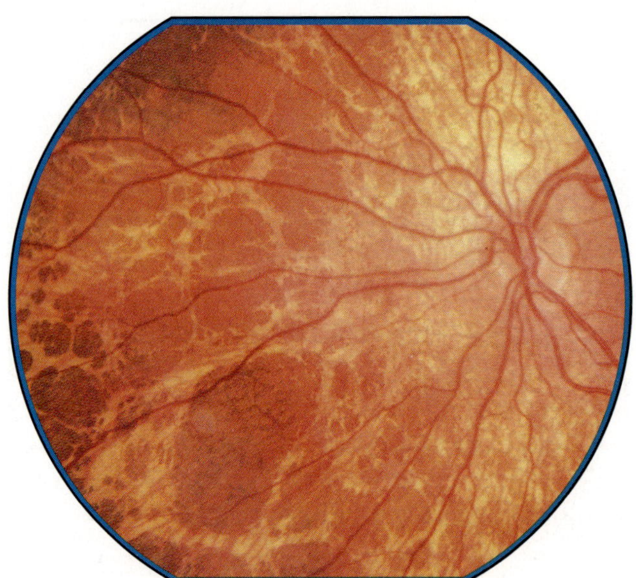

2–91

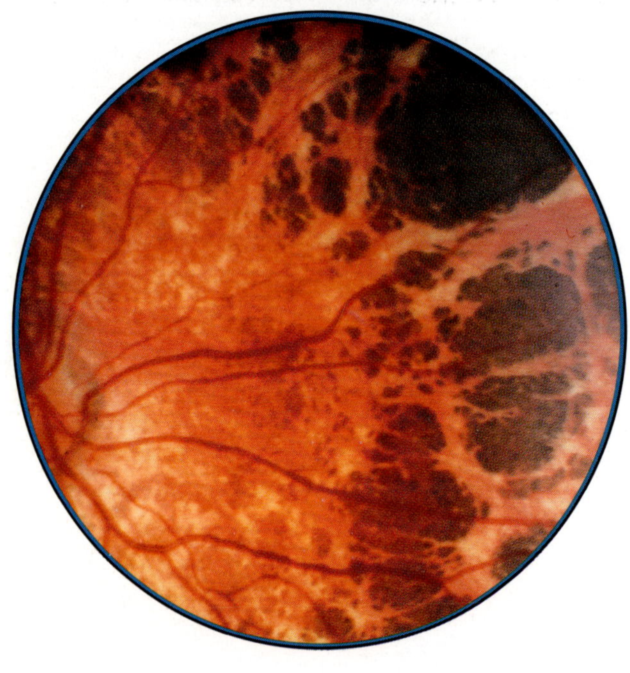

2–92 **2–93**

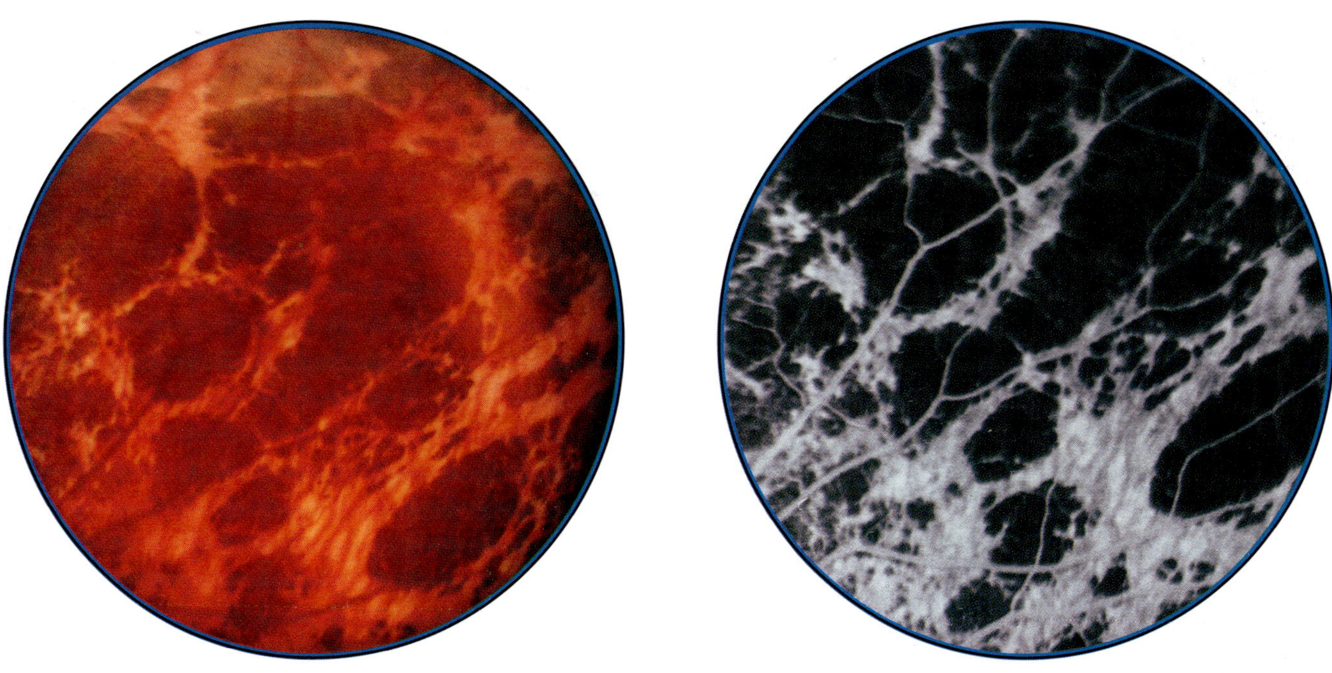

2–89 through 2–93 Carriers of albinism may also be affected. Hyperpigmented beartrack–like lesions may be seen in carriers. Note that the fluorescein angiogram shows blockage in these areas (2–93), as well as increased transmission from the choroid through less pigmented areas. Islands of hypopigmentation are often separated by these deeply pigmented lesions.

2–89 *and* ***2–90,*** *Courtesy of Dr. Jeffrey Shakin.* ***2–91*** *through* ***2–93,*** *Courtesy of Hoger Mietz.*

2–94 CARRIERS OF ALBINISM

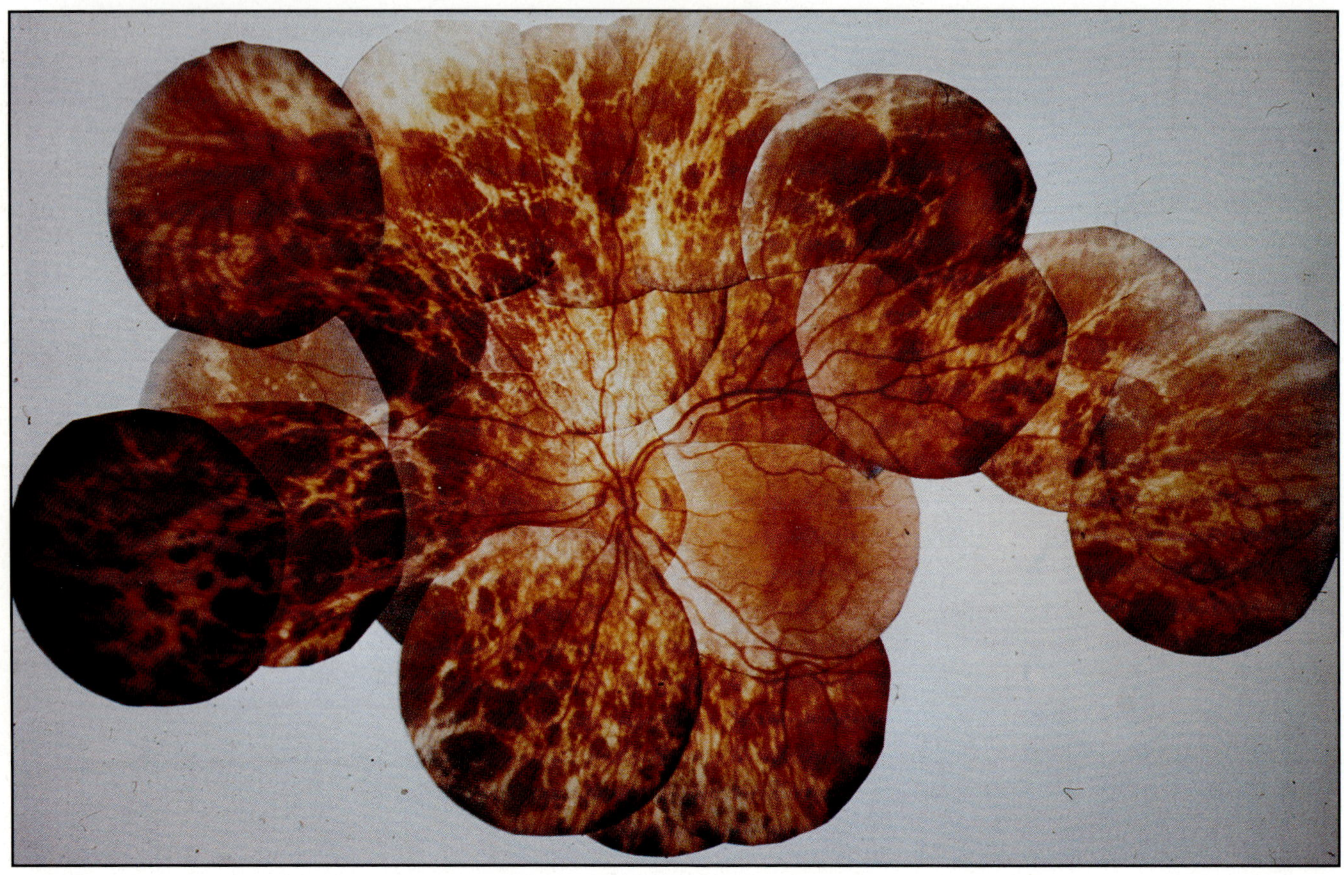

2–94 This montage illustrates the diffuse nature of the bear-track–like changes in this carrier of albinism. Note the hypopigmented areas between the bear-track lesions.

2–94, *Courtesy of Dr. Jeffrey Shakin.*

2–95

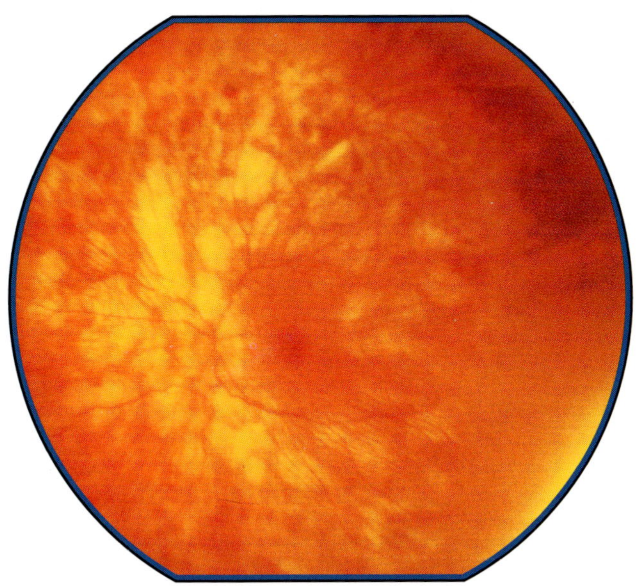

2–96

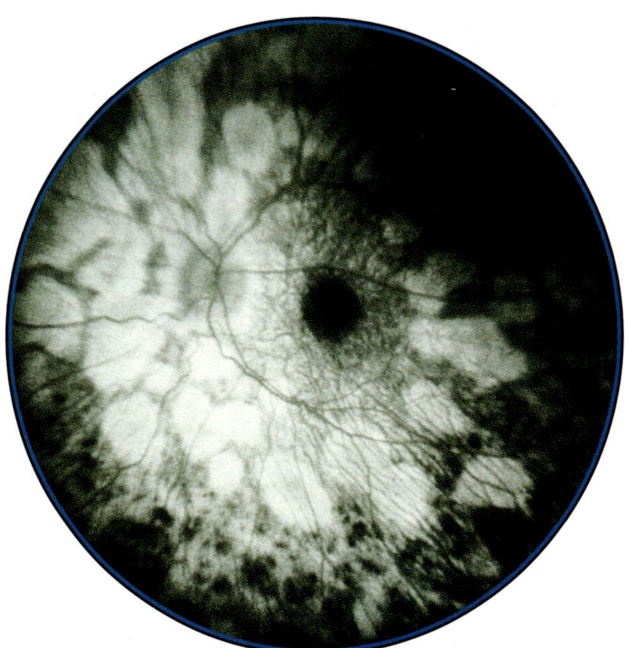

2–97

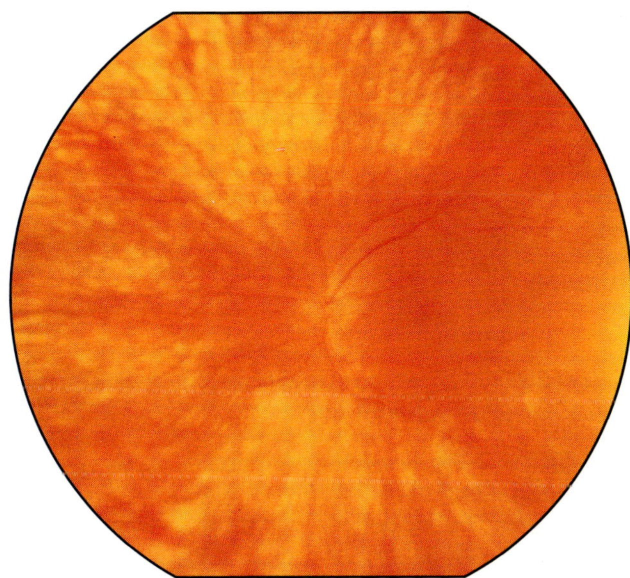

2–95 through 2–97 Other carriers may be affected by a diffuse granular type of lesion. Note the hypopigmented lesions throughout the fundus, which are hyperfluorescent by fluorescein angiography (2–96). These carrier findings are examples of lyonization.

2–95 *through* ***2–97,*** *Courtesy of Dr. Jeffrey Shakin.*

2–98 AICARDI SYNDROME

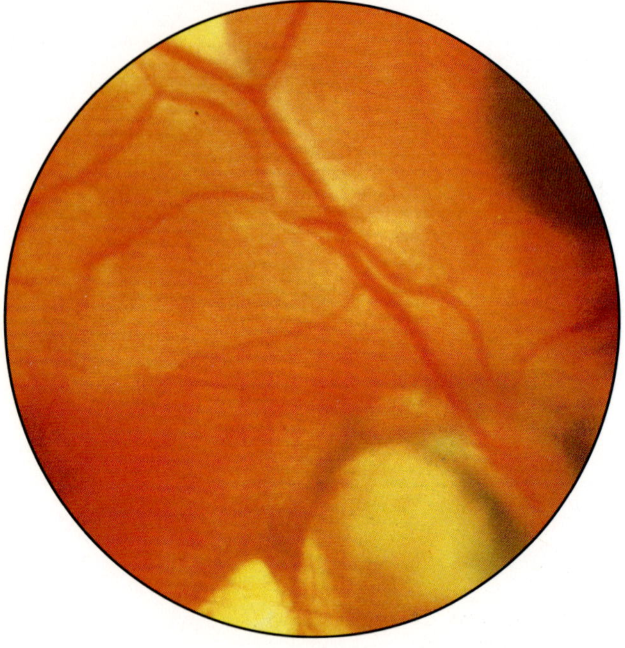

2–99

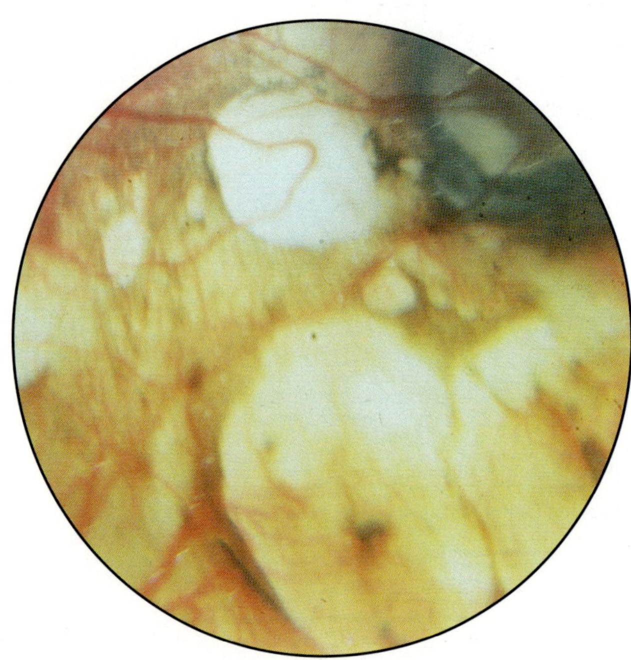

2–100

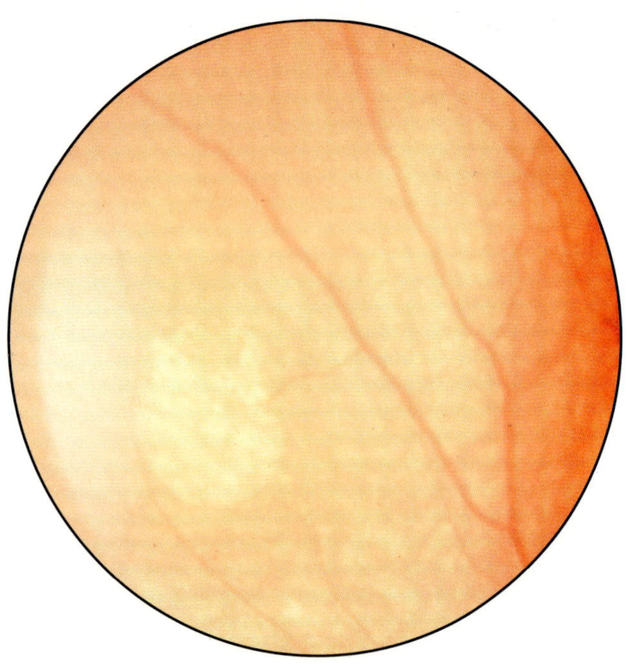

2–98 and 2–99 Infantile spasms, agenesis of the corpus callosum, and a chorioretinopathy are noted in the Aicardi syndrome. Colobomas of the optic nerve and choroid may also occur. The fundus lesions demonstrate well-demarcated areas of whitish lacunae. The fundus may reveal lacunae marginated in some areas by retinal pigment epithelial proliferation. In more advanced cases, atrophic changes prevail throughout. The mutation is probably in the X chromosome. This syndrome is seen only in females, as male offspring usually do not survive.

2–100 Mild pigmentary changes may be noted in carriers of the Aicardi syndrome.

2–98 *and* ***2–99,*** *Courtesy of Dr. Irene Maumenee.* ***2–100,*** *Courtesy of Dr. J. R. Buncic. From Menezes, A, Enzenauer, J, and Buncic, JR: Aicardi syndrome: the elusive mild case, Br J Ophthalmol 78:494–496, 1994.*

Suggested Readings

Appel, SH, and Roses, AD: The macular dystrophies. In Stanbury, JB, Wyngaarden, JS, Fredrickson, DS, Goldstein, JL, and Brown, MS, eds. The metabolic basis of inherited disease, ed 5, New York, 1983, McGraw-Hill, p 1478

Beckerman, BL, and Rapin, I: Ceroid lipofuscinosis, Am J Ophthalmol 80:73, 1975

Crandall, BF, Phillipart, M, Brown, WJ, and Bluestone, DA: Review article: Mucolipidosis IV, Am J Med Genet 12:301, 1982

Deutman, AF, Sengers, RCA, and Trybels, JMF: Gyrate atrophy of the choroid and retina with reticular pigmentary dystrophy and ornithine-ketoacid-transaminase deficiency, Int Ophthalmol 1:49, 1978

DeVenecia, G, and Shapiro, M: Neuronal ceroid lipofuscinosis. A retinal trypsin digest study, Ophthalmology 91:1406, 1984

Evans, SH, Erickson, RP, Kelsch, R, and Peirce, JC: Apparently changing patterns of inheritance in Alport's hereditary nephritis: genetic heterogeneity versus altered diagnostic criteria, Clin Genet 17:285, 1980

Francois, J: Metabolic tapetoretinal degenerations, Surv Ophthalmol 26:293, 1982

Gills, JP, Hobson, R, Hanley, WB, and McKusick, VA: Electroretinography and fundus oculi findings in Hurler's disease and allied mucopolysaccharidoses, Arch Ophthalmol 74:596, 1965

Green, WR: Retina in ophthalmic pathology. In Spencer, WH, eds: Ophthalmic pathology. An atlas and textbook, ed 3, vol 2, Philadelphia, 1985, WB Saunders, p 1034

Konigsmark, BW, and Weiner, LP: The olivopontocerebellar atrophies: a review, Medicine (Baltimore) 49:227, 1970

Ryan, SJ, Knox, DL, Green, WR, and Konigsmark, BW: Olivopontocerebellar degeneration, Arch Ophthalmol 93:169, 1975

Schneider, JA, Wong, V, and Seegmiller, JE: The early diagnosis of cystinosis, J Pediatr 74:114, 1969

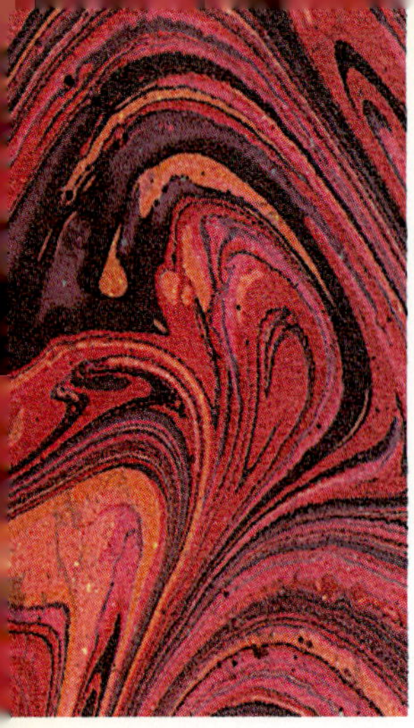

Chapter 3
Hereditary Vitreoretinal Degenerations

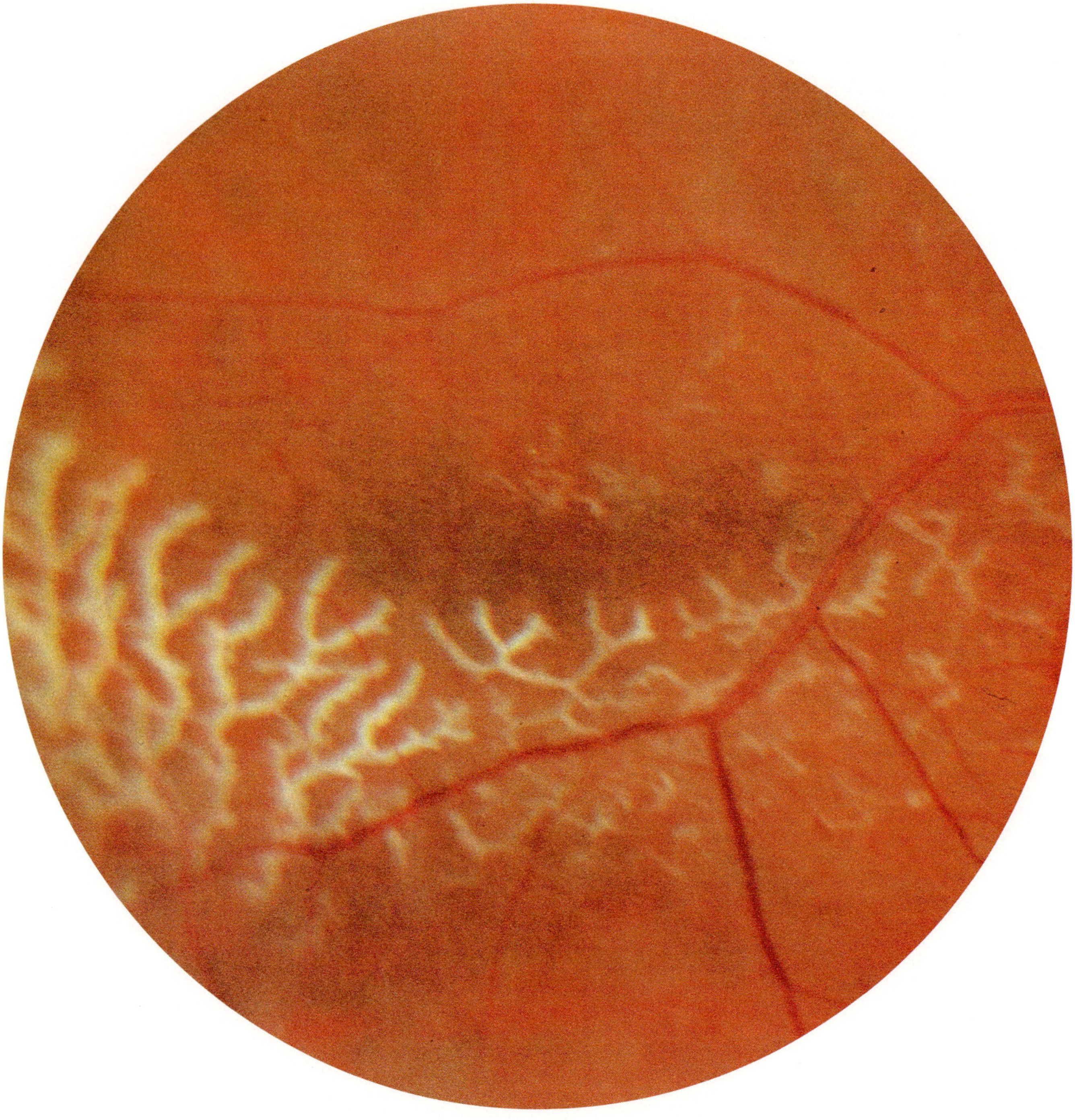

Several hereditary conditions may cause a degeneration of the vitreous and/or retina. These conditions include Wagner's disease, Stickler's disease, and Goldmann-Favre's vitreotapetoretinal degeneration.

3–1 WAGNER'S DISEASE

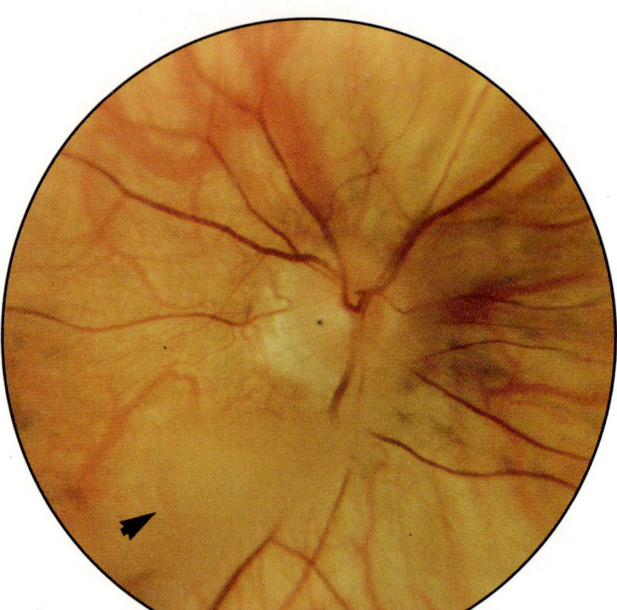

3–2 **3–3**

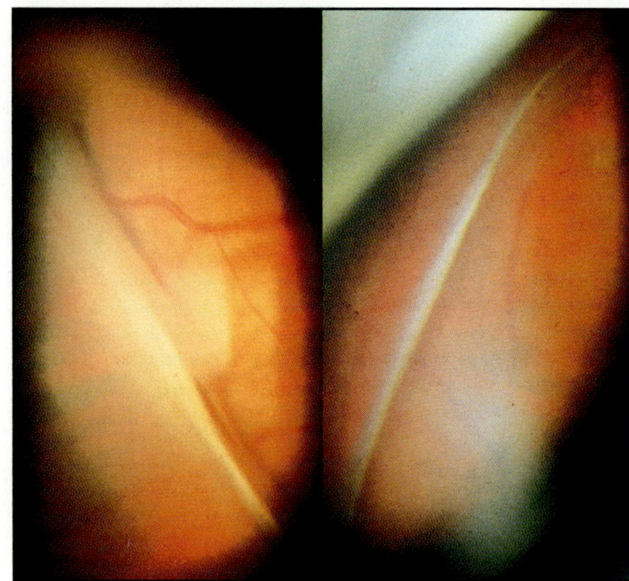

3–4

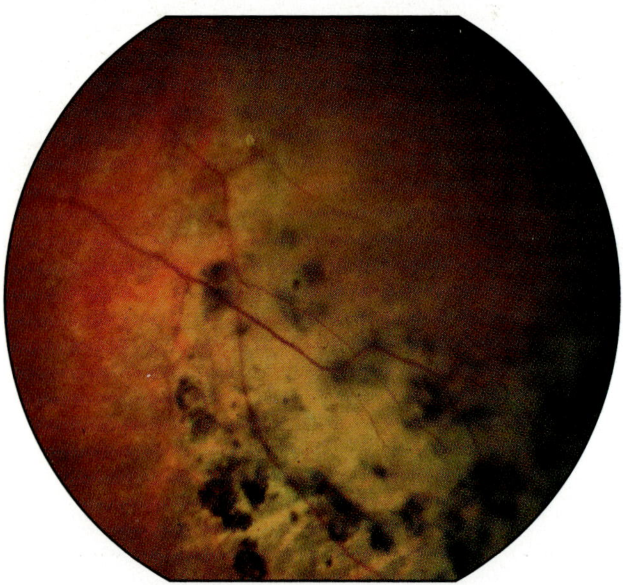

3–1 through 3–4 Wagner's disease consists exclusively of ocular abnormalities, whereas patients with Stickler's syndrome have both ocular and systemic abnormalities. Both are inherited in an autosomal dominant pattern. Wagner's disease consists of myopia, an optically empty vitreous cavity, preretinal avascular membranes (3–1 *[arrowhead]*, 3–2, and 3–3), pigmentation in a vascular distribution (3–4), peripheral vascular sheathing, and chorioretinal atrophy.

3–1 *through* ***3–3,*** *Courtesy of Dr. Irene Maumenee.*

3–5 STICKLER'S SYNDROME

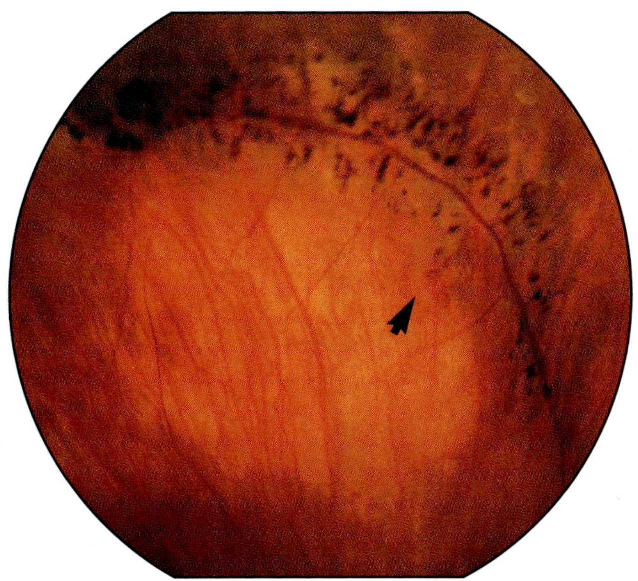

3–6

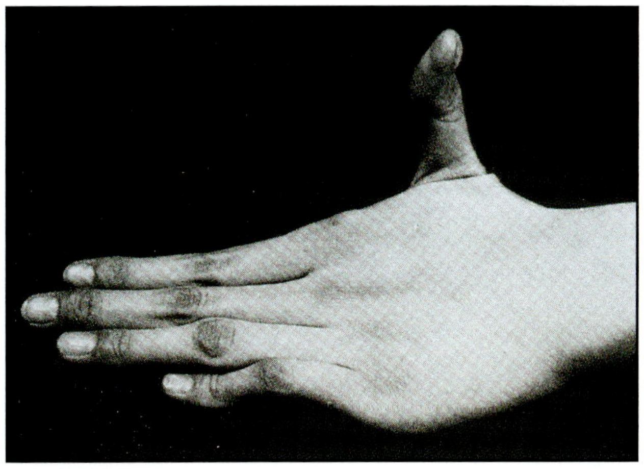

3–7

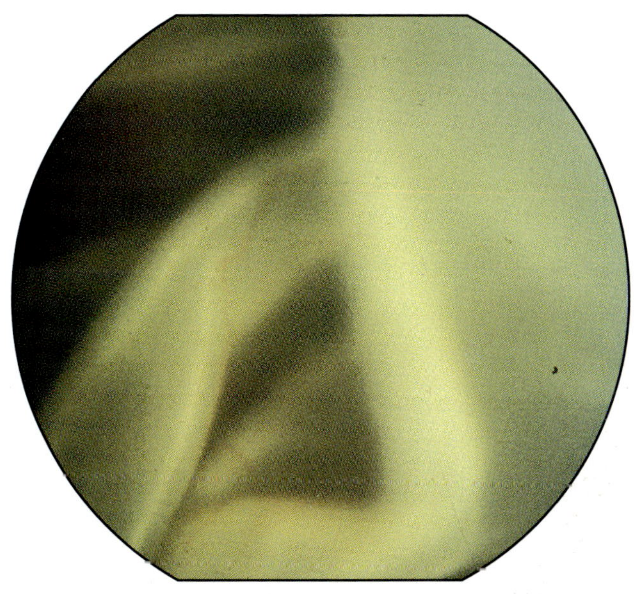

3–5 This patient with Stickler's syndrome has perivascular pigmentary lattice degeneration, a retinal tear *(arrowhead),* and a traction band.

3–6 Stickler's syndrome consists of similar ophthalmic findings to Wagner's syndrome and the following systemic abnormalities: abnormal facial appearance, cleft palate, decreased hearing, and musculoskeletal disease. Loose joints, long fingers, and grooved nails are characteristic skeletal abnormalities noted in Stickler's syndrome.

3–7 Patients with Wagner's disease do not have an increased risk of developing retinal detachment. However, the incidence of retinal detachment is almost 50% in patients with Stickler's syndrome. Affected patients also develop characteristic cataracts in early adulthood.

***3–5, 3–6,** and **3–7,** Courtesy of Dr. Irene Maumenee.*

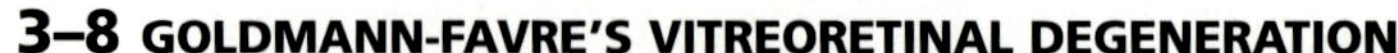

3–8 GOLDMANN-FAVRE'S VITREORETINAL DEGENERATION

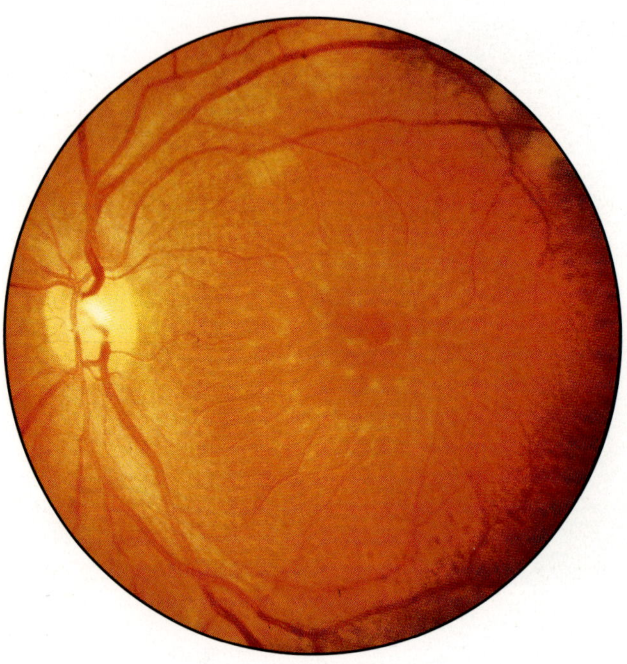

3–8 Goldmann-Favre's vitreoretinal degeneration is a rare bilateral, autosomal recessive disorder. Retinoschisis, vitreous liquefaction, cataract, pigmentary retinal degeneration, and microcystic macular changes are noted. Characteristic cystic changes in the macula are demonstrated in this patient. The cystic changes are sometimes more evident on monochromatic red-free photography. Fluorescein angiography shows fairly symmetric diffuse window defects due to atrophy but no staining into the cystic space.

3–8, *Courtesy of Dr. Irene Maumenee.*

3–9

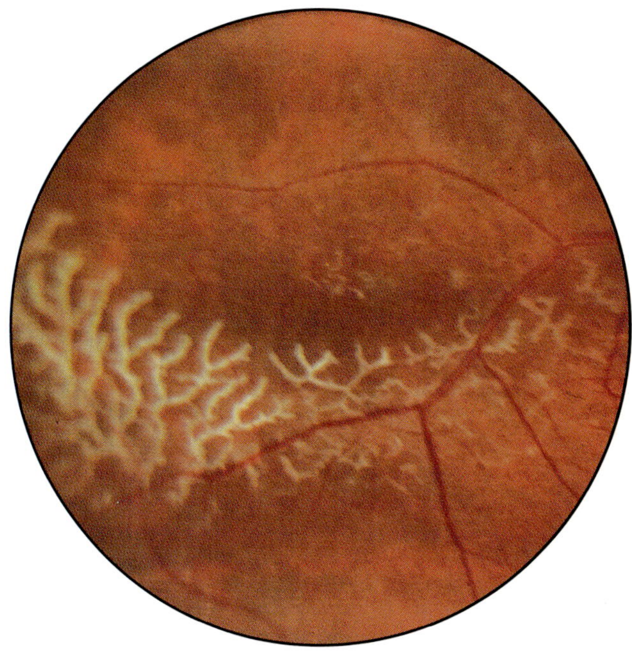

3–10

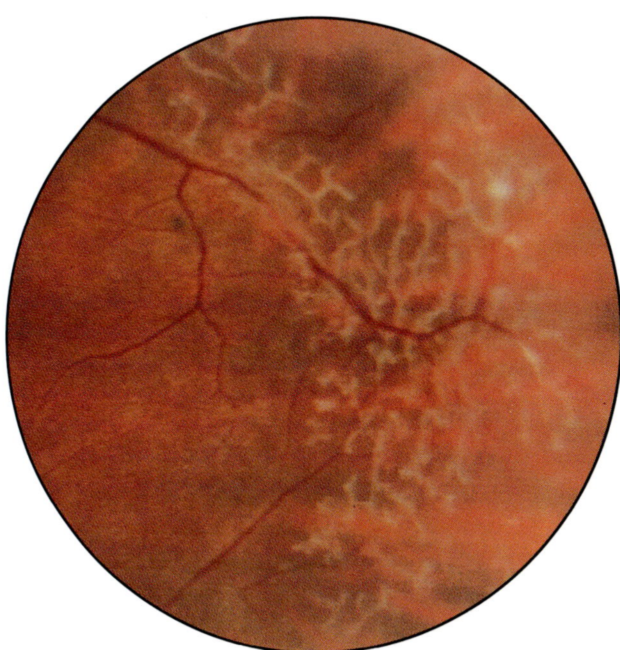

3–11

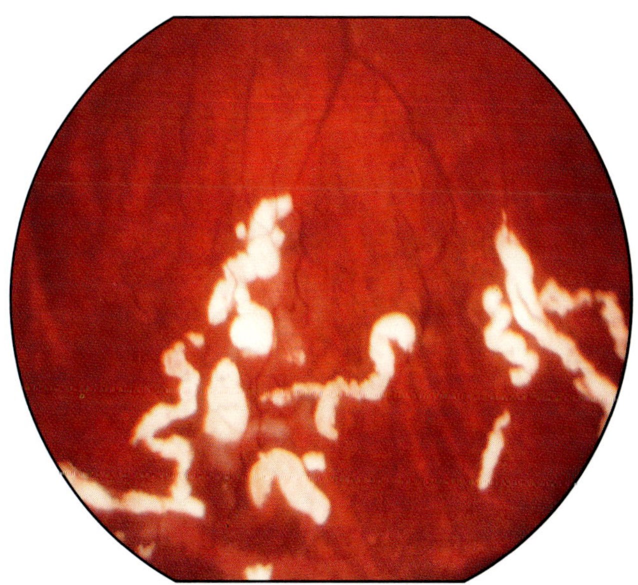

3–9 and 3–10 Peripheral retinoschisis may be lace-like (3–9 and 3–10) and/or have small oval holes in the inner layers. Peripheral retinal vessels may be thinned and irregular.

3–11 Glial proliferation in a wormlike fashion may be noted in the periphery, which extends beneath the inner retinal layer.

3–11, *Courtesy of Dr. Richard Chenoweth.*

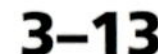

3–12 FAMILIAL EXUDATIVE VITREORETINOPATHY

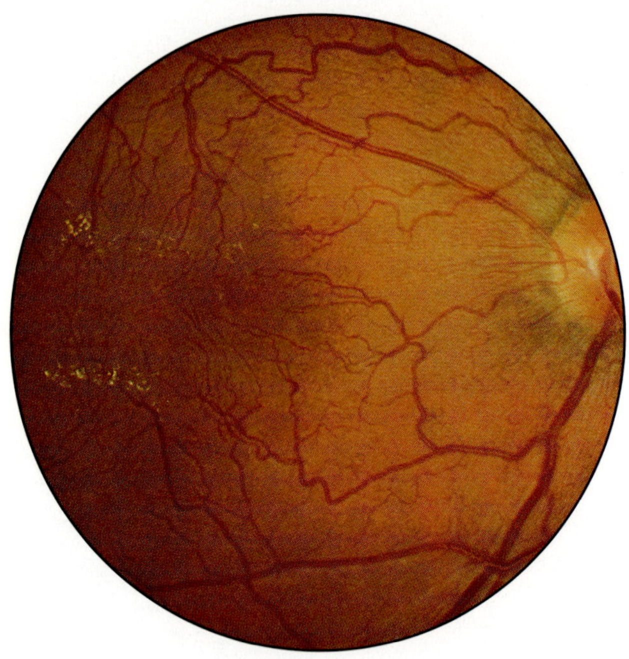

3–13

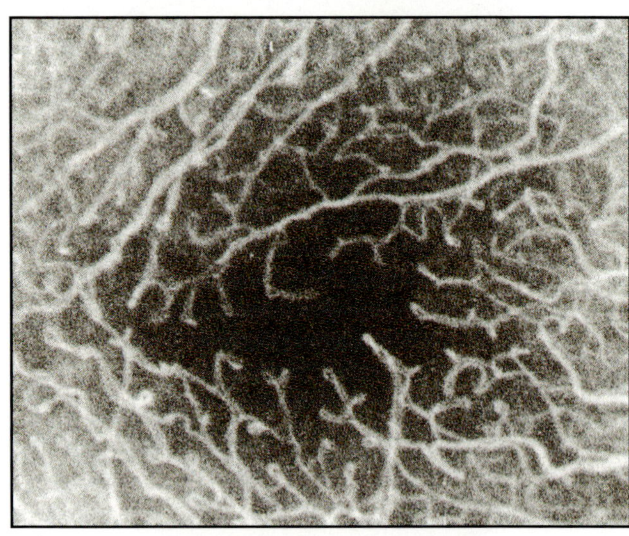

3–14

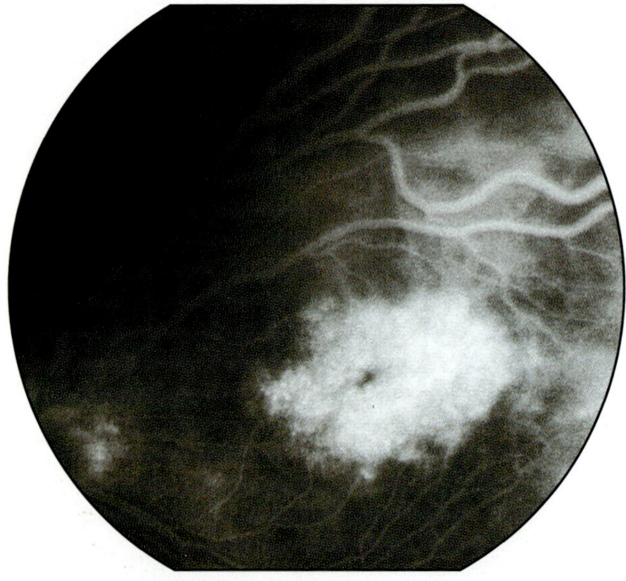

3–12 Familial exudative vitreoretinopathy is an autosomal dominant vitreoretinal degeneration. Prominence and distortion of the retinal capillaries in the macula region with thickening, serous fluid, and lipid exudation can occur in affected patients.

3–13 Fluorescein angiography of the foveal region shows disruption of the foveal ring with dilation, blunting, and distortion of the normal capillary architecture with stretching and pulling of the vessels.

3–14 Cystoid macular edema may also be demonstrated on fluorescein angiography in some cases. These abnormal vessels may leak in the macula and periphery.

***3–12** and **3–13,** Courtesy of Dr. Alessandro Schirru.*

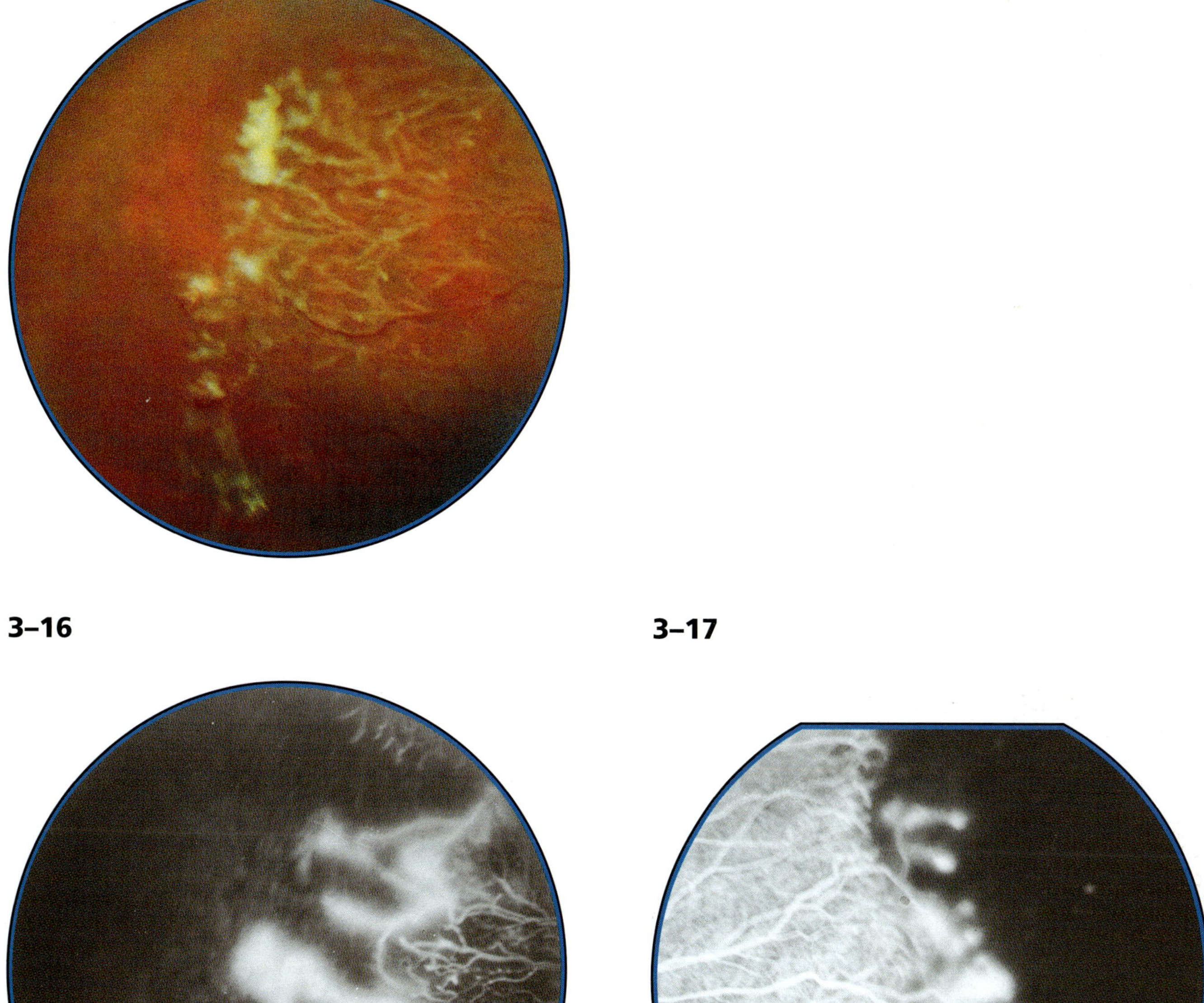

3–15 through 3–17 Peripheral leakage, nonperfusion, and proliferation can be noted. In this case, fibrovascular proliferation appears at the junction between perfused and nonperfused retina in the periphery.

3–18 FAMILIAL EXUDATIVE VITREORETINOPATHY

3-19

3–20

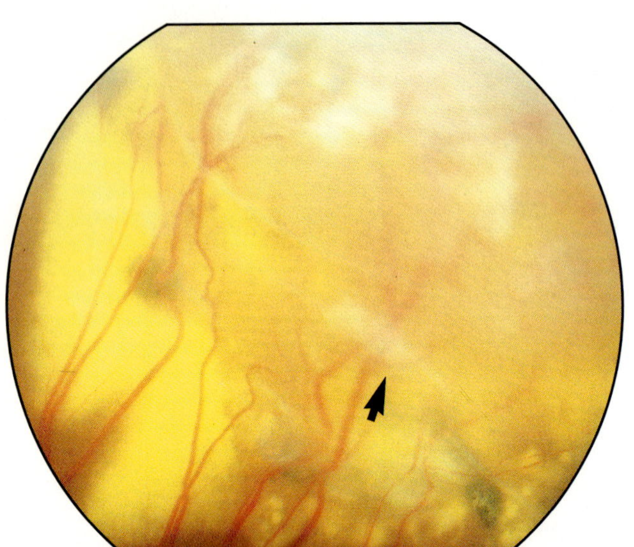

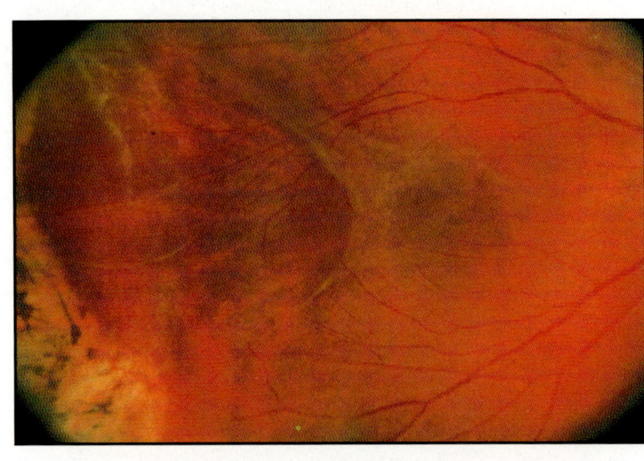

3–21

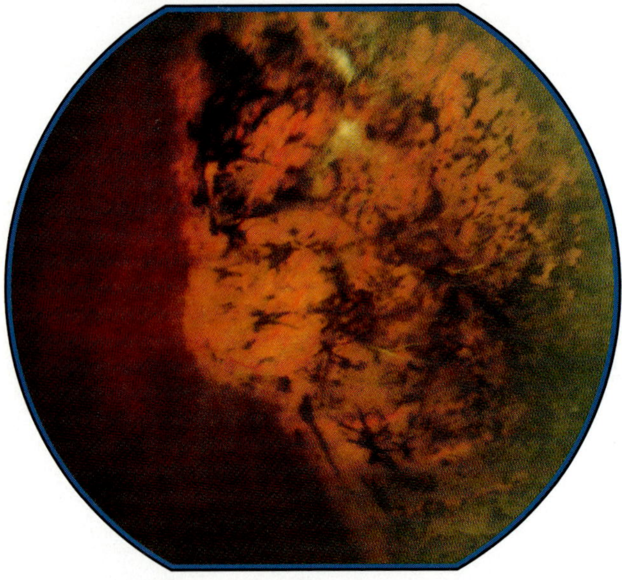

3–22

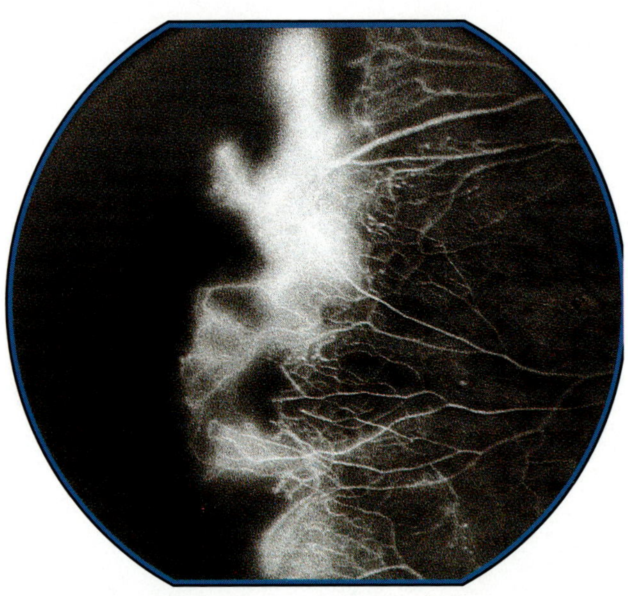

3–18 Extensive subretinal exudation can be demonstrated in advanced cases. A vitreous traction band is also present *(arrowhead)*.

3–19 and 3–20 This 53-year-old male with familial exudative vitreoretinopathy has an epiretinal membrane with temporal dragging of the vessels and fibrovascular proliferation in the temporal periphery of both eyes.

3–21 Retinal pigment epithelial atrophy with secondary pigmentary changes were noted in the temporal periphery of the left eye and suggestive of a spontaneously resolved retinal detachment.

3–22 Fluorescein angiography confirms fibrovascular proliferation and peripheral nonperfusion.

3–19 *through* ***3–22,*** *Courtesy of Drs. Howard and Brian Joondeph.*

Suggested Readings

Ahmad, NN, Ala-Kokko, L, Knowlton, RG, Jimenez, SA, Weaver, EJ, Maguire, JI, Tasman, W, and Prockop, DJ: Stop codon in the procollagen II gene (COL2A1) in a family with the Stickler syndrome (arthro-ophthalmopathy), Proc Natl Acad Sci USA 88:6624–6627, 1991

Alexander, RL, and Shea, M: Wagner's disease, Arch Ophthalmol 74:310–318, 1965

Billington, BM, Leaver, PK, and McLeod, D: Management of retinal detachment in the Wagner-Stickler syndrome, Trans Ophthalmol Soc UK 104:875–879, 1985

Carr, RE, and Siegel, IM: The vitreo-tapeto-retinal degenerations, Arch Ophthalmol 84:436–445, 1970

Fishman, GA, Jampol, LM, and Goldberg, MF: Diagnostic features of the Favre-Goldmann syndrome, Br J Ophthalmol 60:345–353, 1976

Green, WR: Vitreoretinal degenerations. In Spencer, WH, ed: Ophthalmic pathology: an atlas and textbook, ed 3, Philadelphia, 1985, WB Saunders

Maumenee, IH: Vitreoretinal degeneration as a sign of generalized connective tissue diseases, Am J Ophthalmol 88:432–449, 1979

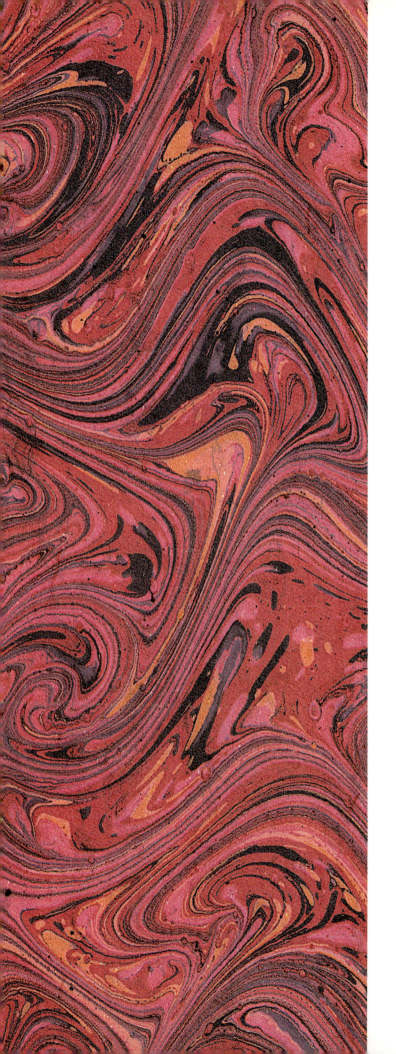

Part II

Tumors of the Retina, Choroid, and Vitreous

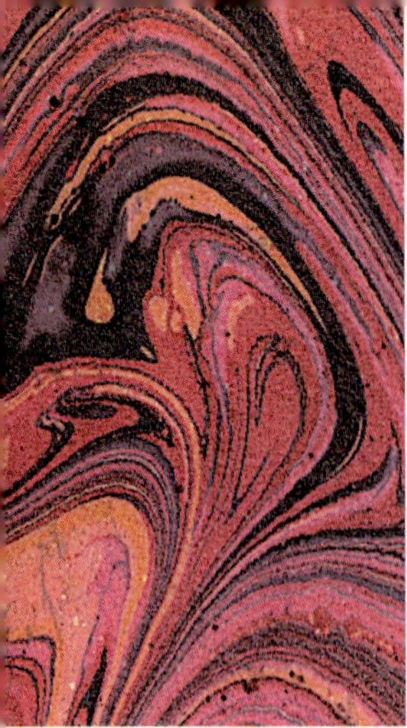

Chapter 4
Retinoblastoma

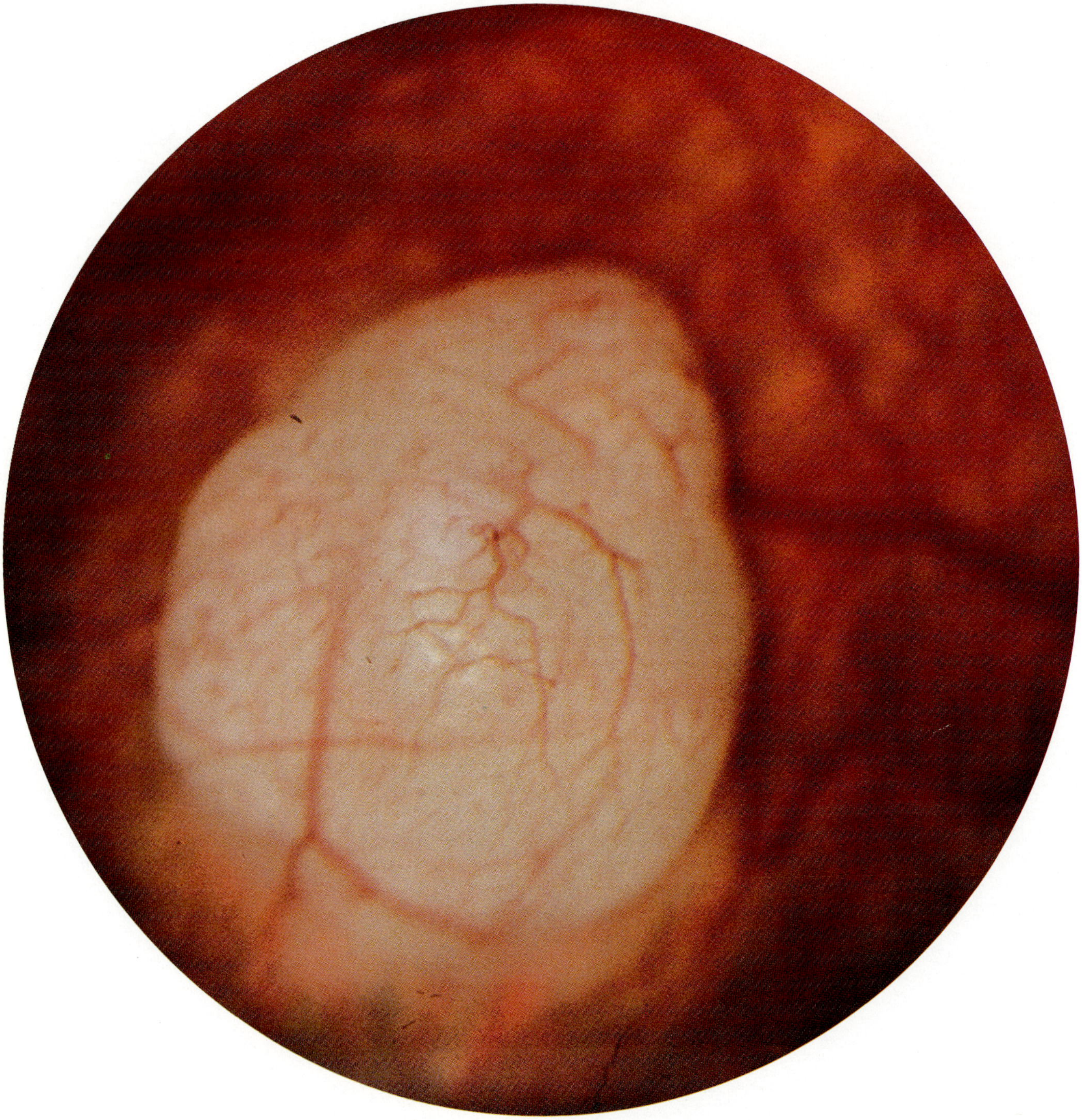

Retinoblastoma is the most common intraocular malignancy of children. Leukocoria and strabismus are common presenting findings.

4–1

4–2

4–3

4–4

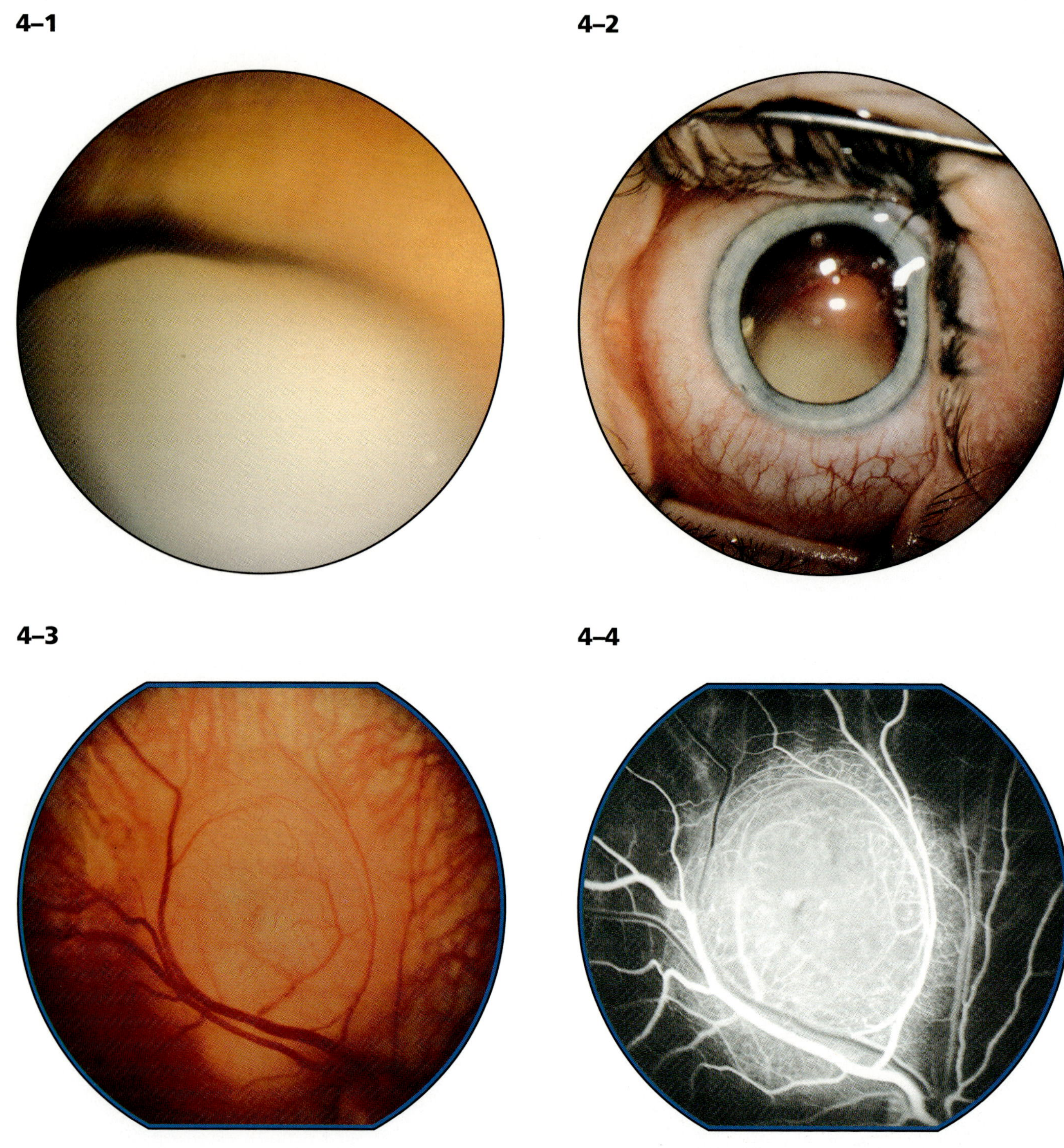

4–1 Retinoblastoma may present as a solid amorphous mass in the vitreous cavity.

4–2 Leukocoria may be an initial sign.

4–3 and 4–4 Retinoblastoma may sometimes be confined to the retina and subretinal areas as demonstrated in this 8-year-old white male. The tumor appears as a fleshy and vascular tumor. Hyperfluorescence of the tumor is demonstrated on the angiogram.

4–1 *through* **4–4,** *Courtesy of Dr. Jerry Shields.*

4–5

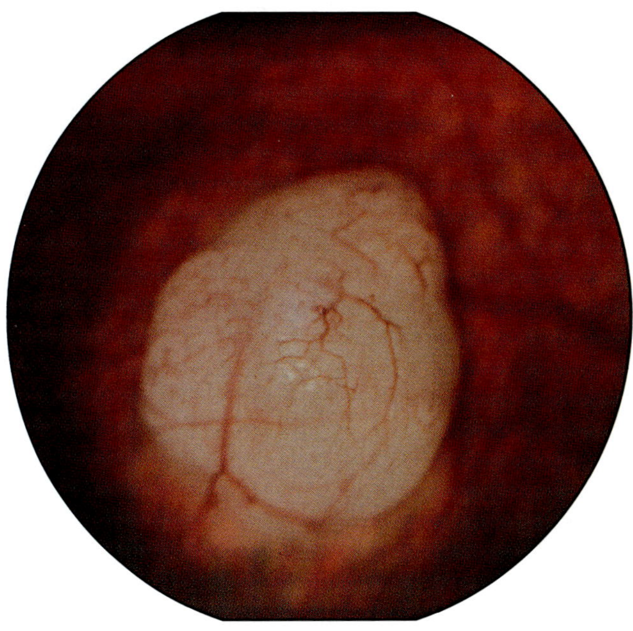

4–6

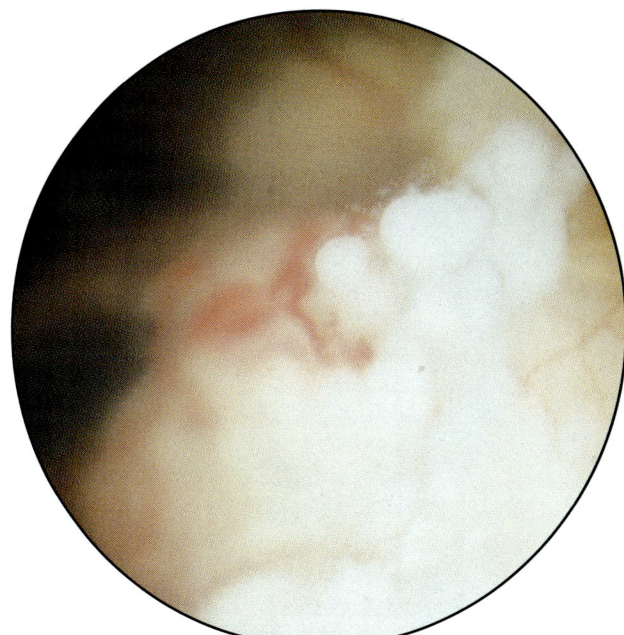

4–7

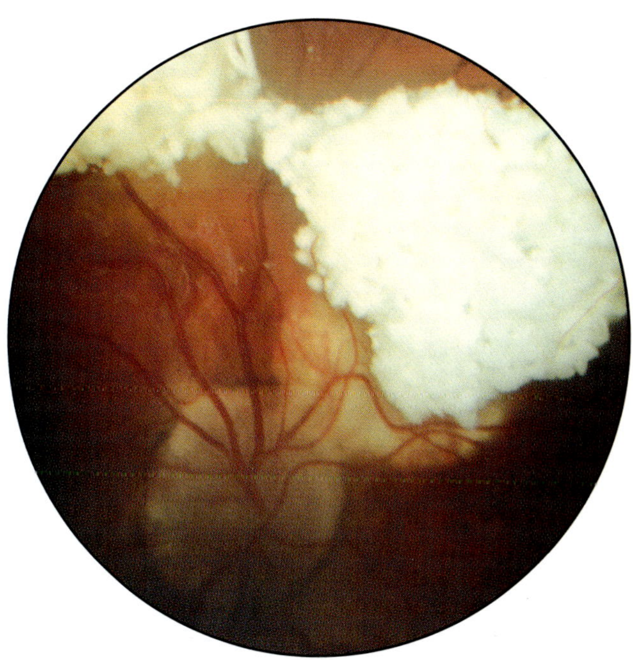

4–5 The tumor may extend outward from the retina into the vitreous.

4–6 In this case large cellular clumps of finely dispersed cells are demonstrated within a cloudy vitreous cavity.

4–7 Retinoblastoma may be managed by external beam radiation in some cases. The regression pattern may resemble cottage cheese.

***4–5, 4–6,** and **4–7,** Courtesy of Dr. Jerry Shields.*

4–8

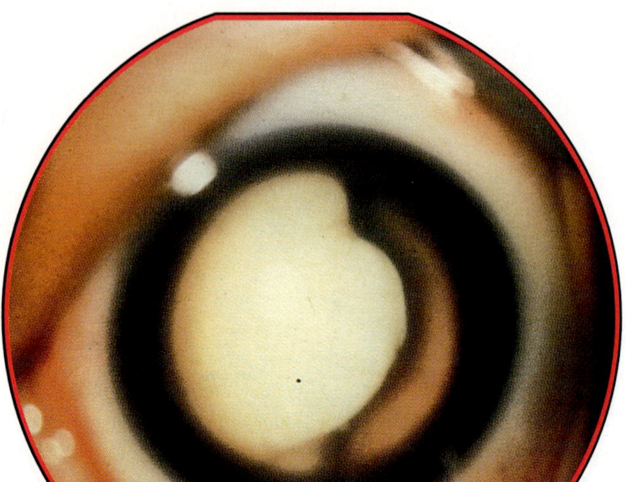

4–9

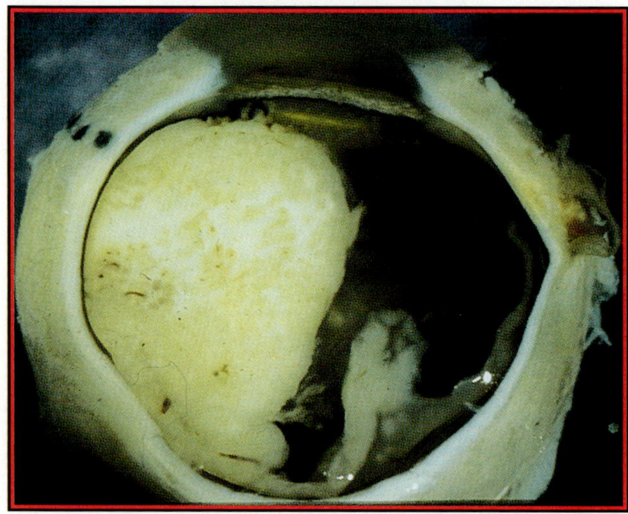

4–10

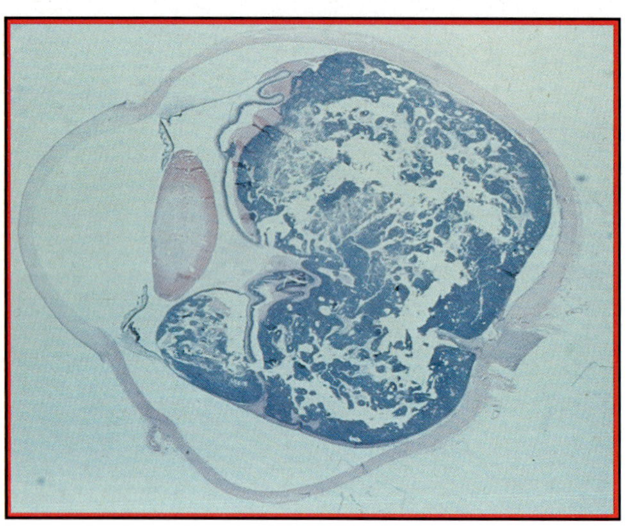

4–8 This patient presented with leukocoria and had an enucleation for presumed retinoblastoma.

4–9 Gross examination reveals a whitish lesion.

4–10 Light microscopy reveals that retinoblastoma fills much of the intraocular contents.

4–10, *Courtesy of Dr. Irene Maumenee.*

4–11

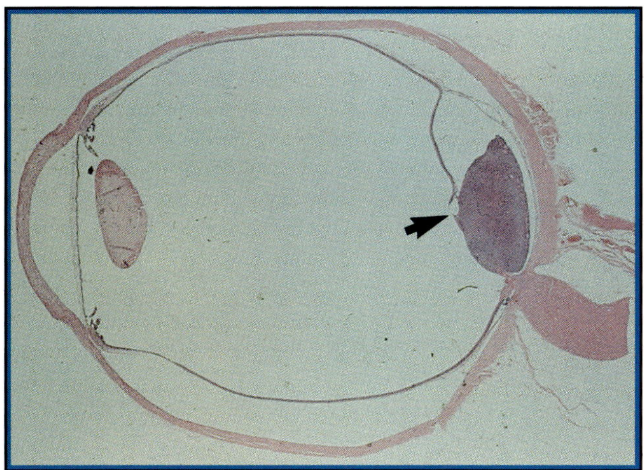

4–12

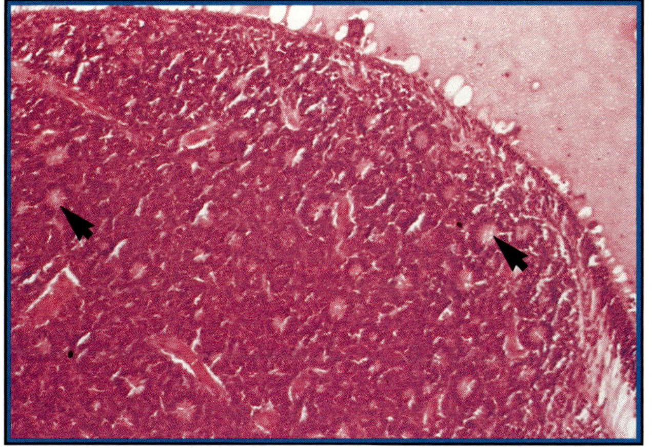

4–13

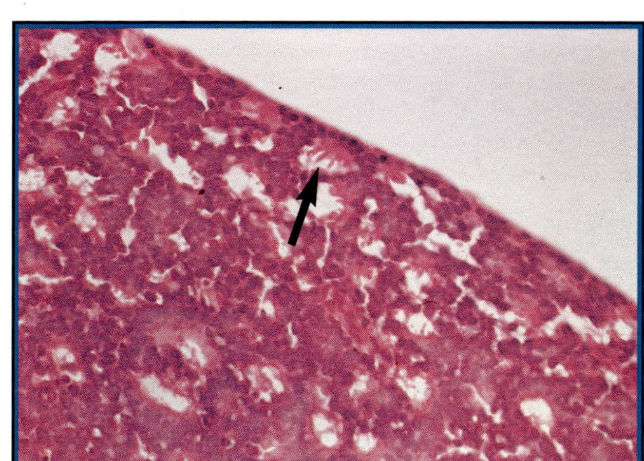

4–11 Retinoblastoma involving the macular area *(arrowhead)* is noted in this 18-month-old female who presented with strabismus.

4–12 and 4–13 Flexner-Wintersteiner rosettes *(arrowheads)* and fleurettes *(arrow)* are present.

Suggested Readings

Abramsom, DH, and Ellsworth, RM: The surgical management of retinoblastoma, Ophthalmic Surg 11:596–598, 1980

Abramson, DH, Ellsworth, RM, Grumbach, N, Sturgis-Buckhout, L, and Halk, BG: Retinoblastoma: correlation between age at diagnosis and survival, J Pediatr Ophthalmol Strabismus 23:174–177, 1986

Abramson, DH, Greenfield, DS, and Ellsworth, RM: Bilateral retinoblastoma. Correlations between age at diagnosis and time course for new intraocular tumors, Ophthalmic Pediatr Genet 13:1–7, 1992

Bader, JL, Miller, RW, Meadows, AT, Zimmerman, LE, Champion, LAA, and Voute, PA: Trilateral retinoblastoma, Lancet 2:582–583, 1980

Benedict, WF, Murphree, AL, Banerjee, A, Spina, CA, Sparkes, MC, and Sparkes, RS: Patient with 13 chromosome deletion: evidence that the retinoblastoma gene is a recessive cancer gene, Science 219:973–975, 1982

Bishop, JM: Molecular themes in oncogenesis, Cell 64:235–248, 1991

Bookstein, R, Lee, YHP, Peccei, A, and Lee, WH: Human retinoblastoma gene: long-range mapping and analysis of its deletion in a breast cancer cell line, Mol Cell Biol 9:1628–1634, 1989

Cowell, JK, Jay, M, Rutland, P, and Hungerford, J: An assessment of the usefulness of electrophoretic variants of esterase-D in the antenatal diagnosis of retinoblastoma in the United Kingdom, Br J Cancer 55:661–664, 1987

Devesa, SS: The incidence of retinoblastoma, Am J Ophthalmol 80:263–265, 1975

Dougherty, TJ: The future of photoradiation therapy in the treatment of cancer, Laser Focus 19:55–57, 1983

Draper, GJ, Heaf, MM, and Kinnier Wilson, LM: Occurrence of childhood cancers among sibs and estimation of familial risks, J Med Genet 14:81–90, 1977

Draper, GJ, Sanders, BM, Brownbill, PA, and Hawkins, MM: Patterns of risk hereditary retinoblastoma and applications to genetic counselling, Br J Cancer 66:211–219, 1992

Dryja, TP, Mukai, S, Petersen, R, Rapaport, JM, Walton, D, and Yandell, DW: Parental origin of mutations of the retinoblastoma gene, Nature 339:556–558, 1989

Eagle, RJ, Shields, JA, Donoso, L, and Milner, RS: Malignant transformation of spontaneously regressed retinoblastoma, retinoma/retinocytoma variant, Ophthalmology 96:1389–1395, 1989

Ellsworth, RM: The management of retinoblastoma, Jpn J Ophthalmol 22-389–395, 1978

Folberg, R, Cleasby, G, Flanagan, JA, Spencer, WH, and Zimmerman, LE: Orbital leiomyosarcoma after radiation therapy for bilateral retinoblastoma, Arch Ophthalmol 101:1562–1565, 1983

Gallie, BL, Ellsworth, RM, Abramsom, DH, and Phillips, RA: Retinoma: spontaneous regression of retinoblastoma or benign manifestation of the mutation? Br J Cancer 45:513–521, 1982

Jakobiec, FA, Tso, MOM, Zimmerman, LE, and Danis, P: Retinoblastoma and intracranial malignancy, Cancer 39:2048–2058, 1977

Lagendijk, JJW: A microwave heating technique for the hyperthermic treatment of tumors in the eye, especially retinoblastoma, Phys Med Biol 27:1313–1324, 1982

McGee, TL, Yandell, DW, and Dryja, TP: Structure and partial genomic sequence of the human retinoblastoma susceptibility gene, Gene 80:119–128, 1989

Murphree, AL, and Benedict, WF: Retinoblastoma: clues to human oncogenesis, Science 223:1028–1033, 1984

Salmonson, PC, Ellsworth, RM, and Kitchin, FD: The occurrence of new retinoblastomas after treatment, Ophthalmology 86:837–843, 1979

Scheffer, H, te Meerman, GJ, Kruize, YCM, van den Berg, AHM, Penninga, DP, Tan, KEWP, der Kinderen, DJ, and Buys, HCM: Linkage analysis of families with hereditary retinoblastoma: nonpenetrance of mutation, revealed by combined use of markers within and flanking the Rb1 gene, Am J Hum Genet 45:252–260, 1989

Shields, JA: Diagnosis and management of intraocular tumors, St Louis, 1983, Mosby–Year Book

Togushida, J, Ishizaki, K, Sasaki, MS, Ikenaga, M, Sugimoto, M, Kotoura, Y, and Yamamuro, T: Chromosomal reorganization for the expression of recessive mutation of the retinoblastoma susceptibility gene in the development of osteosarcoma, Cancer Res 48:3939–3943, 1988

Wiggs, J, Nordenskjöld, M, Yandell, DW, Rapaport, J, Grondin, V, Janson, M, Werelius, B, Petersen, R, Craft, A, Riedel, K, Liberfarb, R, Walton, D, Wilson, W, and Dryja, TP: Prediction of the risk of hereditary retinoblastoma, using DNA polymorphisms within the retinoblastoma gene, N Engl J Med 318:151–157, 1988

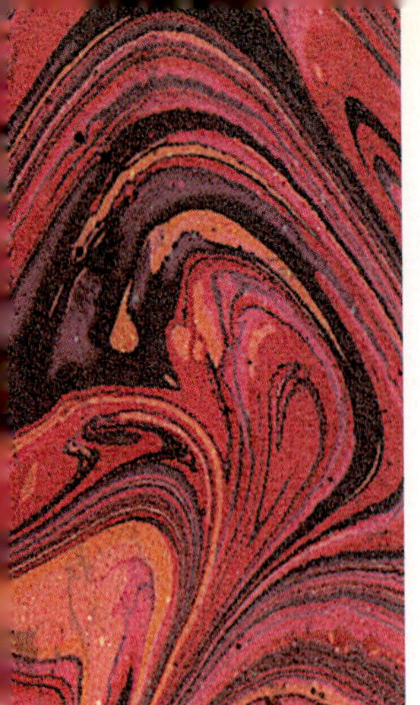

Chapter 5
Cavernous Hemangioma

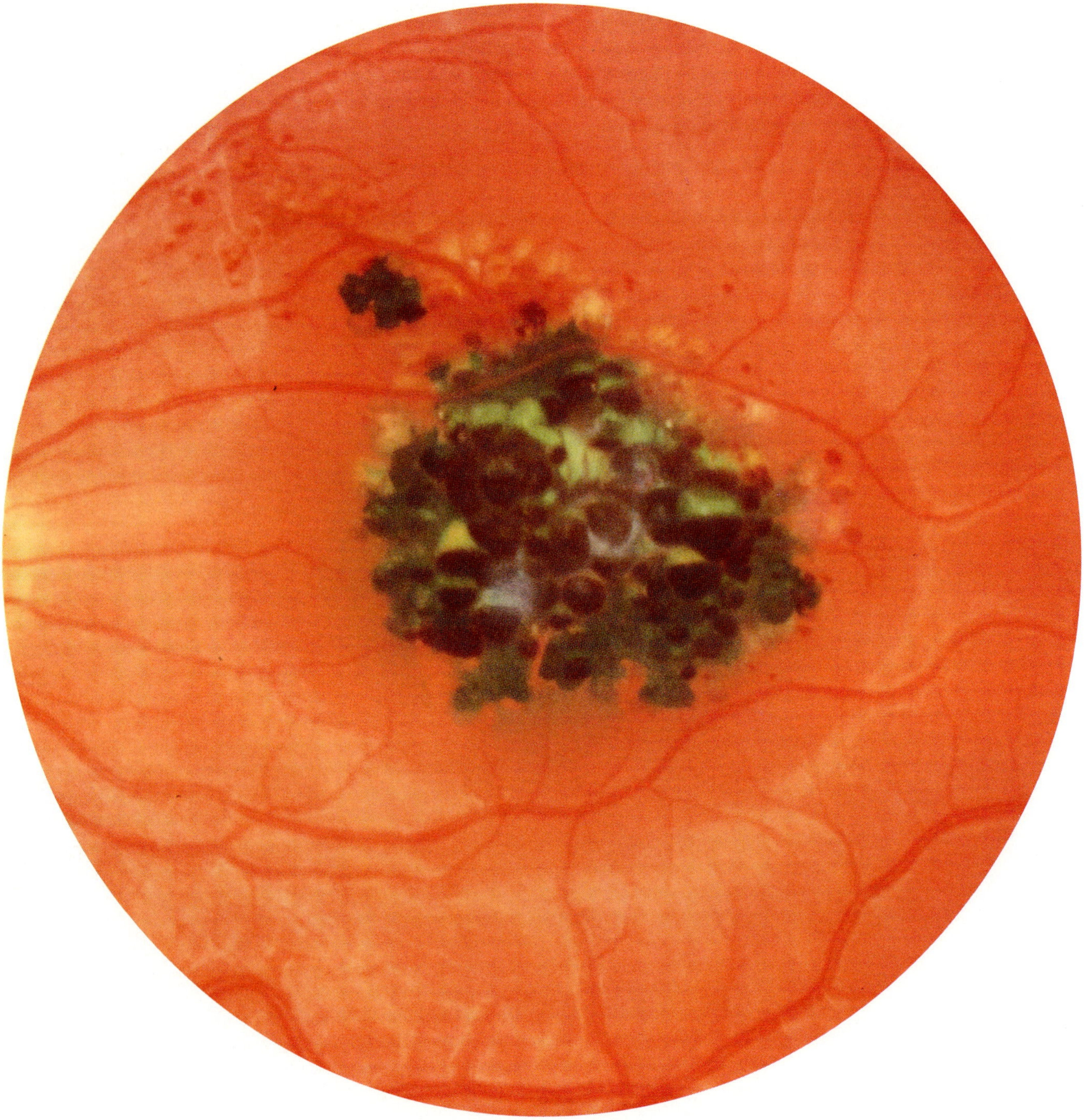

Cavernous hemangiomas of the retina consist of multiple clumps of intraretinal aneurysms. These lesions are usually asymptomatic and rarely cause exudation. Vitreous hemorrhage may occasionally occur. Affected patients may also have central nervous system or cutaneous hemangiomas.

5–1

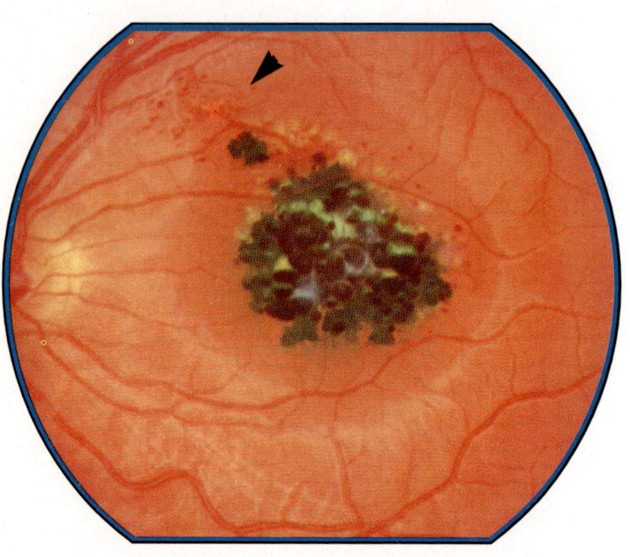

5–2

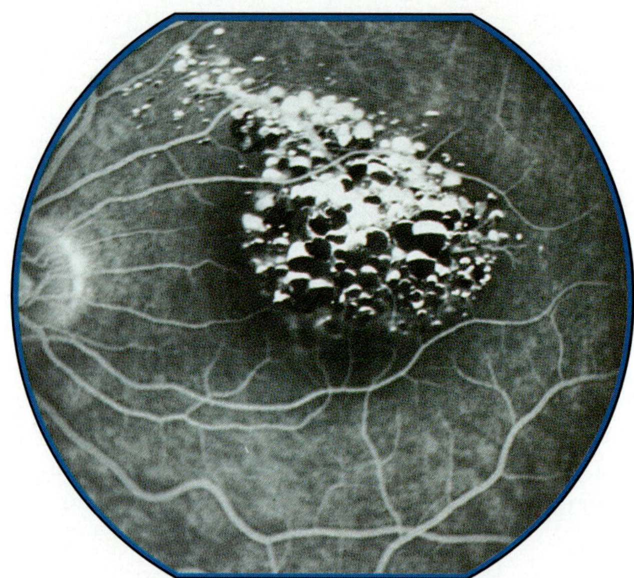

5–3 5–4

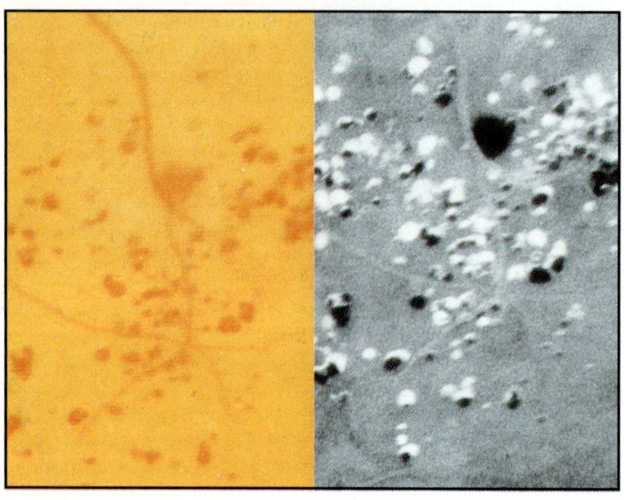

5–1 Cavernous hemangiomas appear as a cluster of grapes. Vascular dilatation and a purplish vascular configuration can be noted. The cavernous vessels vary in size. Note the small lesions supranasally *(arrowhead)* and larger lesions centrally. Some of the large lesions reveal an erythrocytic plasma interface. Pigment epithelial hyperplasia is also noted within the central clump of cavernous vessels.

5–2 The characteristic filling pattern of a cavernous hemangioma can be demonstrated by fluorescein angiography. The vessels are on the venous side of the circulation, but do not leak, and show the plasma erythrocyte interface.

5–3 and 5–4 This classic reddish cavernous hemangioma reveals the characteristic fluorescein angiographic findings. The vascular changes in this patient are scattered rather than clumped.

5–1 *and* ***5–2,*** *Courtesy of Ross Jarrett.*

5–5

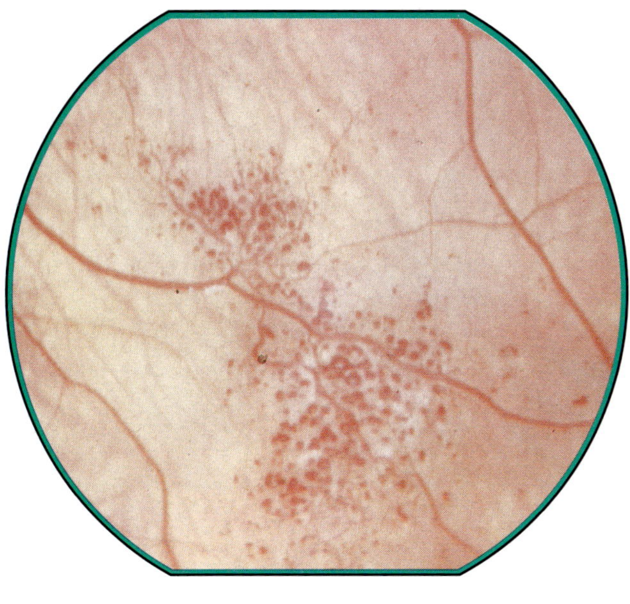

5–6 **5–6A**

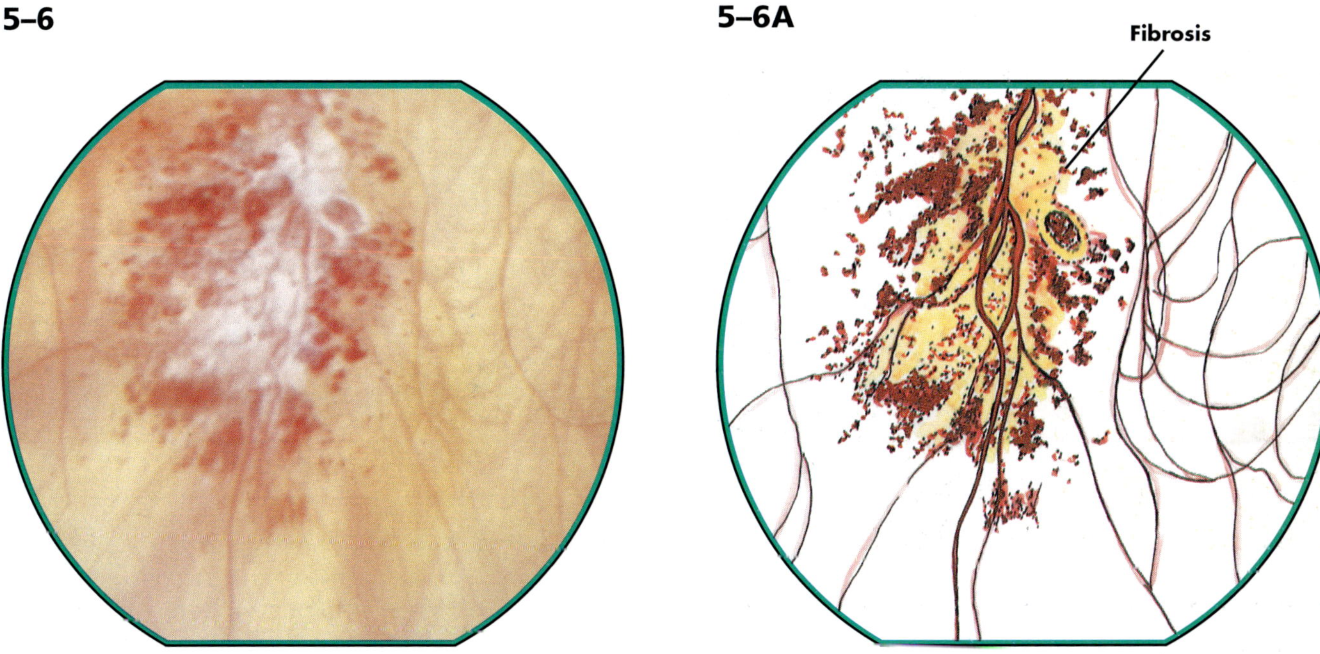

5–5, 5–6, and 5–6A The next series of photographs illustrates a 10-year-old female with bilateral retinal cavernous hemangiomas. Her mother also has a cavernous hemangioma in one eye. Note the extensive fibrosis which is seen in some cases (5–6).

5–5 *and* ***5–6,*** *Courtesy of Dr. Richard Goldberg. From: Goldberg, RE, Pheasant, TR, Shields, JA: Cavernous hemangiomas of the retina, Arch Ophthalmia 97:2321, 1979. Copyright American Medical Association.*

5–7

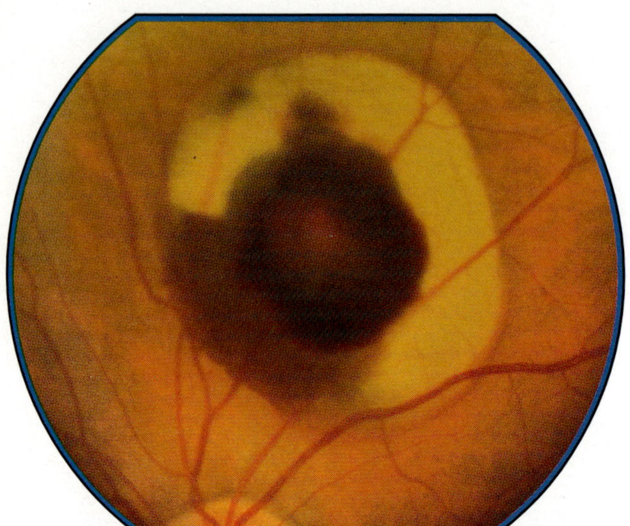

5–8

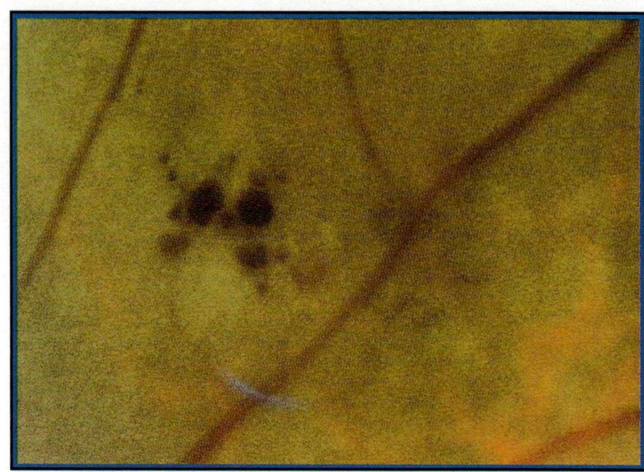

5–9

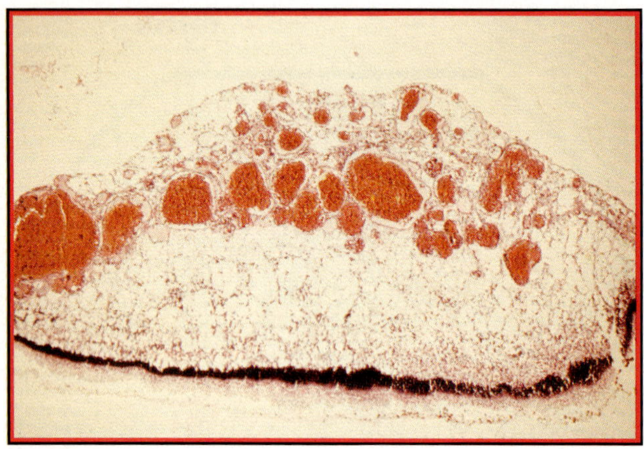

5–9A

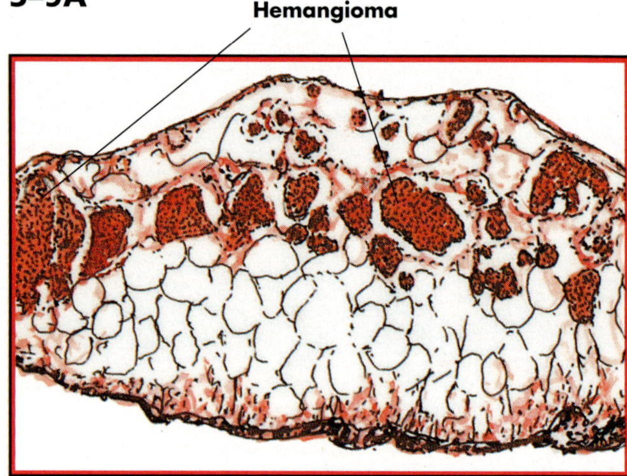

5–10

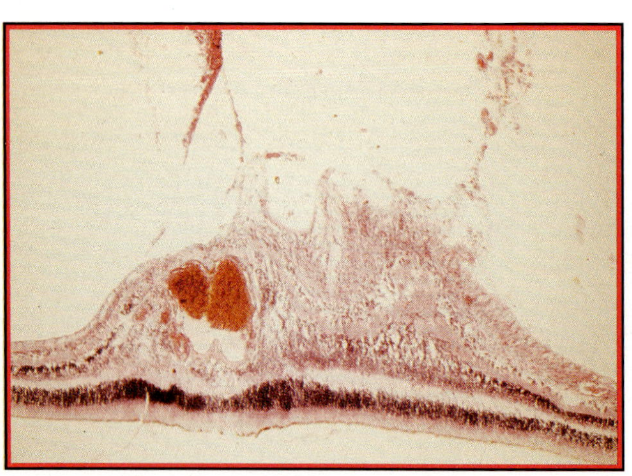

5–7 and 5–8 This patient presented with preretinal, intraretinal, and subretinal hemorrhage, resembling the bleeding pattern seen with retinal arteriolar macroaneurysm. A cavernous hemangioma of the retina was seen after the hemorrhage resolved.

5–9 and 5–9A The retina is greatly thickened by edema and large normal-appearing blood vessels in the inner retinal layers in this histopathologic correlate of a cavernous hemangioma.

5–10 In another area, strands of vitreous with entrapped blood can be seen exerting traction on the retina in the area of a cavernous hemangioma.

5–9 *and* ***5–10,*** *Courtesy of the AFIP. Reprinted with permission from Spencer, W: Ophthalmic pathology: an atlas and textbook, ed 3, Philadelphia, 1985, WB Saunders.*

Suggested Readings

Gass, JDM: Cavernous hemangioma of the retina: A neuro-oculocutaneous syndrome, Am J Ophthalmol 71:799–814, 1971

Gass, JDM: Stereoscopic atlas of macular diseases: diagnosis and treatment, ed 3, St Louis, 1987, Mosby–Year Book, pp 634–639

Goldberg, RE, Pheasant, TR, and Shields, JA: Cavernous hemangioma of the retina: a four-generation pedigree with neurocutaneous manifestations and an example of bilateral retinal involvement, Arch Ophthalmol 97:2321–2324, 1979

Guiffre, G: Cavernous hemangioma of the retina and retinal telangiectasis: distinct or related vascular malformations? Retina 5:221–224, 1985

Lewis, RA, Cohen, MH, and Wise, GN: Cavernous hemangioma of the retina and optic disc and a review of the literature, Br J Ophthalmol 59:422–434, 1975

Reese, AB: Tumors of the eye, ed 2, New York, 1963, Paul B Hoebner

Shields, JA: Diagnosis and management of intraocular tumors, St Louis, 1987, Mosby–Year Book

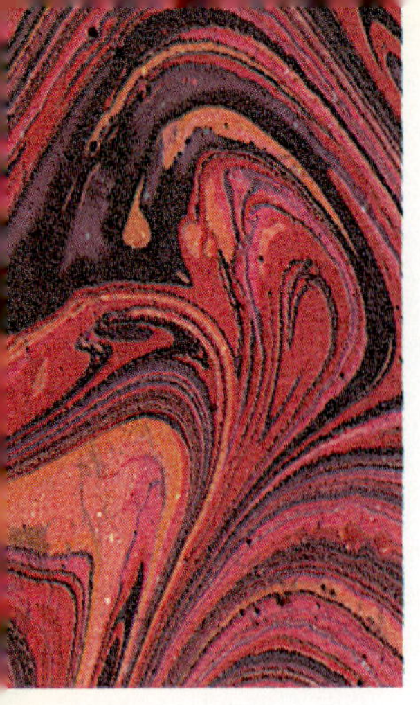

Chapter 6

Capillary Hemangioma of the Retina and von Hippel-Lindau Disease

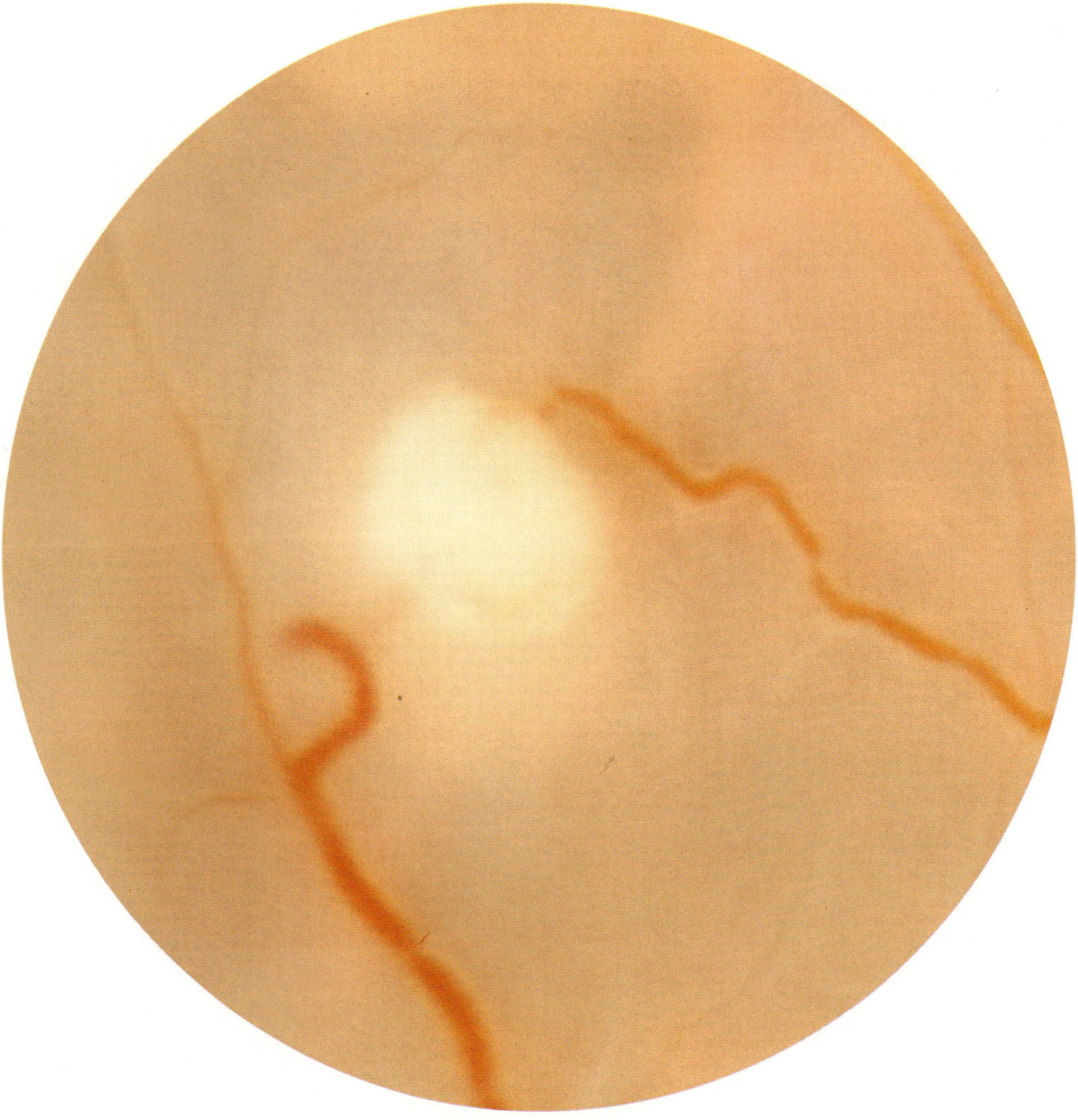

Capillary hemangiomas may be associated with von Hippel-Lindau disease or occur in isolation. Other systemic associations in the autosomal dominant von Hippel-Lindau disorder include hemangioblastomas of the cerebellum, spinal cord, or brain stem; renal cell carcinoma; pheochromocytoma; and benign cysts of the kidney, pancreas, lung, liver, kidney, epididymis, and bone.

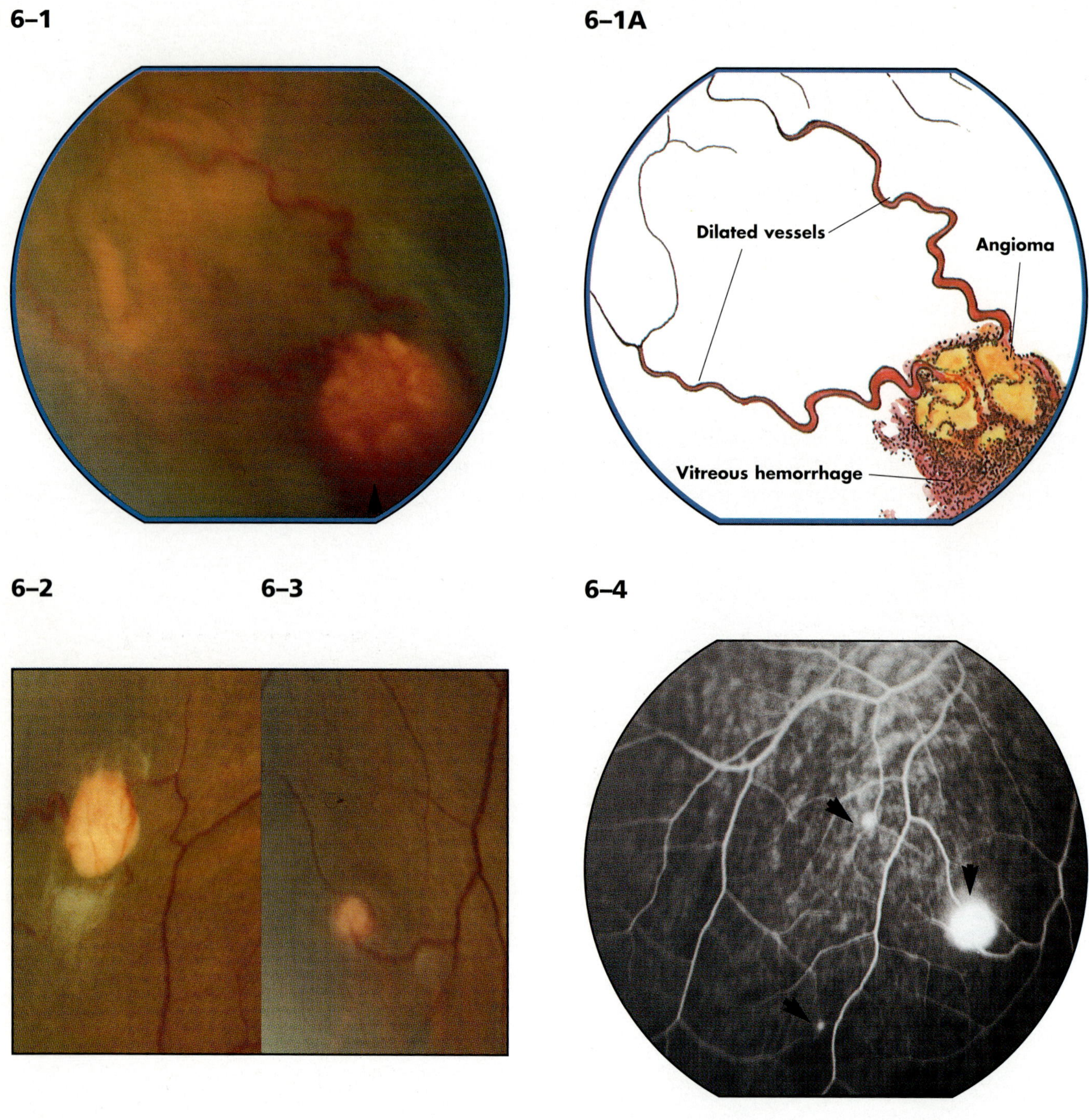

6–1 and 6–1A This capillary hemangioma was associated with the von Hippel-Lindau syndrome. Note the dilated feeding and draining vessels. There is bleeding into the vitreous *(arrowhead)*.

6–2 and 6–3 These patients also have angiomatous lesions associated with von Hippel-Lindau disease. These lesions may be whitish (6–2), pinkish (6–3), large or small.

6–4 Multiple angiomas may be demonstrated by fluorescein angiography, as in this case in which three hyperfluorescent angiomas are noted *(arrowheads)*.

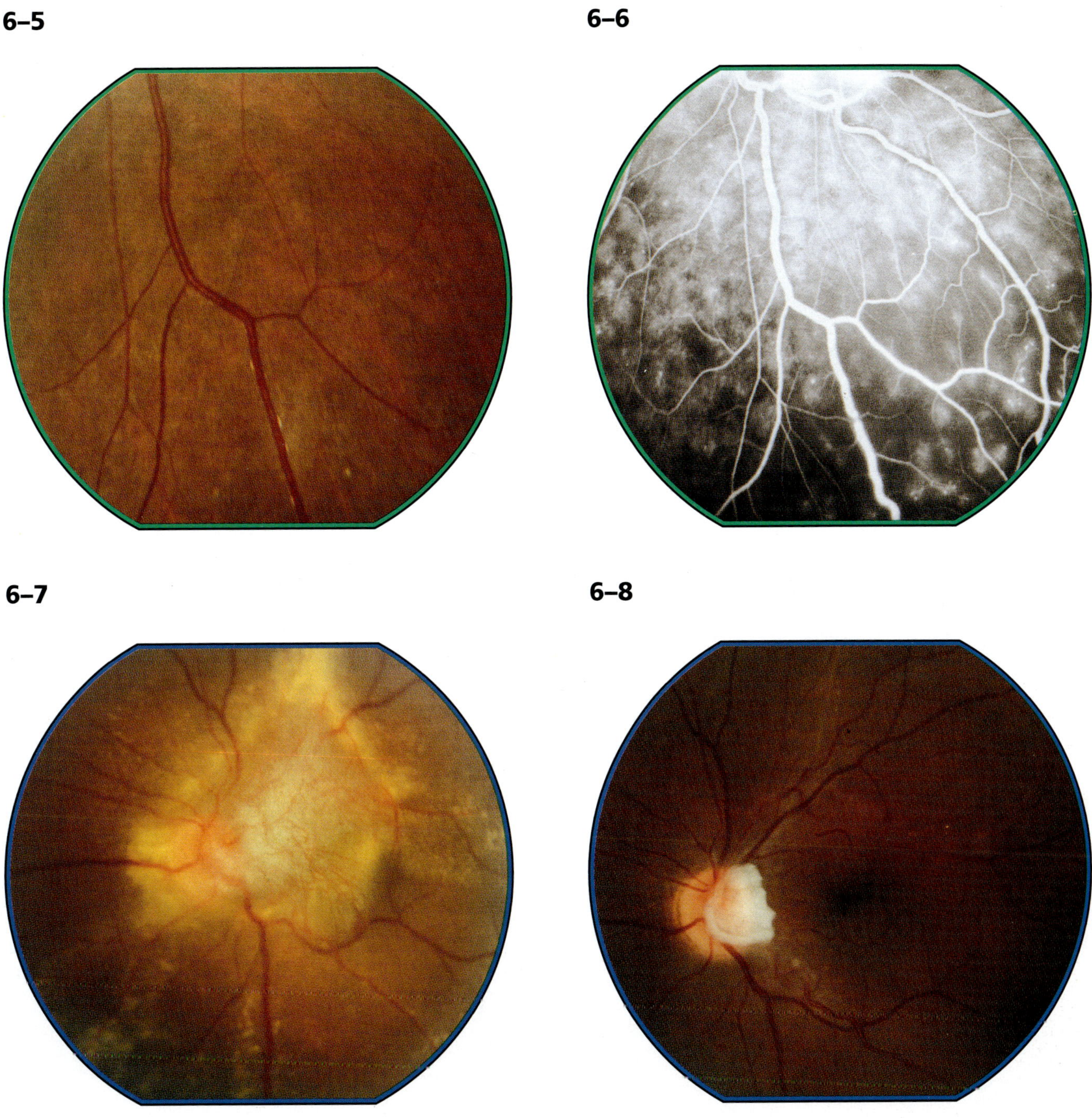

6–5 and 6–6 Fluorescein angiography may demonstrate possible additional small lesions that are not appreciated clinically.

6–7 and 6–8 Fibrovascular proliferation may occur with extensive exudation, leading to a retinal detachment in affected patients. Some fibrovascular proliferation may be indistinguishable from the primary angioma. Note the dilated fine preretinal vessels over the optic disc surrounded by exudative detachment. Vitrectomy was successful in removing the fibrovascular proliferation and reattaching the retina in this case.

***6–7** and **6–8,** Courtesy of Dr. Yale Fisher.*

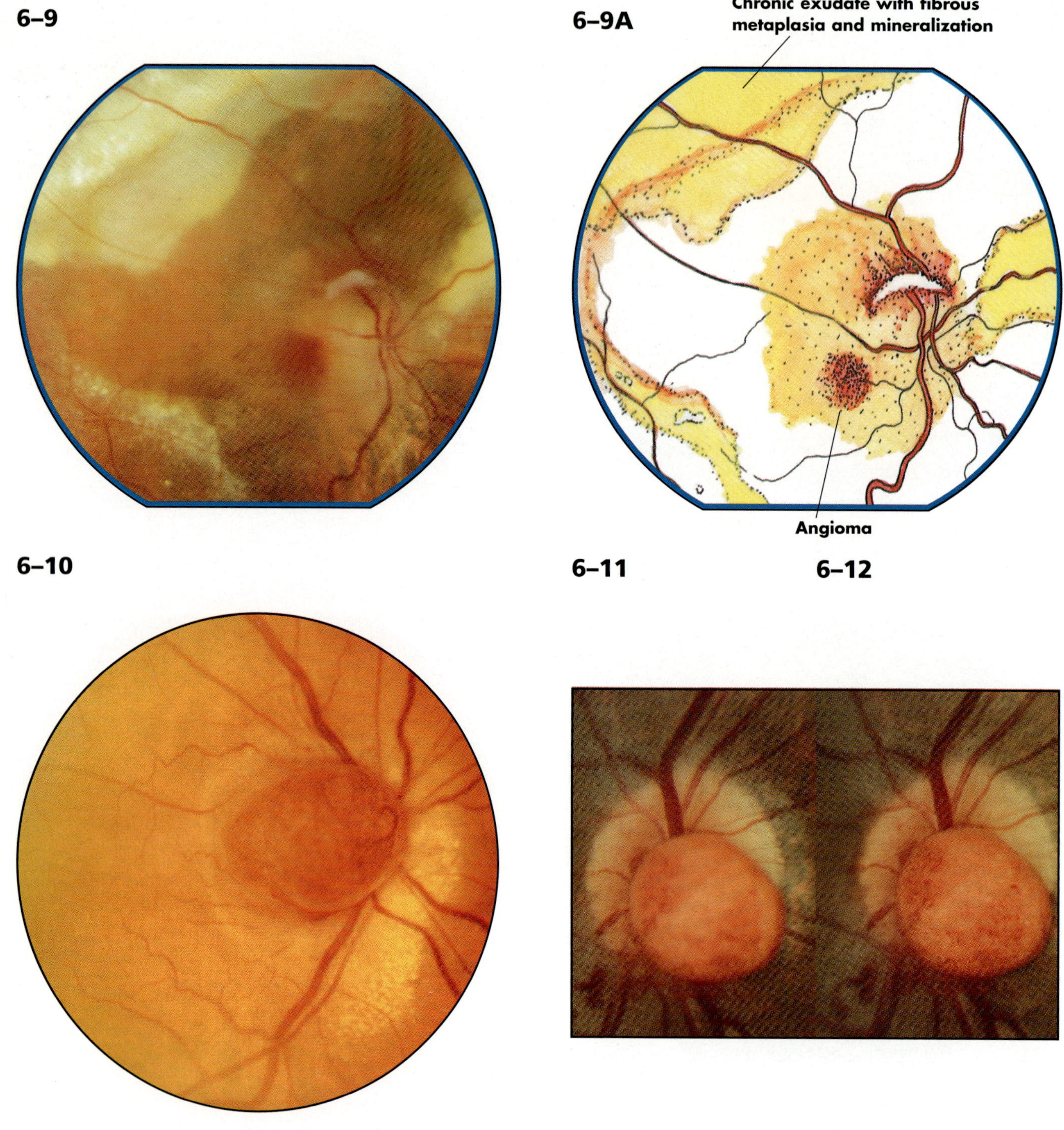

6–9 and 6–9A Massive subretinal exudation may even occur with small angiomatous lesions, as demonstrated in this patient with an angiomatous lesion of the optic disc with endophytic and exophytic growth. Old exudate with fibrous metaplasia and mineralization is noted *(top left of photograph)*.

6–10 Optic disc angiomas can be so large as to obscure the entire optic nerve.

6–11 and 6–12 Another patient demonstrates an angioma at the optic disc *(stereo pair)*.

6–10, *Courtesy of Johnny Justice.* ***6–11*** *and* ***6–12,*** *Courtesy of Mark Williams.*

6–13 **6–14** **6–15**

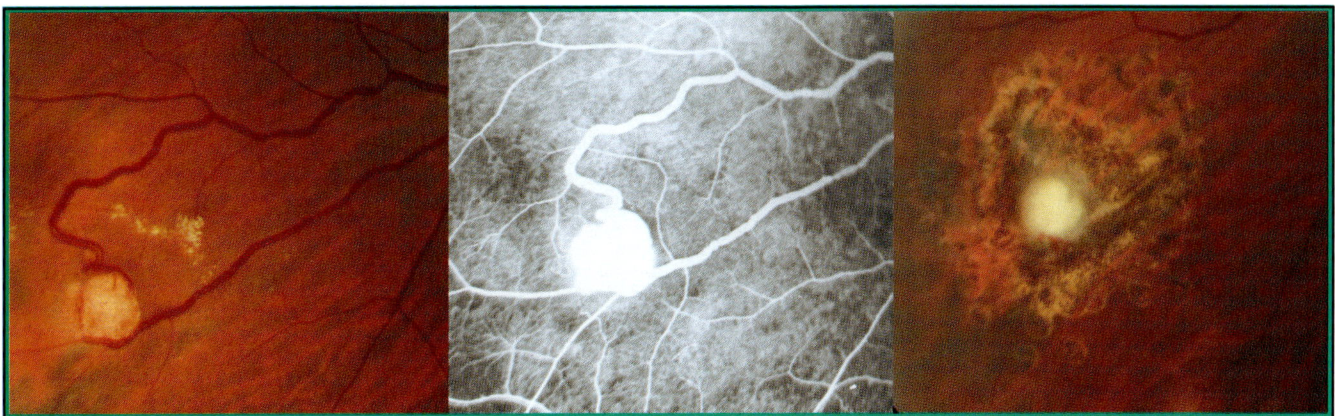

6–16

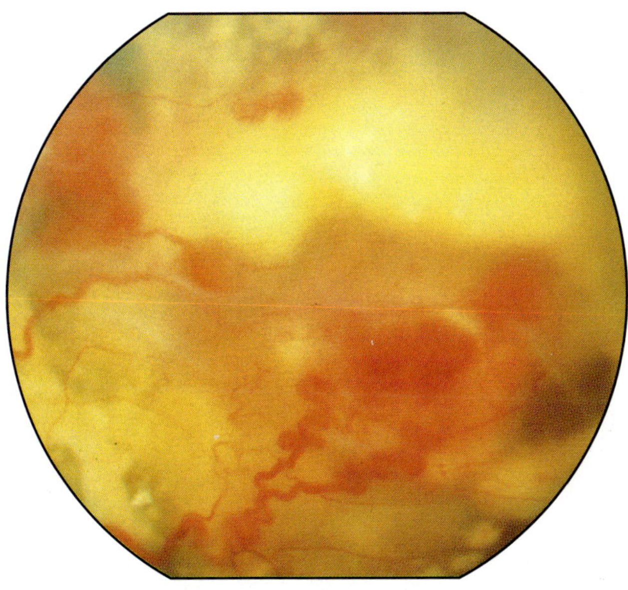

6–13 through 6–15 A small angiomatous lesion is demonstrated in this patient with dilated and beaded feeding vessels. Usually, the draining vessel is larger than the feeding vessel, but there is not much difference in this case. In 6–14, the fluorescein angiogram shows the hyperfluorescent vascular tumor with its feeding and draining vessels. The patient was treated with laser photocoagulation with regression of the lesion (6–15).

6–16 Some lesions may lead to massive exudative detachments as demonstrated in this patient. The angioma is at the end of the tortuous vessels obscured by hemorrhage and exudate.

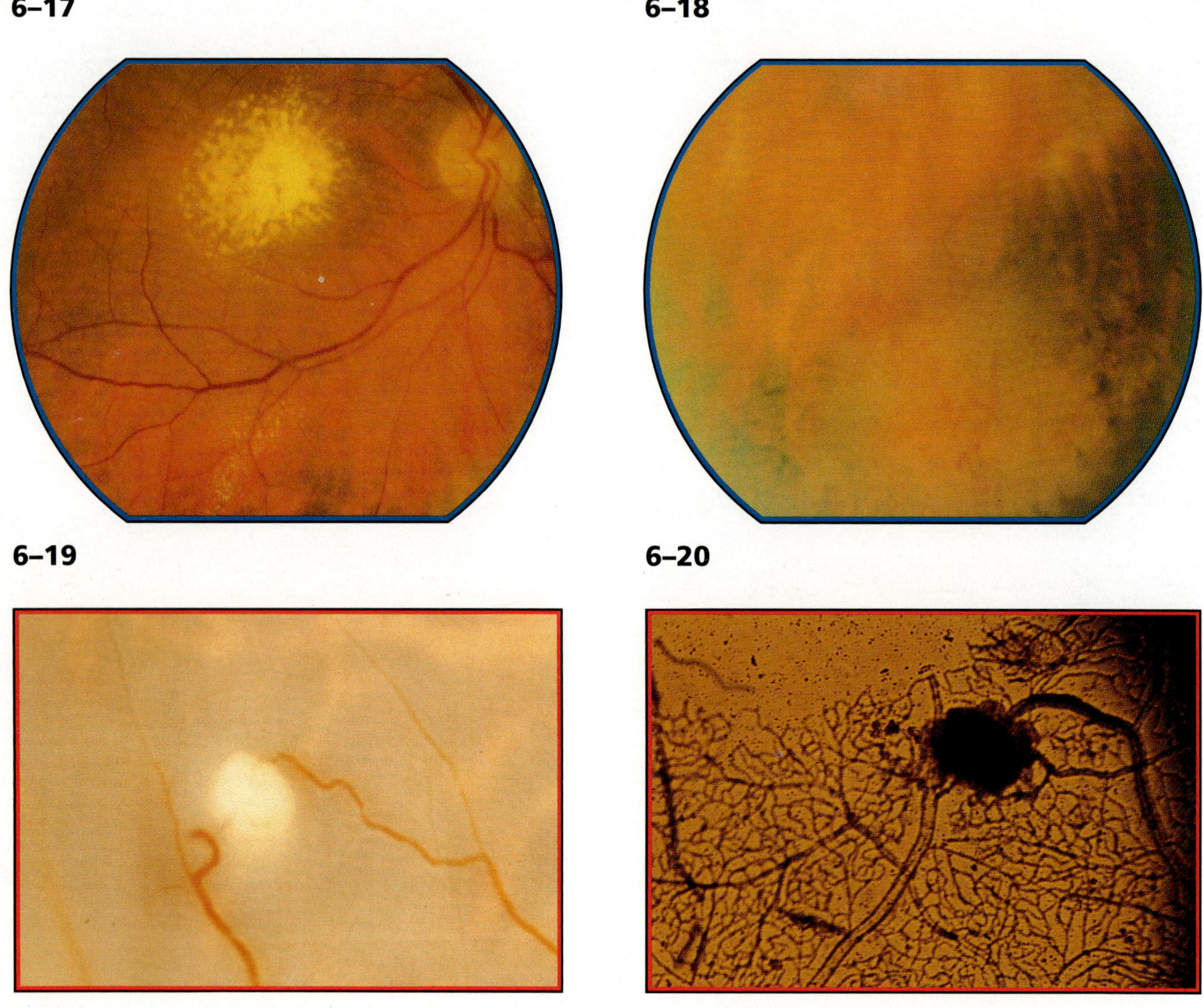

6–17 and 6–18 This patient has an acquired capillary hemangioma. A capillary gray-pink mass is barely visible within a zone of peripheral pigmentary degeneration (6–18). Exudative detachment of the retina with lipid deposition is noted inferiorly. The exudative detachment ascends superiorly to involve the macula with heavy lipid (6–17). The fluorescein study shows a network of fine capillaries with multiple aneurysms and no dilated feeder vessels. These three features differentiate this lesion from that of von Hippel's disease.

6–19 Gross appearance of a capillary hemangioma from a patient with von Hippel-Lindau disease. The retinal angioma has dilated and slightly tortuous afferent and efferent blood vessels.

6–20 Trypsin digest preparation of a similar case shows a small retinal hemangioma.

6–19 *and* ***6–20,*** *From Nicholson, DH, Green, WR, Kenyon, KR: Light and electron microscopic study of early lesions in angiomatous retinae, Am J Ophthalmol 82:193–204, 1976.*

6–21

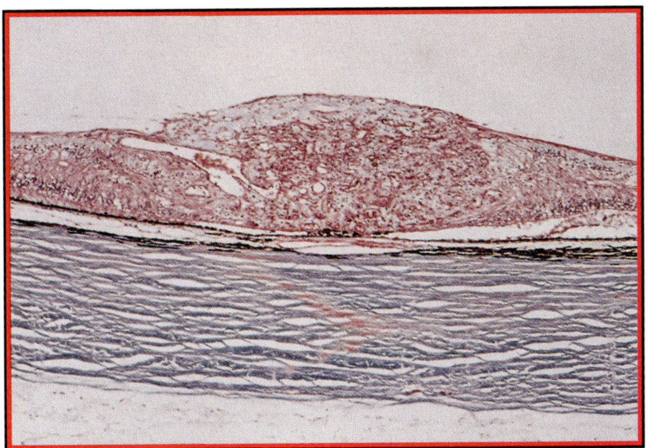

6–22

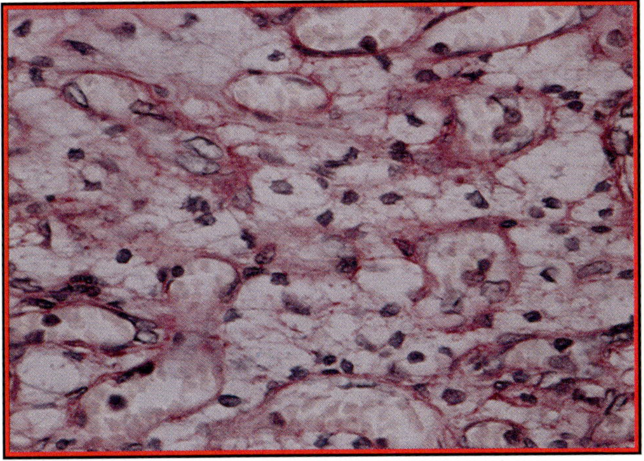

6–23

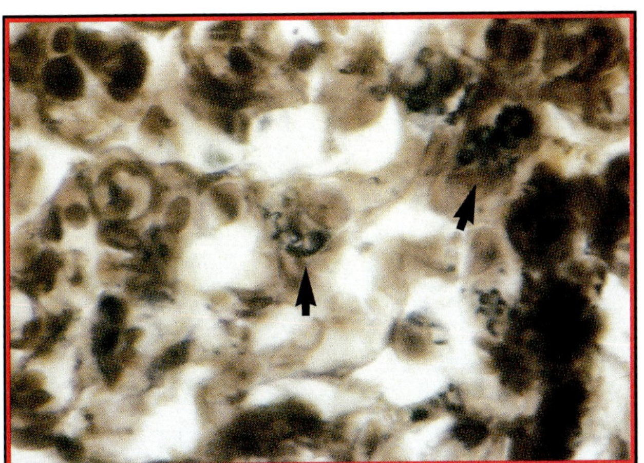

6–21 Light microscopy reveals an angiomatous lesion composed of capillary-like vessels.

6–22 Higher magnification shows the capillary vessels separated by large vacuolated cells.

6–23 Sudan black stain shows lipid deposition, which appears black in this preparation *(arrowheads)*.

6–21 *through* ***6–23,*** *From Nicholson, DH, Green, WR, Kenyon, KR: Light and electron microscopic study of early lesions in angiomatous retinae, Am J Ophthalmol 82:193–204, 1976.*

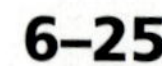

6–24

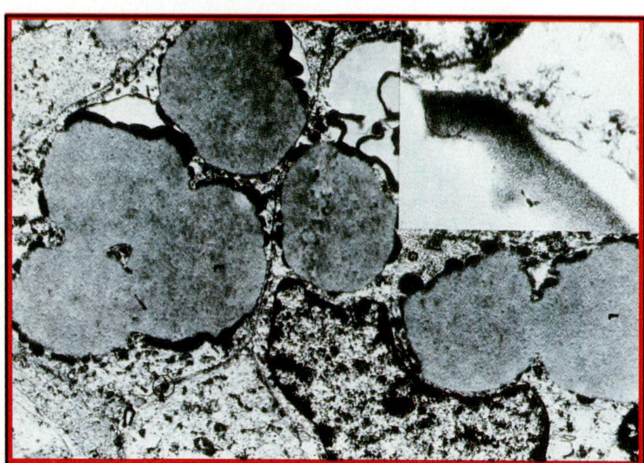

6–25

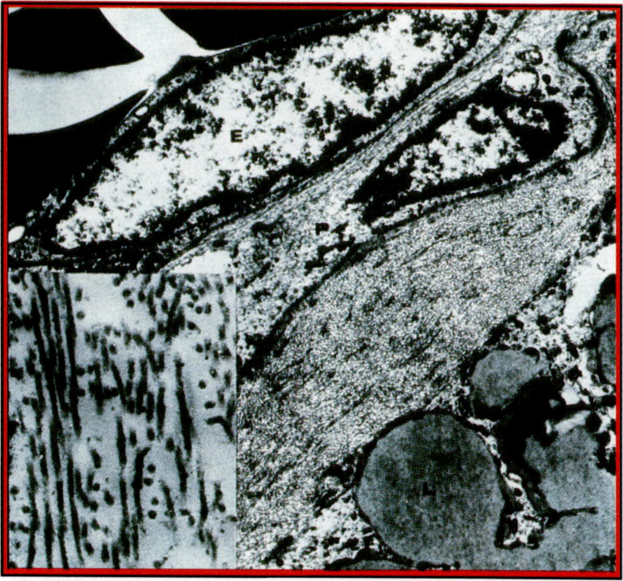

6–26

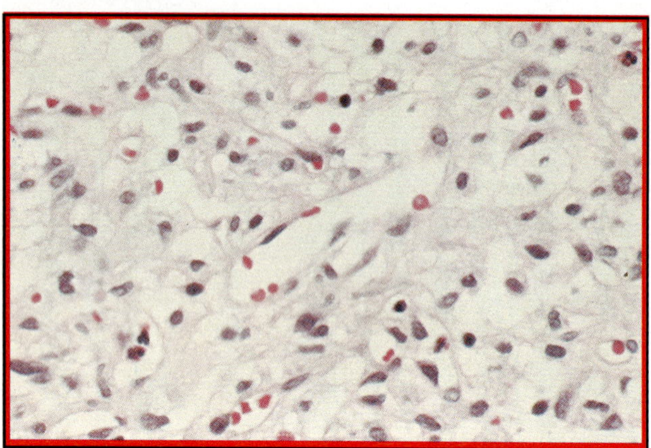

6–24 and 6–25 Electron microscopic appearance of fibrous astrocytes with membrane-bound lipid inclusions.

6–26 This patient also has a cerebellar tumor.

6–24 *and* ***6–25,*** *From Nicholson, DH, Green, WR, Kenyon, KR: Light and electron microscopic study of early lesions in angiomatous retinae, Am J Ophthalmol 82:193–204, 1976.*

Suggested Readings

Annesley, WH, Jr, Leonard, BC, Shields, JA, and Tasman, WS: Fifteen year review of treated cases of retinal angiomatosis, Trans Am Acad Ophthalmol Otolaryngol 83:446–453, 1977

Bonnet, M: Laser treatment for retinal angiomas in von Hippel's disease. In Gitter, KA, Schatz, H, Yannuzzi, LA, and McDonald, HR, eds: Laser photocoagulation of retinal disease: International Laser Symposium of the Macula, San Francisco, 1988, Pacific Medical Press, pp 243–249

Gass, JD, and Braunstein, R: Sessile and exophytic capillary angiomas of the juxtapapillary retina and optic nerve head, Arch Ophthalmol 98:1790–1797, 1980

Goldberg, MF: Clinicopathologic correlation of von Hippel angiomas after xenon arc and argon laser photocoagulation. In Peyman, GA, Apple, DJ, and Sanders, DR, eds: Intraocular tumors, New York, 1977, Appleton-Century-Crofts, pp 219–234

Laatikainen, L, Immonen, I, and Summanen, P: Peripheral retinal angioma-like lesion and macular pucker, Am J Ophthalmol 108:563–566, 1989

Mottow-Lippa, L, Tso, MO, Peyman, GA, and Chejfec, G: Von Hippel angiomatosis. A light, electron microscopic, and immunoperoxidase characterization, Ophthalmology 90:848–855, 1983

Nicholson, DH, Green, WR, and Kenyon, KR: Light and electron microscopic study of early lesions in angiomatosis retinae, Am J Ophthalmol 82:193–204, 1976

Shields, JA, Decker, WL, Sanborn, GE, Augsburger, JJ, and Goldberg, RE: Presumed acquired retinal hemangiomas, Ophthalmology 90:1292–1300, 1983

Watzke, RC, Weingeist, TA, and Constantine, JB: Diagnosis and management of von Hippel-Lindau disease. In Peyman, GA, Apple, DJ, and Sanders, DR, eds: Intraocular tumors, New York, 1977, Appleton-Century-Crofts, pp 199–217

Whitson, JT, Welch, RB, and Green, WR: Von Hippel-Lindau disease: case report of a patient with spontaneous regression of a retinal angioma, Retina (Oct–Dec) 6:253–259, 1986

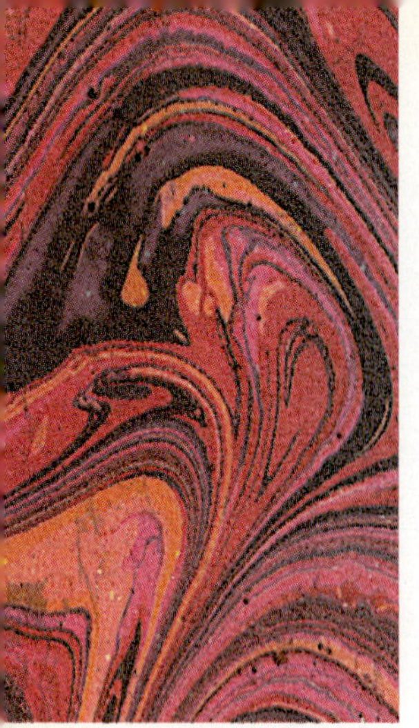

Chapter 7

Tuberous Sclerosis

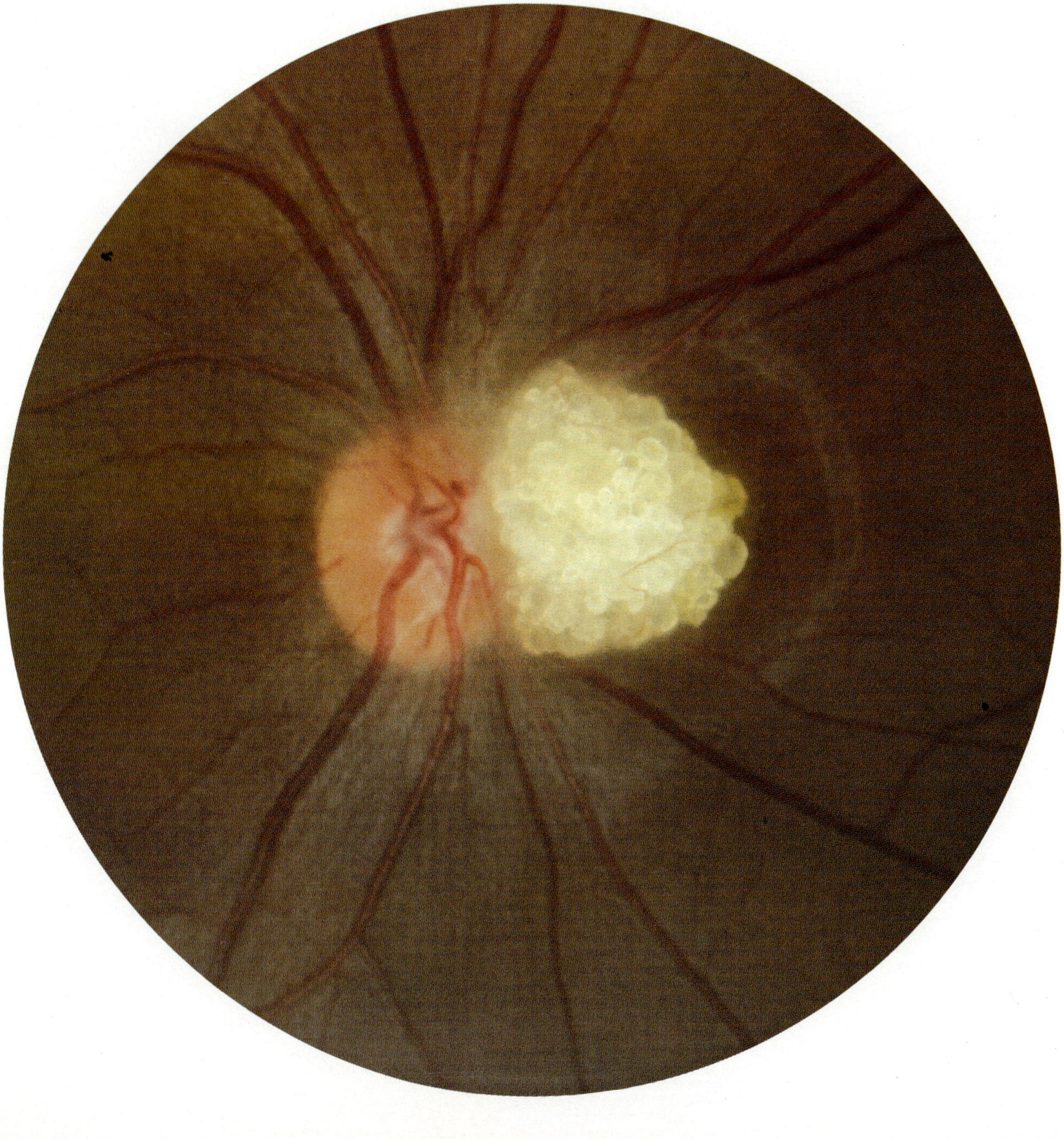

Tuberous sclerosis is a rare syndrome that may affect various organs. Hamartomatous tumors of the central nervous system, skin, viscera, and eye may be noted. This condition is inherited in an autosomal dominant pattern with high variability. Systemic manifestations include seizures, mental retardation, skin abnormalities such as adenoma sebaceum, skeletal abnormalities, and visceral abnormalities. Ocular manifestations include retinal and optic nerve phakomas and ocular adnexal lesions.

7–1

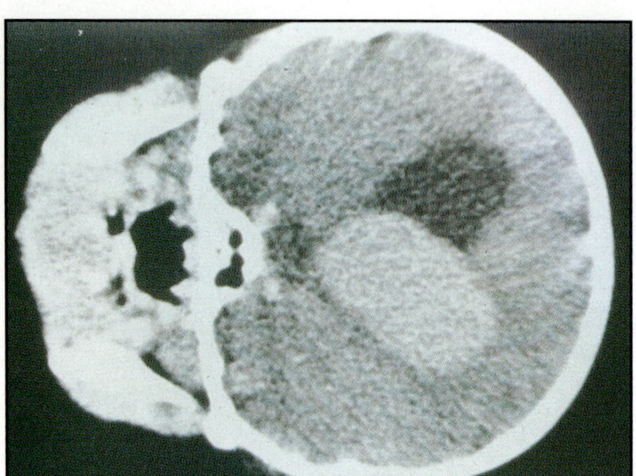

7–2

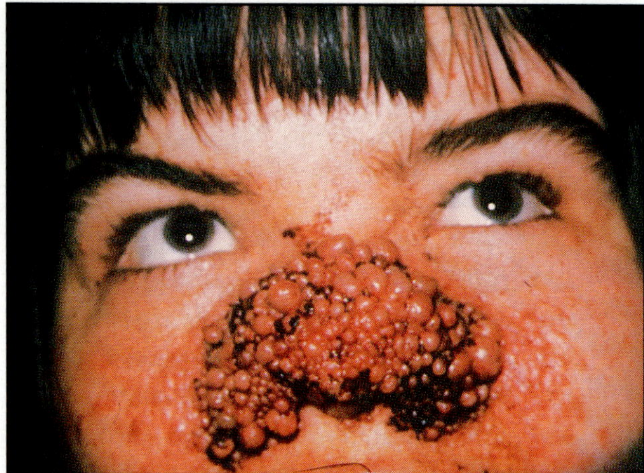

7–3 **7–4** **7–5**

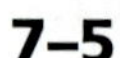

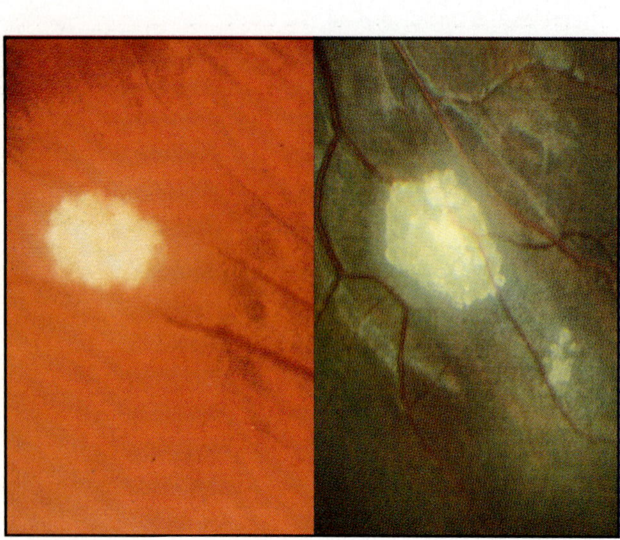

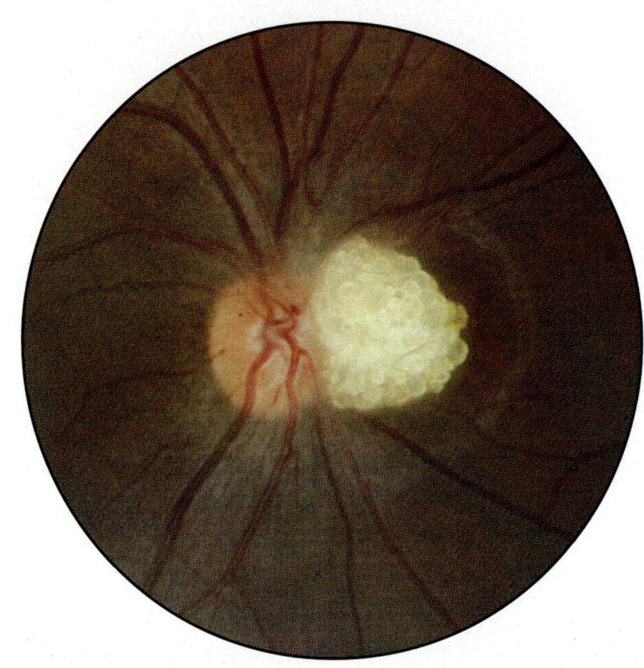

7–1 and 7–2 Tuberous sclerosis is an autosomal dominant condition in which hamartomas occur in the eye, central nervous system, skin, and viscera. Seizures, cerebral calcification (7–1), mental retardation, and skin lesions termed adenoma sebaceum (7–2) are noted in this disorder, which is also known as Bourneville's disease.

7–3 through 7–5 Astrocytic hamartomas of the retina (7–3 and 7–4) or optic disc (7–5) may be present.

7–1 *and* ***7–2,*** *Courtesy of Dr. Irene Maumenee.*

7–6

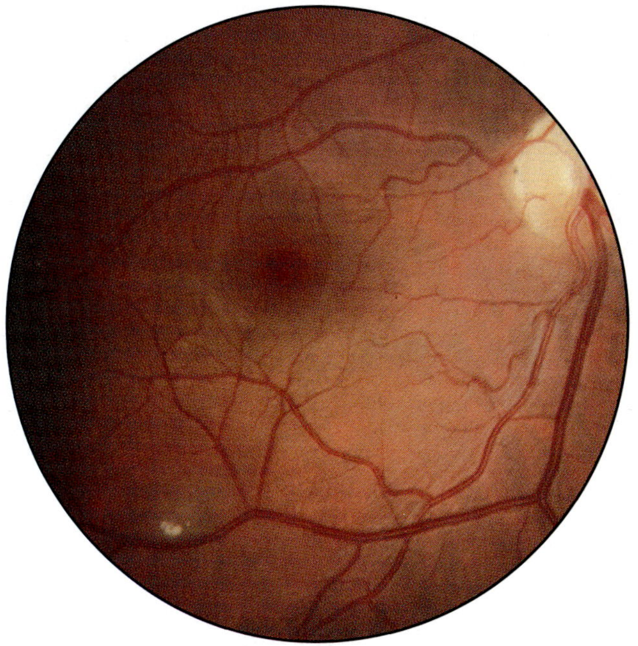

7–7

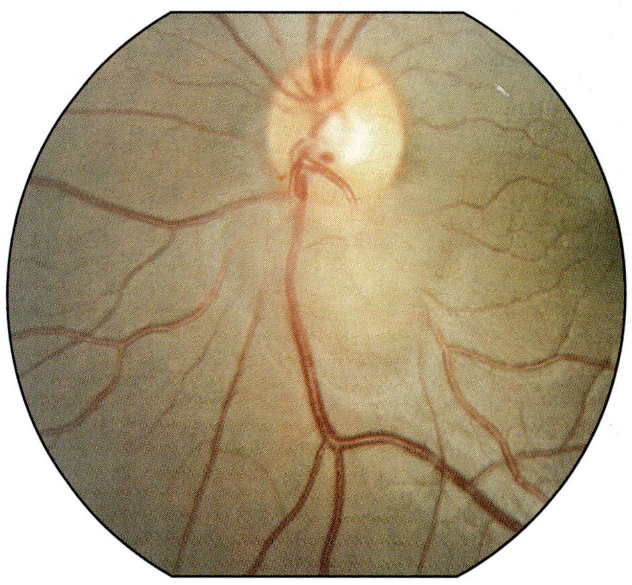

7–8

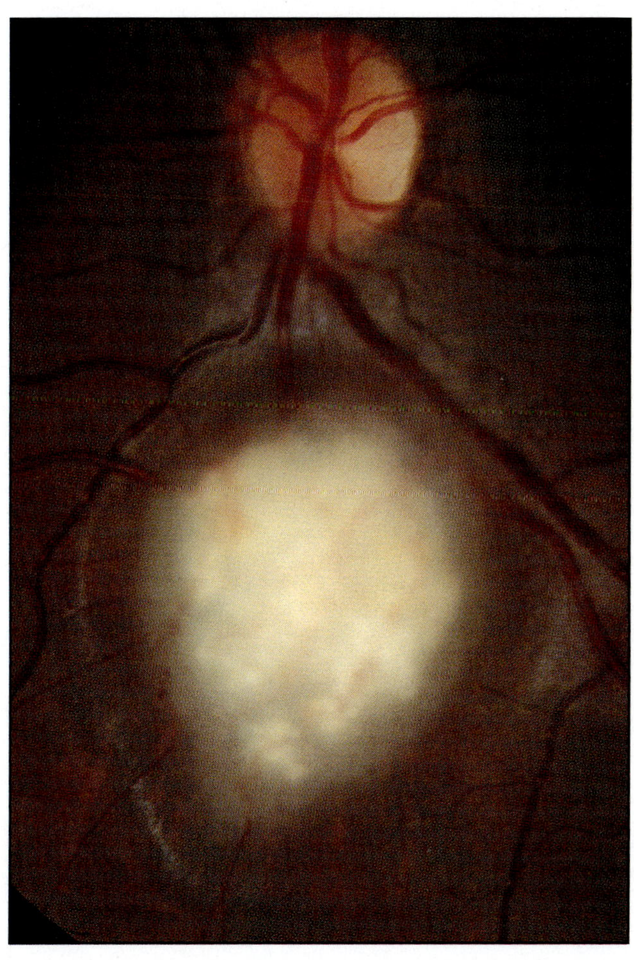

7–6 These lesions may be very small. Although these lesions are usually vascular, glistening, and bumpy, they may be mistaken for pigment epithelium atrophy, fibrous metaplasia, or drusen.

7–7 Note the grayish endophytic astrocytic hamartoma in this patient with tuberous sclerosis. This early lesion has no signs of whitening or calcification.

7–8 This astrocytoma shows a chalky white cheesy central area surrounded by a grayish margin that does not yet show calcification.

7–6, *From Nicholson, DH, and Green, WR: Tumor of the eye, lids and orbit in children. In Harley, RD, ed: Pediatric ophthalmology, Philadelphia, 1975, WB Saunders, p. 923.*

7–9

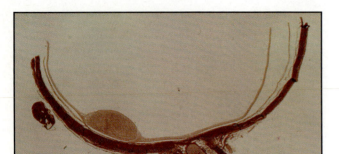

7–10

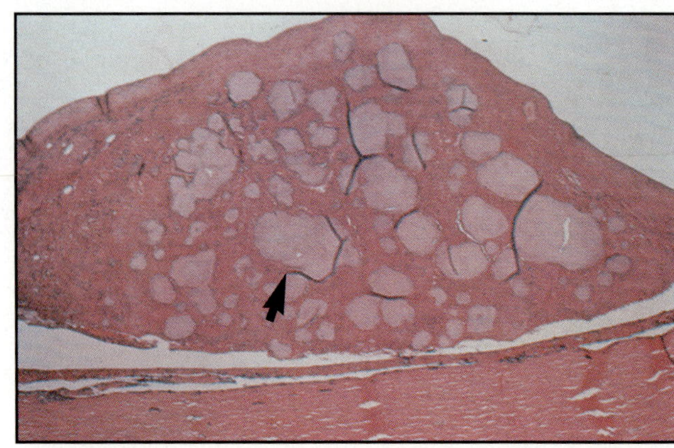

7–11

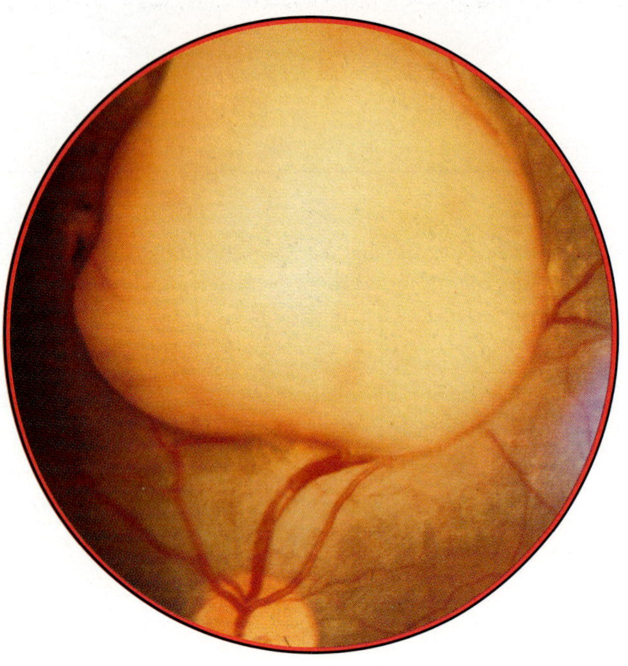

7–12

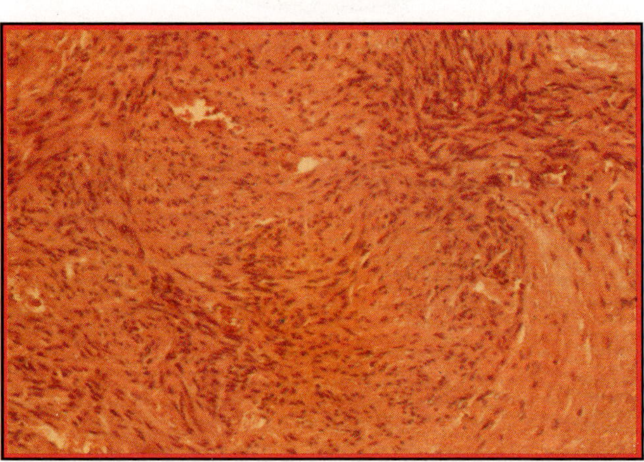

7–9 and 7–10 Retinal glial hamartomas in patients with tuberous sclerosis. These lesions are composed of spindle-shaped cells with areas of calcification *(arrowhead)*.

7–11 and 7–12 Astrocytic hamartomas may also occur isolated in patients who do not have tuberous sclerosis. This elevated whitish yellow amorphous mass was noted growing out from the retina in this patient without tuberous sclerosis (7–11). Histopathology revealed a glial hamartoma composed of elongated fibrous astrocytes containing small nuclei and interlacing cytoplasmic processes (7–12).

***7–11** and **7–12,** Courtesy of Dr. Sergio Cunha.*

7–13

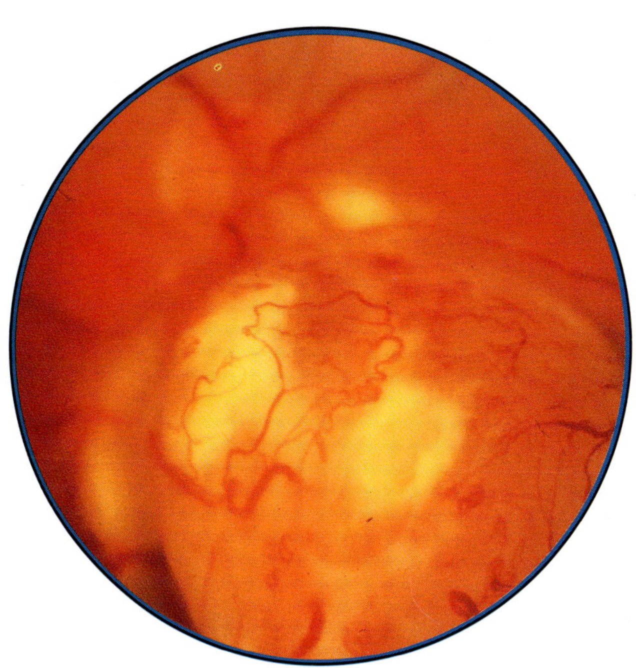

7–14

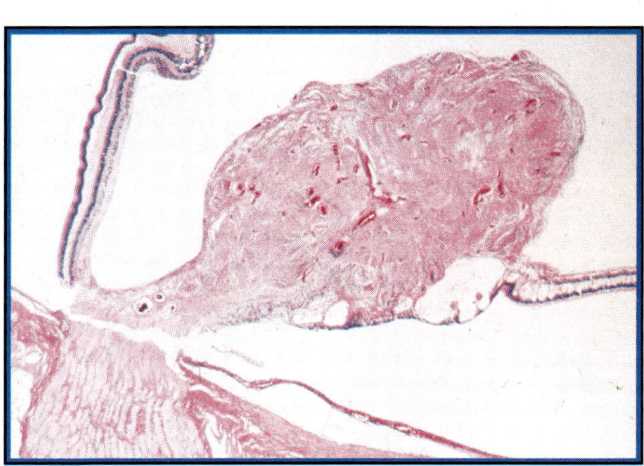

7–13 and 7–14 This patient who also did not have tuberous sclerosis presented with an elevated whitish yellow vascular mass (7–13). Histopathology revealed an astrocytoma (7–14).

***7–13** and **7–14,** Courtesy of Dr. Robert Ramsay.*

Suggested Readings

Barsky, D, and Wolter, JR: The retinal lesions of tuberous sclerosis: an angiogliomatous hamartoma? J Pediatr Ophthalmol 8:261–265, 1971

De Juan, E, Jr, Green, WR, et al: Vitreous seeding by astrocytic hamartoma in a patient with tuberous sclerosis, Retina 4:100–102, 1984

Font, RL, and Ferry, AP: The phakomatoses, Int Ophthalmol Clin 12:1–50, 1972

Fryer, AE, Chalmers, A, Connor, JM, Fraser, I, et al: Evidence that the gene for tuberous sclerosis is on chromosome 9, Lancet 1:659–661, 1987

Gomez, MR: Tuberous sclerosis, New York, 1979, Raven Press

Nyboer, JH, Robertson, DM, and Gomez, MR: Retinal lesions in tuberous sclerosis, Arch Ophthal 94:1277–1280, 1976

Shields, JS: Diagnosis and management of intraocular tumors, St Louis, 1983, Mosby–Year Book, pp 650–656

Williams, R, and Taylor, D: Tuberous sclerosis, Surv Ophthalmol 30:143–153, 1985

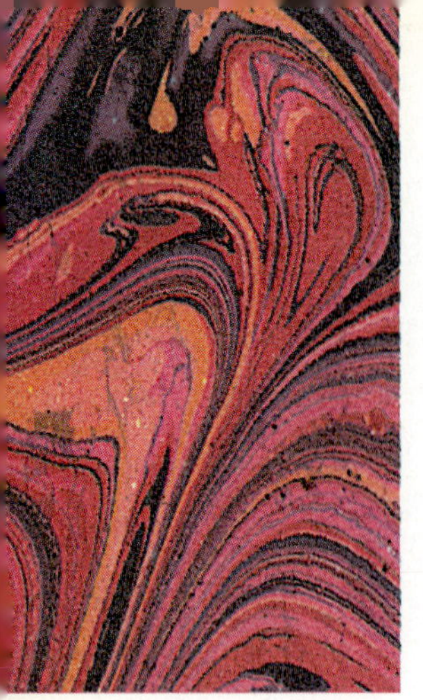

Chapter 8

Other Phakomatoses

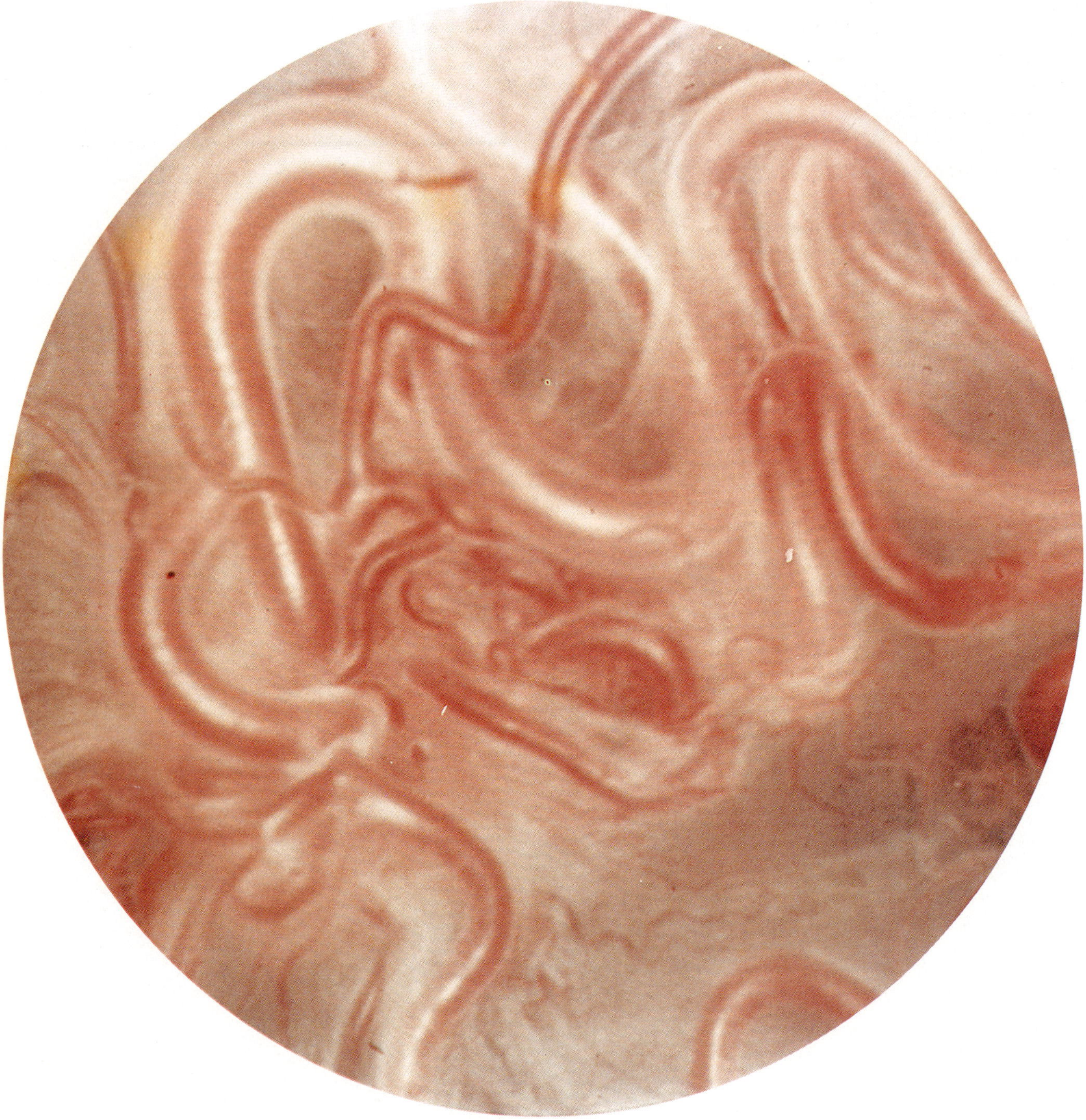

Other phakomatoses besides tuberous sclerosis include the Sturge-Weber syndrome, ataxia-telangiectasia (Louis-Barr syndrome), the Wyburn-Mason syndrome, and neurofibromatosis (von Recklinghausen's disease). Characteristic ophthalmic features may be seen in several of these syndromes. The Sturge-Weber syndrome may show a diffuse choroidal hemangioma. These patients may also have facial vascular lesions, ipsilateral intracranial hemangiomas, a nevus flammus involving the eyelid, anomalous large blood vessels at the conjunctiva and episcleral tissues, malformation of the anterior chamber, and glaucoma. Retinal involvement is not a feature of the Louis-Barr syndrome. The Wyburn-Mason syndrome may have associated abnormal retinal arteriovenous anastomoses. Arteriovenous malformations may also occur in the ipsilateral midbrain. This retinal lesion has also been termed a "racemose hemangioma" since a definite arteriovenous communication cannot always be noted. Neurofibromatosis may show diffuse choroidal involvement or small multifocal whitish lesions in the retina that are termed "astrocytic hamartomas." The astrocytic hamartomas may resemble the lesions of tuberous sclerosis. Larger retinal tumors rarely occur.

8–1 STURGE-WEBER SYNDROME

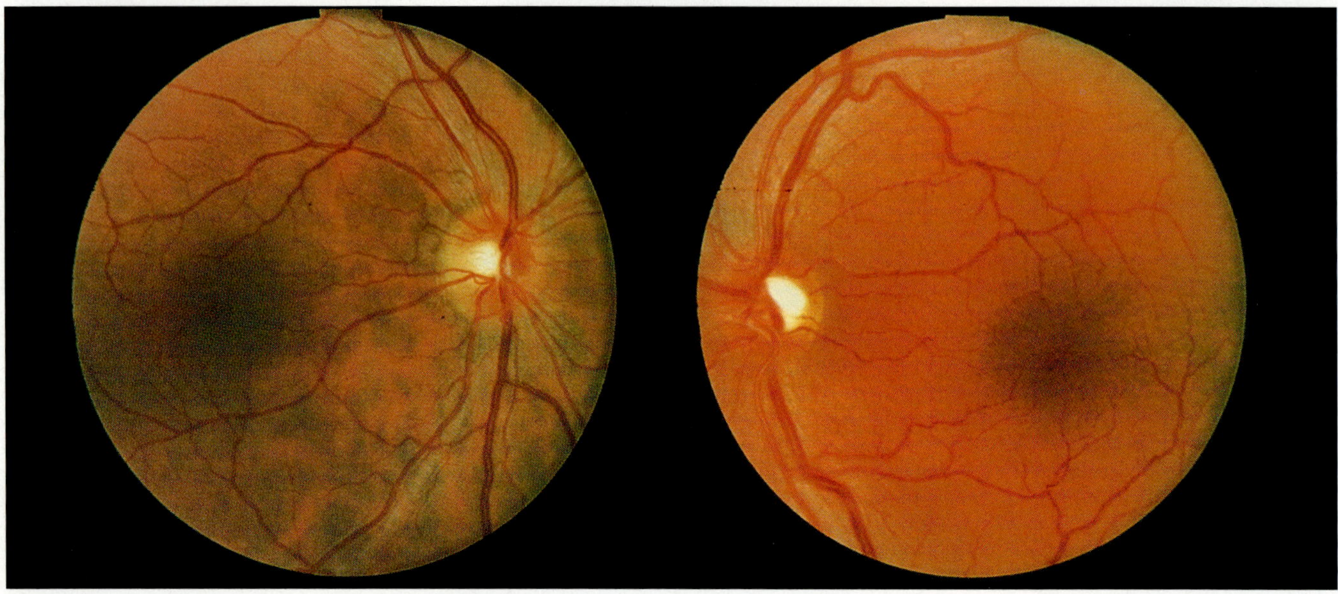

8–2

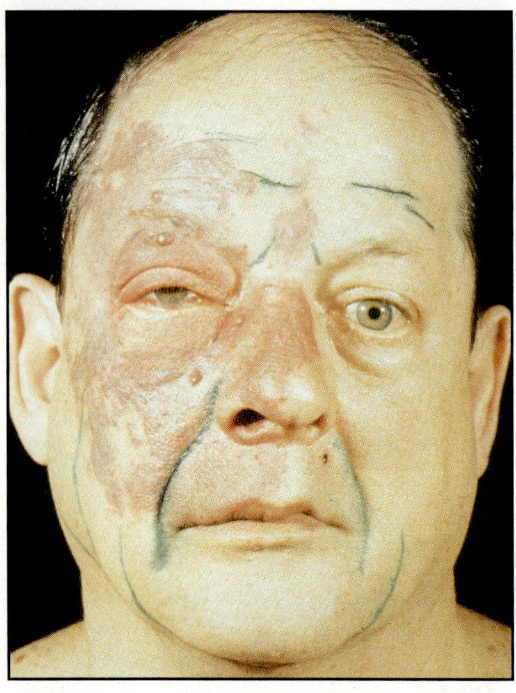

8–1 Diffuse choroidal hemangioma may occur associated with the Sturge-Weber syndrome, which is another one of the phakomatoses. The accompanying photograph shows one eye with a diffuse choroidal hemangioma in comparison to its normal fellow eye. Note the orange reddish color change in the eye with the diffuse hemangioma.

8–2 Weber syndrome also may be seen associated with the classic cutaneous findings of this disorder and/or an intracranial hemangioma.

8–1, *Courtesy of Dr. Thomas Burton.* ***8–2,*** *From Lebwohl, M: Atlas of the skin and systemic disease, New York, 1995, Churchill Livingstone.*

8–3 WYBURN-MASON SYNDROME

8–4

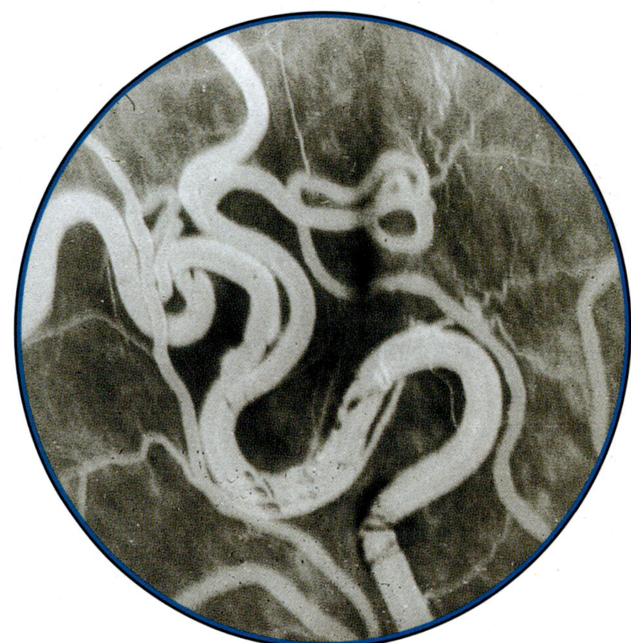

8–5

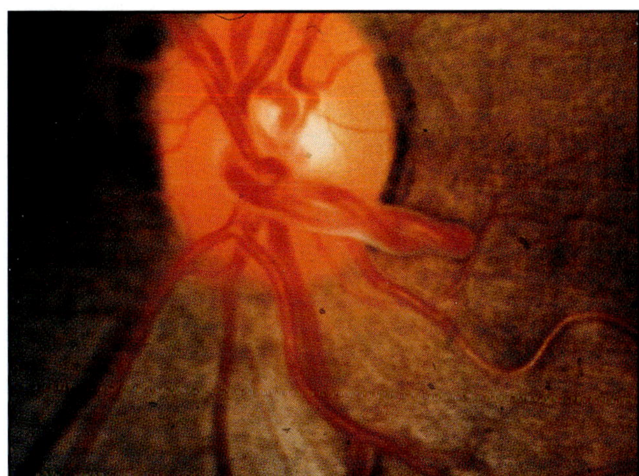

8–3 and 8–4 Patients with the Wyburn-Mason syndrome may have retinal arteriovenous malformations. Fluorescein angiography demonstrates that these vessels do not generally leak unless they become complicated by vascular occlusive changes.

8–5 Congenital arteriovenous shunt vessels, as seen in this patient at the optic disc, may be a forme fruste of the condition.

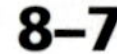

8–6 WYBURN-MASON SYNDROME

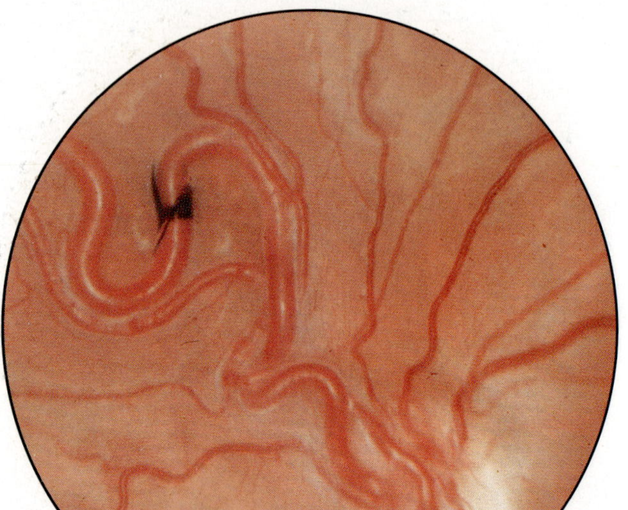

8–7

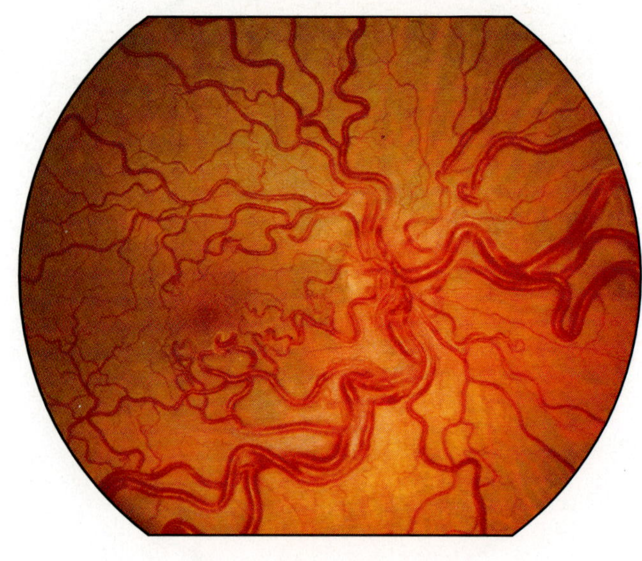

8–6 Pigmentation may sometimes be observed in the abnormal vessels in this disorder.

8–7 Tortuosity and dilatation of the normal vessels as well as malformed vessels may also be noted. Variably sized arteriovenous communications are demonstrated in this patient. Affected patients may have an associated arteriovenous malformation in the midbrain.

8–7, *Courtesy of Ross Jarrett and Neil J. Okun.*

8–8

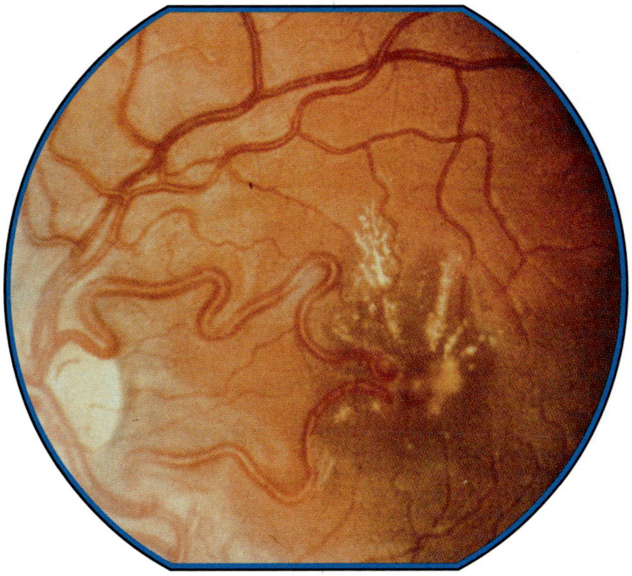

8–9

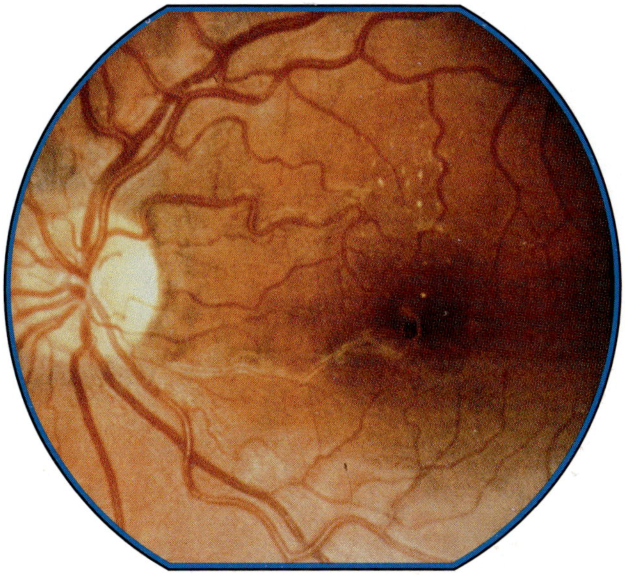

8–10

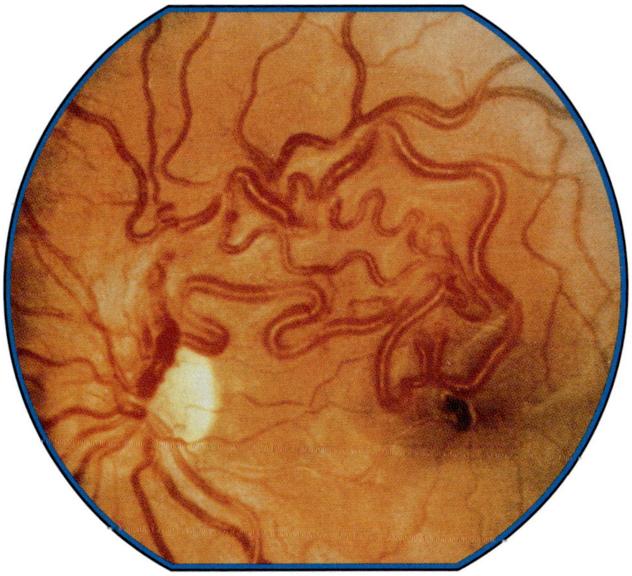

8–11

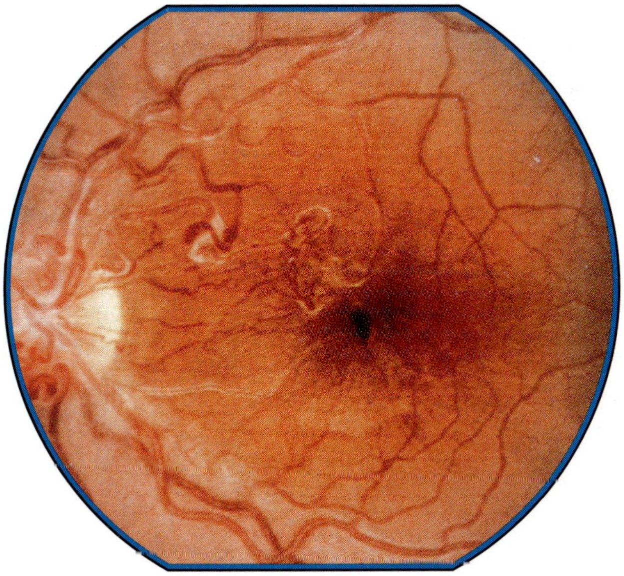

8–8 through 8–10 Rarely, arteriovenous (AV) malformations may show spontaneous regression and then recurrence, as seen in this case with a 17-year follow-up. The patient initially presented with retinal arteriovenous malformations and macular edema. Vascular occlusion of the inferior vessel resulted in sheathing, nonperfusion, and resolution of the exudate. A new AV anastomosis appeared. A hairpin loop is seen connecting the AV segments.

8–11 There was again obstruction of the AV anastomosis with closure of the AV communication and resolution of the edema.

8–8 *through* ***8–11,*** *Courtesy of Dr. Achim Wessing.*

8–12A WYBURN-MASON SYNDROME

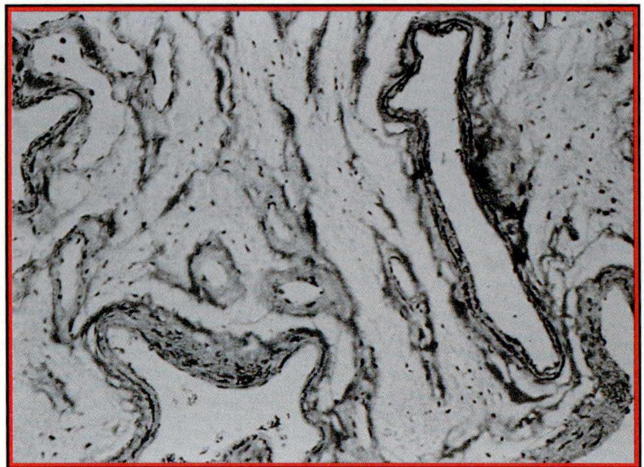

8–12B

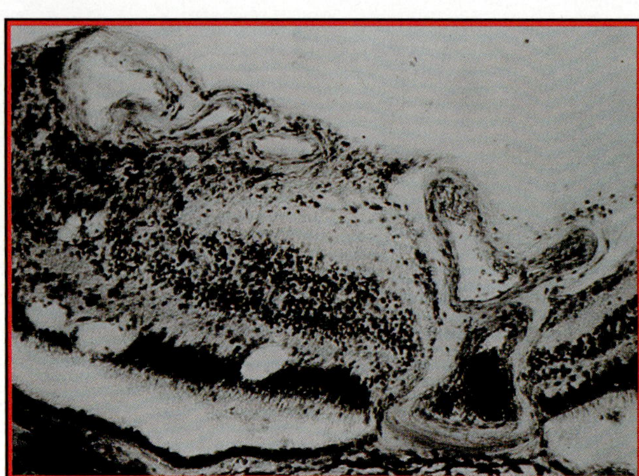

8–13A

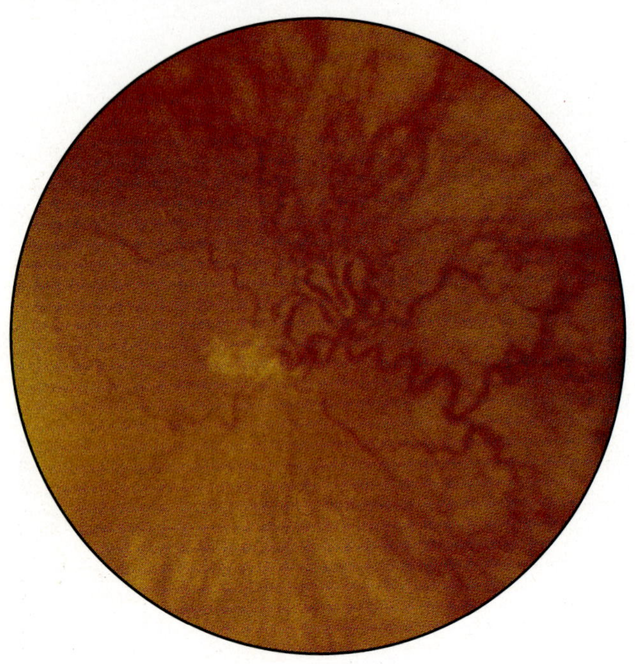

8–13B

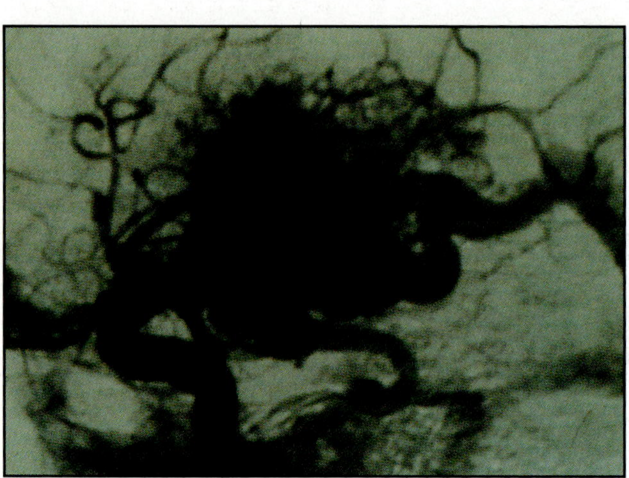

8–12A and 8–12B This patient with the Wyburn-Mason syndrome had an arteriovenous malformation of the optic nerve (8–12A) and retina (8–12B).

8–13A and 8–13B This is a patient with Wyburn-Mason syndrome of the fundus (8–13A) and an intracranial vascular malformation seen with MRI imaging (8–13B).

***8–12A** and **B,** From Cameron, ME and Greer, CH: Congenital arteriovenous aneurysm of the retina: a post mortem report, Br J Ophthalmol 52:768–772, 1968. **8–13A** and **B,** Courtesy of Dr. James Augsberger.*

8–14 NEUROFIBROMATOSIS

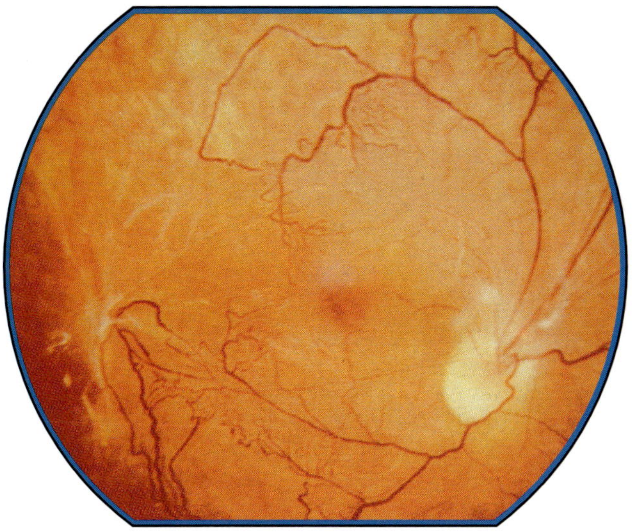

8–15

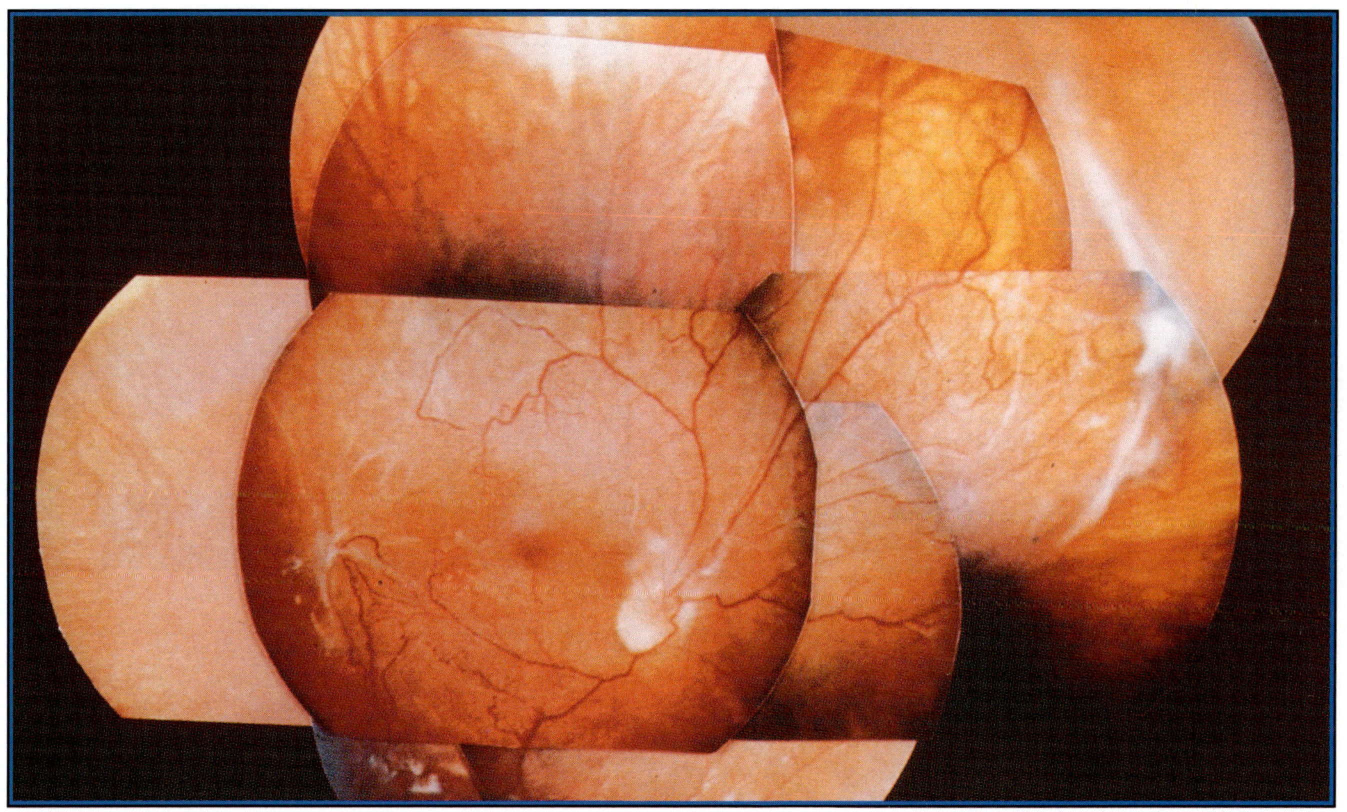

8–14 and 8–15 Patients with neurofibromatosis may have diffuse choroidal involvement, astrocytic hamartomas of the retina, and peripheral retinal vascular occlusions. A loop of AV anastomosis is noted with obliteration of the arteries and veins in the retina. The ischemic retina is associated with widespread preretinal proliferation. Note the islands of nonperfused retina which are present in the posterior pole extending towards the center of the macula and in the periphery.

8–16

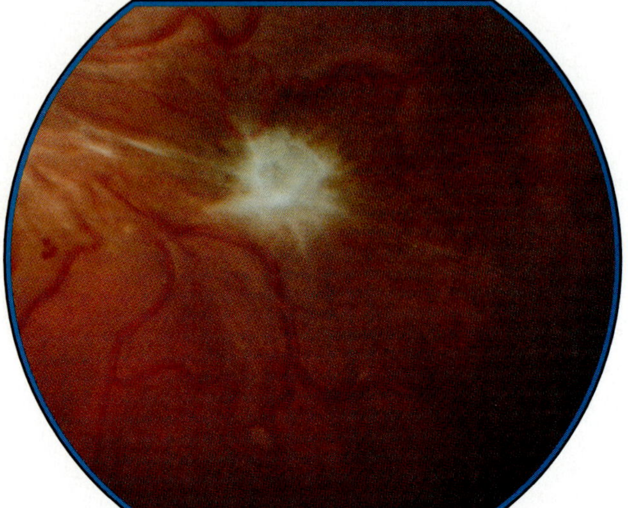

8–17

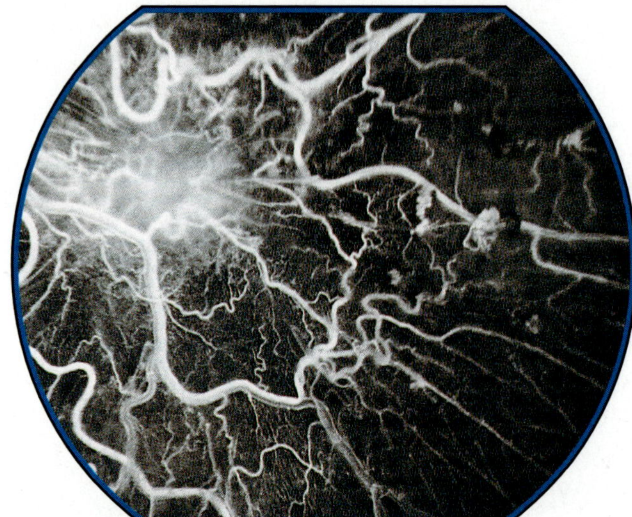

8–18

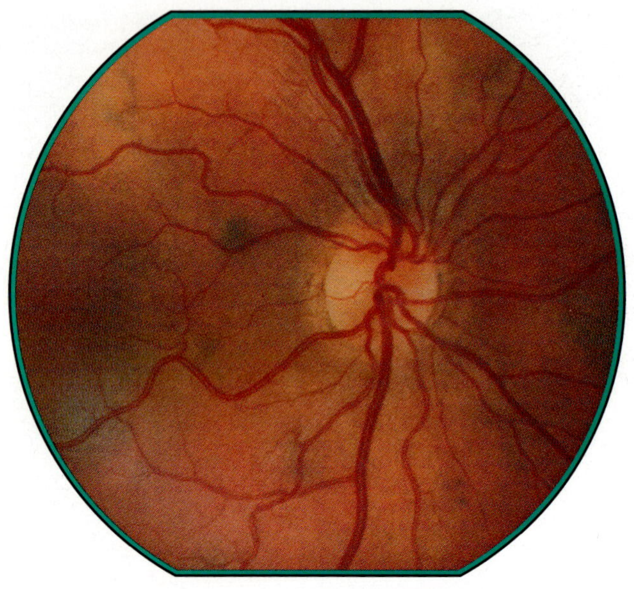

8–19

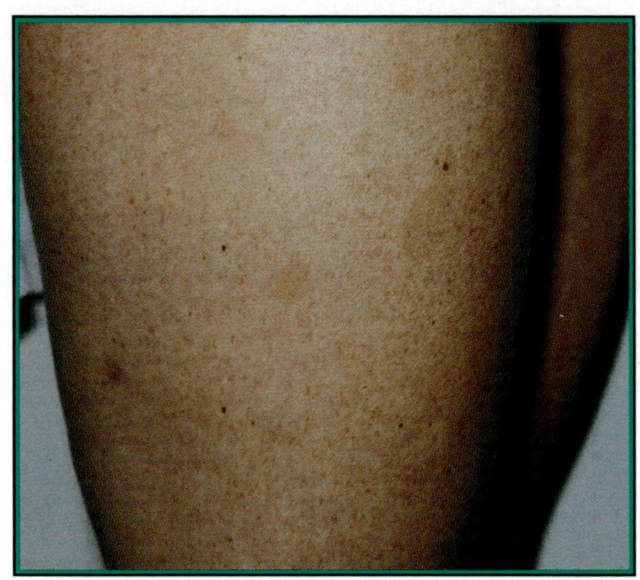

8–20

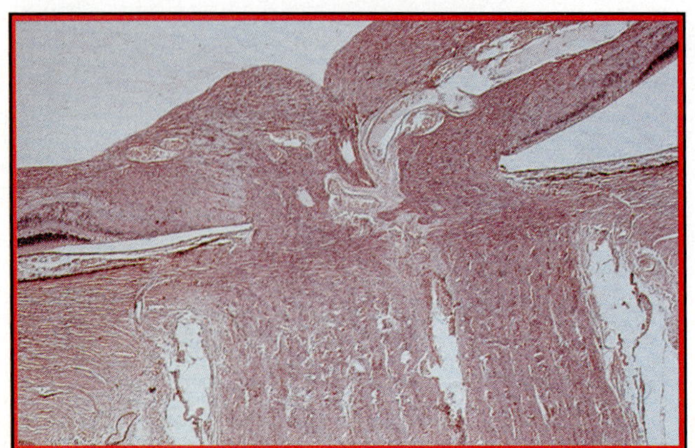

8–16 and 8–17 A hamartoma of the retina is noted in a patient with neurofibromatosis. Note the fibrotic pucker and proliferative vasculature changes with tortuosity.

8–18 and 8–19 This patient with neurofibromatosis has multiple pigmented lesions in the fundus (8–18) and café au lait spots (8–19).

8–20 This glial hamartoma of the optic nerve head is from a patient with neurofibromatosis.

Suggested Readings

Anand, R, Augsburger, JJ, and Shields, JA: Circumscribed choroidal hemangiomas, Arch Ophthalmol 107:1338–1342, 1989

Archer, DB, Deutman, A, Ernest, JT, and Krill, AE: Arteriovenous communications of the retina, Am J Ophthalmol 75:224–241, 1973

Bech, K, and Jensen, OA: On the frequency of co-existing racemose haemangiomata of the retina and brain, Acta Psychiat Neurol Scand 36:47–56, 1961

De Laey, JJ, and Hanssens, M: Vascular tumors and malformations of the ocular fundus, Bull Soc Belge Ophthalmol 225:1–241, 1990

Destro, M, D'Amico, DJ, Gragoudas, ES, Brockhurst, RJ, Pinnolis, MK, Albert, DM, Toppi, TM, and Puliafito, CA: Retinal manifestations of neurofibromatosis. Diagnosis and management, Arch Ophthalmol 109:662–666, 1991

Good, WV, Brodsky, MC, Edwards, MS, and Hoyt, WF: Bilateral retinal hamartomas in neurofibromatosis type 2, Br J Ophthalmol 75:190, 1991

Landau, K, Dossetor, FM, Hoyt, WF, and Muci-Mendoza, R: Retinal hamartoma in neurofibromatosis 2, Arch Ophthalmol 108:328–329, 1990

Mansour, AM, Walsh, JB, and Henkind, P: Arteriovenous anastomoses of the retina, Ophthalmology 94:35–40, 1987

Wallace, MR, Marchuk, DA, Andersen, LB, Letcher, R, Odeh, HM, Saulino, AM, Fountain, JW, Brereton, A, Nicholson, J, Mitchell, AL, Brownstein, BH, and Collins, FS: Type 1 neurofibromatosis gene: identification of a large transcript disrupted in three NF1 patients, Science 249:181–186, 1990

Witschel, H, and Font, RL: Hemangioma of the choroid: a clinicopathologic study of 71 cases and a review of the literature, Surv Ophthalmol 20:415–431, 1976

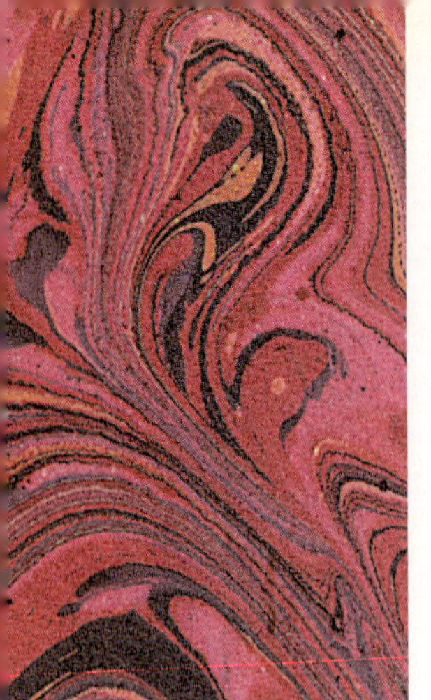

Chapter 9

Melanocytoma of the Optic Nerve Head

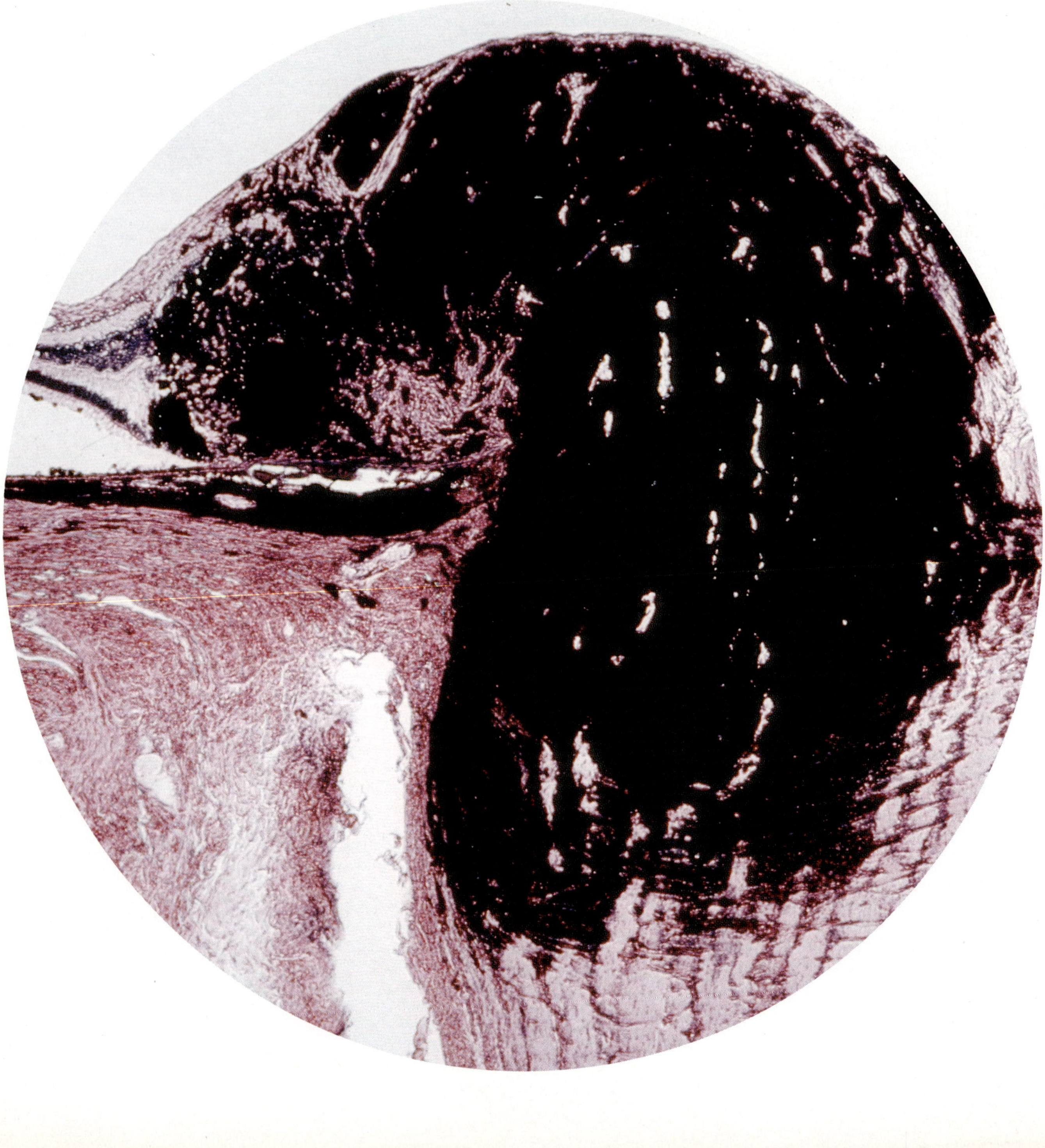

Melanocytomas of the optic nerve head are benign pigmented tumors. It is important to differentiate these lesions from malignant choroidal melanomas. A melanocytoma of the optic nerve is an atypical nevus. It may cause optic disc edema and/or visual field loss. Malignant transformation is exceedingly rare.

9–1

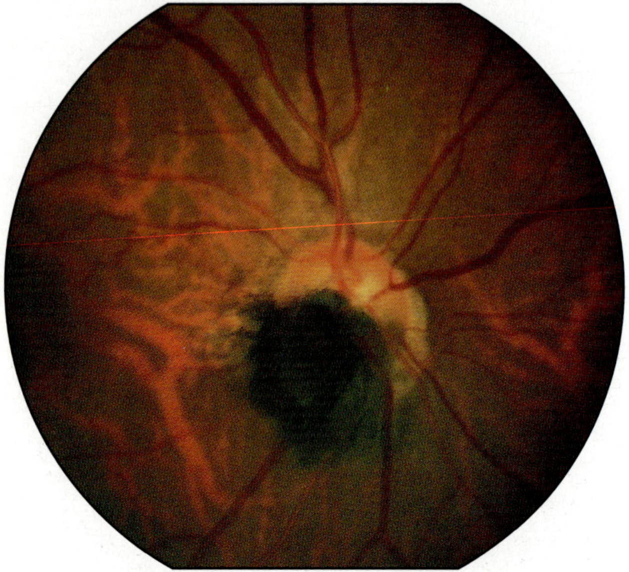

9–2

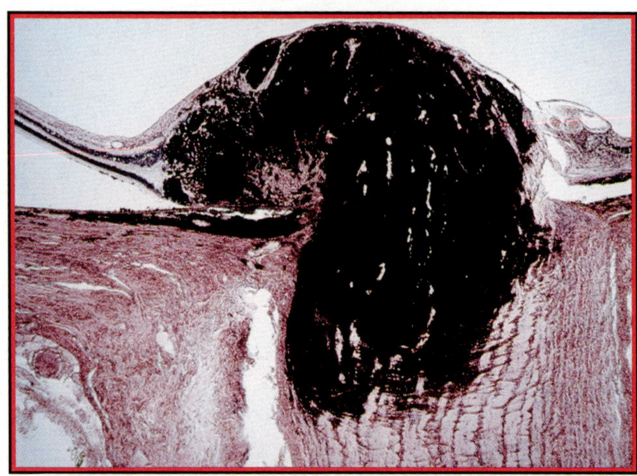

9–3

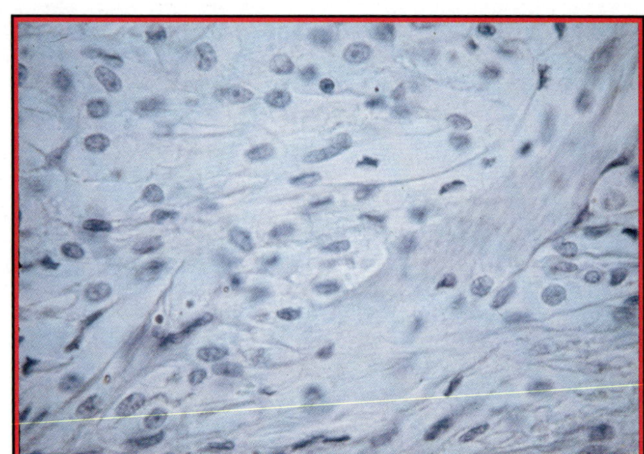

9–1 Melanocytomas are benign densely pigmented tumors that are usually located at the optic nerve head.

9–2 Histopathologic appearance of a melanocytoma involving the optic nerve head, peripapillary retina, and the optic nerve.

9–3 After bleaching of the melanin pigment the cytologic features can be appreciated. The cells have abundant cytoplasm and relatively uniform round or oval nuclei with a small nucleolus.

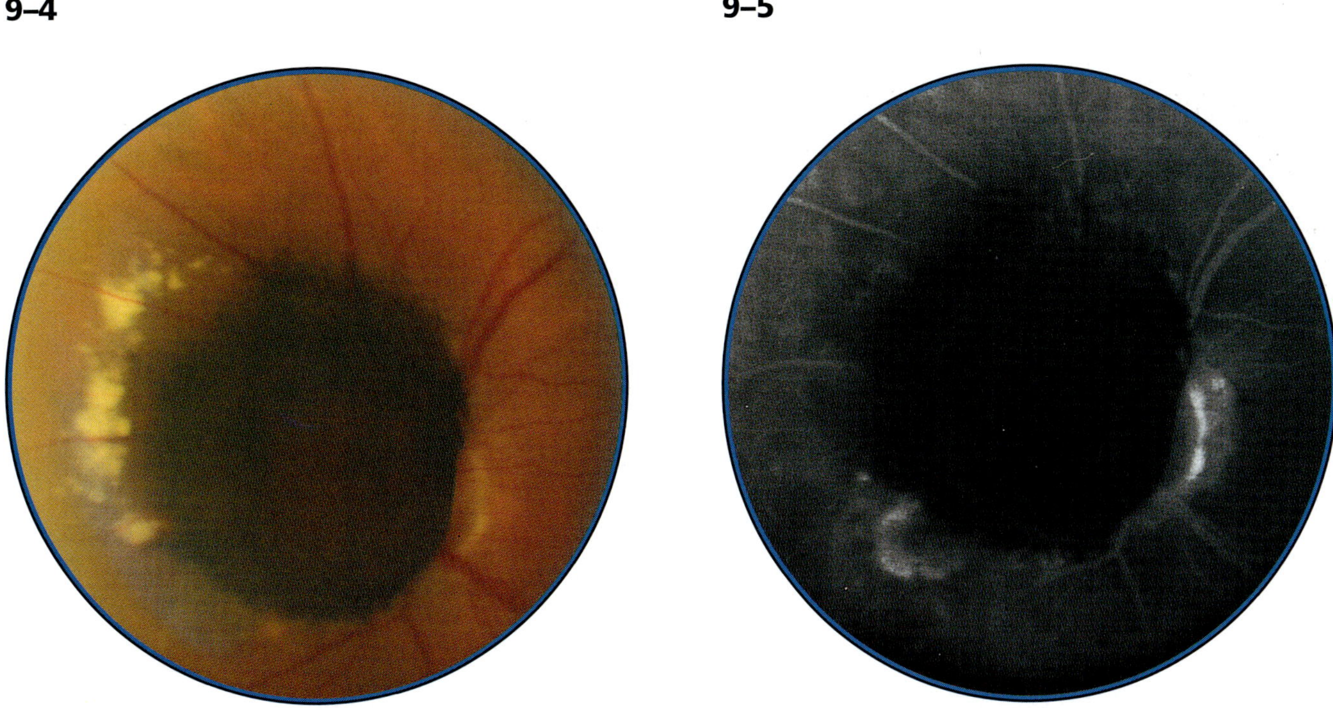

9–4 and 9–5 This patient with a melanocytoma was followed for 22 years and developed choroidal neovascularization at its inferior margin, which is evident as hyperfluorescence on the fluorescein study.

9–6 **9–7**

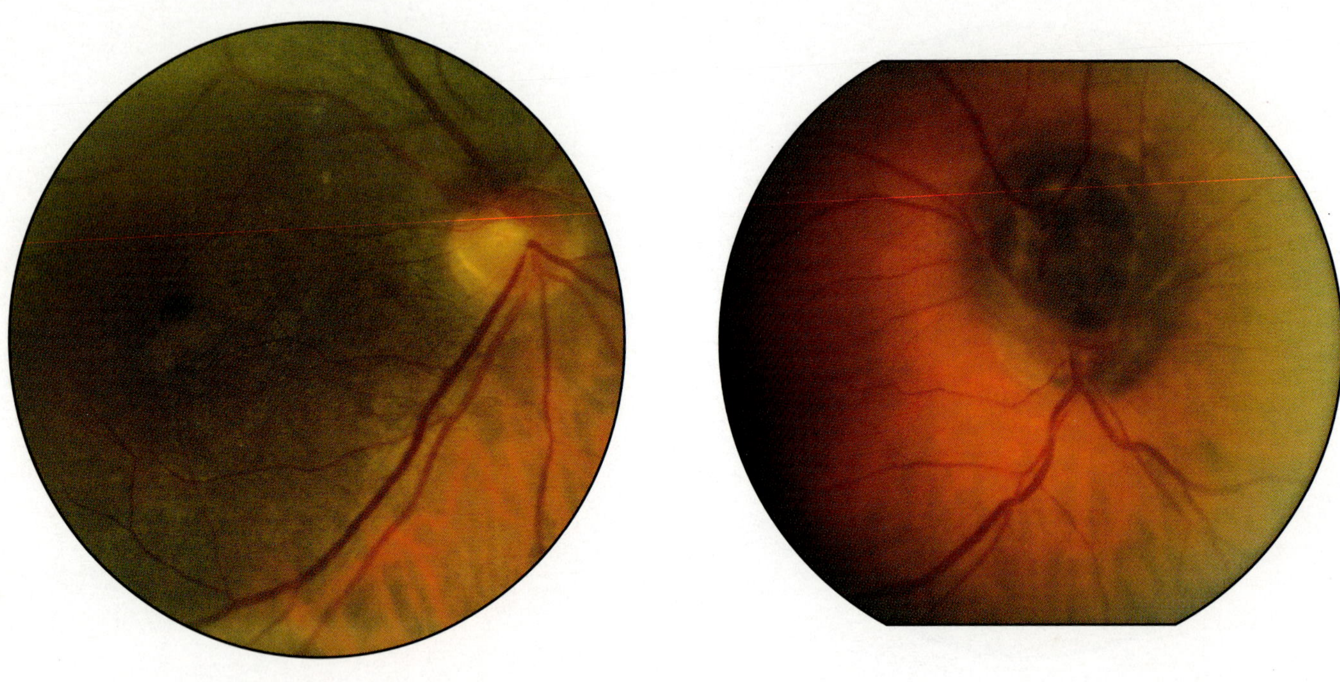

9–6 A melanocytoma may sometimes be more diffuse and extend from the optic disc into the macular region.

9–7 This patient has a retinal pigment epithelium (RPE) adenoma of the optic nerve, which may mimic a melanocytoma. The diagnosis was confirmed by histopathology. It may be very difficult to differentiate an RPE adenoma clinically from a melanocytoma or melanoma.

9–6, *Courtesy of Dr. Jerry Shields.* **9–7,** *Courtesy of Dr. Lee Jampol.*

Suggested Readings

Apple, DJ, Craythorn, JM, Reidy, JJ, Steinmentz, RL, Brady, SE, and Bohart, WA: Malignant transformation of an optic nerve melanocytoma, Can J Ophthalmol 19:320–325, 1984

Erzurum, SA, Jampol, LM, Territo, C, and O'Grady, R: Primary malignant melanoma of optic nerve simulating a melanocytoma, Arch Ophthalmol 110:684–686, 1992

Joffe, L, Shields, JA, Osher, RH, and Gass, JDM: Clinical and follow up studies of melanocytomas of the optic disc, Ophthalmology 86:1067–1078, 1979

Reidy, JJ, Apple, DJ, Steinmetz, RL, Craythorn, JM, Loftfield, K, Gieser, SC, and Brady, SE: Melanocytoma: Nomenclature, pathogenesis, natural history and treatment, Surv Ophthalmol 29:319–327, 1985

Shields, JA: Melanocytoma of the optic nerve. In Shields, JA, ed: Diagnosis and management of intraocular tumors, St Louis, 1983, Mosby–Year Book, Inc

Zografos, L, Uffer, S, Gailloud, C, and Kohli, M: Le mélanome de la papille, nouvelle observation, Klin Monatsbl Augenheilk 180:503–509, 1982

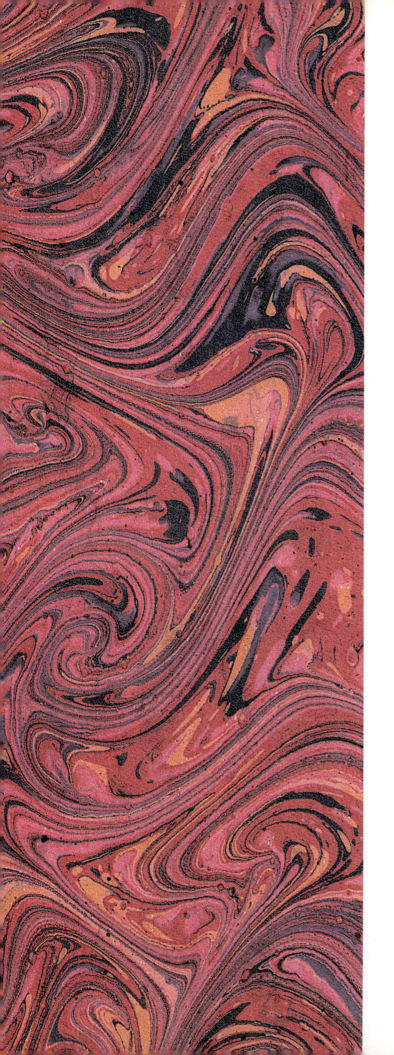

Part III

Tumors of the Retinal Pigment Epithelium

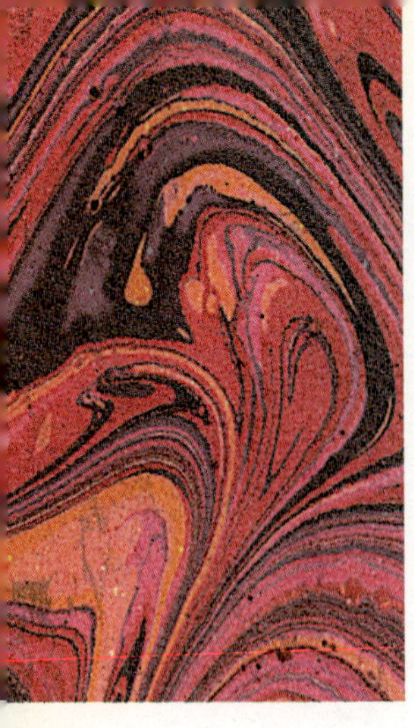

Chapter 10

Congenital Hypertrophy of the Retinal Pigment Epithelium and Other Benign Pigmented Lesions

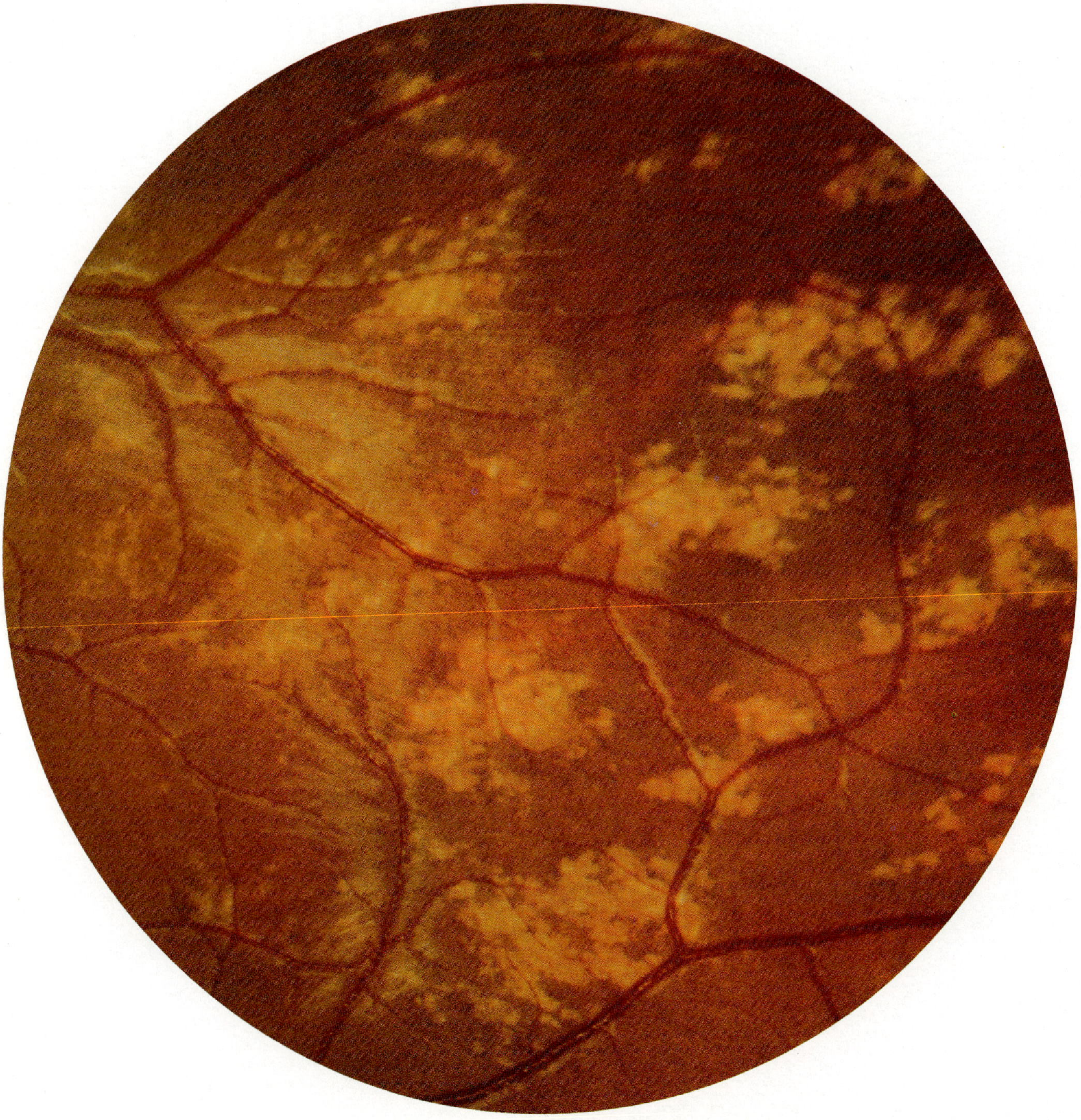

Congenital hypertrophy of the retinal pigment epithelium (CHRPE) is an asymptomatic and benign pigmented lesion of the fundus. Usually these lesions are solitary, round and flat hyperpigmented areas that are well-demarcated. Sometimes a narrow halo of hypopigmented retinal pigment epithelium may be noted. Neither unilateral lesions of CHRPE or grouped pigmentation (bear tracks) have been known to be associated with other ocular or systemic abnormalities. However, multiple and bilateral CHRPE-like lesions have been associated with Gardner's syndrome.

10–1 **10–2**

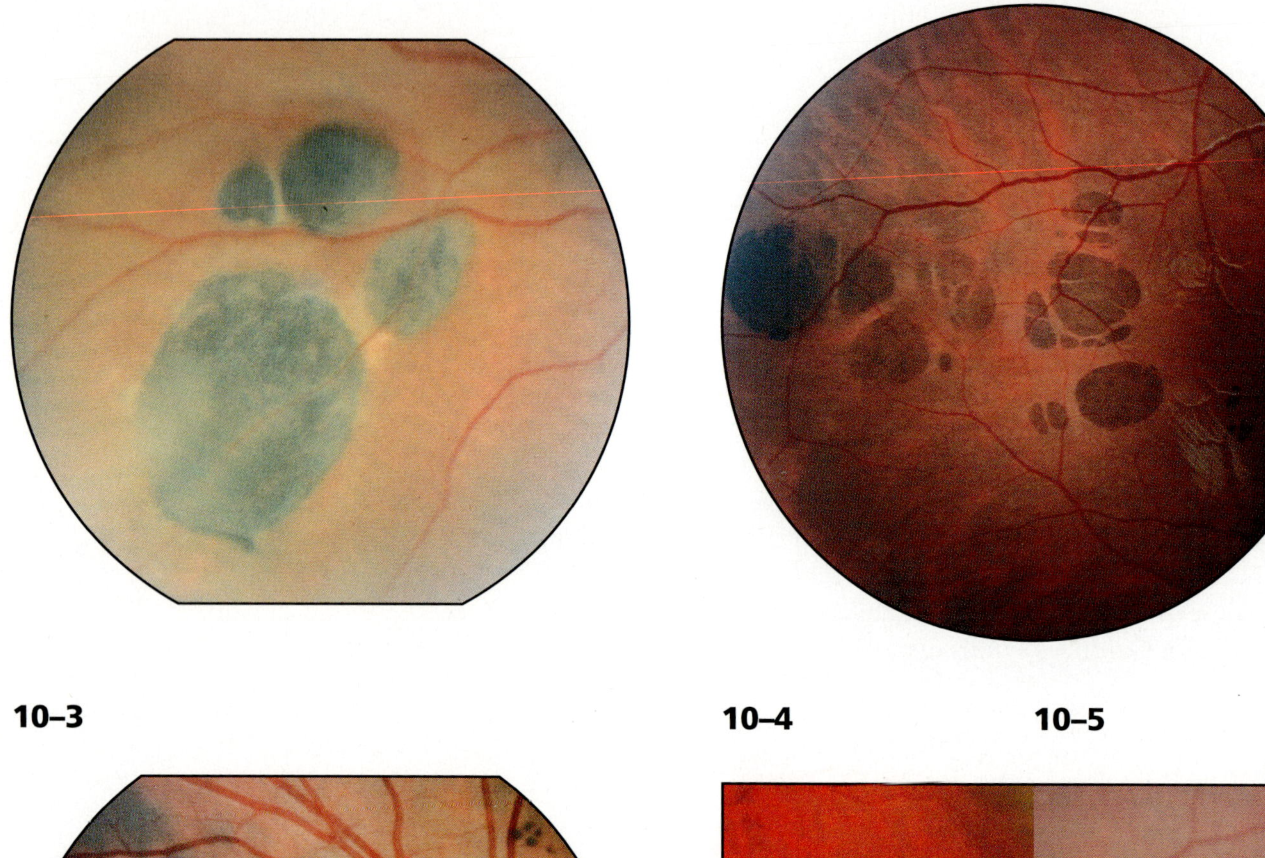

10–3

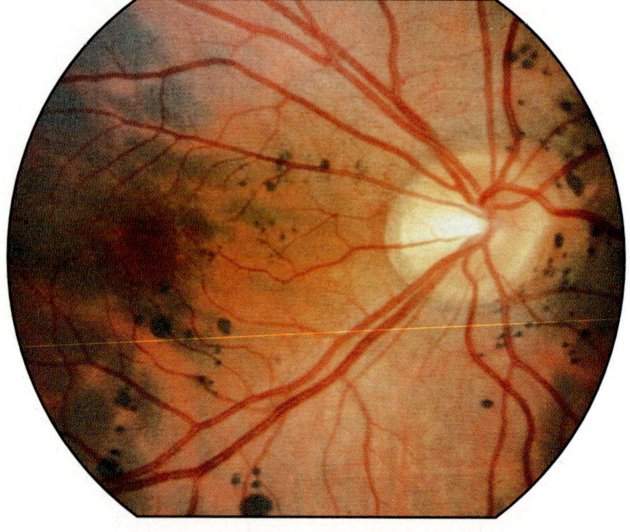

10–4 **10–5**

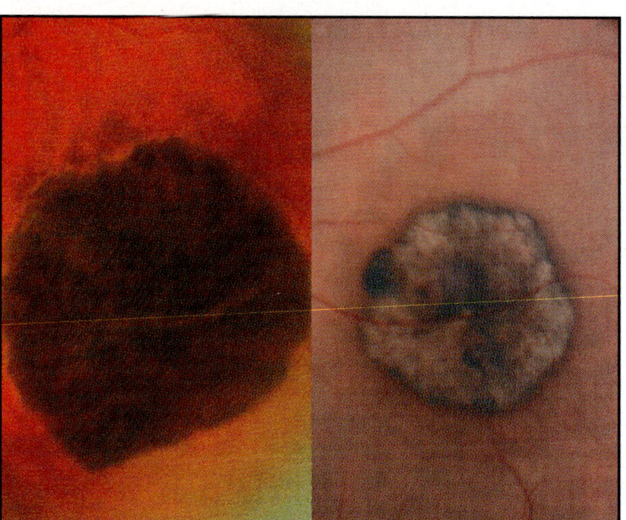

10–1 and 10–2 Bear tracks, congenital hypertrophy of the retinal pigment epithelium, and grouped pigmentation are different terms for congenital lesions of the retinal pigment epithelium. Flat large areas of hyperpigmentation are seen on clinical examination.

10–3 The bear tracks may be multiple in nature and can sometimes be observed around the macular and/or peripapillary region. However, usually they are peripheral in location.

10–4 and 10–5 In some cases, there is hyperpigmentation (10–4) and in other cases atrophy may be noted (10–5).

10–2, *Courtesy of Dr. Jerry Shields.*

10–6

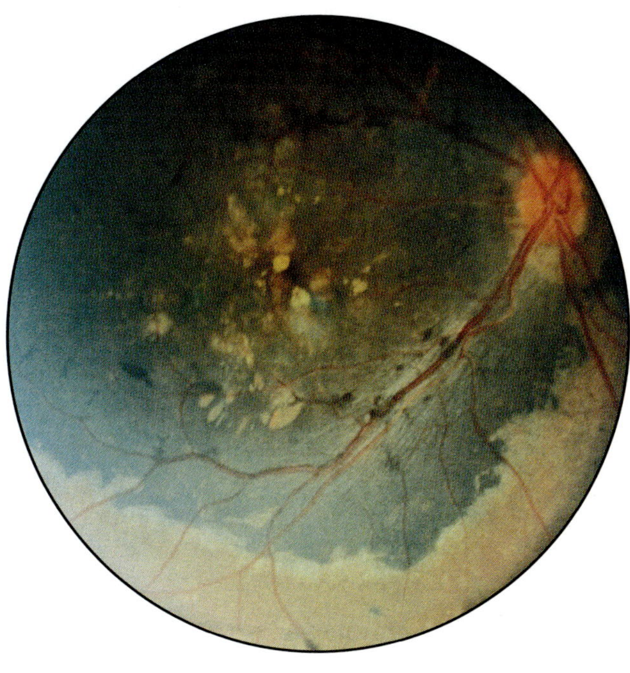

10–7

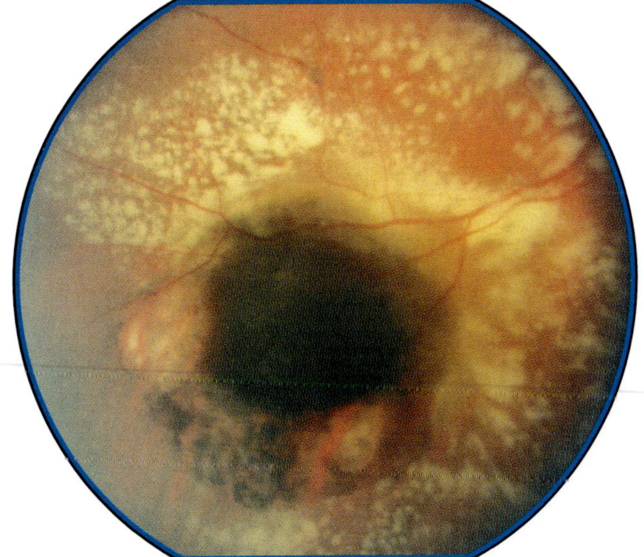

10–8

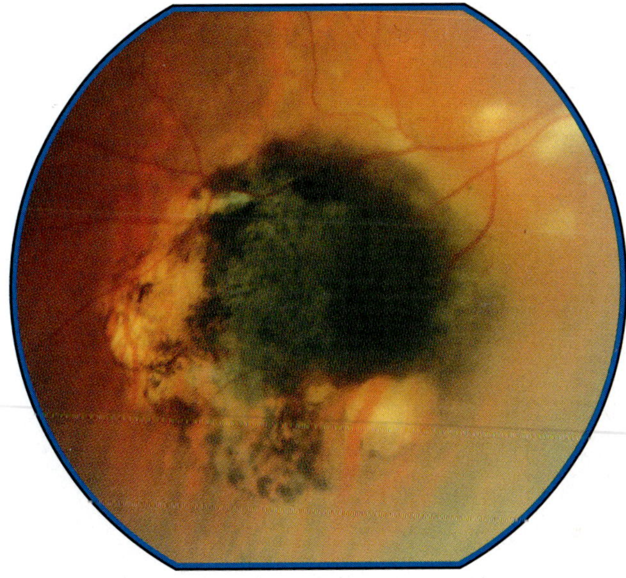

10–6 Hypertrophy of the retinal pigment epithelium (RPE) may sometimes be more diffuse and involve the macular region. A characteristic of RPE hypertrophy is a surrounding halo of atrophy, as demonstrated in this case. These lesions often appear singular as a flat roundish area with variable pigmentation.

10–7 and 10–8 Rarely, choroidal neovascularization secondary to retinal pigment epithelium hypertrophy may be noted, as demonstrated in this case with massive lipid exudation. After laser treatment, the exudation regressed and the detachment resolved.

10–6, *Courtesy of Dr. Evangelos Gragoudas.* ***10–7*** *and* ***10–8,*** *Courtesy of Dr. Mort Rosenthal.*

10–9

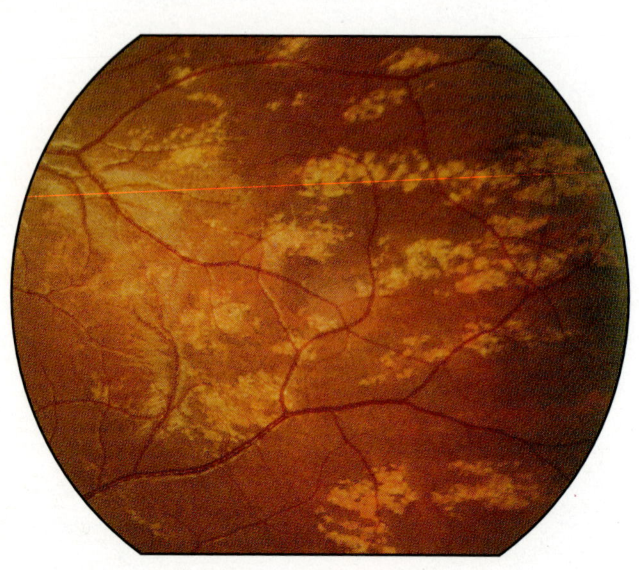

10–10

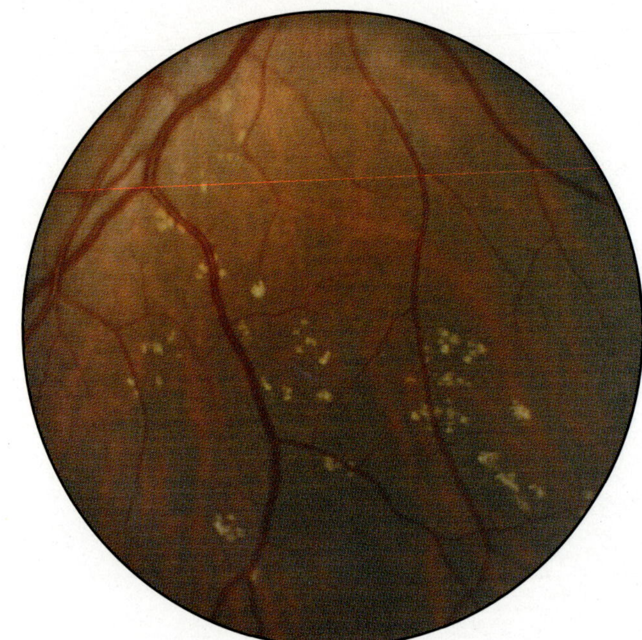

10–11

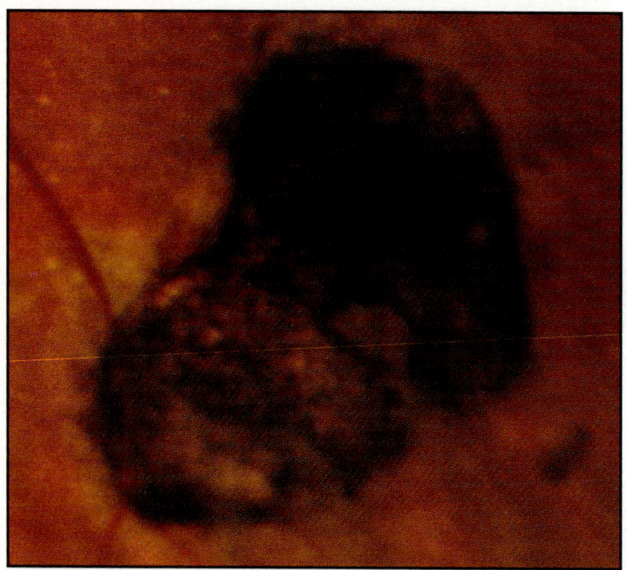

10–12

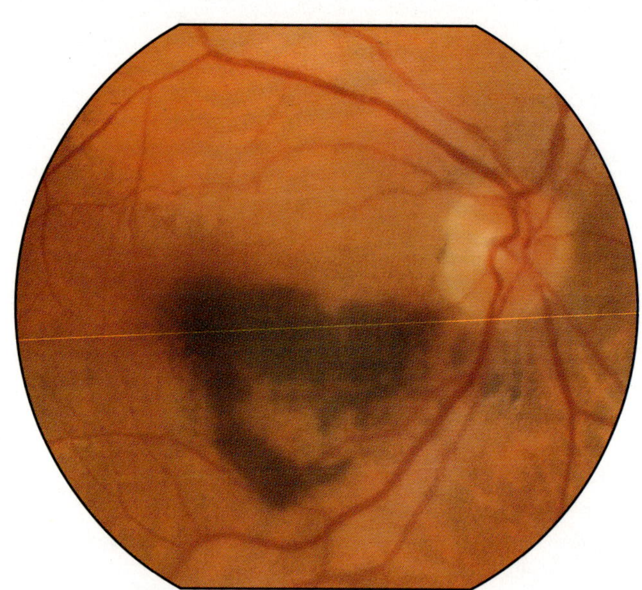

10–9 and 10–10 Bear tracks may be white (the so-called polar bear tracks).

10–11 Reactive hyperplasia of the retinal pigment epithelium may occur secondary to trauma, inflammation, or degeneration.

10–12 Another form of reactive hyperplasia is seen after pigment dispersion following scleral buckling surgery.

10–11, *Courtesy of Dr. Jerry Shields.*

Suggested Readings

Blair, NP, and Trempe, CL: Hypertrophy of the retinal pigment epithelium associated with Gardner's syndrome, Am J Ophthalmol 90:661–667, 1980

Bodmer, WF, Bailey, CJ, Bodmer, J, Bussey, HDR, Ellis A, Gorman, P, Lucibello, FC, Murday, VA, Rider, SH, Scambler, P, Sheer, D, Solomon, E, and Spurr, NK: Localization of the gene for familial adenomatous polyposis on chromosome 5, Nature 328:614–616, 1987

Buettner, H: Congenital hypertrophy of the retinal pigment epithelium, Am J Ophthalmol 79:177–189, 1975

Buettner, H: Congenital hypertrophy of the retinal pigment epithelium in familial polyposis coli, Int Ophthalmol 10:109–110, 1987

Gardner, EJ, and Richards, RC: Multiple cutaneous and subcutaneous lesions occurring simultaneously with hereditary polyposis and osteomatosis, Am J Hum Genet 5:139–148, 1953

Gass, JDM: Focal congenital anomalies of the retinal pigment epithelium, Eye 3:1–18, 1989

Kasner, L, Traboulsi, EI, De la Cruz, Z, and Green, WR: A histopathologic study of the pigmented fundus lesions in familial adenomatous polyposis. Retina (March) 12:35–42, 1992

Lynch, HT, Priluck, I, and Fitzsimmons, ML: Congenital hypertrophy of retinal pigment epithelium in non–Gardner's polyposis kindreds, Lancet 2:333, 1987

Traboulsi, EI, Maumenee, IH, Krush, AJ, Alcorn, D, Giardiello, FM, Burt, RW, Hughes, JP, and Hamilton, SR: Congenital hypertrophy of the retinal pigment epithelium predicts colorectal polyposis in Gardner's syndrome, Arch Ophthalmol 108:525–526, 1990

Traboulsi, EI, Murphy, SF, de la Cruz, ZC, Maumenee, IH, and Green, WR: A clinicopathologic study of the eyes in familial adenomatous polyposis with extracolonic manifestations (Gardner's syndrome), Am J Ophthalmol 110:550–561, 1991

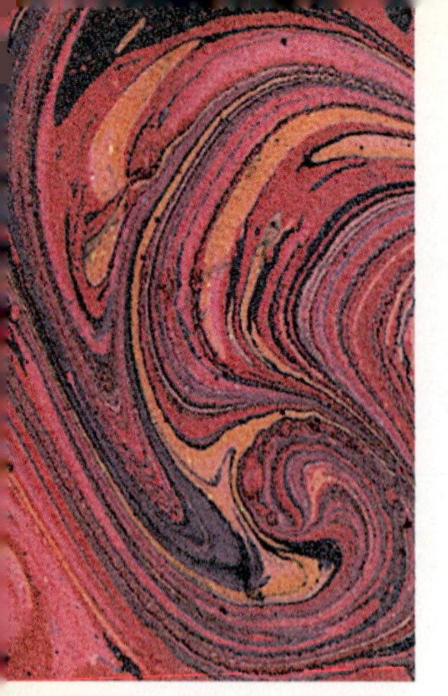

Chapter 11
Combined Hamartoma of the Retina and Retinal Pigment Epithelium

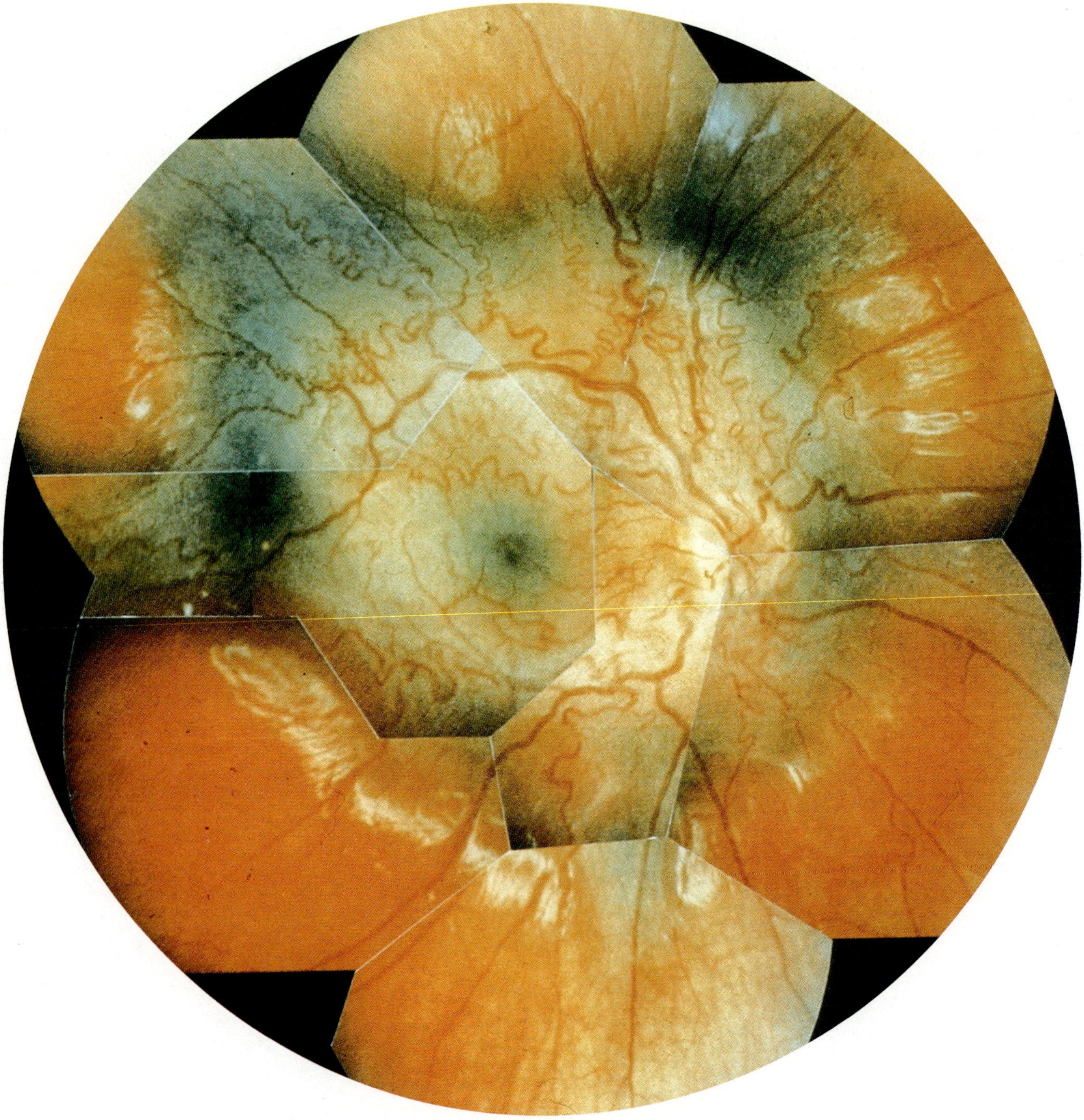

Combined hamartomas of the retina and retinal pigment epithelium are rare benign tumors. They often are pigmented and slightly elevated. In addition, retinal vascular tortuosity and epiretinal membrane formation is common. These lesions are hamartomas, which are benign over-growths of cells that normally occur in the affected area. Thus these lesions contain pigment epithelium, vascular components, and epiretinal membranes. Choroidal neovascularization may be associated with these lesions.

11–1 **11–1A**

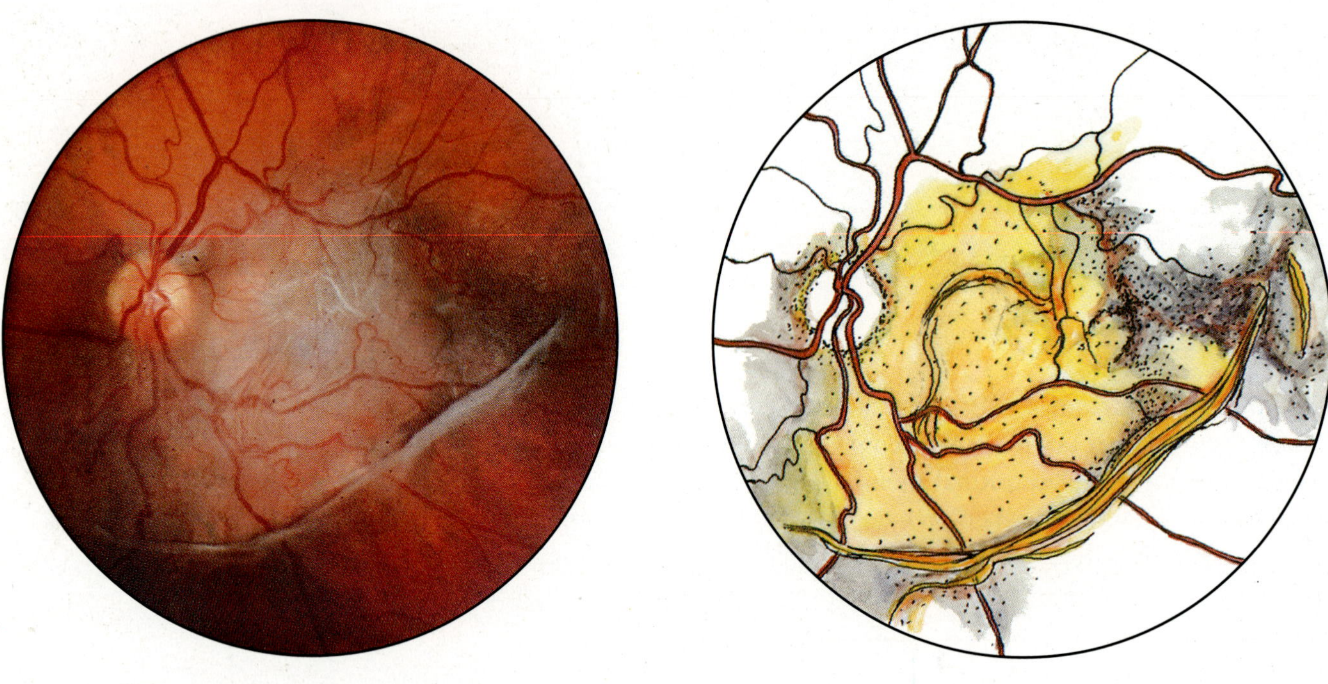

11–1 and 11–1A Combined hamartomas of the retina and retinal pigment epithelium involve all three germinal layers. Hyperpigmentation and tortuous retinal vessels can often be demonstrated. These lesions may progress by alterations in vascular permeability, epiretinal membrane progression, or secondary choroidal neovascularization.

11–1, *Courtesy of Dr. Jeffrey Shakin.*

11–2

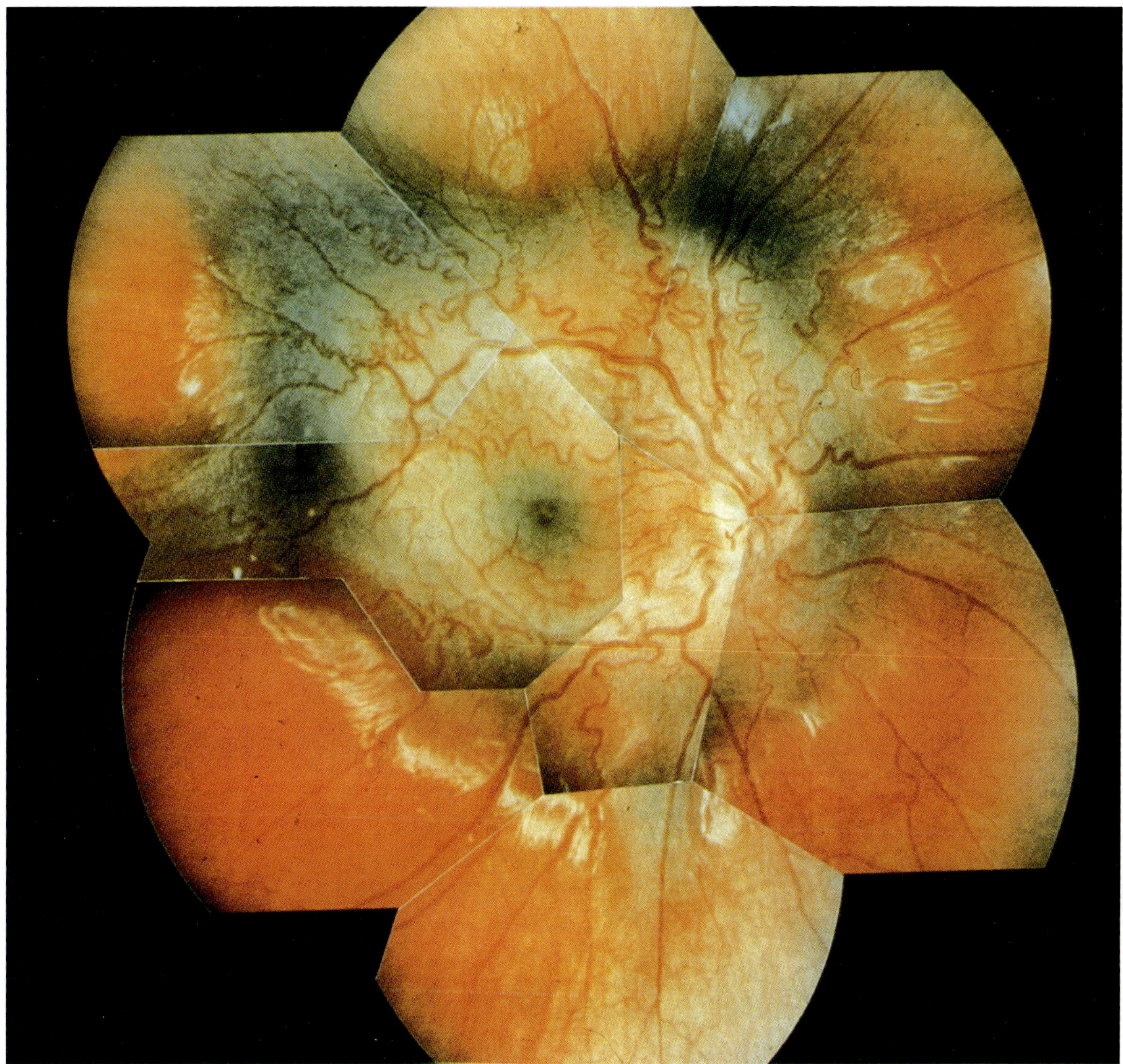

11–2 This patient with an extensive combined hamartoma of the retina and retinal pigment epithelium illustrates hyperpigmentation and marked vascular tortuosity.

11–2, *Courtesy of Dr. Edward B. Mc Lean.*

11–3

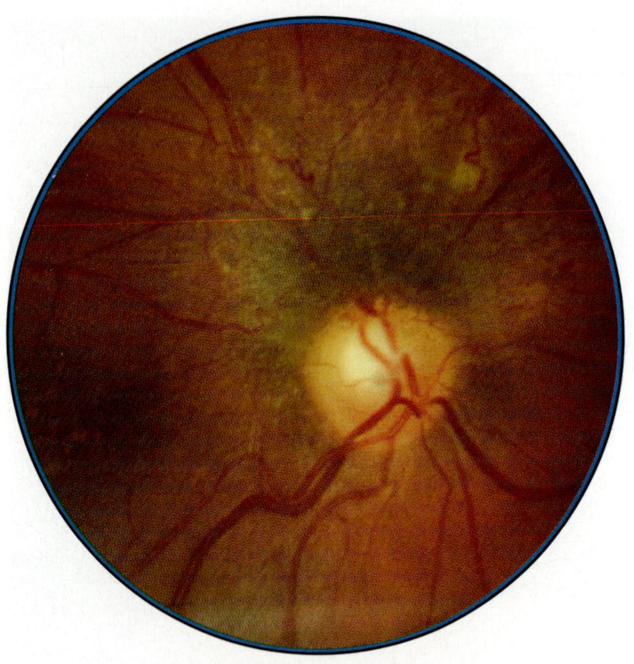

11–4

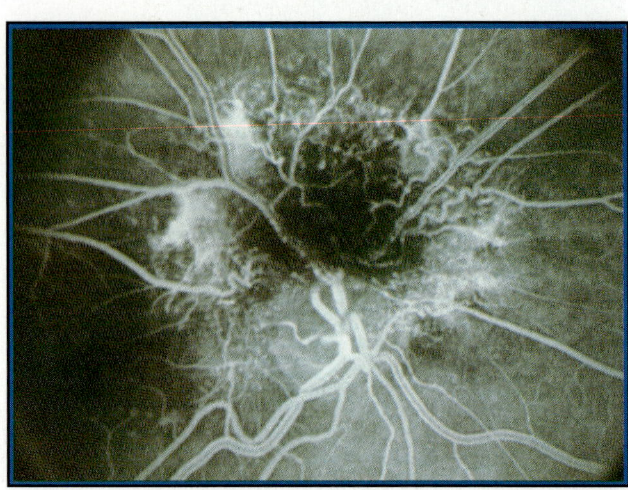

11–5

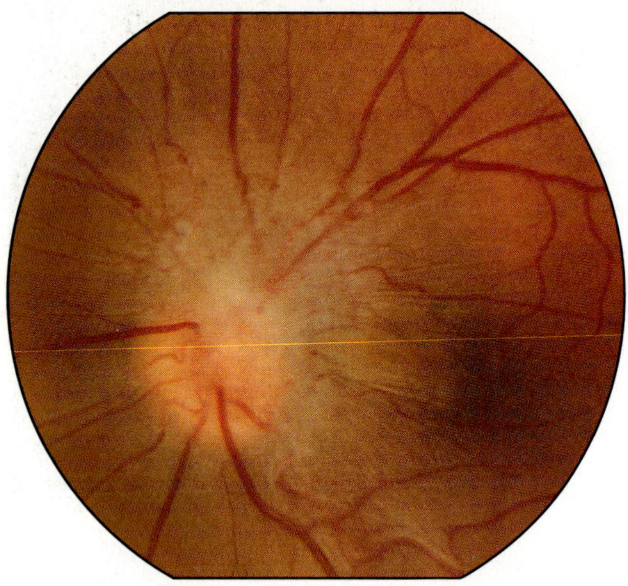

11–3 Hyperpigmentation, thought to be a secondary manifestation, may be more marked in some cases. In this particular case, epiretinal membranes, retinal vessel tortuosity, and hyperpigmentation are demonstrated.

11–4 The fluorescein angiogram illustrates the tortuosity of the vessels. The uncomplicated case does not show vascular staining.

11–5 Traction on the retina from the hamartoma may sometimes occur. In some cases, this traction may lead to folds and/or retinal detachment.

11–3 *and* ***11–4,*** *Courtesy of Dr. Jerry Shields.*

11–6

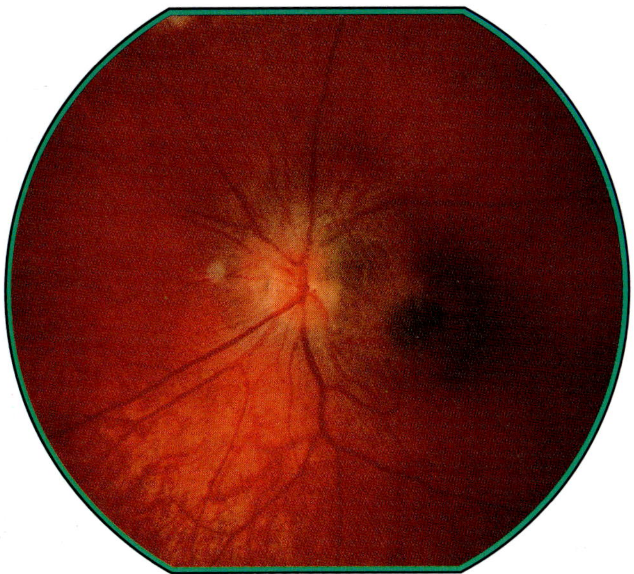

11–7

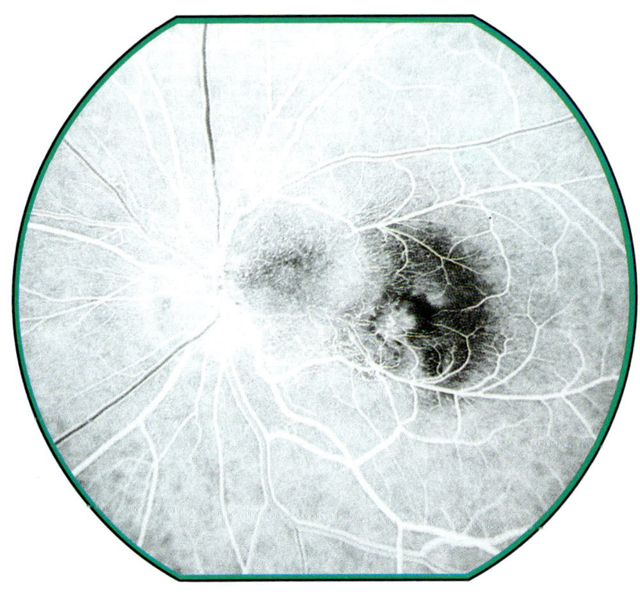

11–8

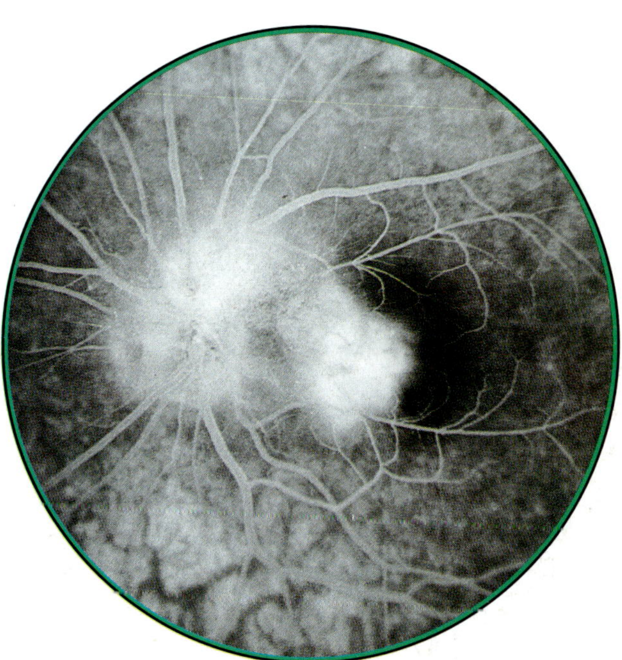

11–6 through 11–8 These hamartomas may sometimes be associated with choroidal neovascularization, as illustrated in this case. The new vessels leak extensively near the fovea.

11–6 *through* ***11–8,*** *Courtesy of Dr. Stuart L. Fine.*

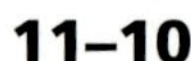

11–9

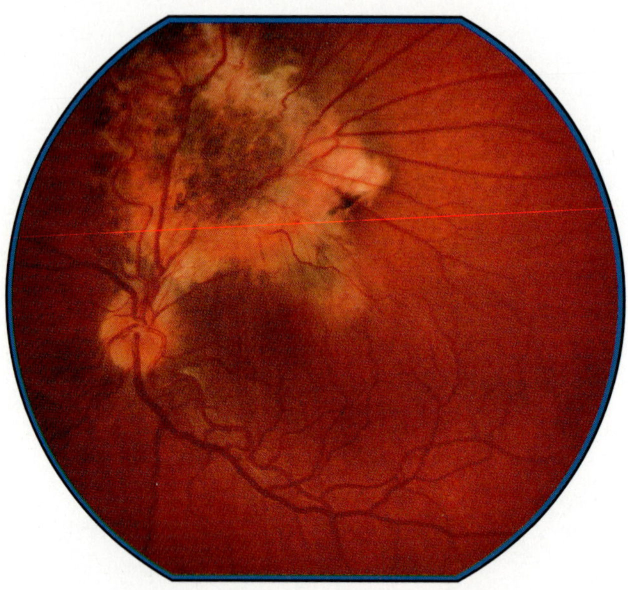

11–10

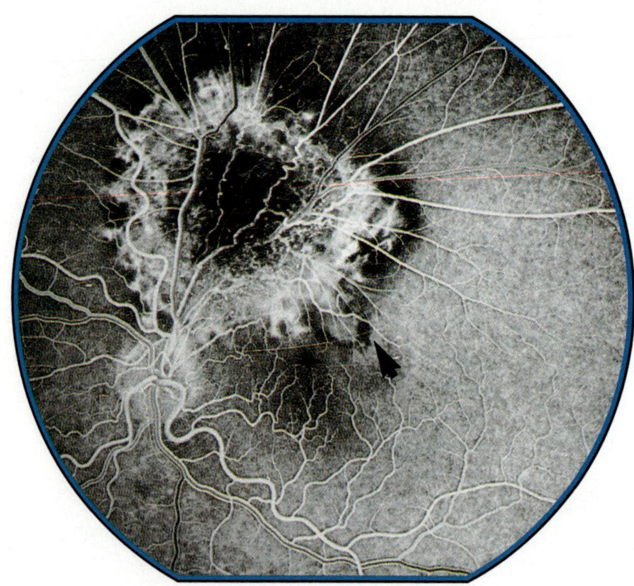

11–11

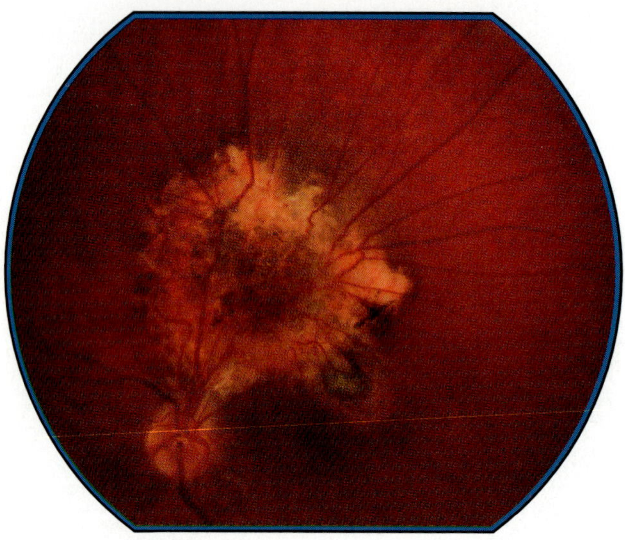

11–9 and 11–10 This patient presented with a combined hamartoma of the retina and retinal pigment epithelium with choroidal neovascularization. Increasing hyperfluorescence indicative of choroidal neovascularization may be observed on the angiogram.

11–11 Laser photocoagulation was applied to the area of the neovascularization. In a report by the Macula Society, approximately 3% of patients with combined hamartomas had associated choroidal neovascularization.

11–12 **11–13**

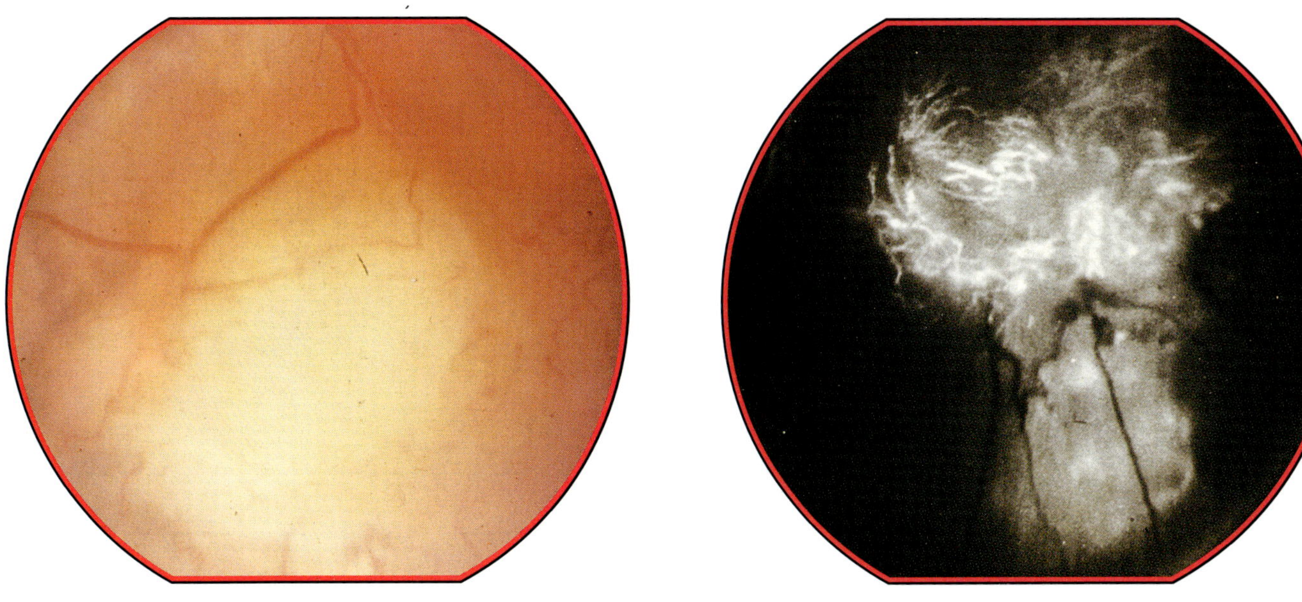

11–12 and 11–13 This 39-year-old white female had a nonpigmented hamartoma of the retina and retinal pigment epithelium.

(Case continued on next page.)

11–14

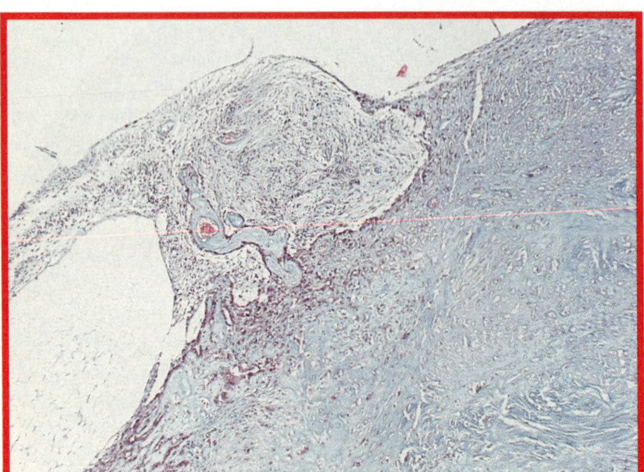

11–15

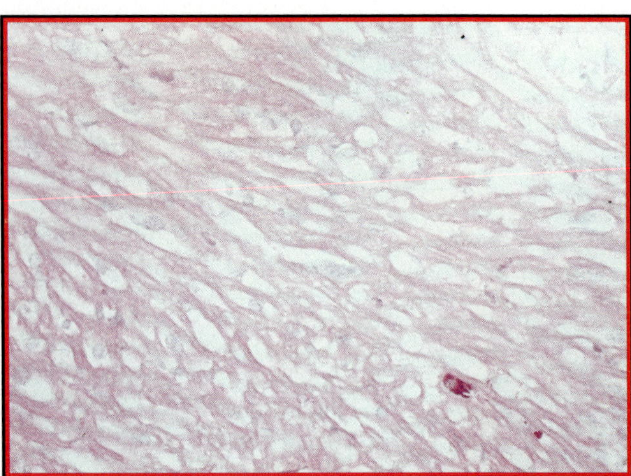

11–14 Histopathologic evaluation reveals retinal pigment epithelial hyperplasia with prominent vascularization in some areas.

11–15 Higher magnification shows multilaminated periodic acid–Schiff positive basement membrane from former hyperplasia of the retinal pigment epithelium.

Suggested Readings

Cosgrove, JM, Sharp, DM, and Bird, AC: Combined hamartoma of the retina and retinal pigment epithelium: The clinical spectrum, Trans Ophthalmol Soc UK 105:106–113, 1986

Friberg, TR, and Gulledge, SL: Hamartomas of the retina and pigment epithelium, Can J Ophthalmol 17:56–60, 1982

Gass, JDM: In discussion of Schachat, AP, Shields, JA, Fine, SL, Sanborn, GE, Weingeist, TA, Valenzuela, RA, and Brucker, AJ, and The Macula Society Research Committee: Combined hamartomas of the retina and retinal pigment epithelium, Ophthalmology 91:1609–1615, 1984

Green, WR: Pathology of the retinal pigment epithelium. In Spencer, WH, ed: Ophthalmic pathology. An atlas and textbook, ed 3, Philadelphia, 1985, WB Saunders

McDonald, HR, Abrams, GW, Burke, JM, and Neuwirth, J: Clinicopathologic results of vitreous surgery for epiretinal membranes in patients with combined retinal and retinal pigment epithelial hamartomas, Am J Ophthalmol 100:806–813, 1985

McLean, EB: Hamartoma of the retinal pigment epithelium, Am J Ophthalmol 82:227–231, 1976

Schachat, AP, Shields, JA, Fine, SL, Sanborn, GE, Weingeist, TA, Valenzuela, RA, and Brucker, AJ, and The Macula Society Research Committee: Combined hamartomas of the retina and retinal pigment epithelium, Ophthalmology 91:1609–1615, 1984

Vogel, MH, and Wessing, A: Die Proliferation des juxtapapillären retinalen Pigmentepithels, Klin Monatsbl Augenheilkd 162:736–743, 1973.

Yannuzzi, LA, Gitter, KA, Schatz, H, and Haining, WM: The macula: A comprehensive text and atlas, Baltimore, 1979, Williams & Wilkins

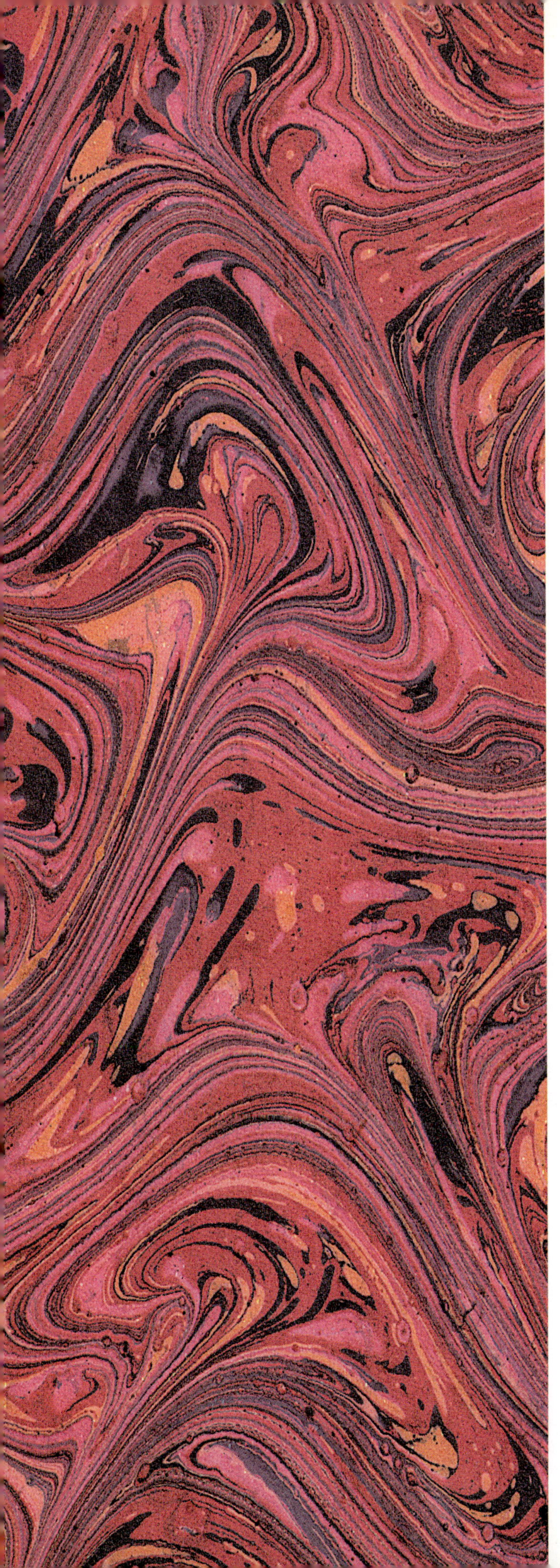

Part IV

Choroidal Melanoma and Other Tumors of the Choroid

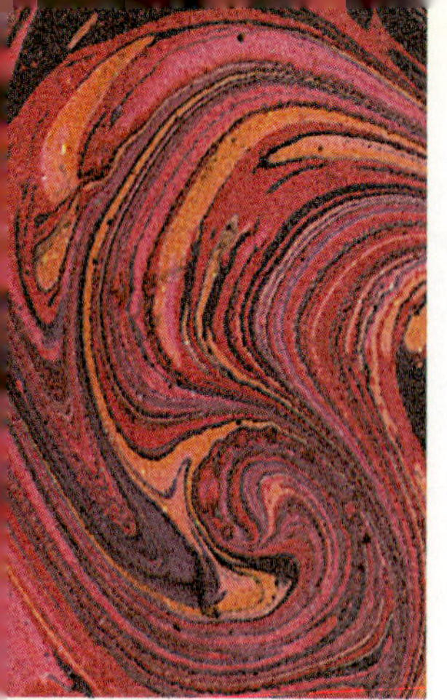

Chapter 12
Choroidal Nevi

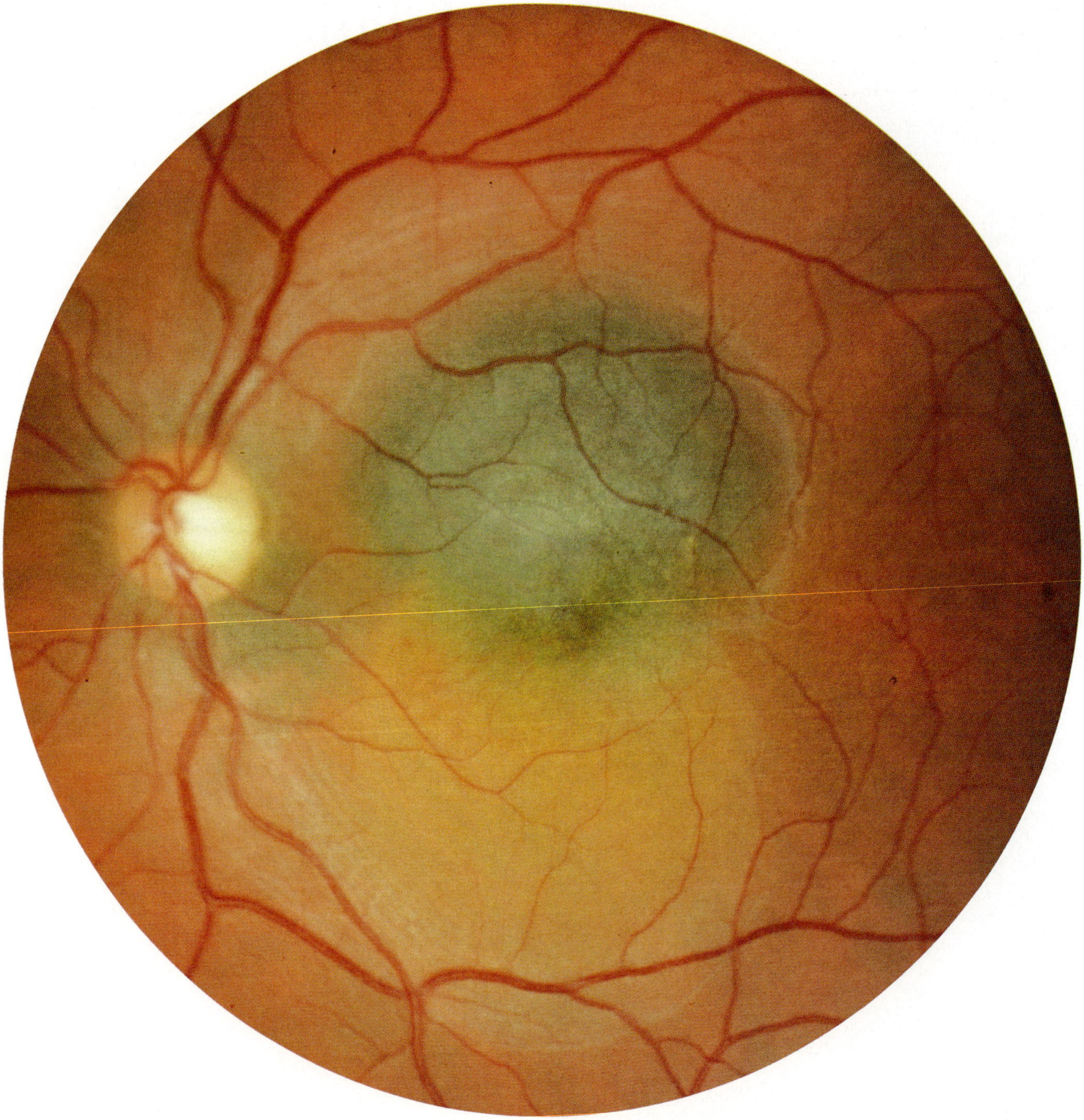

Choroidal nevi are relatively common tumors that consist of benign atypical uveal melanocytes called nevus cells. Rarely malignant transformation to choroidal melanoma will occur.

12–1

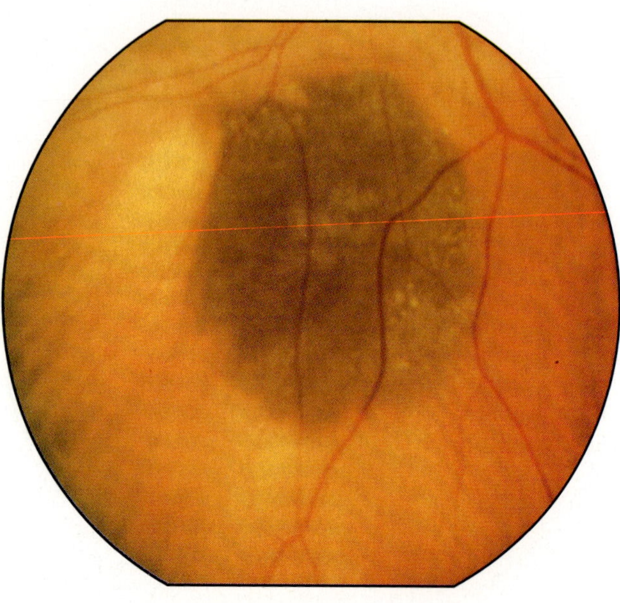

12–2

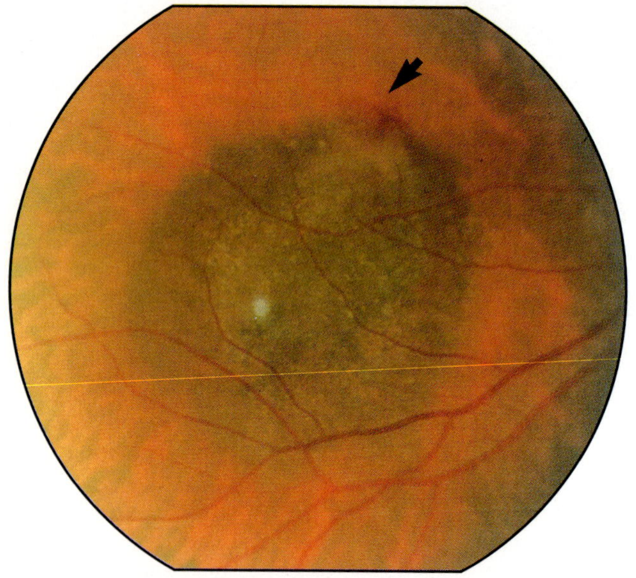

12–3

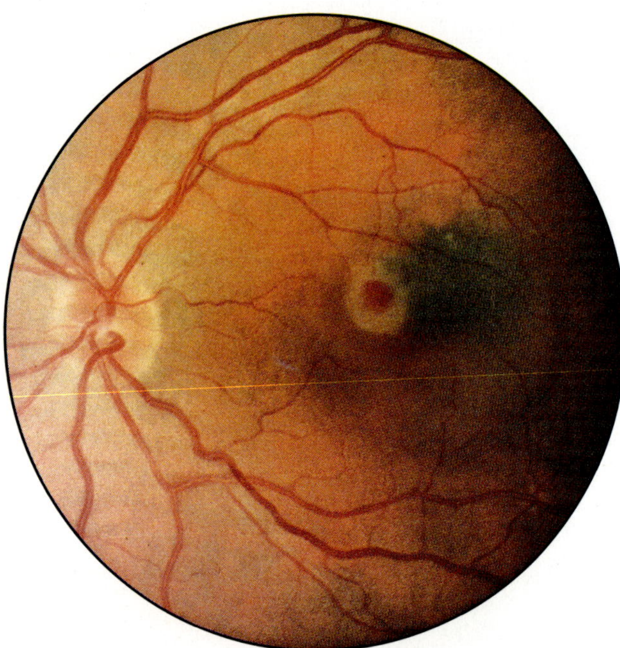

12–1 A choroidal nevus is a relatively flat benign lesion, which is usually pigmented.

12–2 Choroidal nevi may be associated in some cases with choroidal neovascularization. This patient has a choroidal nevus and subretinal hemorrhage secondary to choroidal neovascularization. Notice the subretinal hemorrhage superior to the nevus *(arrowhead)*.

12–3 This patient also presented with choroidal neovascularization and secondary subretinal exudate and hemorrhage. The neovascularization was treated with laser photocoagulation.

12–4

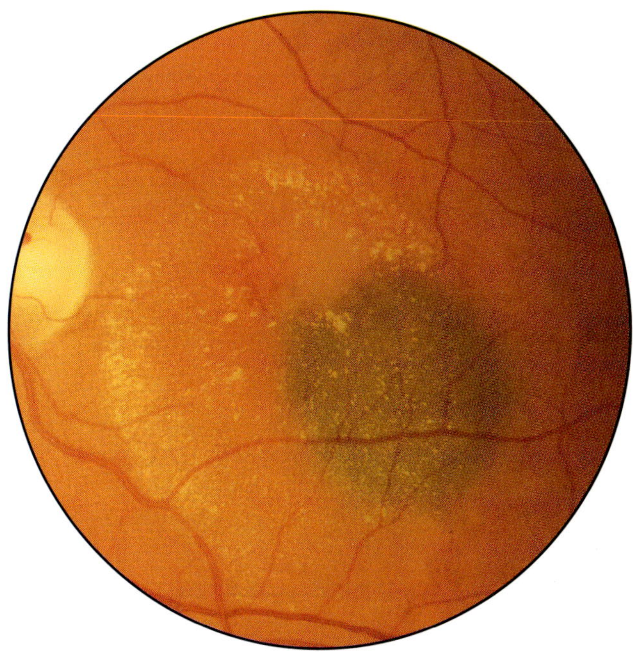

12–5

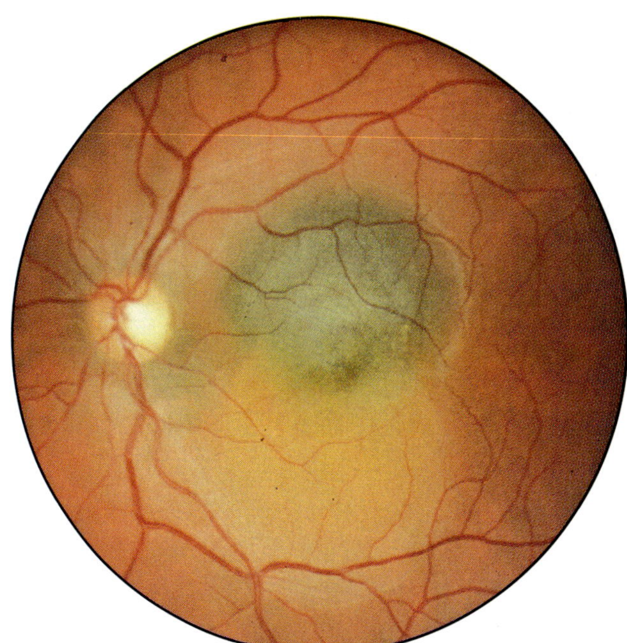

12–6

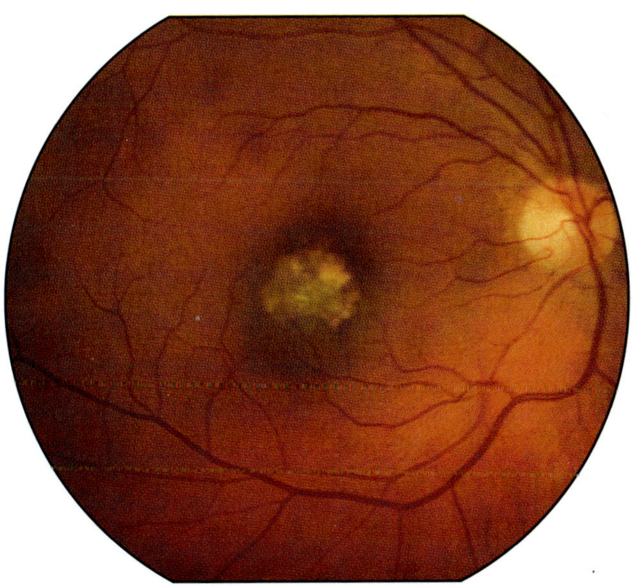

12–4 and 12–5 Serous detachments are seen associated with nevi in these cases.

12–6 Choroidal nevi may have overlying plaques of degeneration secondary to atrophy, drusen, fibrous metaplasia, or fibrovascular scarring. In this patient in whom the lesion was in the macular region, the underlying nevus is somewhat obscured by degenerative changes.

12–5, *Courtesy of Dr. Jerry Shields.*

12–7

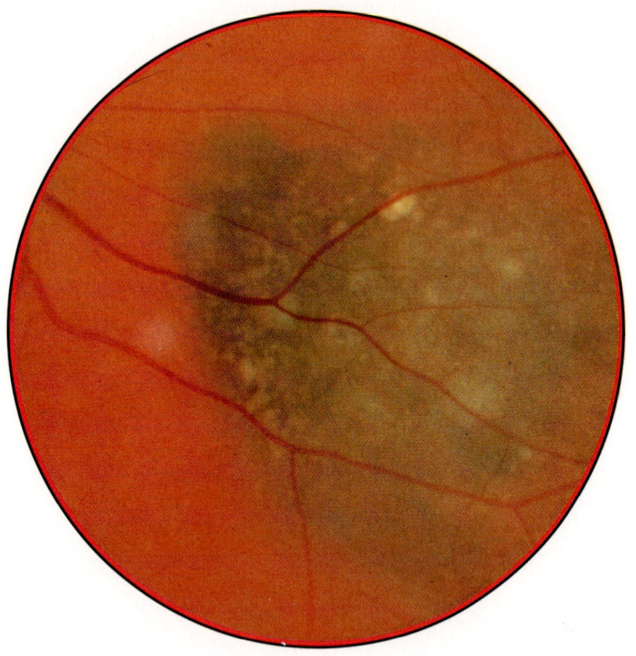

12–8

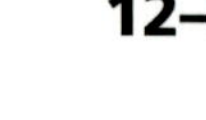

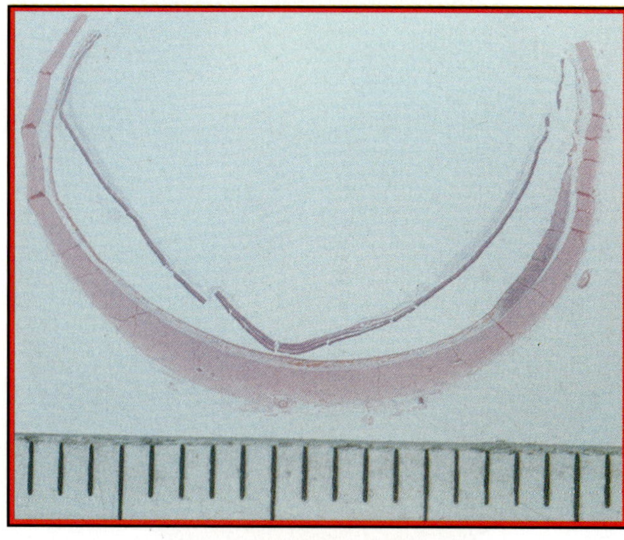

12–9

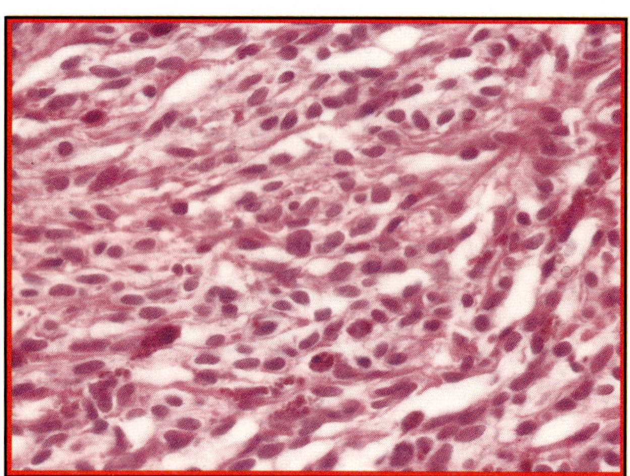

12–7 through 12–9 This patient had an enlarging choroidal nevus with overlying drusen. Microscopic examination reveals uniform nevus cells.

***12–7** through **12–9,** Courtesy of Dr. Gordon Klintworth.*

12–10 **12–11**

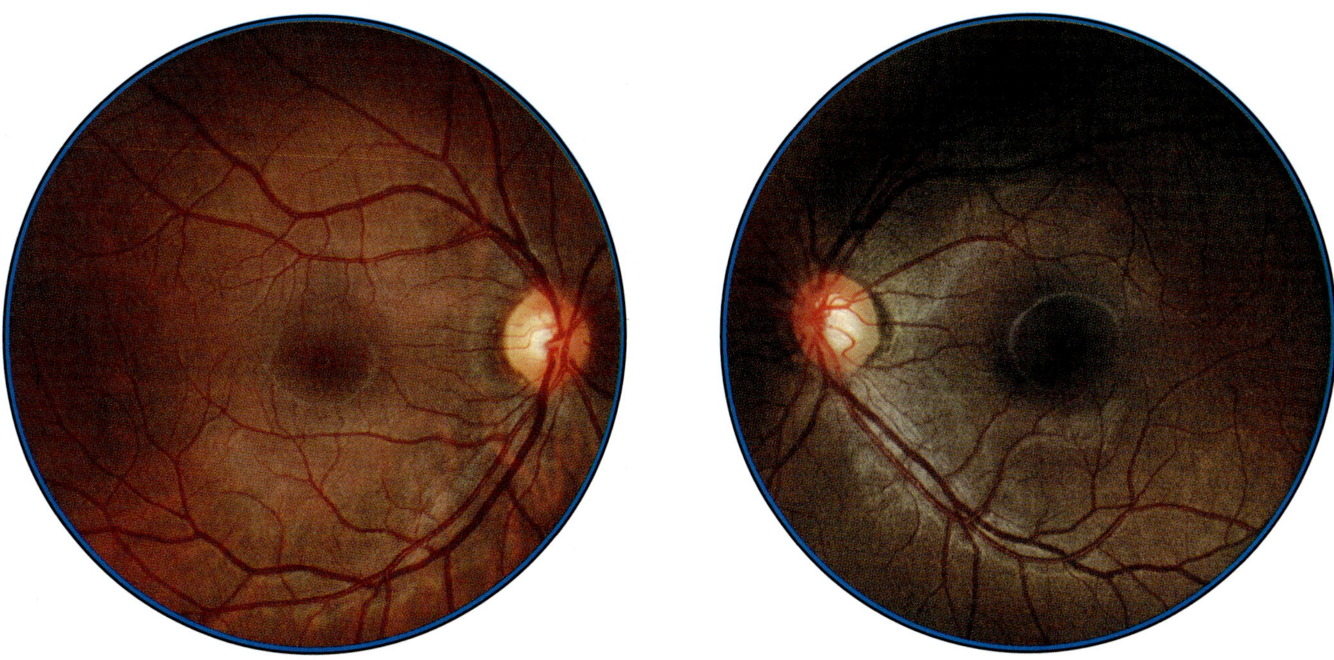

12–10 and 12–11 Ocular melanocytosis shows diffuse hyperpigmentation in the involved eye. The first photograph (12–10) shows the normal fundus of a 24-year-old female. The second photograph (12–11) reveals the fundus of her other eye, which is darker secondary to ocular melanocytosis.

***12–10** and **12–11**, Courtesy of Dr. Jerry Shields.*

Suggested Readings

Albers, EC: Benign melanomas of the choroid and their malignant transformation, Am J Ophthalmol 23:779–783, 1940

Augsburger, JJ, Schroeder, RP, Territo, C, Gamel, JW, and Shields, JA: Clinical parameters predictive of enlargement of melanocytic choroidal lesions, Br J Ophthalmol 73:911–917, 1989

Brown, GC, Shields, JA, and Augsburger, JJ: Amelanotic choroidal nevi, Ophthalmology 88:1116–1121, 1981

Char, DH: Clinical ocular oncology, New York, 1989, Churchill Livingstone

Deutsch, TA, and Jampol, LM: Large druse-like lesions on the surface of choroidal nevi, Ophthalmology 92:73–76, 1985

Folk, JC, Weingeist, TA, Coonan, P, Blodi, CF, Folberg, R, and Kimura, AE: The treatment of serous macular detachment secondary to choroidal melanoma and nevi, Ophthalmology 96:547–551, 1989

Gass, JDM: Problems in the differential diagnosis of choroidal nevi and malignant melanomas, Am J Ophthalmol 83:299–323, 1977

Oosterhuis, JA, and von Winning, CHOM: Naevus of the choroid, Ophthalmologica 178:156–165, 1979

Shields, JA, and Shields, CL: Intraocular tumors: A text and atlas, Philadelphia, 1992, WB Saunders

Yanoff, M, and Zimmerman, LE: Histogenesis of malignant melanomas of the uvea. II. Relationship of uveal nevi to malignant melanomas, Cancer 20:493–507, 1967

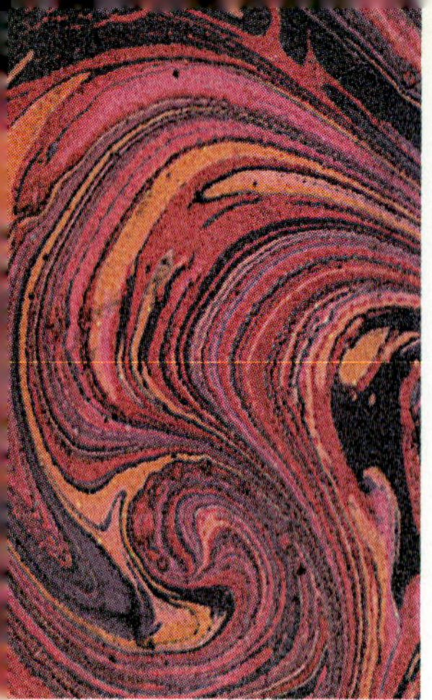

Chapter 13
Choroidal Melanoma

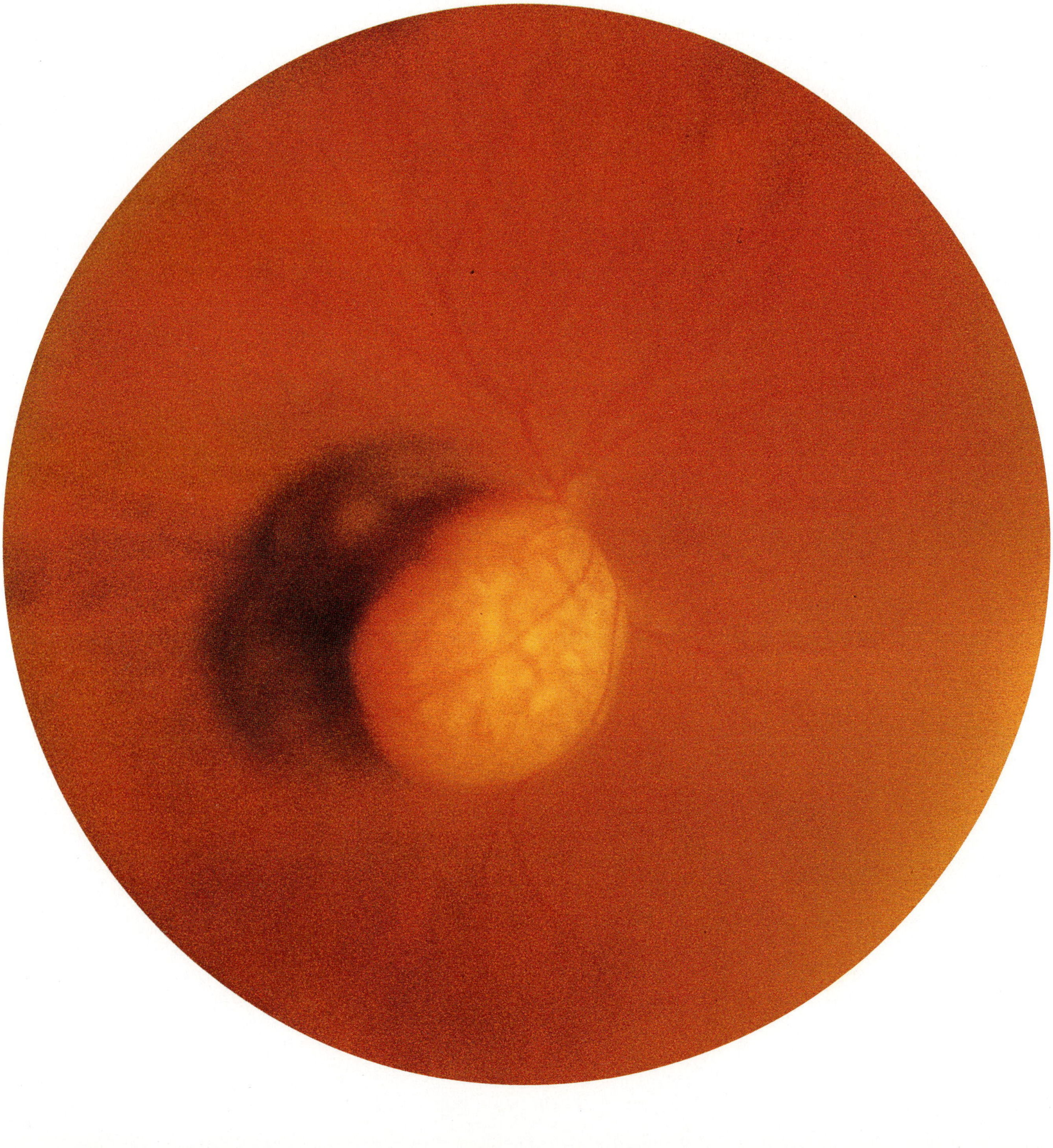

Malignant choroidal melanomas are elevated variably pigmented lesions. Metastasis may occur, especially to the liver. Various treatment modalities including enucleation and radiation therapy are used in these patients.

13–1 13–2

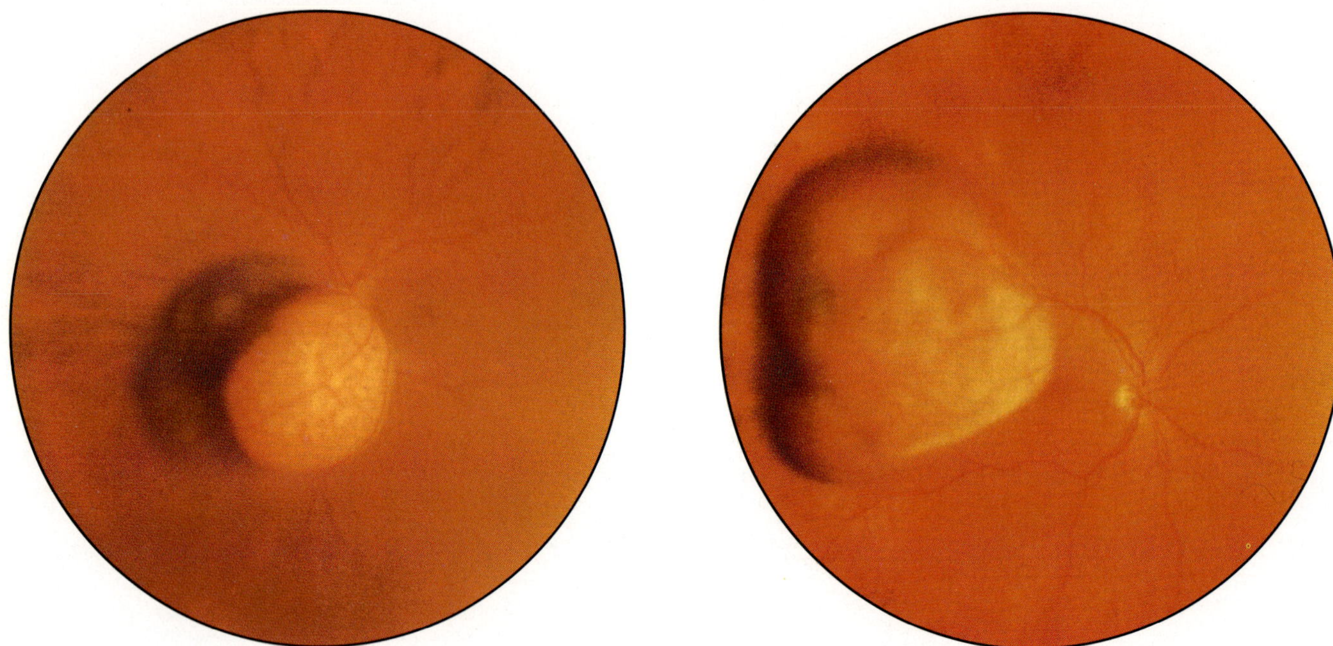

13–3

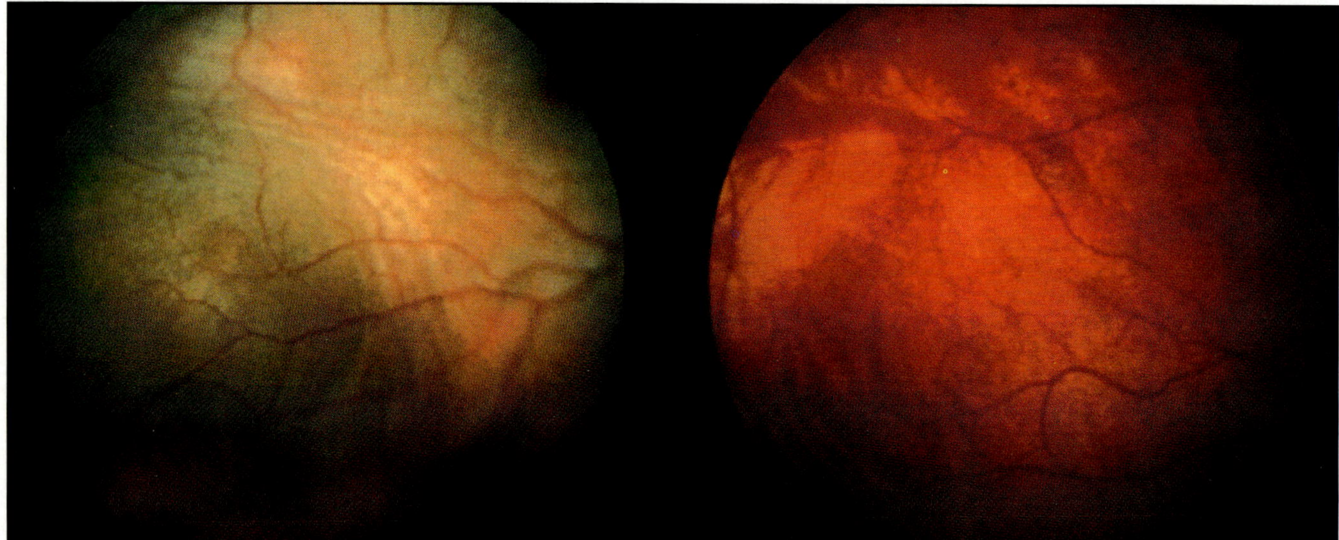

13–1 and 13–2 These wide-field photographs illustrate cases of malignant choroidal melanomas.

13–3 Suprachoroidal hemorrhage following intraocular surgery masquerading as a malignant melanoma. Note the concave margin and the choroidal folds. This patient had spontaneous clearing of the hemorrhage.

***13–1** and **13–2,** Courtesy of Dr. Jerry Shields. **13–3,** Courtesy of Dr. James Augsburger.*

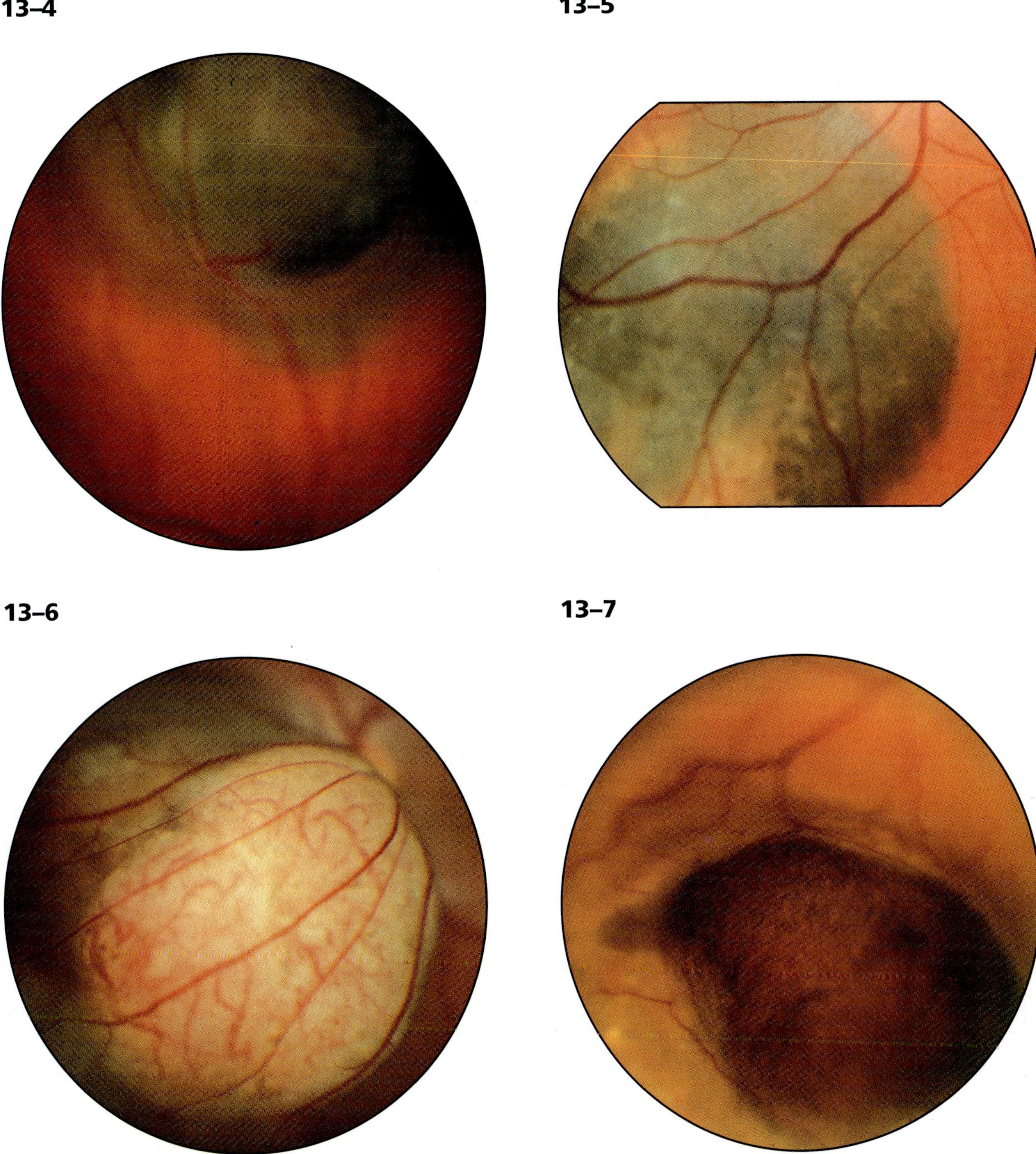

13–4 through 13–6 Choroidal melanomas may be heavily pigmented (13–4), moderately pigmented (13–5), or mostly amelanotic (13–6).

13–7 They may also appear reddish-brown.

13–4 *and* ***13–6,*** *Courtesy of Dr. Jerry Shields.* ***13–5,*** *Courtesy of Dr. Evangelos Gragoudas.*

13–8

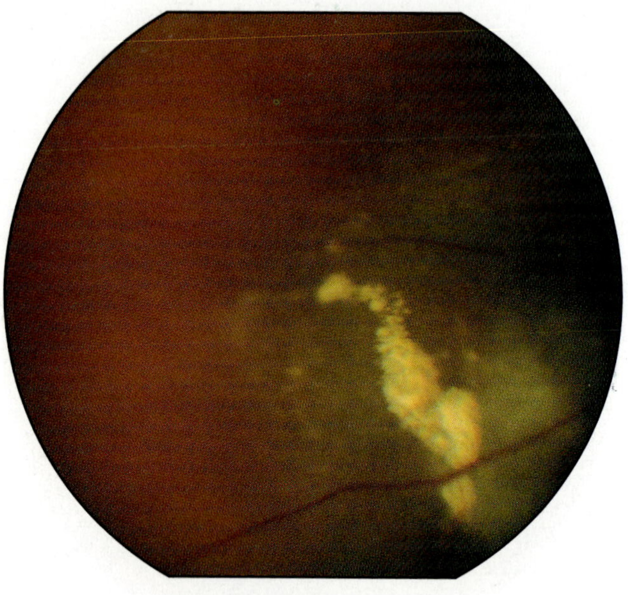

13–9

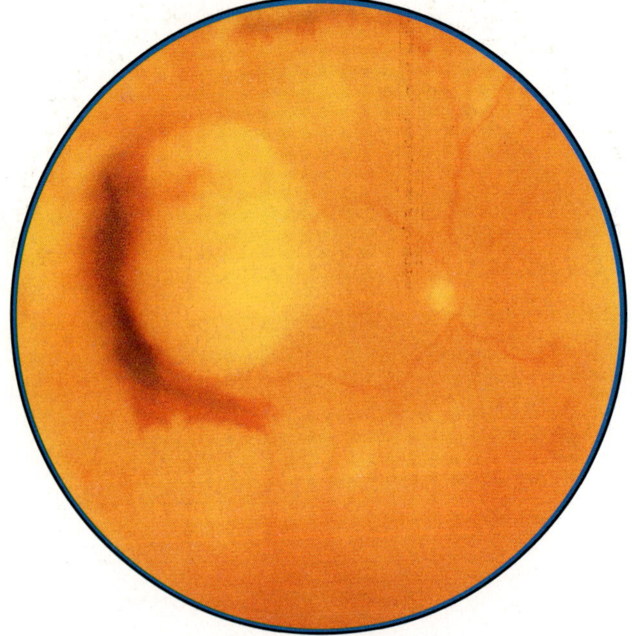

13–10

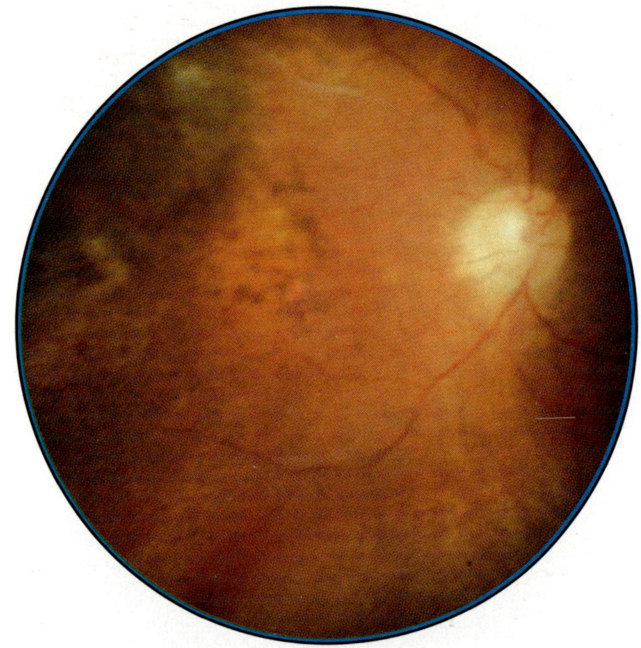

13–8 Choroidal melanomas may sometimes be associated with choroidal neovascularization. In this case the subretinal fluid and lipid is noted outside of the macular region.

13–9 and 13–10 One treatment option for choroidal melanomas is radiation therapy. The first photograph shows a wide-field view of a choroidal melanoma with subretinal hemorrhage. Following plaque irradiation there was regression of the tumor. Retinal pigment epithelial changes and an ischemic retinal vessel along the superior temporal arcade are seen.

***13–9** and **13–10,** Courtesy of Dr. Jerry Shields.*

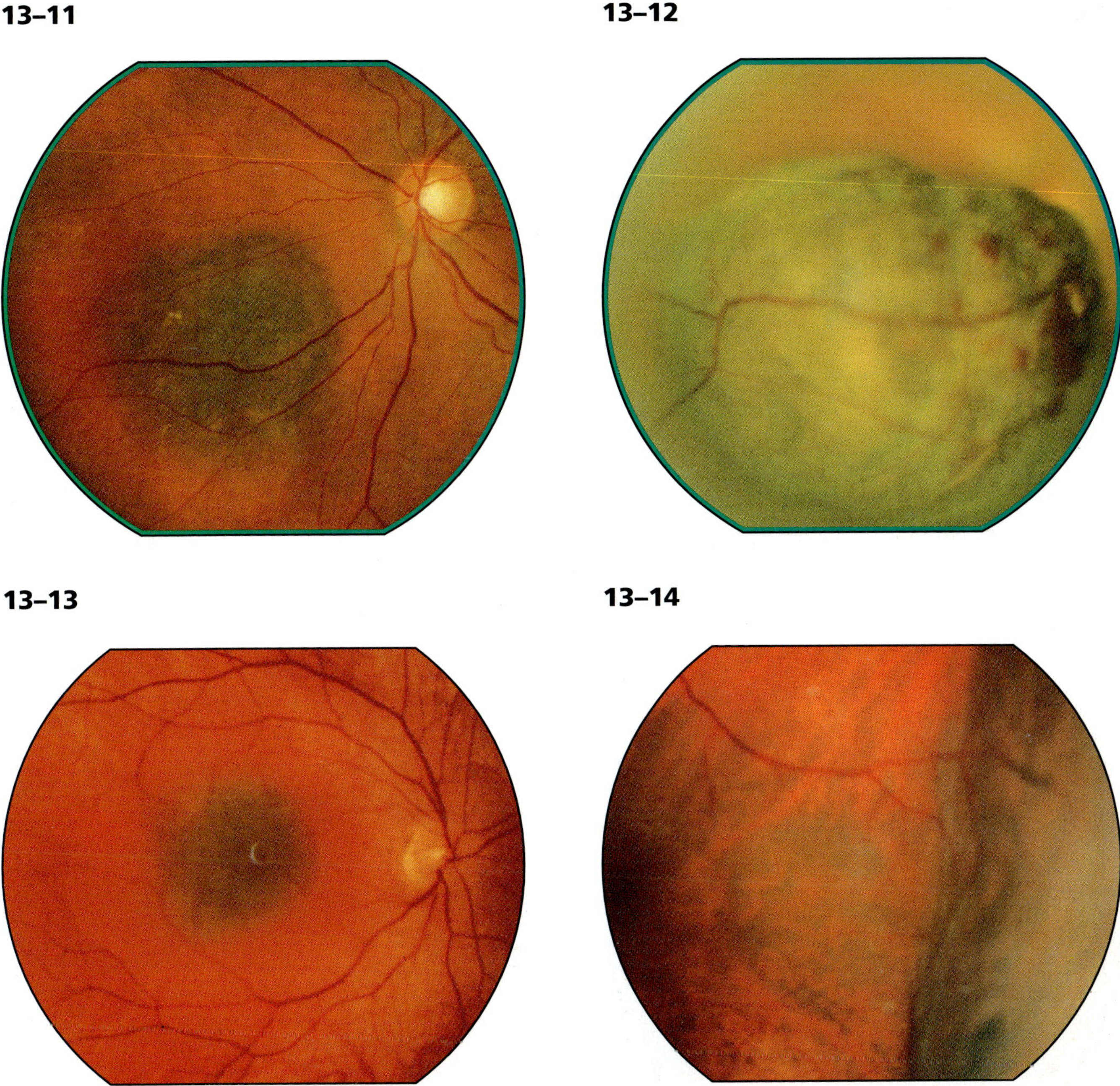

13–11 and 13–12 Choroidal nevi must be carefully followed since they may rarely undergo transformation into a malignant choroidal melanoma, as in this case in which the patient was followed every 6 months for 11 years. The choroidal nevus (13–11) appeared flat only a few months before its transformation into an elevated malignant choroidal melanoma (13–12).

13–13 This patient had a metastatic lesion to the choroid from skin melanoma. This choroidal lesion is associated with an overlying and dependent serous detachment and is difficult to distinguish from a choroidal melanoma. A complete medical history and physical examination are essential in patients with choroidal melanoma to ascertain that the disease does not represent metastatic disease.

13–14 Choroidal detachments may sometimes be confused with choroidal melanomas. Ultrasound is useful in distinguishing difficult cases.

***13–11** and **13–12,** Courtesy of Dr. Yale Fisher. **13–13,** Courtesy of Dr. Evangelos Gragoudas.*

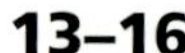

13–15

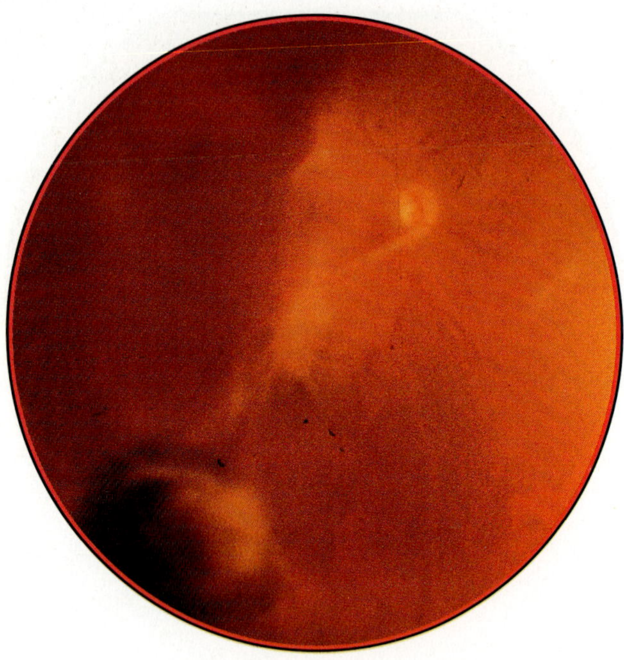

13–16

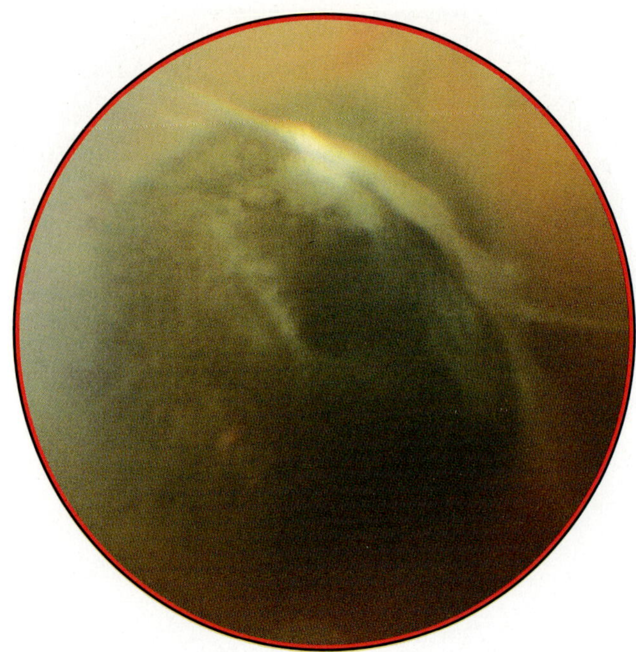

13–17

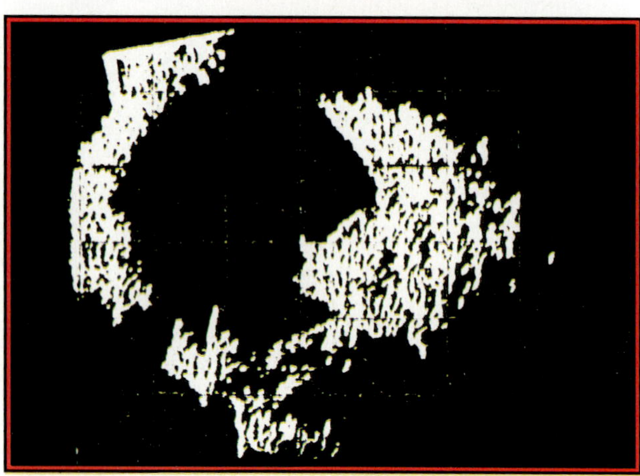

13–15 and 13–16 Retinal pigment epithelial adenomas are rare benign tumors that can be misdiagnosed as malignant choroidal melanomas. This 46-year-old black female had 2/200 vision in the right eye. Ophthalmoscopy revealed a severe macular pucker with preretinal fibrosis extending from the macula to a jet-black tumor at the inferotemporal equator. The tumor was 10 mm in diameter and 6 mm in height. It appeared to arise abruptly from the outer retina rather than from the choroid.

13–17 Ultrasonography showed a highly elevated mass that was internally heterogeneous and showed a strong acoustic shadow. The initial clinical and ultrasonic findings of this lesion were consistent with retinal pigment epithelial adenoma. A pars plana vitrectomy was performed with peeling of the premacular membrane. Visual acuity improved postoperatively to 20/200. *(Case continues on next page, Figures 13–18 through 13–20.)*

***13–15** through **13–17**, Courtesy of Dr. Alexander Irvine.*

13–18

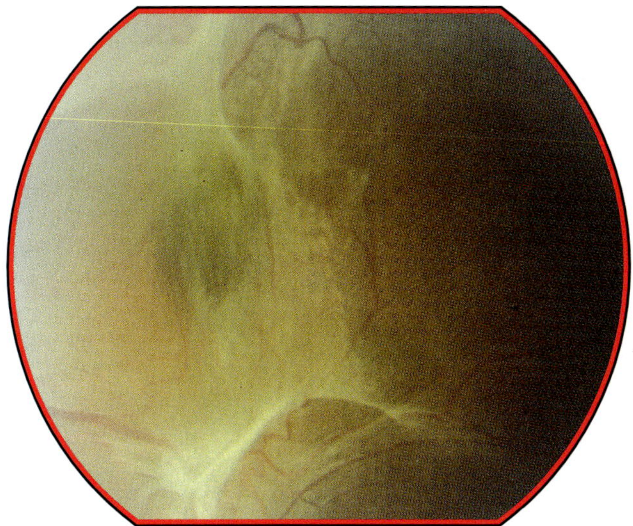

13–19

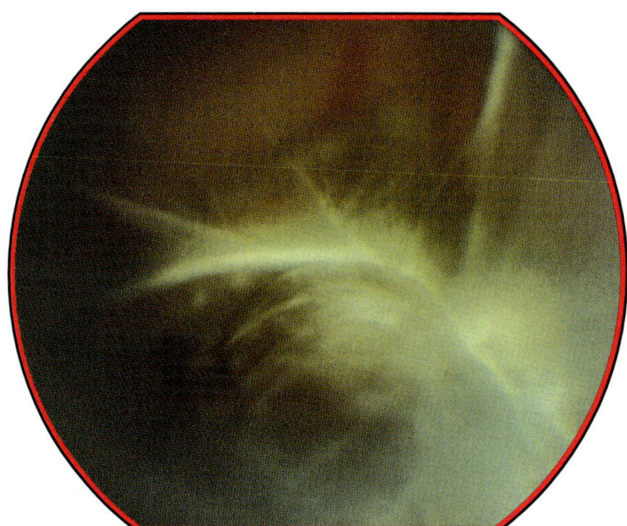

13–20

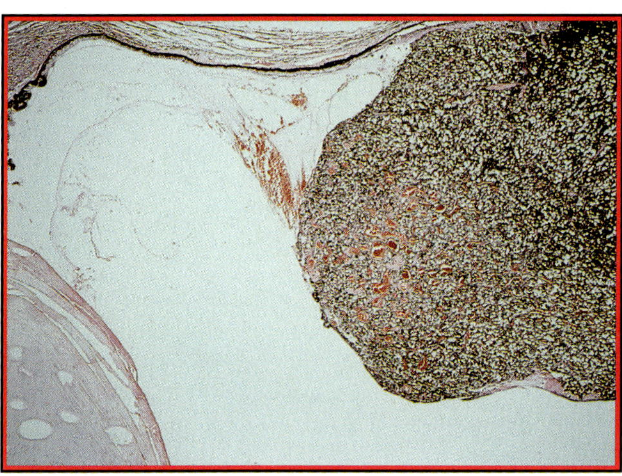

13–18 and 13–19 The preretinal fibrosis, however, rapidly recurred. Within 6 months, the vision had fallen to counting fingers. The patient developed an increasingly dense cataract and ultrasonography showed that the height of the lesion had increased. Since it was believed that this lesion might be malignant, a fine-needle biopsy was performed. The needle biopsy was considered equivocal and possibly consistent with malignancy. The eye was thus enucleated.

13–20 On histopathologic examination, a well-circumscribed ovoid dark brown tumor is seen arising from the retinal pigment epithelium (RPE). The tumor is composed of tubules and layers of uniformly heavily pigmented cuboidal and polyhedral cells with round oval nuclei, inconspicuous nucleoli, and no mitotic figures. Small vacuoles with hyaluronidase-sensitive mucopolysaccharide were also noted. The tumor cells were pigmented with large ovoid granules similar to the pigment granules in the normal retinal pigment epithelium. Anteriorly the tumor was highly vascularized. The histopathologic findings were consistent with a diagnosis of retinal pigment epithelial adenoma. This case shows the difficulty that may be encountered in differentiating such RPE adenomas from malignant choroidal melanomas.

13–18 *through* ***13–20,*** *Courtesy of Dr. Alexander Irvine.*

13–21

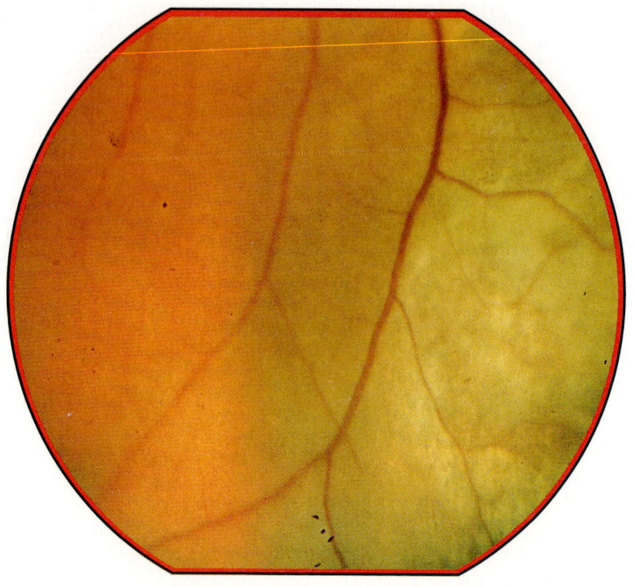

13–22

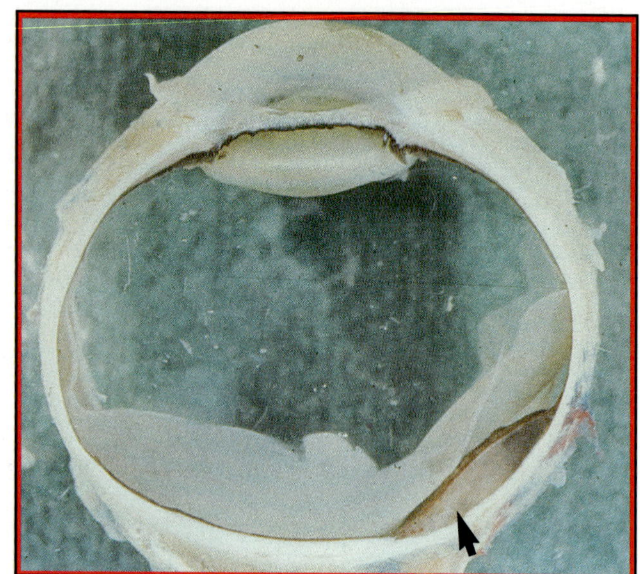

13–23

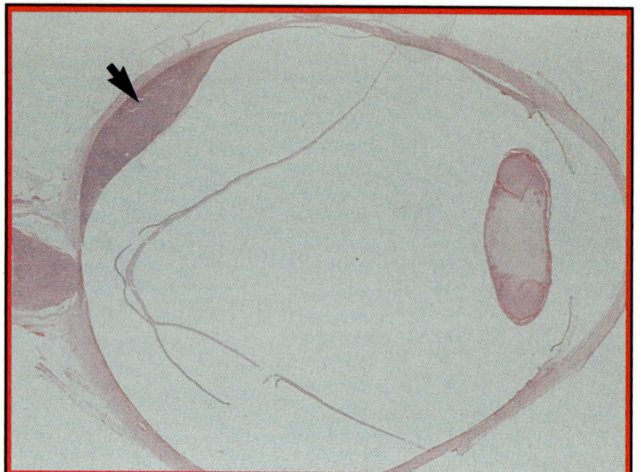

13–24

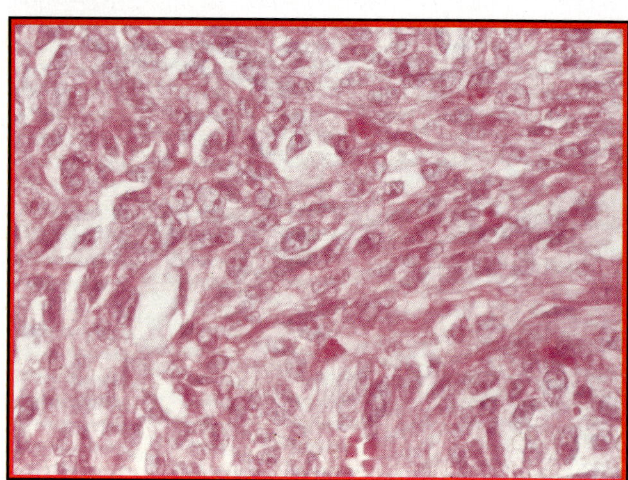

13–21 This case is a clinicopathologic correlation of a patient with a malignant melanoma of the choroid.

13–22 Gross examination shows the elevated brownish choroidal tumor *(arrowhead)*.

13–23 On cross-section a 10-mm diameter x 2.0-mm thick tumor is noted *(arrowhead)*.

13–24 A malignant choroidal melanoma with a mixed cell type is demonstrated on higher magnification.

Suggested Readings

Annesley, WH: Peripheral exudative hemorrhagic chorioretinopathy, Trans Am Ophthalmol Soc 78:321, 1980

Barr, CC, Sipperly, JO, and Nicholson, DH: Small melanomas of the choroid, Arch Ophthalmol 96:1580, 1978

Char, DH: Management of small choroidal melanomas, Surv Ophthalmol 22:377–386, 1978

Char, DH, Stone, RD, Irvine, AR, Crawford, JB, Hilton, GF, Lonn, LI, and Schwartz, A: Diagnostic modalities in choroidal melanoma: sensitivity, specificity, and reproductibility, Am J Ophthalmol 89:223–230, 1980

Ferry, AP: Lesions mistaken for malignant melanoma of the posterior uvea. A clinicopathologic analysis of 100 cases with ophthalmoscopically visible lesions, Arch Ophthalmol 72:463, 1964

Font, RL, Spaulding, AG, and Zimmerman, LE: Diffuse malignant melanoma of the uveal tract: a clinicopathologic report of 54 cases, Trans Am Acad Ophthalmol Otolaryngol 72:877–895, 1968

Gass, JDM: Problems in the differential diagnosis of choroidal nevi and malignant melanomas, Trans Am Acad Ophthalmol Otolaryngol 83:19–48, 1985

Jensen, OA: Malignant melanomas of the uvea in Denmark 1943–1952. A clinical, histopathological, and prognostic study, Acta Ophthalmol (Copenh) 75:1, 1963

Margo, CE, and McLean, IW: Malignant melanoma of the choroidal and ciliary body in black patients, Arch Ophthalmol 102:77–79, 1984

McLean, IW, Foster, WD, and Zimmerman, LE: Uveal melanoma: location, size, cell type, and enucleation as risk factors in metastasis, Hum Pathol 13:123, 1982

Michelson, JB, Felberg, NT, and Shields, JA: Evaluation of metastatic cancer to the eye, Arch Ophthalmol 95:692–697, 1977

Schachat, AP, Robertson, DM, Mieler, WF, Schwartz, D, Augsburger, JJ, Schatz, H, and Gass, JDM: Sclerochoroidal calcification, Arch Ophthalmol 110:196–199, 1992

Shields, JA: Diagnosis and management of intraocular tumors, St Louis, 1983, Mosby–Year Book, p 373

Shields, JA, Augsburger, JJ, Brady, LW, and Day, JL: Cobalt plaque therapy of posterior uveal melanomas, Ophthalmology 89:1201, 1982

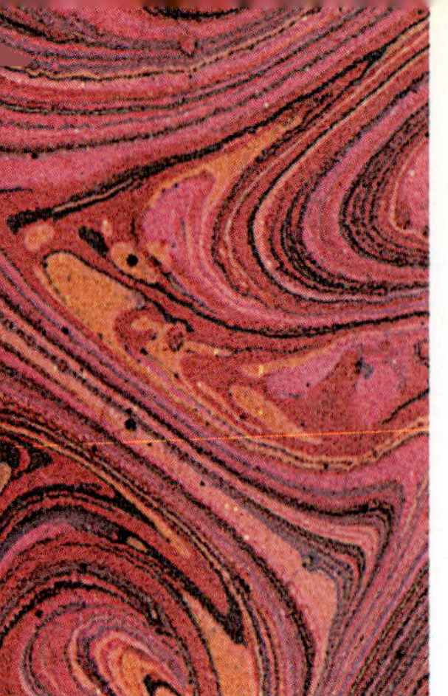

Chapter 14

Choroidal Metastasis

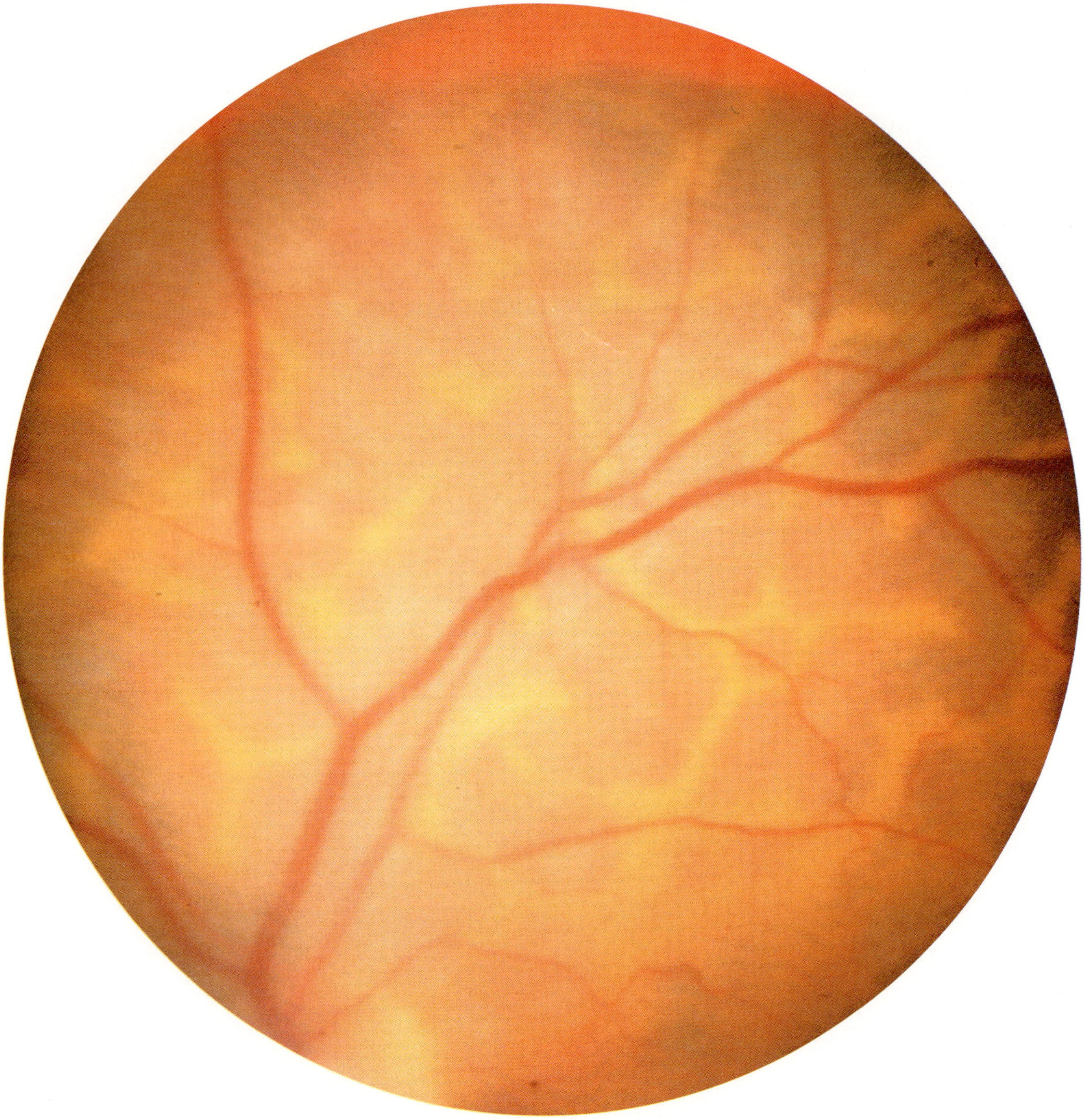

Metastatic tumors are the most common intraocular malignancies, and the choroid is the most common site for intraocular metastasis. When the choroidal metastasis is from the breast the great majority of patients will have a prior history of breast carcinoma. However, when bronchiogenic carcinoma is the source of the choroidal metastasis, often the lung cancer has not been previously diagnosed. The most common primary sites of choroidal metastasis are breast, lung, and gastro-intestinal tract.

14–1 BREAST METASTASIS

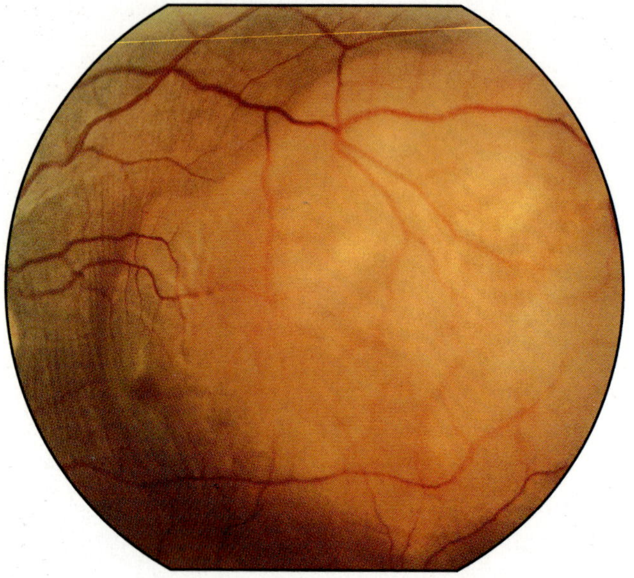

14–1A

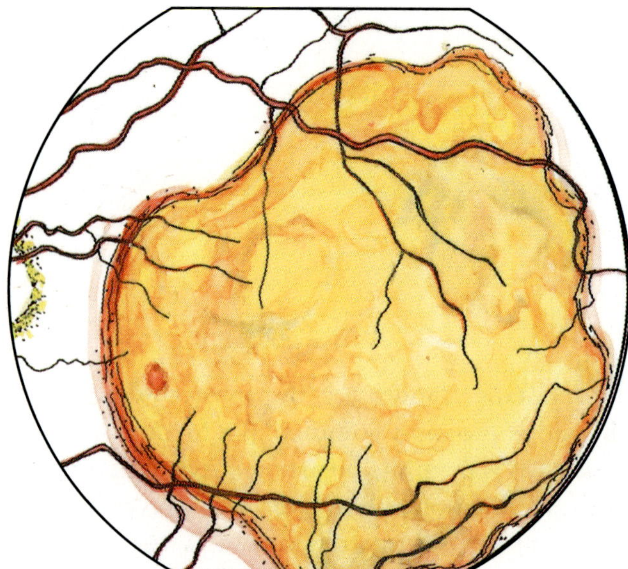

14–2

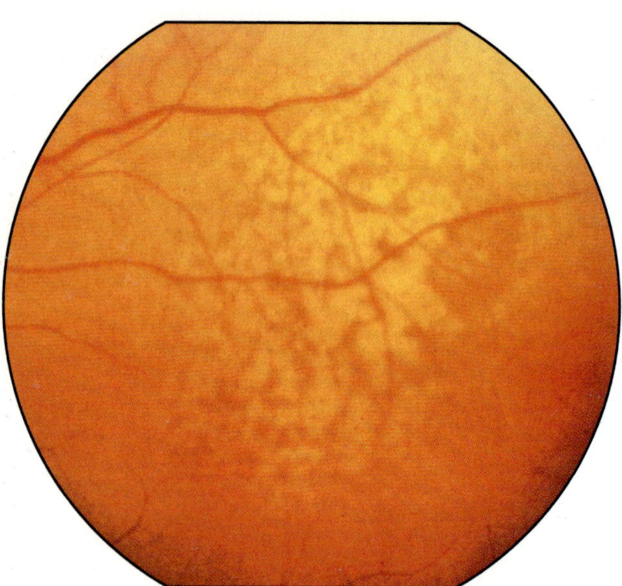

14–3

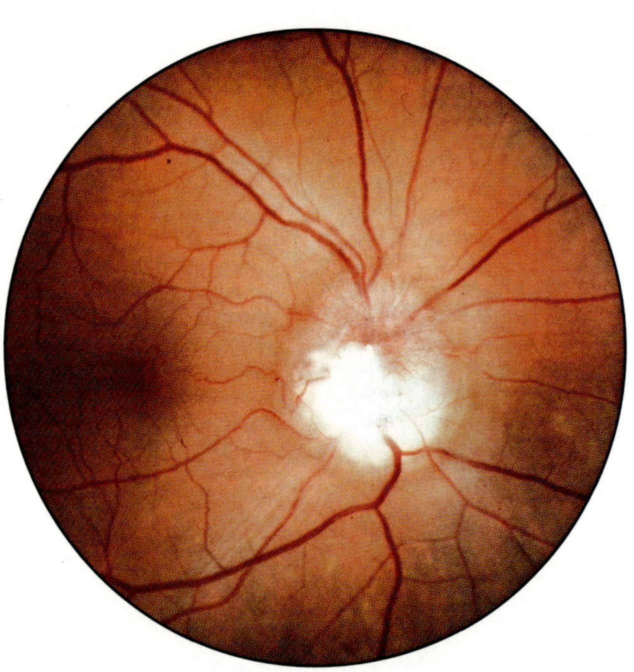

14–1, 14–1A, and 14–2 Breast metastasis to the choroid is usually noted in patients with a history of breast cancer or mastectomy. A serous detachment with whitish clumps and retinal folds may be noted in some cases (14–1) and in other cases a leopard-like configuration may be seen (14–2).

14–3 Breast cancer may sometimes metastasize to the optic nerve.

14–1, *Courtesy of Dr. Evangelos Gragoudas.* ***14–2,*** *From Guyer, DR, et al: Indocyanine-green angiography of intraocular tumors, Semin Ophthalmol (Dec) 1993. Courtesy of Dr. Evangelos Gragoudas.* ***14–3,*** *Courtesy of Dr. Jeffrey Shakin.*

14–4

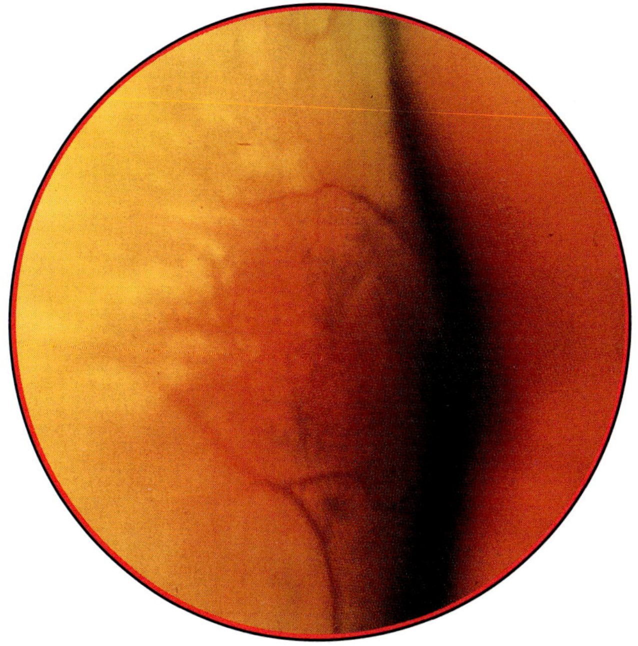

14–5

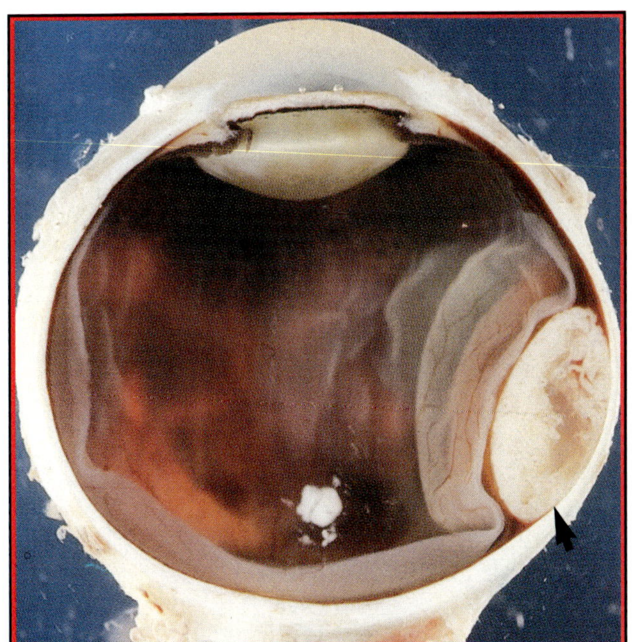

14–6

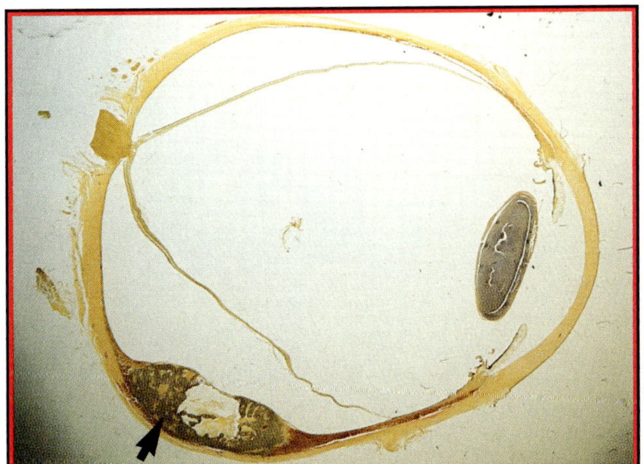

14–7

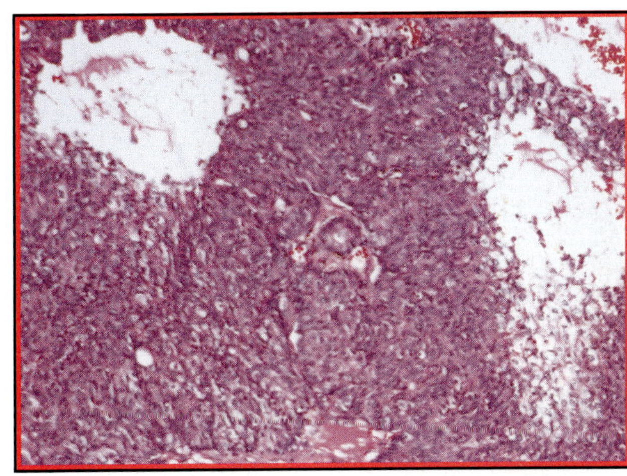

14–4 through 14–7 This case is a clinicopathologic correlation of a patient with metastatic breast carcinoma. The clinical photograph reveals a solid detachment of the retina. Histopathologic examination reveals a whitish choroidal mass *(arrowhead)* with a central area of necrosis (14–5 and 14–6), which is composed of neoplastic cells arranged in an acinar pattern (14–7).

14–8 LUNG METASTASIS

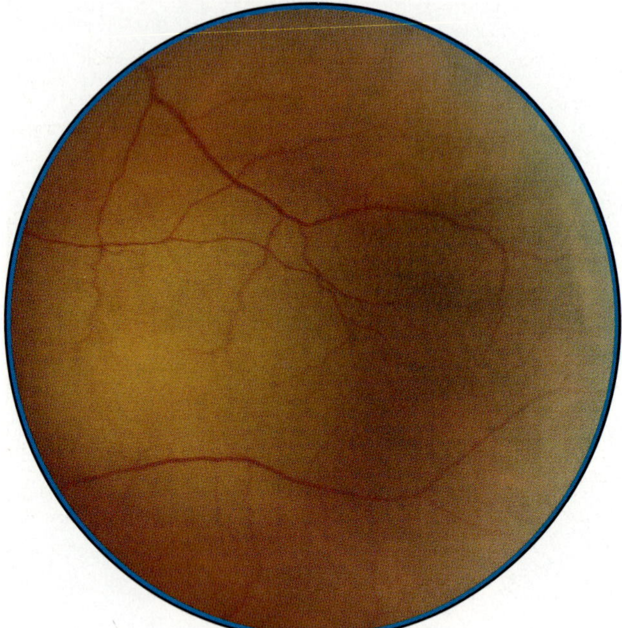

14–9

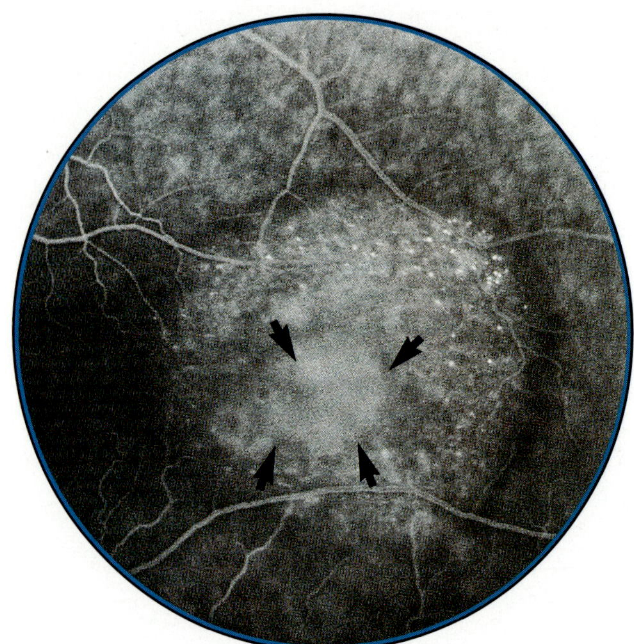

14–10

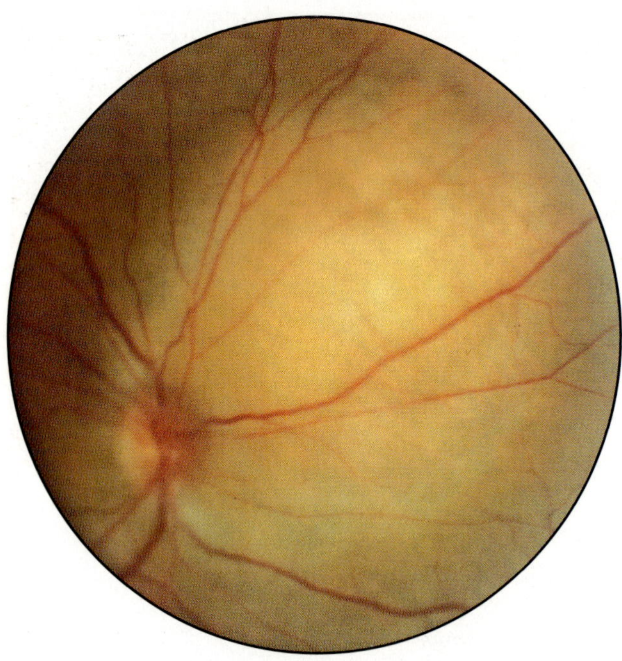

14–8 through 14–10 Patients with lung metastasis to the choroid often do not have a documented past history of lung cancer. Note the whitish-yellow elevated mass in this patient. The fluorescein angiogram shows staining of a small serous pigment epithelial detachment overlying the tumor *(arrowheads)*. The multiple hyperfluorescent spots are believed to represent invasion and alteration of the retinal pigment epithelium by the tumor cells. A serous macular detachment with solid yellowish-white material may also be noted (14–10).

14–10, *Courtesy of Dr. Jerry Shields.*

14–11 BRONCHIAL CARCINOID

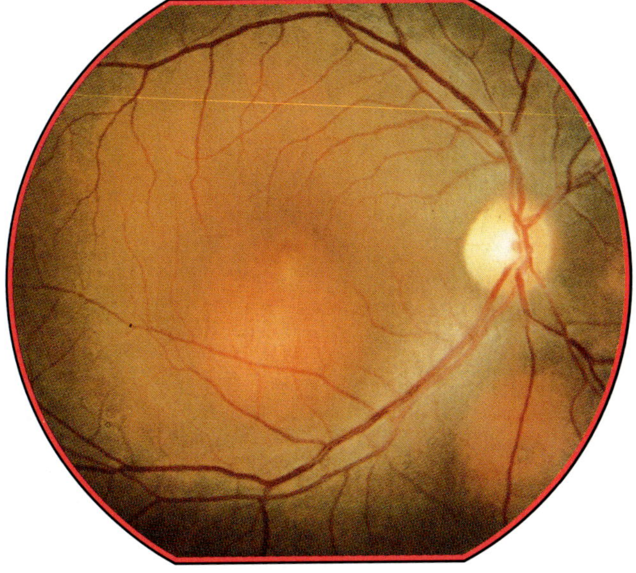

14–12

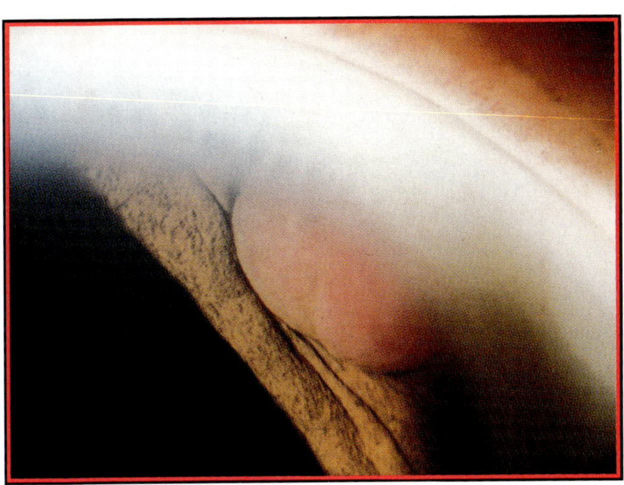

14–13

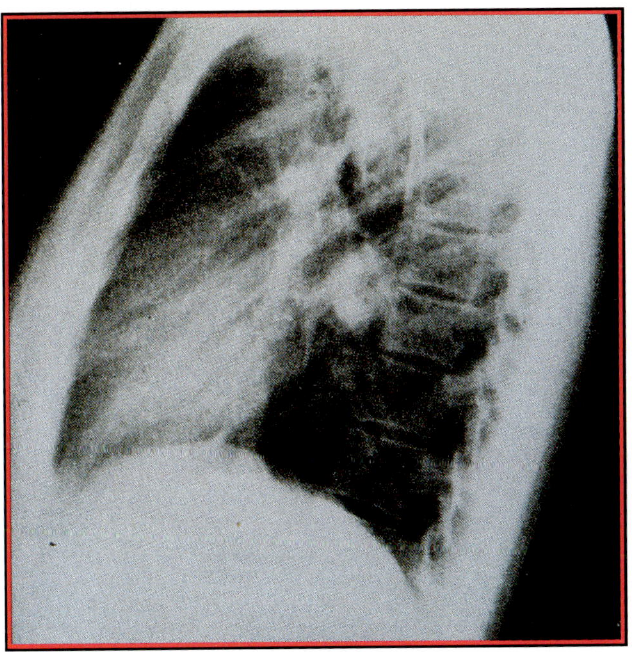

14–14

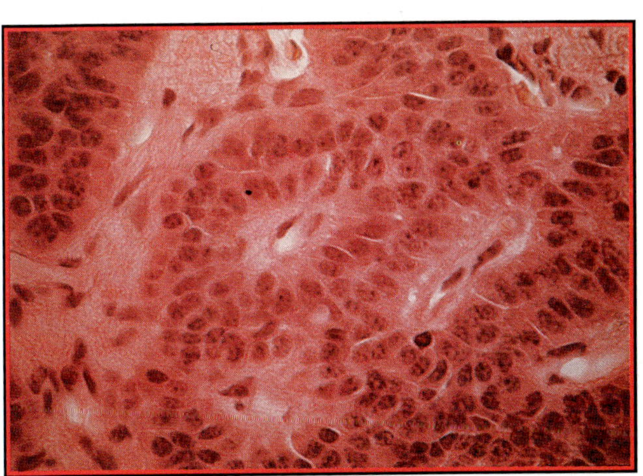

14–11 through 14–14 Bronchial carcinoids may rarely metastasize to the choroid, as in this patient. Multifocal, slightly elevated, reddish orange nodules can be seen (14–11), as well as metastatic lesions to the iris and anterior chamber (14–12). Chest x-ray (14–13) reveals the bronchial lesion. A lung biopsy confirmed bronchial carcinoid (14–14).

14–11 *through* ***14–14,*** *Courtesy of Dr. Evangelos Gragoudas.* ***14–11,*** *From Guyer, DR, et al: Indocyanine-green angiography of intraocular tumors, Semin Ophthalmol (Dec) 1993.*

BILATERAL DIFFUSE UVEAL MELANOCYTIC PROLIFERATION (BDUMP)

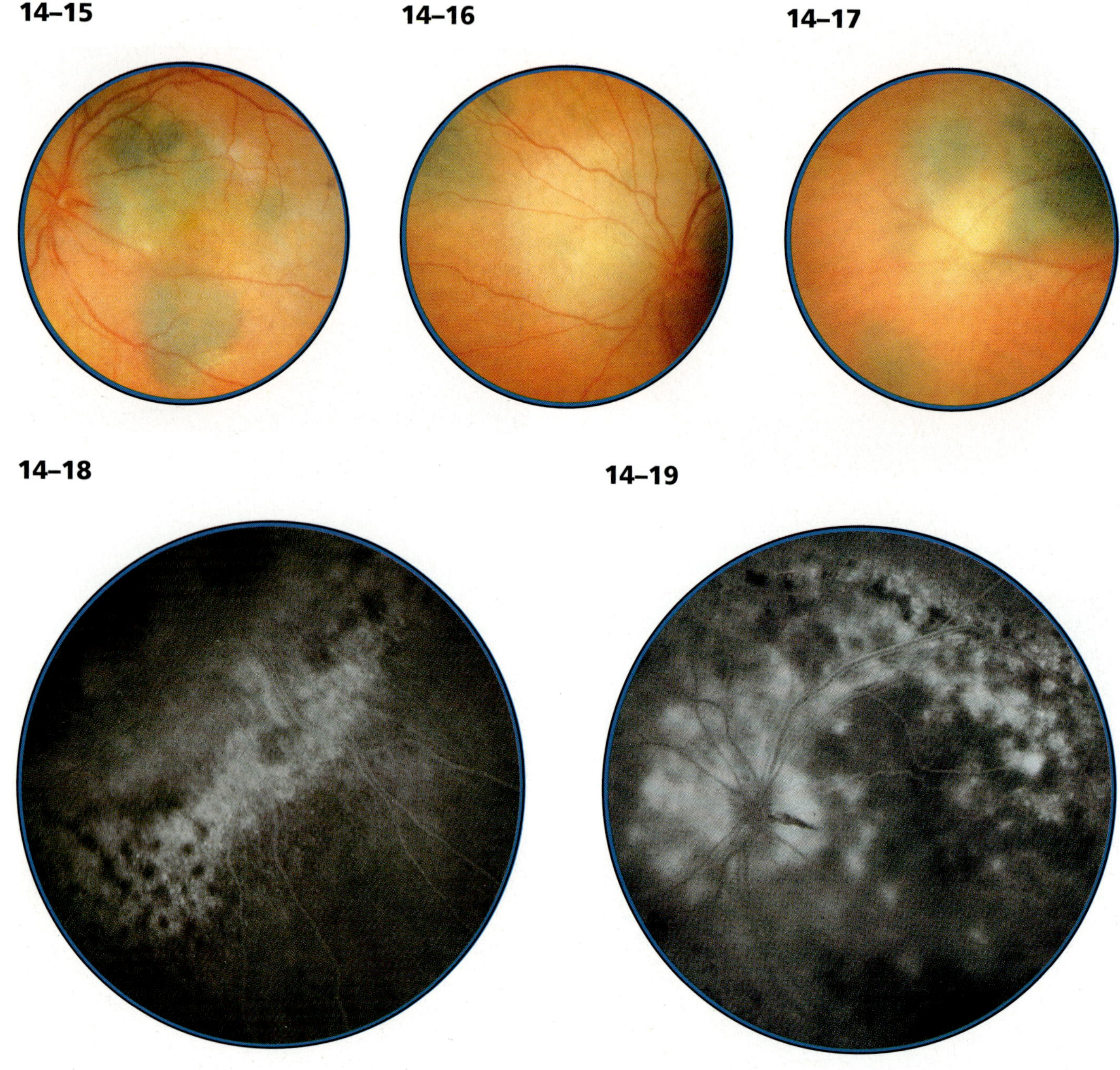

14–15 through 14–19 Bilateral diffuse uveal melanocytic proliferation (BDUMP) is a condition in which diffuse uveal thickening due to spindle-shaped melanocytes occurs. Associated systemic neoplasms are noted in these patients, including cancers of the ovary, lung, pancreas, gallbladder, colon, and kidney. Multiple faint orange spots or elevated pigmented choroidal masses are observed in the fundus. This 60-year-old male had bilateral, slightly elevated pigmented uveal masses with an overlying exudative detachment and lipid deposition. He was found to have renal adenocarcinoma. Multifocal leaks of the retinal pigment epithelium are noted on the fluorescein study.

***14–15** through **14–19,** Courtesy of Dr. Arch McNamara.*

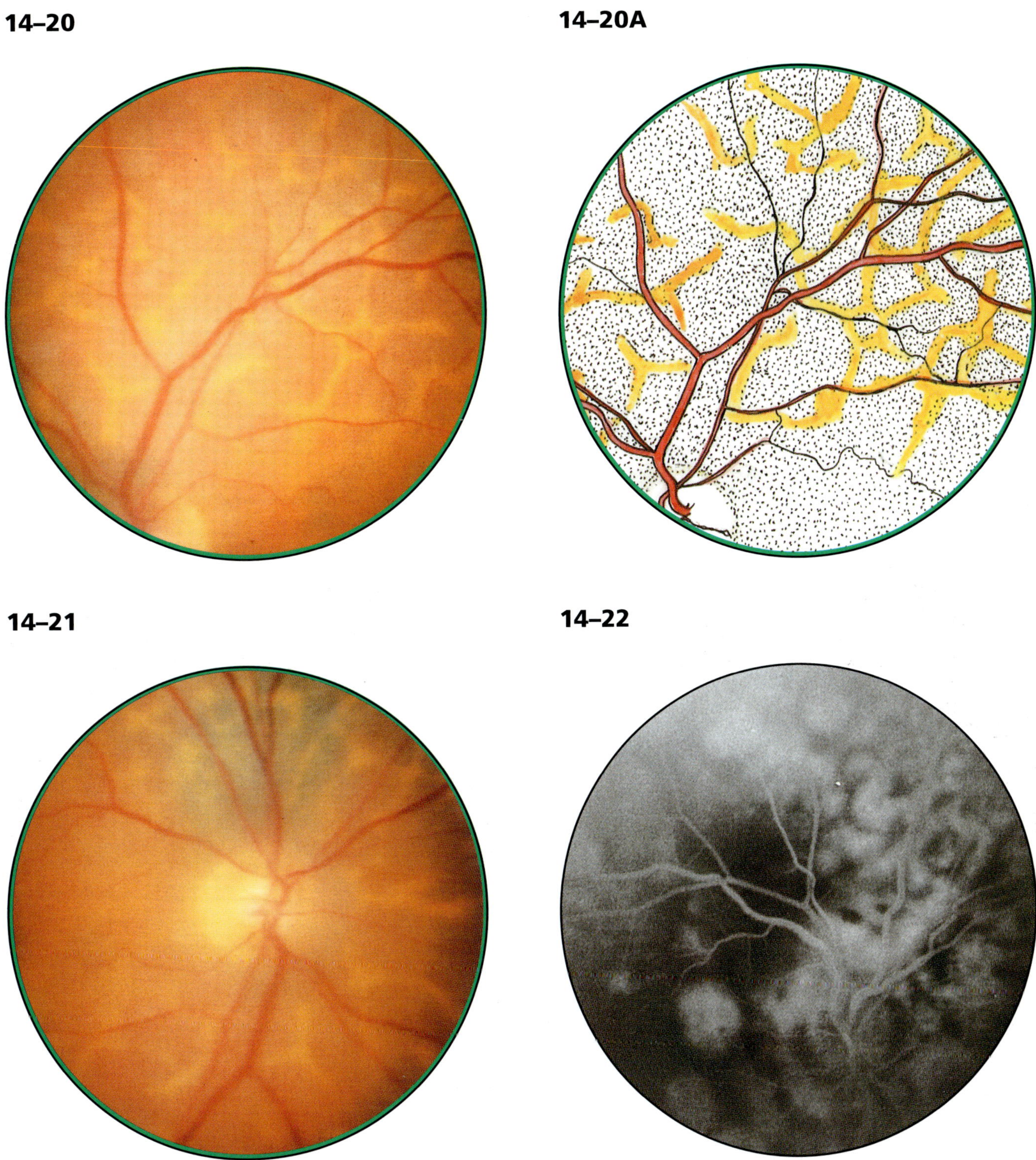

14–20, 14–20A, and 14–21 This patient also has BDUMP with polygonal yellowish-orange lesions. These lesions may or may not be seen over the melanotic masses (14–20 and 14–21).

14–22 Fluorescein findings in another patient with BDUMP illustrate multiple islands of staining that correspond to the orange pigmentary disturbances seen clinically.

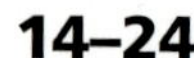

14–23 CANCER-ASSOCIATED RETINOPATHY

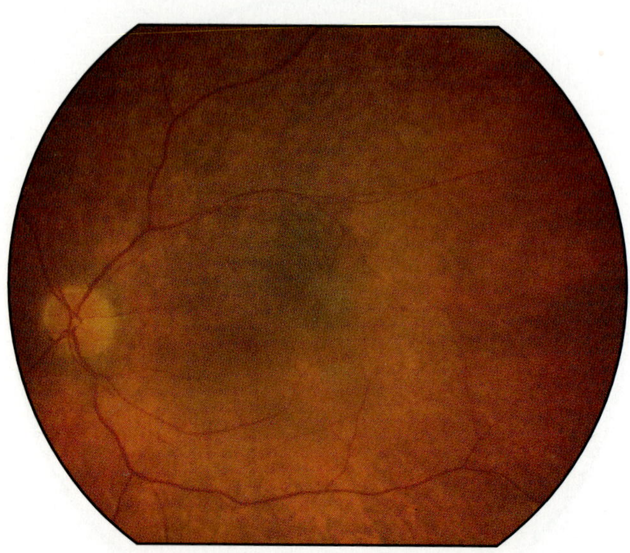

14–24

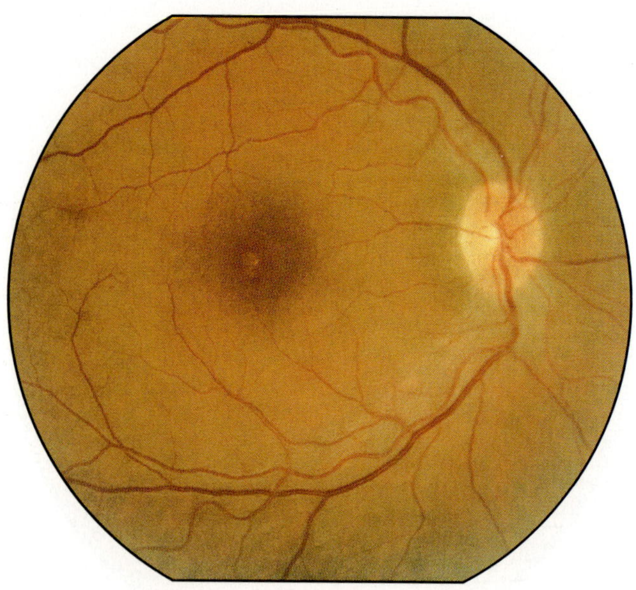

14–23 This patient has vessel attenuation, generalized retinal pigment epithelial thinning, and granularity. Often fundus findings may be minimal or nondetectable in this cancer-associated retinopathy. The medical workup revealed a systemic cancer.

14–24 This patient has a paraneoplastic cone degeneration with normal rod function and a visual acuity of hand motions. An area of foveal atrophy is noted. She had an associated endometrial cancer.

14–23, *Courtesy of Dr. William Mieler.* ***14–24,*** *Courtesy of Dr. Cynthia MacKay.*

Suggested Readings

Bell, RM, Bullock, JD, and Albert, DM: Solitary choroidal metastasis from bronchial carcinoid, Br J Ophthalmol 59:155–163, 1975

Brady, LW, Shields, JA, Augsburger, JJ, and Day, JL: Malignant intraocular tumors, Cancer 49:578–585, 1982

Burmeister, BH, Benjamin, CS, and Childs, WJ: The management of metastases to eye and orbit from carcinoma of the breast, Aust NZ J Ophthalmol 18:187–190, 1990

Castro, PA, Albert, DM, Wang, WJ, and Ni, C: Tumors metastatic to the eye and adnexa, Int Ophthalmol Clin 22:189–223, 1982

Dobrowsky, W: Treatment of choroid metastases, Br J Radiol 61:140–142, 1988

Griffin, JD, and Garnick, MB: Eye toxicity of cancer chemotherapy: a review of the literature, Cancer 48:1539–1549, 1981

Merrill, CF, Kaufman, DI, and Dimitrov, NV: Breast cancer metastatic to the eye is a common entity, Cancer 68:623–627, 1991

Shakin, EP, Shields, JA, and Augsburger, JJ: Metastatic cancer to the uvea and optic disc. An analysis of two hundred cases, Second International Meeting on Diagnosis and Treatment of Intraocular Tumors, Nyon, Switzerland, November 1987

Shields, JA: Diagnosis and management of intraocular tumors, St Louis, 1983, Mosby–Year Book

Stephens, RF, and Shields, JA: Diagnosis and management of cancer metastatic to the uvea: a study of 70 cases, Ophthalmology 86:1336–1349, 1979

Thatcher, N, and Thomas, PRM: Choroidal metastases from breast carcinoma: a survey of 42 patients and the use of radiation therapy, Clin Radiol 26:549–553, 1975

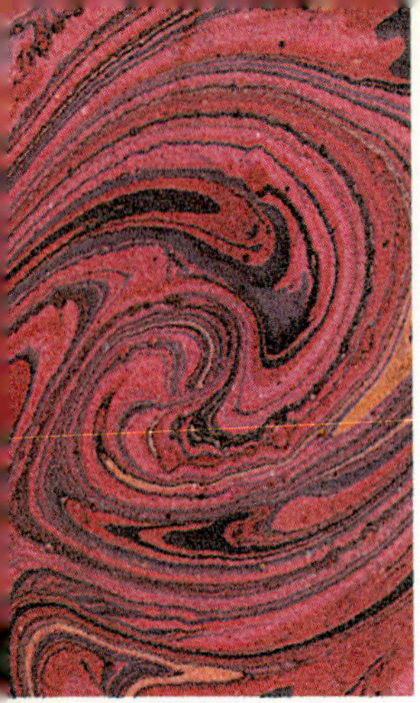

Chapter 15
Choroidal Osteomas

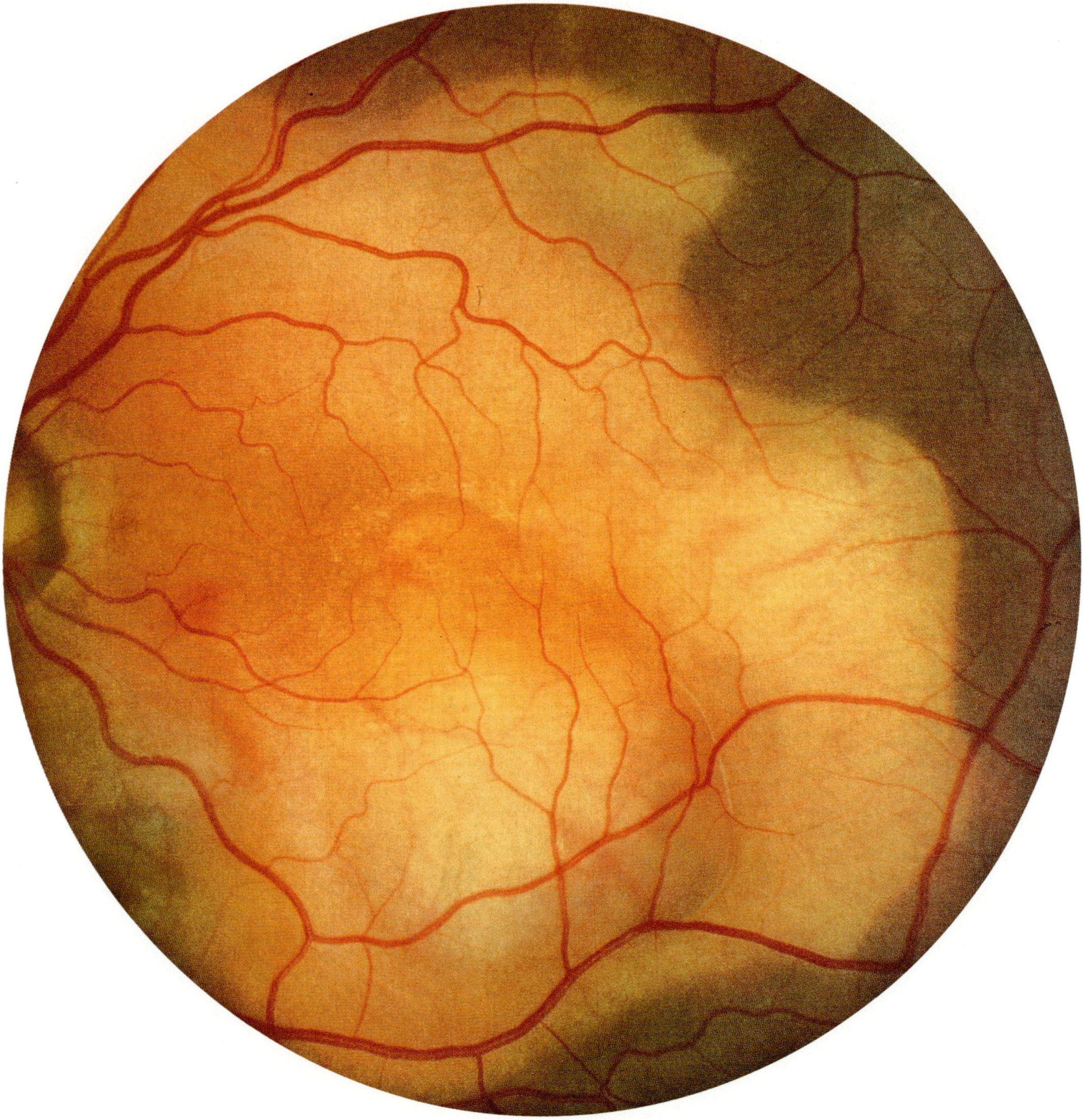

Choroidal osteomas are benign bony tumors. They may show osteoclastic activity, osteoblastic growth, or develop choroidal neovascularization.

15–1

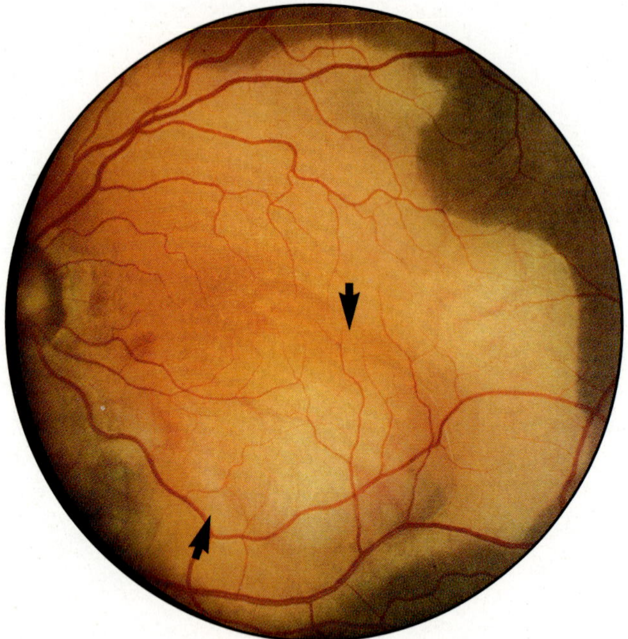

15–2 **15–2A**

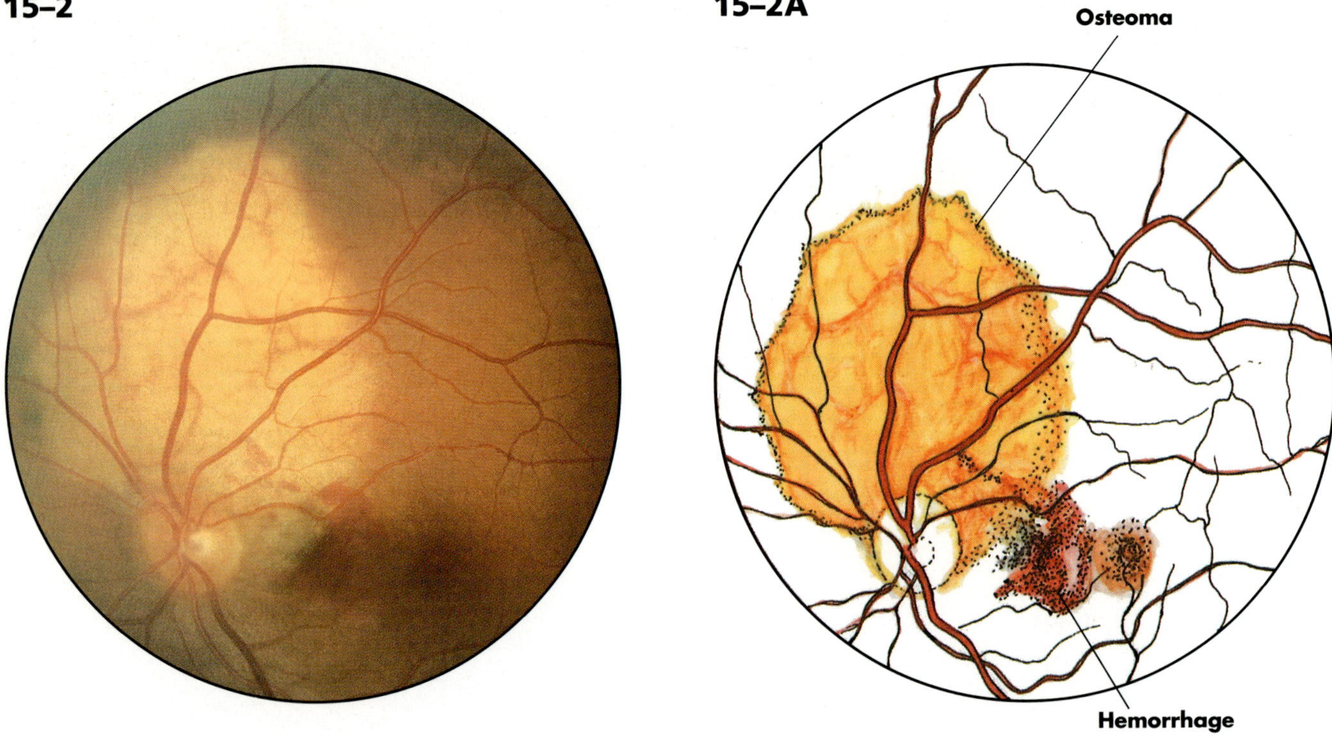

15–1 Choroidal osteomas are often seen in young white females. Pseudopod borders with wedged-shaped edges are often noted with coarse yellowish bony changes. This patient also has an overlying exudative detachment in the central macula (*arrowheads*).

15–2 and 15–2A The osteomas may be associated with subretinal hemorrhage due to choroidal neovascularization.

15–1, *Courtesy of Dr. Jerry Shields.*

15–3

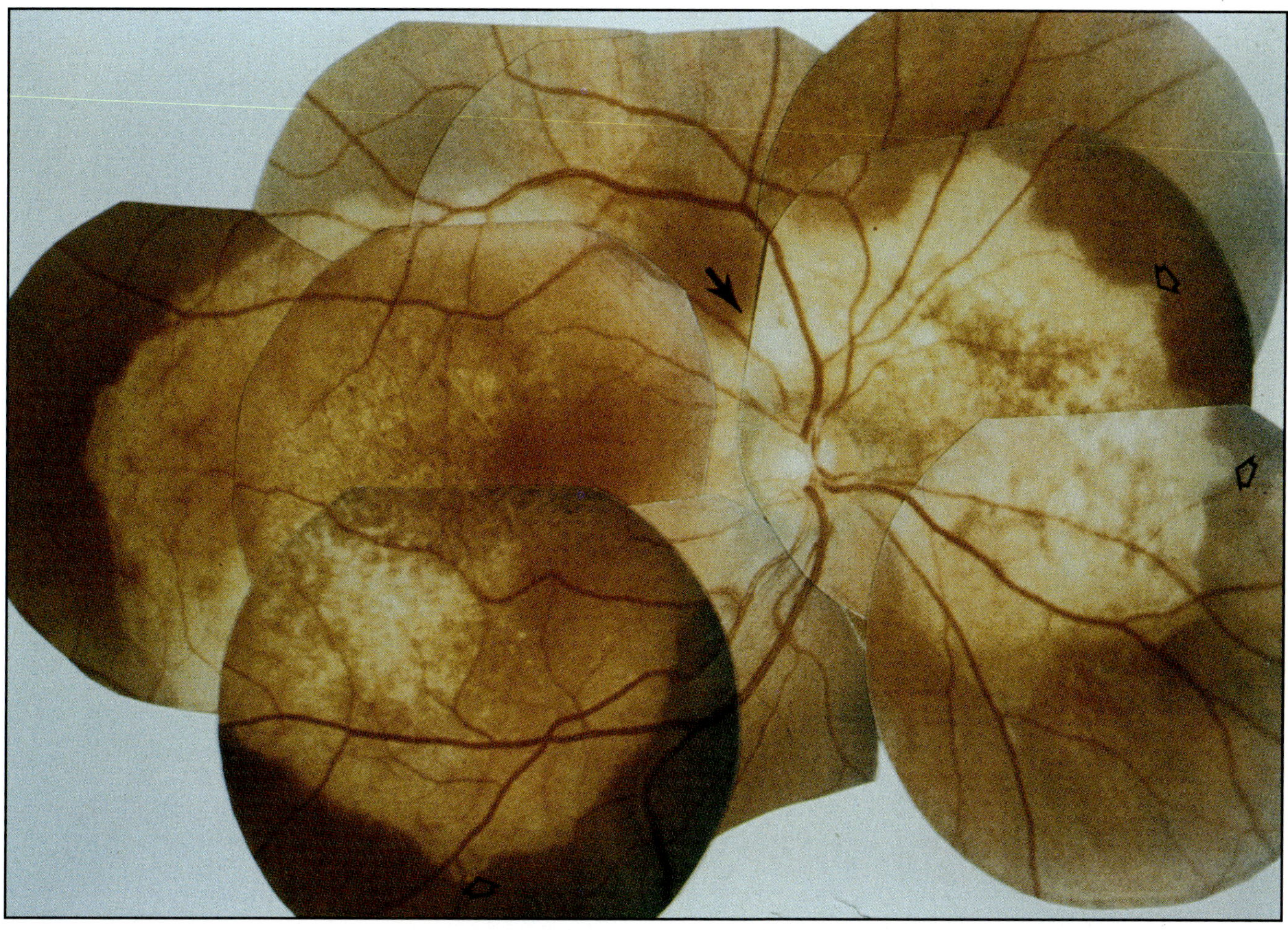

15–3 The montage shows an eye with an extensive choroidal osteoma that extends with a wedge-shaped growth pattern toward the periphery *(arrows)*.

15 3, *Courtesy of Dr. Jerry Shields.*

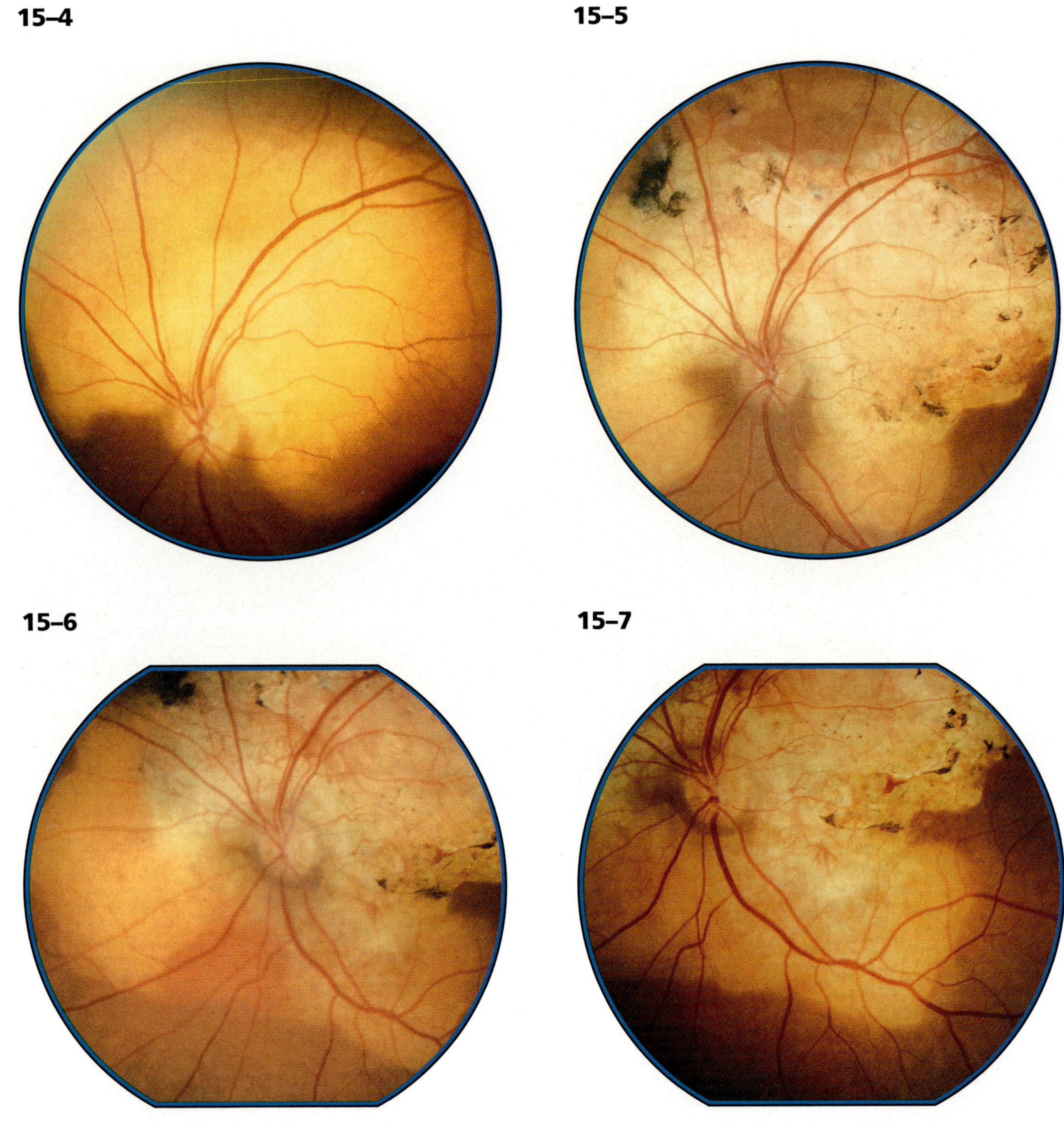

15–4 through 15–7 This series of photographs illustrates progressive growth of a choroidal osteoma. The patient initially had a lesion demonstrating pure osteoblastic activity (15–4). Note the sparing of the inferior juxtapapillary area. Seven years later, there is osteoclastic activity with retinal pigment epithelial hyperplasia and scarring in the superior portion of the lesion (15–5). There has also been some marginal osteoblastic activity superiorly. Note extension of the lesion inferiorly. Subretinal hemorrhage is also present (15–6). Four years later, there is continued osteoblastic activity inferior to the disc (15–7).

15–8

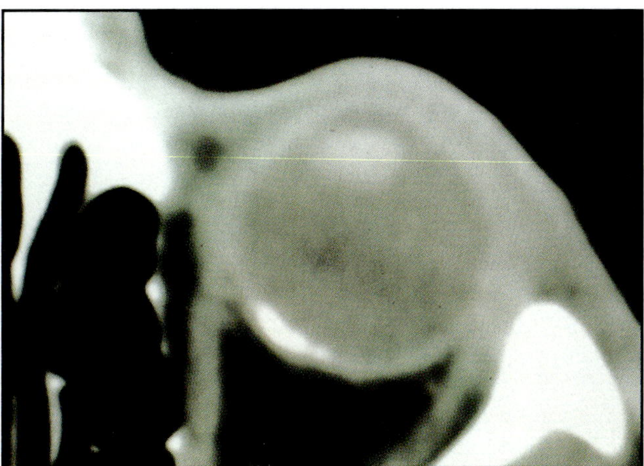

15–9

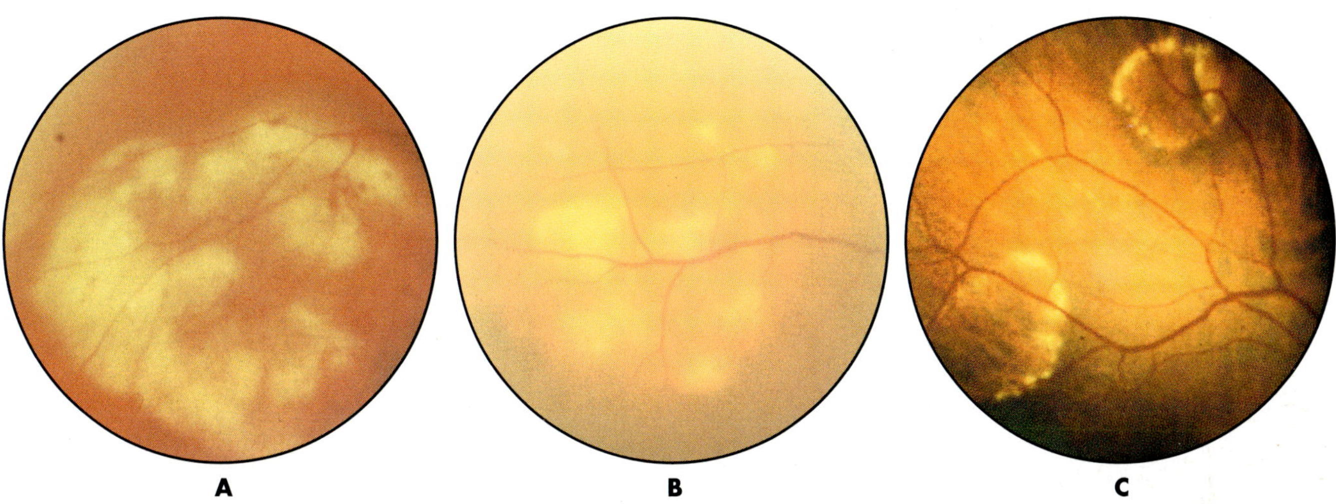

15–8 A choroidal osteoma is illustrated by a CAT scan.

15–9 In the differential diagnosis of ocular calcification is the benign condition of uveoscleral calcification. Yellowish irregular subretinal nodules are noted in these cases.

15–9A, *Courtesy of Dr. Andrew Schachat.* ***15–9B,*** *Courtesy of Dr. John Killian.* ***15–9C,*** *Courtesy of Dr. James Augsberger.*

15–10

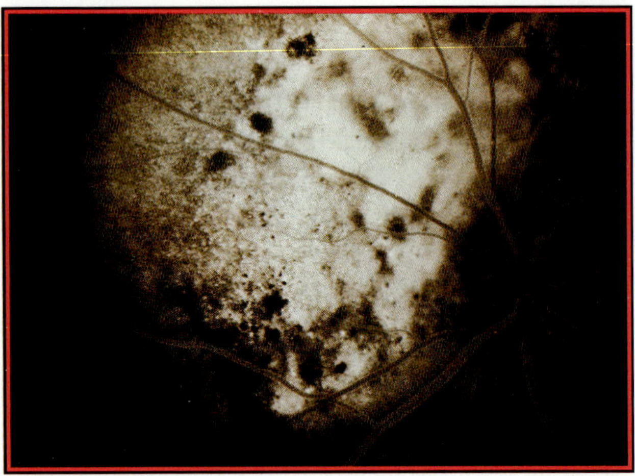

15–11

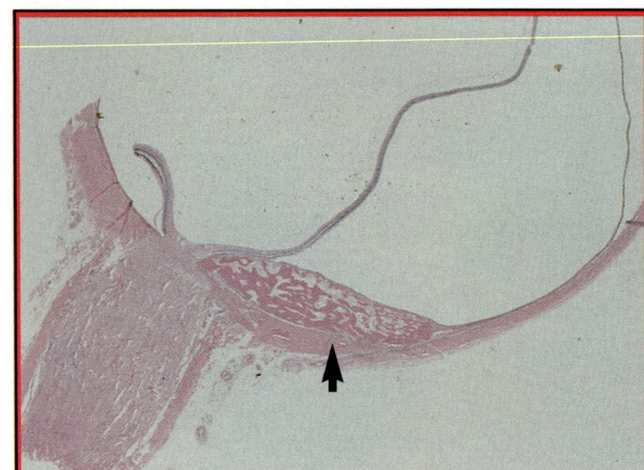

15–12

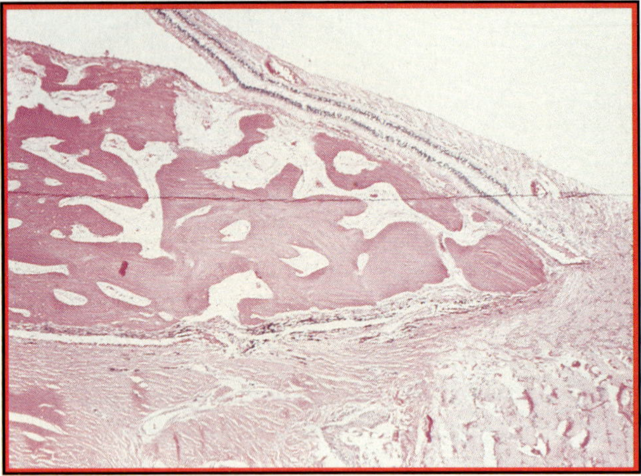

15–13

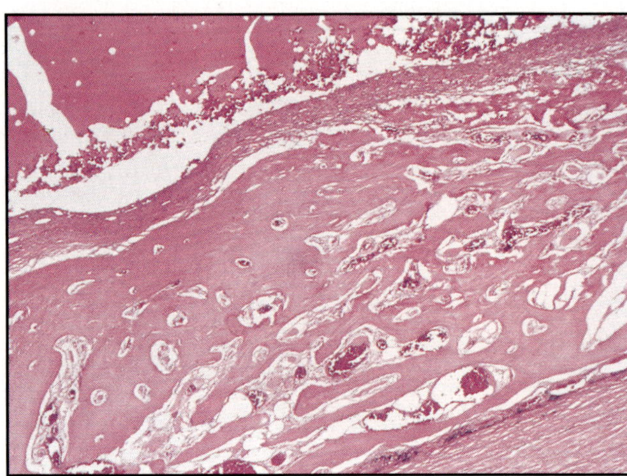

15–10 through 15–13 This clinicopathologic correlation of a patient with a choroidal osteoma demonstrates the histopathologic features of this disorder. The clinical photograph shows a peripapillary choroidal osteoma. On cross-sectional examination, a choroidal osteoma is noted near the optic disc *(arrowhead)*. Higher magnification shows that the lesion is composed of compact bone. Light microscopy from another case shows that the bony material is intermingled with vascular components.

***15–10** and **15–13,** From Font, R, et al: EOPS 1976.*

Suggested Readings

Augsburger, JJ, Shields, JA, and Rife, CJ: Bilateral choroidal osteoma after nine years, Can J Ophthalmol 14:281–284, 1979

Avila, MP, El-Markabi, H, Azzolini, C, Jalkh, AE, Burns, D, and Weiter, JJ: Bilateral choroidal osteoma with subretinal neovascularization, Ann Ophthalmol 16:381–385, 1984

Coston, TO, and Wilkinson, CP: Choroidal osteoma, Am J Ophthalmol 86:368–372, 1978

Gass, JDM: New observations concerning choroidal osteomas, Int Ophthalmol 1:71–84, 1979

Green, WR: Uveal tract. In Spencer, WH, Font, RL, Green, WR, Howes, EL, Jr, Jakobiec, FA, and Zimmerman, LE, eds: Ophthalmic pathology: An atlas and textbook, vol 3, Philadelphia, 1985, WB Saunders

Katz, RS, and Gass, JD: Multiple choroidal osteomas developing in association with recurrent orbital inflammatory pseudotumor, Arch Ophthalmol 101:1724–1727, 1983

Kline, LB, Shalka, HW, Davidson, JD, and Wilmes, FJ: Bilateral choroidal osteomas associated with fatal systemic illness, Am J Ophthalmol 93:192–197, 1982

Schachat, AP, Robertson, DM, Mieler, WF, Schwartz, D, Augsburger, JJ, Schatz, H, and Gass, JDM: Sclerochoroidal calcification, Arch Ophthalmol 110:196–199, 1992

Shields, CL, Shields, JA, and Augsburger, JJ: Review: Choroidal osteoma, Surv Ophthalmol 33:17–27, 1988

Shields, JA: Diagnosis and management of intraocular tumors, St Louis, 1983, Mosby–Year Book

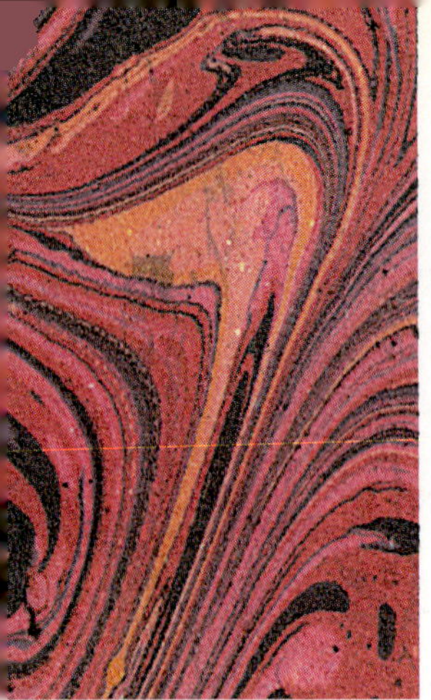

Chapter 16
Choroidal Hemangioma

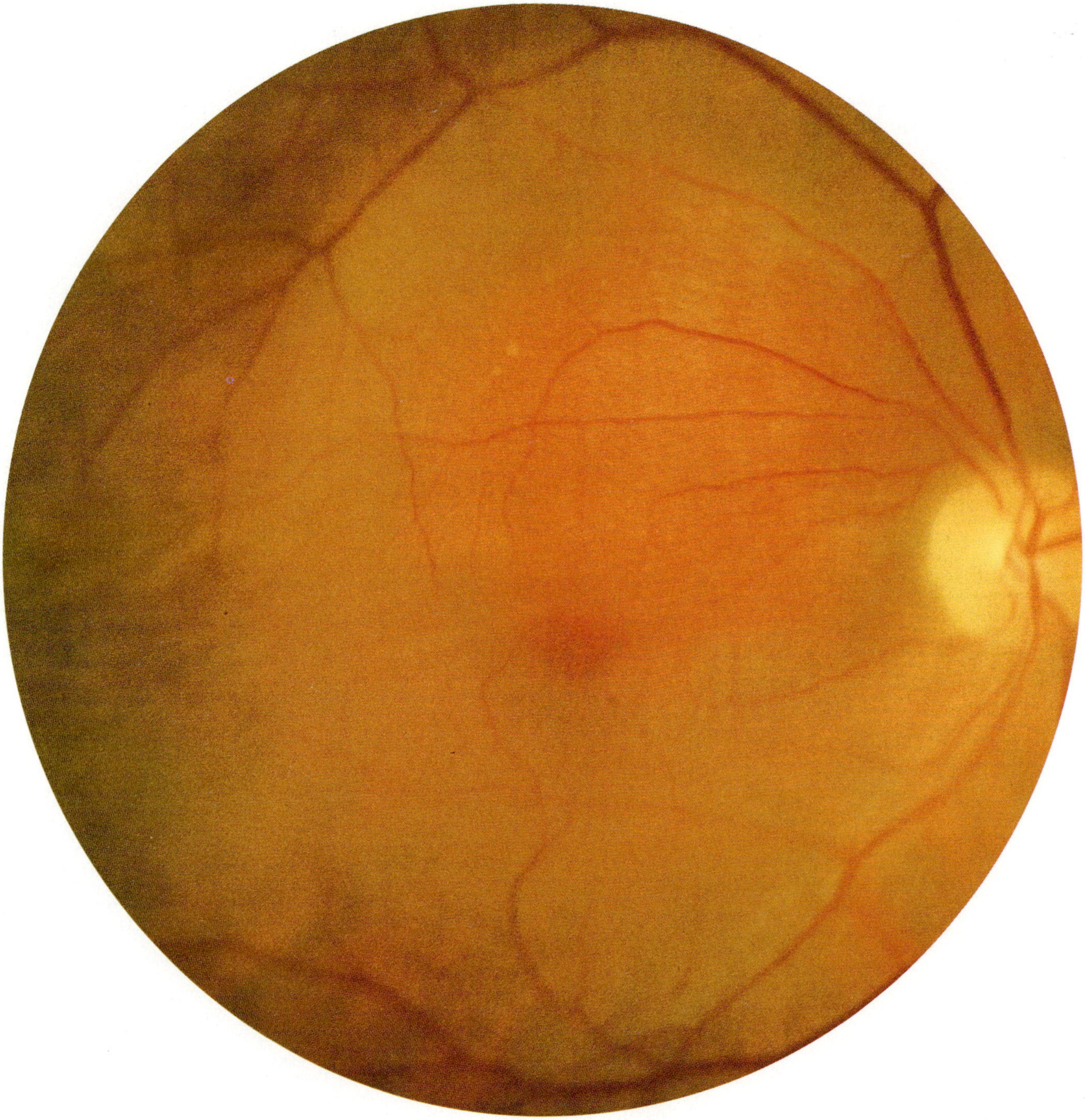

Choroidal hemangiomas are benign vascular lesions. They may be focal or diffuse in nature.

16–1

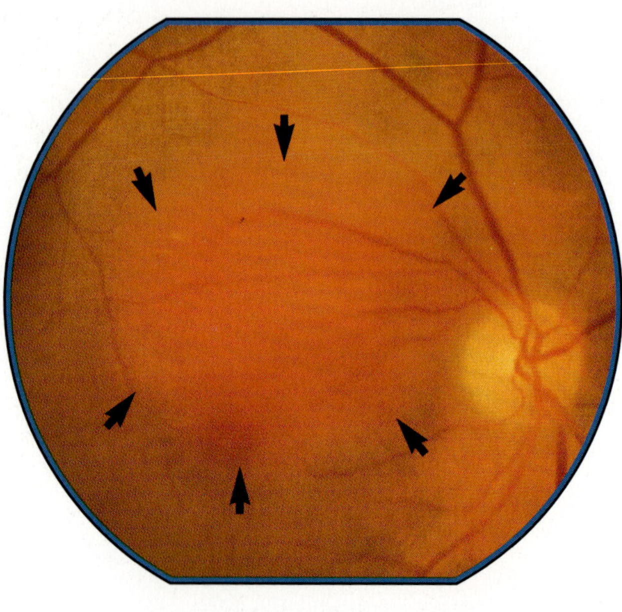

16–2

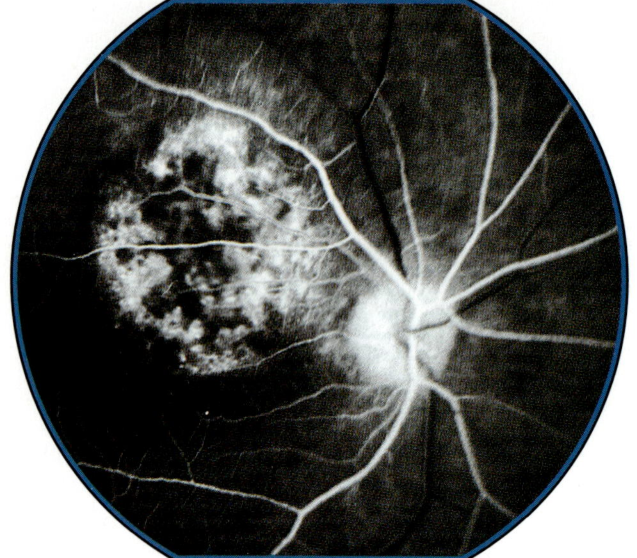

16–3

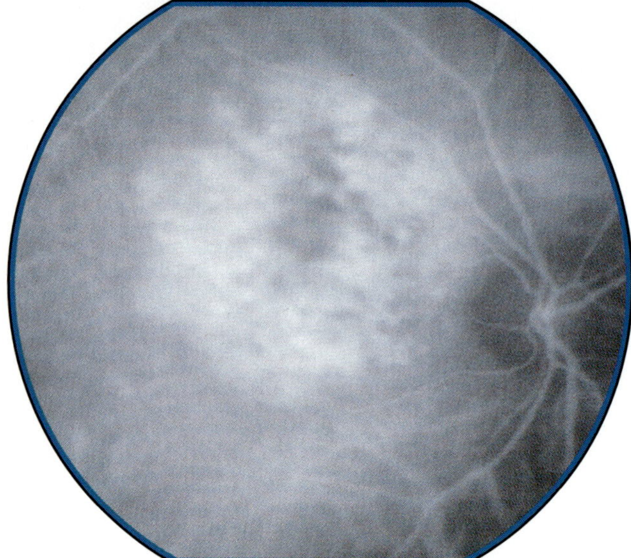

16–1 through 16–3 This patient has a focal choroidal hemangioma. Note the reddish discoloration of this choroidal lesion *(arrowheads)*. These tumors are hyperfluorescent by fluorescein angiography during the choroidal phase. Indocyanine-green (ICG) angiography shows an intensely hyperfluorescent lesion with a speckled body and stellate borders.

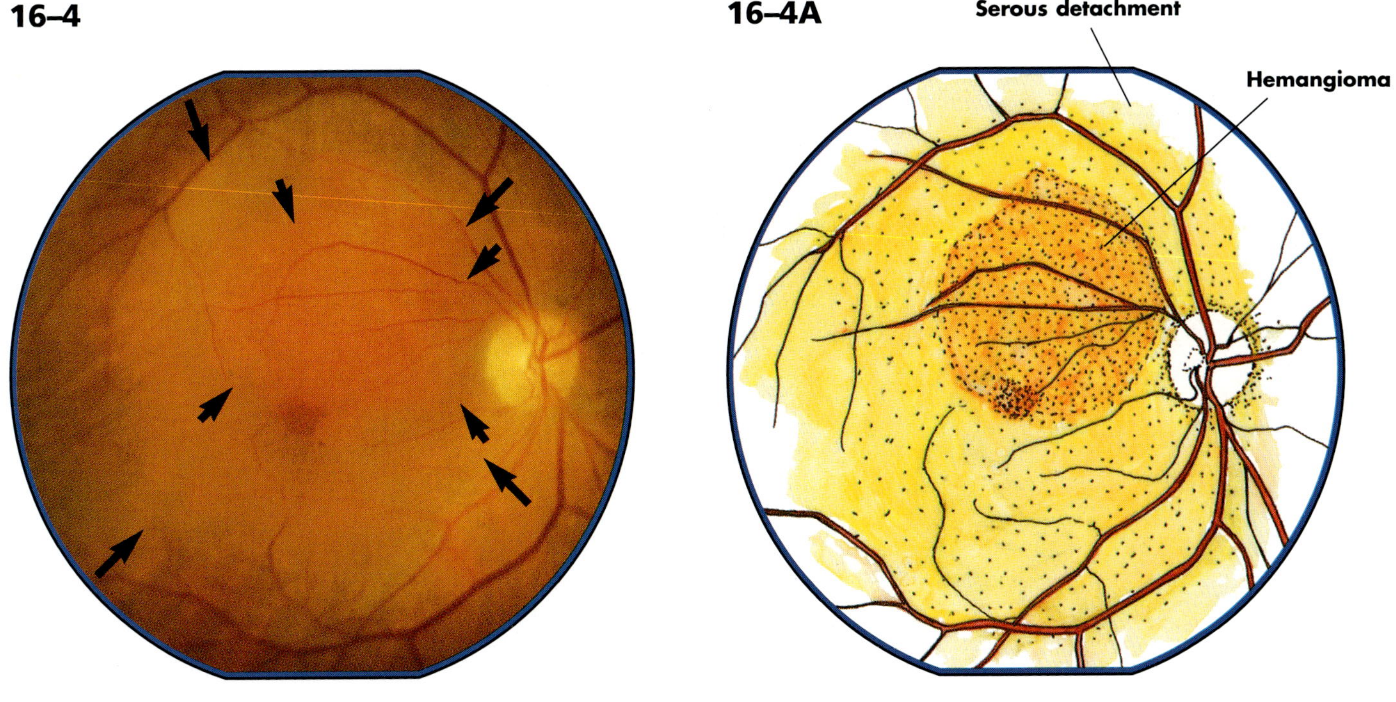

16–4 and 16–4A These vascular tumors *(arrowheads)* may show secondary serous detachment *(arrows)*.

16–5

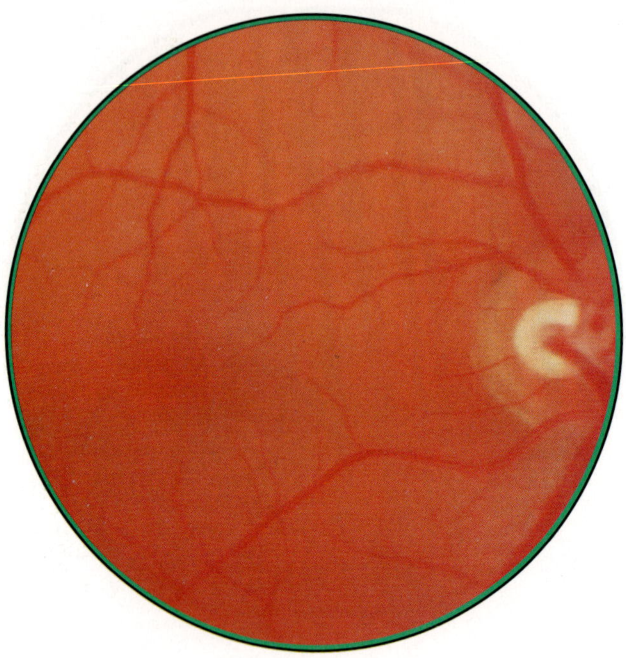

16–6

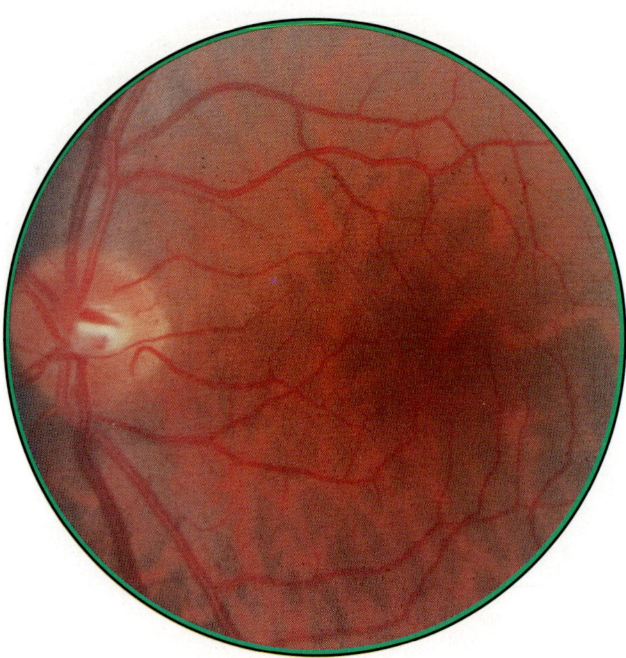

16–5 and 16–6 A diffuse choroidal hemangioma may be demonstrated in association with the Sturge-Weber syndrome. The first photograph shows the abnormal right fundus. Note the reddish choroidal background, the obscuration of the normal choroidal large vessel pattern, and pronounced cupping of the optic disc due to the diffuse choroidal vascular tumor. The second photograph is the same patient's normal left fundus.

***16–5** and **16–6,** Courtesy of Dr. Jerry Shields.*

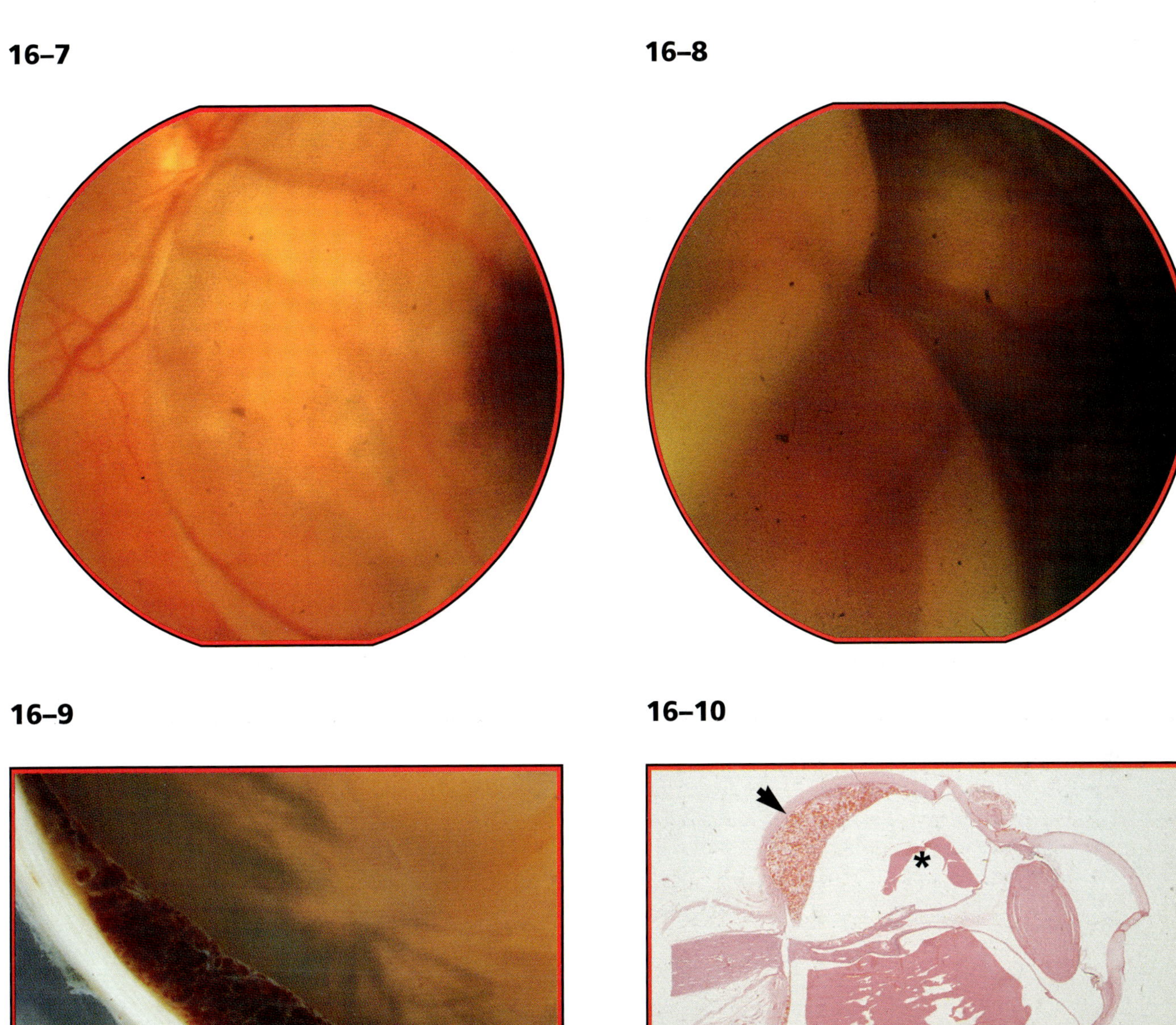

16–7 and 16–8 This patient had a localized choroidal hemangioma with a secondary massive bullous detachment.

16–9 Gross examination shows the reddish vascular nature of the tumor.

16–10 Light microscopy reveals a choroidal hemangioma *(arrow)*, as well as a large retinal detachment *(asterisks)*.

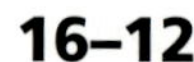

16–11

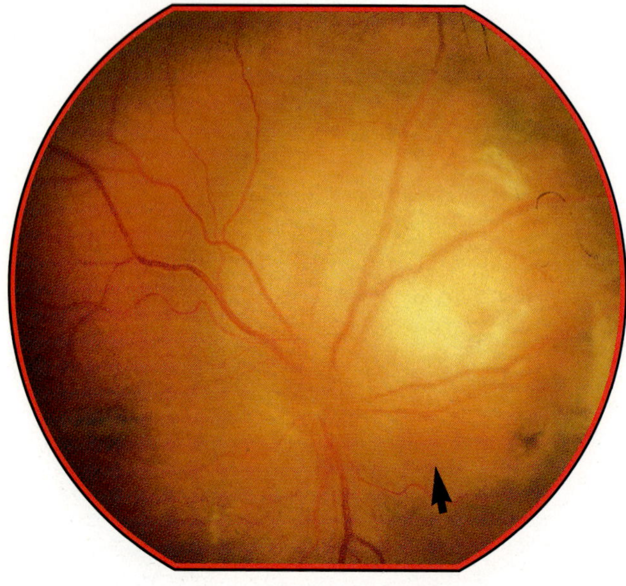

16–12

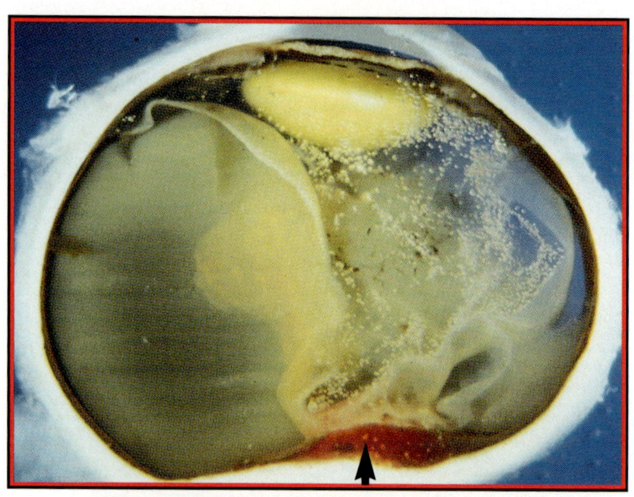

16–13

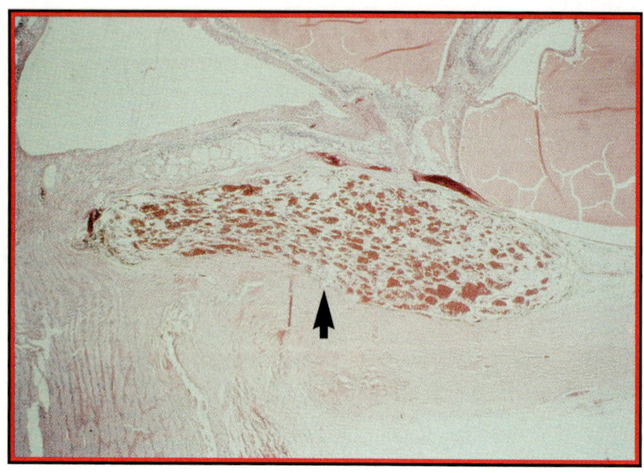

16–14

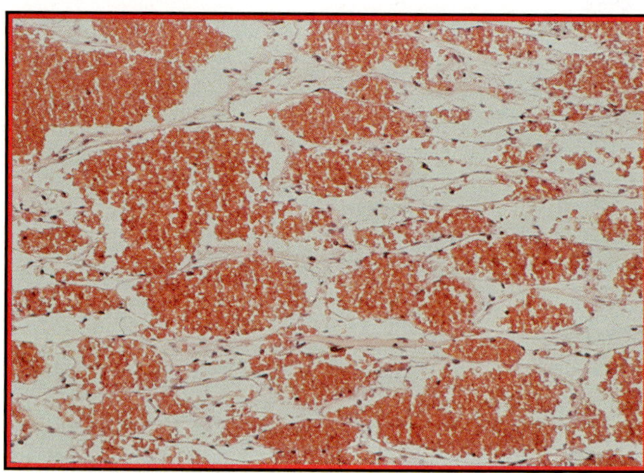

16–11 through 16–14 This case is a clinicopathologic correlation of a patient with a choroidal hemangioma. The patient had a whitish-yellow peripapillary lesion with a suggestion of reddish discoloration inferiorly *(arrowhead)*. Gross examination reveals a choroidal hemangioma *(arrowhead)*. Light microscopy reveals the choroidal hemangioma *(arrowhead)* to be composed of large vascular channels.

16–11 *through* ***16–14,*** *Courtesy of Dr. Jerry Shields.*

16–15

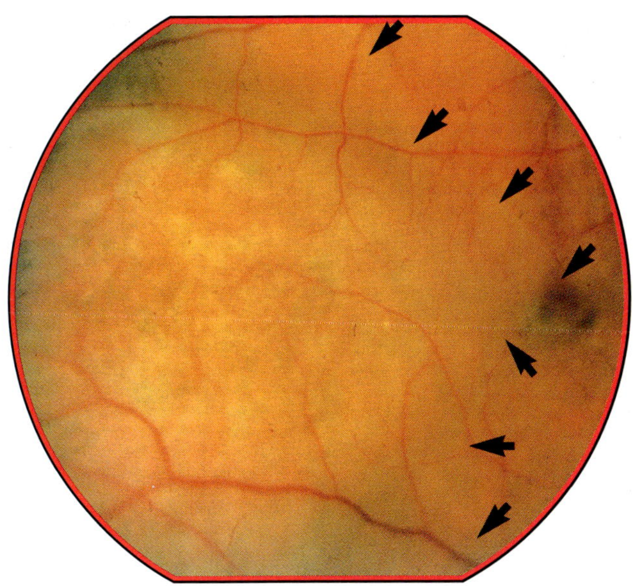

16–16

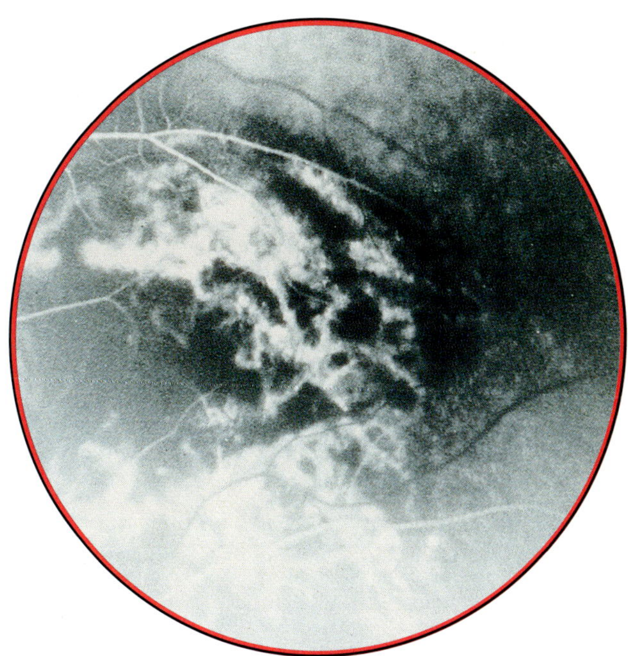

16–17

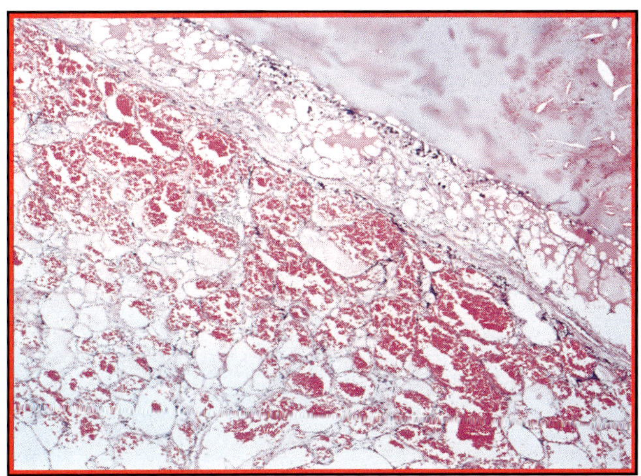

16–15 through 16–17 This patient also had a whitish and reddish elevated lesion with retinal detachment *(arrowheads)*. A pigmentary degeneration is noted at the fovea. Fluorescein angiography shows hyperfluorescence consistent with a vascular lesion. Light microscopy reveals a characteristic choroidal hemangioma with large vascular channels.

16–15 *through* ***16–17,*** *Courtesy of Dr. Henry Ring.*

Suggested Readings

Augsburger, JJ, Shields, JA, and Moffatt, KP: Circumscribed choroidal hemangiomas. Long-term visual prognosis, Retina 1:56–61, 1981

Chishold, IH, and Blach, RK: Choroidal hemangioma, a diagnostic and therapeutic problem, Trans Ophthalmol Soc UK 93:161–169, 1973

Coleman, DJ, Abramson, DH, Jack, RL, and Franzen, LA: Ultrasonic diagnosis of tumors of the choroid, Arch Ophthalmol 91:344–354, 1974

Gass, JDM: Differential diagnosis of intraocular tumors. A stereoscopic presentation, St Louis, 1974, Mosby–Year Book, pp 114–129

Reese, AB: Tumors of the eye, ed 3, Hagerstown, MD, 1976, Harper & Row Publishers, pp 277–282

Shields, JA, and Shields, CL: Intraocular tumor. A text and atlas, Philadelphia, 1992, WB Saunders, pp 240–252

Shields, JA, and Zimmerman, LE: Lesions simulating malignant melanoma of the posterior uvea, Arch Ophthalmol 89:466–471, 1973

Zografos, L, Gailloud, C, and Bercher, L: Irradiation treatment of choroidal hemangiomas, J Fr Ophthalmol 12:797–807, 1989

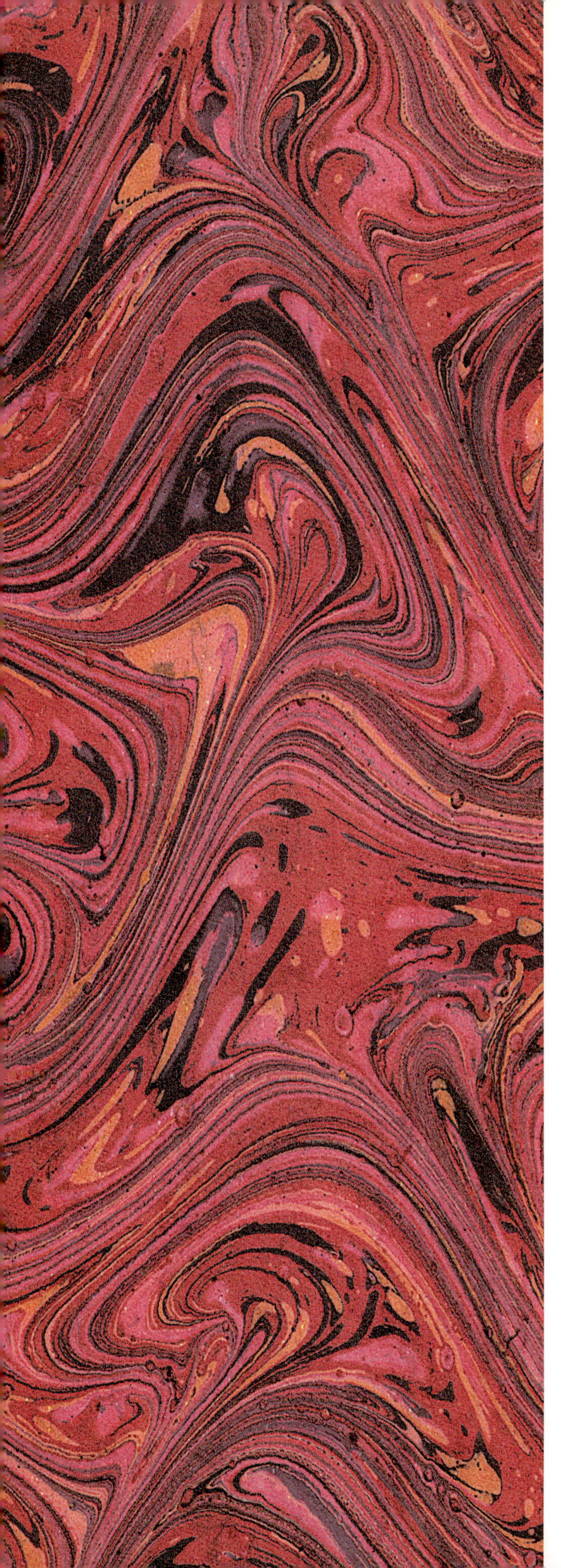

Part V

Intraocular Lymphoid Tumors

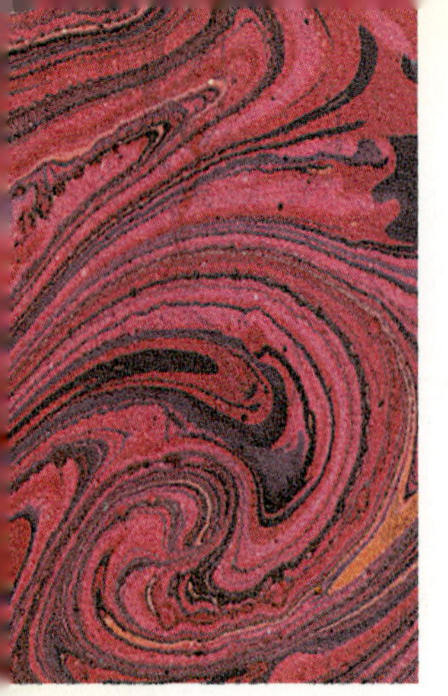

Chapter 17

The Leukemias and the Lymphomas

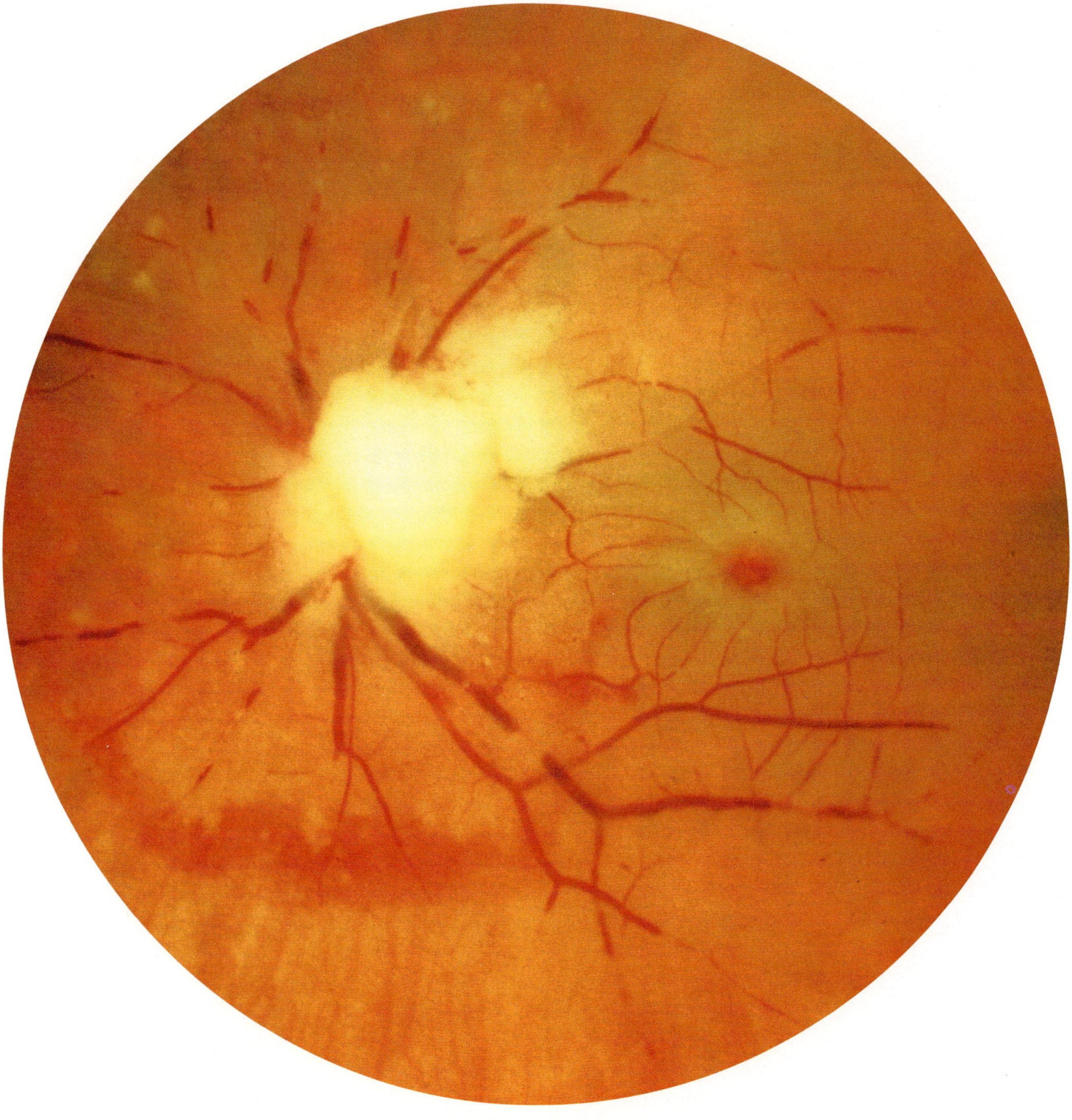

Leukemic retinopathy consists of intraretinal hemorrhages, white-centered hemorrhages, cotton-wool spots, and leukemic infiltrates. Lymphoma may also present in the eye often as a vitritis or infiltrate.

17–1 LEUKEMIA

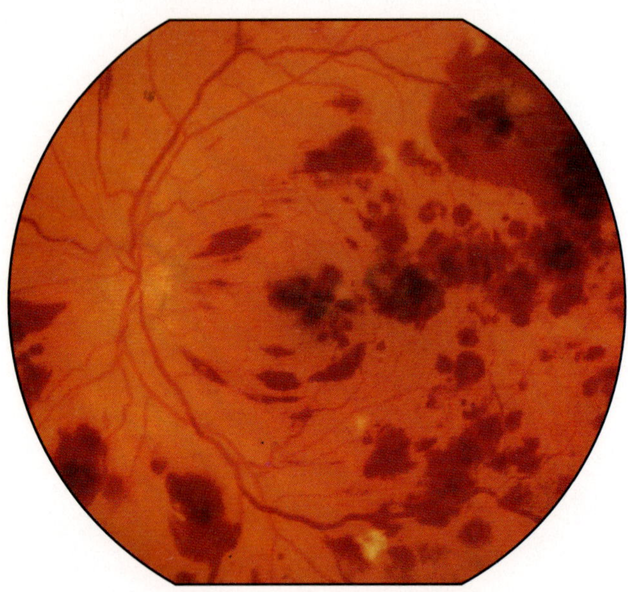

17–2

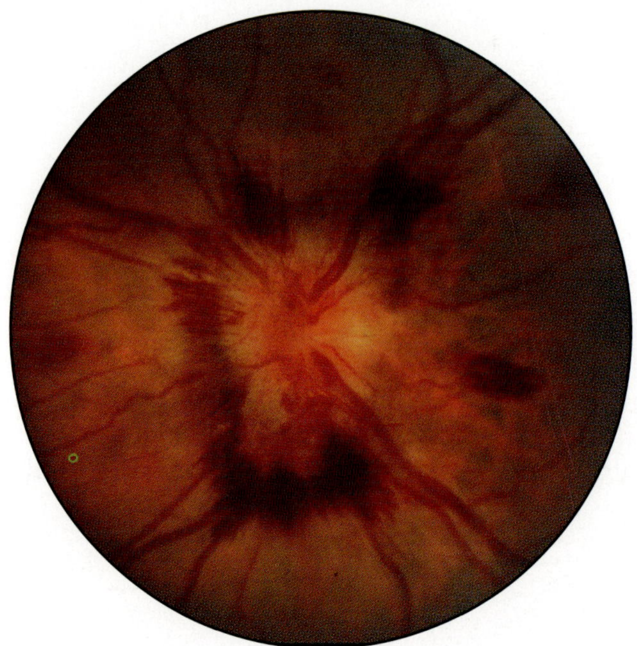

17–3

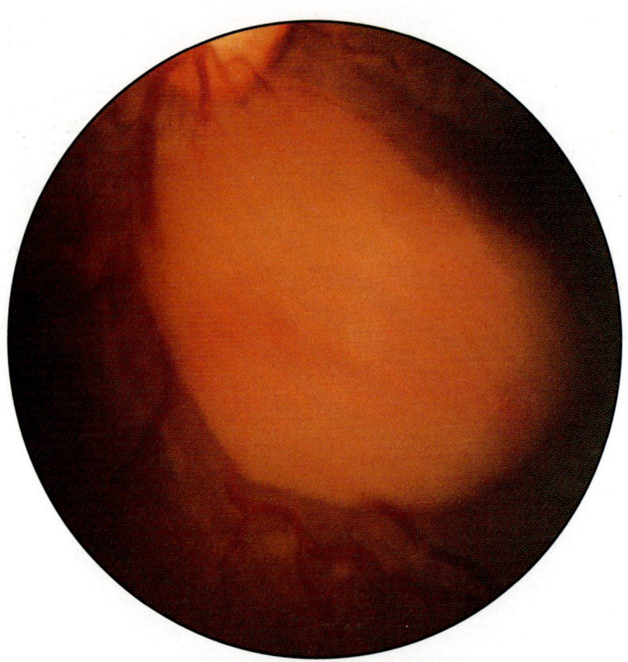

17–1 Leukemia may affect the retina or choroid. Leukemic retinopathy consists of intraretinal hemorrhages, white-centered hemorrhages (Roth's spots), and cotton-wool spots.

17–2 Optic disc edema may also be noted.

17–3 Leukemic infiltration may rarely occur in the fundus.

17–3, *From Ryan, SJ: Retina, ed 2, St Louis, 1994, Mosby–Year Book. Courtesy of Dr. Andrew Schachat.*

17–4

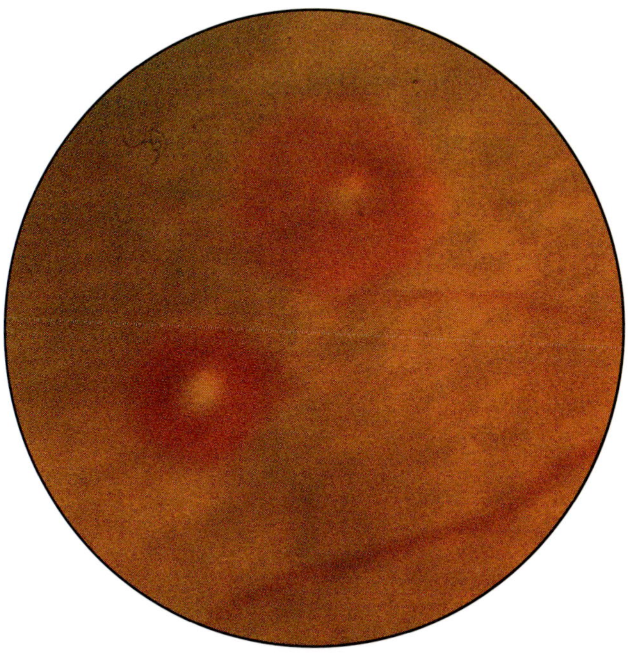

17–5

17–5A

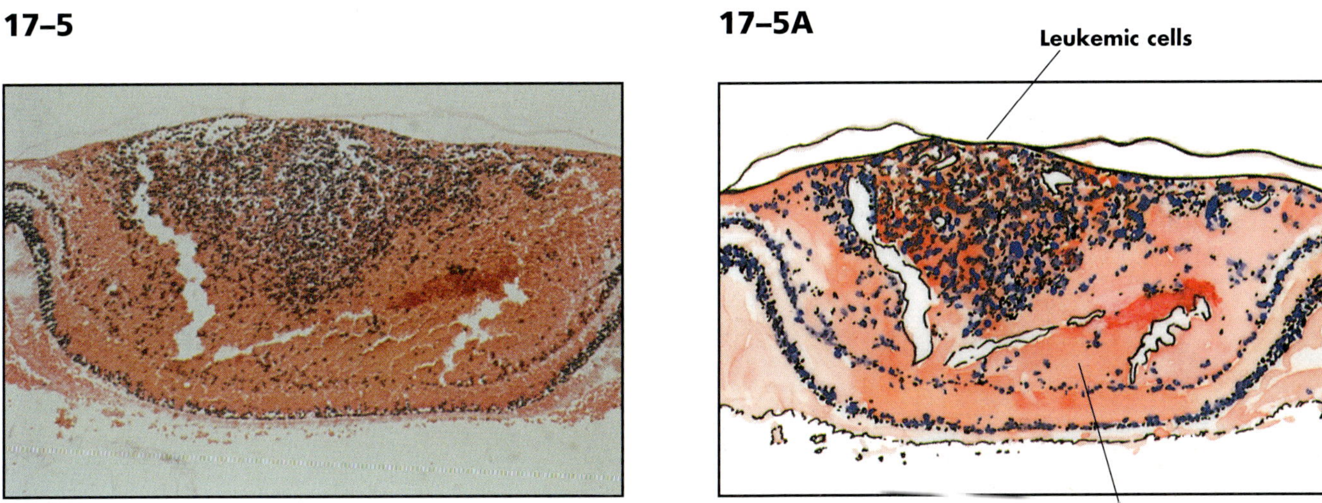

17–4 Opthalmoscopic appearance of white-centered retinal hemorrhages (Roth spots).

17–5 and 17–5A White-centered hemorrhage with the center containing leukemic cells.

17–5, *From Green, WR and McLean, IW: Retina. In Spencer, WH, ed: Ophthalmic pathology, ed 4, Philadelphia, 1996, WB Saunders.*

17–6

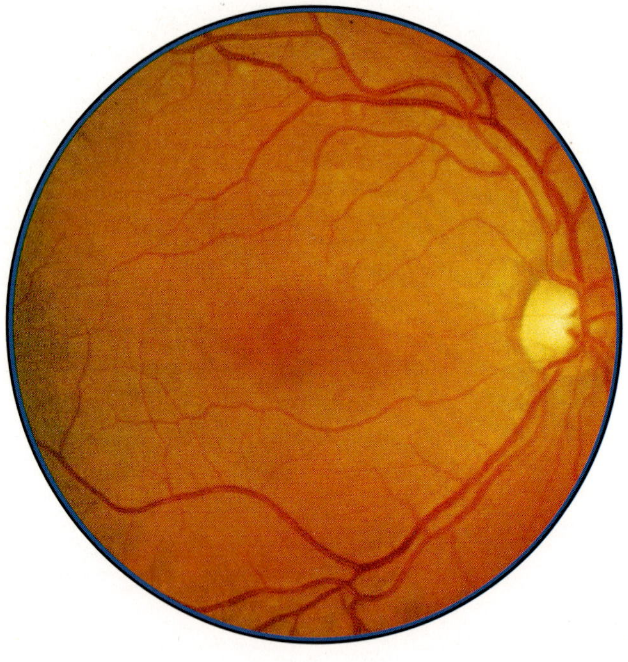

17–7

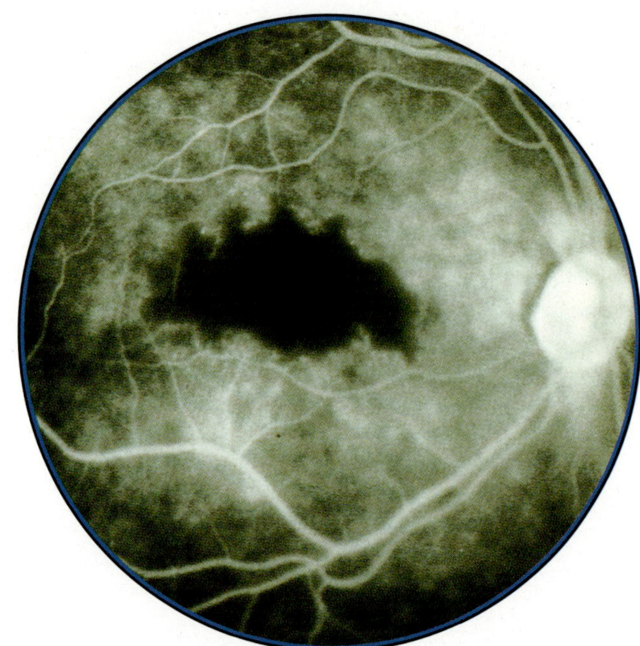

17–8A

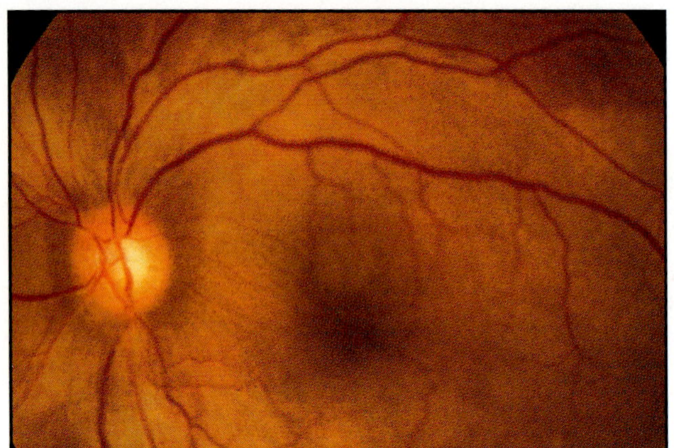

17–8B

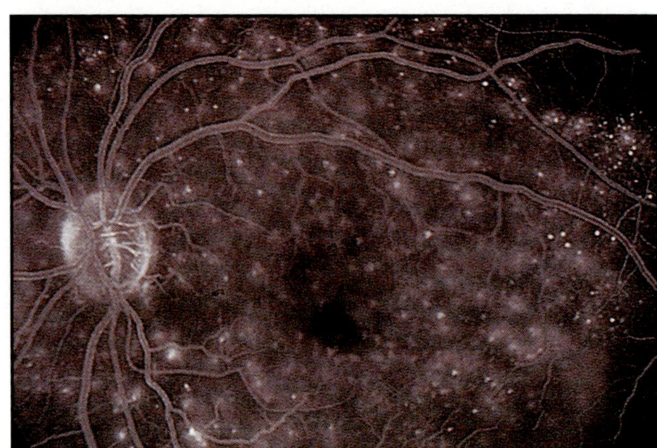

17–6 and 17–7 Leukemia rarely may show retinal vasculature changes including leakage and ischemia of the macula.

17–8A and B This patient with leukemia has a whitish-yellowish infiltrative lesion (17–8A). Fluorescein angiography reveals multiple hyperfluorescent spots (17–8B).

__17–6__ and __17–7,__ From Minnella, A, Yannuzzi, LA, Slakter, J, and Rodriguez, A: Bilateral perifoveal ischemia associated with chronic granulocytic leukemia, Arch Ophthalmol 106:1170, 1988. Copyright 1988, American Medical Association. __17–8A__ and __B,__ Courtesy of Dr. Richard Rosen.

17–9

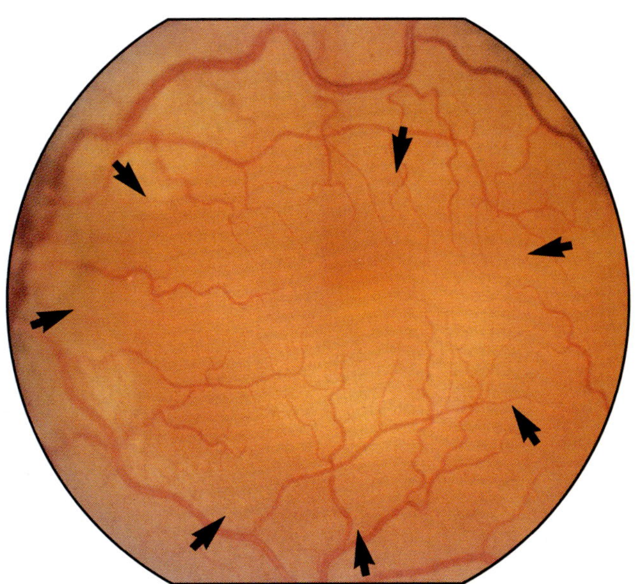

17–10

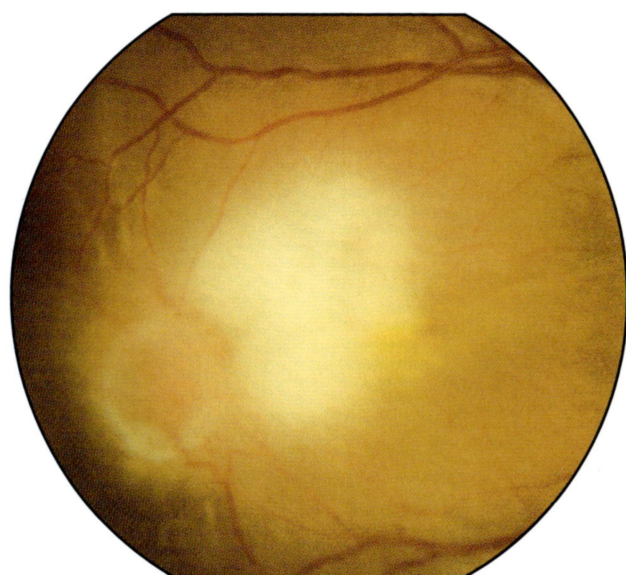

17–9 In this leukemic patient, a serous detachment is noted. Multifocal leakage was noted by fluorescein angiography in this case, which resembled a Harada's-like detachment of the macula.

17–10 This patient with leukemia developed an opportunistic infection with vitritis and a fluffy white chorioretinal lesion. Toxoplasma was identified in this case.

17–9, *Courtesy of Dr. Stuart L. Fine.* ***17–10,*** *Courtesy of Dr. H. Jay Wisnicki.*

17–11 LYMPHOMA

17–12

17–13

17–14

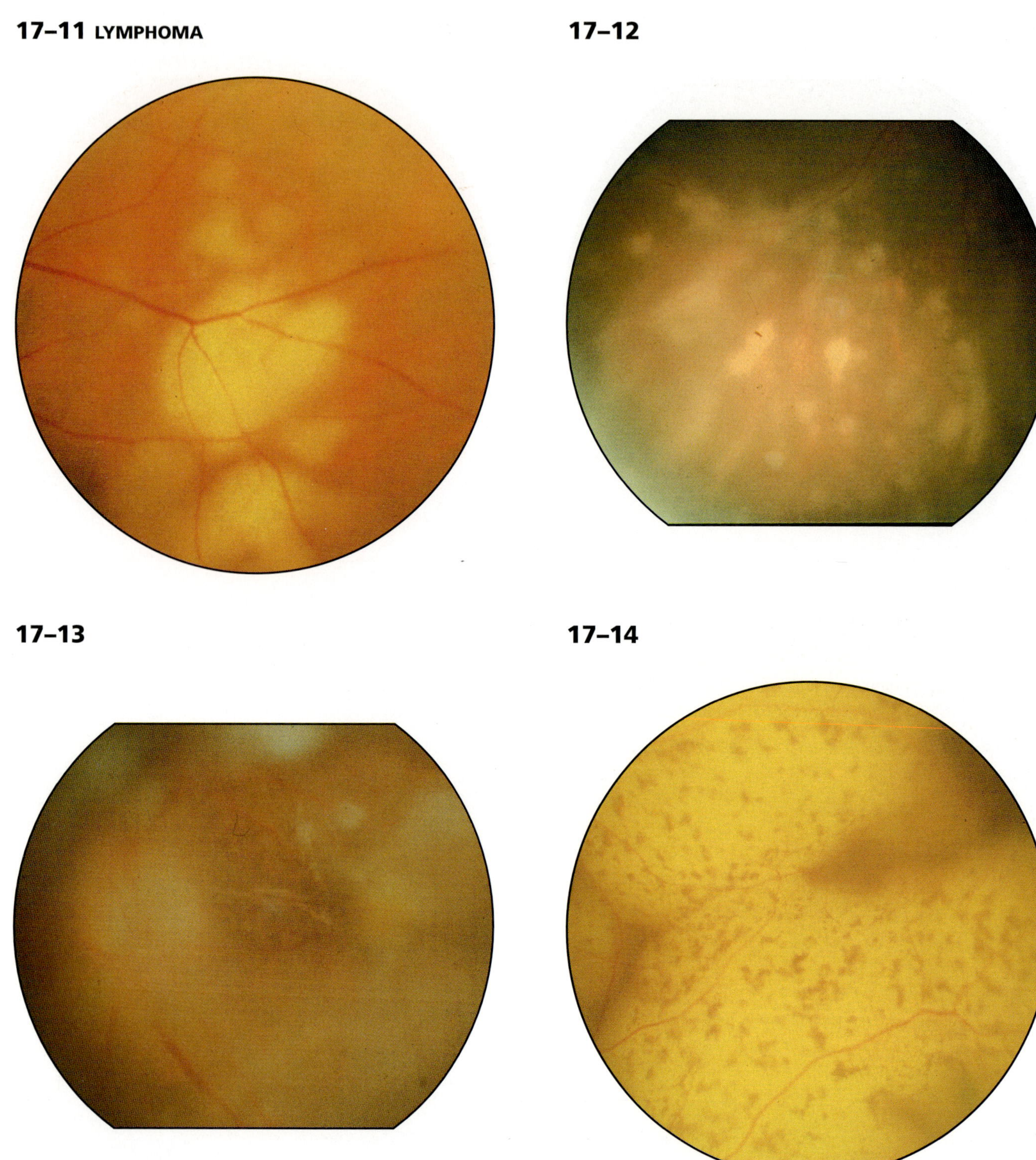

17–11 and 17–12 Large-cell lymphoma or so-called reticulum cell lymphoma may appear as deep whitish-yellow variably sized subretinal infiltrates (17–11). Retinal vasculitis and vitritis may also be noted (17–12).

17–13 Severe overlying vitritis is common in patients with large-cell lymphoma.

17–14 A leopard-type pattern may also be seen as in this patient with large subretinal infiltrative lesions.

17–15

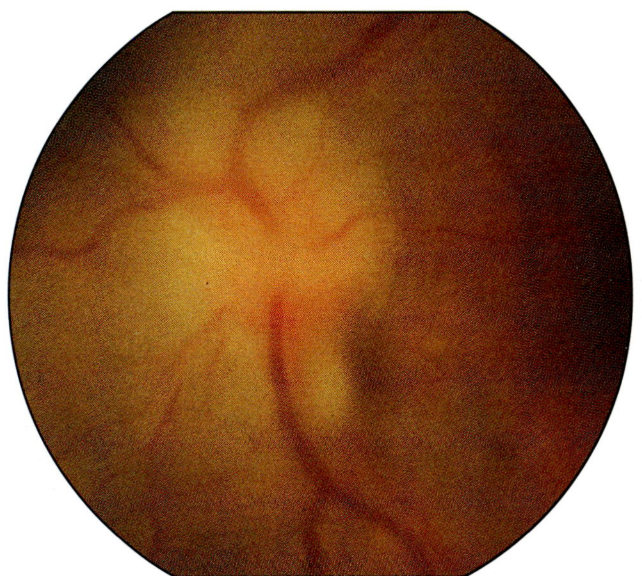

17–16

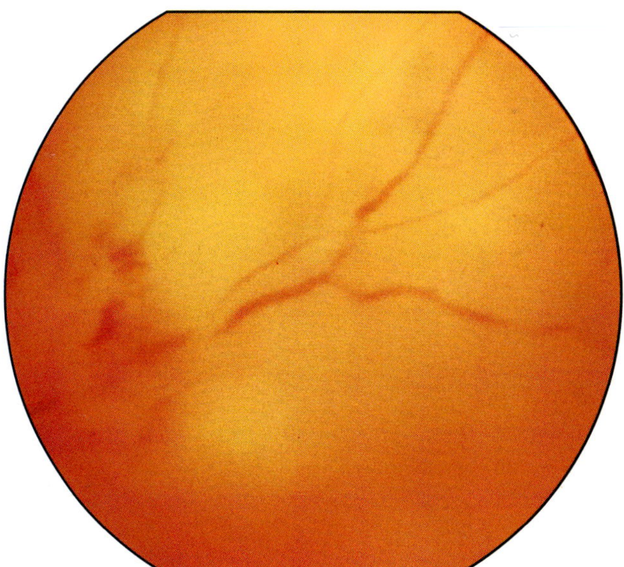

17–17

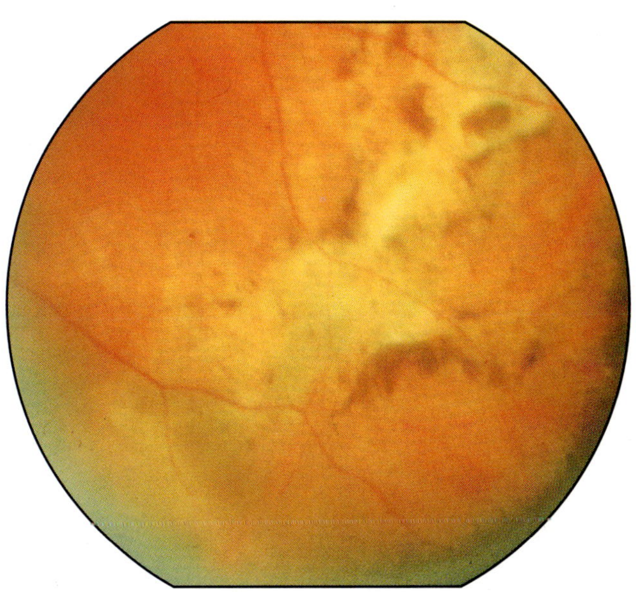

17–15 Burkitt's lymphoma may also occasionally involve the eye with multifocal chorioretinal spots, vitritis, and optic nerve infiltration.

17–16 A creamy white deep lesion with secondary hemorrhage is observed in this patient with ocular lymphoma.

17–17 This case shows scarring that developed in areas of tumor detachments of the retinal pigment epithelium.

17–17, *From Barr, CC, Green, WR, Payne, JW, Knox, DO, and Thompson, RL: Intraocular reticulum cell sarcoma: clinicopathologic study of four cases and review of literature, Surv Ophthalmol 19:224–239, 1975.*

17–18 LYMPHOMA

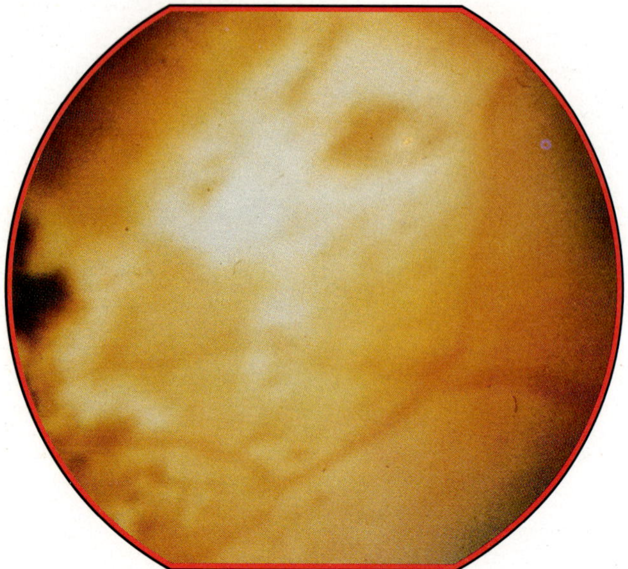

17–19

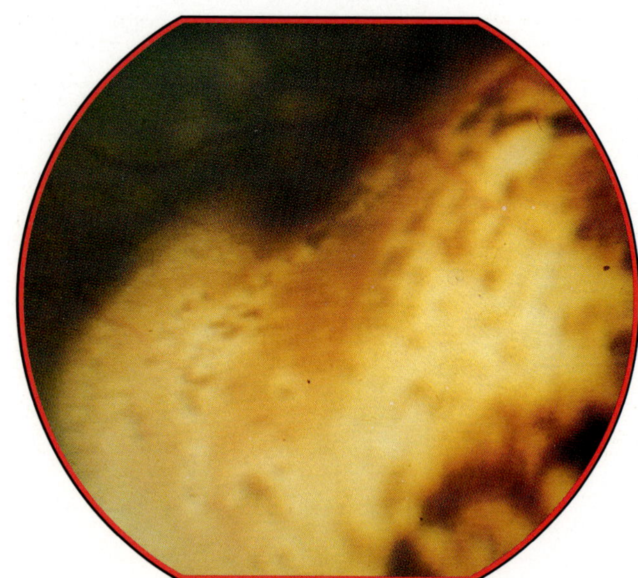

17–20

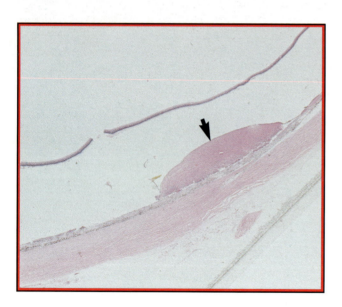

17–18 This case is a clinicopathologic correlation of a patient with ocular lymphoma. Postmortem findings of this 46-year-old female showed tumor in all organs except the brain. A large subretinal pigment epithelium mass in the superior fundus of the right eye was noted with satellite lesions 6 months after the onset of symptoms.

17–19 A large partially pigmented subretinal mass was also noted temporal to the macula in the left eye 4 months after initial symptoms.

17–20 On histopathologic examination, a large area of pigment epithelial detachment secondary to necrotic tumor was noted *(arrowhead)*.

17–18 *through* ***17–20,*** *From Barr, CC, Green, WR, Payne, JW, Knox, DO, and Thompson, RL: Intraocular reticulum cell sarcoma: clinicopathologic study of four cases and review of literature, Surv Ophthalmol 19:224–239, 1975.*

(Case continued on next page.)

17–21

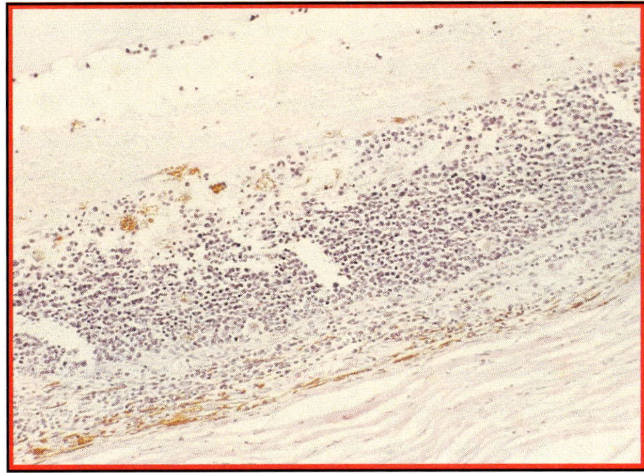

17–22

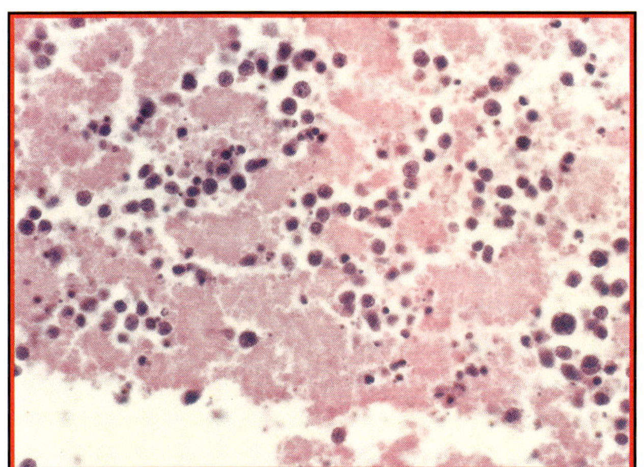

17–23

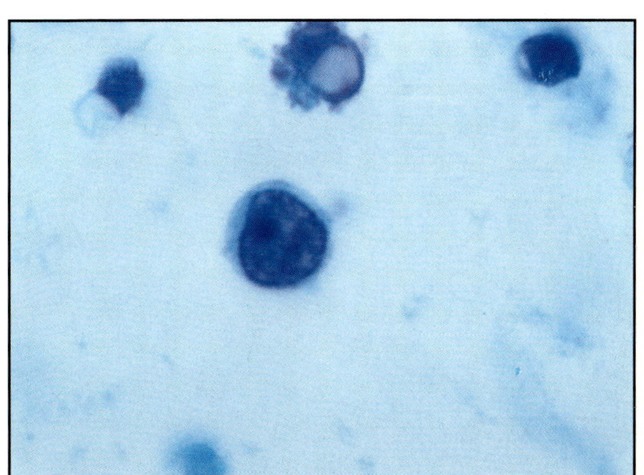

17–21 and 17–22 Higher power view of retinal pigment epithelial detachment by tumor and necrotic debris. The choroid was free of tumor.

17–23 Cytopathologic evaluation of surgically removed vitreous can be useful in the diagnosis of ocular lymphoma. This photograph shows a vitrectomy specimen consisting of characteristic lymphoma cells with scant cytoplasm, nucleolus, and nuclear membrane abnormalities.

17–21 *and* ***17–22,*** *From Barr, CC, Green, WR, Payne, JW, Knox, DO, and Thompson, RL: Intraocular reticulum cell sarcoma: clinicopathologic study of four cases and review of literature, Surv Ophthalmol 19:224–239, 1975.*

17–24 LYMPHOMA

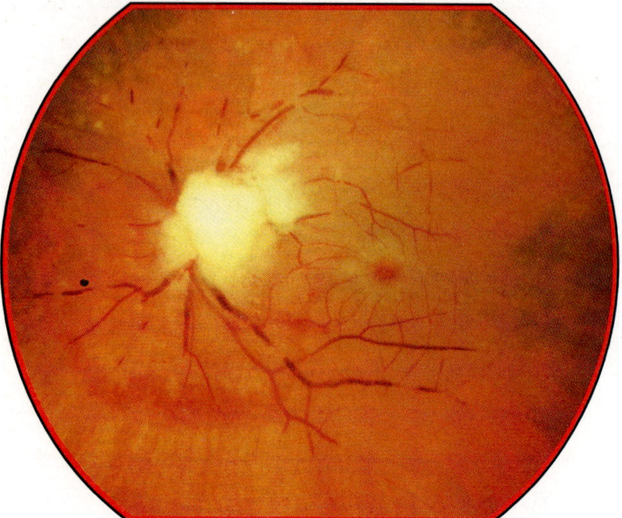

17–25

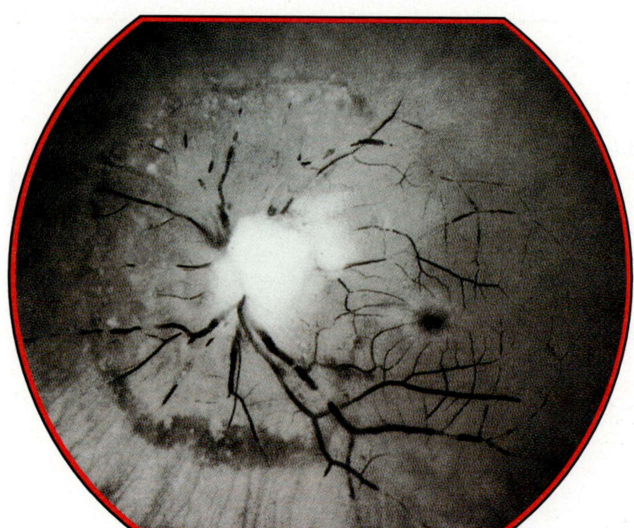

17–26

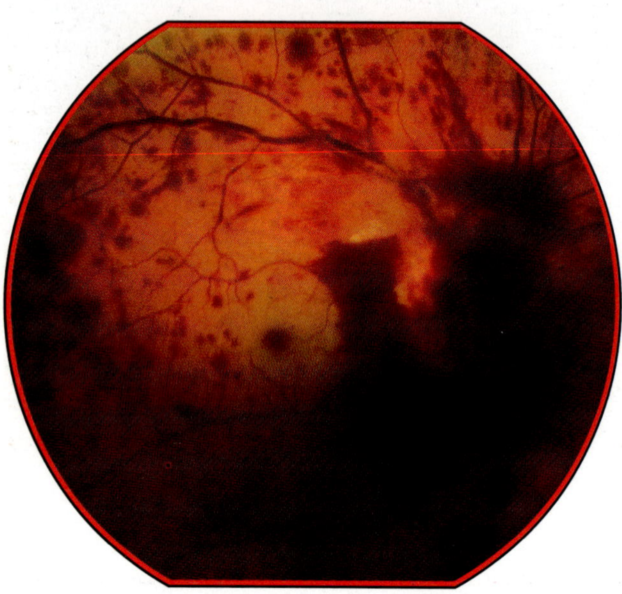

17–24 through 17–26 This 57-year-old white female with non-Hodgkins lymphoma presented with no light perception in both eyes. There was a markedly swollen optic nerve head, a cherry-red spot and vascular nonperfusion of most of the retina in the left eye (17–24). Capillary nonperfusion with attenuated and disrupted blood vessels was noted for 360° (17–24 and 17–25). The right eye demonstrated combined central retinal vein and artery occlusions.

17–24 *through* ***17–26,*** *From Green, WR, et al: Bilateral ischemic optic neuropathy and retinal vascular occlusions associated with lymphoma and sepsis, Ophthalmology 97:882–888, 1990.*

(Case continued on next page.)

17–27

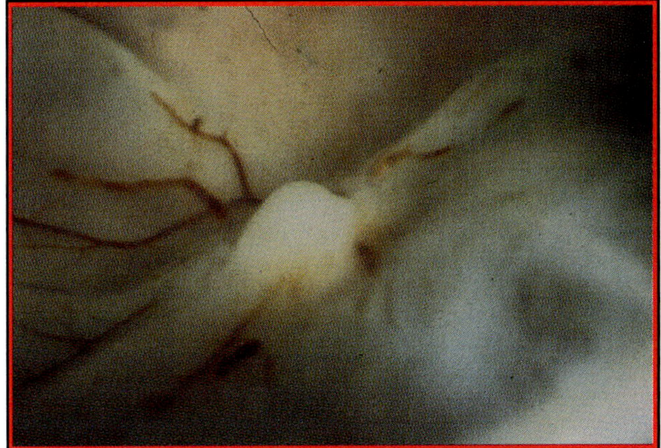

17–28

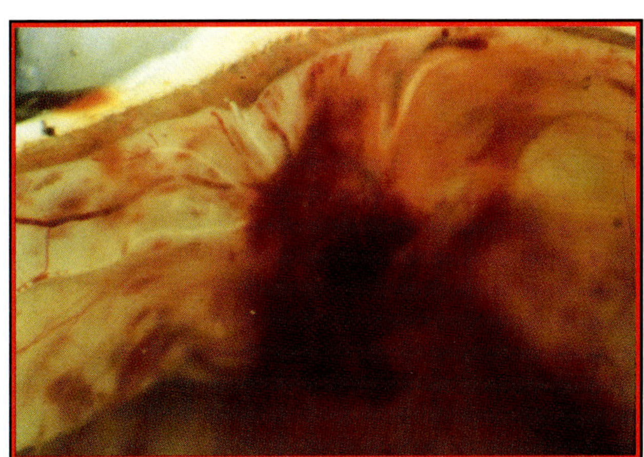

17–29

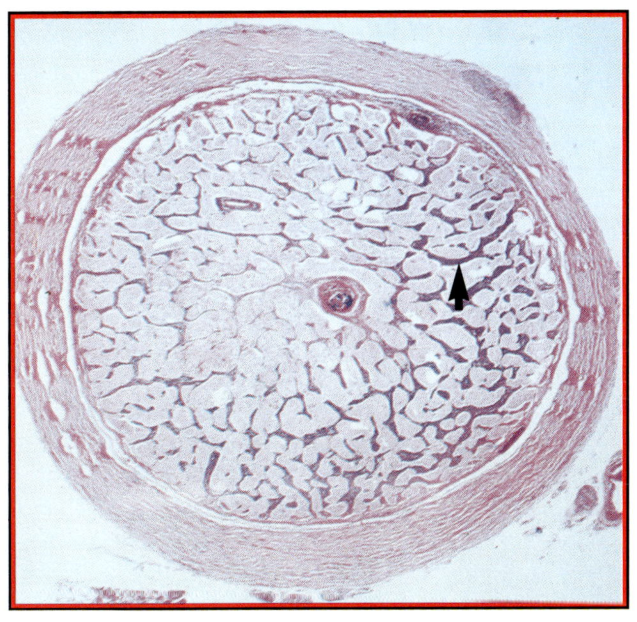

17–30

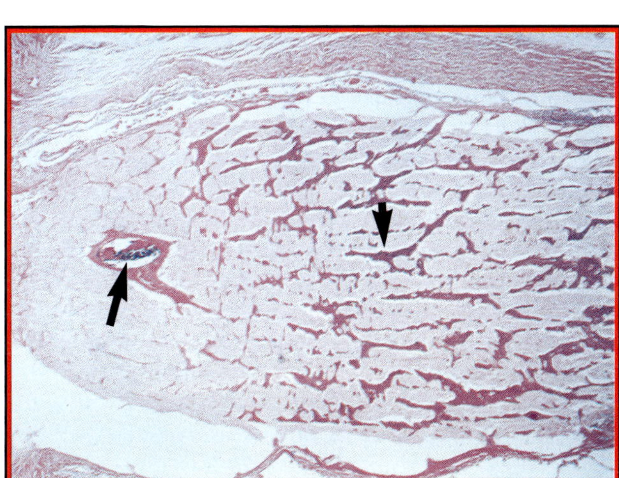

17–27 through 17–30 The patient died secondary to sepsis. Gross examination of the left eye reveals a markedly swollen optic nerve head. Hemorrhage and occluded retinal vessels are noted throughout the fundus of the right eye. Light microscopy reveals tumor invasion of the optic nerve *(arrowhead)* and septic emboli in the central retinal vessels *(arrow)*.

***17–27** through **17–30,** From Green, WR, et al: Bilateral ischemic optic neuropathy and retinal vascular occlusions associated with lymphoma and sepsis, Ophthalmology 97:882–888, 1990.*

17–31 BENIGN LYMPHOID HYPERPLASIA

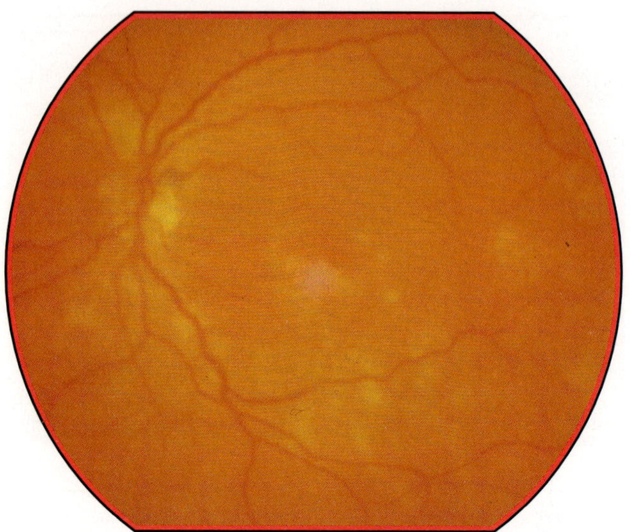

17–32

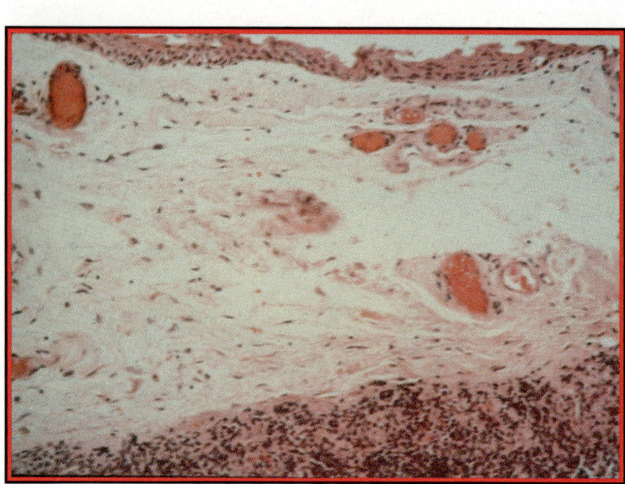

17–31 Patients with benign lymphoid hyperplasia may also demonstrate focal whitish-yellow choroidal lesions.

17–32 Histopathologic examination of a conjunctival biopsy disclosed a monomorphic infiltrate of well-differentiated lymphocytes.

17–31 *and* ***17–32,*** *Courtesy of Dr. Evan Sachs.*

Suggested Readings

Al-Hazza, SAF, Green, WR, and Mann, RB: Uveal involvement in systemic angiotropic large cell lymphoma: microscopic and immunohistochemical studies, Ophthalmol 100 (June): 961–965, 1993

Allen, RA, and Straatsma, BA: Ocular involvement in leukemia and allied disorders, Arch Ophthalmol 66:490–508, 1961

Barr, CC, Green, WR, Payne, JW, Knox, DL, Jensen, AD, and Thompson, RL: Intraocular reticulum cell sarcoma: a clinicopathologic study of four cases and review of the literature, Surv Ophthalmol 19:224–238, 1975

Barr, CC, and Joondeph, HC: Retinal periphlebitis as the initial clinical finding in a patient with Hodgkin's disease, Retina 3:253–257, 1983

Belmont, JB, Michelson, JB, and Bordin, GM: Ocular inflammation associated with chronic lymphocytic leukemia, J Ocul Ther Surg 4:125–129, 1985

Brihayeian Gerrtruyden, M: Retinal lesions in Hodgkin's disease, Arch Ophthalmol 56:94–99, 1956

Char, DH, Ljung, B, Deschenes, J, and Miller, TR: Intraocular lymphoma: immunological and cytological analysis, Br J Ophthalmol 72:905–911, 1988

Diddie, KR, Schanzlin, DJ, Mausolf, FA, Minckler, DS, and Trousdale, MD: Necrotizing retinitis caused by opportunistic virus infection in a patient with Hodgkin's disease, Am J Ophthalmol 88:668–673, 1979

Freeman, LN, Schachat, AP, Knox, DL, Michels, RG, and Green, WR: Clinical features, laboratory investigations, and survival in ocular reticulum cell sarcoma, Ophthalmology 94:1631–1939, 1987

Guyer, DR, Schachat, AP, Vitale, S, Markowitz, JA, Braine, H, Burke, PJ, Karp, JE, and Graham, M: Leukemic retinopathy: relationship between fundus lesions and hematologic parameters at diagnosis, Ophthalmology 96:860–864, 1989

Karp, LA, Zimmerman, LE, and Payne, T: Intraocular involvement in Burkitt's lymphoma, Arch Ophthalmol 85:295–298, 1971

Kincaid, MC, and Green, WR: Ocular and orbital involvement in leukemia, Surv Ophthalmol 27:211–232, 1983

Knapp, AJ, Gartner, S, and Henkind, P: Multiple myeloma and its ocular manifestations, Surv Ophthalmol 31:343–351, 1987

Lang, GK, Surer, JL, Green, WR, Finkelstein, D, Michels, RG, and Maumenee, AE: Ocular reticulum cell sarcoma. Clinicopathologic correlation of a case with multifocal lesions, Retina 5:79–86, 1985

Lewis, RA, and Clark, RB: Infiltrative retinopathy in systemic lymphoma, Am J Ophthalmol 79:48–52, 1975

Lopez, PF, Sternberg, P, Dabbs, CK, Vogler, WR, Crocker, I, and Kalin, NS: Bone marrow transplant retinopathy, Am J Ophthalmol 112:635–646, 1991

Michels, RG, Knox, DL, Erozan, VS, and Green, WR: Intraocular reticulum cell sarcoma: diagnosis by pars plana vitrectomy, Arch Ophthalmol 93:1331–1335, 1975

Minnella, A, Yannuzzi, LA, Slakter, J, and Rodriguez, A: Bilateral perifoveal ischemia associated with chronic granulocytic leukemia, Arch Ophthalmol, 106:1170, 1988

Ridley, ME, McDonald, HR, Sternberg, P, Blumenkranz, MS, Zarbin, MA, and Schachat, AP: Retinal manifestations of ocular lymphoma (reticulum cell sarcoma), Ophthalmology 99:1153–1161, 1992

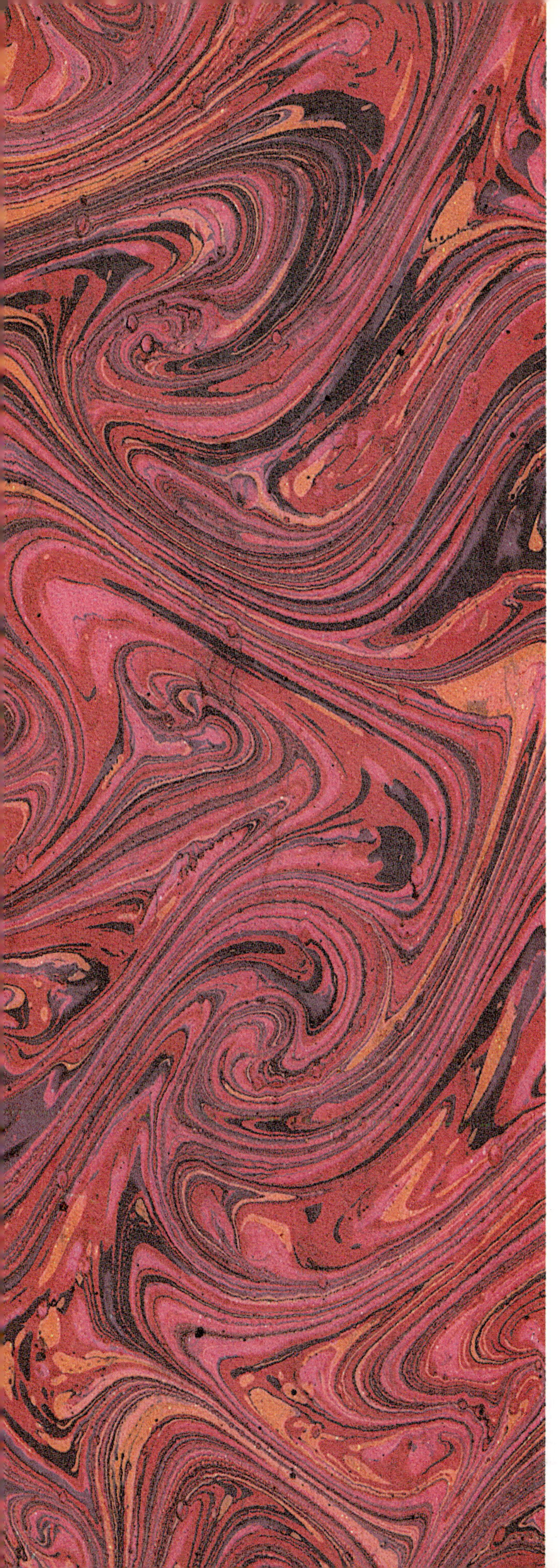

Part VI

Macular Diseases

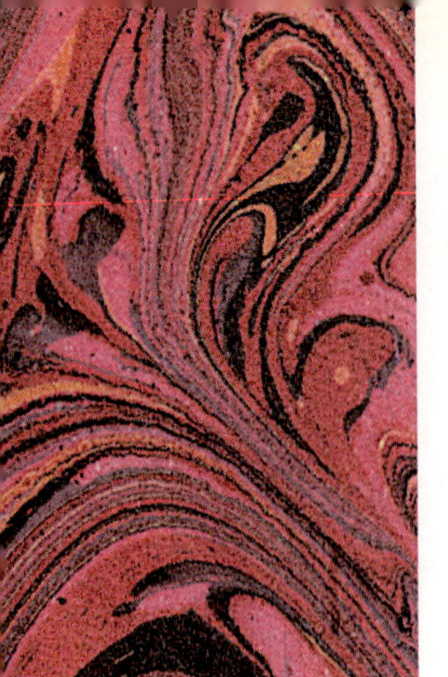

Chapter 18
Age-Related Macular Degeneration

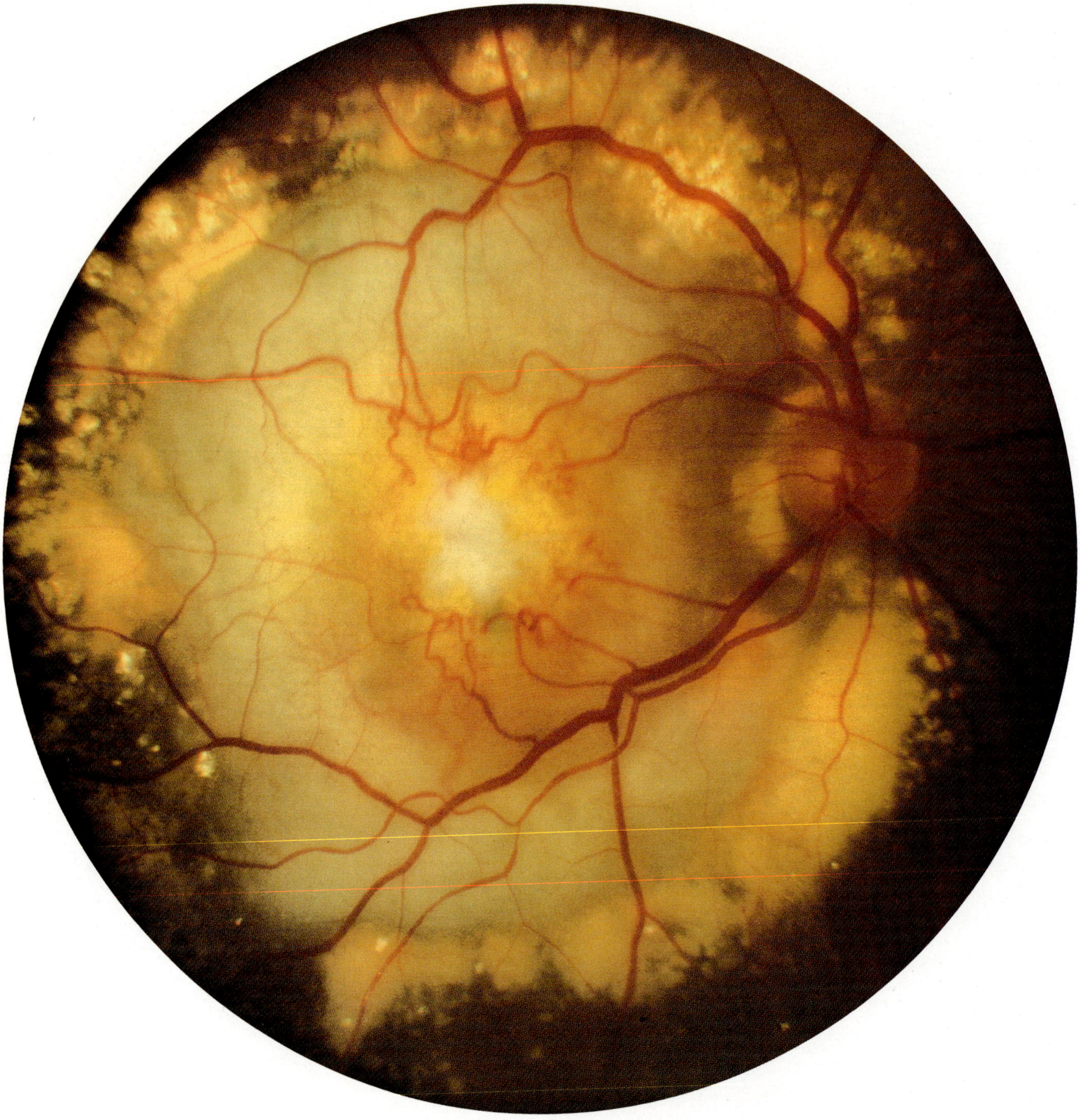

Age-related macular degeneration is the most common cause of irreversible blindness in the Western world. Various reports suggest that between 6% and 10% of people between 65 and 74 years of age and between 19% and 30% of people over 75 years of age have this condition. Several risk factors have been identified including age, sex, hereditary, light irides, cigarette smoking, cardiovascular disease, and environment factors such as light toxicity and nutrition. Thus, the condition appears to be multifactorial. The most important factor, however, is the aging process.

There are two types of age-related macular degeneration. The atrophic, or dry form, of the condition includes drusen and geographic atrophy and is responsible for approximately 90% of cases. Although the exudative, or wet form of the disease is only present in approximately 10% of cases, it is responsible for approximately 90% of the severe vision loss associated with macular degeneration.

The earliest finding of this condition is drusen, which are deposits of extracellular material between the basement membrane of the retinal pigment epithelium and Bruch's membrane. Several types of drusen have been identified including hard drusen or nodular drusen, soft drusen, and cuticular drusen. Soft drusen predispose to exudative changes and may represent small serous pigment epithelial detachments.

Geographic atrophy, which consists of retinal pigment epithelial changes, also may occur as part of nonexudative macular degeneration.

Exudative age-related macular degeneration with abnormal blood vessel growth or choroidal neovascularization is the major cause of severe vision loss in this disease. Other forms of exudative macular degeneration in addition to choroidal neovascularization include retinal pigment epithelial detachments, retinal pigment epithelial rips or tears, disciform scars, and rarely vitreous hemorrhage. Well-delineated or classic choroidal neovascularization identified by fluorescein angiography may be eligible for laser photocoagulation, which can decrease the risk of severe vision loss by approximately 50%. However, recurrences are common and occur in approximately 50% to 60% of treated cases.

Unfortunately, the great majority of patients with exudative maculopathy have poorly defined or occult choroidal neovascularization in which the fluorescein angiogram cannot image the neovascularization well enough to permit laser photocoagulation. Occult choroidal neovascularization may be divided into cases with or without pigment epithelial detachments. Digital indocyanine-green videoangiography is a new technique that may benefit some of these patients with occult neovascularization. Antiangiogenic drugs may be an alternative treatment for such patients in the near future.

Non-exudative Macular Degeneration

18–1 DRUSEN

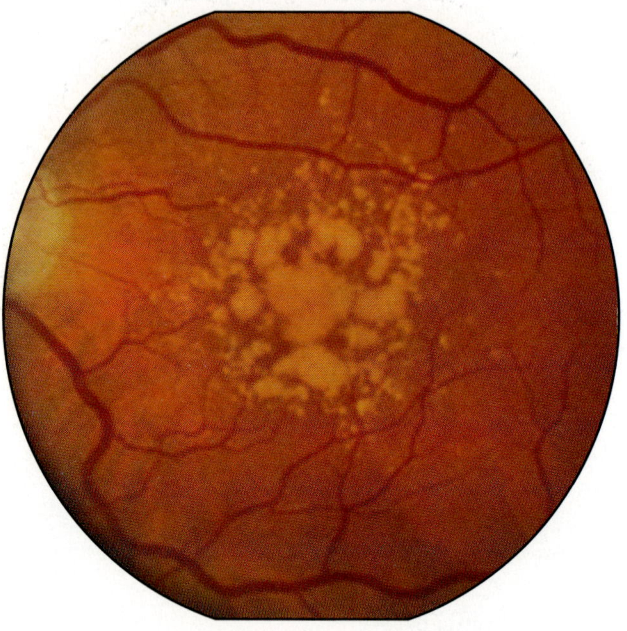

18–2 18–3

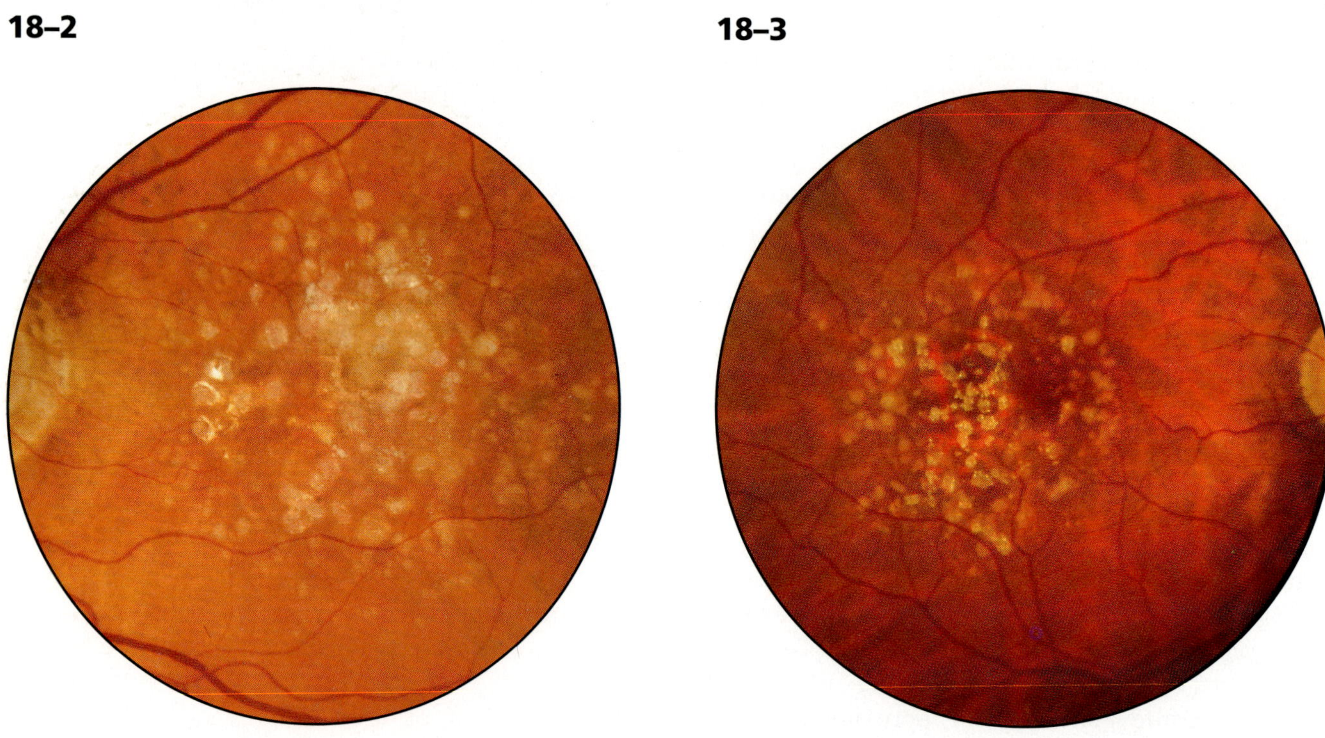

18–1 Drusen are the earliest form of age-related macular degeneration. Drusen may be hard or nodular, soft or diffuse or cuticular. Risk factors for exudative maculopathy include confluency of drusen and retinal pigment epithelium hyperpigmentation. The first patient has hard drusen as well as larger soft or diffuse drusen, which are seen centrally in this case.

18–2 and 18–3 Mineralization of drusen can sometimes occur.

18–1, *Courtesy of Mark Croswell.*

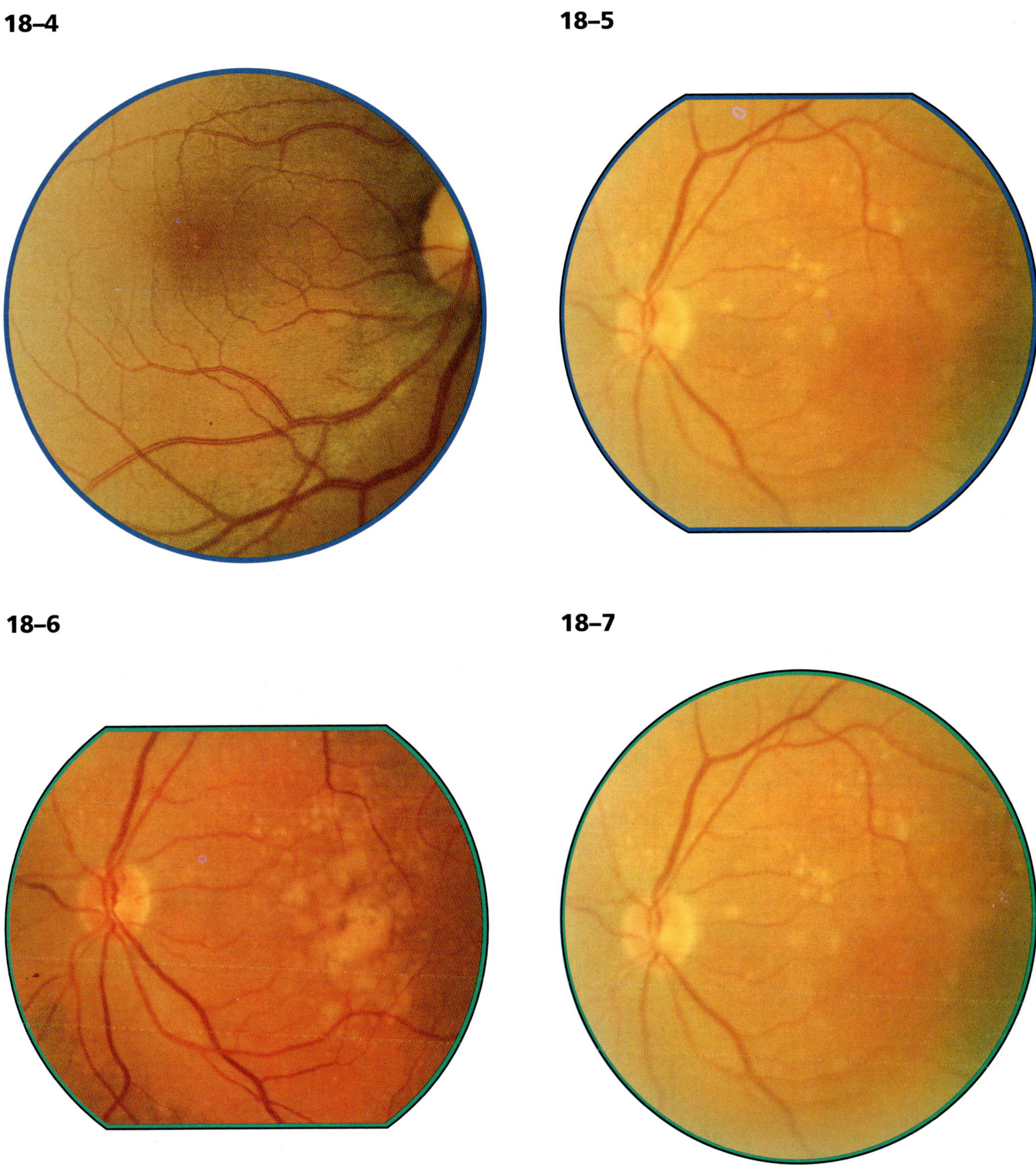

18–4 and 18–5 Drusen are usually bilateral and symmetric, however, in this case, marked asymmetry of the drusen can be appreciated when comparing the patient's two eyes.

18–6 and 18–7 Drusen can rarely disappear spontaneously as seen in this case. The second photograph shows the same eye approximately 2.5 years later.

18–8 PATHOLOGY: DRUSEN

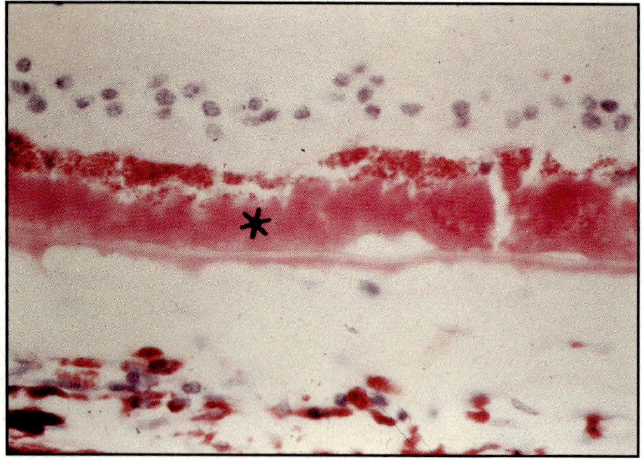

18–9

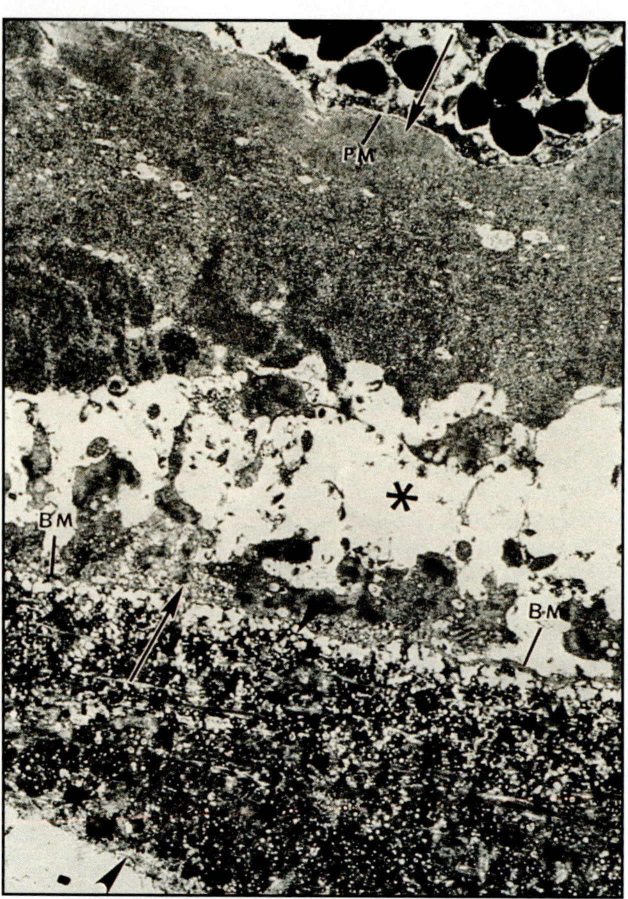

18–8 Early histopathologic changes of age-related macular degeneration include diffuse thickening of the inner portion of Bruch's membrane, which consists of basal laminar and linear deposits. Basal laminar deposits are located between the attenuated retinal pigment epithelium and the basement membrane of the retinal pigment epithelium *(asterisk)*.

18–9 Ultrastructural analysis reveals that the basal laminar deposits (between the arrows) are located between the plasma membrane (PM) and the basement membrane (BM) of the retinal pigment epithelium and consist mostly of wide-spaced collagen. A cleavage in this material *(asterisk)* led to early detachment. Vesicular material (basal linear deposit) is present throughout Bruch's membrane (between arrowheads).

***18–8** and **18–9**, From Green, WR, Enger, C: Age-related macular degeneration histopathologic studies. The 1992 Lorenz E. Zimmerman Lecture, Ophthalmology 100:1519–1535, 1993.*

18–10

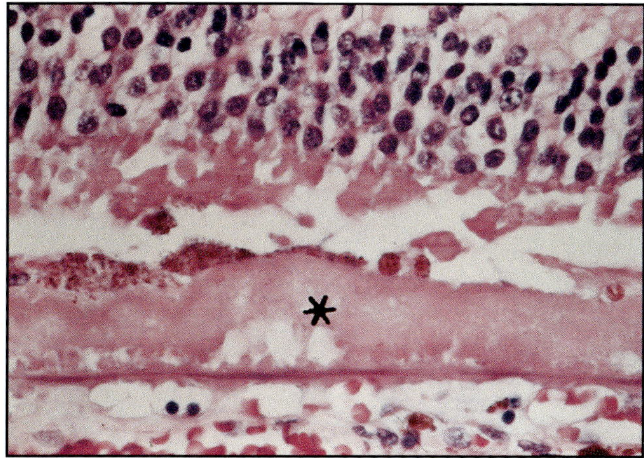

18–11

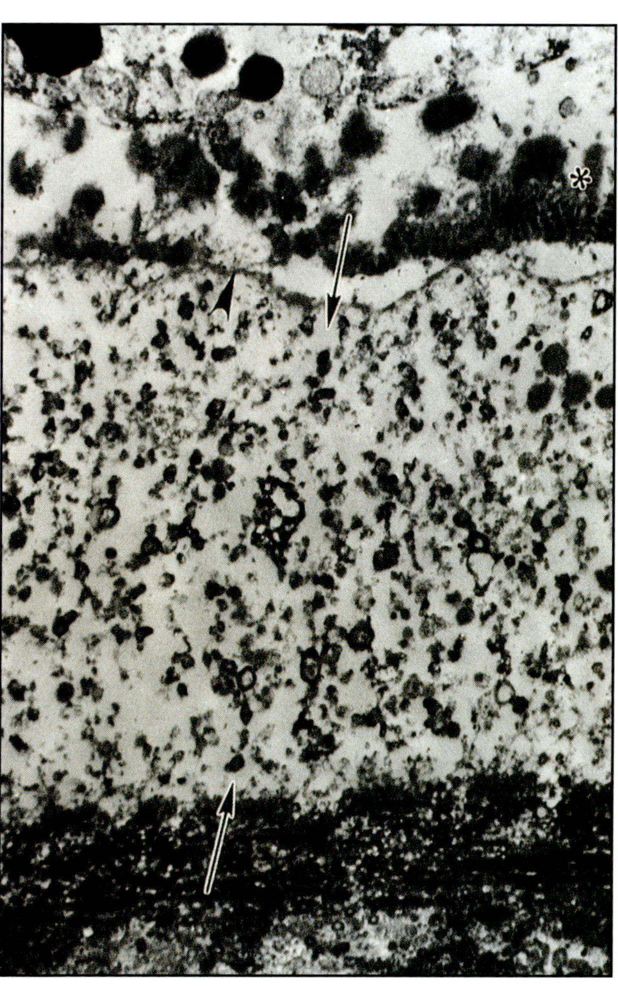

18–10 Basal linear deposits, or diffuse drusen, cause diffuse thickening of the inner aspect of Bruch's membrane *(asterisk)*.

18–11 Electron microscopic analysis of basal linear deposits shows that this material is composed of coated and noncoated vesicular material (between the arrows) located between the retinal pigment epithelium basement membrane *(arrowhead)* and the remainder of Bruch's membrane. Wide-spaced collagen (basal laminar deposit) *(asterisk)* is noted internal to the retinal pigment epithelium basement membrane *(arrowhead)*.

***18–10** and **18–11,** From Green, WR, Enger, C: Age-related macular degeneration histopathologic studies. The 1992 Lorenz E. Zimmerman Lecture, Ophthalmology 100:1519–1535, 1993.*

18–12 DRUSEN

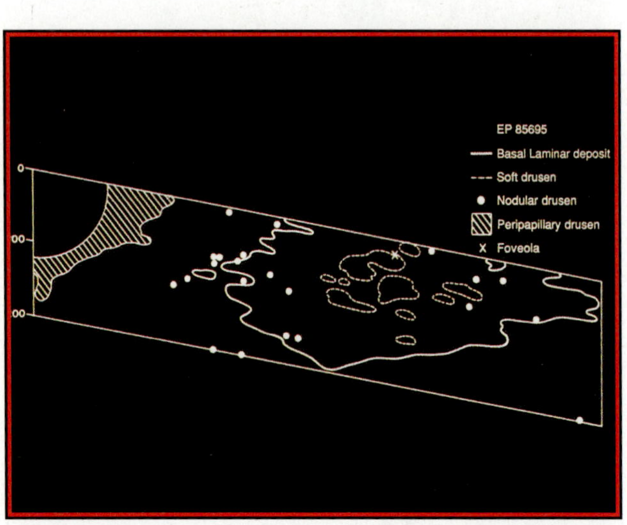

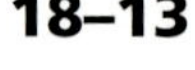

18–13

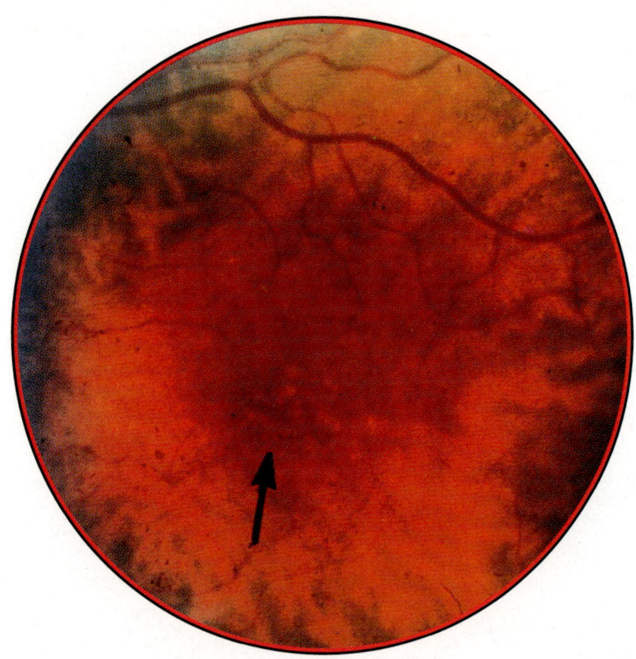

18–12 through 18–15 This case illustrates the clinicopathologic features of soft drusen due to the localized accumulation of basal linear deposit. The clinical photograph shows the soft drusen *(arrow)*. A two-dimensional reconstruction map from the study of serial sections depicts the relationships of the soft drusen, extent of basal laminar deposit, and rare scattered nodular drusen. Histopathologic examination reveals a localized detachment *(asterisk)* of the intact retinal pigment epithelium and a thin layer of basal laminar deposit *(arrow)*. Ultrastructurally, the soft druse consists of a localized accumulation of basal linear material (between the arrows and insert C) located between the retinal pigment epithelial basement membrane (BM) and the remainder of Bruch's membrane. A thin layer of basal laminar deposit (between arrowheads and insert B) is noted between the intact retinal pigment epithelium and its basement membrane. The detachment of the basal linear deposit *(asterisk)* is probably artifact (cc, choriocapillaris). Higher-power magnification of the basal laminar deposits with widespread collagen with a periodicity of 100 nm (insert B). Higher-power view of the basal linear deposits with granular and vesicular material (insert C).

18–12 *through* ***18–15,*** *From Green, WR, Enger, C: Age-related macular degeneration histopathologic studies. The 1992 Lorenz E. Zimmerman Lecture, Ophthalmology 100:1519–1535, 1993.*

18–14

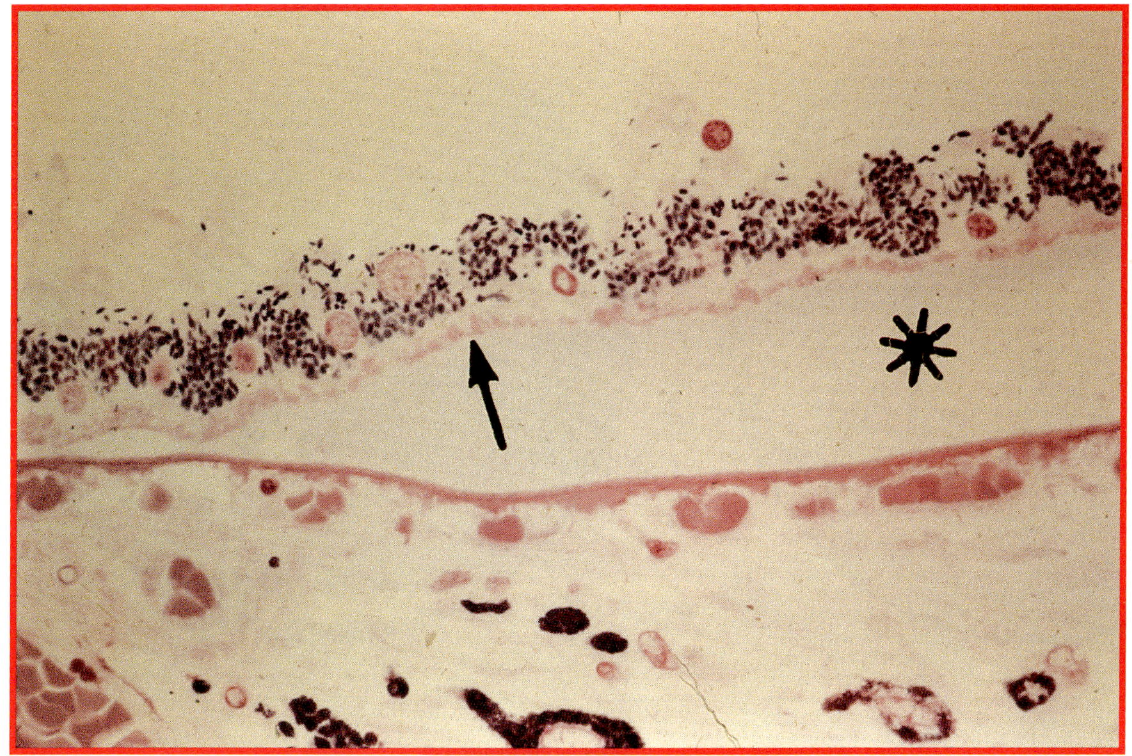

18–15

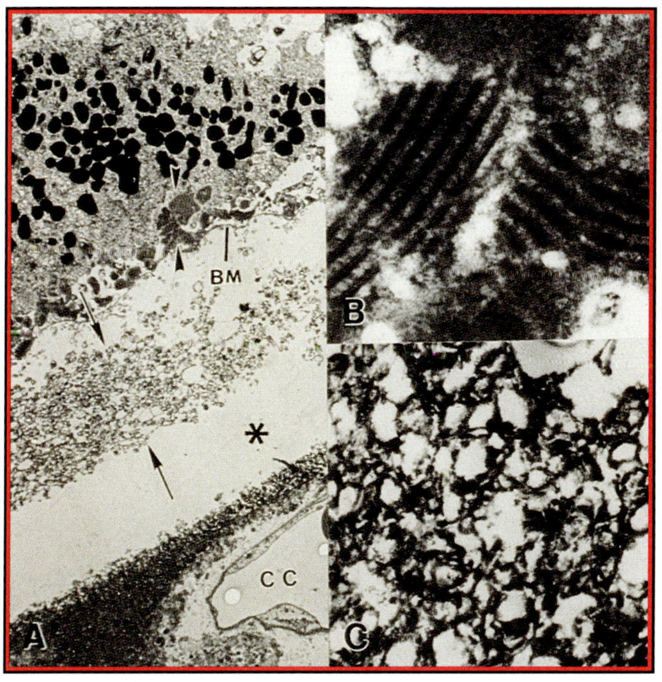

18–16 GEOGRAPHIC ATROPHY

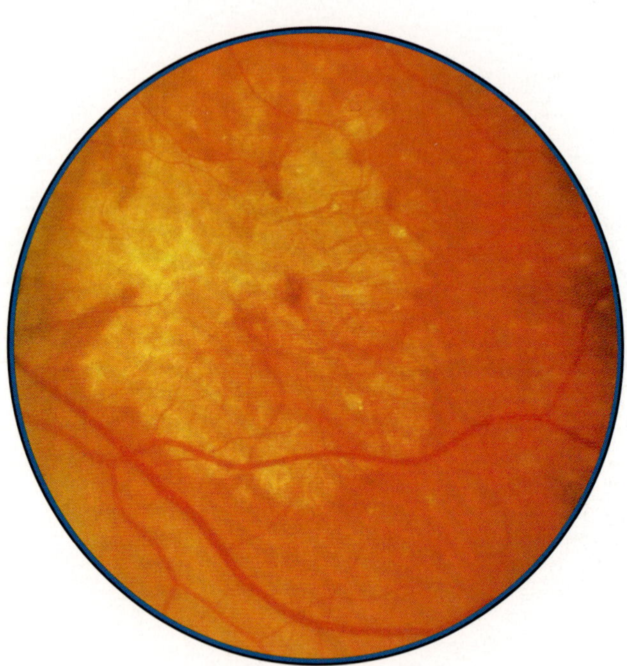

18–17

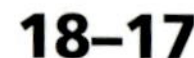

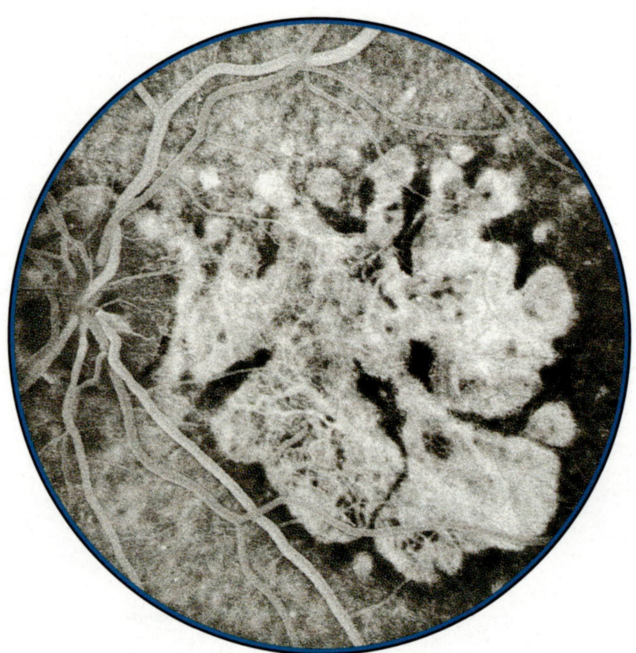

18–16 and 18–17 Atrophic, geographic, or areolar atrophy may be seen in the dry form of macular degeneration. Retinal pigment epithelial atrophy can be noted in these cases. Window defects are noted on the corresponding fluorescein angiogram.

18–16 *and* ***18–17,*** *Courtesy of Dr. Neil Bressler and the Wilmer Reading Center, copyright Wilmer Reading Center, 1994.*

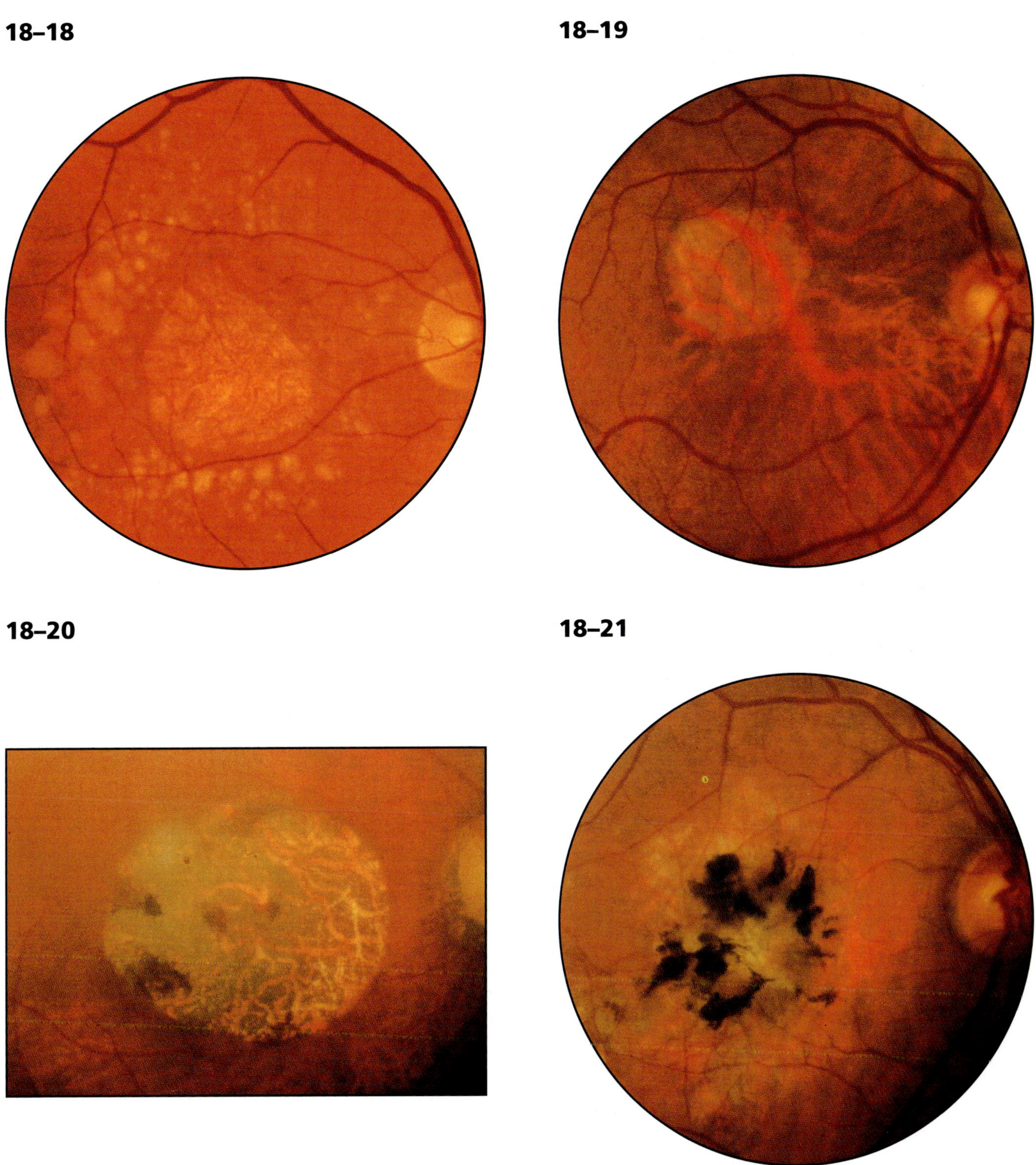

18–18 through 18–21 Geographic atrophy can appear primarily as hypopigmentation with (18–18) or without (18–19) associated drusen or varying degrees of hyperpigmentation and metaplasia (18–21).

18–22 EVOLUTION OF GEOGRAPHIC ATROPHY

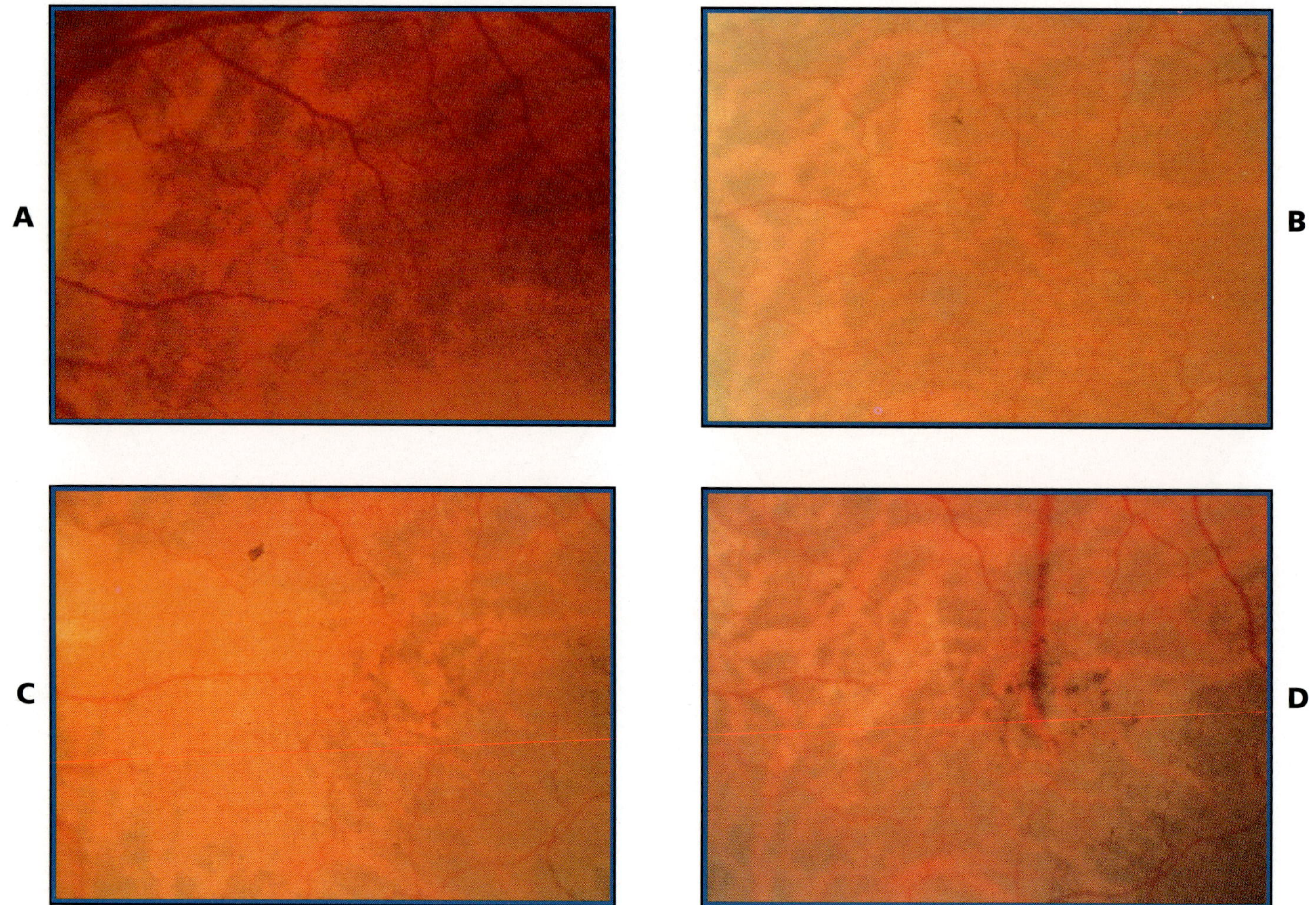

18–22 and 18–23 These photographs illustrate the evolution of age-related geographic atrophy over 16 years. The first frame shows the normal fundus seen in a tigroid pattern *(18–22, A)*; vision is 20/15. The second frame shows the patient five years later with drusen faintly visible *(18–22, B)*; vision at this time is 20/20. A ring of pigment clumping later is noted to develop around the center of the fovea *(18–22, C)*. Two years later, the pigment clumping around fixation has increased *(18–22, D)*; vision is still 20/20. At this point, the choroidal vasculature pattern is still prominent. Two years later, the patient fixates between the two small areas of atrophy that have developed *(18–23, A and B)*. Pigment clumping and small drusen are spreading outward. The surrounding incipient atrophy corresponds to the area of geographic atrophy that develops subsequently. One year later the atrophic area involves fixation; vision has dropped to 20/200 *(18–23, C)*. Later, the atrophy has almost doubled in area *(18–23, D)*; vision is 20/400. The choroidal atrophy has caused exposed vessels to appear white.

18–23

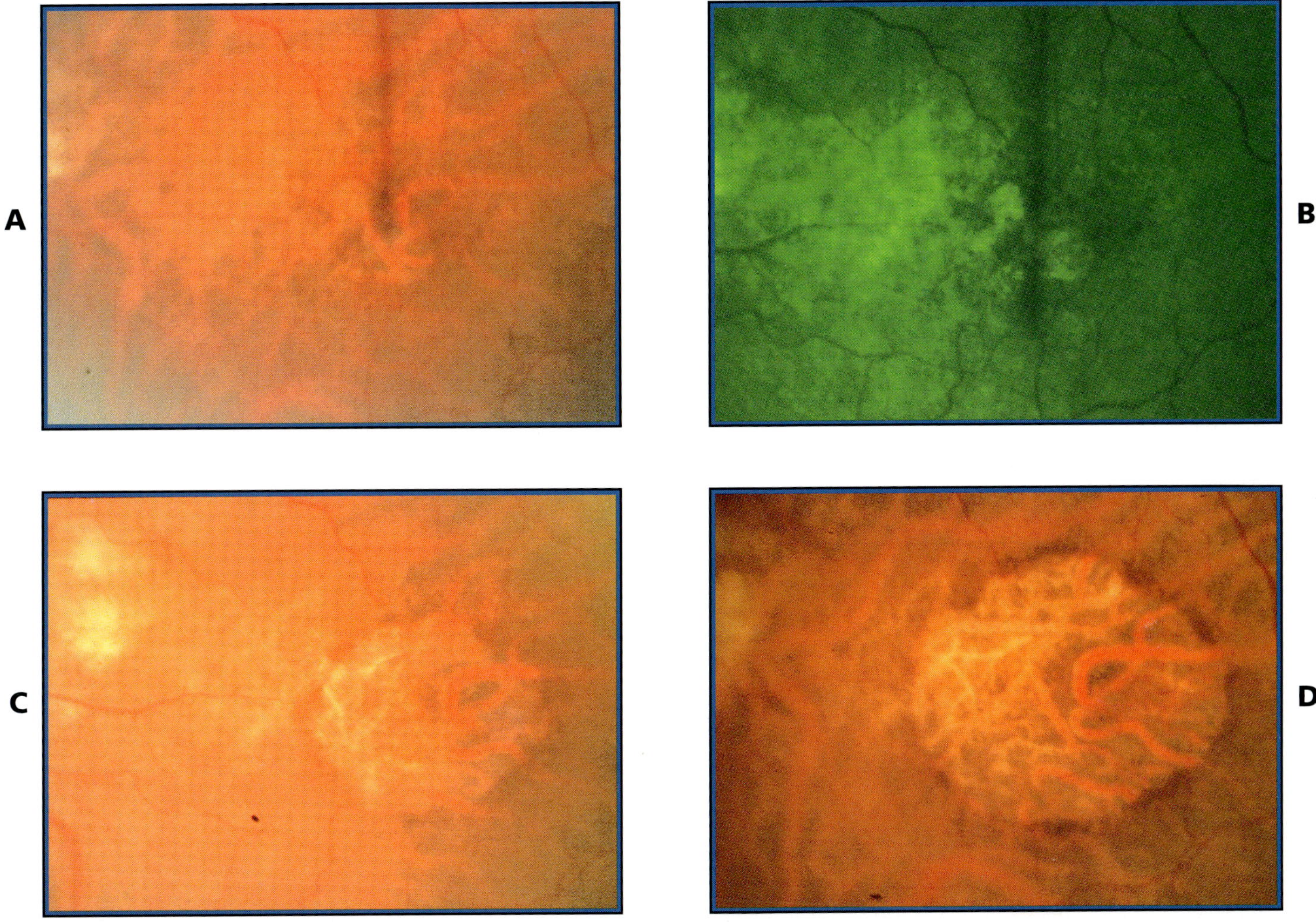

18–24 GEOGRAPHIC ATROPHY

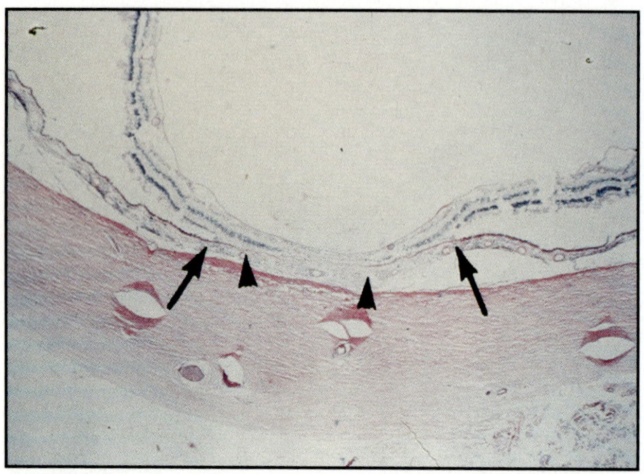

18–25

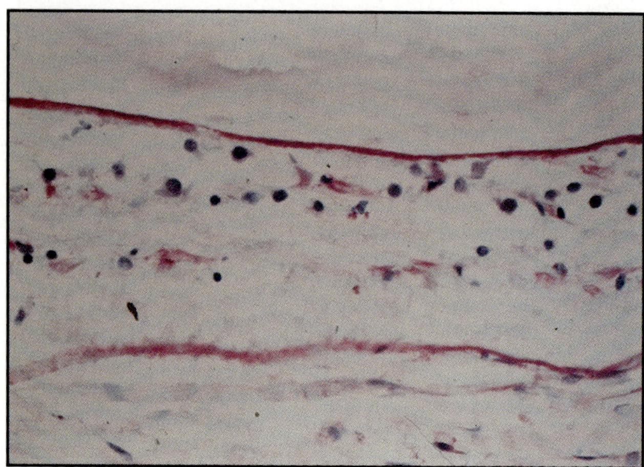

18–26

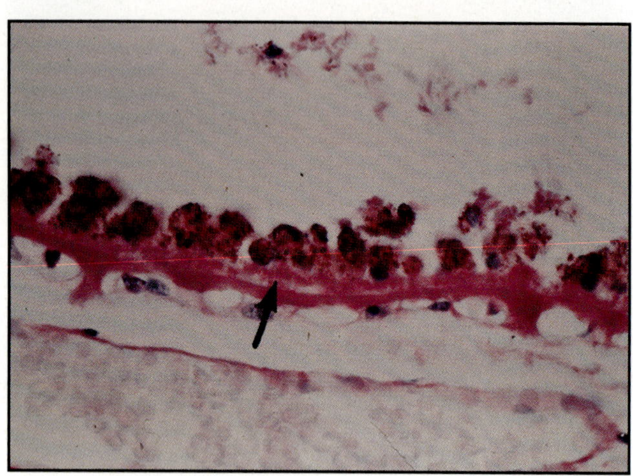

18–24 through 18–26 This histopathologic correlation of an eye with geographic atrophy reveals total retinal pigment epithelial and photoreceptor cell atrophy in a 2-mm central area (between arrows) (18–24). Centrally there is loss of basal laminar deposits (18–24 between arrowheads and 18–25). Basal laminar deposits are present outside this area *(arrow)*.

***18–24** through **18–26,** From Green, WR, and Enger, C: Age-related macular degeneration histopathologic studies. The 1992 Lorenz E. Zimmerman Lecture, Ophthalmology 100:1519–1535, 1993.*

Exudative Macular Degeneration

18–27 CHOROIDAL NEOVASCULARIZATION

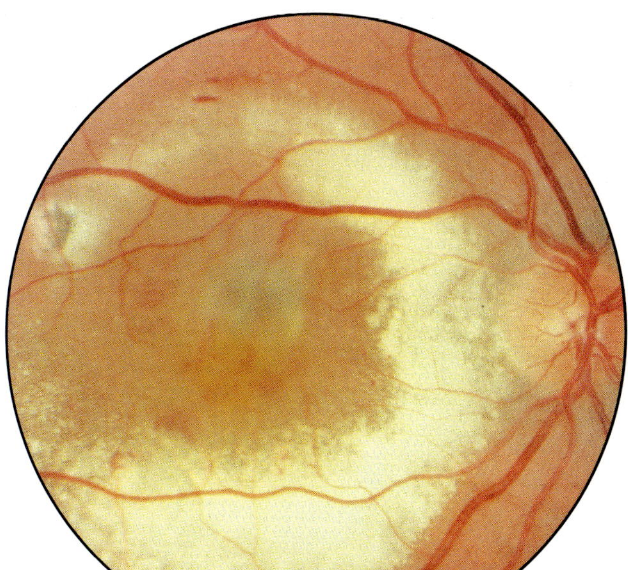

18–27A

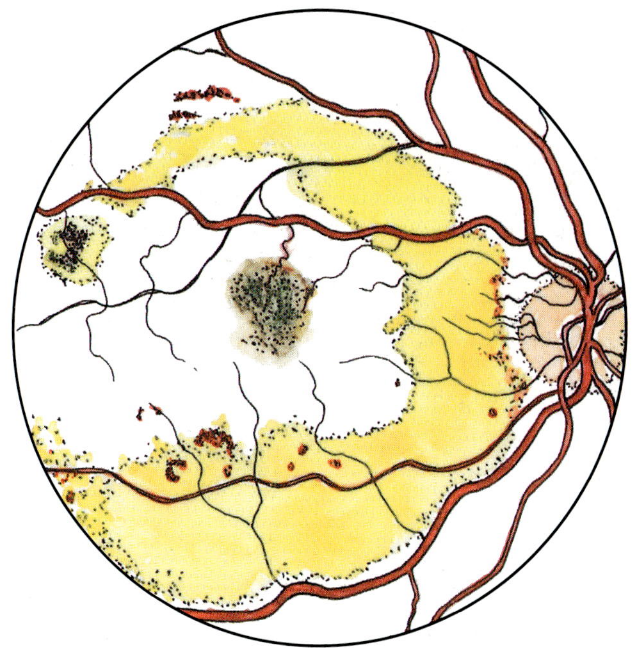

18–28

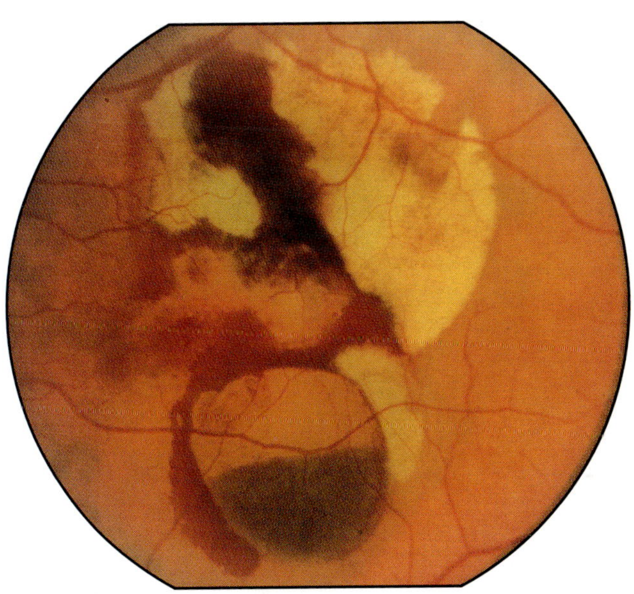

18–27 and 18-27A Exudative maculopathy is caused by choroidal neovascularization. A grayish-green choroidal neovascular membrane is seen (18–27). Early in the exudative process, subretinal fluid, hemorrhage and lipid appear secondary to the neovascularization.

18–28 Subretinal hemorrhage secondary to choroidal neovascularization is present in the next patient. A pigment epithelial detachment is noted inferiorly. Hemoglobinized and dehemoglobinized blood is present.

18–28, *Courtesy of Mark Croswell.*

18–29 CHOROIDAL NEOVASCULARIZATION

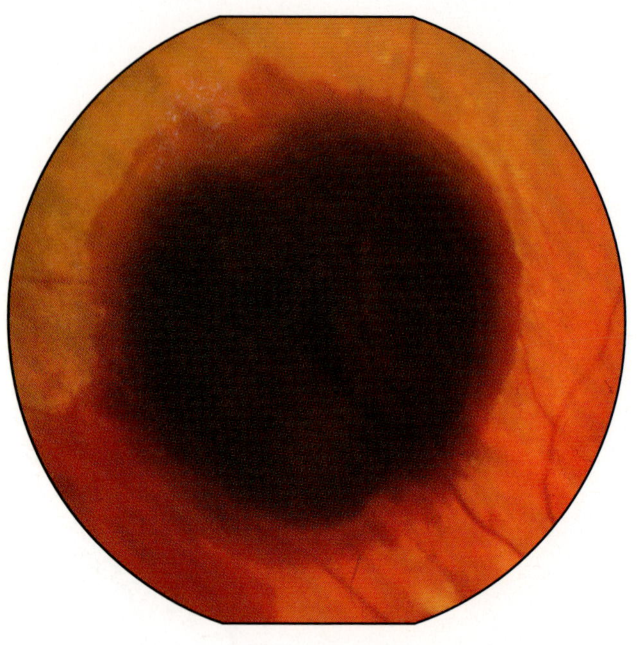

18–30

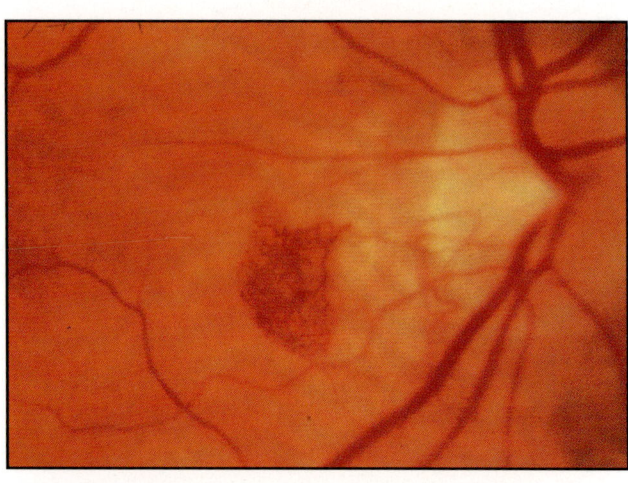

18–31

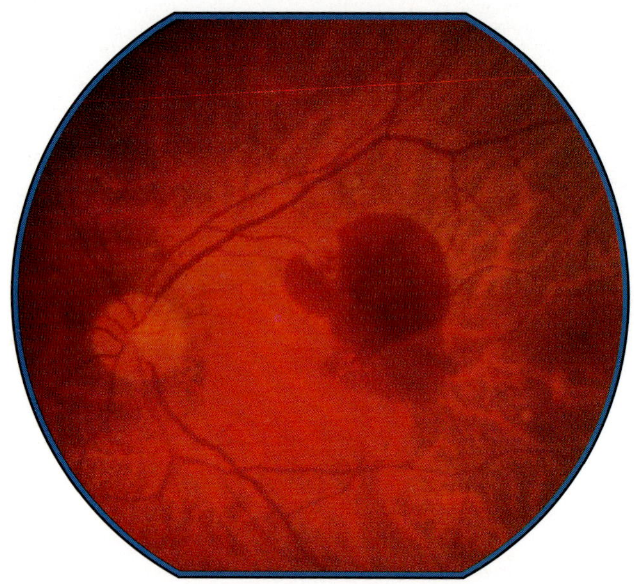

18–32

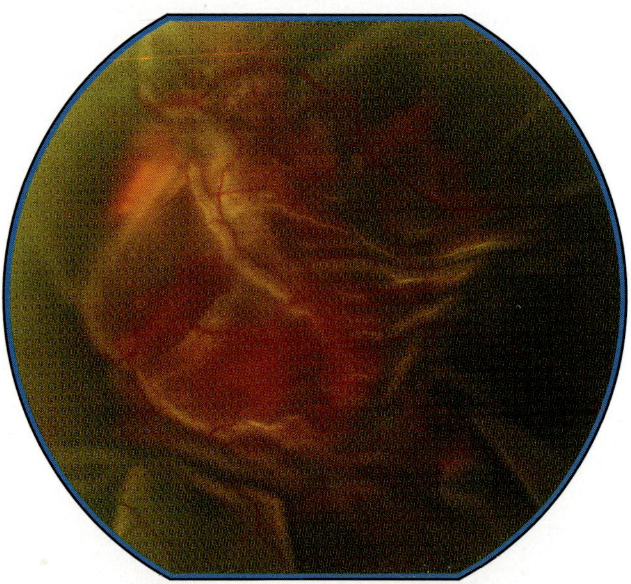

18–29 More extensive subretinal hemorrhage can also occur and give the appearance of a pseudomelanoma.

18–30 Rarely, "pure" choroidal neovascularization can occur without overlying exudation, as demonstrated in this case.

18–31 and 18–32 This patient had subretinal hemorrhage from subfoveal choroidal neovascularization (18–31), and 7 weeks later developed massive hemorrhagic exudation with bullous detachment (18–32). The fundus at this point has the appearance of a pseudomelanoma, but the earlier photograph showing subfoveal neovascularization was helpful in confirming the diagnosis of macular degeneration.

18–33 DISCIFORM SCARS

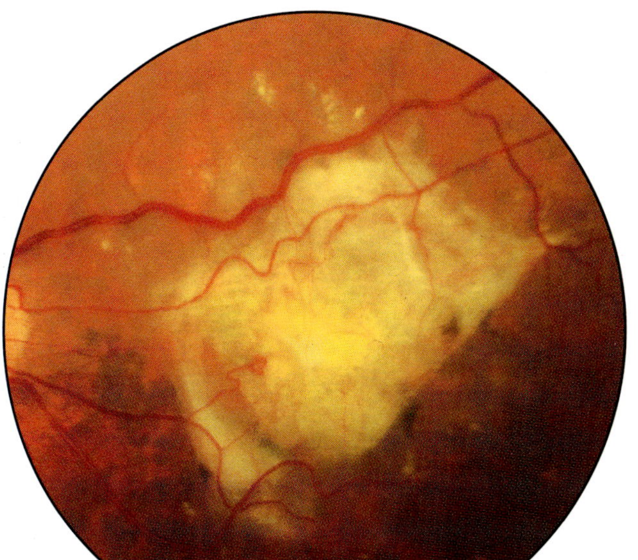

18–34

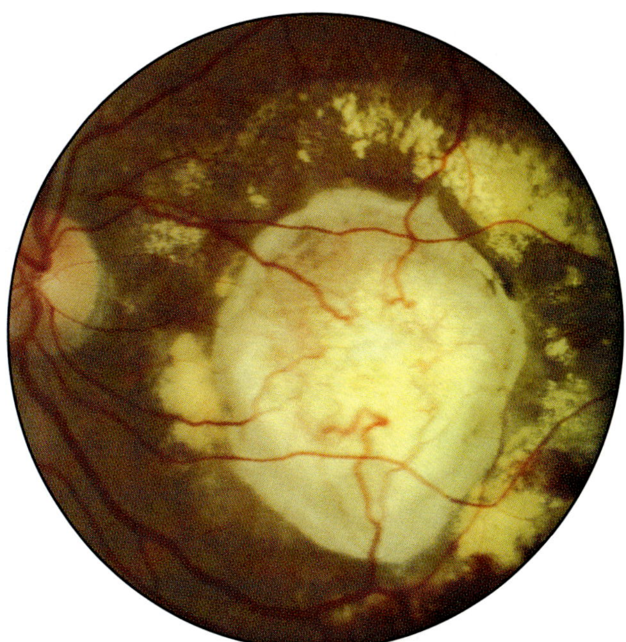

18–35

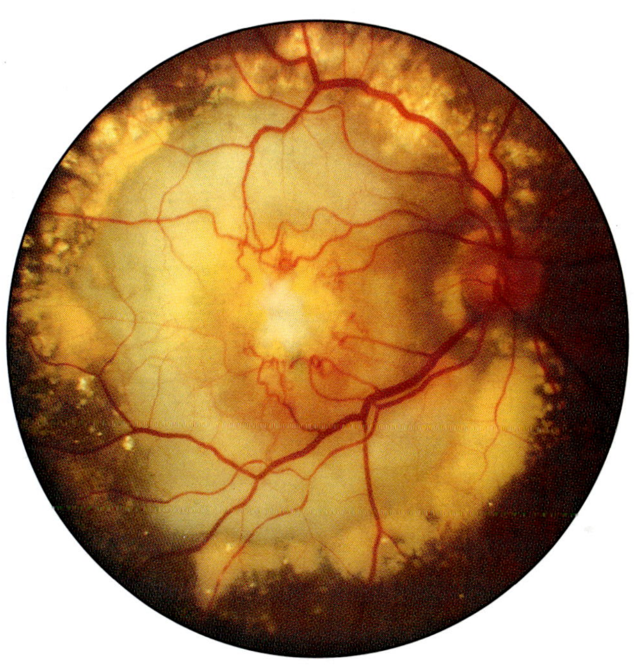

18–33 through 18–35 The end result of choroidal neovascularization is disciform scarring. Anastomosis between the retinal and choroidal circulations can sometimes be seen (18–34 and 18–35).

18–36 RARE SPONTANEOUS RESOLUTION OF CNV 18–37

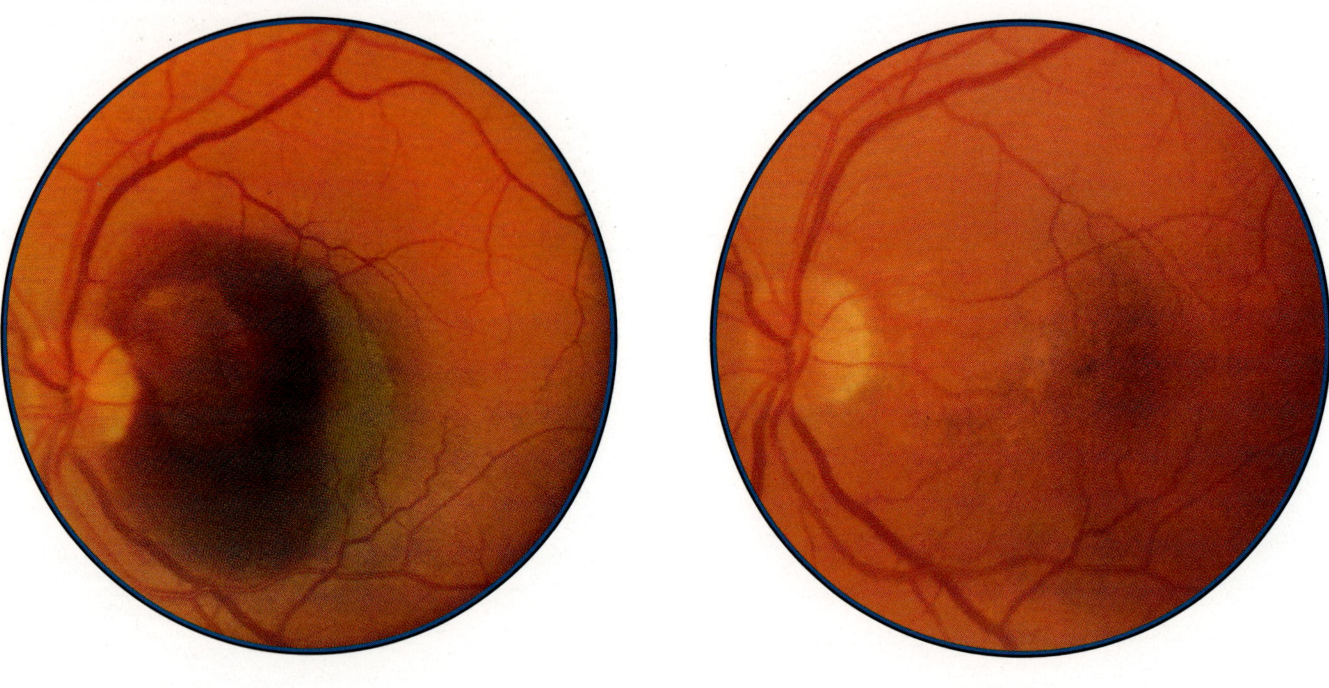

18–36 This patient presented with subretinal hemorrhage that obscured the foveal region.

18–37 Rarely, spontaneous regression of the hemorrhage can occur.

18–38 WELL-DEFINED (CLASSIC) CNV

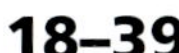

18–39

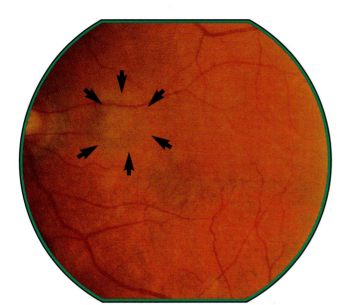

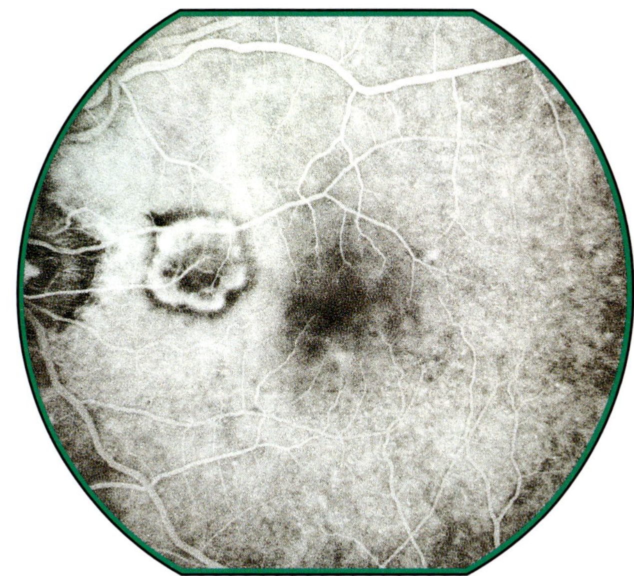

18–40

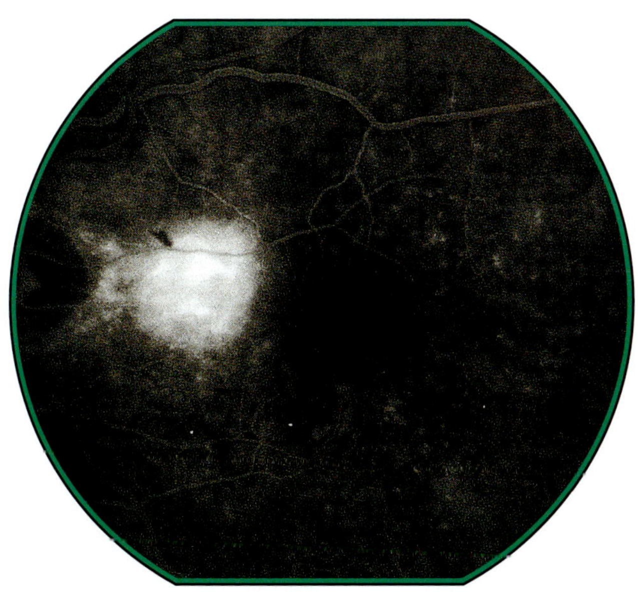

18–38 A minority of patients with choroidal neovascularization have well-defined or classic choroidal neovascularization. This patient has subretinal fluid and hemorrhage with a classic grayish-green neovascular membrane superonasal to the macula *(arrowheads)*.

18–39 and 18–40 Fluorescein angiography confirms the well-defined, extrafoveal choroidal neovascular membrane, which can be treated with laser photocoagulation. Note how the neovascularization demonstrates increasing hyperfluorescence (18–40). Unfortunately, well-delineated classic choroidal neovascularization, which is potentially treatable, occurs in less than 15% of patients with exudative maculopathy.

***18–38** and **18–40,** Courtesy of Dr. Neil Bressler and the Wilmer Reading Center, copyright Wilmer Reading Center, 1994.*

18–41 POORLY-DEFINED (OCCULT) CNV

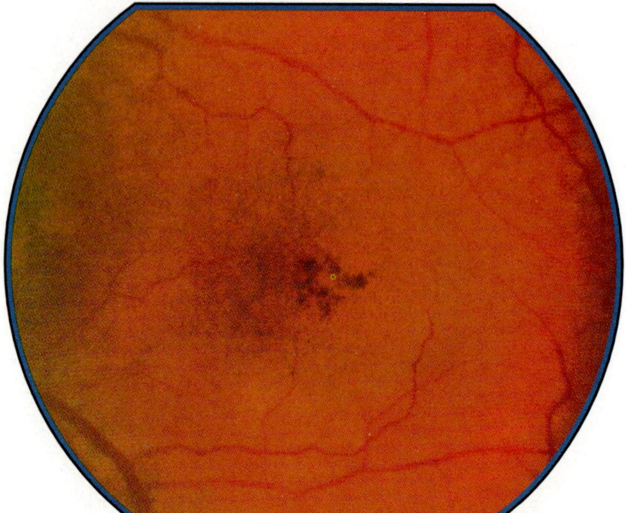

18–42

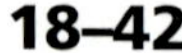

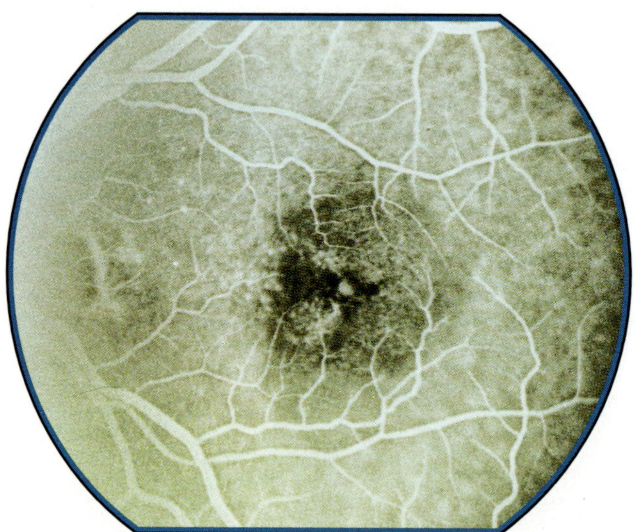

18–43

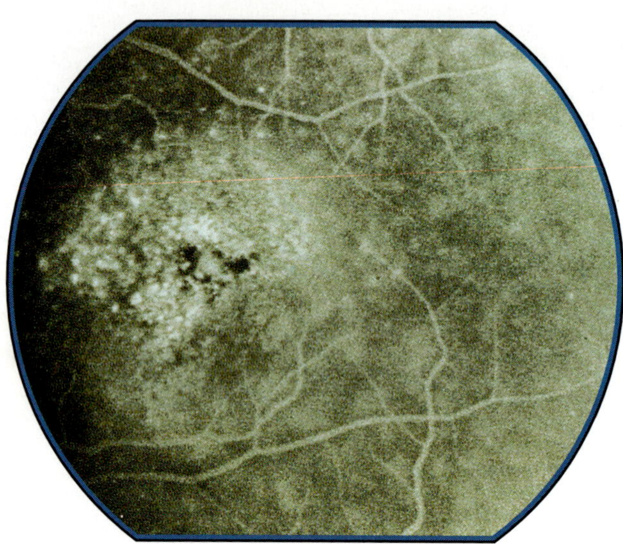

18–41 through 18–43 The fundus photograph demonstrates an area of subretinal fluid extending through the foveal center with evidence of pigment migration in the central portion of the lesion. The early phase of the angiogram in stereo demonstrates an area of irregular elevation of the retinal pigment epithelium, a fibrovascular pigment epithelial detachment. The nasal portion of the irregularly elevated area shows more bright hyperfluorescence than the temporal portion of the lesion. Overlying the irregularly elevated retinal pigment epithelium is evidence of hyperfluorescent dye filling the subretinal space fairly homogeneously, most evident inferior to the irregularly elevated retinal pigment epithelium. In the late phase of the angiogram, bright hyperfluorescence is noted throughout the area of irregular elevation of the retinal pigment epithelium, and more obvious dye accumulation in the subretinal space is noted inferior to the irregularly elevated retinal pigment epithelium. This area of irregular elevation of the retinal pigment epithelium represents fibrovascular pigment epithelial detachment, a form of occult choroidal neovascularization (CNV).

***18–41** through **18–43,** Courtesy of Dr. Neil Bressler and the Wilmer Reading Center, copyright Wilmer Reading Center, 1994.*

18–44

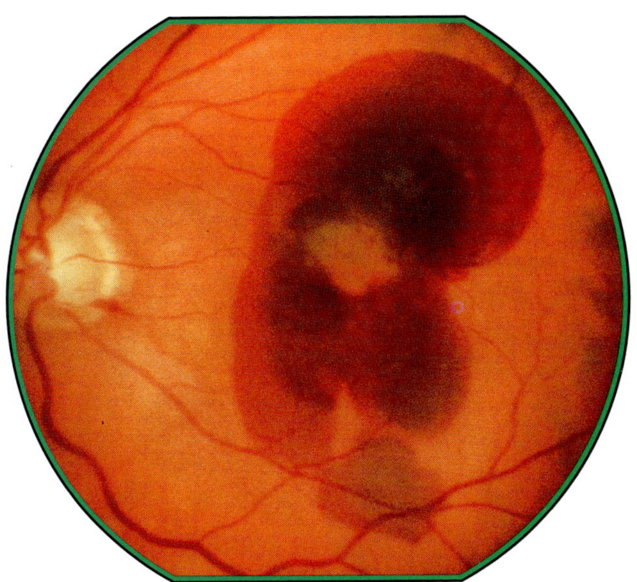

18–45

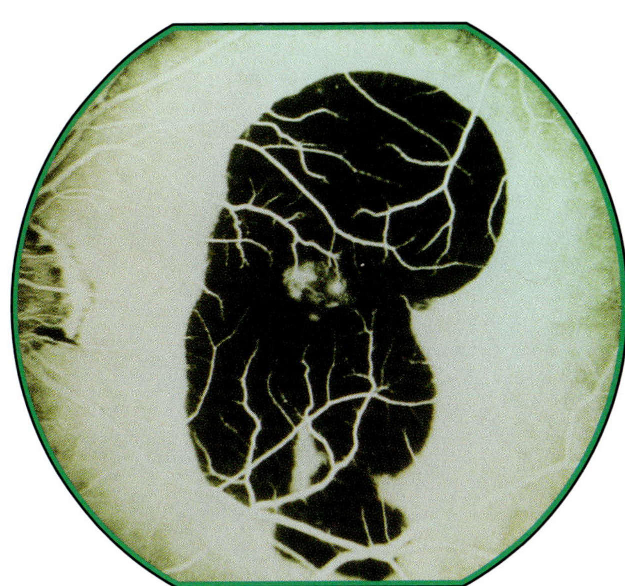

18–44 and 18–45 Poorly-defined choroidal neovascularization may show overlying blockage on the fluorescein angiogram secondary to subretinal hemorrhage, as demonstrated in this case. The color photograph shows subretinal hemorrhage (18–44) and the corresponding fluorescein angiogram (18–45) shows hypofluorescence secondary to the blood. A treatable choroidal neovascular membrane cannot be imaged by fluorescein angiography due to the blockage.

__18–44__ and __18–45__, Courtesy of Dr. Neil Bressler and the Wilmer Reading Center, copyright Wilmer Reading Center, 1994.

18–46 POORLY DEFINED CNV

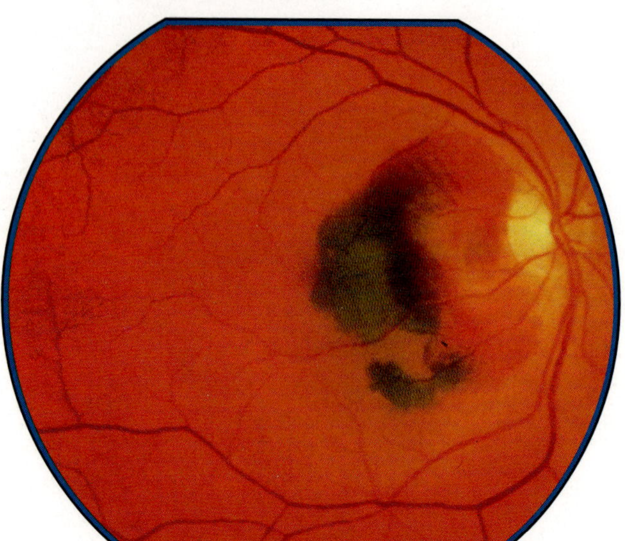

18–47

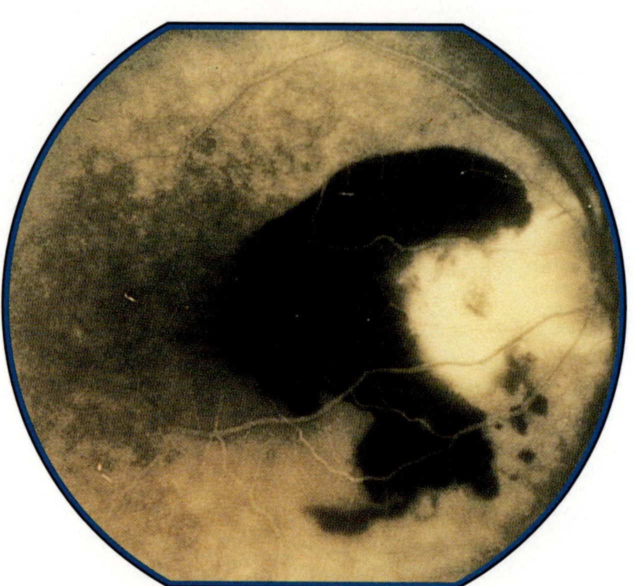

18–46 This patient has subretinal hemorrhage involving the fovea with an acute drop in vision in his only eye to 20/200.

18–47 Fluorescein angiography shows hyperfluorescence near the optic disc, consistent with choroidal neovascularization, and much blockage secondary to the hemorrhage. This patient has a poorly-defined choroidal neovascular membrane since the extent of neovascularization cannot be fully appreciated by fluorescein angiography due to the blocked areas. Digital indocyanine-green (ICG) videoangiography is a new adjunctive technique to fluorescein angiography for imaging occult or poorly-defined choroidal neovascularization. Since ICG is active in the near infrared range and has a high protein binding capacity, its special properties confer certain advantages over sodium fluorescein in imaging such eyes. ICG can penetrate better through overlying subretinal hemorrhage and serosanguinous fluid than sodium fluorescein in some cases.

***18–46** and **18–47,** From Slakter, JS, et al: A pilot study of indocyanine-green videoangiography guided laser photocoagulation of occult choroidal neovascularization in age-related macular degeneration, Arch Ophthalmol 112:465–472, 1994.*

(Case continued on next page.)

18–48 ICG

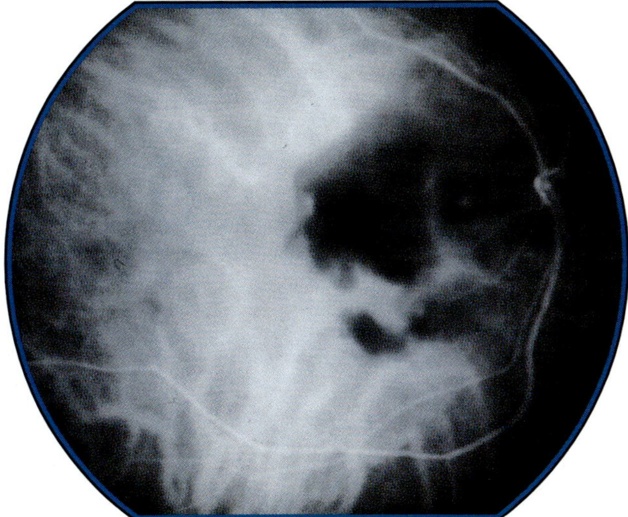

18–49

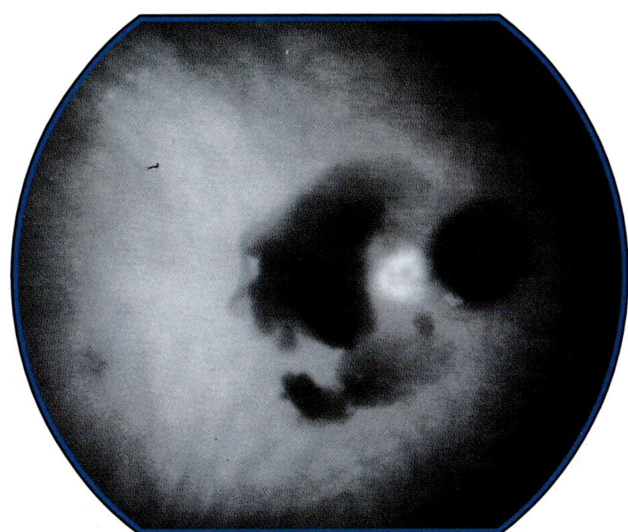

18–50

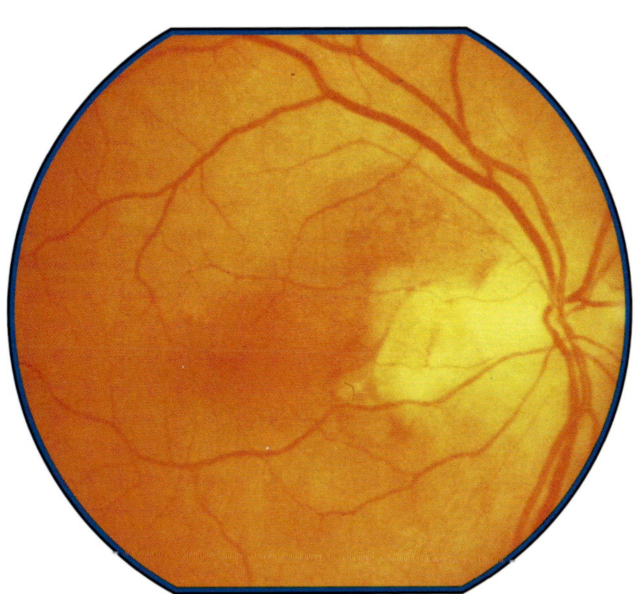

18–48 and 18–49 The same patient's ICG angiogram demonstrates a focal area of hyperfluorescence in an extrafoveal location. Notice how the ICG angiogram shows a focal well-defined lesion, which was poorly defined on the fluorescein angiogram.

18–50 This area was photocoagulated using ICG guidance, with resolution of the subretinal hemorrhage and neovascularization, and a dramatic improvement in visual acuity to 20/30.

***18–48** through **18–50,** From Slakter, JS, et al: A pilot study of indocyanine-green videoangiography guided laser photocoagulation of occult choroidal neovascularization in age-related macular degeneration, Arch Ophthalmol 112:465–472, 1994.*

18–51 POORLY DEFINED CNV AND ICG

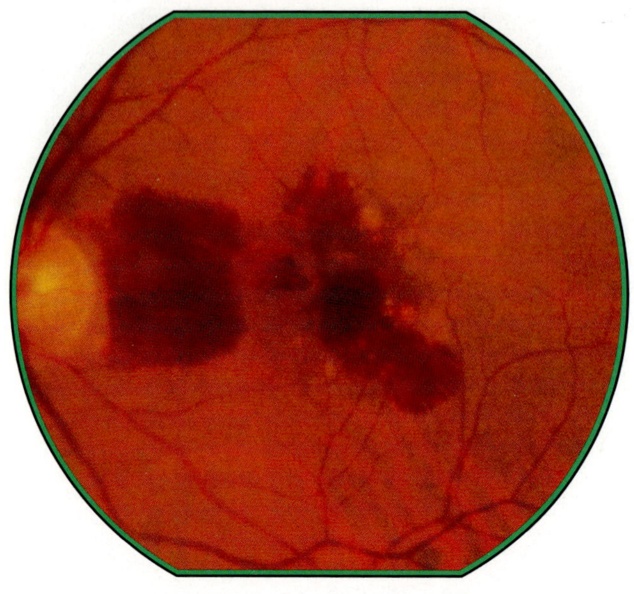

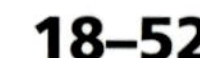

18–52

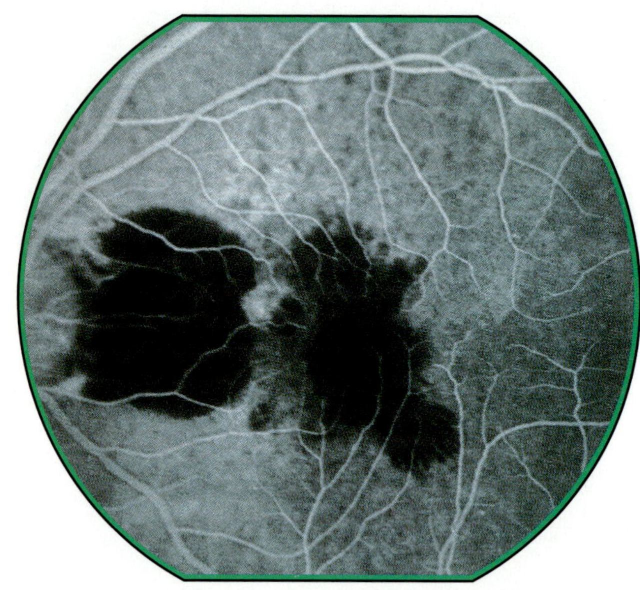

18–53

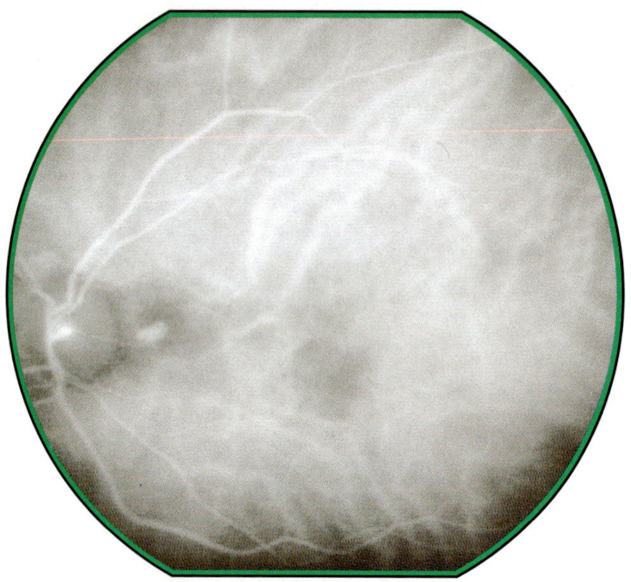

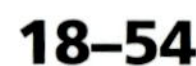

18–54

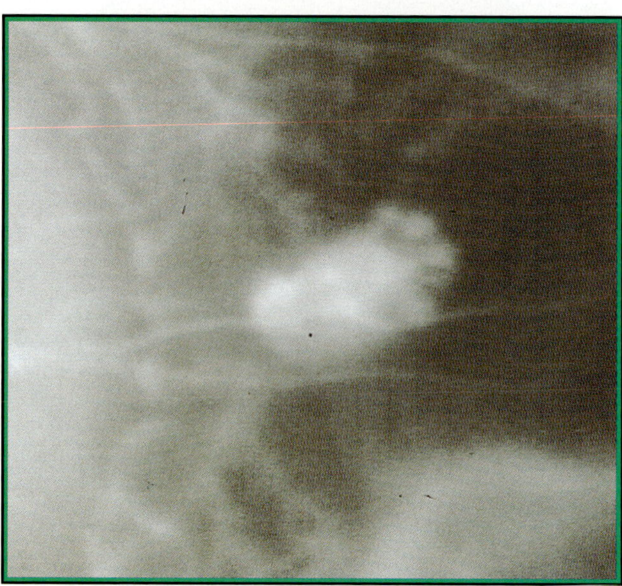

18–51 and 18–52 This patient also has occult choroidal neovascularization. Note the subretinal hemorrhage (18–51), which causes blockage on the fluorescein angiogram (18–52). An area of juxtafoveal neovascularization was suspected on the fluorescein study (18–52).

18–53 and 18–54 Digital ICG videoangiography reveals an area of neovascularization adjacent to the optic disc. Note that this area is nasal to the suspicious area on the fluorescein angiogram.

(Case continued on next page.)

18–55

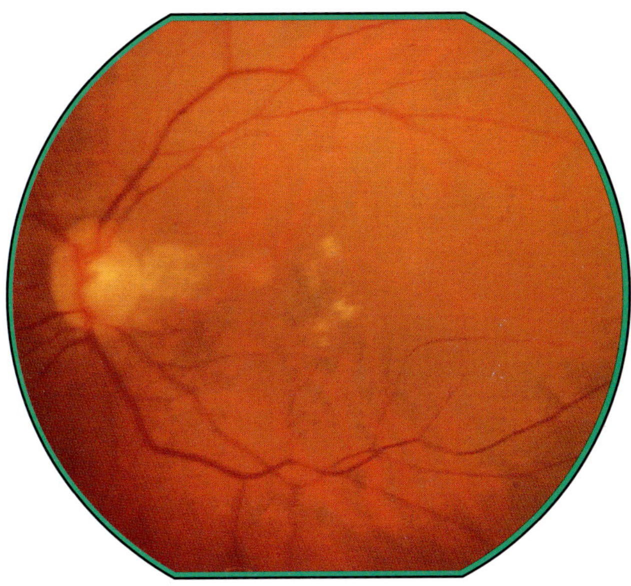

18–56

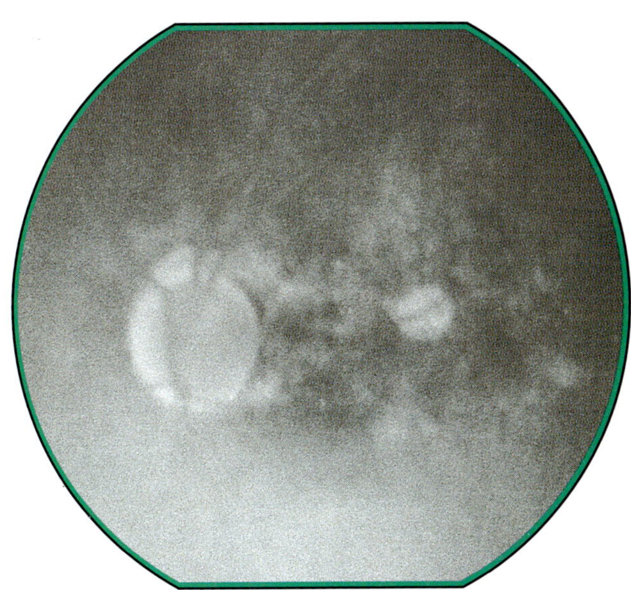

18–55 ICG-guided laser photocoagulation was performed with resolution of the exudative findings.

18–56 Fluorescein angiography performed postoperatively revealed that the suspicious area was actually an atrophic region with underlying leakage from the peripapillary neovascularization.

18–51 *through* ***18–56,*** *From Guyer, DR, et al: Digital indocyanine-green videoangiography of occult choroidal neovascularization, Ophthalmology 101:1727–1735, 1994.*

18–57 POORLY DEFINED CNV AND ICG

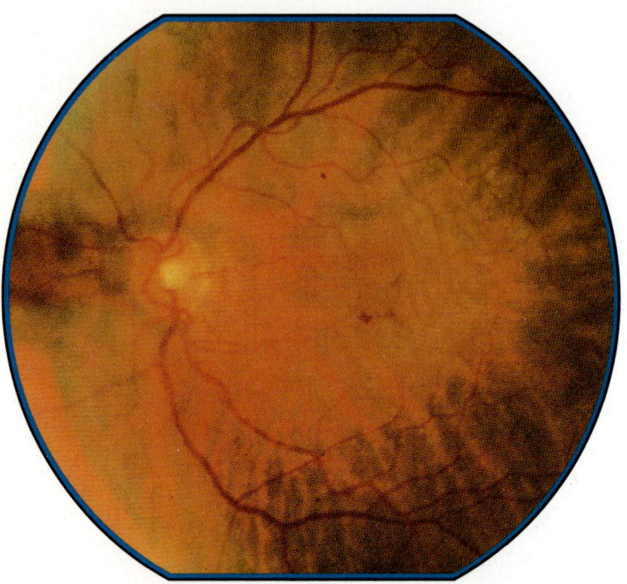

18–58

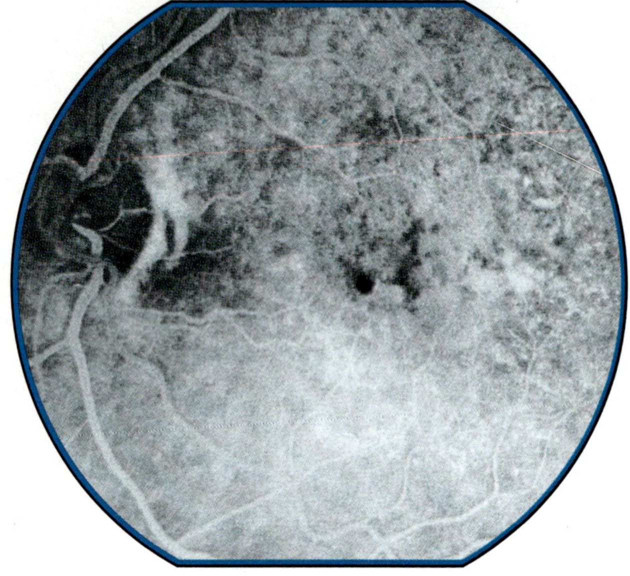

18–59

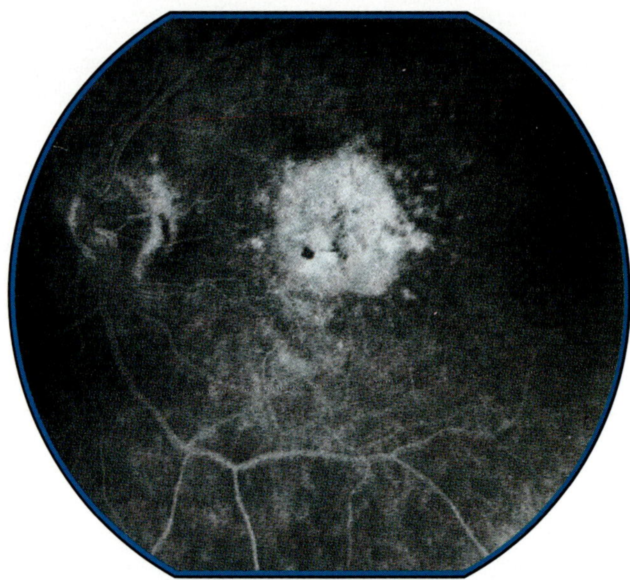

18–57 This patient also has choroidal neovascularization with subretinal hemorrhage and fluid.

18–58 and 18–59 Fluorescein angiography reveals occult neovascularization.

(Case continued on next page.)

18–60 **18–61**

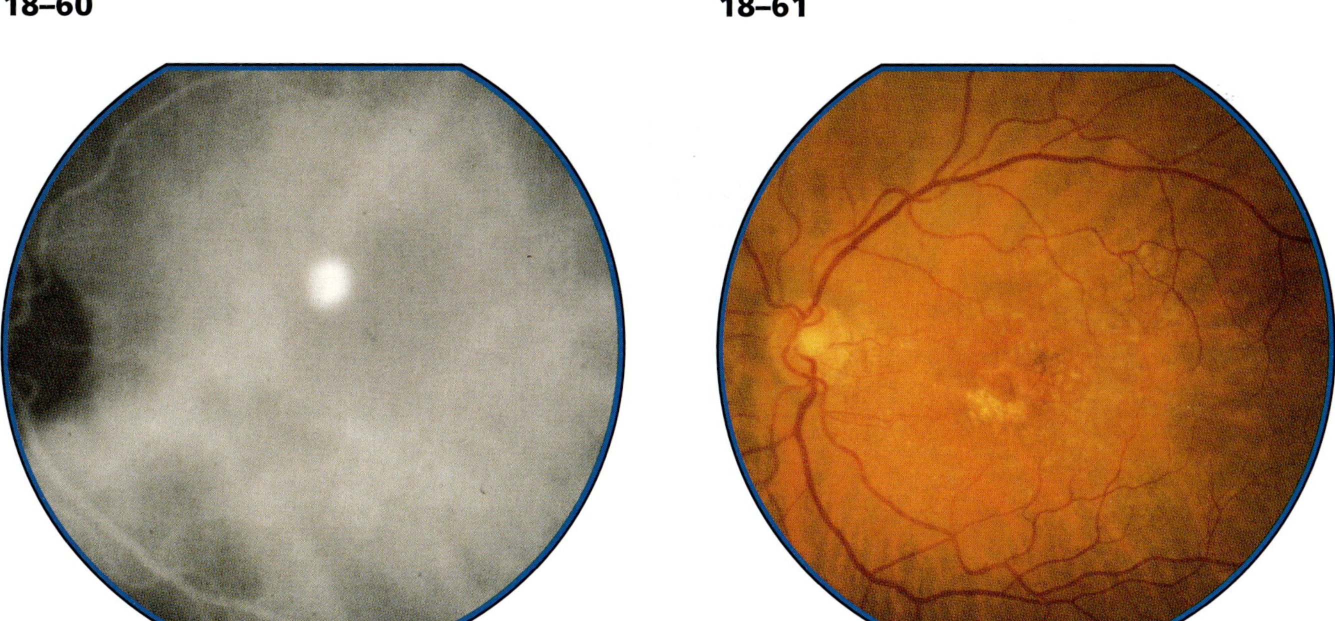

18–60 and 18–61 Digital ICG videoangiography reveals a focal "hot spot" (18–60), which was photocoagulated under ICG guidance with resolution of the exudation (18–61).

Differential Diagnosis: Other Causes of CNV

18–62 PSEUDOTUMOR CEREBRI

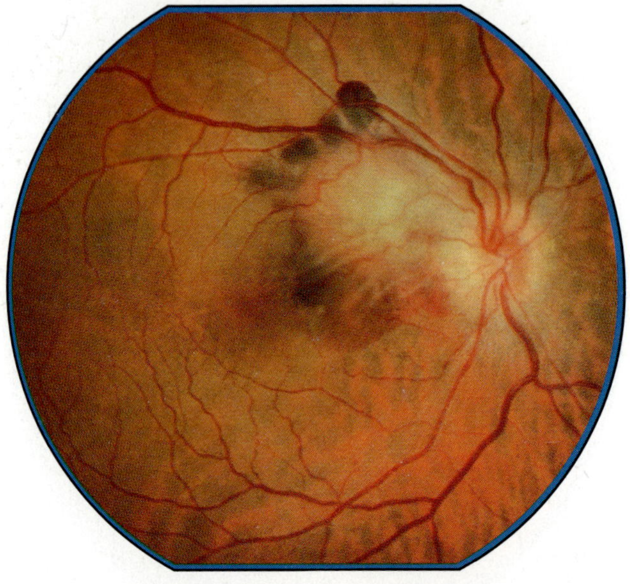

18–63

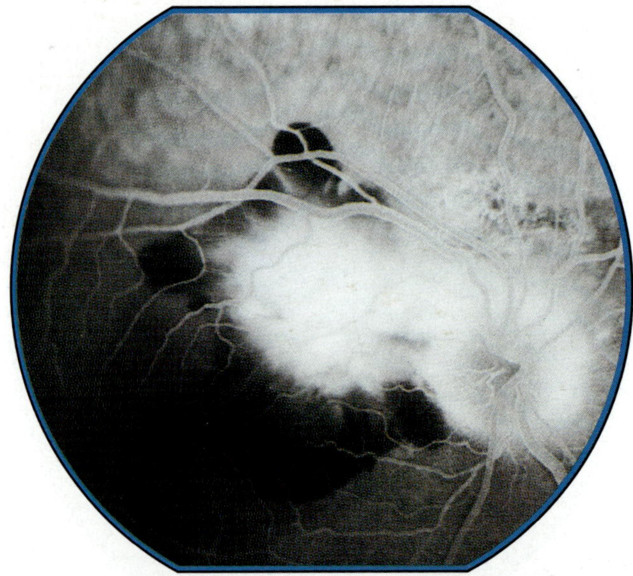

18–64 IDIOPATHIC

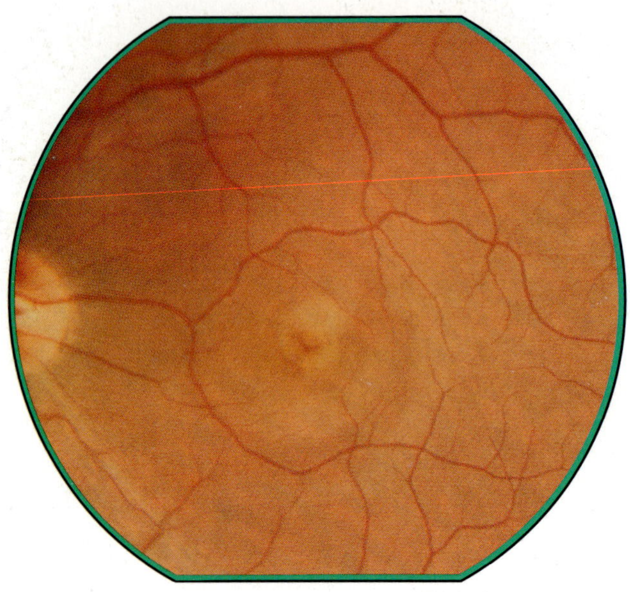

18–65

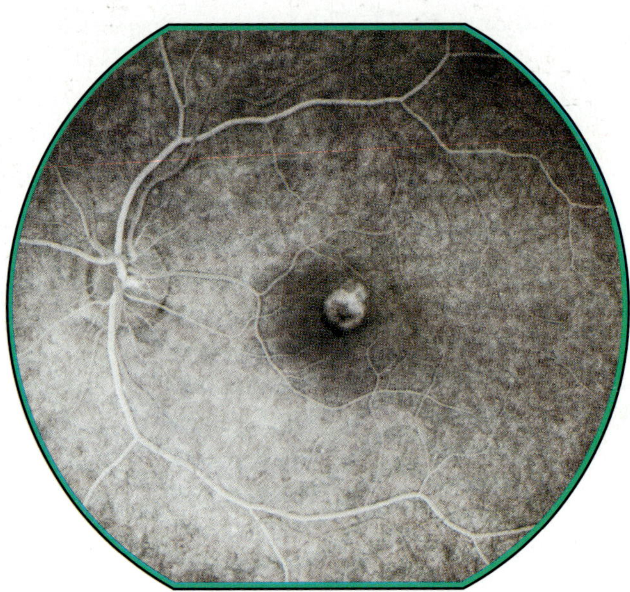

18–62 and 18–63 There are many other causes of choroidal neovascularization other than age-related macular degeneration. Some of these are addressed in the sections on myopia and the presumed ocular histoplasmosis syndrome. This patient shows optic disc edema with secondary subretinal fluid and hemorrhage. The fluorescein angiogram reveals choroidal neovascularization. This patient has optic disc edema secondary to pseudotumor cerebri with secondary choroidal neovascularization, which rarely may occur in these patients.

18–64 and 18–65 Another form of choroidal neovascularization is idiopathic. This type is often seen in young patients in which there is no other cause for the neovascularization.

18–62 *and* ***18–63,*** *Courtesy of Dr. Gary Brown.*

18–66 SEPTIC EMBOLI

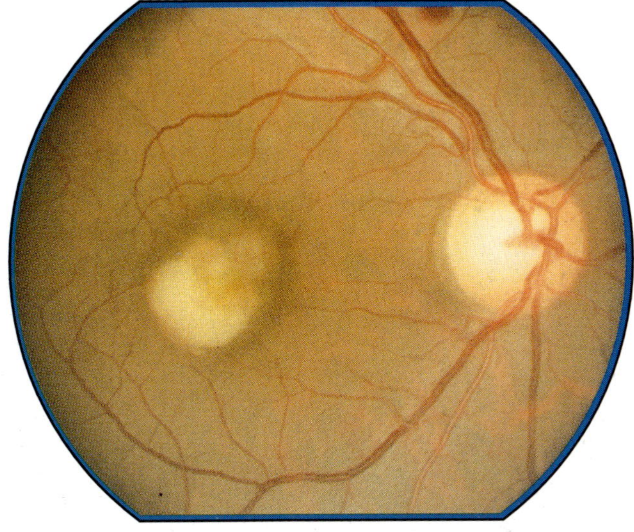

18–67

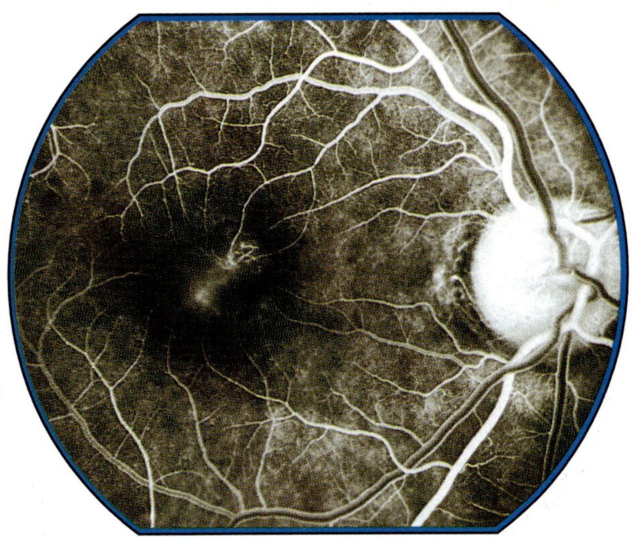

18–68

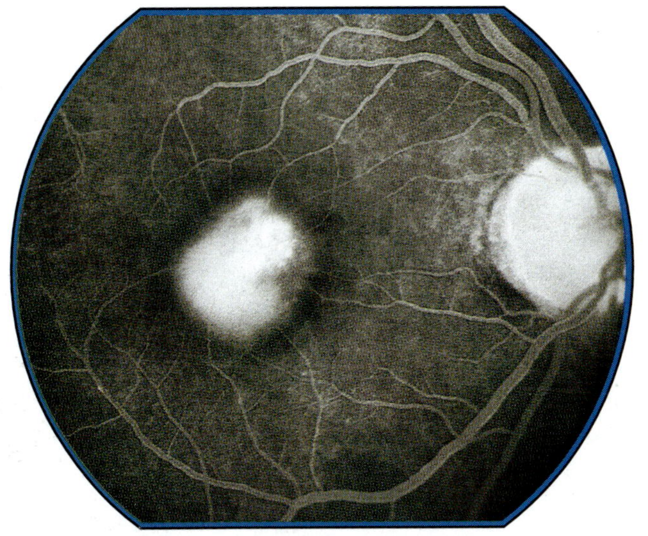

18–69

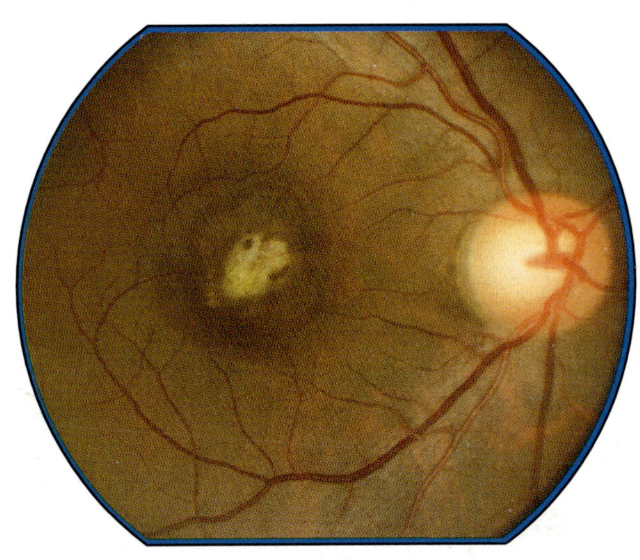

18–70

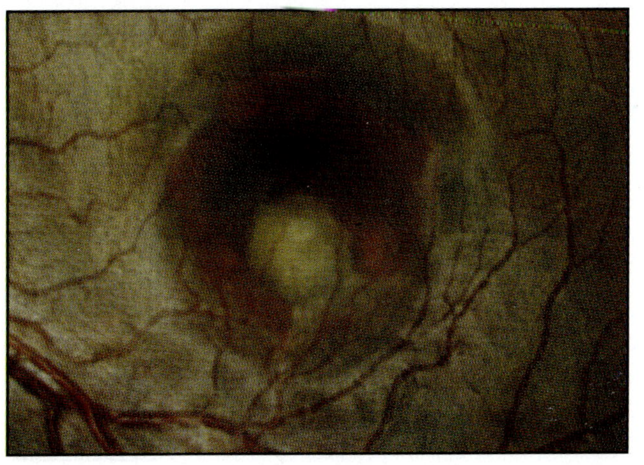

18–66 through 18–69 Metastatic choroidal abscess and choroidal neovascularization membrane associated with *Staphylococcus aureus* endocarditis in a heroin user.

18–70 This rare association of septic embolization and choroiditis with choroidal neovascularization is also demonstrated in this 13-year-old female with subacute bacterial endocarditis.

18–66 *through* ***18–69,*** *Courtesy of Dr. Gustavo E. Coll and Dr. Hilel Lewis. From Coll, GE, and Lewis, H: Metastatic choroidal abscess and choroidal neovascular membrane associated with* Staphylococcus aureus *endocarditis in a heroin user, Retina, 14(3):256–259, 1994.*

18–71 **PATHOLOGY: CNV**

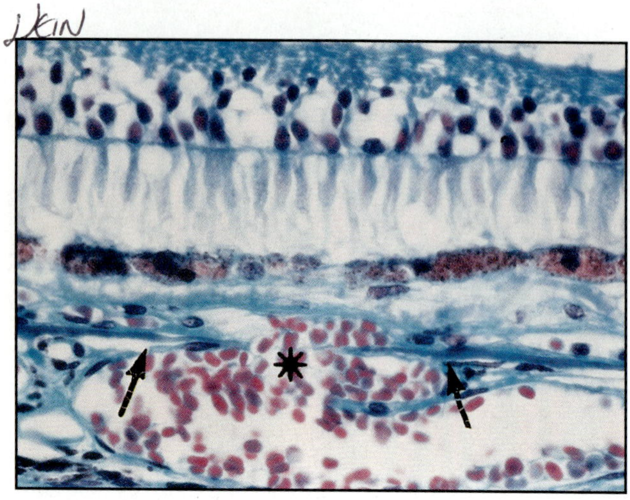

18–71A

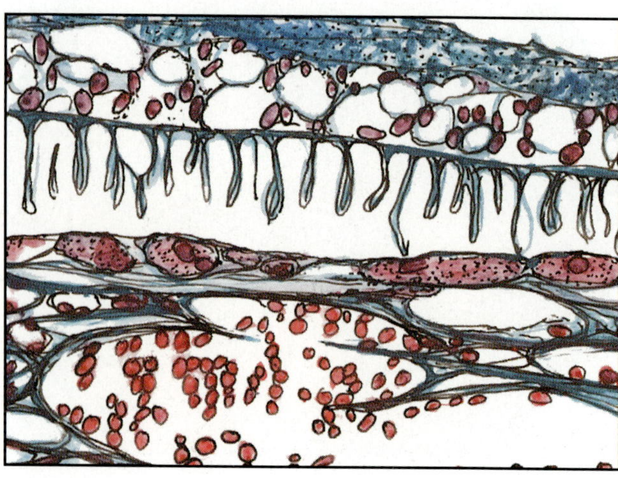

18–72

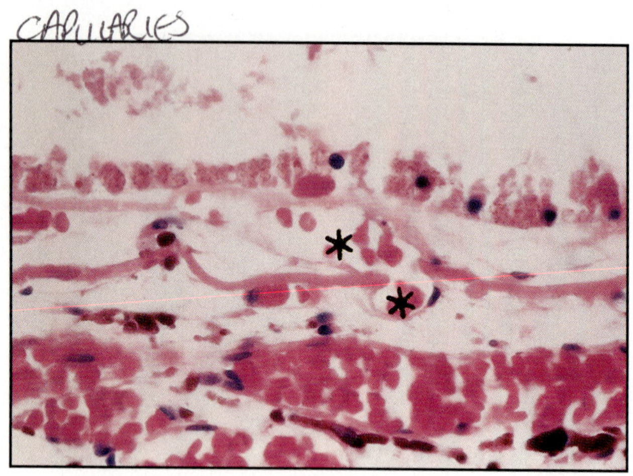

18–73

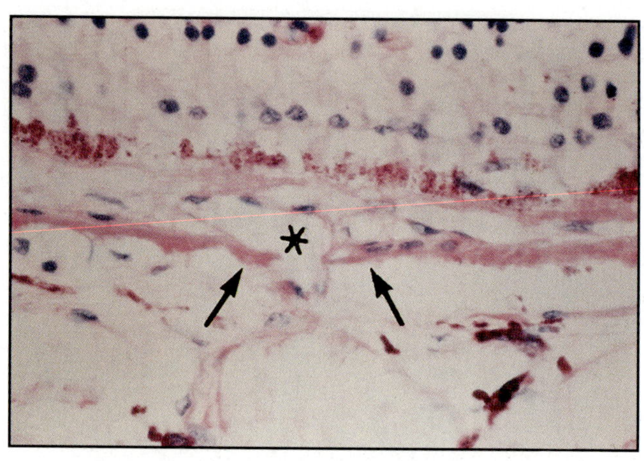

18–74

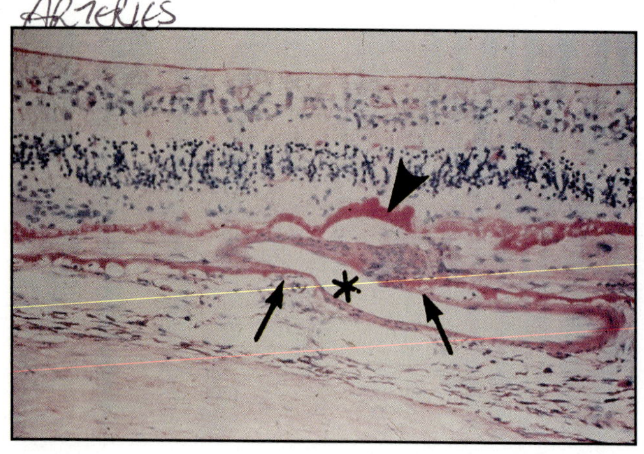

18–71 and 18–71A, through 18–74 These photographs show histopathologic examples of choroidal neovascularization where veins (18–71), capillaries (18–72 and 18–73), and arteries (18–74) extend through defects in Bruch's membrane. In these examples, arrows delineate defects in Bruch's membrane. Asterisks show areas of choroidal neovascularization that invade the subretinal pigment epithelial space. Arrowhead shows areas of basal laminar deposit.

18–71 *through* ***18–74,*** *From Green, WR, and Enger, C: Age-related macular degeneration histopathologic studies. The 1992 Lorenz E. Zimmerman Lecture, Ophthalmology 100:1519–1535, 1993.*

18–75 PATHOLOGY: SCARS

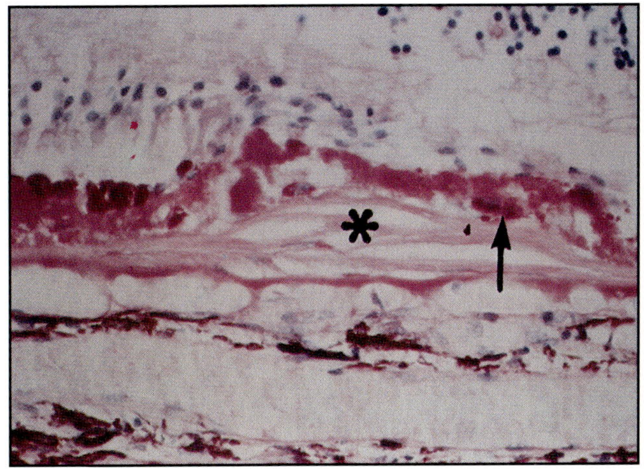

18–75A

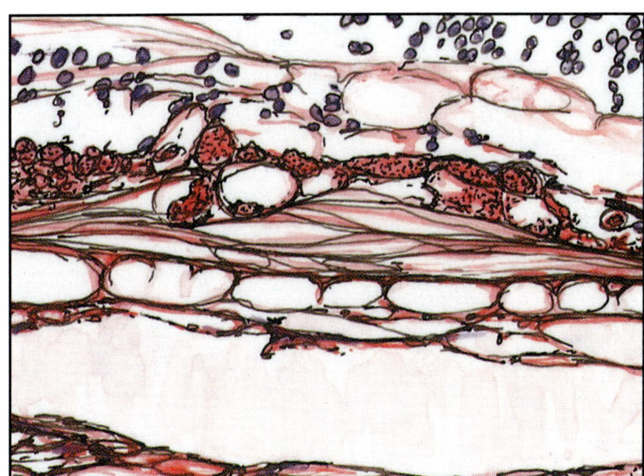

18–76

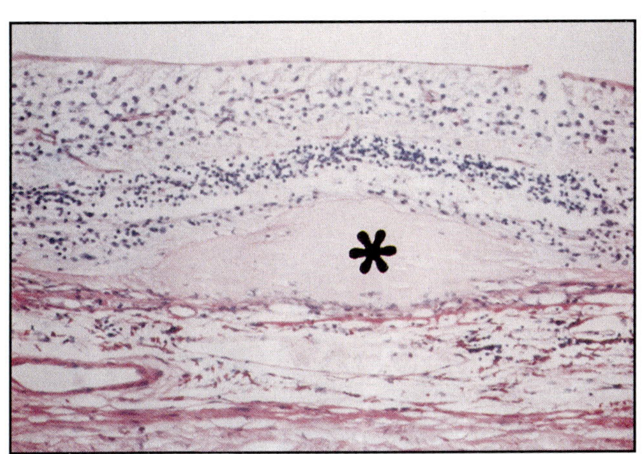

18–75 and 18–75A This histopathologic case is an example of a thin subretinal pigment epithelial fibrocellular disciform scar *(asterisk)* located between basal laminar deposit *(arrow)* and the remainder of Bruch's membrane. The retinal pigment epithelium and photoreceptors are atrophic except for a small area to the left.

18–76 This example demonstrates a subretinal disciform scar *(asterisk)* in which there is total loss of the photoreceptor cell layer. The retinal pigment epithelium is atrophic.

***18–75** and **18–76,** From Green, WR, and Enger, C: Age-related macular degeneration histopathologic studies. The 1992 Lorenz E. Zimmerman Lecture, Ophthalmology 100:1519–1535, 1993.*

18–77 PATHOLOGY: SCARS

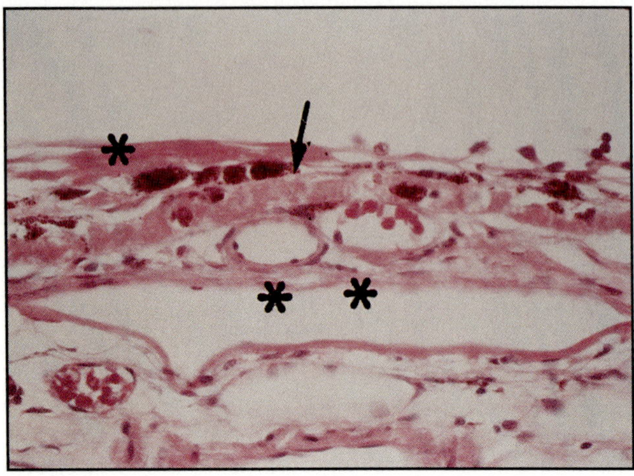

18–77A

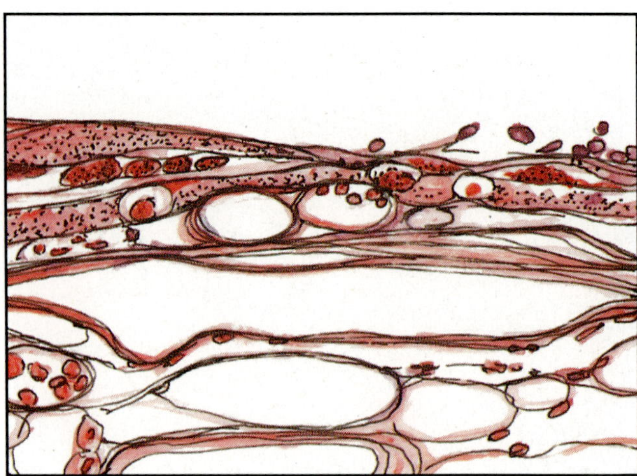

18–78

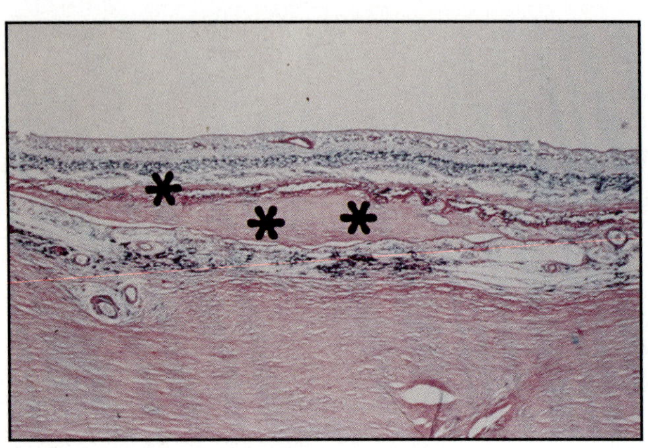

18–77 and 18–77A A two-component disciform scar is noted in this example. Basal laminar deposits *(arrow)* separate the thinner, nonvascularized subretinal component *(single asterisk)* from the thicker, vascularized intra–Bruch's membrane component *(double asterisks)*. Residual retinal pigment epithelium is present. There is a moderate-to-complete loss of the photoreceptor cell layer.

18–78 This example also shows a two-component disciform scar. Residual basal laminar deposits separate the thinner, nonvascularized subretinal component *(single asterisks)* from the thicker vascularized intra–Bruch's membrane component *(double asterisk)* of the scar.

***18–77** and **18–78,** From Green, WR, and Enger, C: Age-related macular degeneration histopathologic studies. The 1992 Lorenz E. Zimmerman Lecture, Ophthalmology 100:1519–1535, 1993.*

18–79 PIGMENT EPITHELIAL DETACHMENTS

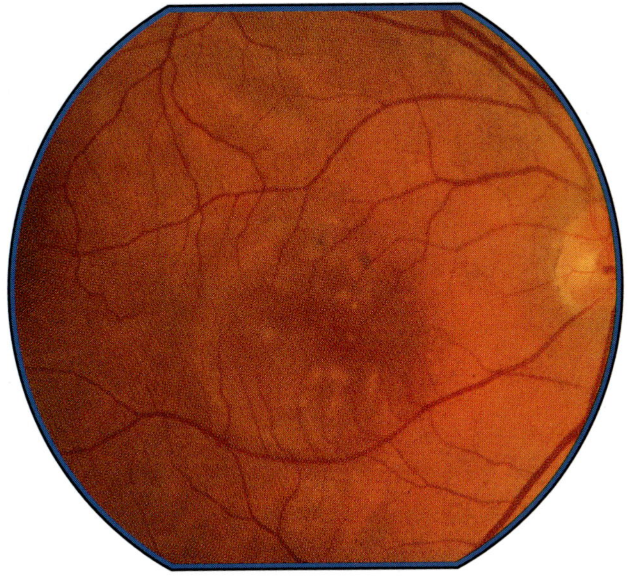

18–80

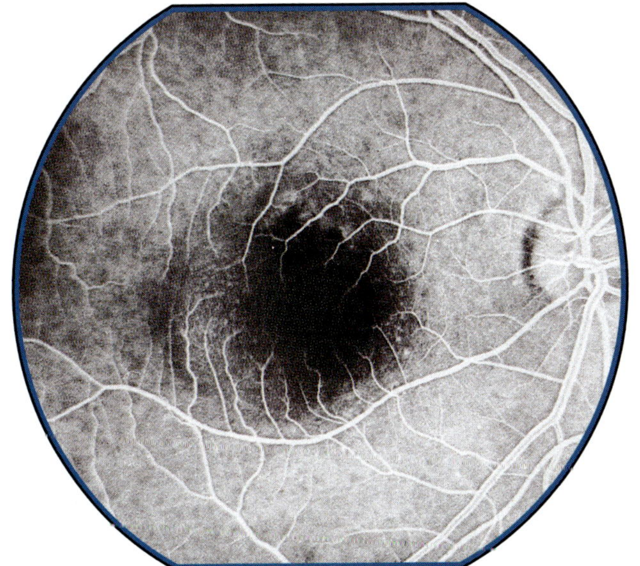

18–81

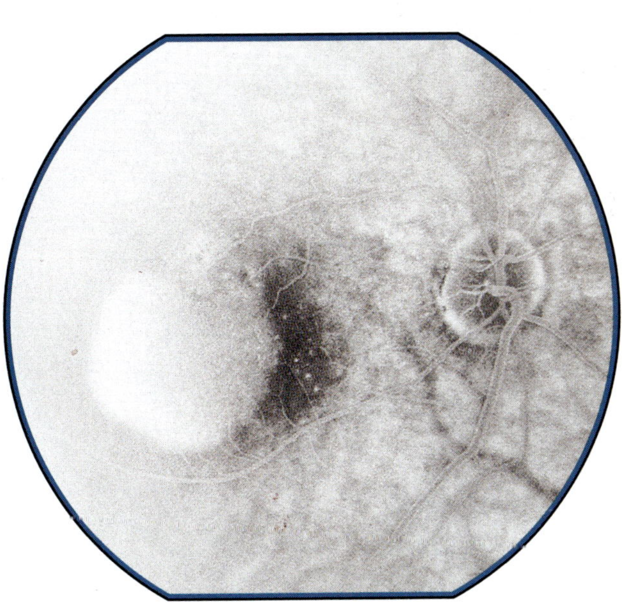

18–79 through 18–81 Pigment epithelial detachments are observed in a subgroup of patients with exudative macular degeneration. They consist of a domelike elevation of the pigment epithelium with serous fluid. Usually, these detachments are neovascularized. This patient presented with a pigment epithelial detachment. Fluorescein angiography demonstrates increasing hyperfluorescence of the pigment epithelial detachment.

(Case continued on next page.)

18–82 PED AND ICG

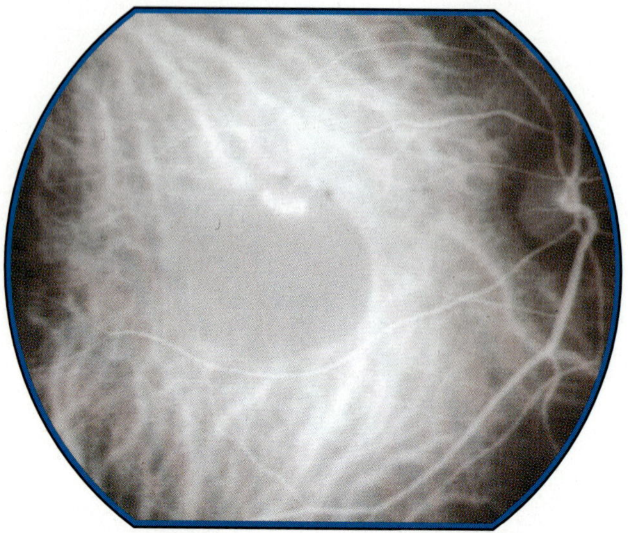

18–83

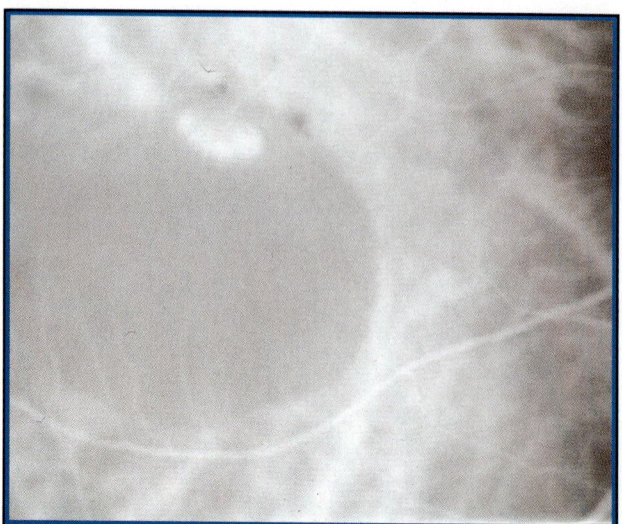

18–84

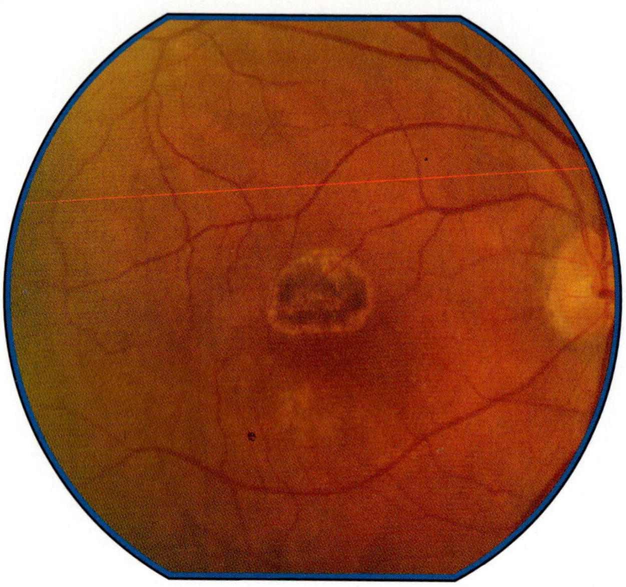

18–82 and 18–83 Digital ICG angiography can separate the hyperfluorescent neovascularized portion of the pigment epithelial detachment from the hypofluorescent serous component.

18–84 ICG-guided laser photocoagulation was applied to the neovascularization with resolution of the detachment.

18–85

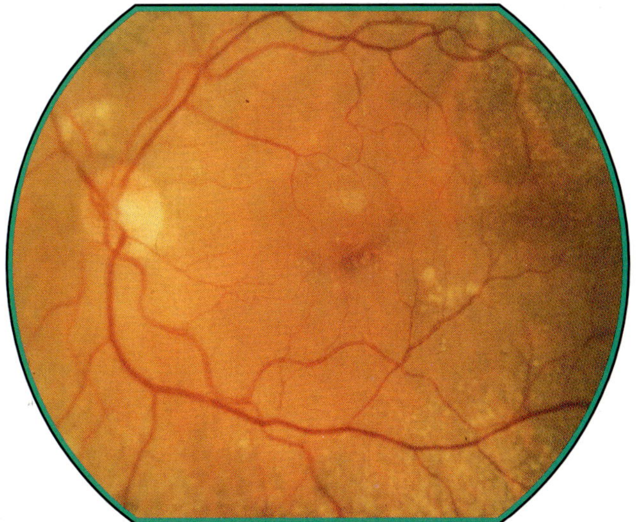

18–86

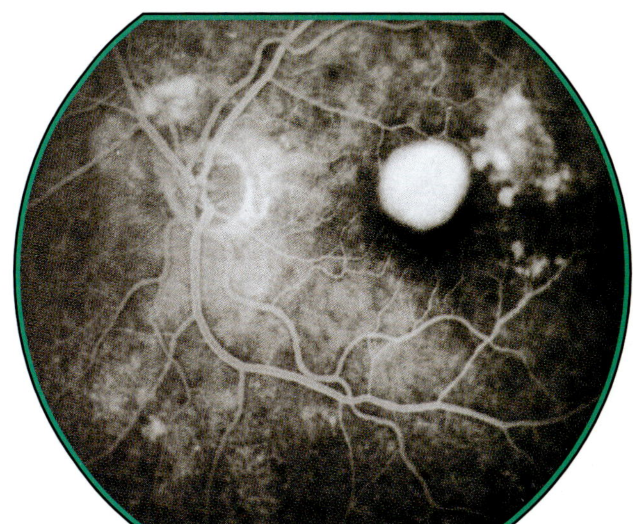

18–87

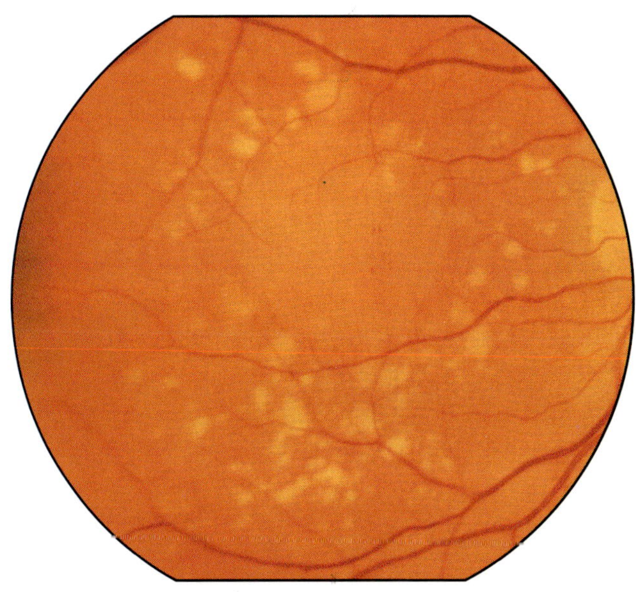

18–85 and 18–86 This patient has drusen and a pigment epithelial detachment (18–85) with the characteristic increasing hyperfluorescence on the fluorescein angiogram (18–86).

18–87 This patient has a markedly elevated pigment epithelial detachment with drusen.

18–88 PIGMENT EPITHELIAL DETACHMENTS

18–89

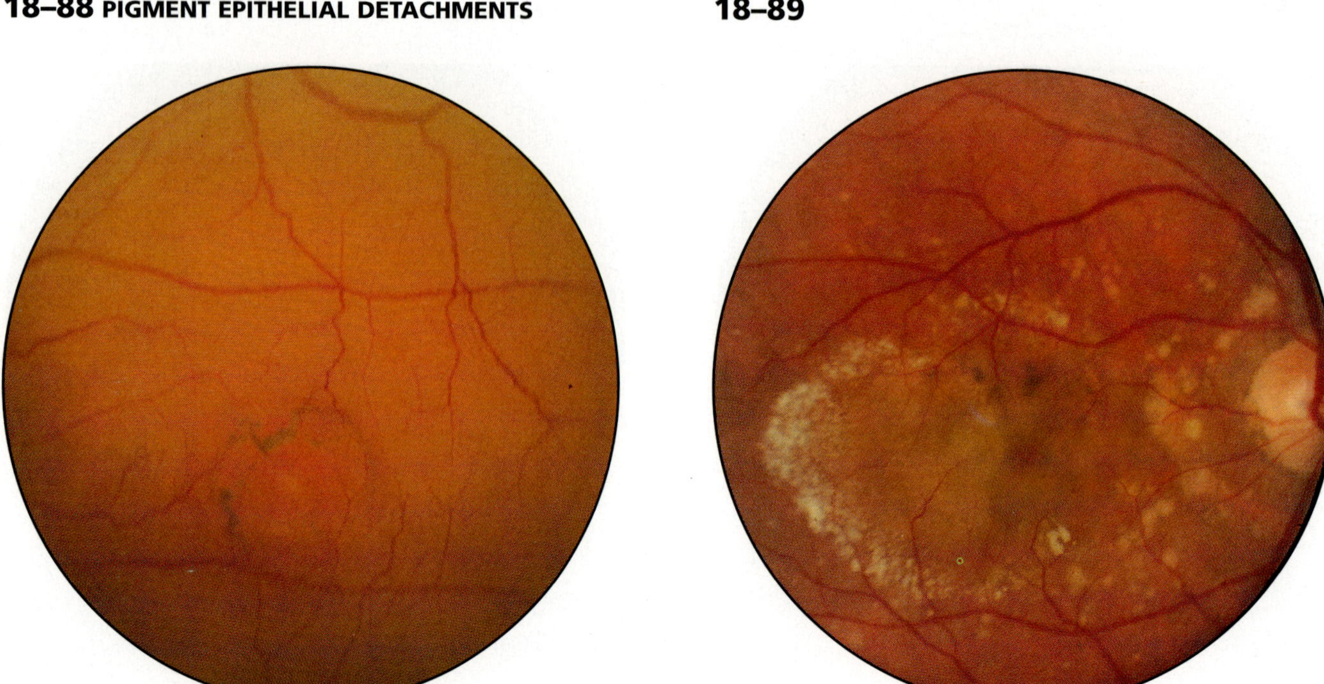

18–88 and 18–89 Chronic retinal pigment epithelial detachments may demonstrate persistent detachment with pigmentation (18–88) or lipid exudation (18–89).

18–90

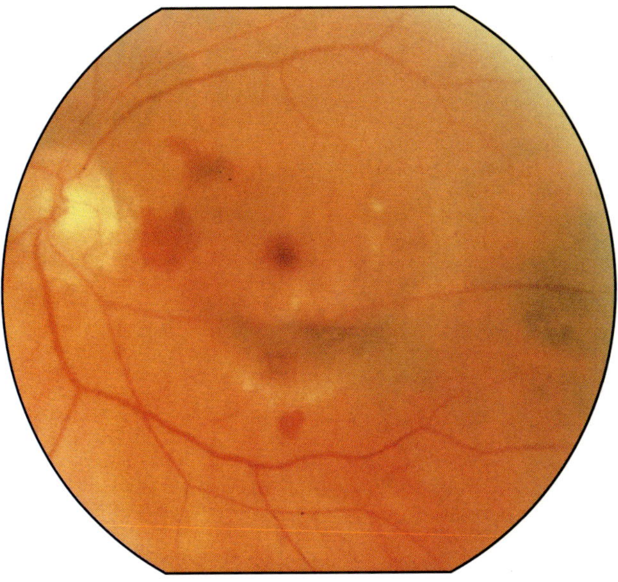

18–91

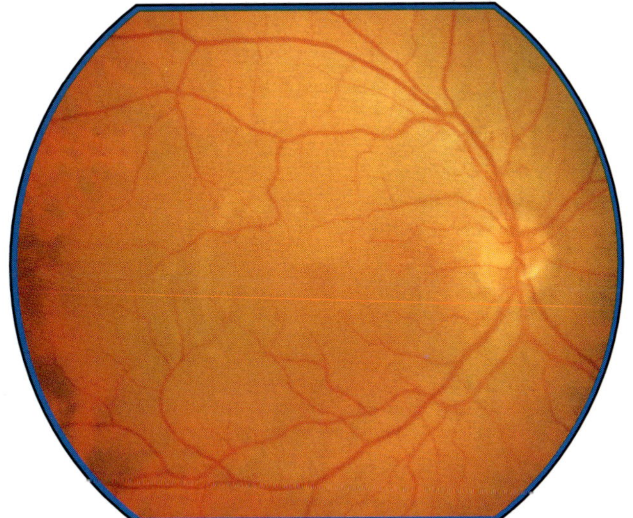

18–92

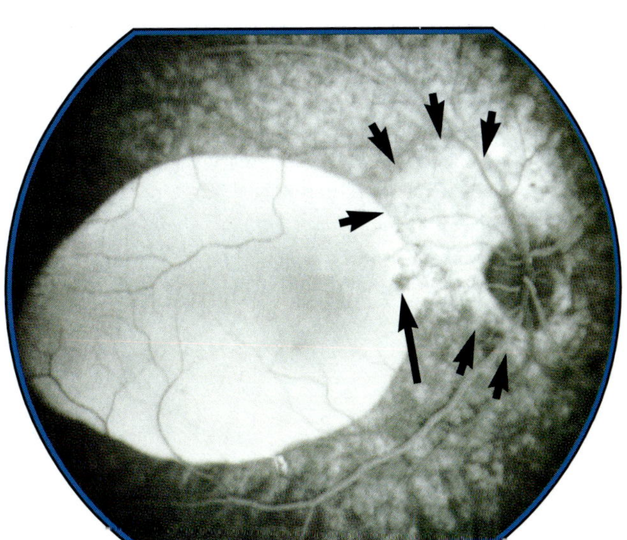

18–90 Hemorrhagic pigment epithelial detachments commonly occur.

18–91 and 18–92 This patient has an extremely large pigment epithelial detachment. Note how well the fluorescein angiogram delineates the detachment. There is a shallow thickening in the peripapillary region consistent with occult neovascularization *(arrowheads)*. The actively proliferating neovascularization is seen in silhouette emerging from the occult vessels into the subpigment epithelial space *(arrow)*.

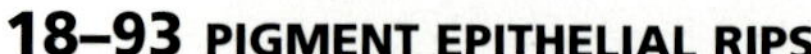

18–93 PIGMENT EPITHELIAL RIPS

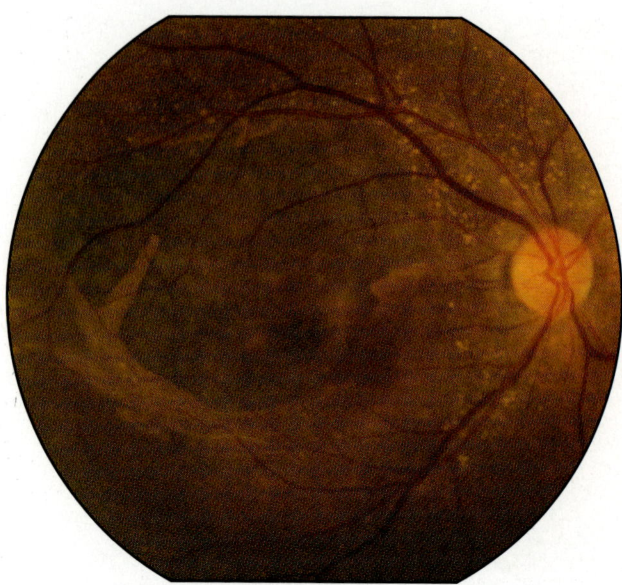

18–93 This patient has an unusually large spontaneous pigment epithelial rip (tear) in the central macula. The pigment epithelium has retracted inferiorly where there are folds or a corrugated effect. The inferior margin of the rip may also be seen to form a coiling effect from the subpigment epithelial tangential traction induced by presumed choroidal neovascularization. The superior and nasal margin of the rip actually show a flapping effect as these edges suspend in the subneurosensory retinal space. Widespread drusen are evident outside the rip, but these are not evident beneath the elevated pigment epithelium. Within the rip itself, scattered residual drusenoid material may be seen as irregular, soft orange deposits that were not displaced with the contracted pigment epithelium.

18–94 **18–95**

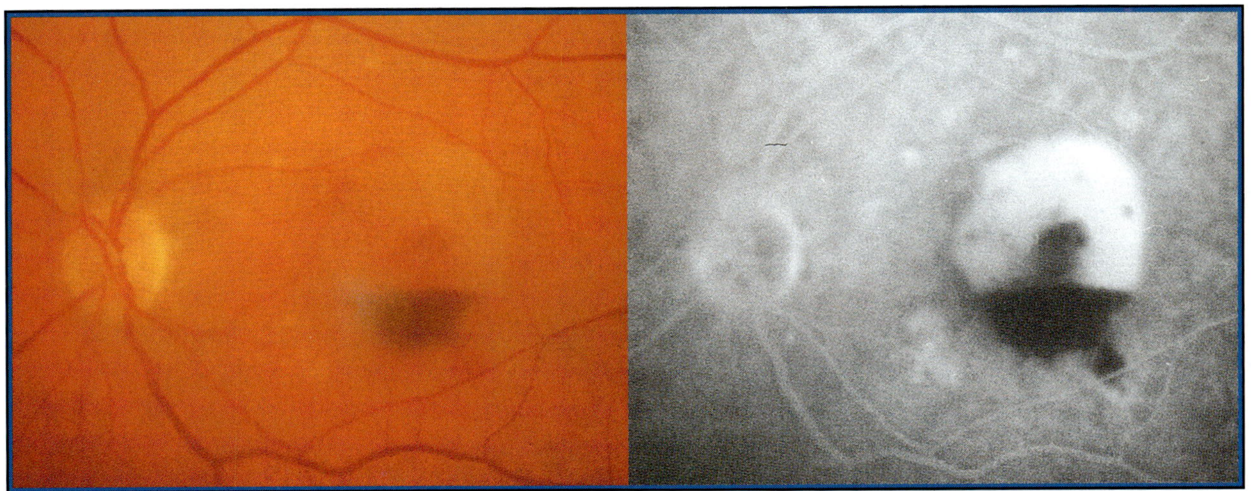

18–96 **18–97**

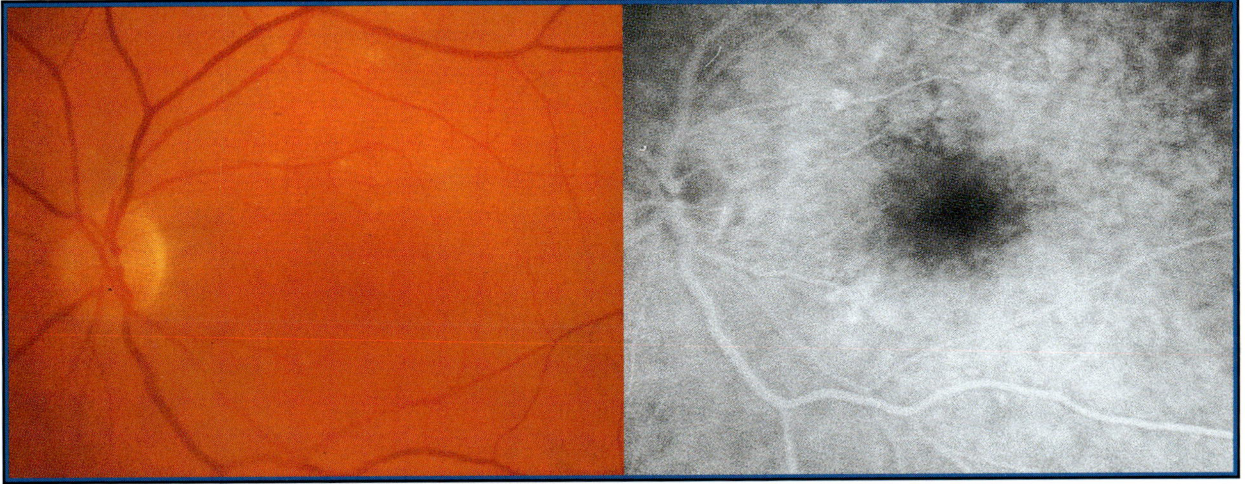

18–94 through 18–97 In rare situations, pigment epithelial detachments may spontaneously improve. This patient had a hemorrhagic pigment epithelial detachment. Five months later, spontaneous resolution of the pigment epithelial detachment with improvement on the fluorescein angiogram is noted.

***18–94** through **18–97**, Courtesy of Dr. Alfredo Pece.*

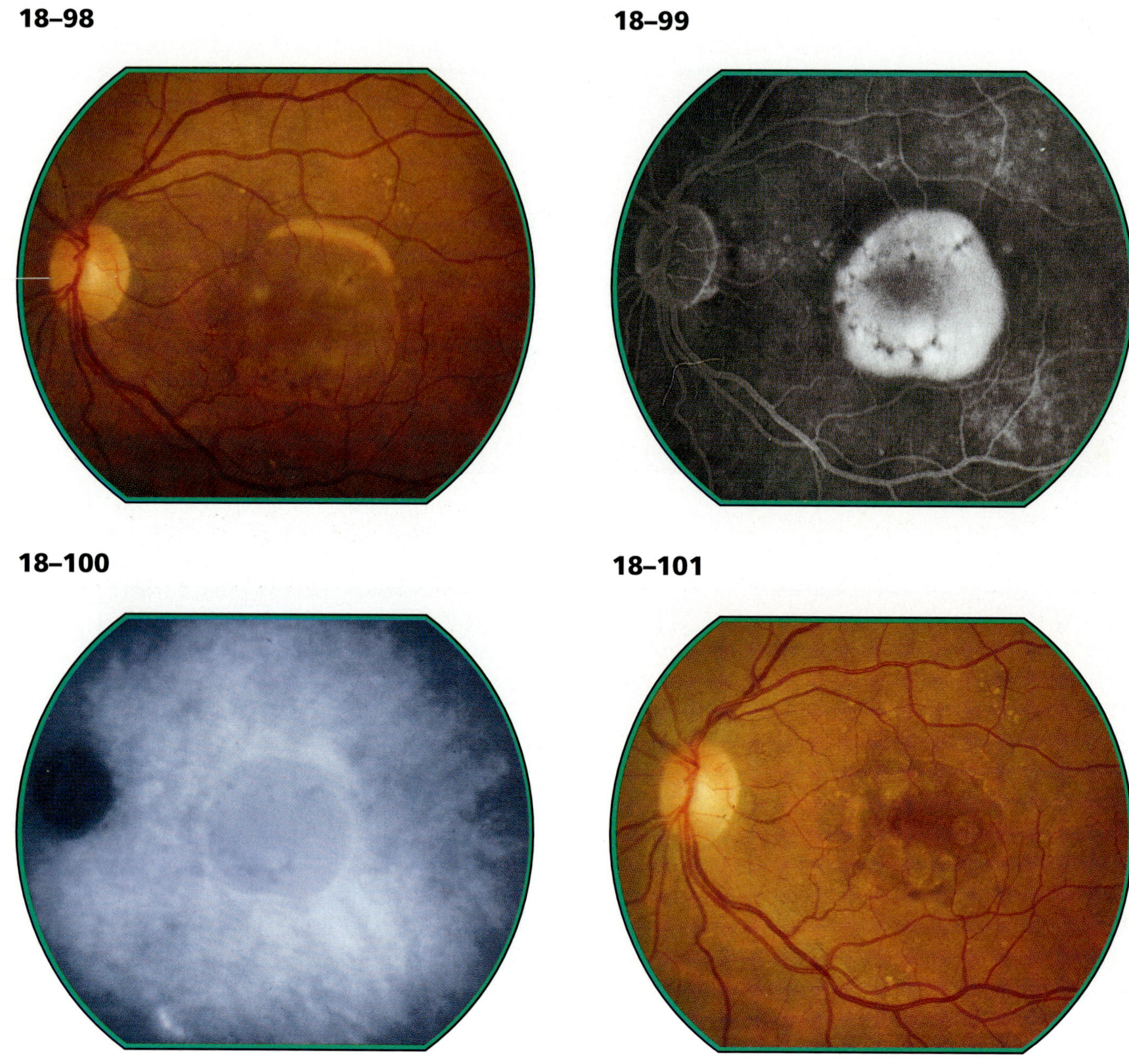

18–98 through 18–101 Pigment epithelial detachments may be purely serous. The fluorescein angiogram demonstrates hyperfluorescence. However, ICG angiography is more useful in demonstrating that the pigment epithelial detachment is nonvascularized. Mild grid laser photocoagulation flattened the detachment.

18–102 RPE RIPS

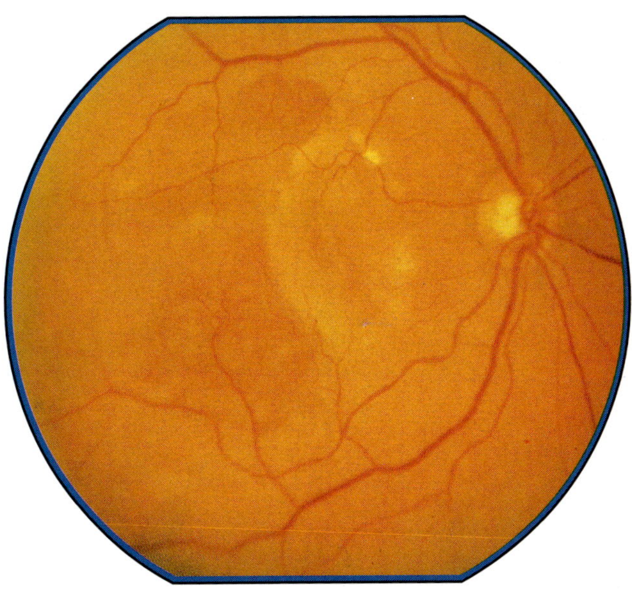

18–103

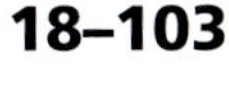

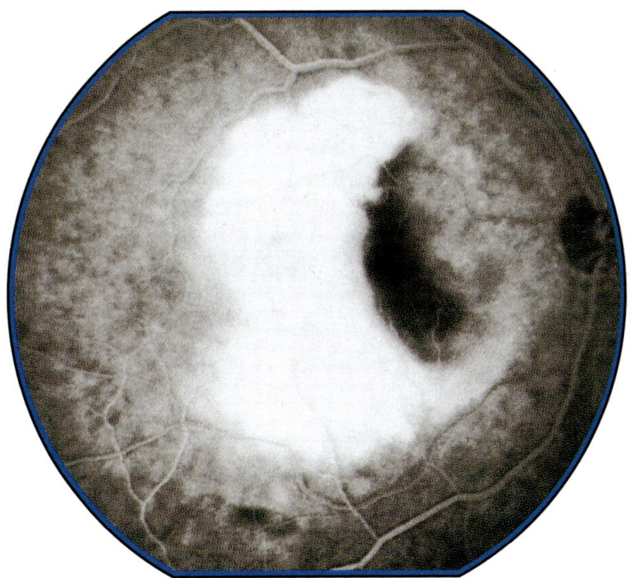

18–102 Rips or tears of the retinal pigment epithelium may occur spontaneously or following laser photocoagulation treatment. Clinically, one can appreciate the rolled edge of the rip as well as the area devoid of tissue.

18–103 Fluorescein angiography reveals hyperfluorescence in the exposed area of the rip and blockage in the area of the redundant rolled tissue.

18–104 PIGMENT EPITHELIAL RIPS **18–105**

18–106 **18–107**

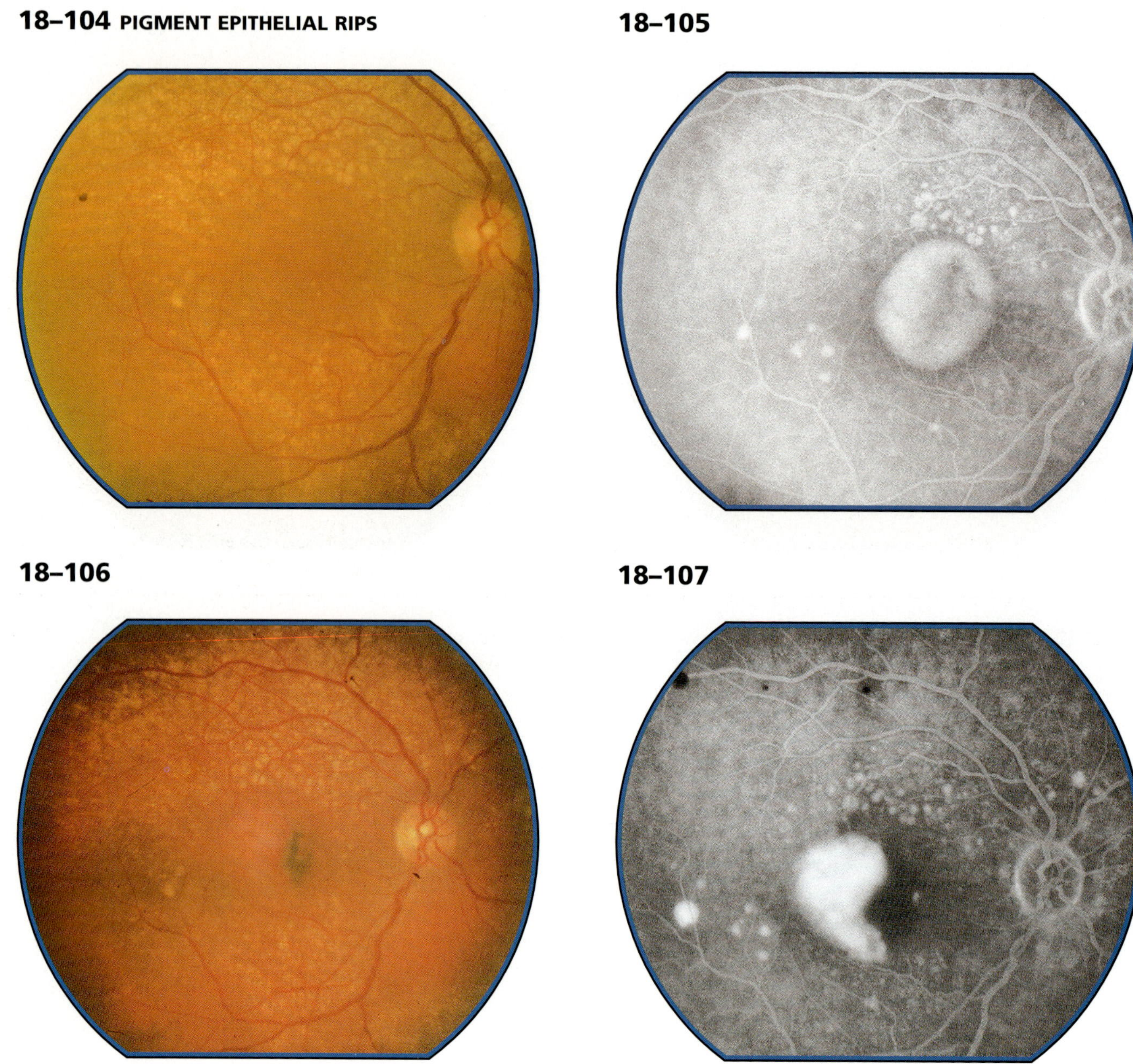

18–104 through 18–107 This patient has a pigment epithelial detachment in the right eye with associated drusen and characteristic hyperfluorescence on the fluorescein angiogram. The patient had a rip of the retinal pigment epithelium in the other eye. Approximately 1 year later, a rip of the pigment epithelium spontaneously occurred in the right eye. Clinically, an area of bare choroid can be demonstrated as well as a rolled-over edge of retinal pigment epithelium. Fluorescein angiography confirms the rip. The hyperfluorescent area shows the underlying choroid. The nasal area of blockage reveals the rolled-over retinal pigment epithelium. This patient was asymptomatic and maintained a visual acuity of 20/25.

18–108

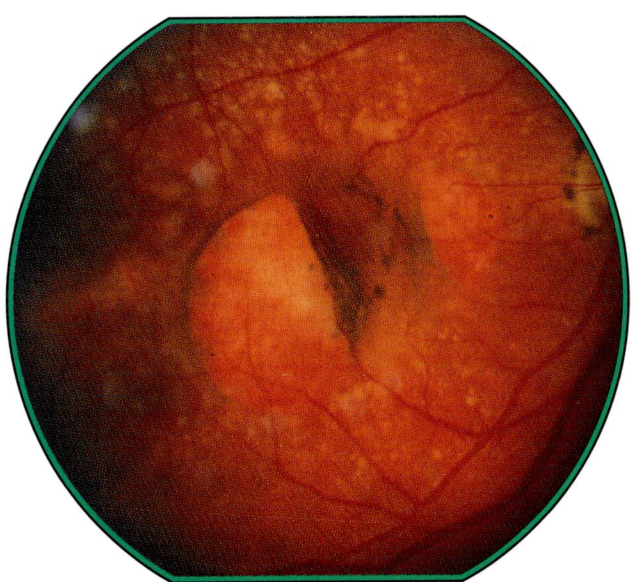

18–109

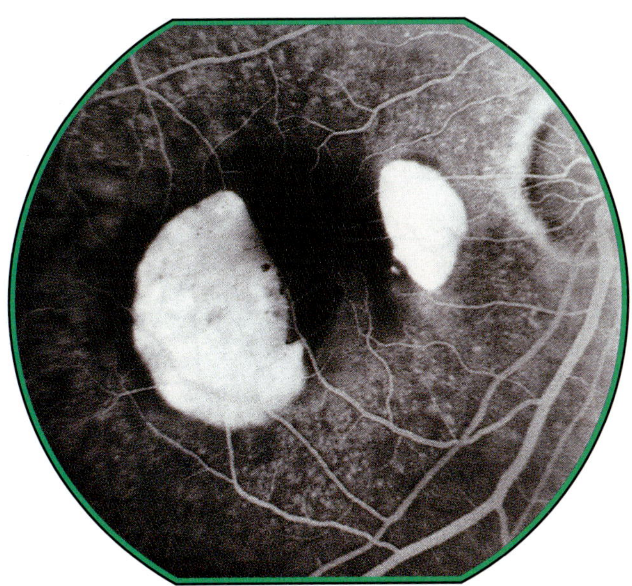

18–108 and 18–109 This patient has a double rip of the retinal pigment epithelium. A central area is noted that corresponds to the rolled edges of the retinal pigment epithelium. On each side is a rip that shows the exposed choroid. Fluorescein angiography confirms the double rip.

***18–108** and **18–109**, Courtesy of Dr. Jeffrey Shakin.*

18–110 **PIGMENT EPITHELIAL RIPS**

18–111

18–112

18–113

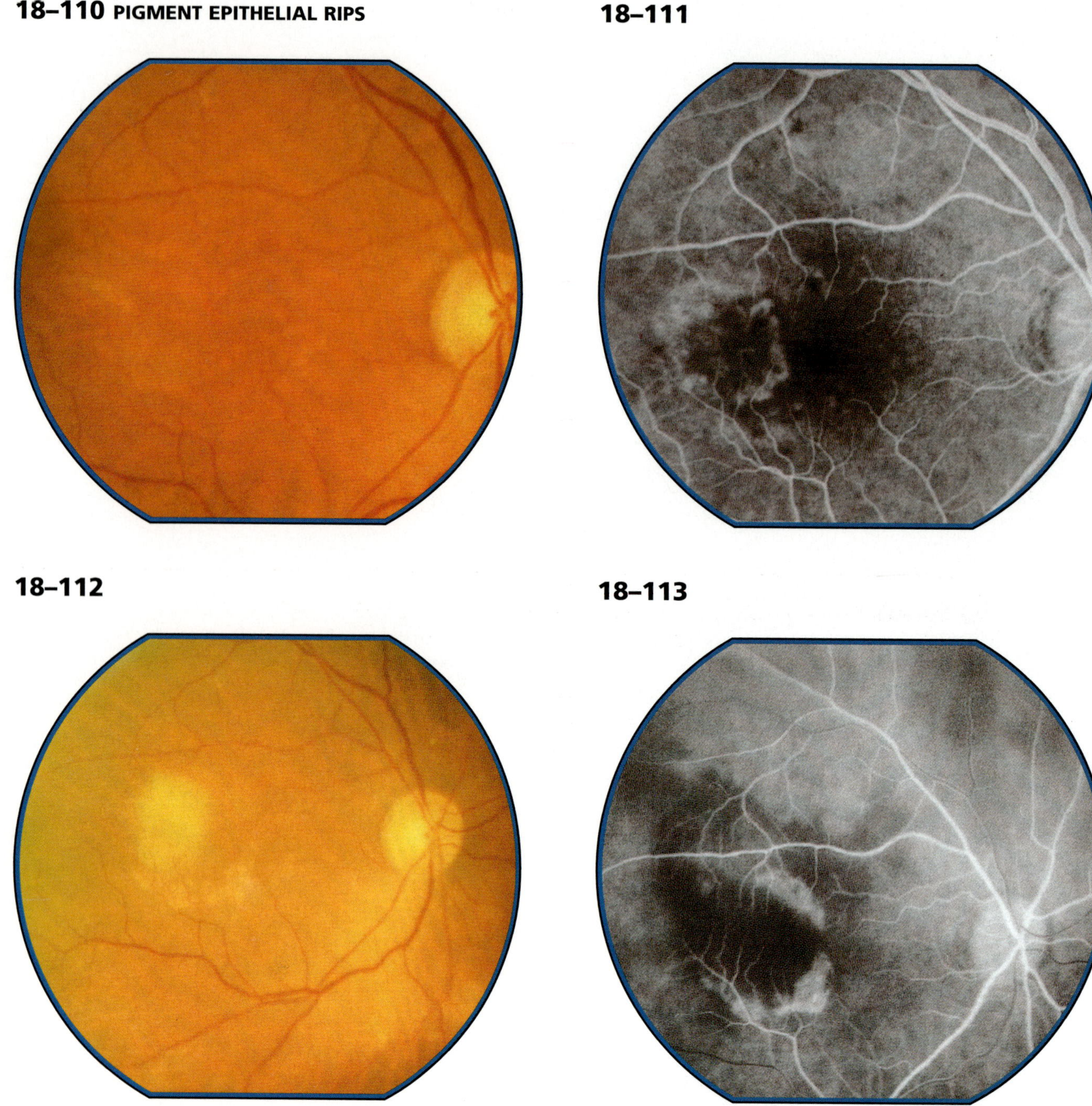

18–110 through 18–113 Rips of the retinal pigment epithelium may also occur following laser photocoagulation therapy. This patient has subretinal fluid (18–110) and a well-defined area of choroidal neovascularization by fluorescein angiography (18–111). Laser photocoagulation was applied to the area of neovascularization. Adjacent to the laser scar is an area of retinal pigment epithelium that is beginning to rip. Fluorescein angiography confirms the rip.

(Case continued on next page.)

18–114

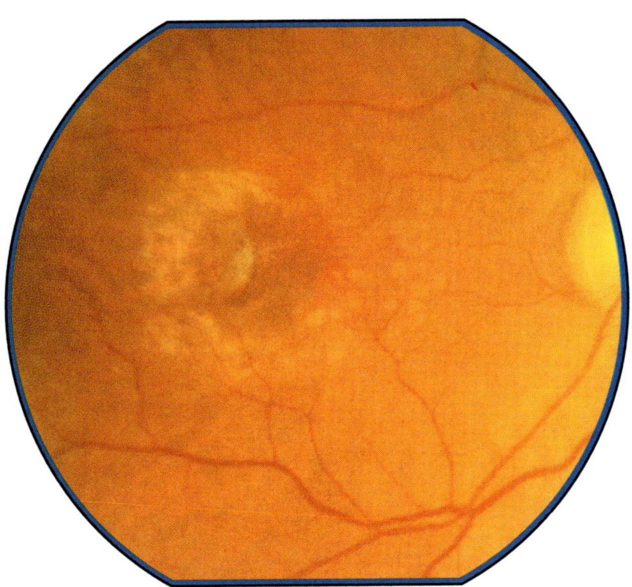

18–115

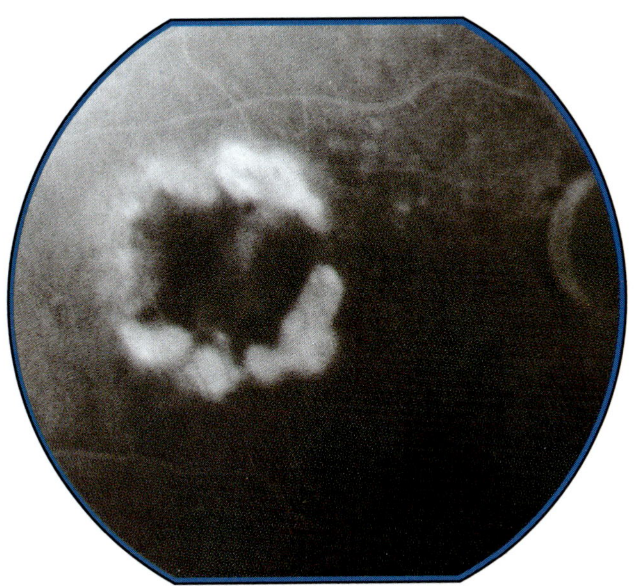

18–114 and 18–115 Six weeks later, the rip is more extensive, becoming circumferential, as noted clinically (18–114) and by fluorescein angiography (18–115). Visual acuity, however, is still 20/40.

18–116 IDIOPATHIC POLYPOIDAL VASCULOPATHY

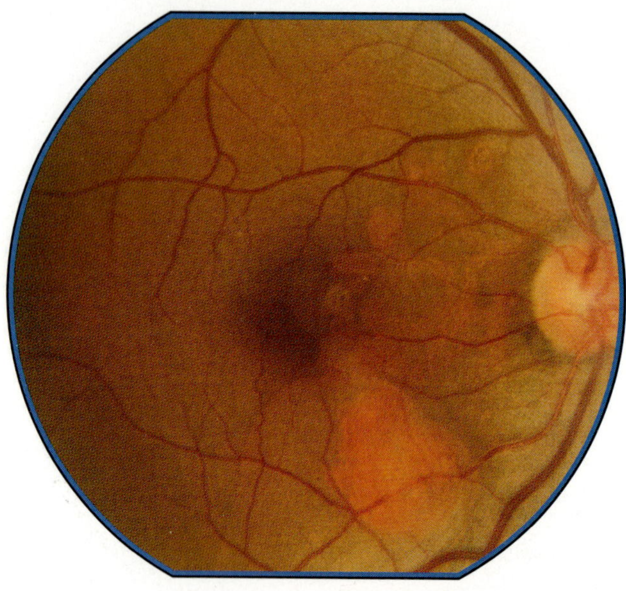

18–117

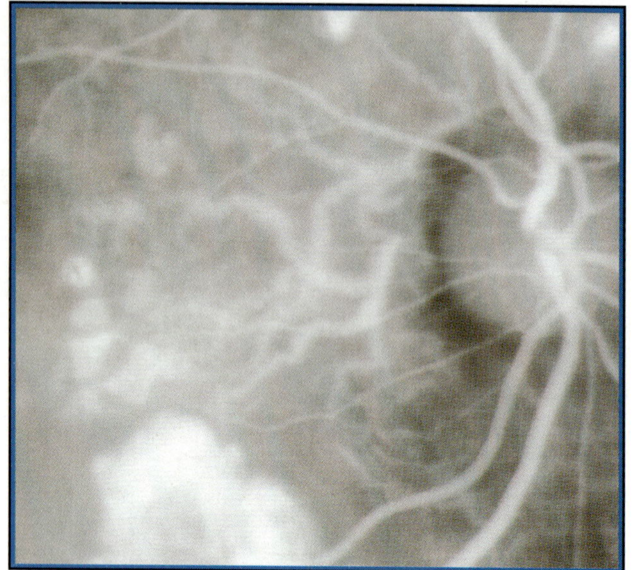

18–118

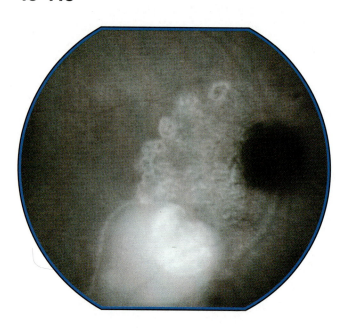

18–116 A variant of macular degeneration is idiopathic polypoidal vasculopathy, which is often seen in younger patients. In this condition, there is a choroidal lesion consisting of dilated vessels ending in polypoidal aneurysmal excrescences that cause recurrent serous and hemorrhagic detachments. The natural history of this disease is more favorable than age-related macular degeneration, and patients often have spontaneous remissions and exacerbations. The clinical photograph shows the characteristic aneurysmal dilatation with the secondary serous and hemorrhagic exudation noted in this disease.

18–117 and 18–118 ICG angiography illustrates the dilated choroidal vessels.

18–119 VITELLIFORM DEGENERATION AND CUTICULAR DRUSEN

18–120

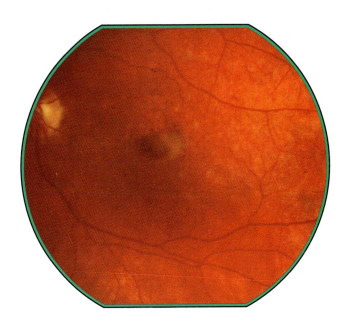

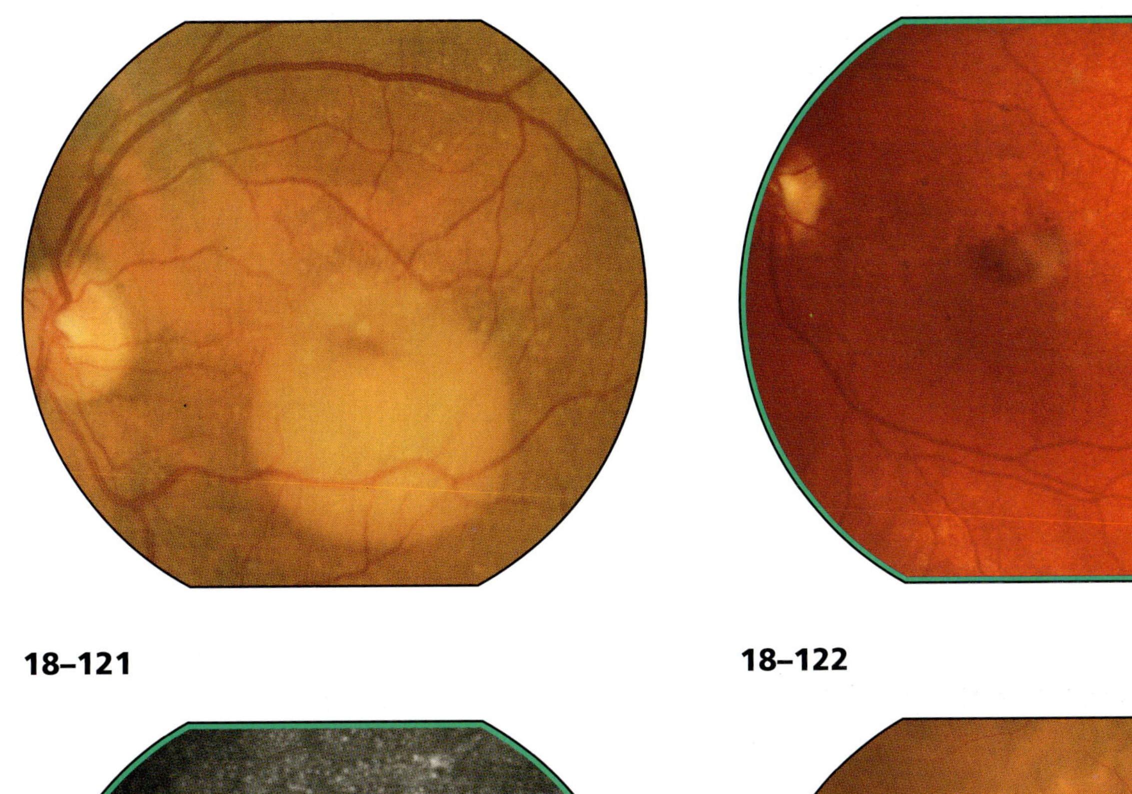

18–121

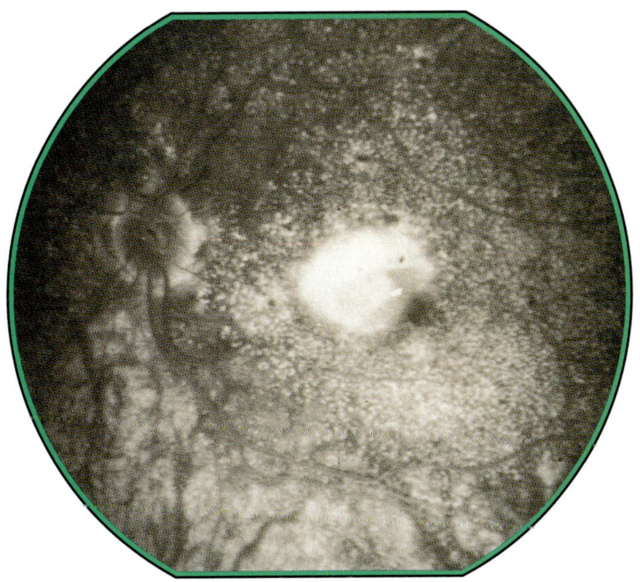

18–122

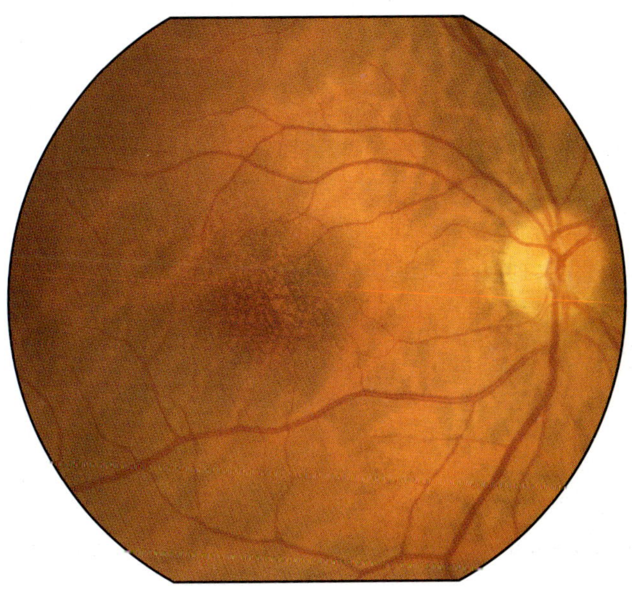

18–119 Vitelliform degeneration with associated cuticular drusen is a hereditary form of macular degeneration. A yellowish vitelliform-like lesion can be seen bilaterally in these patients. This condition is often seen in younger individuals. These patients must be carefully observed for choroidal neovascularization.

18–120 and 18–121 Cuticular drusen are often associated with these vitelliform detachments. This patient has an exudative pigmentary detachment and cuticular drusen. Note that the cuticular drusen are best demonstrated by fluorescein angiography.

18–122 This patient also has fine cuticular drusen.

Suggested Readings

Bird, AC: Pathogenesis of retinal pigment epithelial detachment in the elderly: the relevance of Bruch's membrane change, Doyne Lecture, Eye 5:1–12, 1991

Bressler, NM, Bressler, SB, and Gragoudas, ES: Clinical characteristics of choroidal neovascular membranes, Arch Ophthalmol 105:209–213, 1987

Bressler, NM, Bressler, SB, Seddon, JM, Gragoudas, ES, and Jacobson, LP: Drusen characteristics in patients with exudative versus non-exudative age-related macular degeneration, Retina 8:108–114, 1988

Bressler, SB, Silva, JC, Bressler, NM, Alexander, J, and Green, WR: Clinicopathologic correlation of occult choroidal neovascularization in age-related macular degeneration, Arch Ophthalmol (June) 110:827–832, 1992

Chuang, MD, and Bird, AC: The pathogenesis of tears of the retinal pigment epithelium, Am J Opthalmol 105:285–290, 1988

Coscas, G, and Soubrane, G: Photocoagulation des néovaisseaux sous-rétiniens dans la dégénérescence maculaire sénile par laser à argon, Résultats de l'étude randomisée de 60 cas, Bull Mem Soc Fr Ophthalmol 94:149–154, 1982

Dastgheib, K, Bressler, SB, and Green, WR: Clinicopathologic correlation of laser lesion expansion after treatment of choroidal neovascularization, Retina 13:345–352, 1993

de Juan, Jr, and Machemer, R: Vitreous surgery for hemorrhagic and fibrous complications of age-related macular degeneration, Am J Ophthalmol 105:25–29, 1988

El Baba, F, Green, WR, Fleischmann, J, Finkelstein, D, and de la Cruz, Z: Clinicopathologic correlation of lipidization and detachment of the retinal pigment epithelium, Am J Ophthalmol (May) 101:576–583, 1986

Eye Disease Case–Control Study Group: Antioxidant status and neovascular age-related macular degeneration, Arch Ophthalmol 111:104–109, 1993

Eye Disease Case–Control Study Group: Risk factors for neovascular age-related macular degeneration, Arch Ophthalmol 110:1701–1708, 1992

Ferris, FL, III: Senile macular degeneration: review of epidemiologic features, Am J Epidemiol 118:132–151, 1983

Freund, KP, Yannuzzi, LA, and Sorenson, JA: Age-related macular degeneration and choroidal neovascularization, Am J Ophthalmol, 115:786–791, 1993

Gass, JDM: Serous retinal pigment epithelial detachment with a notch: a sign of occult choroidal neovascularization, Retina 4:205–220, 1984

Green, WR: Clinicopathologic studies of treated choroidal neovascular membranes: a review and report of two cases, Retina (July–Sept) 11:328–356, 1991

Green, WR, and Enger, C: Age-related macular degeneration histopathologic studies: the 1993 Lorenz E. Zimmerman Lecture, Ophthalmol 100 (Oct):1519–1535, 1993

Green, WR, and Key, SN, III: Senile macular degeneration: a histopathologic study, Trans Am Ophthalmol Soc 75:180–254, 1977

Green, WR, McDonnell, PJ, and Yeo, JH: Pathologic features of senile macular degeneration, Ophthalmology 92:615–627, 1985

Guyer, DR, et al: Digital indocyanine-green videoangiography of occult choroidal neovascularization, Ophthalmology 101:1727–1735, 1994

Guyer, DR, Adamis, AP, Gragoudas, ES, Folkman, J, Slakter, JS, and Yannuzzi, LA: Systemic antiantiogenic therapy for choroidal neovascularization, Arch Ophthalmol 110:1383–1384, 1992

Guyer, DR, Fine, SL, Maguire, MG, Hawkins, BS, Owens, SL, and Murphy, RP: Subfoveal choroidal neovascular membranes in age-related macular degeneration: visual prognosis in eyes with relatively good initial visual acuity, Arch Ophthalmol 104:702–705, 1986

Kenyon, KR, Maumenee, AE, Ryan, SJ, Whitmore, PV, and Green, WR: Diffuse drusen and associated complications, Am J Ophthalmol 100:119–128, 1985

Macular Photocoagulation Study Group: Argon laser photocoagulation for neovascular maculopathy after five years: results from randomized clinical trials, Arch Ophthalmol 109:12109–12114, 1991

Macular Photocoagulation Study Group: Laser photocoagulation of subfoveal neovascular lesions in age-related macular degeneration: results of a randomized clinical trial, Arch Ophthalmol 109:1220–1231, 1991

Macular Photocoagulation Study Group: Laser photocoagulation of subfoveal recurrent neovascular lesions in age-related macular degeneration: results of a randomized clinical trial, Arch Ophthalmol 109:1232–1241, 1991

Macular Photocoagulation Study Group: Subfoveal neovascular lesions in age-related macular degeneration: guidelines for evaluation and treatment in the Macular Photocoagulation Study, Arch Ophthalmol 109:1241–1257, 1991

Macular Photocoagulation Study Group: Five-year follow-up of fellow eyes of patients with age-related macular degeneration and unilateral extrafoveal choroidal neovascularization, Arch Ophthalmol 111:1189–1199, 1993

Macular Photocoagulation Study Group: Laser photocoagulation of subfoveal neovascular lesions of age-related macular degeneration: updated findings from two clinical trials, Arch Ophthalmol 111:1200–1209, 1993

Maguire, P, and Vine, AK: Geographic atrophy of the retinal pigment epithelium, Am J Ophthalmol 102:621–625, 1986

Moorfields Macular Study Group: Treatment of senile disciform macular degeneration: a single blind randomized trial by argon laser photocoagulation, Br J Ophthalmol 66:745–753, 1982

Morgan, CM, and Schatz, H: Atrophic creep of the retinal pigment epithelium after focal macular photocoagulation, Ophthalmology 96:96–103, 1989

Pauleikhoff, D, Harper, CA, Marshall, J, and Bird, AC: Aging changes in Bruch's membrane: a histochemical and morphologic study, Ophthalmology 97:171–178, 1990

Sarks, JP, Sarks, SH, and Killingsworth, M: Evolution of geographic atrophy of the retinal pigment epithelium, Eye 2:552–577, 1988

Sarks, SH: Aging and degeneration in the macular region: a clinico-pathological study, Br J Ophthalmol 60:324–341, 1976

Small, ML, Green, WR, Alpar, JJ, and Drewry, RE, Jr: Senile macular degeneration: a clinicopathologic correlation of two cases with neovascularization beneath the retinal pigment epithelium, Arch Ophthalmol 94:601–607, 1976

Sorenson, JA, Yannuzzi, LA, and Shakin, JL: Recurrent subretinal neovascularization, Ophthalmology, vol 92, 1059–1074, 1985

Yannuzzi, LA: Krypton red laser of subretinal neovascularization, Retina, pp 29–46, 1982

Yannuzzi, LA, and Friedman, R: Age-related macular degeneration, NY: Macula Foundation MEETH, 1987

Yannuzzi, LA, and Friedman, R: Age-related macular degeneration, Bull NY Acad Med 64(9):995–1013, 1988

Yannuzzi, LA, and Shakin, J: Krypton red laser photocoagulation of the ocular fundus, Retina 2:1–14, 1982

Yannuzzi, L, Slakter, J, Sorenson, J, Guyer, D, and Orlock, D: Digital indocyanine green videoangiography and choroidal neovascularization, Retina, vol 12, pp 191–223, 1992

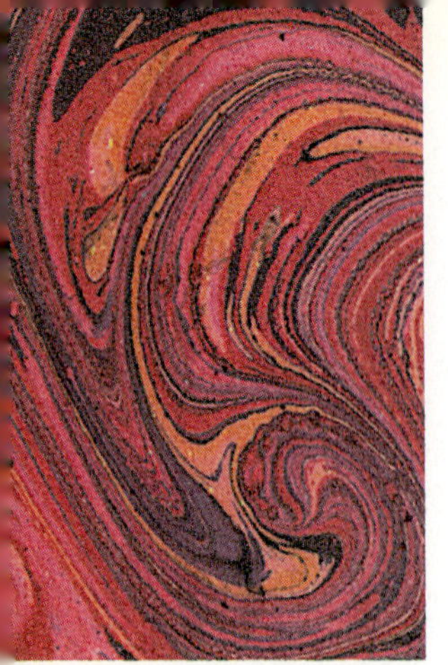

Chapter 19
Degenerative Myopia

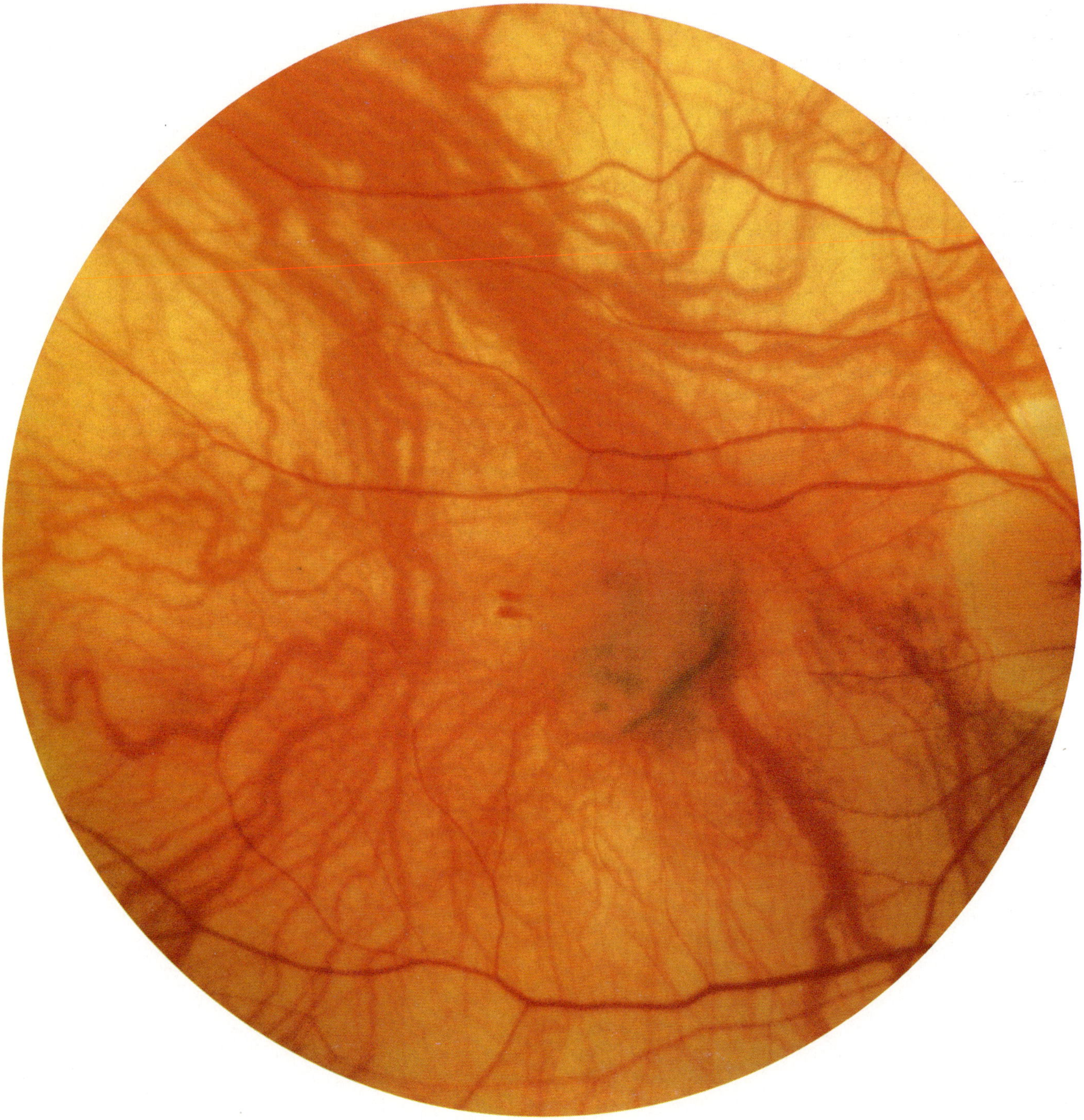

Degenerative or pathologic myopia is a major cause of blindness worldwide. Pathologic myopia may produce macular degeneration, lacquer cracks, choroidal neovascularization, and disciform scars.

Degenerative myopia is usually defined as changes greater than 6 spherical diopters. The condition is usually due to increased axial length.

Degenerative myopia can have several ophthalmologic findings. The optic disc appears tilted. Temporally, an oval area of hypopigmentation may occur, which is called the conus or temporal crescent. Posterior staphyloma may also be noted. The retinal pigment epithelium and choroid are thinned in myopia. Thus, the underlying choroidal vessels can be better appreciated. Later in life, patients with posterior staphylomas have a higher incidence of chorioretinal atrophy. These atrophic areas may coalesce into larger lesions with time. Breaks in Bruch's membranes, which are called lacquer cracks, are common in degenerative myopia. Lacquer cracks are fine yellowish-white, usually horizontal breaks in Bruch's membrane. Lacquer cracks may be associated with choroidal neovascularization. A lacquer crack may extend and cause a macular hemorrhage unassociated with choroidal neovascularization. These hemorrhages usually resolve with time.

A Fuchs' spot is a dark spot in the macula of a patient with degenerative myopia. These pigmented or hemorrhagic lesions represent choroidal neovascularization in a myopic patient. Choroidal neovascularization is believed to occur in approximately 5% to 10% of patients with myopia. Laser photocoagulation can be considered for some of these patients. Lacquer cracks in atrophic areas suggest a poor prognosis for patients with degenerative or pathologic myopia. These eyes are at risk of choroidal neovascularization.

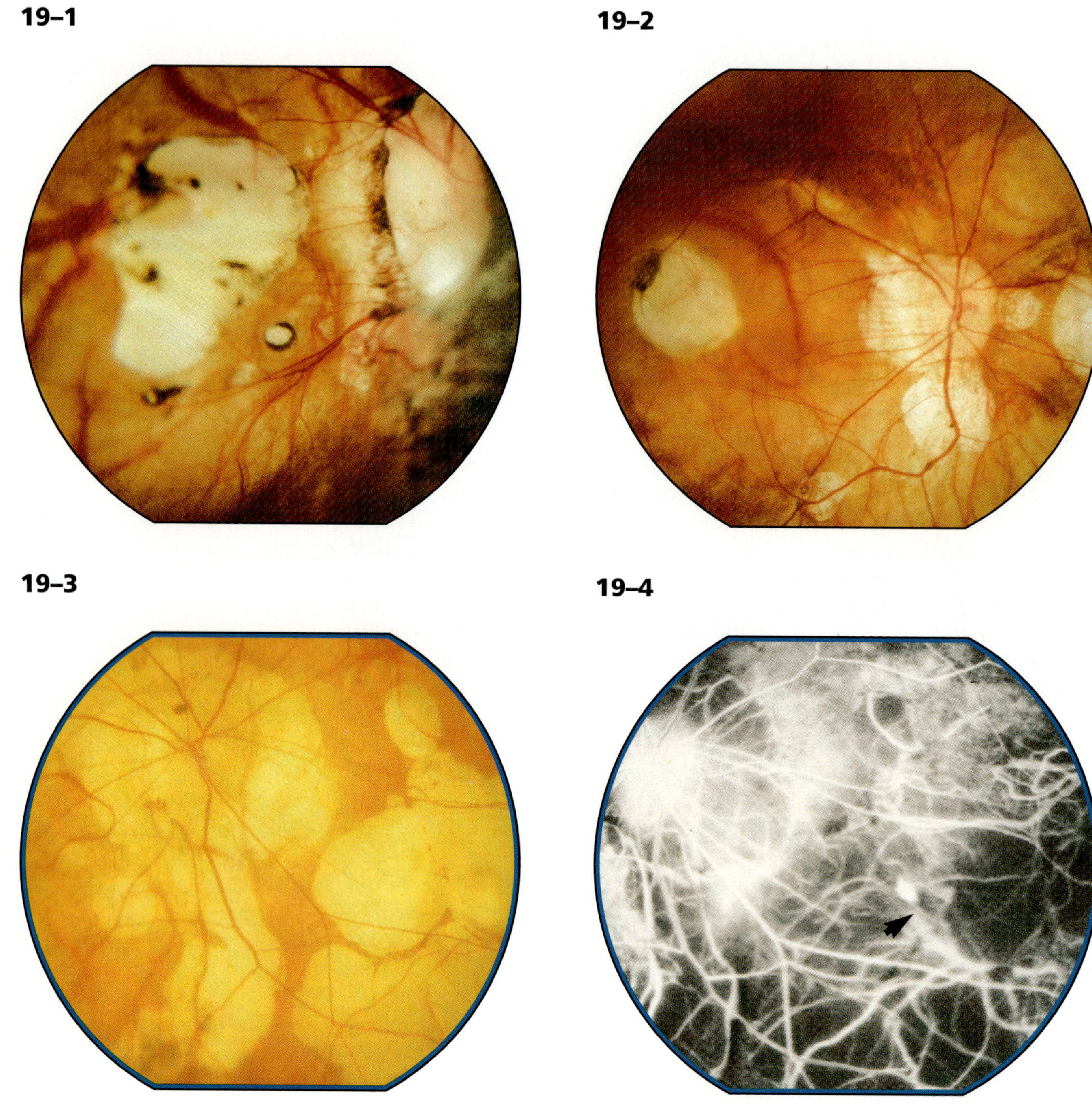

19–1 and 19–2 The typical features of degenerative myopia are demonstrated in these patients, including a peripapillary conus, a tilted disc, chorioretinal atrophy, and retinal pigment epithelial hyperplasia. Various areas of the photographs are out of focus because of photographic difficulties due to the staphyloma. Focal areas of atrophy can also be noted in the macular region. The underlying choroid can be better visualized due to thinning.

19–3 and 19–4 A faint subfoveal disciform scar has faded and is indistinguishable from the atrophic areas in this patient. The fluorescein study confirms the neovascularization *(arrowhead)*.

19–5

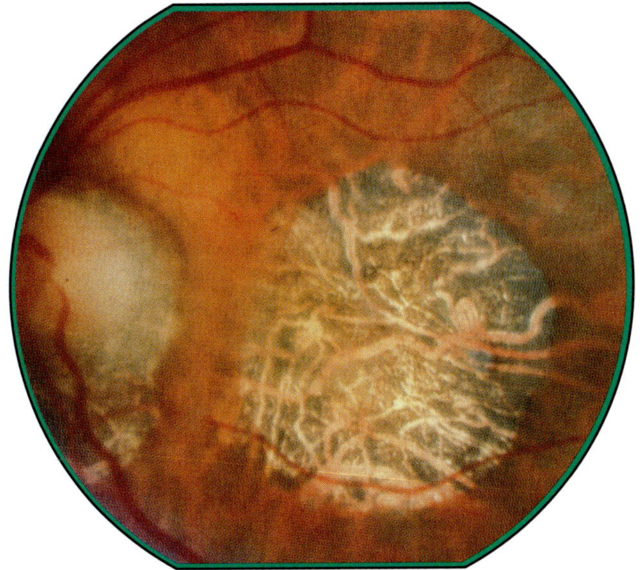

19–6

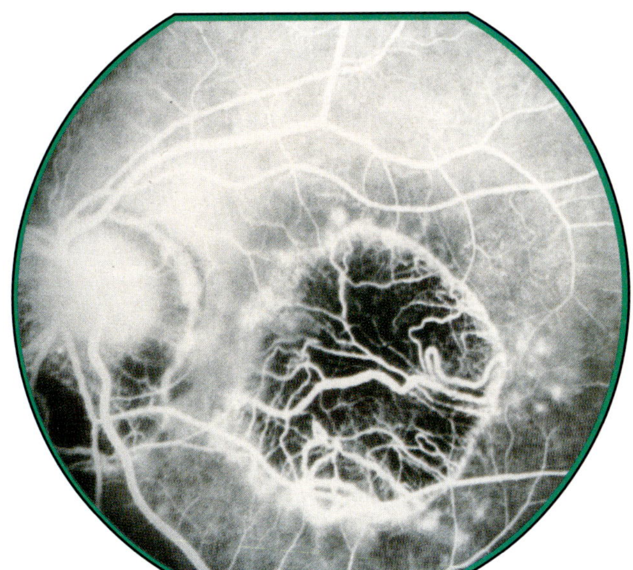

19–7

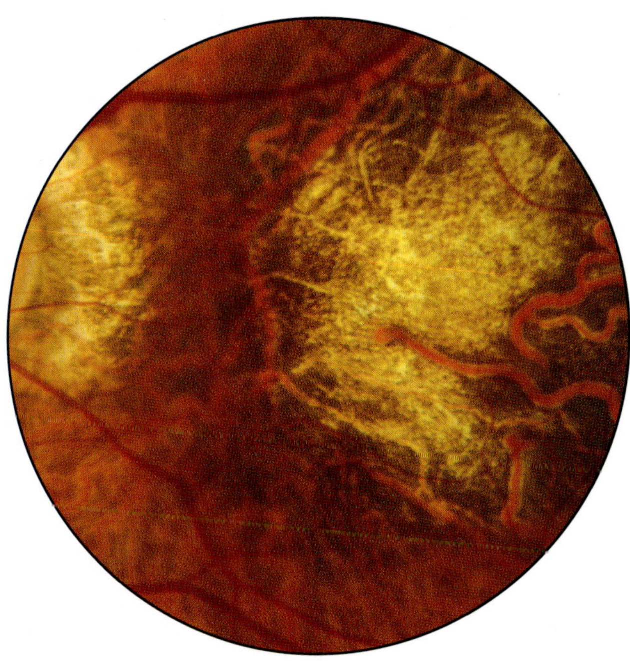

19–5 through 19–7 A more coarse and fine atrophy in the macula can also be seen in these patients. The retinal pigment epithelial and choriocapillaris atrophy expose larger choroidal vessels on the fluorescein study.

19–8

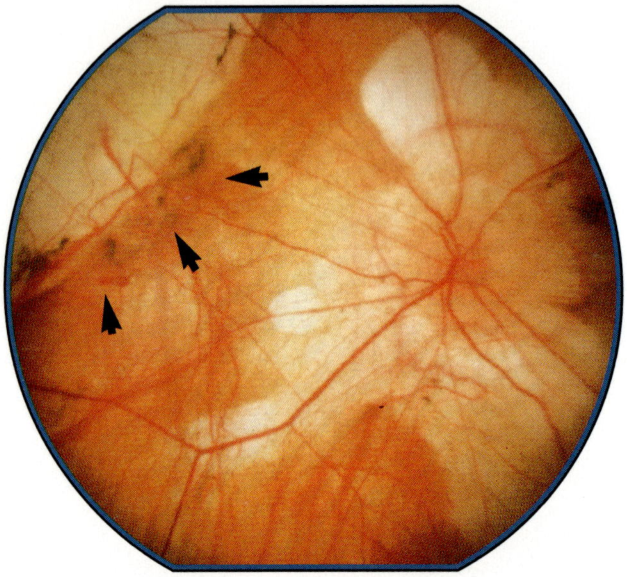

19–8A

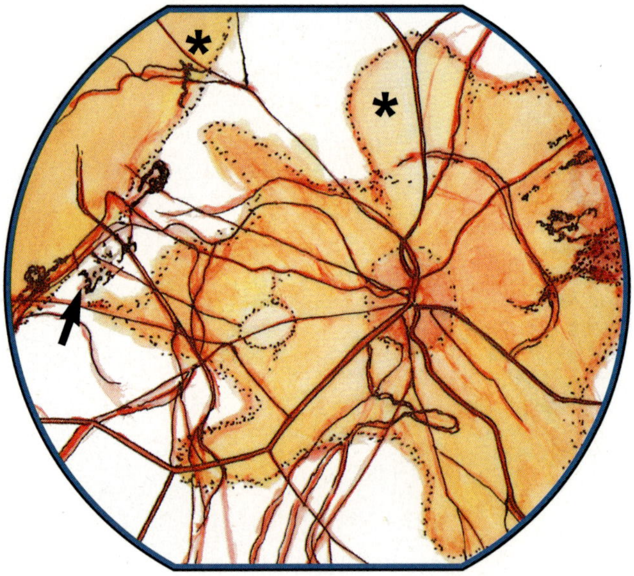

19–9

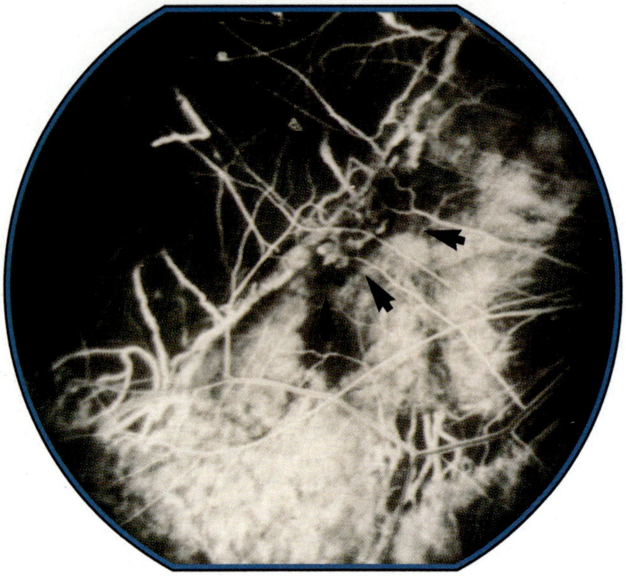

19–10

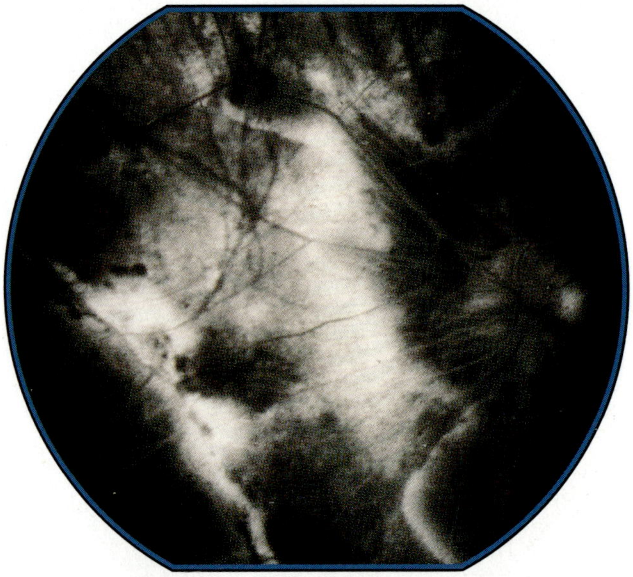

19–8 and 19–8A Subretinal hemorrhage due to choroidal neovascularization can be observed in the margin of zonal atrophy in this myopic patient *(arrowheads). Asterisks,* atrophy; *small arrows,* hemorrhage and neovascularization.

19–9 The fluorescein study shows early lacy fluorescence at the margin of the atrophy *(arrowheads).*

19–10 Late staining of the neovascularization is evident, which must be differentiated from the brush-fire hyperfluorescence produced by the normal choriocapillaris through partially atrophic retinal pigment epithelium in the nasal macula.

19–11

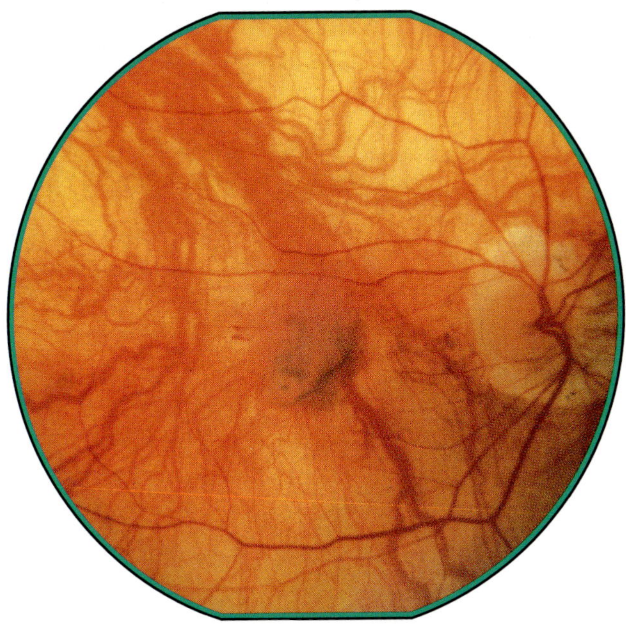

19–12

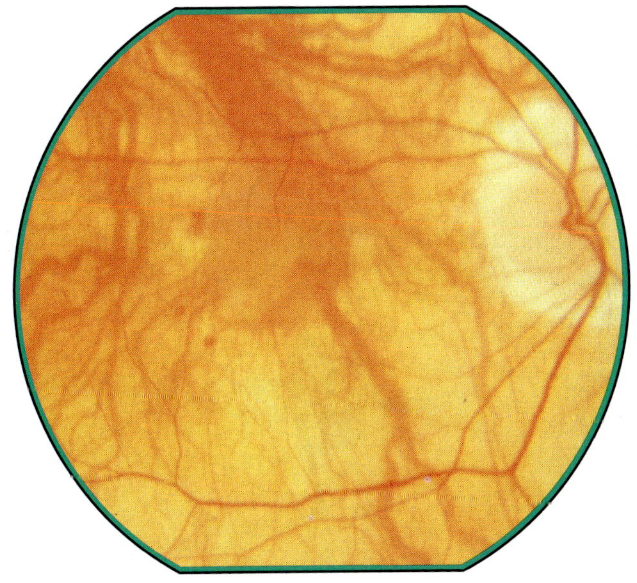

19–13

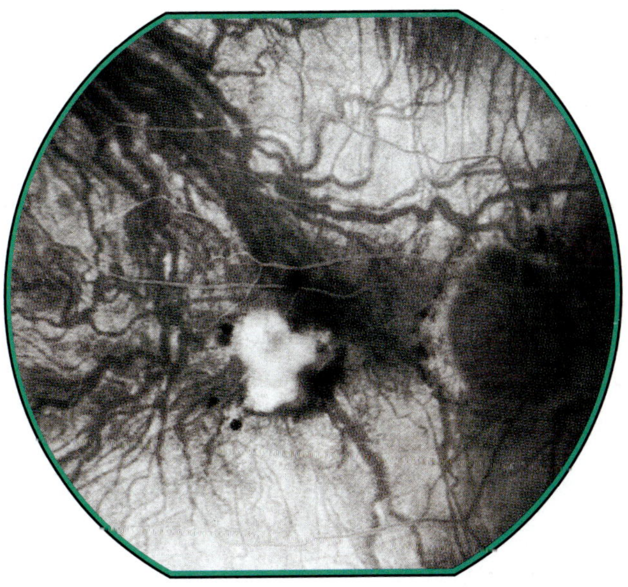

19–11 In this case, pigment epithelial proliferation produces a more characteristic pigmentary Fuchs' spot.

19–12 The choroidal neovascularization or a Fuchs' spot and hemorrhage at another time in this same patient with pathologic myopia is not associated with hyperpigmentation.

19–13 The fluorescein angiogram confirms the choroidal neovascularization in the absence of clinically evident pigmentation.

19–14

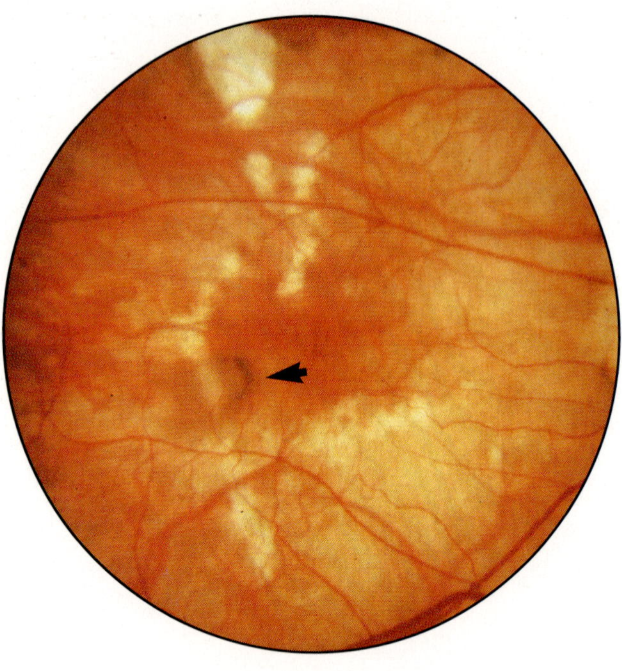

19–15

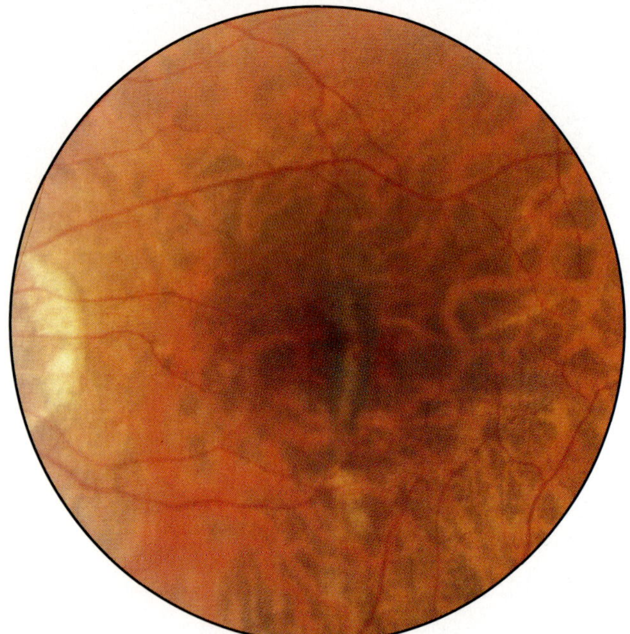

19–15A

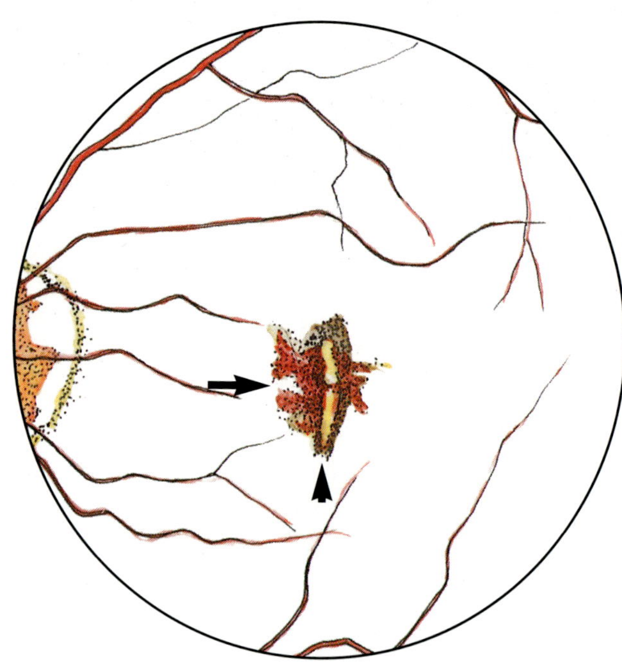

19–14 Fuchs' spots *(arrowhead)* typically occur in lacquer cracks.

19–15 and 19–15A Lacquer cracks *(arrowhead)* can sometimes be oriented vertically. In this case, the Fuchs' spot follows the course of the lacquer crack, with proliferation of the vessels and hemorrhage *(arrow)* at its edges. Note the hemorrhage across the crack.

19–16

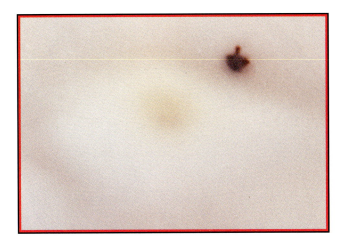

19–17

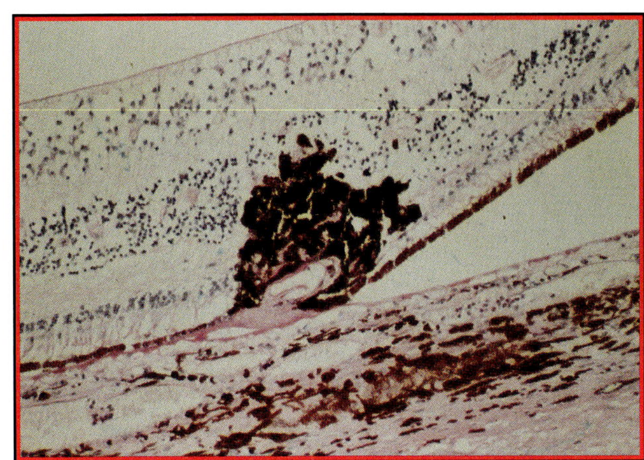

19–18

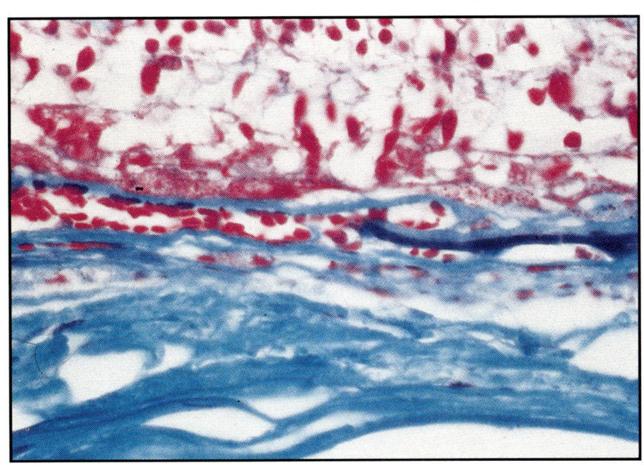

19–16 and 19–17 Gross (19–16) and microscopic (19–17) appearance of a Fuchs' spot near the fovea with choroidal neovascular tissue surrounded by hyperplastic retinal pigment epithelium (19–17).

19–18 An area shows a lacquer crack with a discontinuity of Bruch's membrane and choroidal neovascularization.

19–16 *and* ***19–17,*** *Reprinted with permission from Green, WR: Retina. In Spencer, WH, ed: Ophthalmic pathology. An atlas and textbook, vol 2, Philadelphia, 1985, WB Saunders, p 920.*

19–19

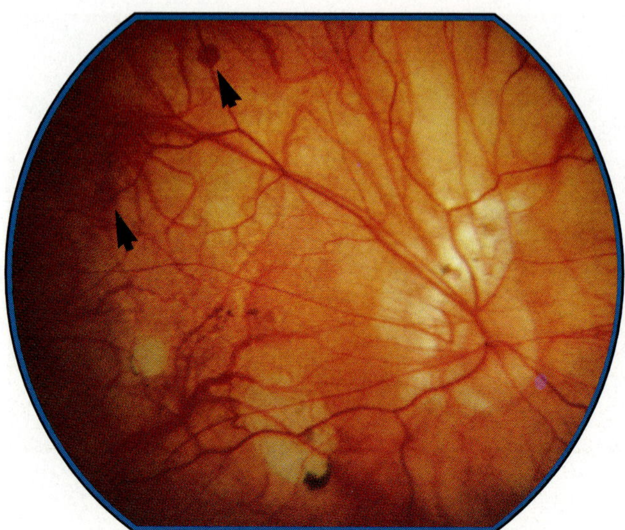

19–20

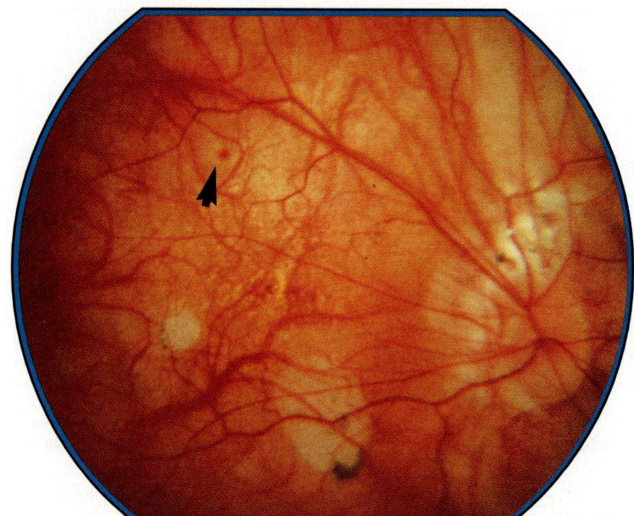

19–21

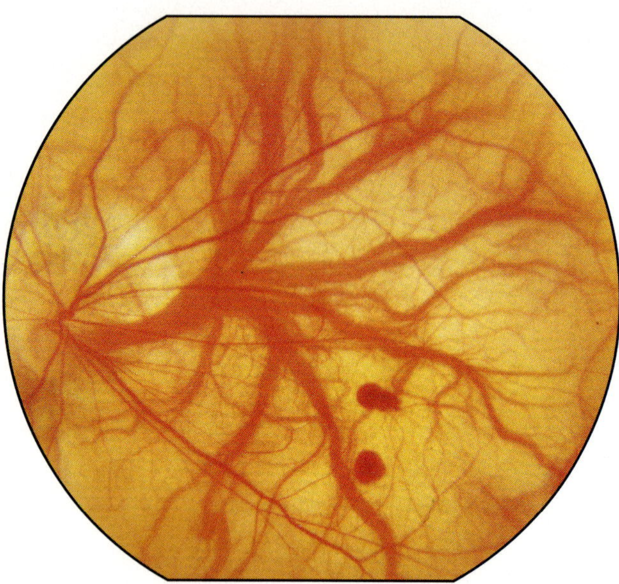

19–19 and 19–20 In some cases, the subretinal hemorrhages *(arrowheads)* in myopia spontaneously resolve, compared with the exudative process that occurs with age-related macular degeneration. This patient has 4 hemorrhages (19–19) which spontaneously resolved (19–20). The patient developed another small hemorrhage at a different site (19–20). This patient had 14 such hemorrhages that resolved spontaneously over approximately 10 years.

19–21 Note the thinned myopic fundus in this patient, who also had subretinal hemorrhage that spontaneously resolved. There is also a large posterior ciliary artery.

19–22

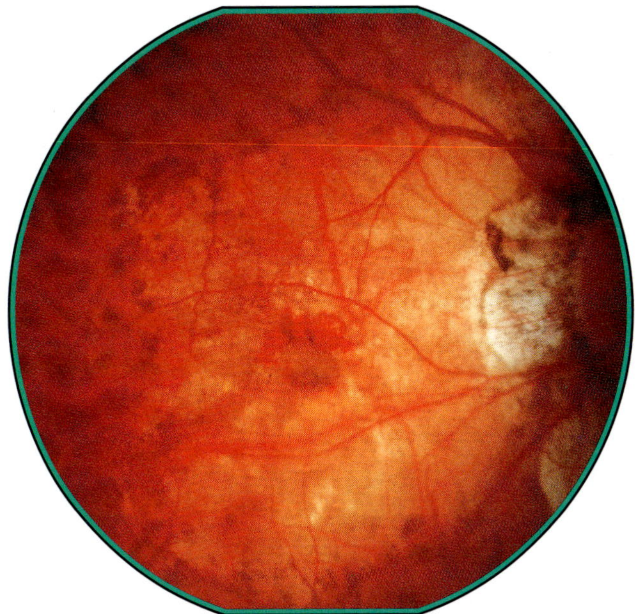

19–23

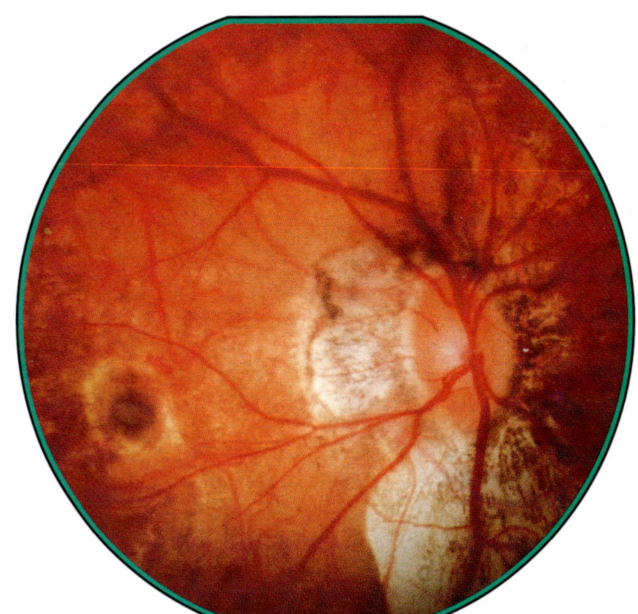

19–24

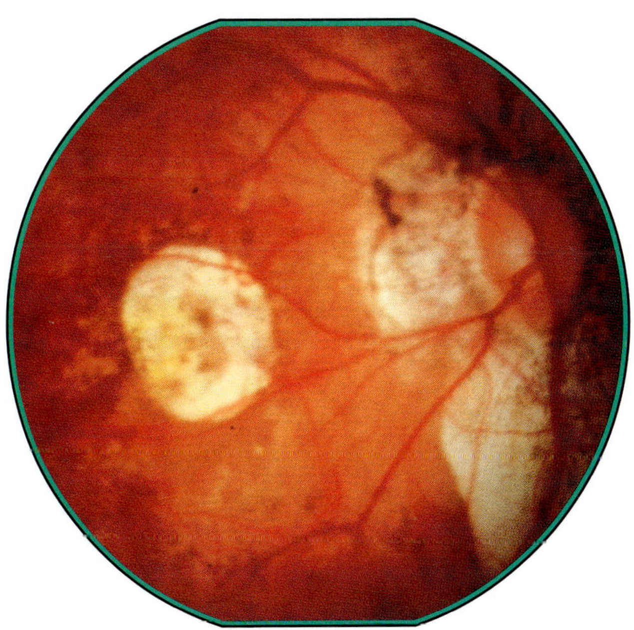

19–22 and 19–23 Progressive atrophy following laser photocoagulation can often be demonstrated in patients with exudative myopic degeneration. This patient presented with subretinal hemorrhage secondary to choroidal neovascularization due to myopia. Note the pigmented Fuchs' spot margined by hemorrhage. Laser photocoagulation was applied to this lesion.

19–24 With time, there was progression of the size of the laser scar. However, the natural course of myopic degeneration also may show progression of atrophic areas, as demonstrated in the next case.

19–25 **19–26**

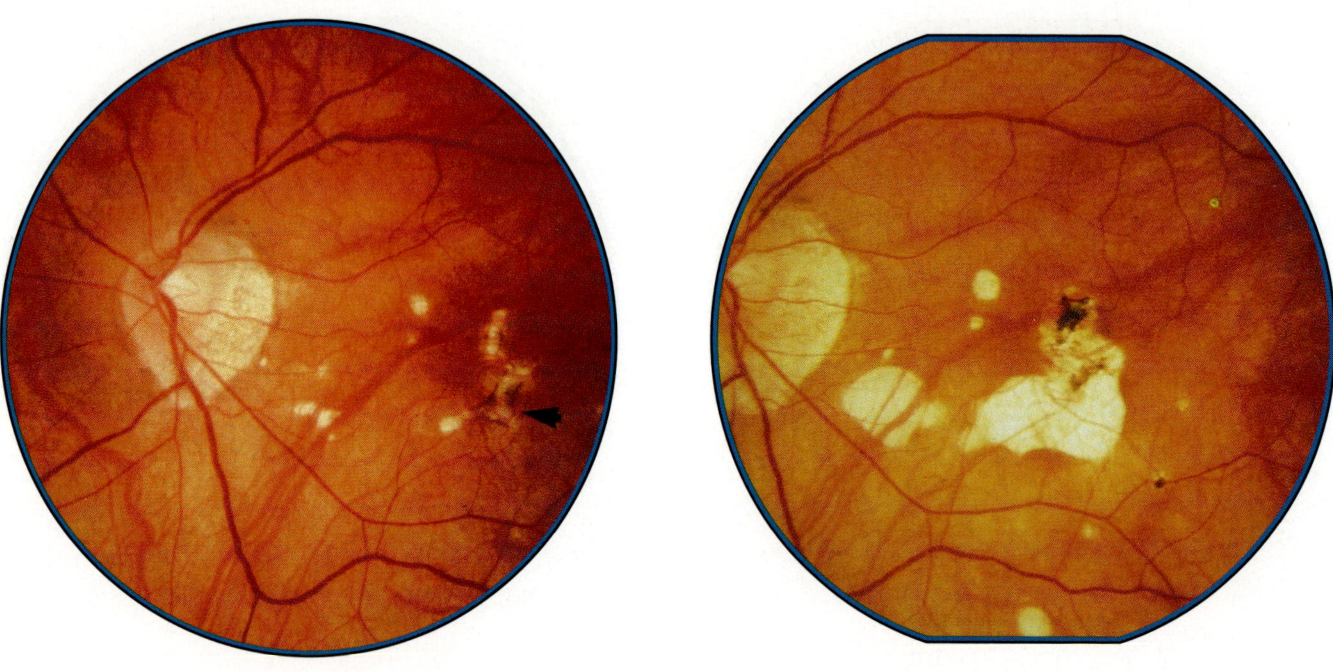

19–25 This patient presented with peripapillary myopic degeneration and a focal area of choroidal neovascularization *(arrowhead)*.

19–26 With time, the areas of atrophic degeneration increased in size, particularly contiguous with the neovascularization.

19–27 **19–28**

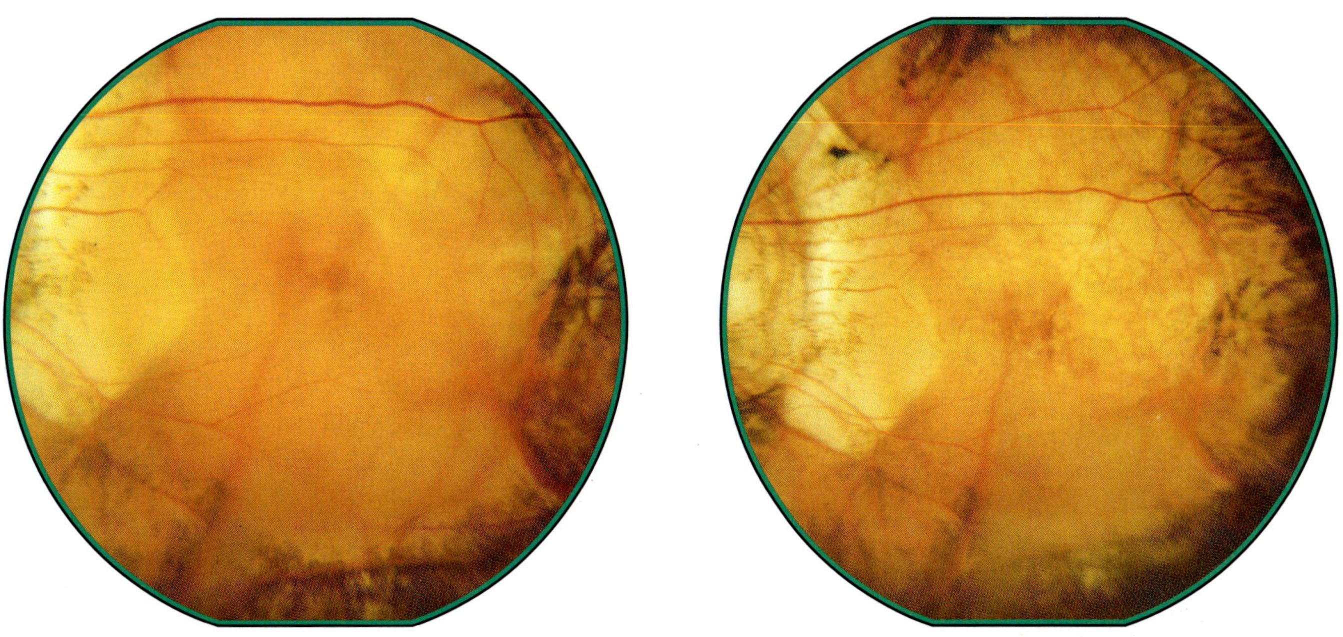

19–27 Myopia may also lead to tractional retinal detachments, as in this case. Note the detachment of the posterior pole.

19–28 Vitrectomy was performed with reattachment of the retina and improvement in visual acuity.

19–27 *and* ***19–28,*** *Courtesy of Dr. Yale L. Fisher.*

19–29 **19–30**

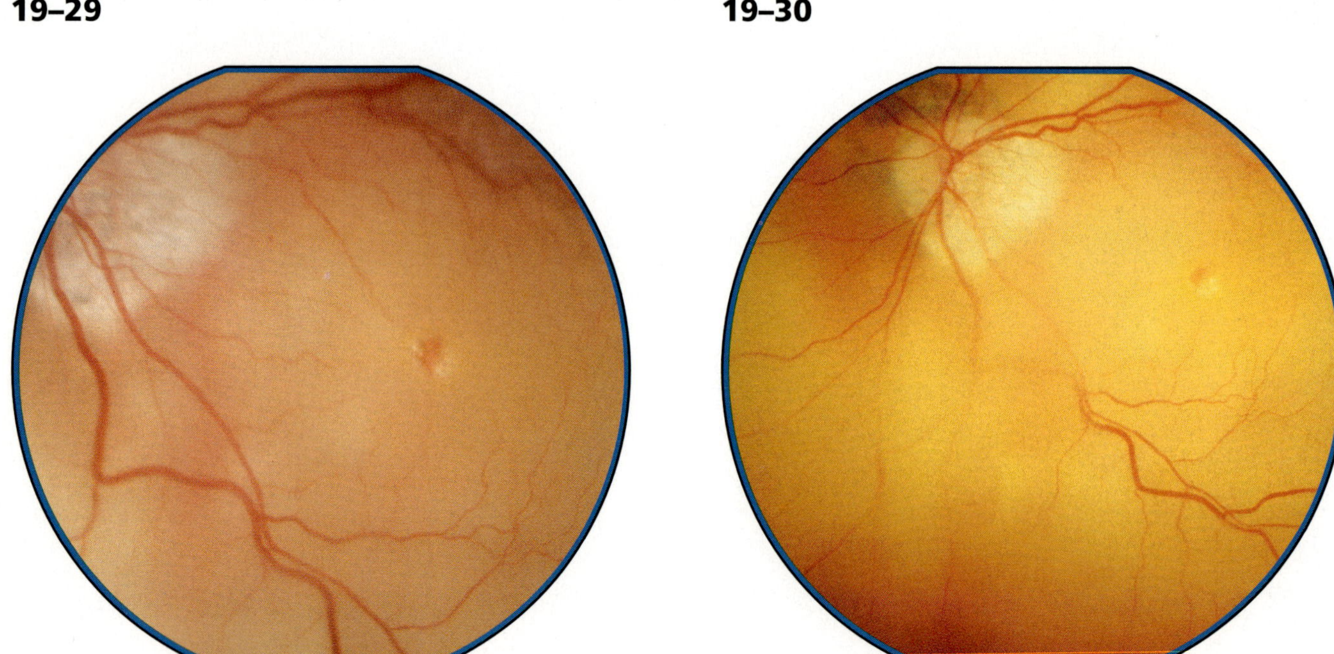

19–29 and 19–30 This patient has myopia with a macular hole and secondary retinal detachment. Note the myopic conus, macular hole and retinal detachment.

19–29 *and* ***19–30,*** *Courtesy of Dr. Stanley Chang.*

Suggested Readings

Avila, MP, Weiter, JJ, Jalkh, AE, Trempe, CL, Pruett, RC, and Schepens, CL: Natural history of choroidal neovascularization in degenerative myopia, Ophthalmology 91:1573–1581, 1984

Brancato, R, Menchini, U, Pece, A, Capoferri, C, Avanza, P, and Radrizzani, E: Dye laser photocoagulation of macular subretinal neovascularization in pathological myopia, Int Ophthalmol 11:235–238, 1988

Brancato, R, Pece, A, Avanza, P, and Raddrizzani, E: Photocoagulation scar expansion after laser therapy for choroidal neovascularization in degenerative myopia, Retina 10:239–243, 1990

Curtin, BJ: "The myopias": basic science and clinical management, Philadelphia 1985, Harper & Row Publishers

Green, JL, and Rabb, MF: Degeneration of Bruch's membrane and retinal pigment epithelium, Int Ophthalmol Clin 21:27–50, 1981

Grossniklaus, HE, and Green, WR: Pathologic findings in pathologic myopia, Retina 12:127–133, 1992

Jalkh, AE, Weiter, JJ, Trempe, CL, Pruett, RC, and Schepens, CL: Choroidal neovascularization in degenerative myopia: role of laser photocoagulation, Ophthalmic Surg 18:721–725, 1987

Milch, FA, Yannuzzi, LA, and Rudick, AJ: Pathologic myopia and subretinal hemorrhages, Ophthalmology 94 (Suppl):117, 1987

Rabb, MF, Garron, I, and La Franco, FP: Myopic macular degeneration, Int Ophthalmol Clin 21:51–69, 1981

Soubrane, G, Pison, J, Bornert, P, Perrenoud, F, and Coscas, G: Néovaisseaux sous–rétiniens de la myopie dégénérative: résultats de la photocoagulation, Bull Soc Ophthalmol Fr 86:269–272, 1986

Sperduto, RD, Seigel, D, Roberts, J, and Rowland, M: Prevalence of myopia in the United States, Arch Ophthalmol 101:405–407, 1983

Wallman, J, Turkel, J, and Trachtman, J: Extreme myopia produced by modest change in early visual experience, Science 201:1249–1254, 1978

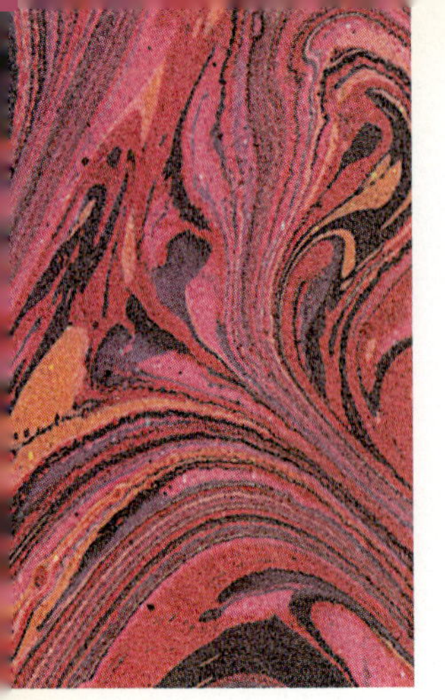

Chapter 20

Central Serous Chorioretinopathy

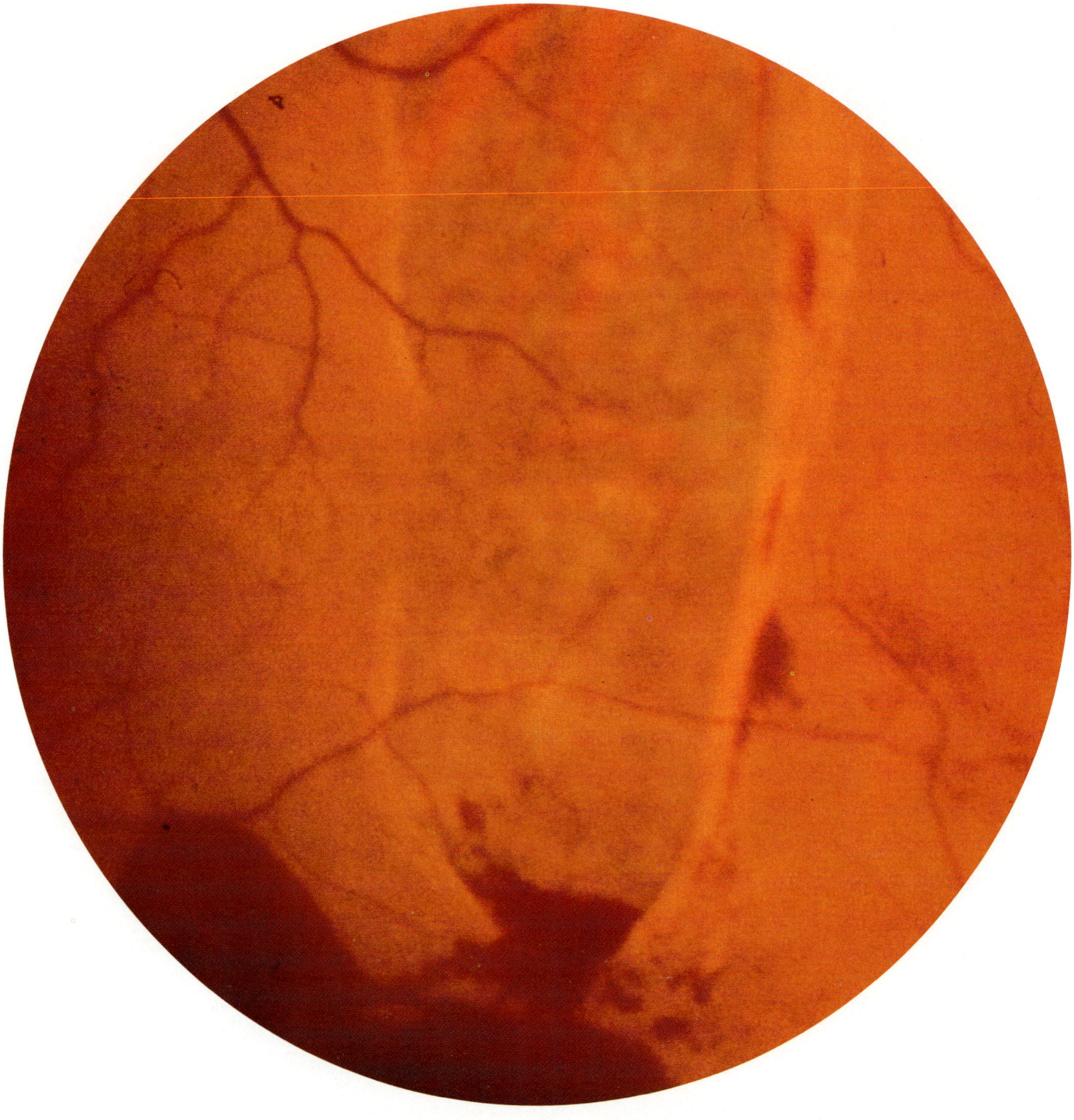

Central serous chorioretinopathy is a condition usually seen in younger patients in which a neurosensory retinal detachment is noted with or without an associated pigment epithelial detachment. The condition has been associated with a "type A" personality, and a similar picture has been induced in monkeys after intravenous epinephrine injection. Recent work with digital indocyanine-green videoangiography suggests that choroidal hyperpermeability may be important in the pathogenesis of this disorder. Unlike choroidal neovascularization secondary to age-related macular degeneration, subretinal hemorrhage is usually not noted in this condition. Rarely, chronic detachment, retinal pigment epithelial changes, or secondary choroidal neovascularization can be seen. Even rarer, deep intraretinal hemorrhage may be associated with this condition due to stretching of the blood vessels. The condition usually spontaneously regresses within several months. Approximately one-third to one-half of patients will have a recurrence.

20–1

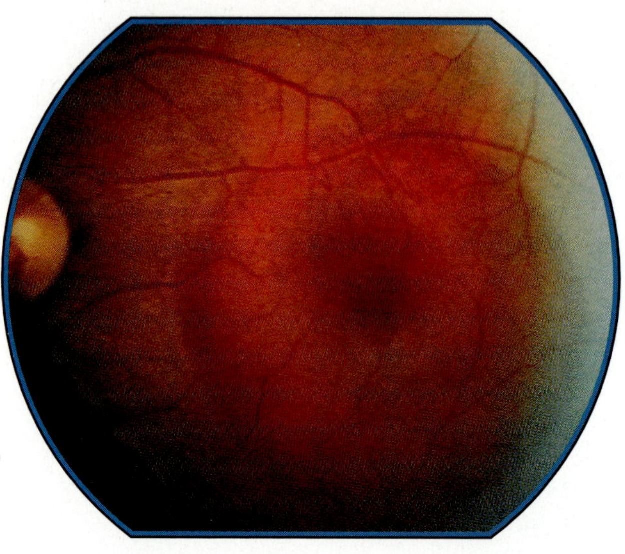

20–2

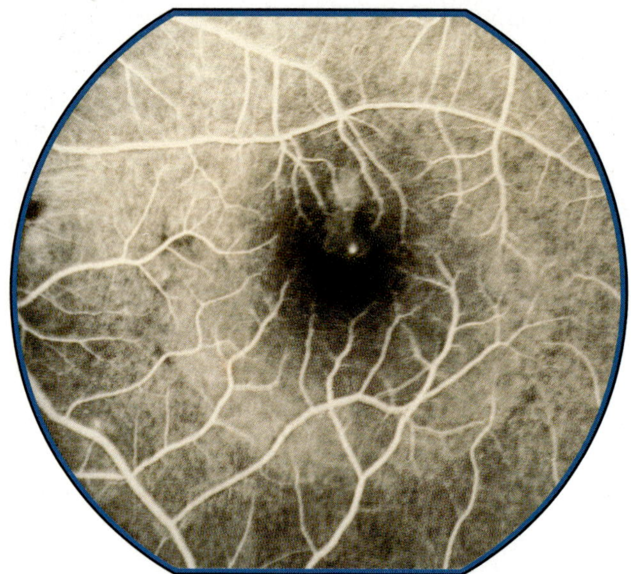

20–3

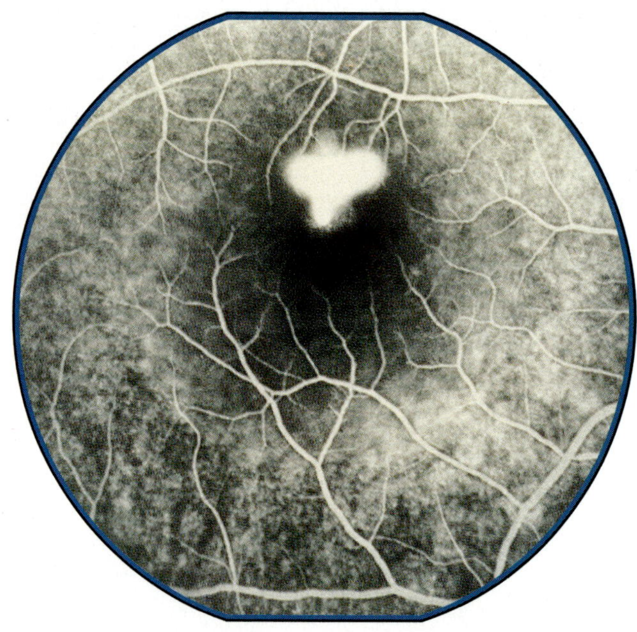

20–1 through 20–3 This patient has a serous macular detachment with the characteristic fluorescein angiographic findings of central serous chorioretinopathy. Early in the study, a pinpoint area of hyperfluorescence is noted (20–2), which leads to the characteristic smokestack configuration (20–3). Only approximately 15% to 20% of patients with central serous chorioretinopathy have this characteristic smokestack appearance.

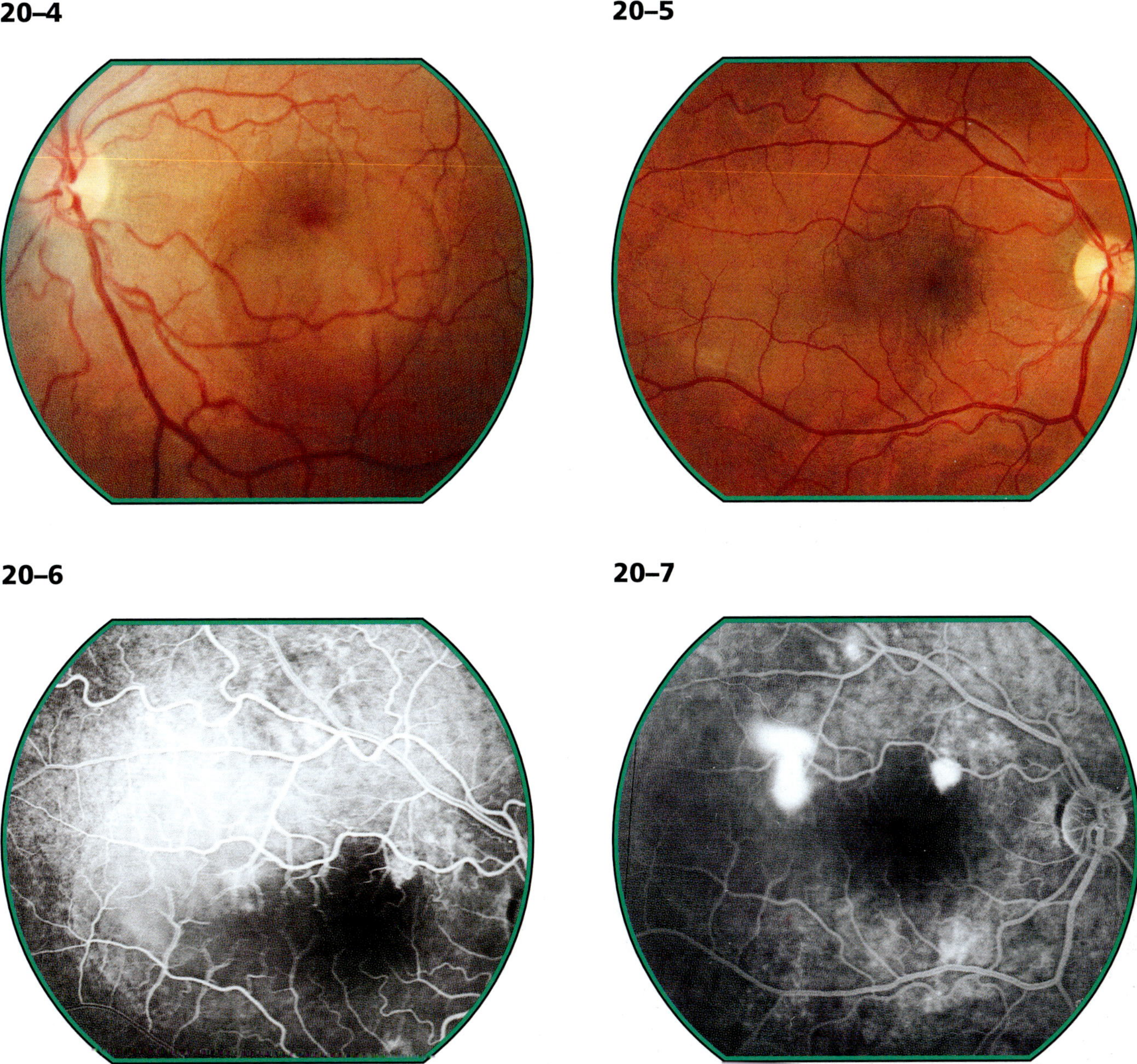

20–4 and 20–5 Another patient demonstrates central serous chorioretinopathy in both eyes.

20–6 and 20–7 The fluorescein angiogram shows a smokestack leak temporal to the macula and several pigment epithelial detachments. The pigment epithelial detachments show faintly increasing hyperfluorescence on the fluorescein angiogram.

20–6 *and* ***20–7,*** *From Guyer, DR, et al: Digital indocyanine-green videoangiography of central serous chorioretinopathy, Arch Ophthalmol 112:1057–1062, 1994. Copyright 1994, American Medical Association.*

(Case continued on next page.)

20–8 CSC–ICG

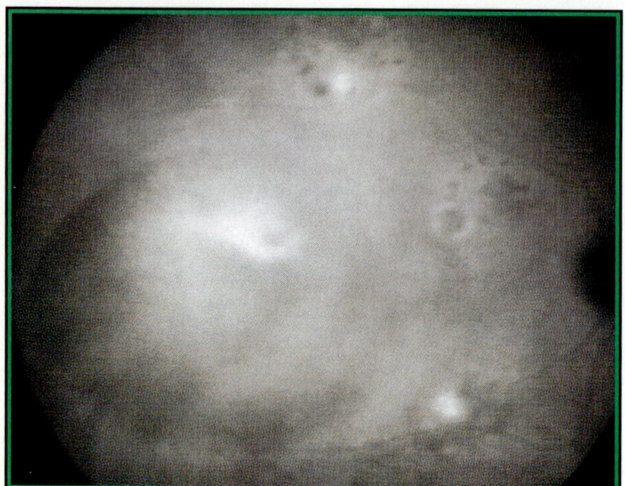

20–9

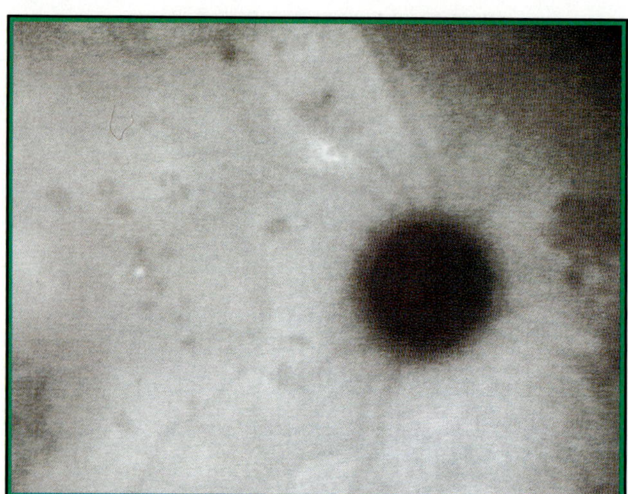

20–10

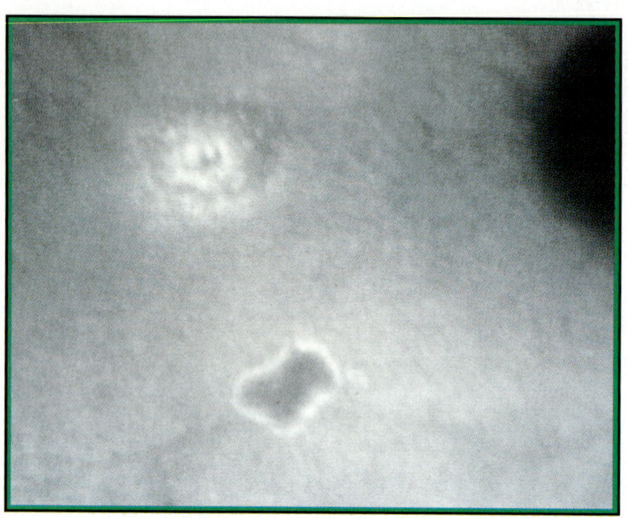

20–8 through 20–10 Digital indocyanine-green (ICG) videoangiography findings suggest that pigment epithelial detachments may be more common in this disorder and that the condition may thus be more diffuse than previously believed. Note the multiple pigment epithelial detachments on the ICG angiogram with their characteristic late central hypofluorescent region surrounded by a rim of hyperfluorescence.

20–8 *through* ***20–10,*** *From Guyer, DR, et al: Digital indocyanine-green videoangiography of central serous chorioretinopathy, Arch Ophthalmol 112:1057–1062, 1994. Copyright 1994, American Medical Association.*

20–11

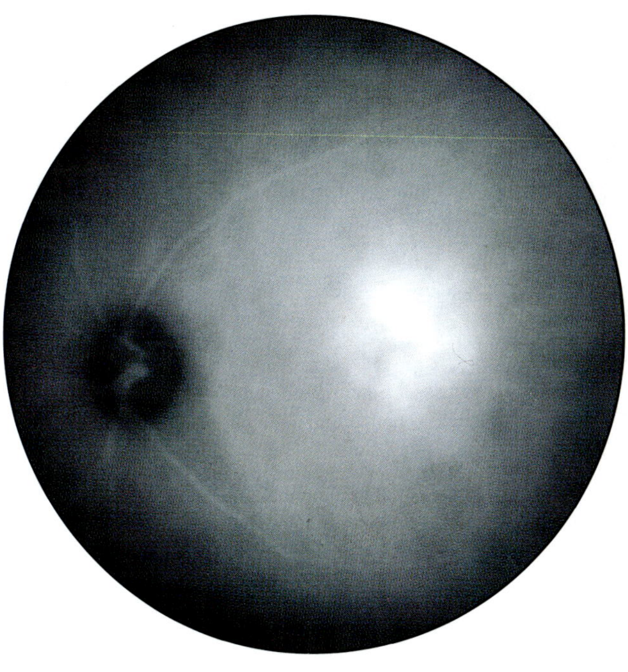

20–12

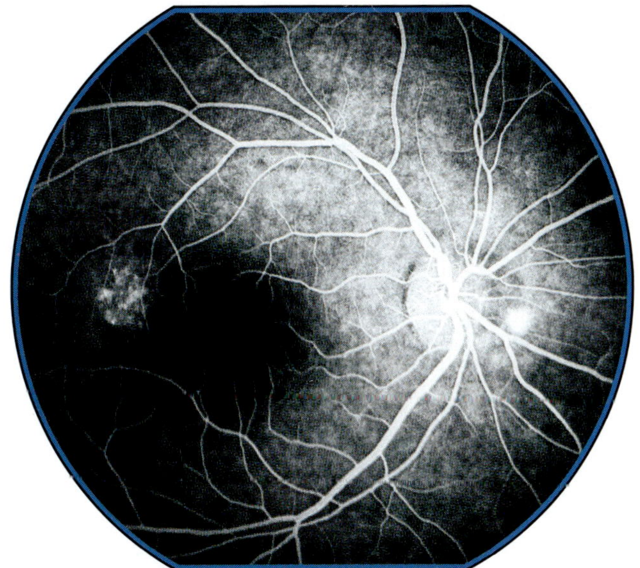

20–13

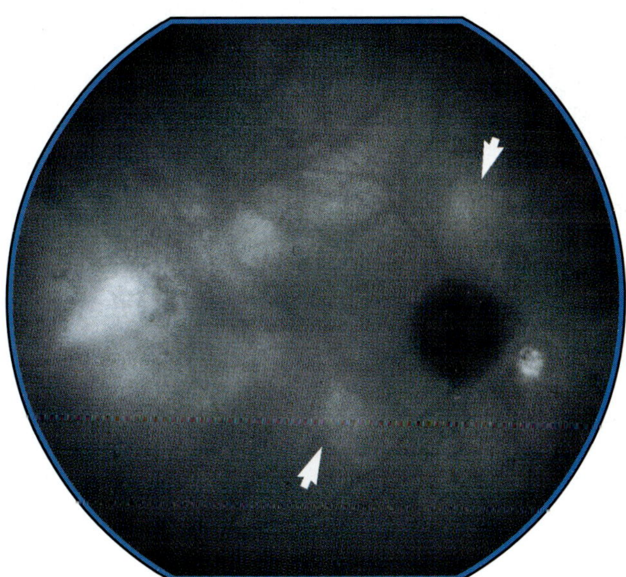

20–11 through 20-13 ICG angiography also reveals choroidal hyperpermeability around active leakage sites (20–11) and in areas that appear normal by clinical examination and fluorescein angiography *(arrowheads)* (20–12, fluorescein angiogram; 20–13, ICG angiogram).

20–11 *through* ***20–13,*** *From Guyer, DR, et al: Digital indocyanine-green videoangiography of central serous chorioretinopathy, Arch Ophthalmol 112:1057–1062, 1994. Copyright 1994, American Medical Association.*

20–14 FIBRIN

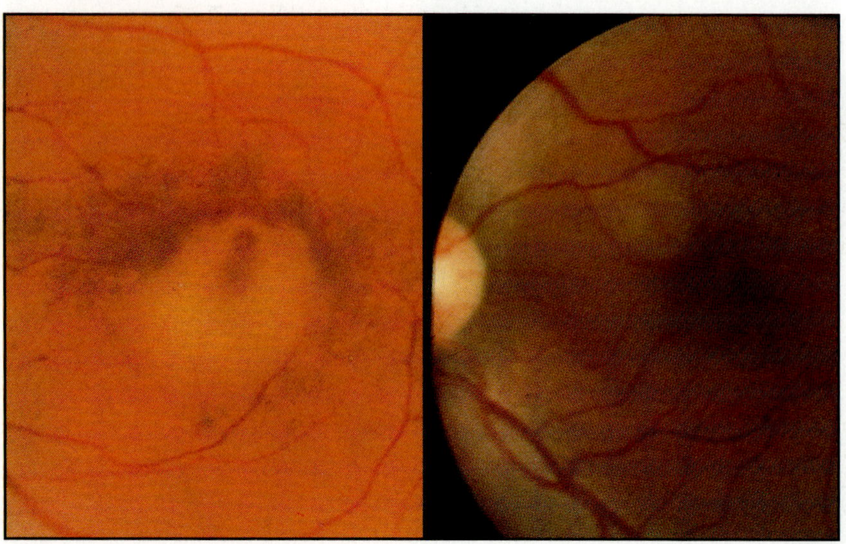

20–15 ORGAN TRANSPLANTATION

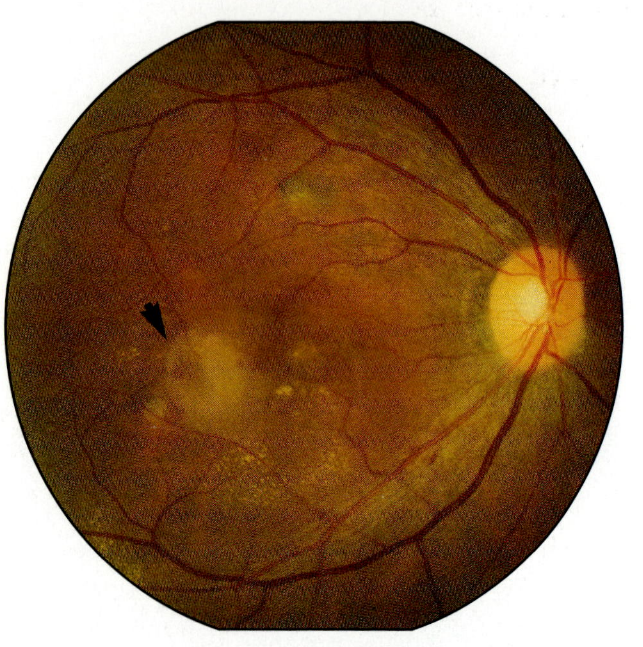

20–16 CHRONIC CHANGES

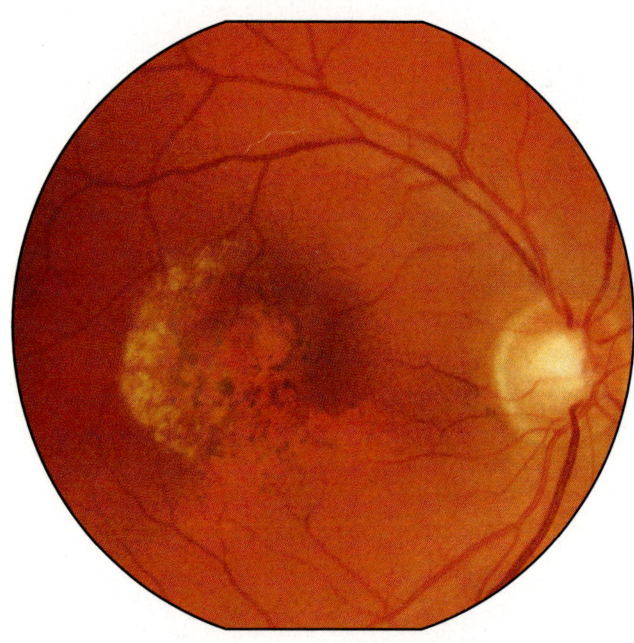

20–14 Fibrin deposition may be noted in some patients. It often masks an underlying serous retinal pigment epithelium (RPE) detachment.

20–15 Organ transplantation may sometimes be associated with a central serous chorioretinopathy-like picture, as in this patient. Note the serous fluid and fibrin *(arrowhead)* noted in this patient after organ transplantation.

20–16 Chronic signs of central serous chorioretinopathy may include persistent serous detachment with exudation, pigmentation, atrophy and fibrous metaplasia, as seen in this case.

20–17 RPE DECOMPENSATION

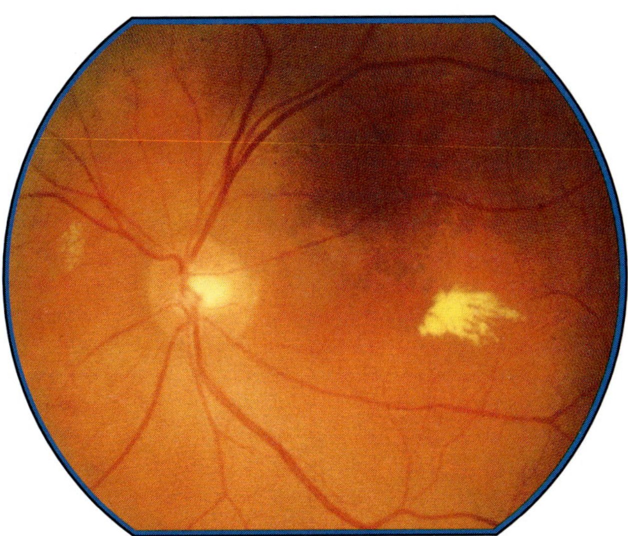

20–18

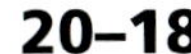

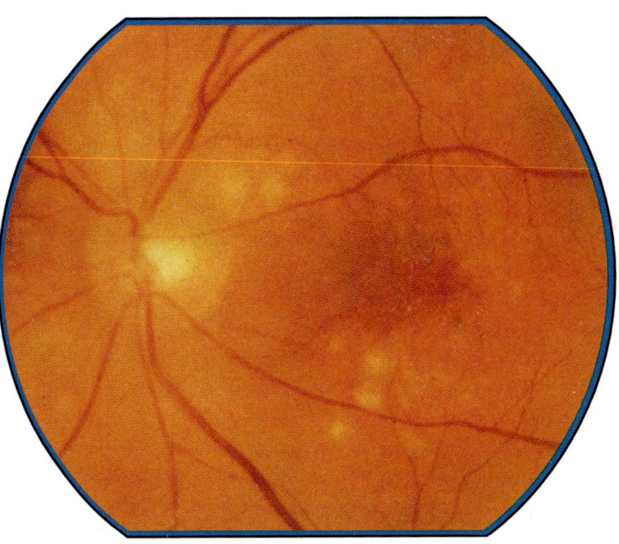

20–17 and 20–18 Chronic lipid exudation is also present in this case of diffuse RPE decompensation (20–17), which was successfully treated with mild grid laser photocoagulation (20–18).

***20–17** and **20–18**, From Lebwohl, M: Atlas of the skin and systemic disease, New York, 1995, Churchill Livingstone.*

20–19 RPE BLOWOUT

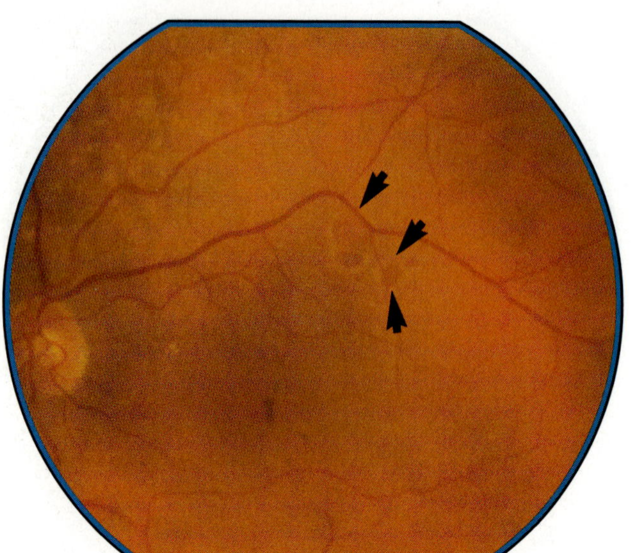

20–20

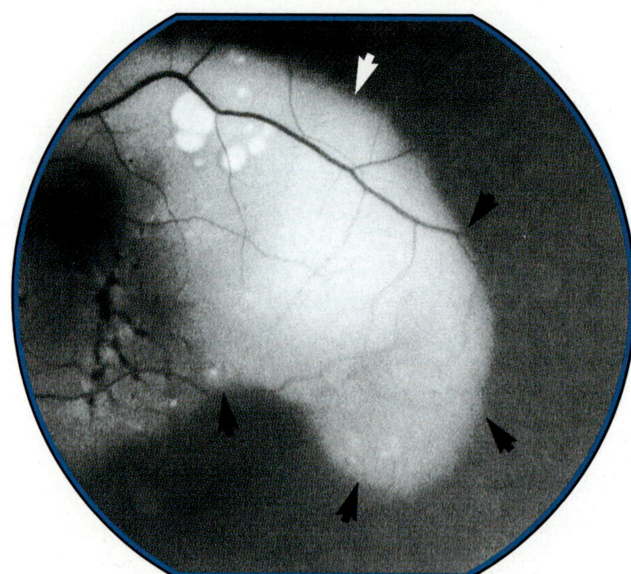

20–21 GIANT RIP

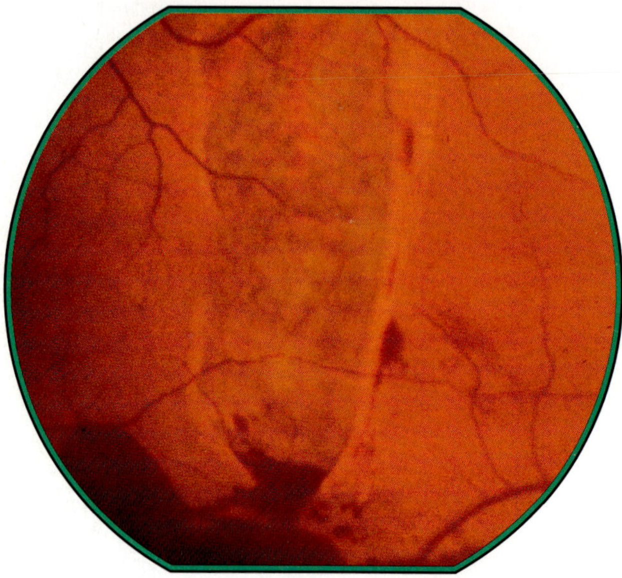

20–22

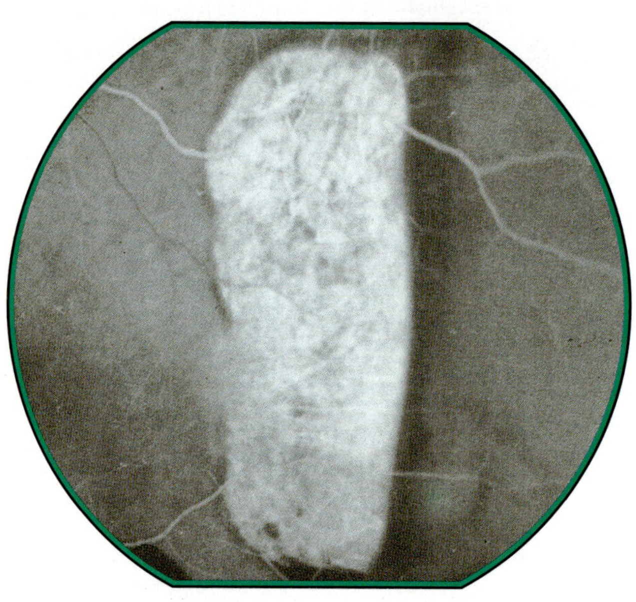

20–19 and 20–20 This patient with central serous chorioretinopathy developed holes *(arrowheads)* in a large retinal pigment epithelial detachment. These represent "blowouts" of the retinal pigment epithelium detachment. The holes are accentuated in the fluorescein study since the subretinal pigment epithelial staining is not masked by intact retinal pigment epithelium. The pigment epithelial detachment *(arrowheads)* is unusually large.

20–21 and 20–22 Rarely, a giant rip of the retinal pigment epithelium can be seen in patients with severe central serous chorioretinopathy. In this case, the giant rip was associated with hemorrhage. The characteristic fluorescein angiographic findings of a retinal pigment epithelium rip were also noted. Although hemorrhage was present, choroidal neovascularization was never found. Rips like this are at risk of occurring in patients with central serous chorioretinopathy and systemic steroid administration.

***20–21** and **20–22,** Courtesy of Dr. Stuart Green.*

20–23 SPONTANEOUS HEMORRHAGE

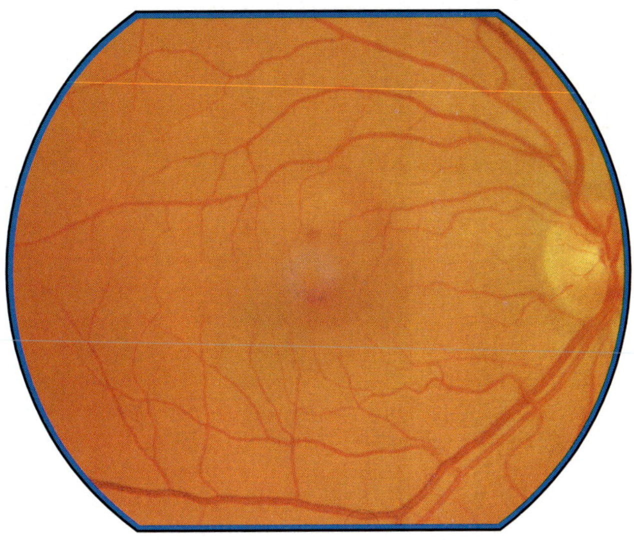

20–24

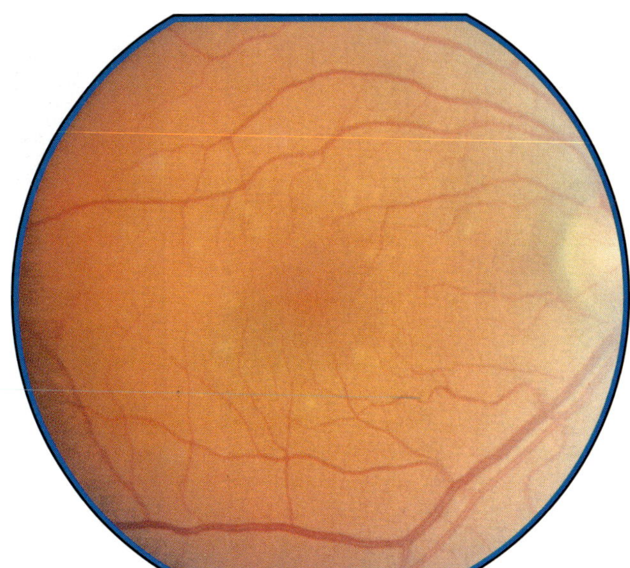

20–25 RPE CHANGES

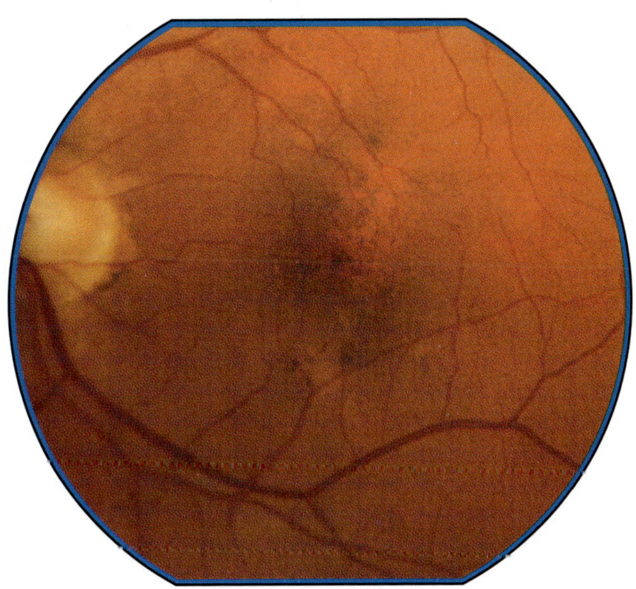

20–23 Central serous chorioretinopathy does not typically present with hemorrhage. In fact, the presence of hemorrhage often suggests underlying choroidal neovascularization. Choroidal neovascularization can rarely be associated with central serous chorioretinopathy. However, some patients with central serous chorioretinopathy can have a subretinal hemorrhage secondary to stretching of the retinal pigment epithelium on the choriocapillaries and passage of a small amount of blood into the subretinal space.

20–24 This type of hemorrhage resolves spontaneously with time as seen here.

20–25 Retinal pigment epithelial changes can often be seen in the other eye or in other areas of the fundus of the same eye and represent the resolved or healed stage of previous acute episodes of central serous chorioretinopathy.

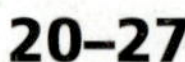

20–26 TRACTS

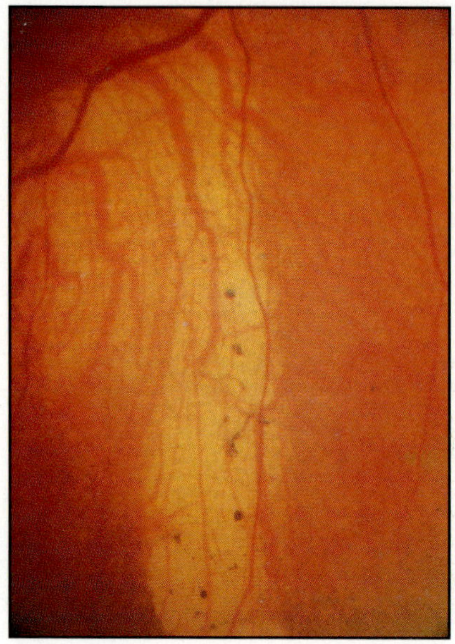

20–27

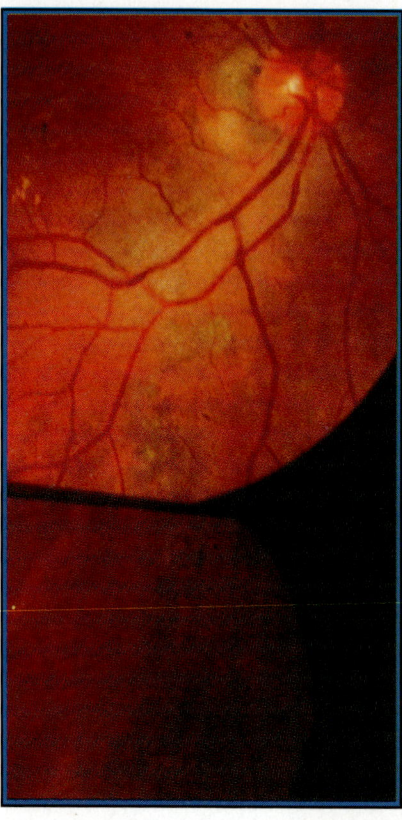

20–28

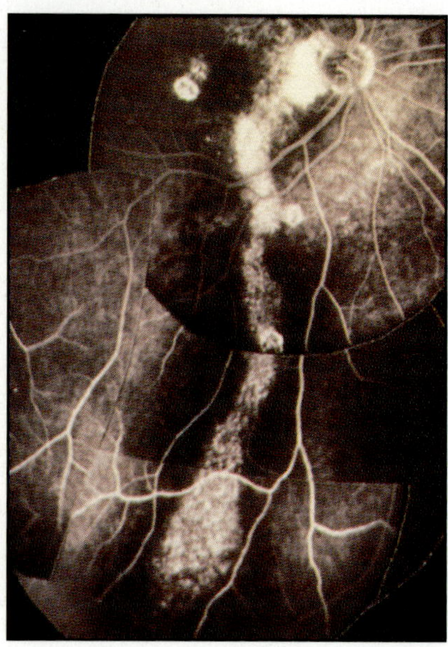

20–26 through 20–28 Often atrophic tracts can be seen inferiorly in patients with central serous chorioretinopathy. Note that the fluorescein angiogram better delineates the tract that extends inferiorly (20–28). Also note that these tracts may be hypopigmented (20–26) or hyperpigmented (20–27).

20–29

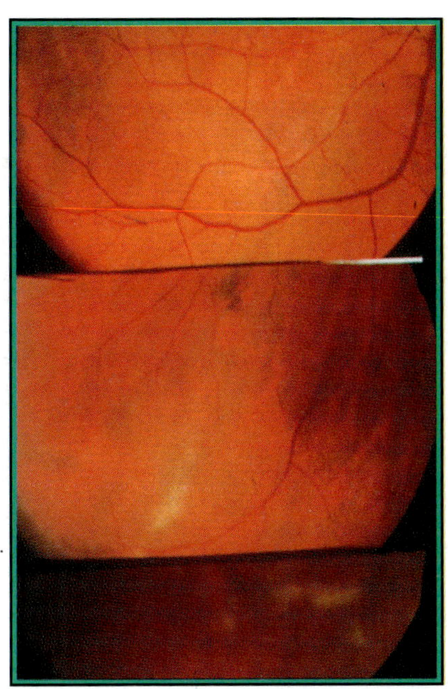

20–30

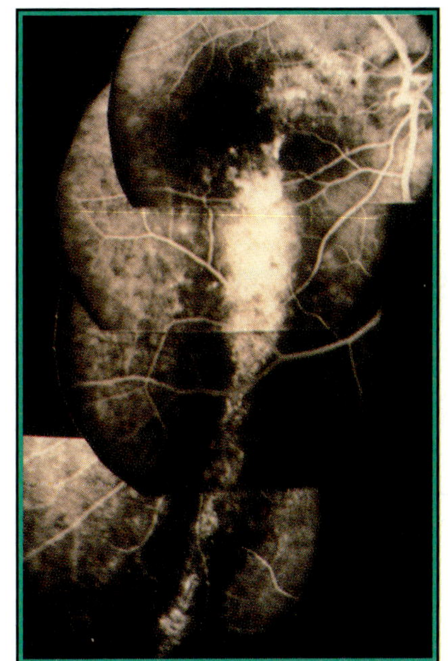

20–31

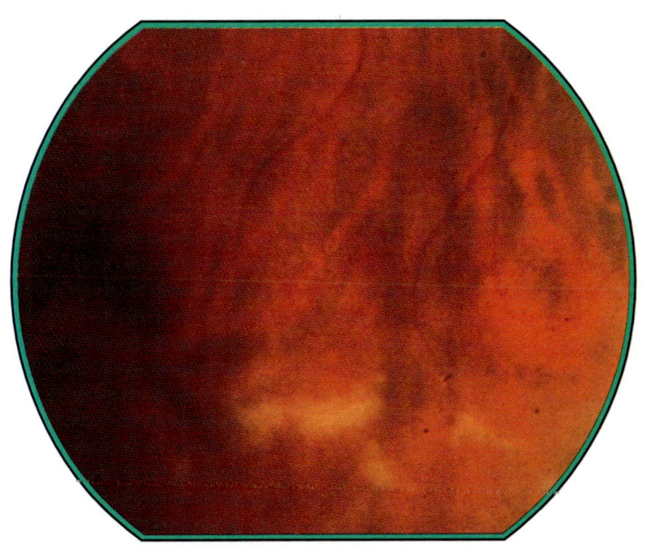

20–32

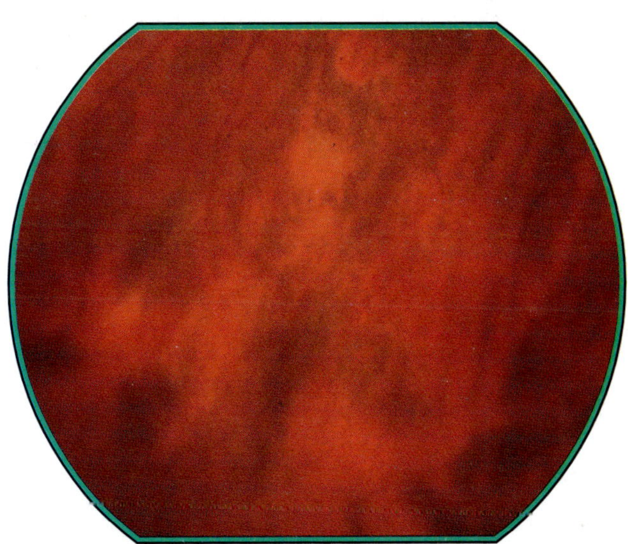

20–29 and 20–30 This patient with central serous chorioretinopathy has an atrophic retinal pigment epithelial tract and a dependent detachment. The retinal capillaries in the region of the inferior peripheral detachment are telangiectatic and leaky. Window defects are noted along the course of the tract on the fluorescein angiogram. At least two focal areas of retinal pigment epithelium leakage in the macula account for the neurosensory detachment.

20–31 The inferior dependent detachment of the same patient reveals lipid deposition and serous retinal elevation.

20–32 In the same patient, laser photocoagulation of the RPE leaks in the macula resulted in resolution of the macular detachment, secondary inferior peripheral dependent detachment, and associated lipid deposition. Visual acuity improved from 20/50 to 20/30.

***20-29** through **20–32,** From Yannuzzi, LA, ed: Central serous chorioretinopathy in laser photocoagulation of the macula, Philadelphia, 1989, JB Lippincott, p 8.*

20–33 CSC–CNV

20–34

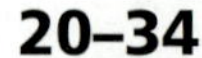

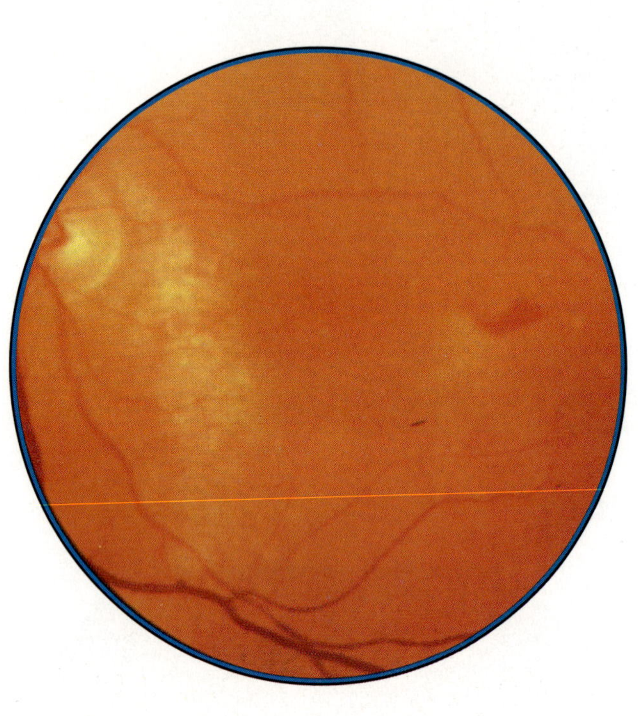

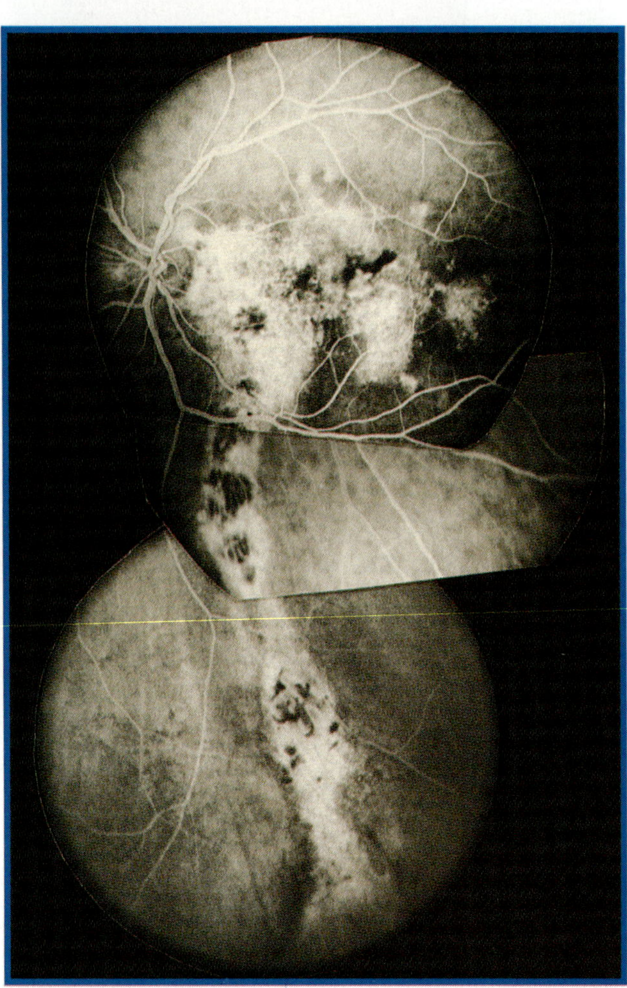

20–33 and 20–34 This patient has recurrent acute central serous chorioretinopathy with a focal area of secondary choroidal neovascularization. Note the atrophic tract beginning at the temporal juxtapapillary area extending into the inferior retina. Also note the dirty gray subretinal pigmentary disturbance in the temporal juxtafoveal region with hemorrhage at its margin, which represents a choroidal neovascular membrane (20–33).

20–33 *and* ***20–34,*** *From Yannuzzi, LA, ed: Central serous chorioretinopathy in laser photocoagulation of the macula, Philadelphia, 1989, JB Lippincott, p 8.*

20–35 BULLOUS DETACHMENT

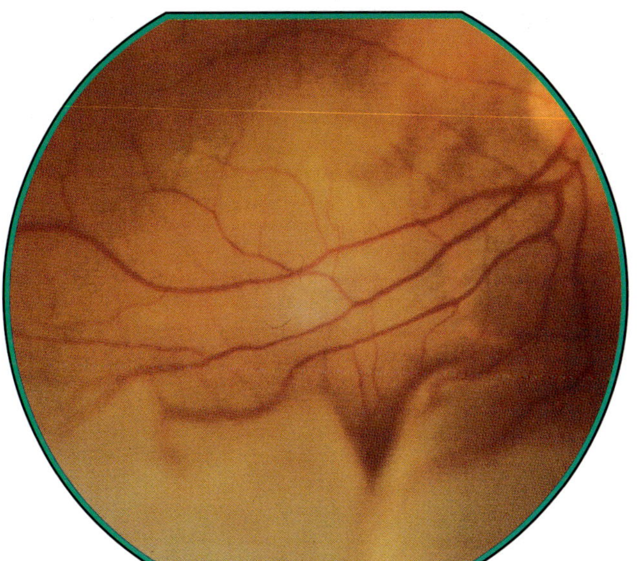

20–36

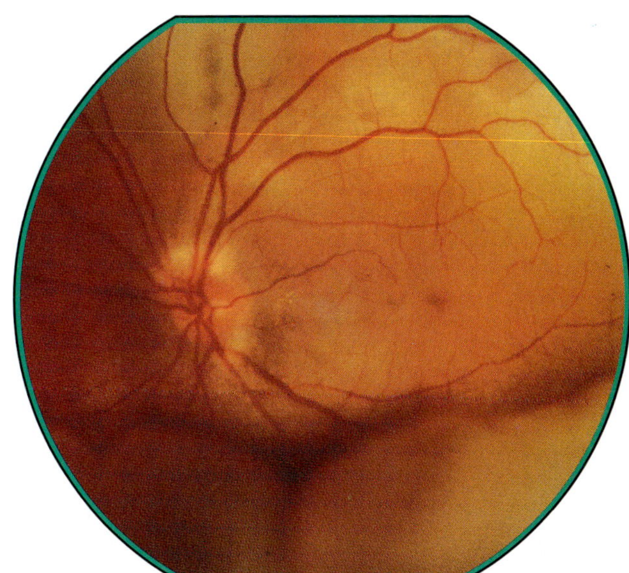

20–37

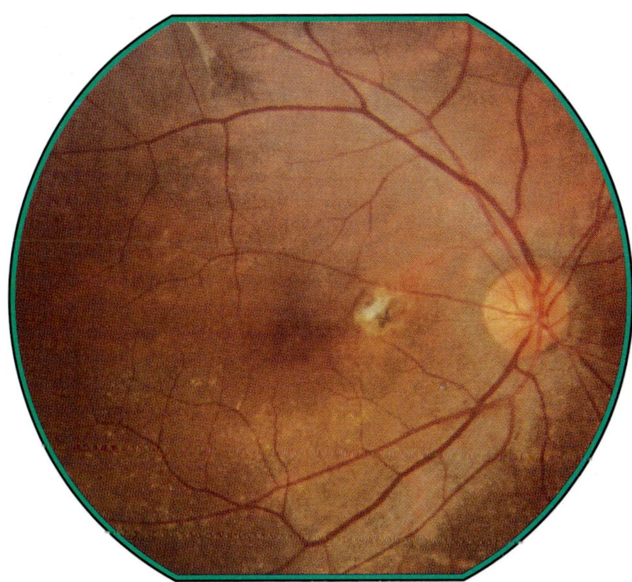

20–38

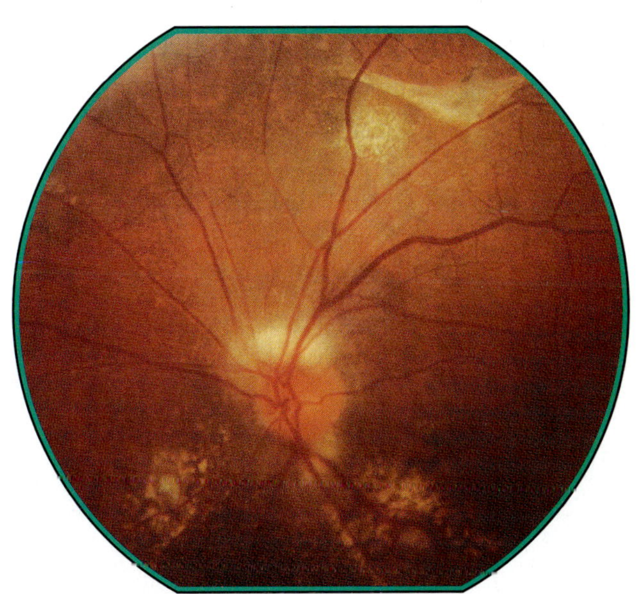

20–35 and 20–36 This patient has massive bullous detachment secondary to central serous chorioretinopathy. He also has fibrin deposition.

20–37 and 20–38 Atrophic and pigmentary changes, fibrous metaplasia, and subretinal fibrosis were noted after resolution.

20–35 *through* ***20–38,*** *Courtesy of Drs. Richard Rosen and Joseph Walsh.*

20–39 MEMBRANOPROLIFERATIVE GLOMERULONEPHRITIS TYPE II

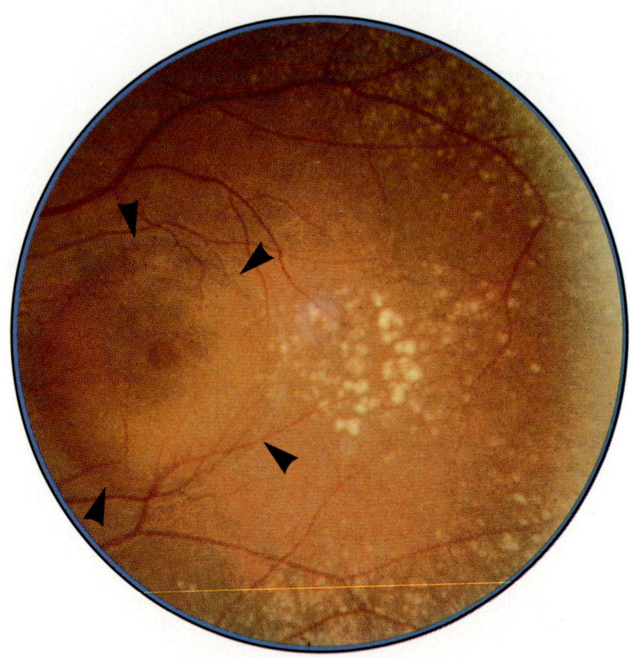

20–39A

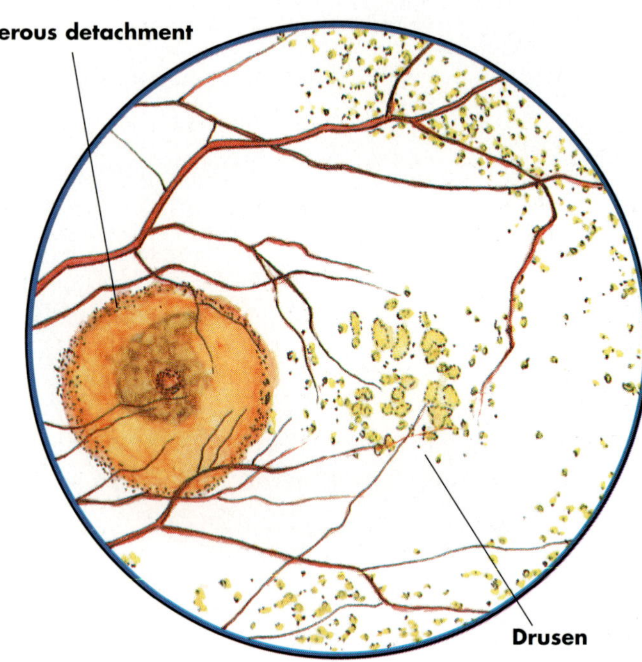

20–40

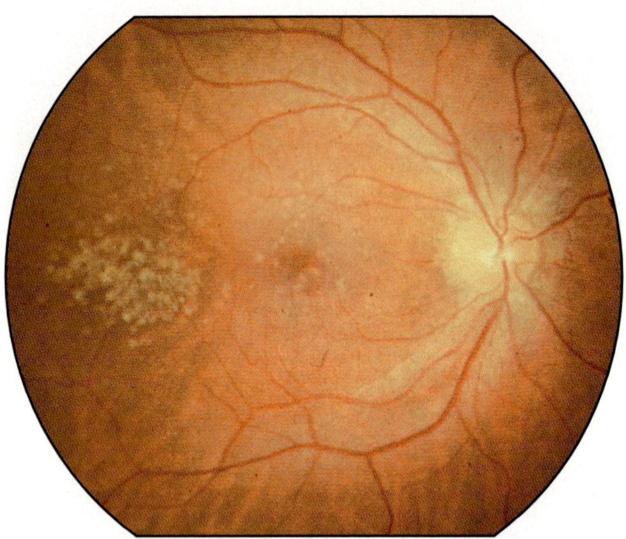

20–39 and 20–39A This 36-year-old patient has the unusual condition of dense-deposit or basal laminar drusen retinopathy secondary to membranoproliferative glomerulonephritis type II associated with serous detachment of the neurosensory retina *(arrowheads)* in the peripheral retina.

20–40 Another patient with glomerulonephritis illustrates dense-deposit or basal laminar drusen retinopathy.

***20–39** and **20–40,** From Ulbig, MRW, et al: Membranoproliferative glomerulonephritis type II associated with central serous retinopathy, Am J Ophthalmol 116:410–413, 1993.*

Suggested Readings

Gass, JDM: Pathogenesis of disciform detachment of the neuroepithelium: I. General concepts and classification, Am J Ophthalmol 63:573–585, 1967

Gass, JDM: Stereoscopic atlas of macular diseases, St Louis, 1970, Mosby–Year Book

Gass, JDM: Bullous retinal detachment: an unusual manifestation of idiopathic central serous choroidopathy, Am J Ophthalmol 75:810–821, 1973

Guyer, DR, et al: Digital indocyanine-green videoangiography of central serous chorioretinopathy, Arch Ophthalmol 112:1057–1062, 1994.

Ie, D, Yannuzzi, LA, Spaide, RF, Rabb, MF, Blair, NP, and Daly, MJ: Subretinal exudative deposits in central serous chorioretinopathy, Brit J Ophthalmology 77:349–353, 1993

Jalkh, AE, Jabbour, N, Avila, MP, Trempe, CL, and Schepens, CL: Retinal pigment epithelium decompensation II. Laser treatment, Ophthalmology 91:1549–1553, 1984

Klein, ML, van Buskirk, EM, Friedman, E, Gragoudas, E, and Chandra, S: Experience with nontreatment of central serous choroidopathy, Arch Ophthalmol 91:247–250, 1974

Marmor, M: New hypothesis on the pathogenesis: a treatment of serous retinal detachment, Graefes Arch Clin Exp Ophthalmol 226:548–552, 1988

Piccolino, F: Central serous chorioretinopathy: some considerations on pathogenesis, Ophthalmology 182:204–210, 1981

Schatz, H, Yannuzzi, LA, and Gitter, K: Subretinal neovascularization following Argon laser photocoagulation treatment for central serous chorioretinopathy, Trans Am Acad Ophthalmol 83:893–906, 1977

Spitznas, M: Central serous chorioretinopathy, Ophthalmology 87(8S):88, 1980

Spitznas, M: Pathogenesis of central serous retinopathy working hypothesis, Graefes Arch Clin Exp Ophthalmol 324, 1986

Spitznas, M, and Huke, J: Number, shape and topography age points in acute type I central serous retinopathy, Graefes Clin Exp Ophthalmol 225:437–440, 1987

Vatzke, RC, Burton, TC, and Leaverton, PE: Ruby laser photocoagulation therapy of central serous retinopathy. Part 1: A controlled clinical study. Part II: Factors affecting prognosis, Trans Am Acad Ophthalmol Otolaryngol, 78:OP205–OP211, 1974

Watzke, RD, Burton, TC, and Woolson, RF: Direct and indirect photocoagulation of central serous choroidopathy, Am J Ophthalmol 88:914–918, 1979

Wessing, A: Changing concept of central serous retinopathy treatment, Trans Am Acad Ophthalmol Otolaryngol 77:27, 1973

Yannuzzi, LA: Type A behavior and central serous chorioretinopathy, Trans Am Ophthalmol Soc 84:799–845, 1986

Yannuzzi, LA: Type–A behavior and central serous chorioretinopathy, Retina 7:111–131, 1987

Yannuzzi, LA, Shakin, JL, Fisher, YL, and Altomonte, M: Peripheral retinal detachments and retinal pigment epithelial atrophic tracts secondary to central serous pigment epitheliopathy, Ophthalmology 91:1553–1572, 1984

Yannuzzi, LA, Shakin, JL, Fisher, YL, and Altomonte, M: Retinal pigment epithelial atrophic tracts and dependent retinal detachments secondary to central serous pigment epitheliopathy, Ophthalmology 91(12), (Dec) 1984

Yannuzzi, LA, Slakter, JS, Kaufman, SR, and Gupta, K: Laser treatment of diffuse retinal pigment epitheliopathy, Eur J Ophthalmol 2(3):103–114, 1992

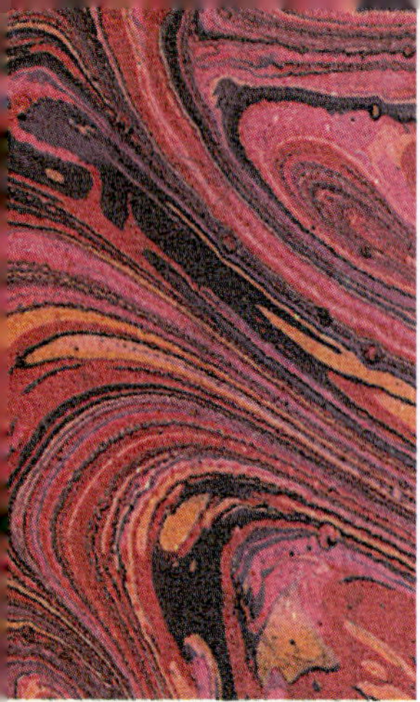

Chapter 21

Macular Holes

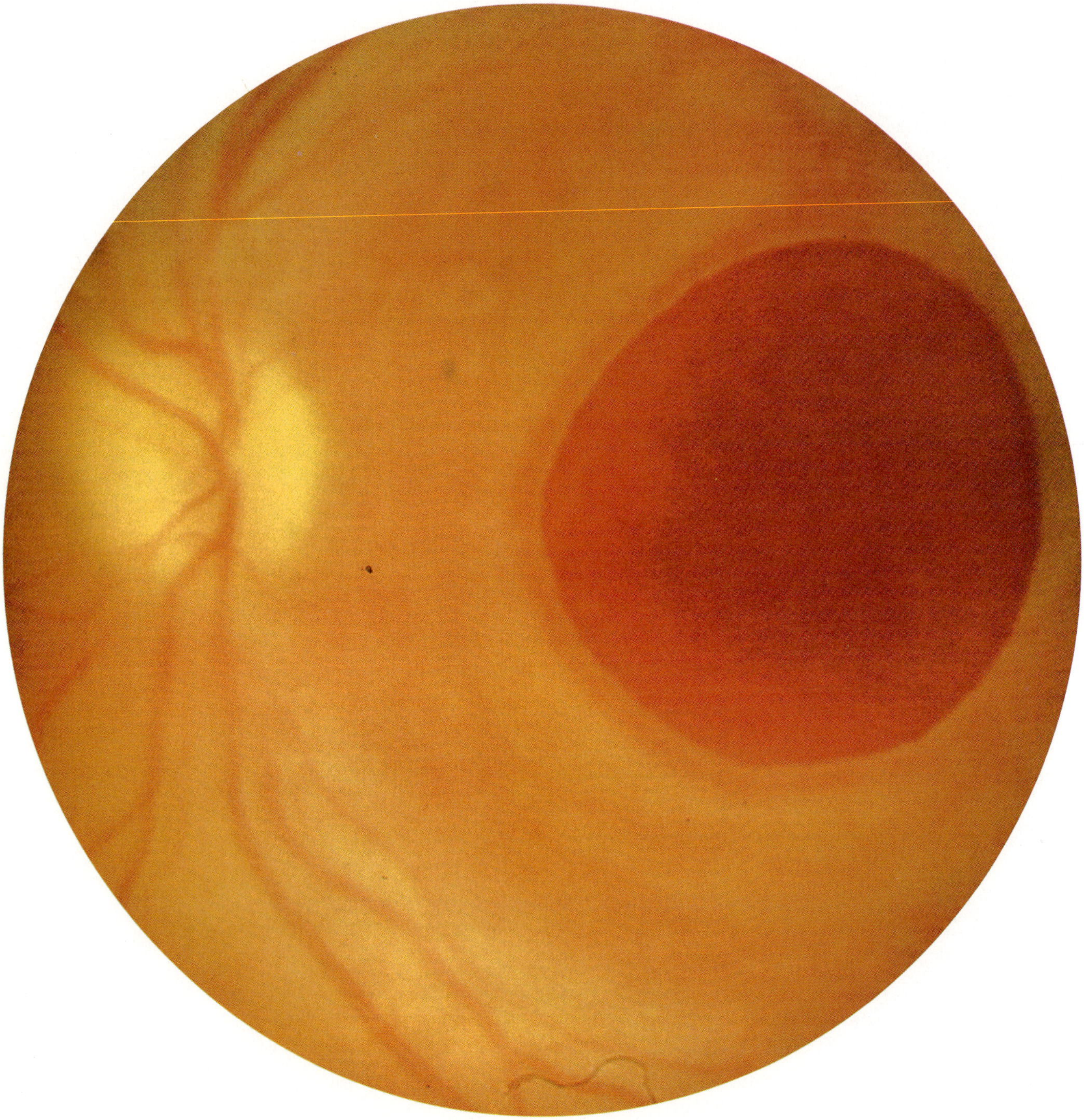

Idiopathic macular holes and their precursor lesions are usually noted in elderly females. The condition is due to tangential traction on the prefoveal cortical vitreous. Gass has recently suggested a new classification system with stage 1 lesions (pre-macular hole lesions), stage 2 lesions (early eccentric holes), and stages 3 and 4 lesions (full-thickness macular holes). Pars plana vitrectomy can flatten the macular hole in many cases, often with improvement in visual acuity.

21–1

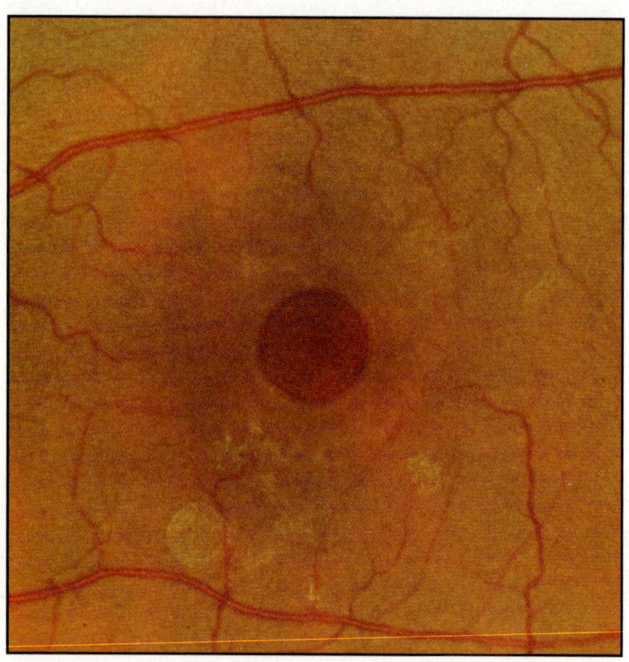

21–2

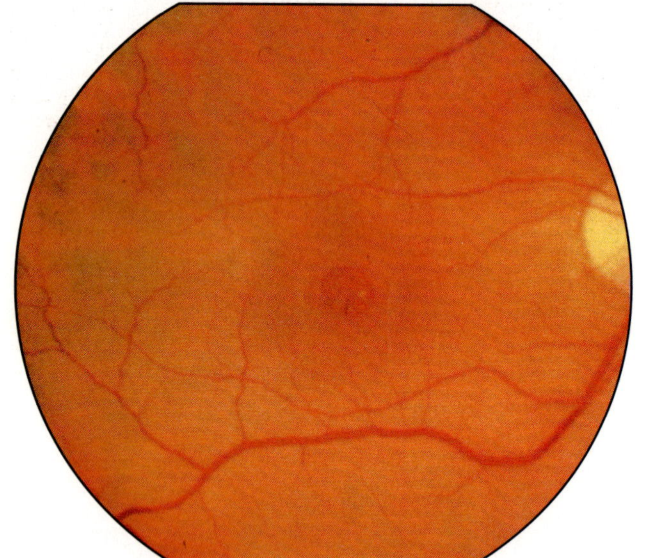

21–2A

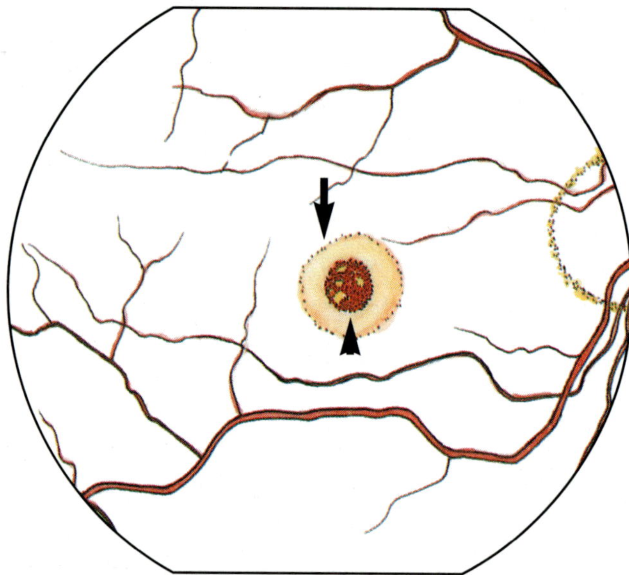

21–1, 21–2, and 21–2A Idiopathic full-thickness macular holes (*arrowhead* in 21–2A) consist of an area devoid of retinal tissue, a cuff of surrounding subretinal fluid (*arrow* in 21–2A), and often yellowish deposits at the level of the retinal pigment epithelium in the hole.

21–1, *From Guyer, DR, and Gragoudas, ES: Idiopathic macular holes. In Albert, D, and Jakobiec, F, eds: Principles and practices of ophthalmology, Philadelphia, 1993, WB Saunders.*

21–3

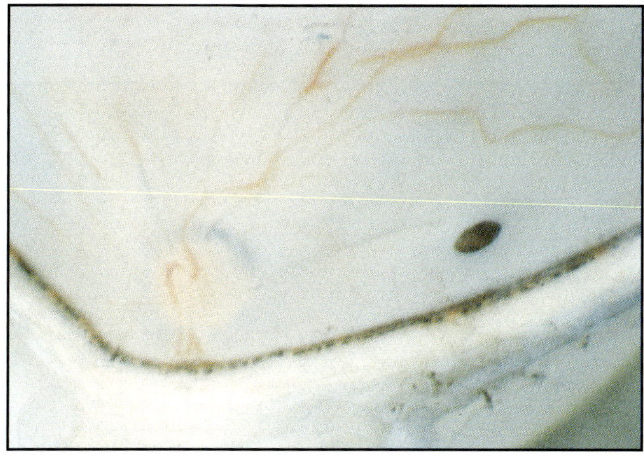

21–4

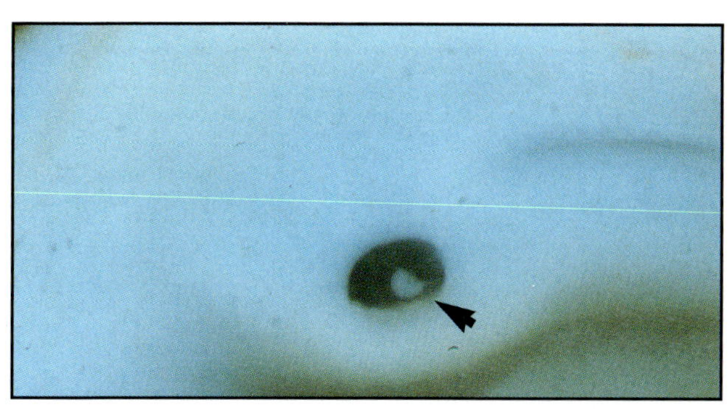

21–5

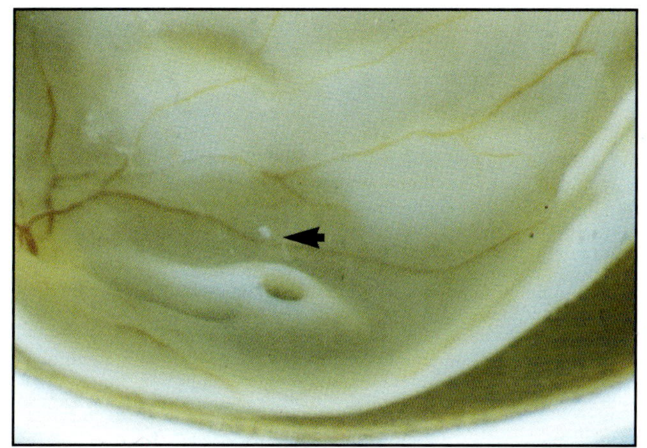

21–6

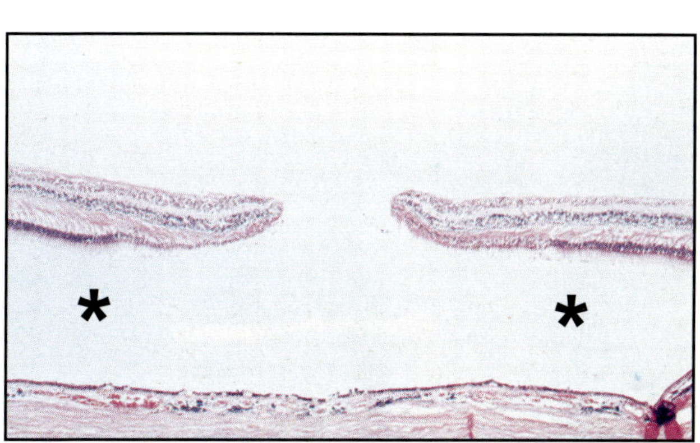

21–7

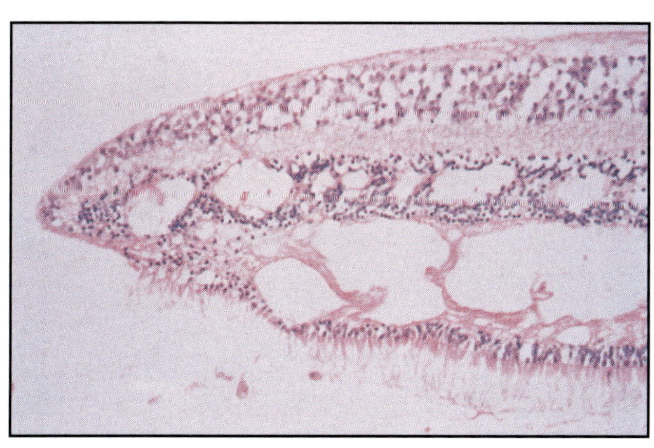

21–3 through 21–7 Histopathologic examination often reveals an overlying operculum *(arrowheads)* (21–3 through 21–5), an area of surrounding detachment *(asterisks)* (21–6), and cystoid macular edema (21–7). Variable degeneration of the photoreceptors is also noted (21–7).

21–6 *and* ***21–7,*** *From Guyer, DR, Green, WR, de Bustros, S, and Fine, SL: Histopathologic features of idiopathic macular holes and cysts, Ophthalmology 97:1045–1051, 1990.*

21–8 RARE SPONTANEOUS RESOLUTION

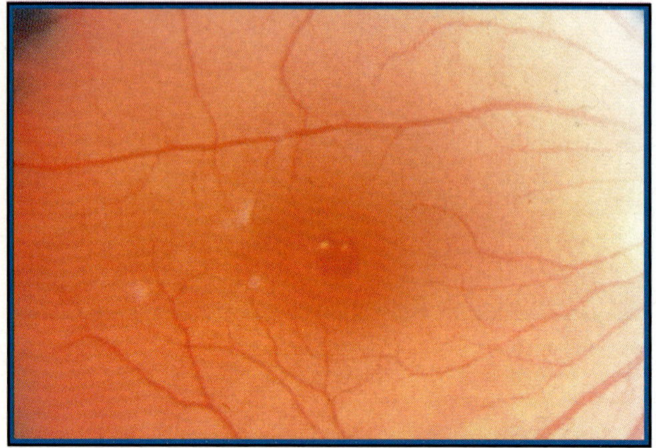

21–9

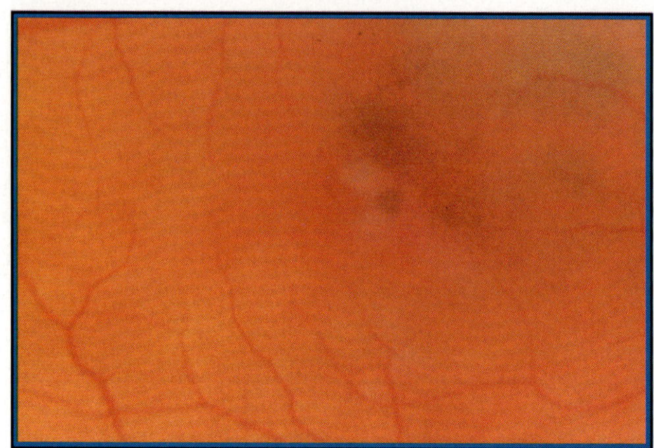

21–10

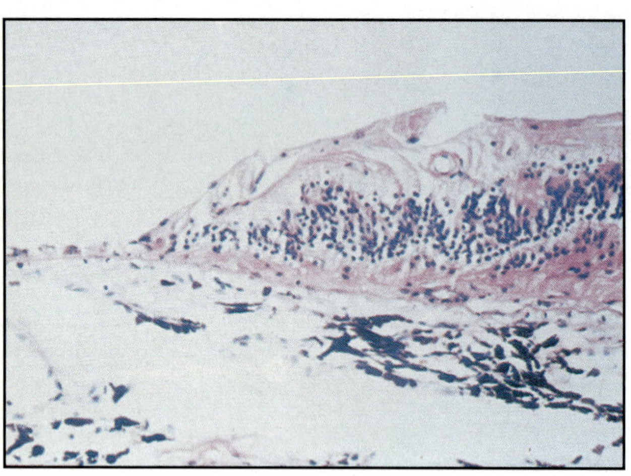

21–8 and 21–9 The natural history of idiopathic full-thickness macular holes is poor. Rarely, a full-thickness macular hole (21–8) may show spontaneous resolution (21–9). In this case, the visual acuity improved and a flat reddish lesion was noted (21–9).

21–10 A possible histopathologic correlate of this flat resolved lesion has also been observed in histopathologic examination. In this case of a presumed resolved macular hole, there is no cystoid macular edema and there is an adhesion between the retina and Bruch's membrane.

21–8 and 21–9, From Guyer, DR, de Bustros, S, et al: The natural history of idiopathic macular holes and cysts, Arch Ophthalmol 110:1264–1268. Copyright 1992 American Medical Association.

21–11 VITRECTOMY FOR MACULAR HOLES

21–12

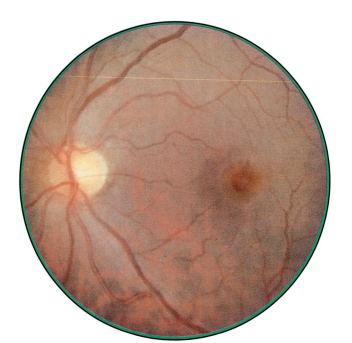

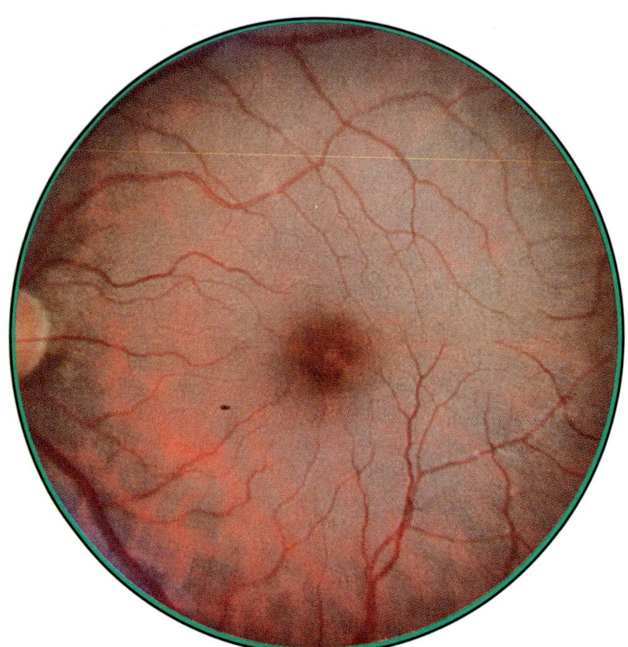

21–13 DEMARCATION LINES

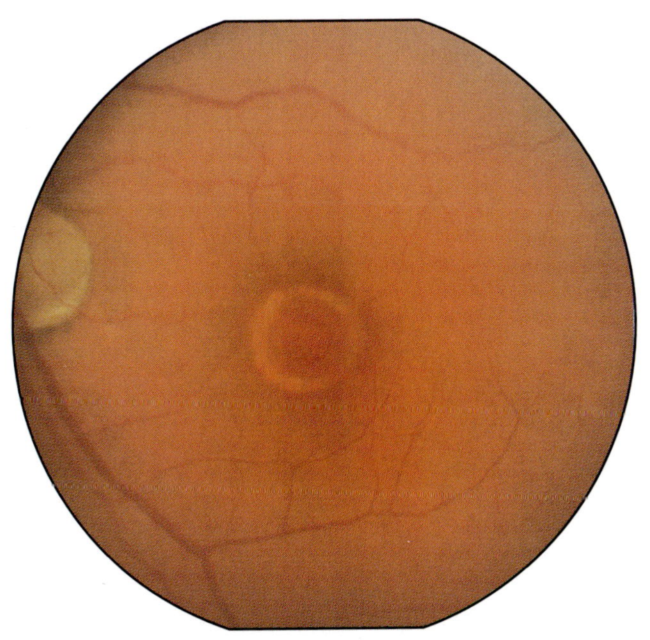

21–14 ATROPHIC CHANGES

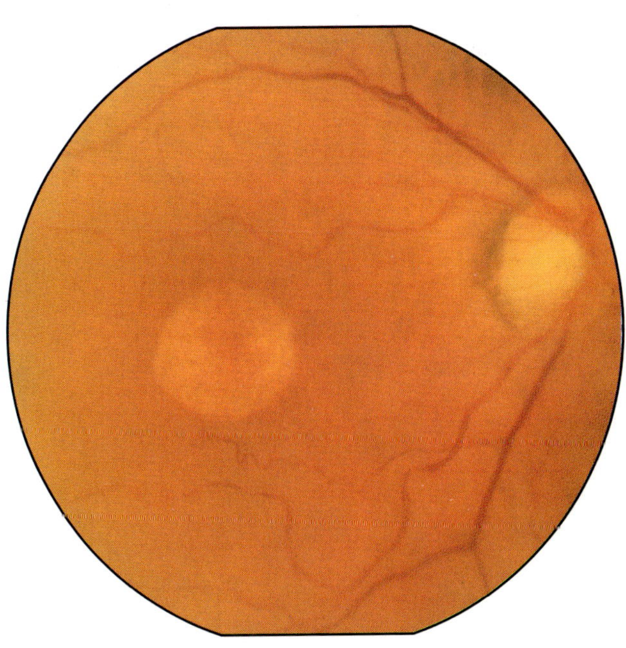

21–11 and 21–12 Flattening and resolution of macular holes can sometimes be accomplished by pars plana vitrectomy (21–11, preoperative photograph; 21–12, postoperative photograph).

21–13 and 21–14 Macular holes may occasionally show demarcation lines (21–13) or atrophic changes (21–14).

21–11 and 21–12, Courtesy of Dr. Neil Kelly. From Kelly, NE, and Wendel, RT: Vitreous surgery for idiopathic macular holes: results of a pilot study, Arch Ophthalmol 109:654-659, 1991. Copyright 1991 American Medical Association.

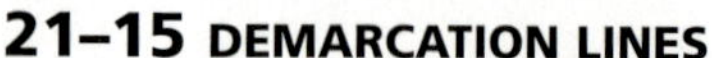

21–15 DEMARCATION LINES

21–16

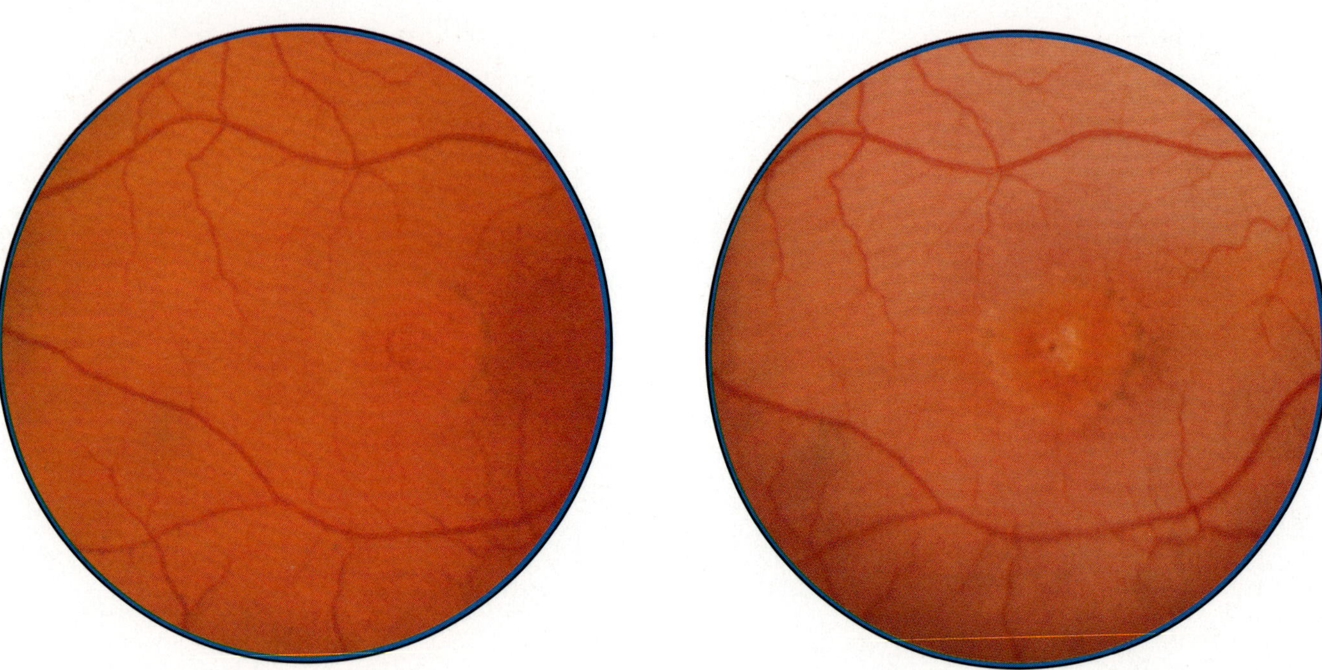

21–15 and 21–16 The demarcation line may sometimes be seen better postoperatively (21–15, preoperatively; 21–16, postoperatively).

21–15 *and* ***21–16,*** *Courtesy of Dr. Neil Kelly.*

21–17 PREMACULAR HOLE LESIONS

21–18

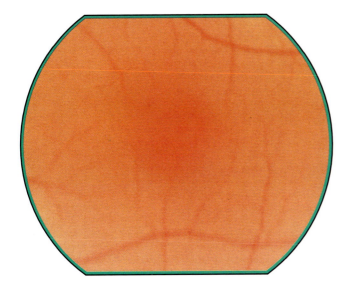

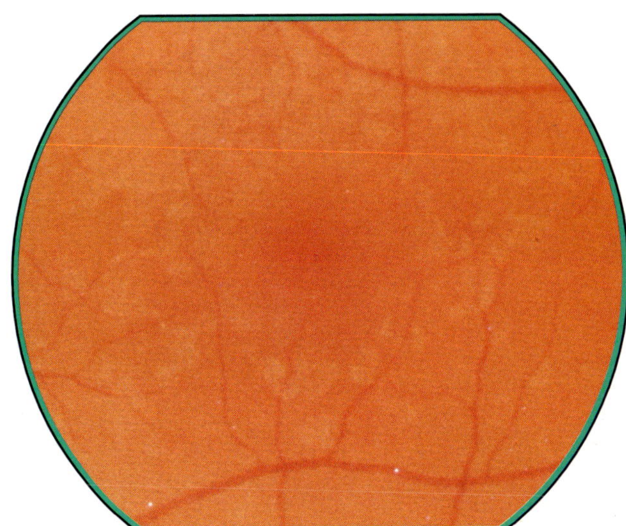

21–19 OTHER CAUSES OF MACULAR HOLES

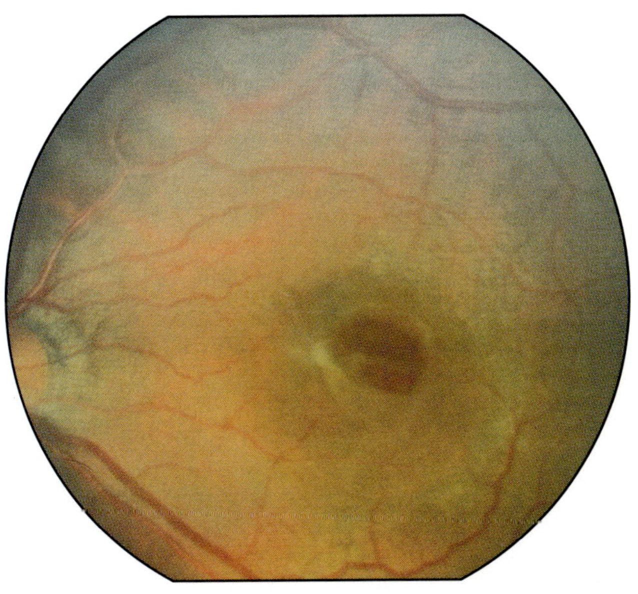

21–20

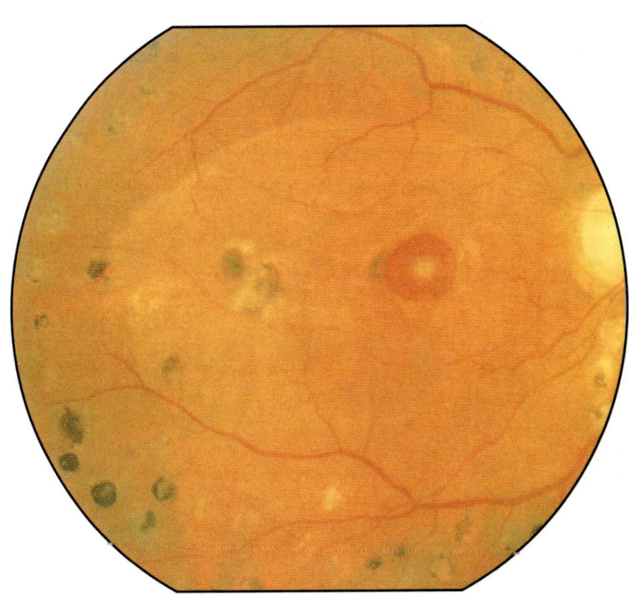

21–17 and 21–18 Premacular hole lesions have been termed macular cysts, involutional macular thinning, or stage 1 lesions. Stage 1a lesions have yellow spots, and stage 1b lesions have a yellow ring, as demonstrated in this patient. This patient had resolution of the yellow ring and improvement in visual acuity from 20/80 to 20/30 sixteen months later. Natural series studies report that anywhere from 33% to 80% of premacular hole lesions will show such spontaneous resolution.

21–19 and 21–20 Macular holes may be associated with other conditions such as trauma (21–19), myopia, optic nerve pits, or after laser photocoagulation for diabetic retinopathy (21–20).

21–17 *and* ***21–18,*** *From Guyer, DR, de Bustros, S, et al: The natural history of idiopathic macular holes and cysts, Arch Ophthalmol 110:1264–1268, 1992. Copyright 1992 American Medical Association.*

21–21 SECONDARY DETACHMENT

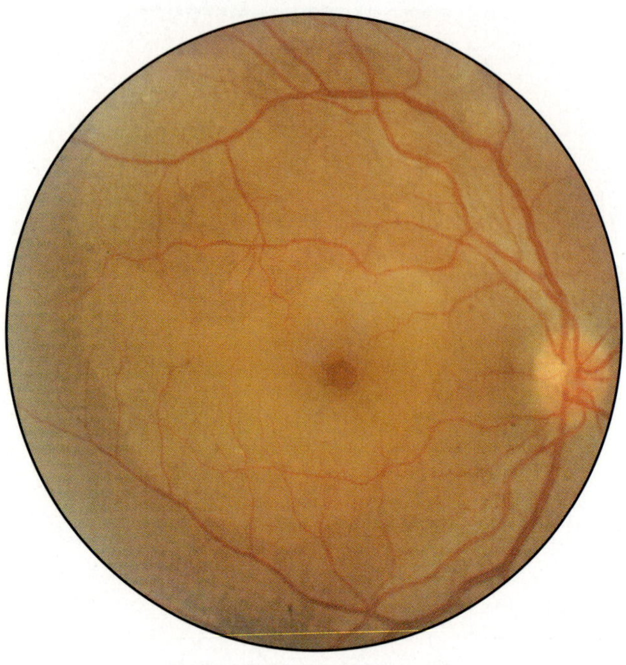

21–22 TRAUMA

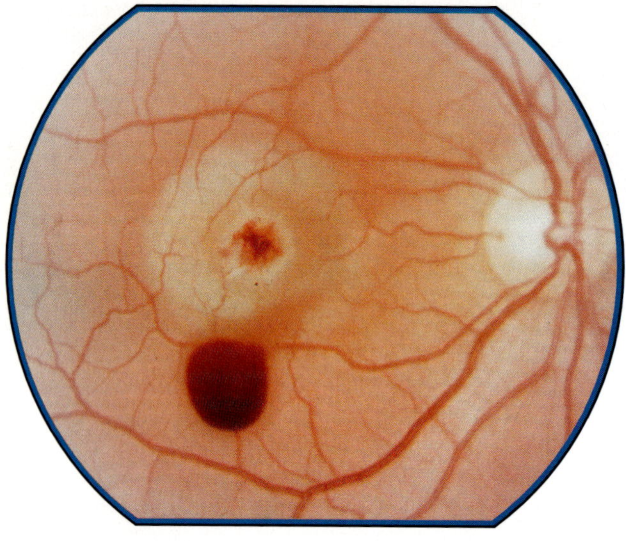

21–23

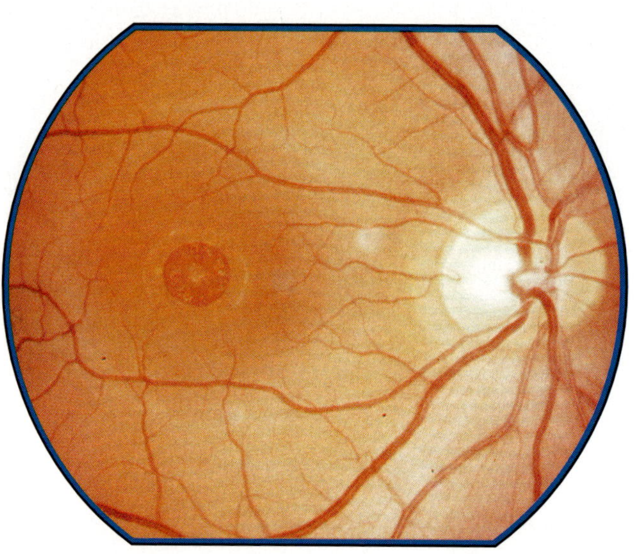

21–21 Macular holes can also lead to secondary detachments of the posterior pole in cases of trauma and myopia.

21–22 and 21–23 This patient had accidental direct exposure to a laser in a physics laboratory. Acutely a hemorrhagic macular lesion is noted with additional hemorrhage inferiorly. Retinal whitening is also present (21–22). Three months later, a full-thickness macular hole is noted (21–23).

***21–22** and **21–23,** Courtesy of Dr. Donald Frambach.*

21–24 MICROMACULAR HOLE

21–25 GIANT MACULAR HOLE

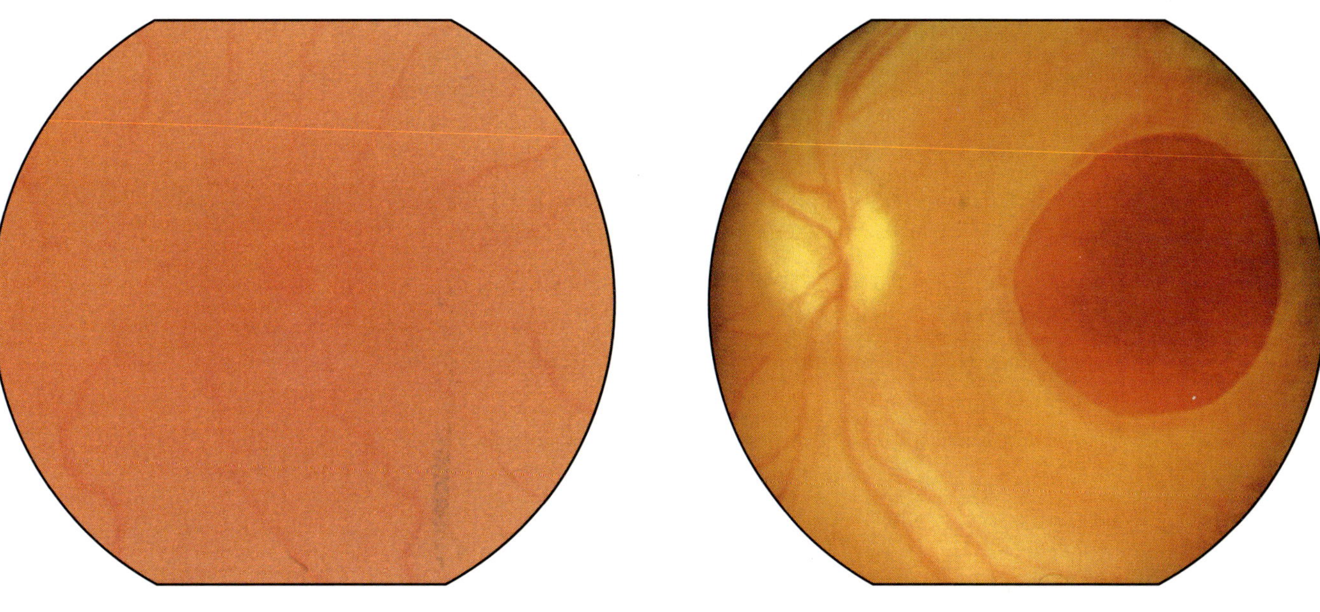

21–24 and 21–25 Micromacular holes (21–24) or giant macular holes (21–25) also may occur. Giant macular holes are often due to trauma.

Suggested Readings

Aaberg, TM: Macular holes: a review, Surv Ophthalmol 139–162, 1970

Blankenship, GW: Treatment of myopic macular holes and detachment with liquid vitreous–intravitreal gas exchange. In Blankenship, GW, Binder, S, Gonvers, M, and Stirpe, M, eds: Basic and advanced vitreous surgery, vol 2, New York, 1986, Springer–Verlag

Fisher, Y, Slakter, J, Yannuzzi, L, and Guyer, D: A prospective natural history study in kinetic ultrasound evaluation of idiopathic macular holes, Ophthalmology 101:5–11, 1994

Fisher, YL, Slakter, JS, Friedman, RA, and Yannuzzi, LA: Kinetic ultrasound evaluation of the posterior vitreoretinal interface, Ophthalmology 98:1135–1138, 1991

Fisher, YL, Slakter, JS, and Yannuzzi, LA: Idiopathic macular hole: the natural course of the fellow eye (in press)

Frangieh, GT, Green, WR, and Engel, HM: A histopathologic study of macular holes and cysts, Retina 1:311–336, 1981

Funata, M, Wendel, RT, De la Cruz, Z, and Green, WR: Clinicopathologic study of bilateral macular holes treated with pars plana vitrectomy and gas tamponade, Retina 12:289–298, 1992

Gass, JDM: Lamellar macular hole: a complication of cystoid macular edema after cataract extraction—a clinicopathologic case report, Trans Am Ophthalmol Soc 73:231–250, 1975

Gass, JDM: Stereoscopic atlas of macular diseases: diagnosis and treatment, ed 3, St Louis, 1987, Mosby–Year Book

Guyer, DR, DeBustros, S, Diener–West, M, and Fine, SL: The natural history of idiopathic macular holes and cysts, Invest Ophthalmol Vis Sci 3(suppl):155, 1989

Guyer, DR, DeBustros, S, Diener–West, M, and Fine, SL: Observations on patients with idiopathic macular holes and cysts, Arch Ophthalmol 110:1264–1268, 1992

Guyer, DR, and Green, WR: Idiopathic macular holes and precursor lesions. In: Franklin, RM: Proceedings of the symposium on retina and vitreous, New Orleans Academy of Ophthalmology, New Orleans, LA, Kugler Publications, New York, 1993, pp 135–162

Guyer, DR, Green, WR, de Bustros, S, and Fine, SL: Histopathologic features of idiopathic macular holes and cysts, Ophthalmology 97:1045–1051, 1990

Kelly, NE, and Wendel, RT: Vitreous surgery for idiopathic macular holes. Results of a pilot study, Arch Ophthalmol 109:654–659, 1991

Madreperla, SA, Geiger, GL, Funata, M, de la Cruz, Z, and Green, WR: Clinicopathologic correlation of a macular hole treated by cortical vitreous peeling and gas tamponade, Ophthalmology 101:682–686, 1994

Morgan, CM, and Schatz, H: Idiopathic macular holes, Am J Ophthalmol 99:437–444, 1985

Watzke, RC: Acquired macular disease. In Duane's clinical ophthalmology, vol 3, New York, Harper & Row

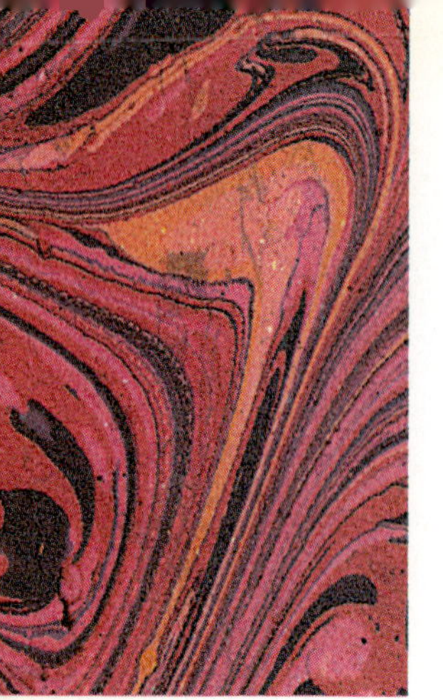

Chapter 22

Macular Dystrophies

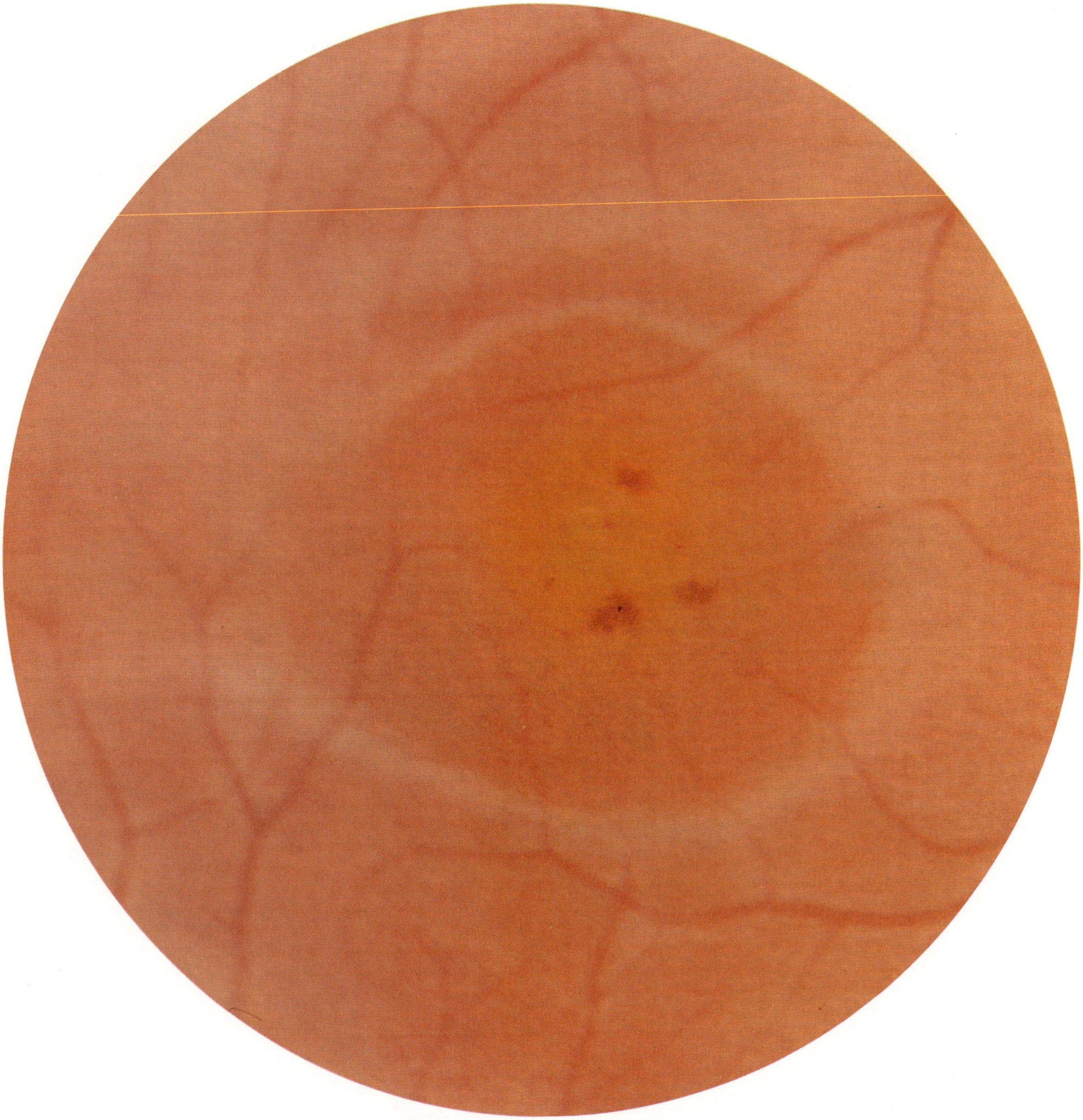

Various dystrophies may have characteristic macular findings. These conditions include X-linked juvenile retinoschisis, cone dystrophy, Stargardt's disease or fundus flavimaculatus, Best's disease, reticular dystrophy of the retinal pigment epithelium or Sjögren's disease, benign concentric annular macular dystrophy, and Sorsby's pseudoinflammatory macular dystrophy.

22–1 SPIELMEYER-VOGT-BATTEN DISEASE

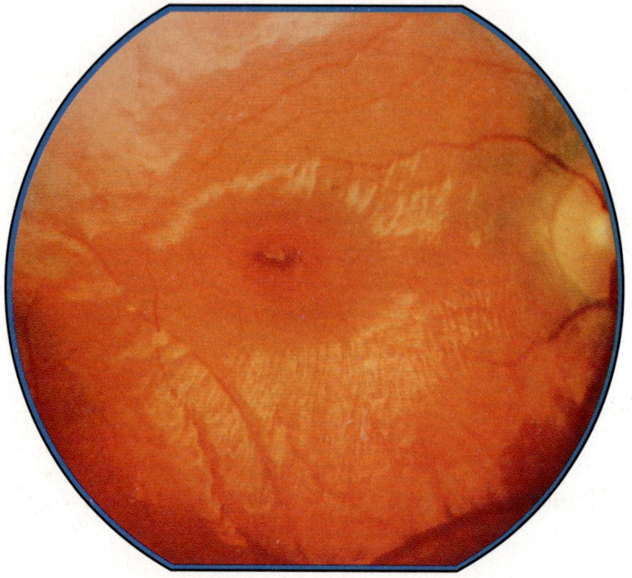

22–2

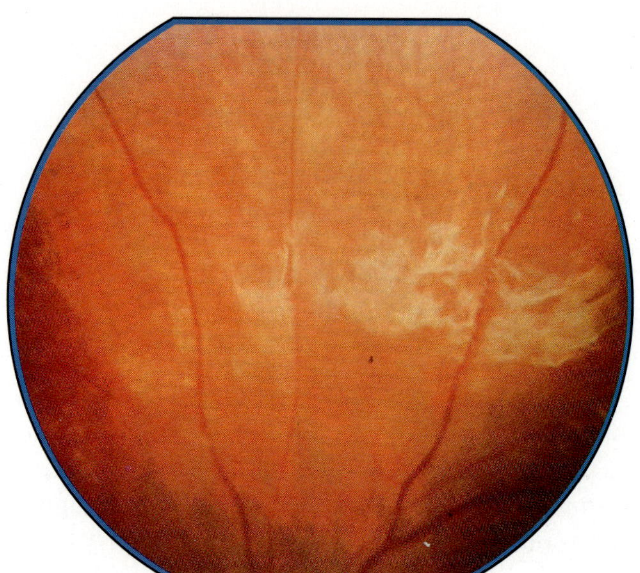

22–3

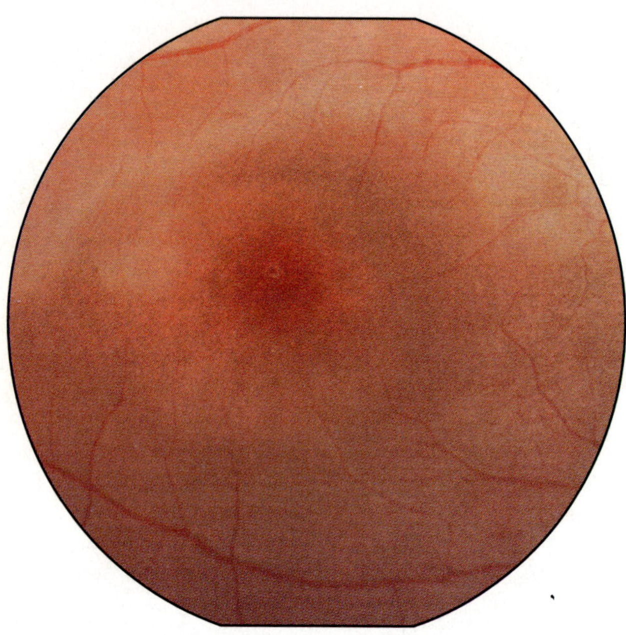

22–1 through 22–3 Spielmeyer-Vogt-Batten disease is a type of ceroid lipofuscinosis. Affected patients may have macular and pigmentary changes, including a bull's eye maculopathy, internal limiting membrane wrinkling, pigmentary changes, and attenuated vessels.

22–1 *and* ***22–2,*** *Courtesy of Dr. Gary Abrams.* ***22–3,*** *From Ryan, SJ: Retina, ed 2, St Louis, 1994, Mosby–Year Book. Courtesy of Bateman, Lang, and Maumenee.*

22–4 **JUVENILE X-LINKED RETINOSCHISIS** **22–5**

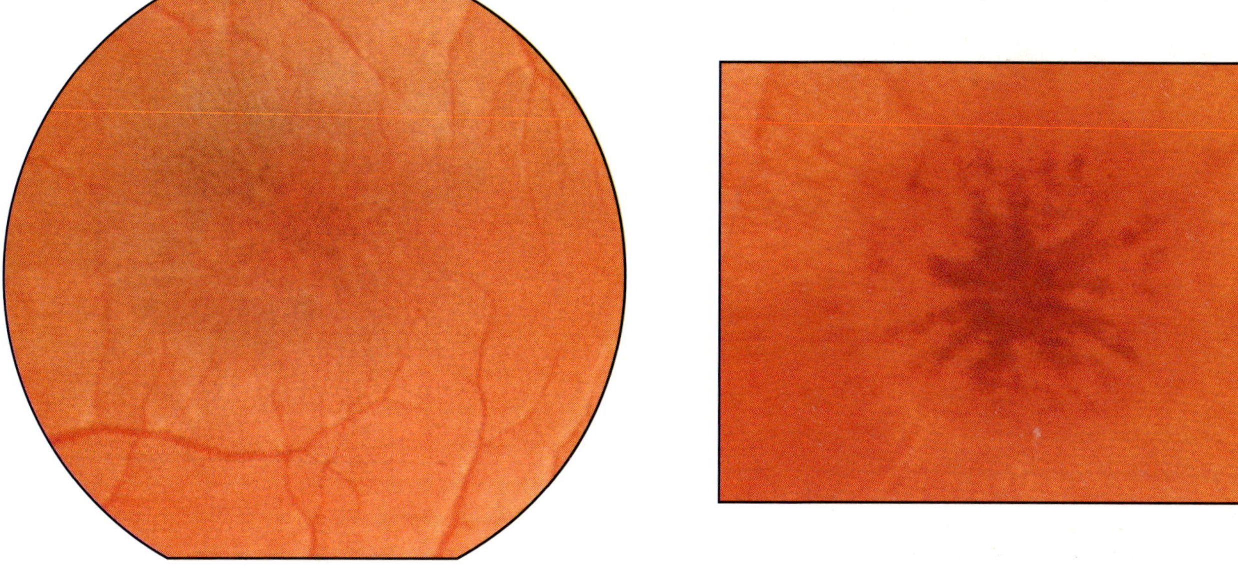

22–6 **22–7**

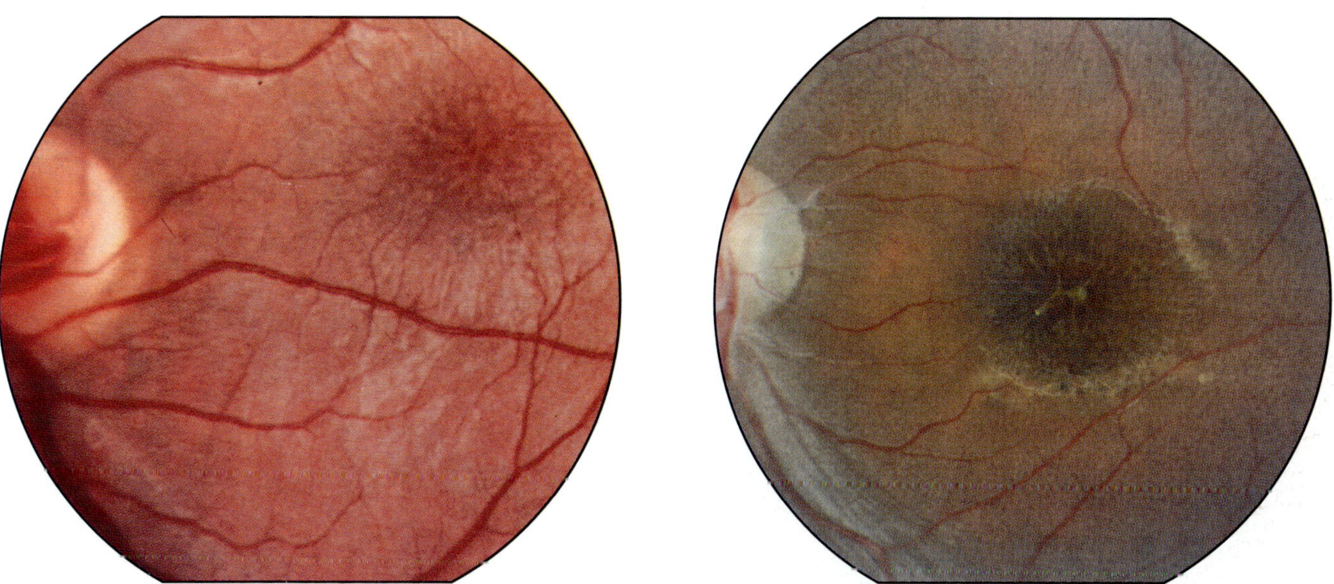

All patients with this condition have foveal retinoschisis. Retinoschisis may also occur in the retinal periphery in approximately 50% of cases. The abnormality of the fovea appears to be congenital. We know of one case that showed spontaneous resolution of the macular findings.

22–4 through 22–7 The first four photographs in this series illustrate the macula appearance of juvenile X-linked retinoschisis. The macula has a characteristic spoke-wheel appearance. Ectopic maculae are commonly seen in this disorder (22–6).

22–4, *Courtesy of Dr. Harry Flynn.* ***22–5,*** *Courtesy of Wills Eye Hospital.* ***22–7,*** *Courtesy of Drs. Ron Carr and Ken Noble.*

22–8 JUVENILE X-LINKED RETINOSCHISIS

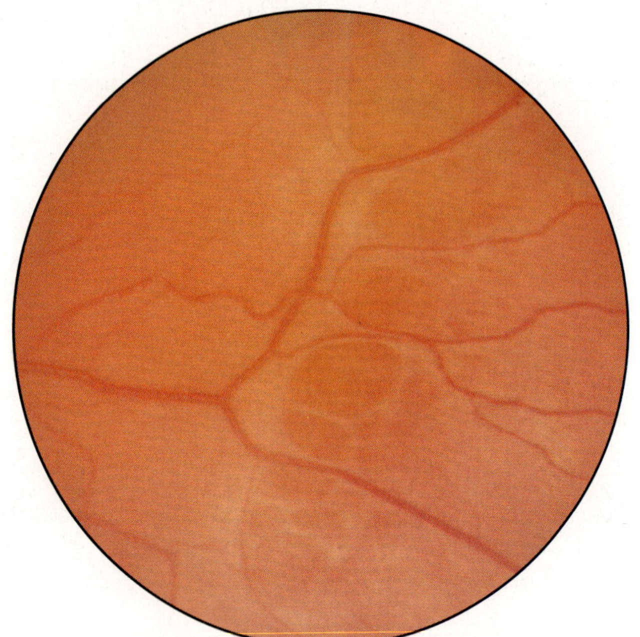

22–9

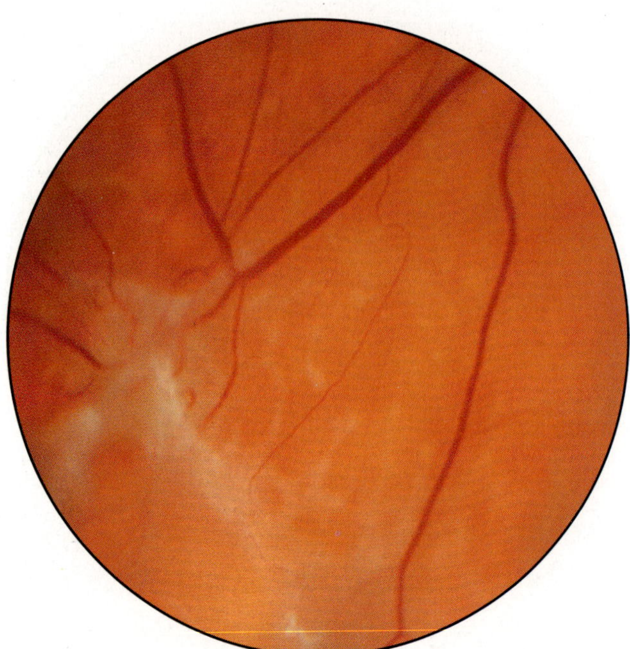

22–10

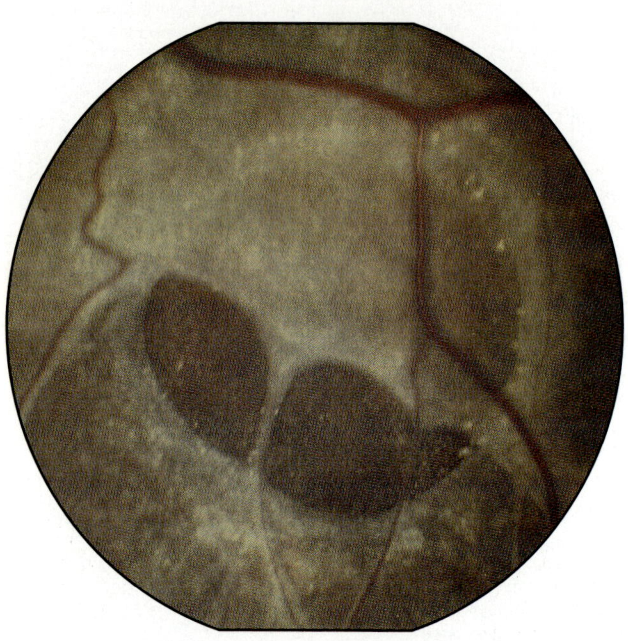

22–8 through 22–10 The next three photographs reveal the peripheral findings in this disorder, including superficial retinal holes and white dendritic figures. Electroretinopathy in these patients reveal a decreased B-wave.

22–8 *and* ***22–9,*** *Courtesy of Drs. Ron Carr and Ken Noble.*

22–11

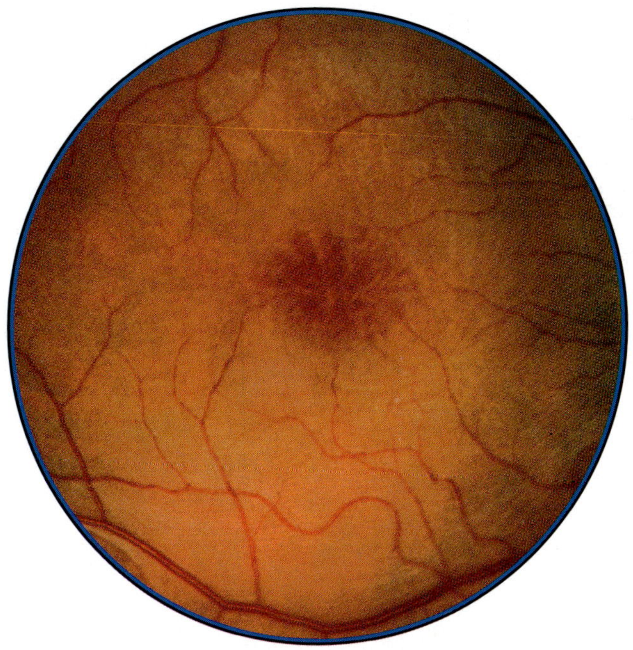

22–12

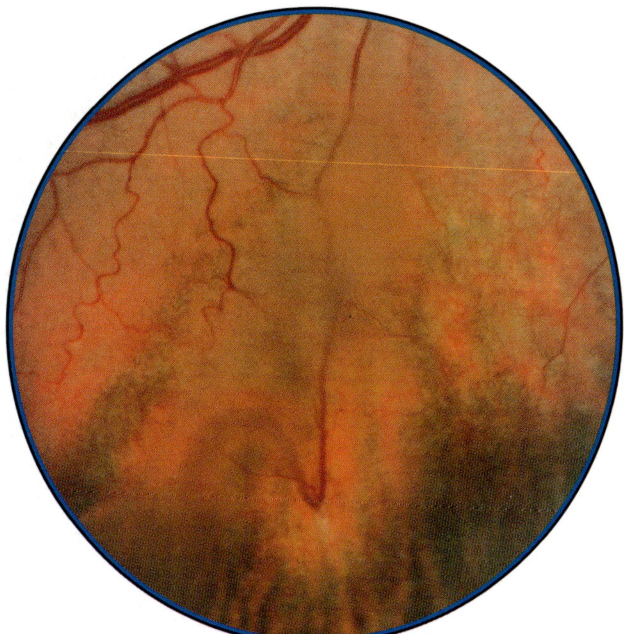

22–13

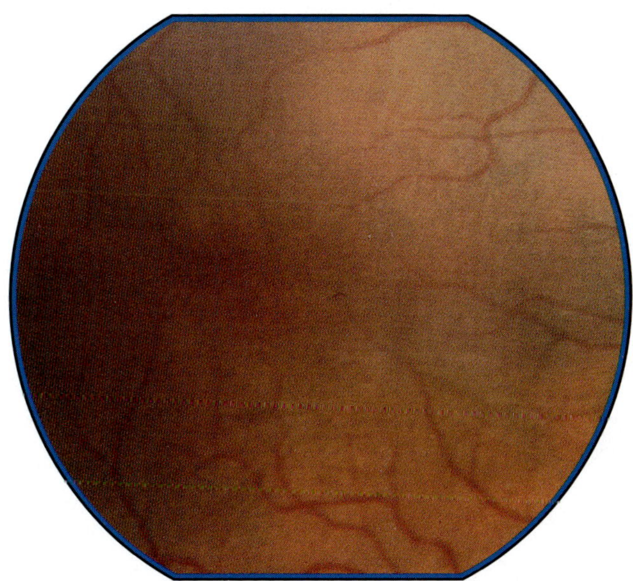

22–11 and 22–12 This patient has the characteristic schisis findings in the macula with a slightly ectopic fovea (22–11) as well as schisis in the periphery (22–12).

22–13 This patient experienced resolution of the schisis findings in the macular region, an unusual occurrence. Note that the macular changes have closed or disappeared following a posterior vitreous detachment 2 years later, with only some internal limiting membrane changes noted.

22–11 *through* ***22–13,*** *Courtesy of Dr. Harold Weissman.*

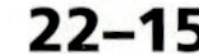

22–14 FUNDUS FLAVIMACULATUS

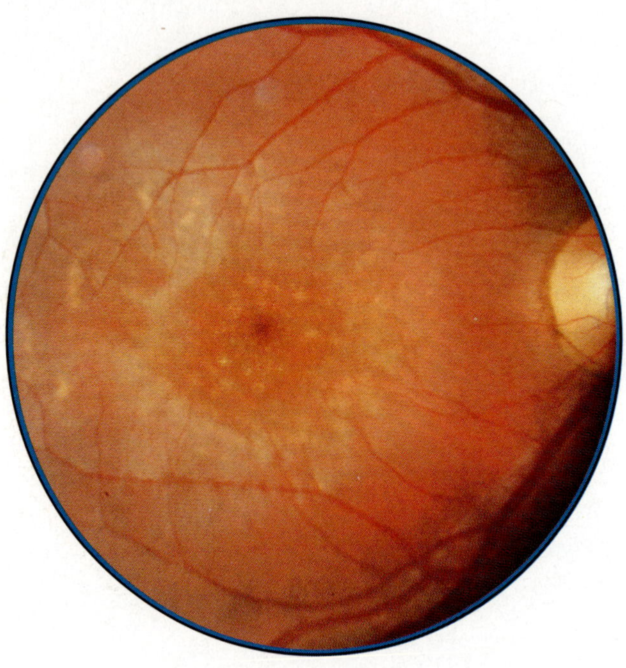

22–15

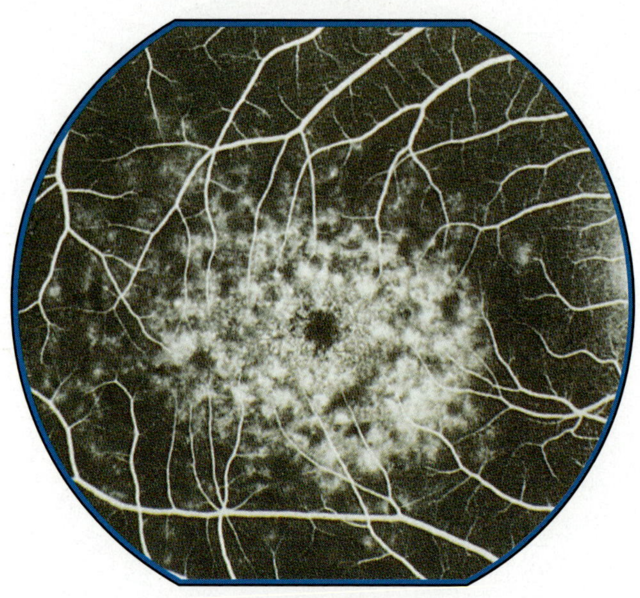

Fundus flavimaculatus or Stargardt's disease is an atrophic macular dystrophy with flecks. These flecks have a characteristic pisiform shape, and the macula has a "beaten-bronze" pattern. The characteristic fluorescein angiographic pattern is the dark or silent choroid, which is due to lipofuscin accumulation. This condition is usually inherited in an autosomal recessive pattern.

22–14 This patient illustrates the classic clinical macular findings of Stargardt's disease, or fundus flavimaculatus, which includes a polymorphic sheen, macular granularity, a hyperpigmented fovea, and flecks. The macula lesion is characteristic in these patients and was first described as Stargardt's disease.

22–15 The classic fluorescein angiographic appearance of fundus flavimaculatus is the dark or silent choroid.

22–16 **22–17**

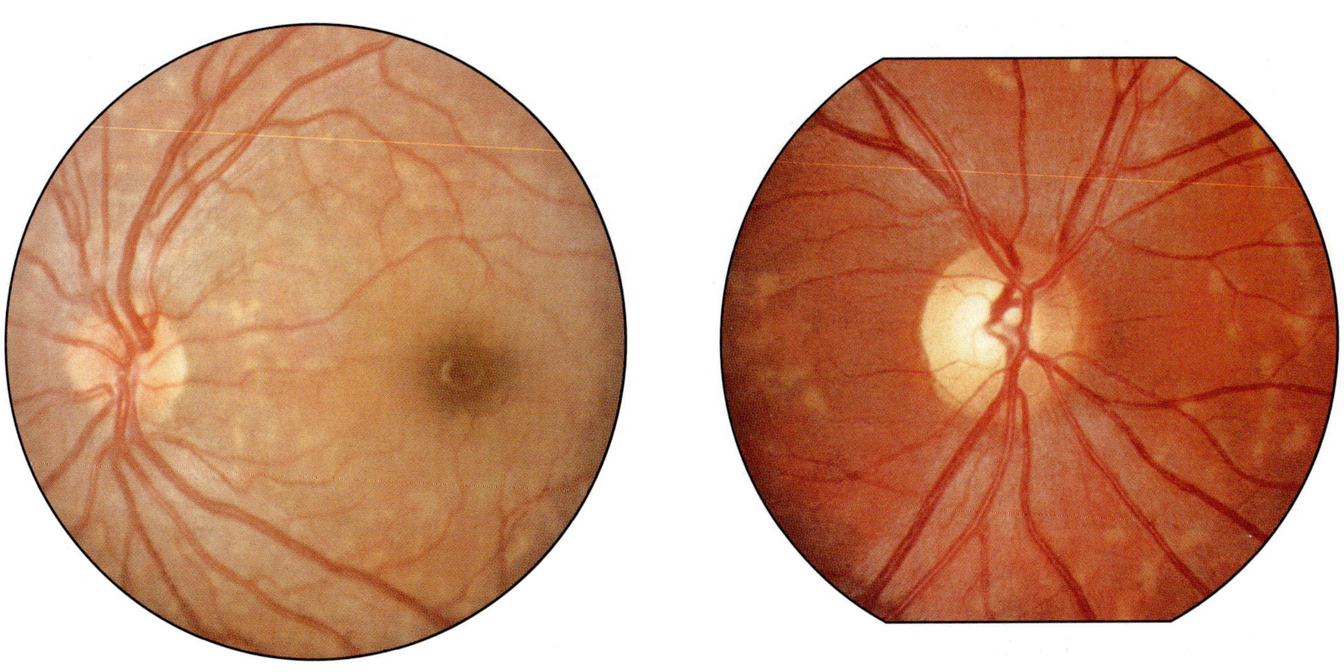

22–16 This patient also has fundus flavimaculatus. Notice the flecks as well as the macular lesion.

22–17 The pisiform-like fundus lesions of fundus flavimaculatus can be observed around the disc in this case.

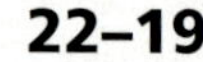

22–18 FUNDUS FLAVIMACULATUS

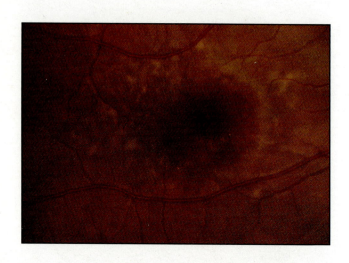

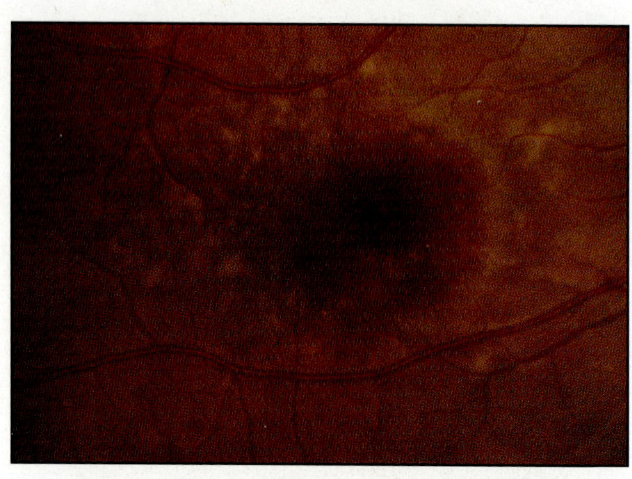

22–19

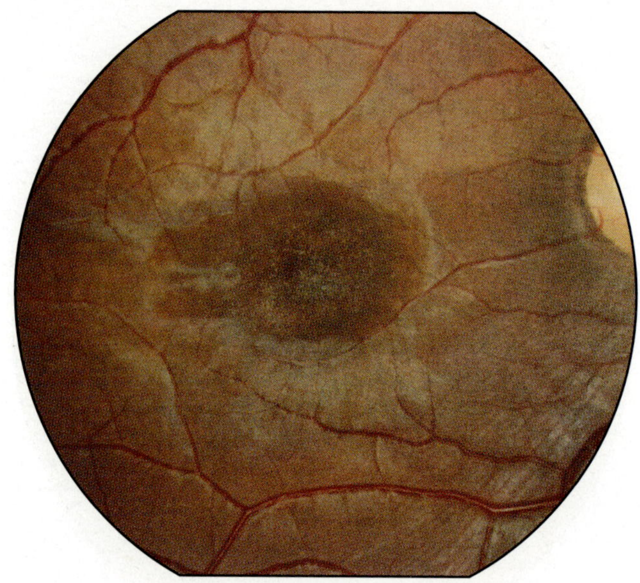

22–20

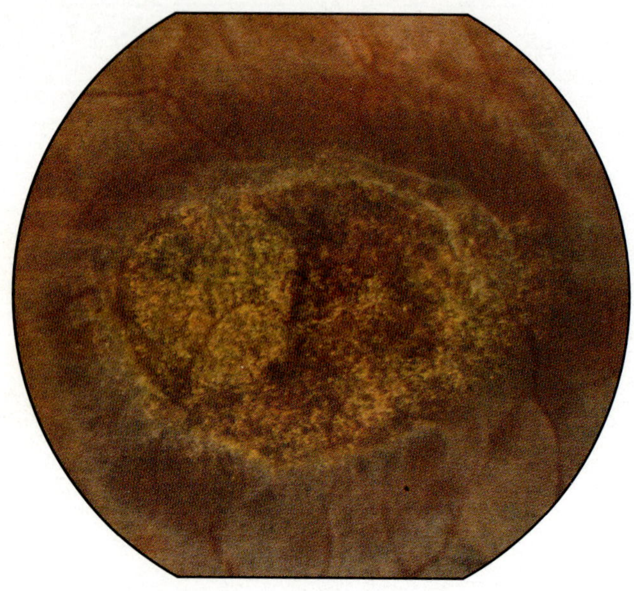

22–21

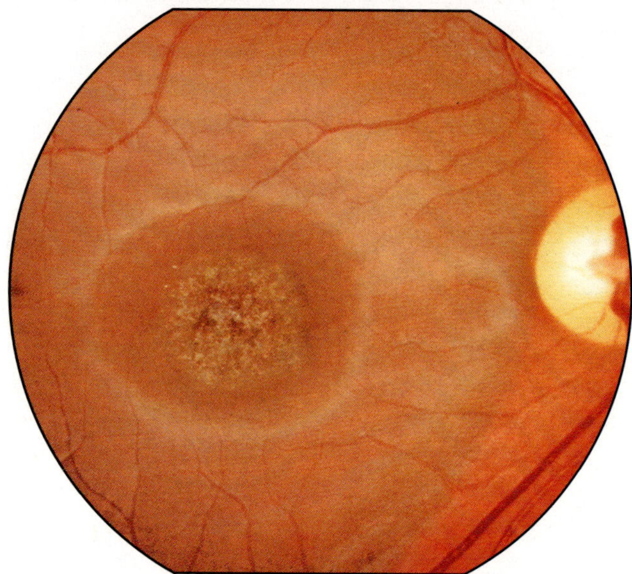

22–18 The typical appearance of the macula in Stargardt's disease is a mild pigment granularity surrounded by regular yellowish-white deep flecks.

22–19 Sometimes the pigmentary abnormalities can be mild and unassociated with these whitish flecks.

22–20 Other cases have a more pronounced pigmentary macular change, and in these cases the tapetal-like reflexes are referred to as having a "beaten-bronze" or polychromatic appearance.

22–21 The classic granularity to the macular lesion in Stargardt's disease is illustrated without flecks in this case.

22–18 *through* ***22–20,*** *Courtesy of Drs. Ron Carr and Ken Noble.*

22–22

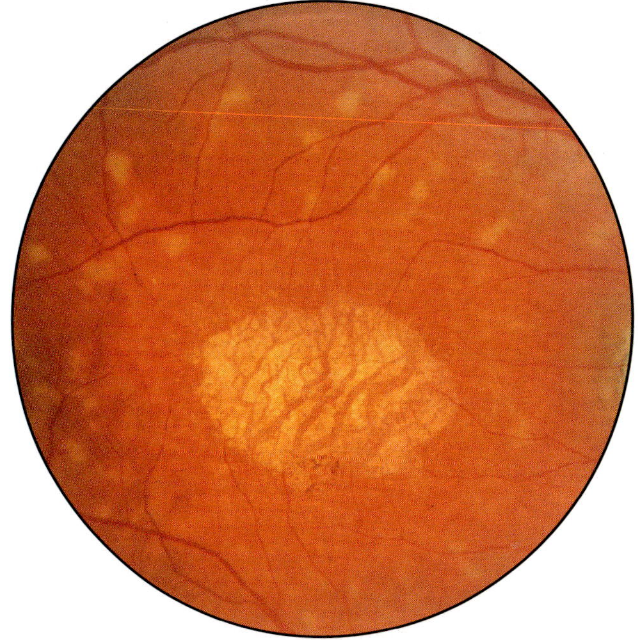

22–23

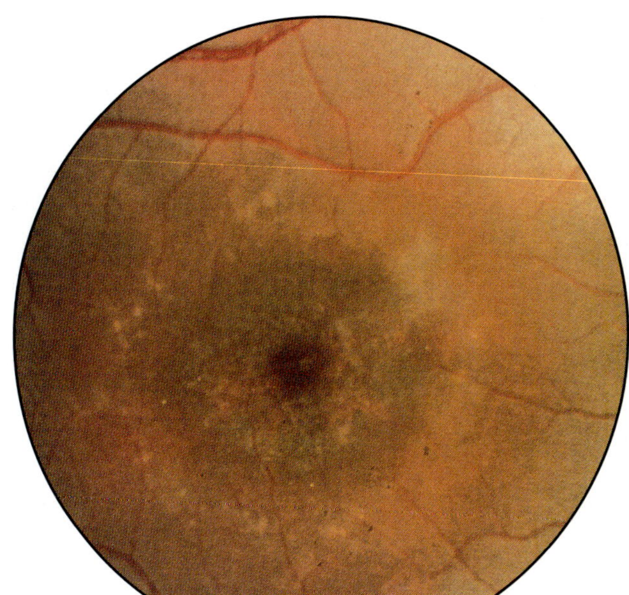

22–24

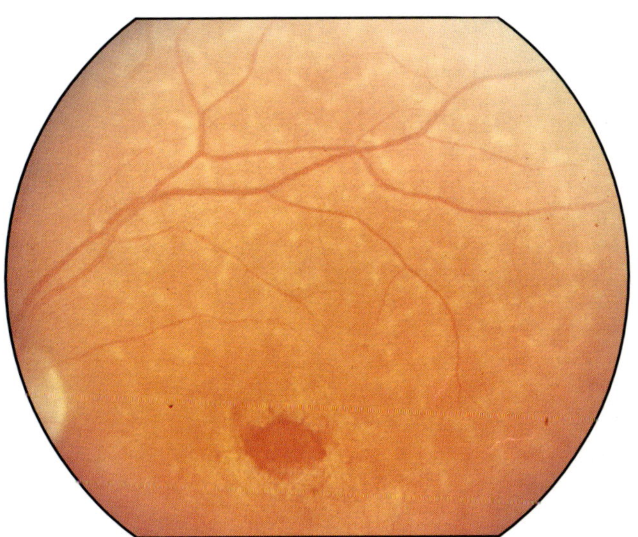

22–22 The macular lesion in time will become associated with atrophy, which is extreme in this patient. Notice the fleck-like lesions in the posterior pole.

22–23 An atypical maculopathy associated with fundus flavimaculatus is illustrated in this patient, in which there is a bull's eye ring.

22–24 This patient also has an atypical fundus appearance. Notice the pisiform-like whitish lesions and the reddish appearance to the macular lesion.

***22–22** and **22–23**, Courtesy of Drs. Ron Carr and Ken Noble.*

22–25 FUNDUS FLAVIMACULATUS

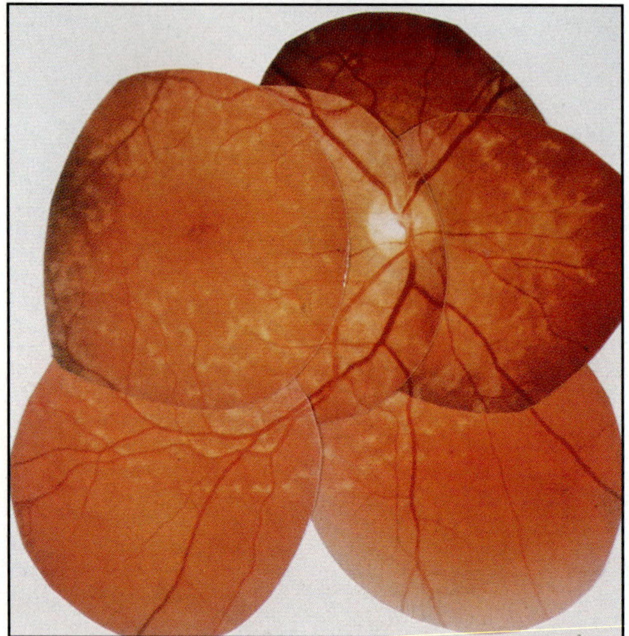

22–26

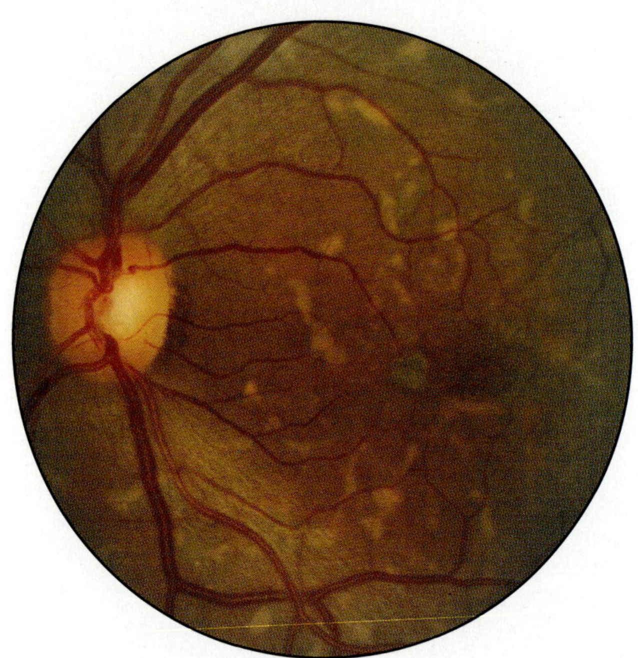

22–25 The yellowish-white flecks in fundus flavimaculatus can be demonstrated in the posterior pole, nasal to the optic disc and peripheral to the temporal vessel arcades.

22–26 Larger flecks can be observed in this patient, as well as a focal area of foveal atrophy.

22–27 through 22–31 Clinicopathologic correlation of a patient with fundus flavimaculatus. The patient has the characteristic yellow flecks and macula abnormalities. Light microscopy reveals atrophy of the retina and retinal pigment epithelium (RPE) in the foveal region. Adjacent retinal pigment epithelial cells are greatly distended with lipofuscin. Pigmented cells with lipofuscin present in the subretinal space correspond to the flecks observed ophthalmoscopically.

22–25 *and* ***22–26,*** *Courtesy of Drs. Ron Carr and Ken Noble.* ***22–27*** *through* ***22–31,*** *From Lopez, PF, Maumenee, IH, de la Cruz, Z, and Green, WR: Autosomal-dominant fundus flavimaculatus: clinicopathologic correlation, Ophthalmology 97:798–809, 1990.*

22–27

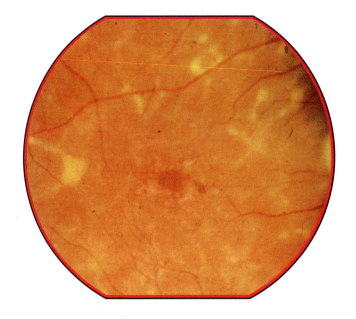

22–28

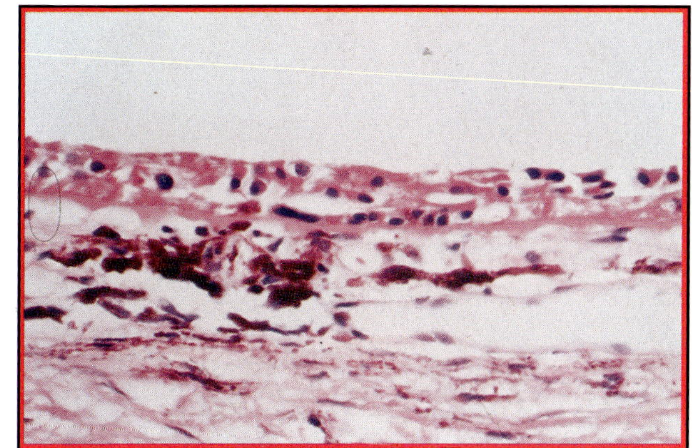

22–29

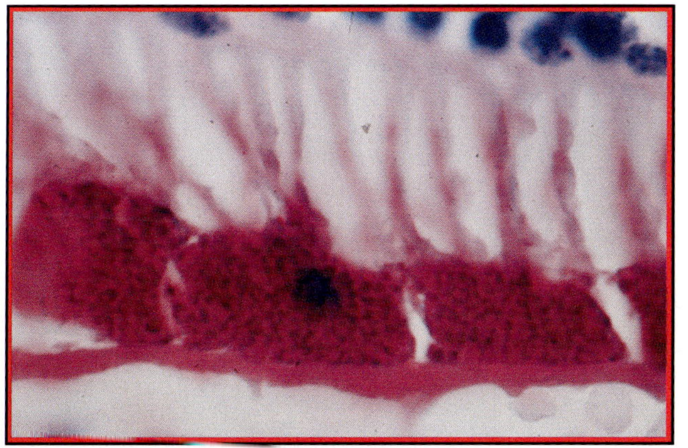

22–30

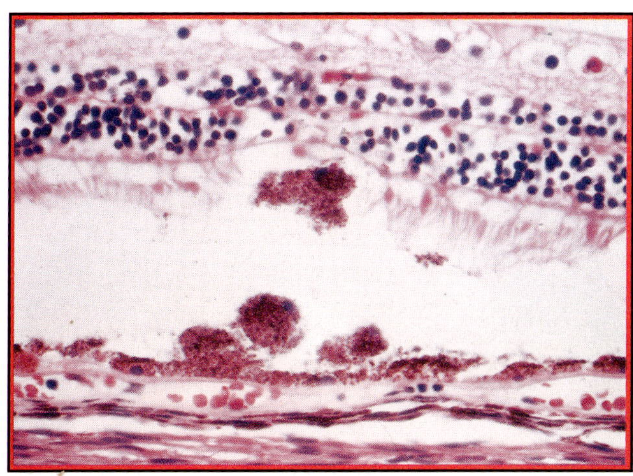

22–31

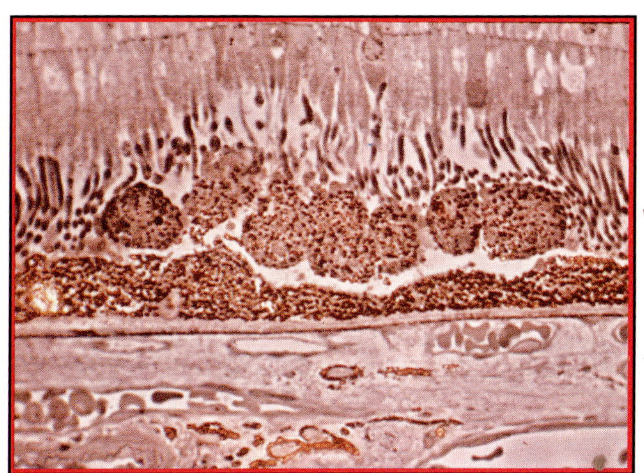

22–32 BEST'S DISEASE

22–32A

22–33

22–34

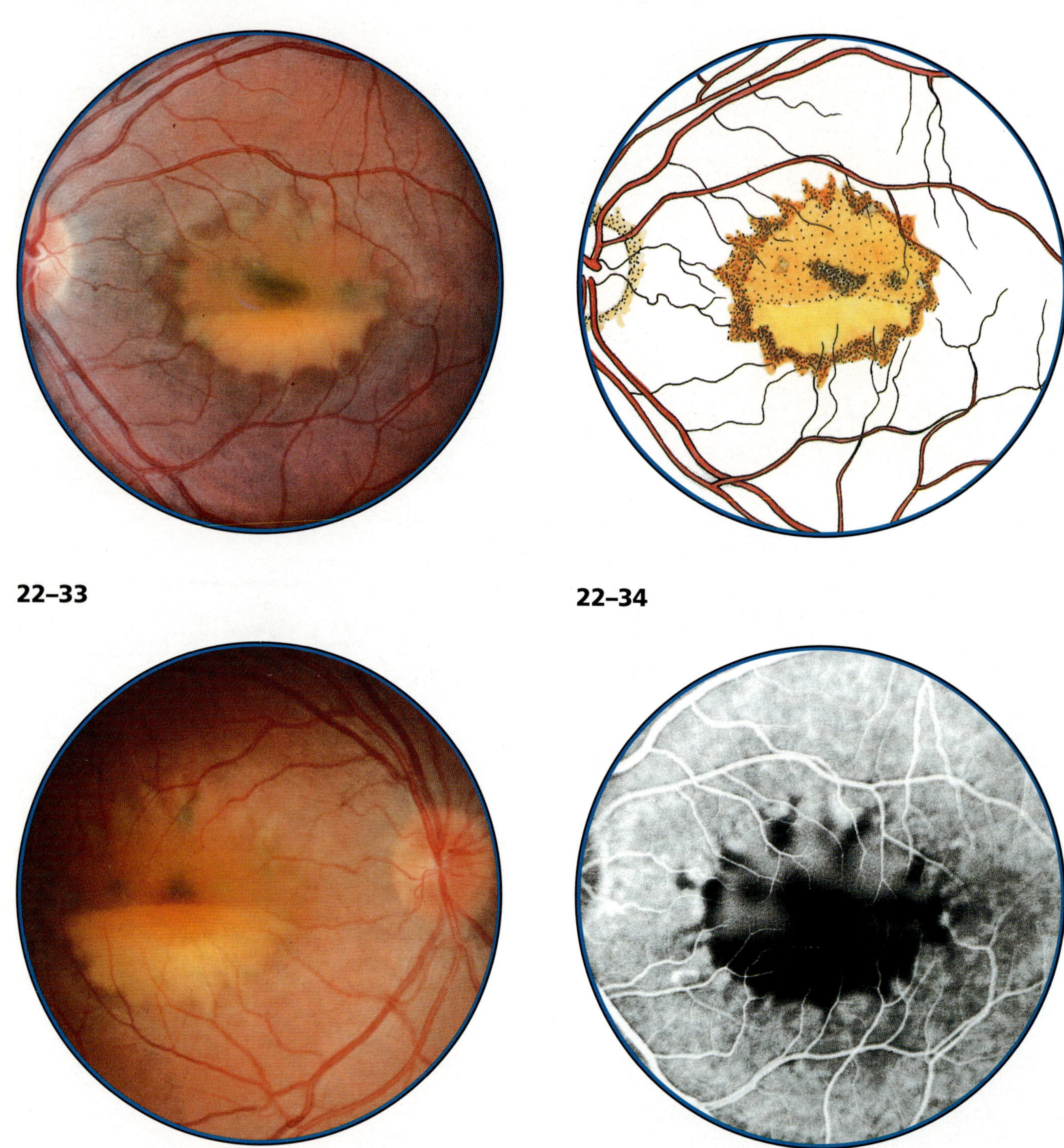

22–32, 22–32A, and 22–33 This patient with Best's disease illustrates the stellate-like borders characteristic of this disorder. Lipofuscin deposition is noted inferiorly in both eyes.

22–34 Fluorescein angiography of the preceding patient with Best's disease shows blockage in the area of lipofuscin deposition.

22–35 NATURAL HISTORY: STAGE I

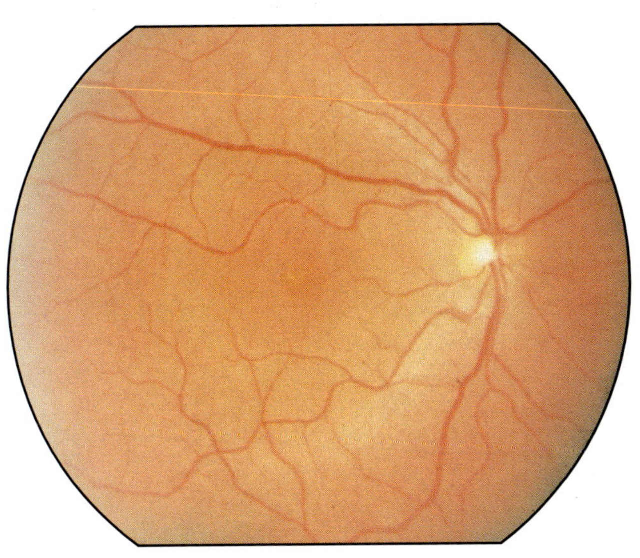

22–36

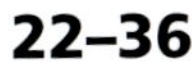

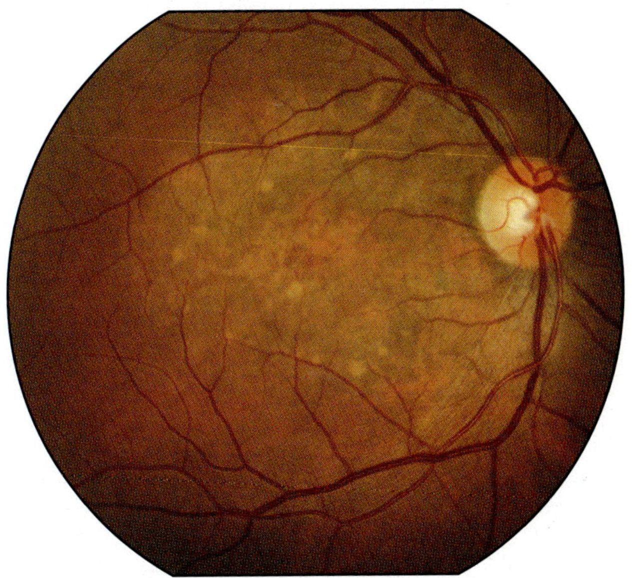

22–35 and 22–36 The following fundus photographs (22–35 through 22–46) illustrate the natural history of macular lesions in Best's vitelliform macular dystrophy. Stage I lesions show a mild degree of foveal pigment mottling and nonspecific hypopigmentation.

22–35, *From Fishman, G, et al: Ophthalmology 100:1668, 1993. Courtesy of Dr. Gerald Fishman.*

Best's Disease

22–37 NATURAL HISTORY: STAGE II

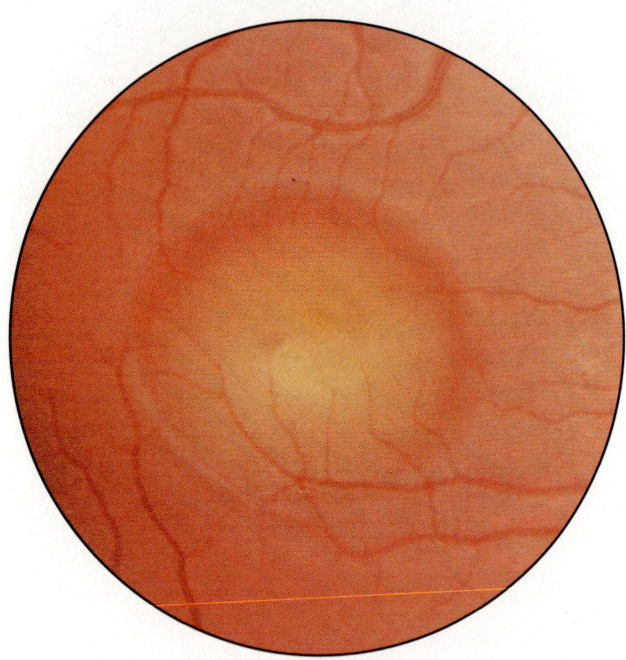

22–38

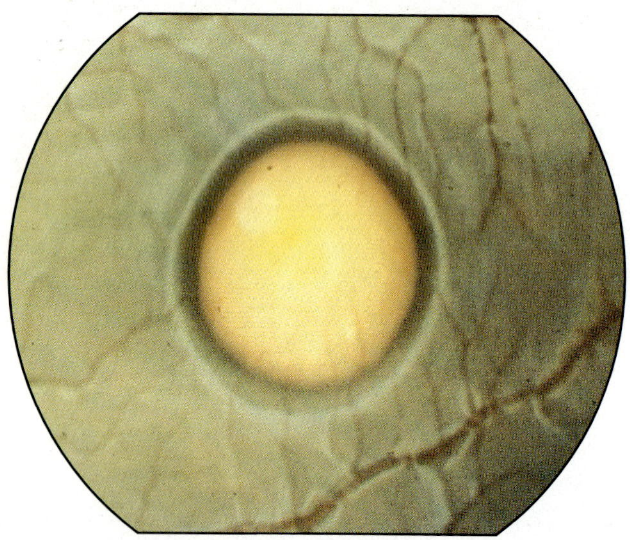

22–39

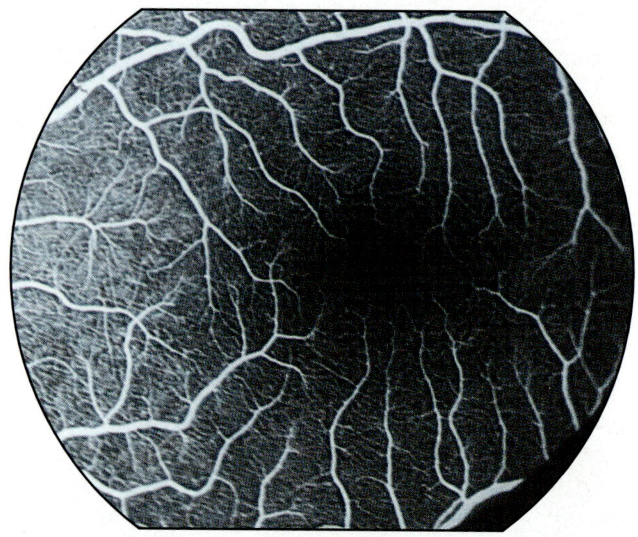

22–37 In stage II lesions, the typical vitelliform or egg yolk lesion can be appreciated.

22–38 The intact egg yolk stage has a dramatic appearance made even more so in view of this patient's normal 20/20 vision.

22–39 The angiogram at this stage may be normal. In other cases, blocked transmission may correspond to the lesion.

22–37, *From Fishman, G, et al: Ophthalmology 100:1668, 1993. Courtesy of Dr. Gerald Fishman.* ***22–38*** *and* ***22–39,*** *Courtesy of Drs. Ron Carr and Ken Noble.*

22–40 NATURAL HISTORY: STAGE IIIA

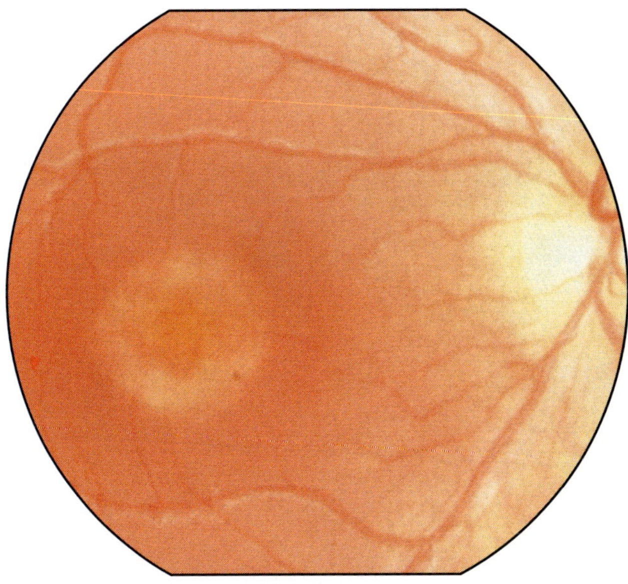

22–41 NATURAL HISTORY: STAGE IIIB

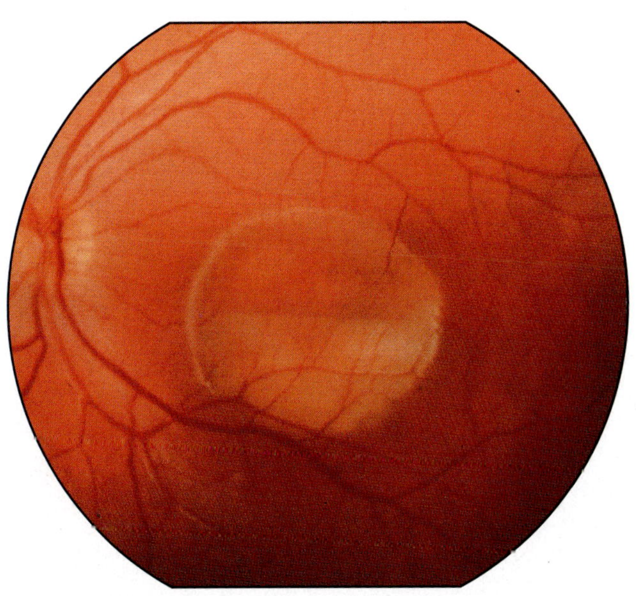

22–42

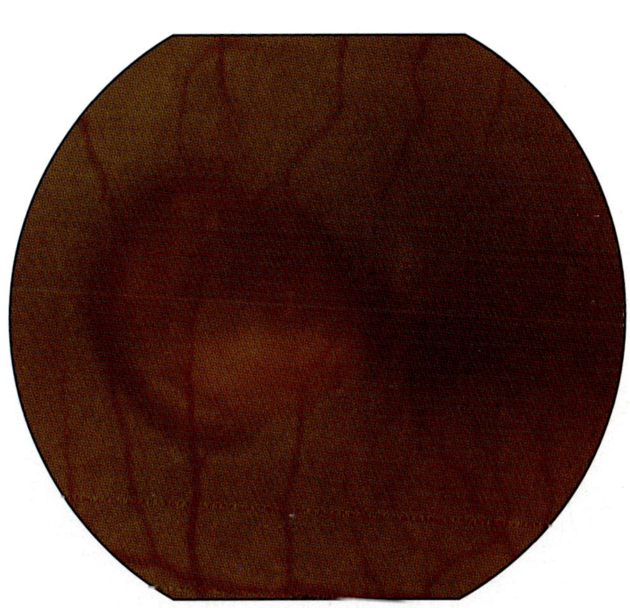

22–40 In stage IIIa lesions, a scrambled or "fried egg" appearance is noted.

22–41 and 22–42 The pseudohypopyon lesion in which the yellow material develops a layered appearance is seen in stage IIIb lesions.

22–40 *and* ***22–41,*** *From Fishman, G, et al: Ophthalmology 100:1668, 1993. Courtesy of Dr. Gerald Fishman.* ***22–42,*** *Courtesy of Drs. Ron Carr and Ken Noble.*

Best's Disease

22–43 NATURAL HISTORY: STAGE IIIC

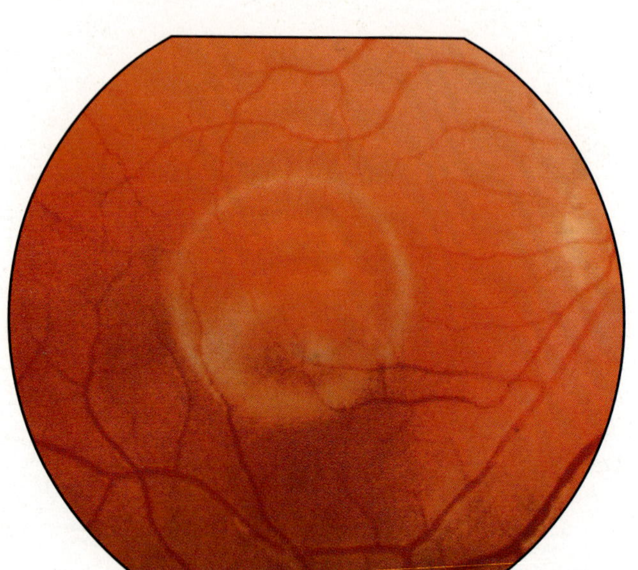

22–44 NATURAL HISTORY: STAGE IIID

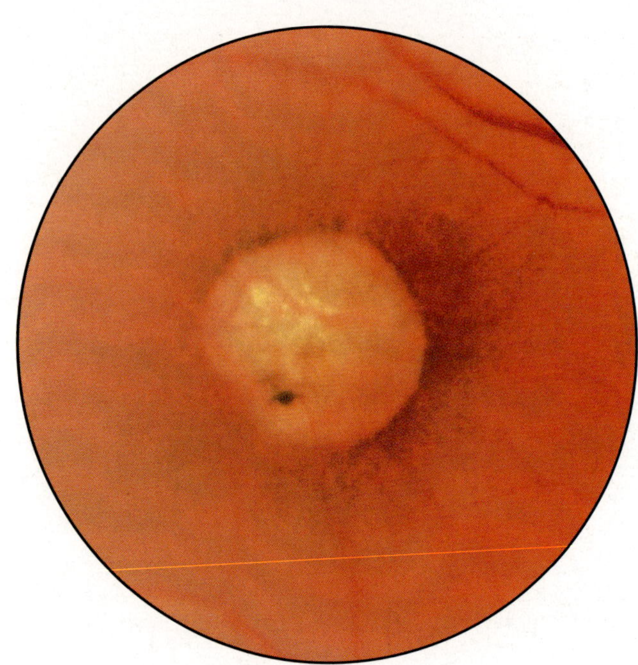

22–45 NATURAL HISTORY: STAGE IV

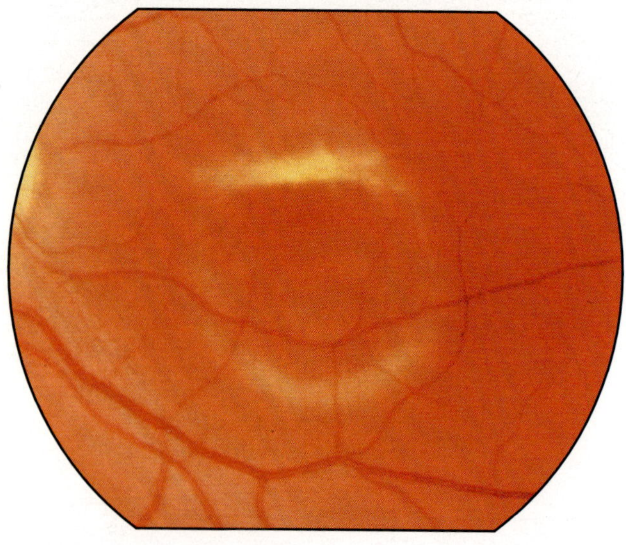

22–46

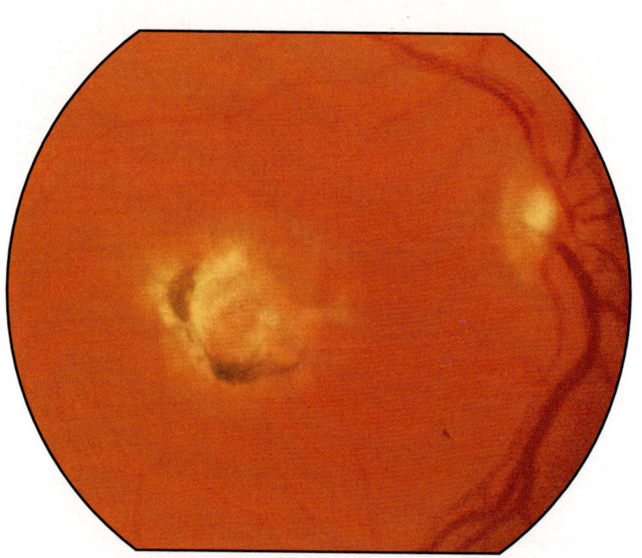

22–43 In stage IIIc lesions, only a sparse amount of the yellowish vitelliform material remains.

22–44 Stage IIId lesions are similar to stage IIIc lesions except that the choriocapillaris is also atrophic.

22–45 and 22–46 In stage IV lesions, fibrotic, gliotic-appearing scar tissue is noted in addition to resorption of the vitelliform material.

***22–43** through **22–46,** From Fishman, G, et al: Ophthalmology 100:1668, 1993. Courtesy of Dr. Gerald Fishman.*

22–47 BEST'S AND CNV

22–48

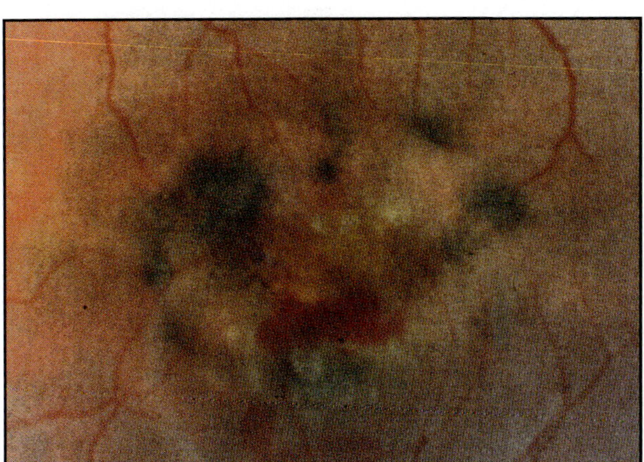

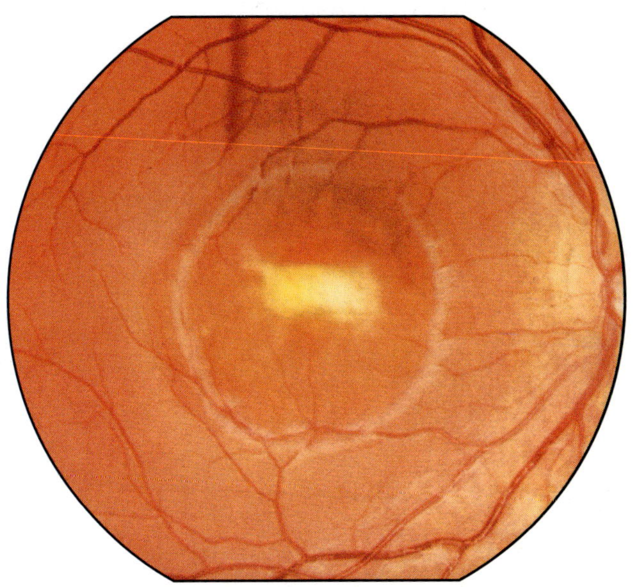

22–47 This patient with Best's disease has subretinal hemorrhage secondary to choroidal neovascularization.

22–48 This patient had Best's disease with choroidal neovascularization which spontaneously regressed into a scar.

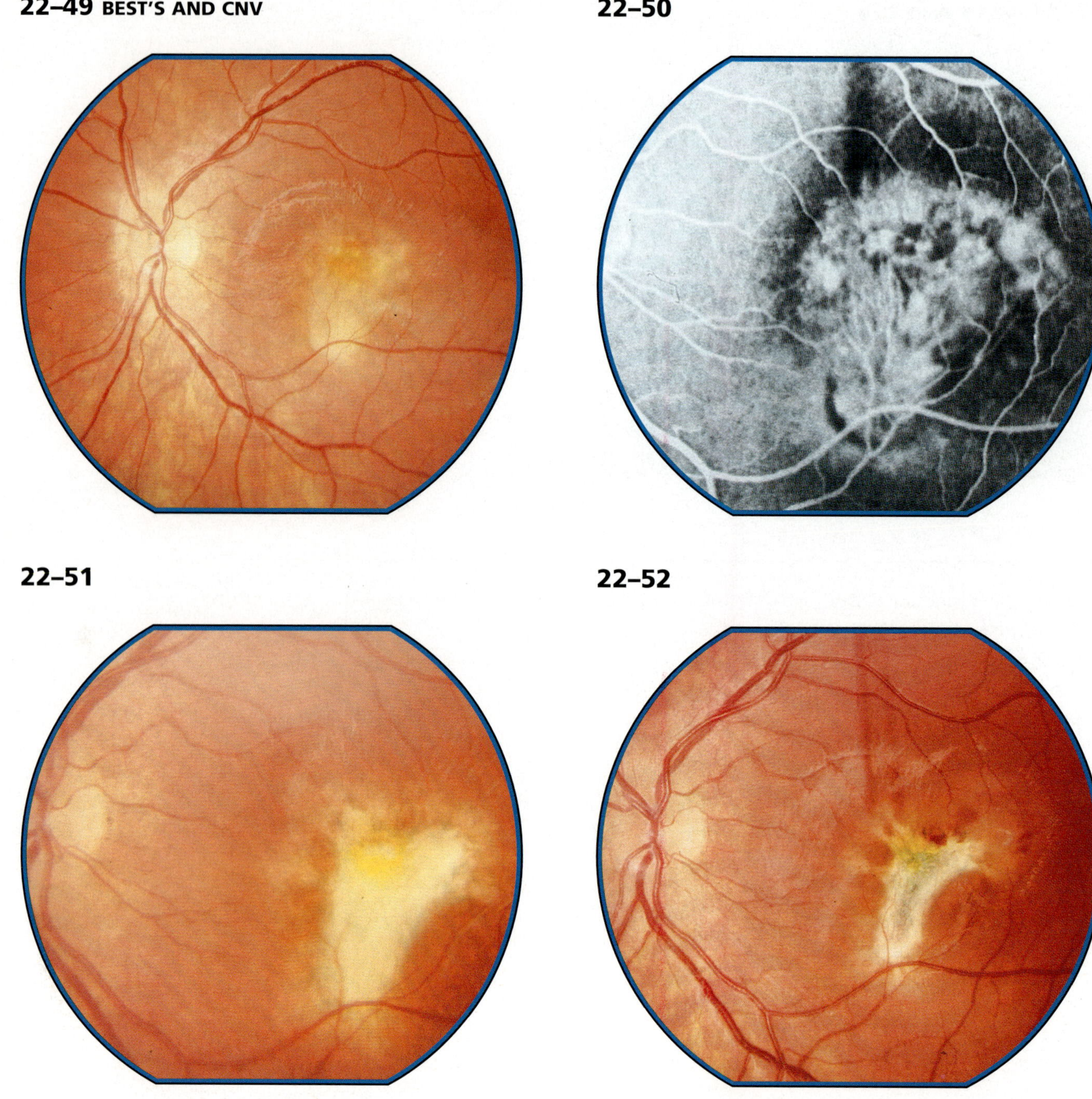

22–49 and 22–50 22–49 was the fellow eye of 22–48 on p. 307. The patient developed choroid neovascularization, which is seen better with fluorescein angiography (22–50).

22–51 and 22–52 One month later (22–51) and three months later (22–52) there is spontaneous regression and scar formation and improvement of the visual acuity to 20/30.

22–53 MULTIFOCAL BEST'S DISEASE

22–54

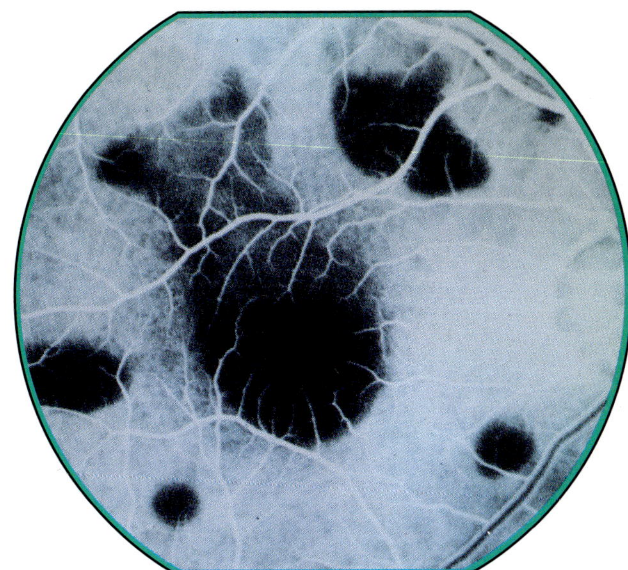

22–55

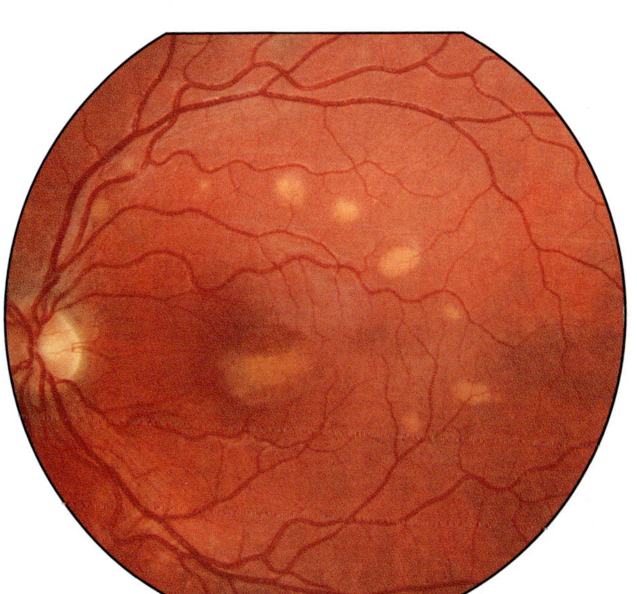

22–56

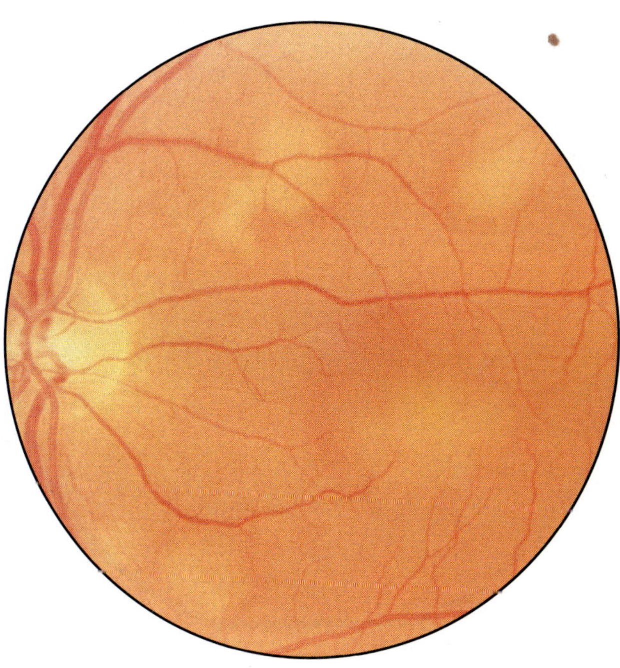

22–53 and 22–54 Multifocal lesions can sometimes be seen with Best's disease. The fluorescein angiogram of this last case reveals blockage secondary to lipofuscin in the various lesions (22–54).

22–55 This case illustrates another patient with multifocal Best's disease. Note the pseudohypopyon macular lesion as well as satellite lesions.

22–56 Another patient illustrates multiple focal lesions in Best's disease.

***22–53** and **22–54,** Courtesy of Dr. Tom Weingeist.*

22–57 MULTIFOCAL BEST'S DISEASE

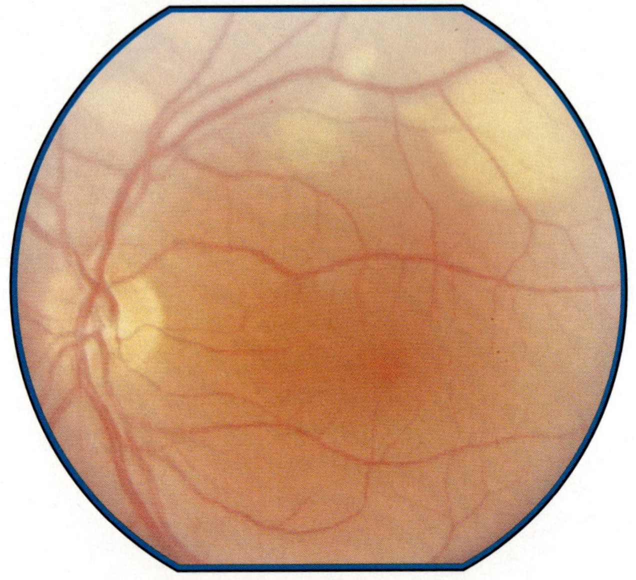

22–58

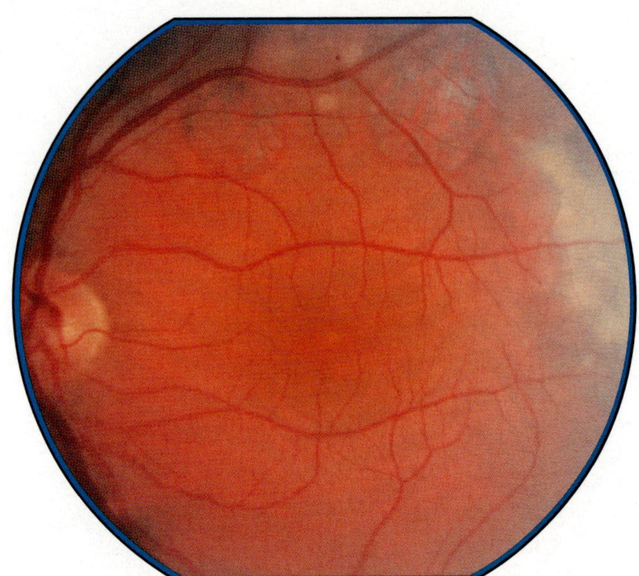

22–59

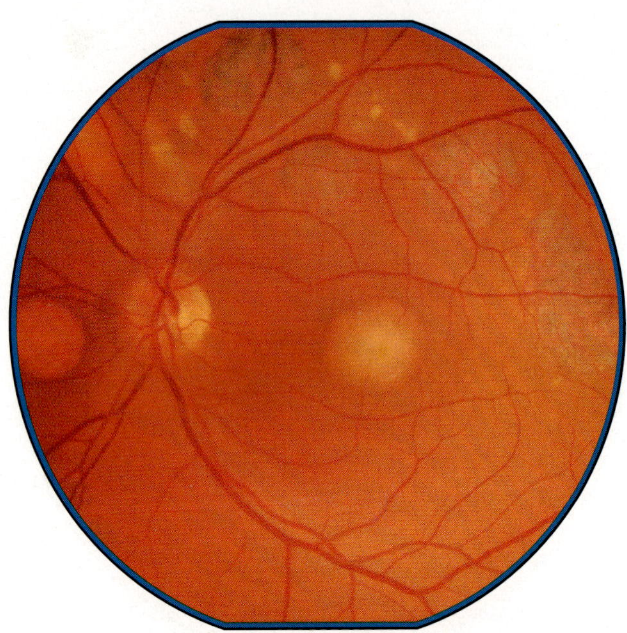

22–57 This patient had multifocal Best's disease with minimal initial involvement of the macula. Visual acuity was 20/20.

22–58 Five years later, many of the multifocal lesions have regressed and a minimal yellowish change is noted in the macular region.

22–59 Seven years after the initial presentation, the multifocal lesions have regressed further, and a characteristic egg yolk lesion is noted in the macular region. Vision at this time is 20/25.

22–57 *through* ***22–59,*** *Courtesy of Dr. Stephen Ryan.*

22–60

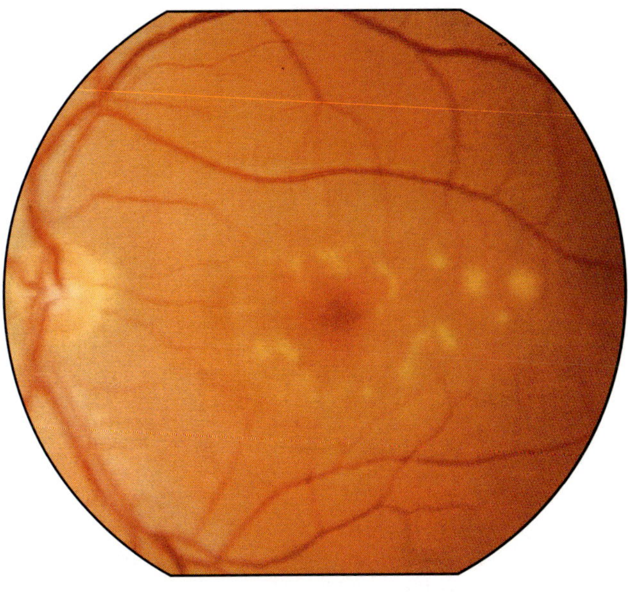

22–61

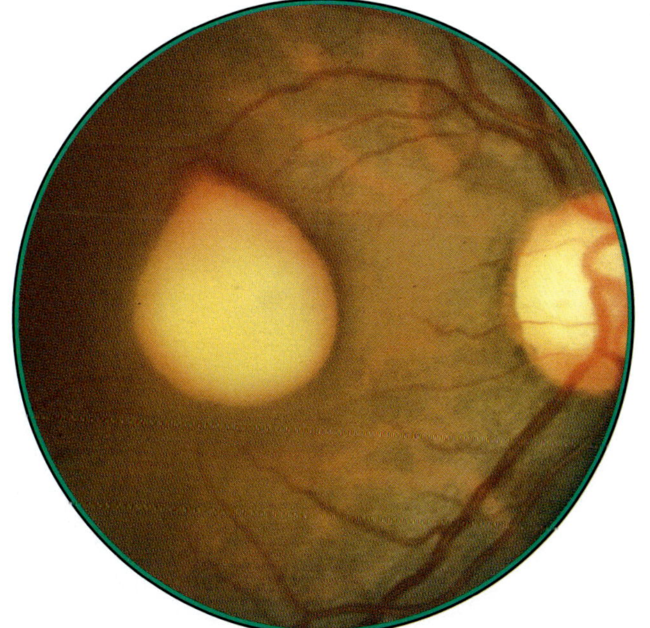

22–62

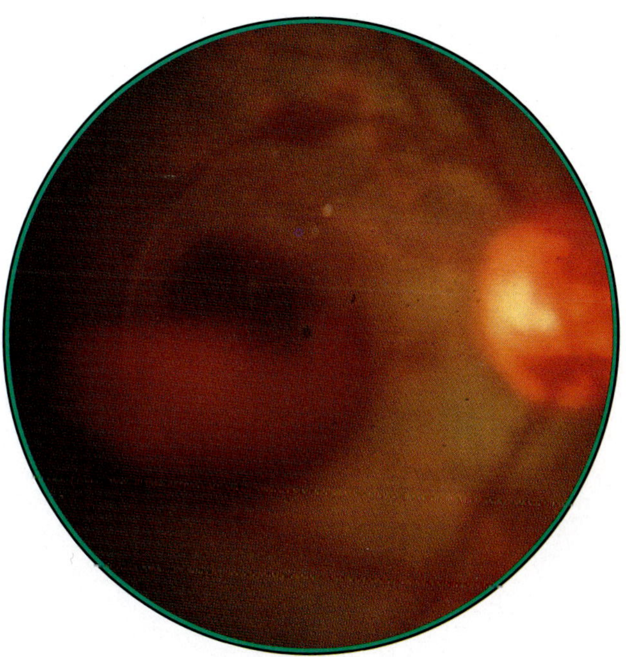

22–60 This patient with Best's disease has flecks with a mineralized-like appearance.

22–61 and 22–62 The differential diagnosis of Best's disease includes resolving subhyaloid hemorrhage, such as in this case. A yellowish lesion resembling the egg yolk lesion of Best's disease is seen as dehemoglobinization of the blood occurs. The second photograph shows the initial subhyaloid hemorrhage. The unilaterality of this case was inconsistent with Best's disease.

22–63 BEST'S DISEASE–CPC

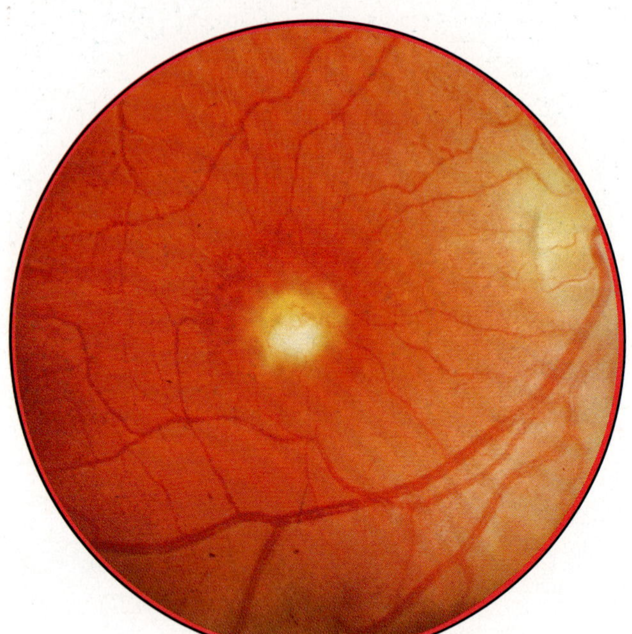

22–64

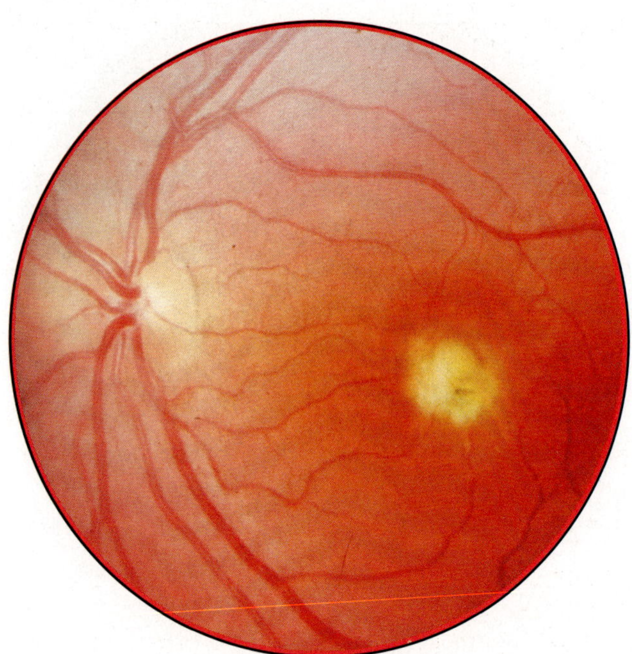

22–65

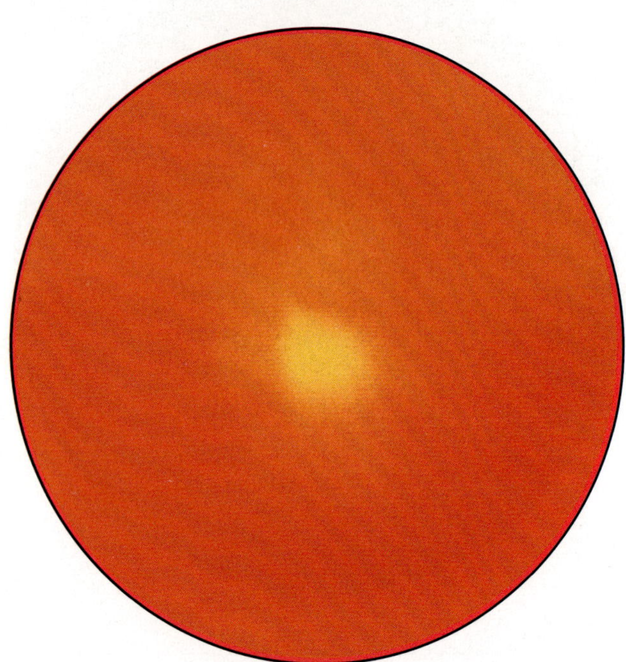

22–63 This case is a clinicopathologic correlation of an 80-year-old woman with Best's disease.

22–64 and 22–65 An 8-year-old niece of the proband also had the condition.

22–63 *through* ***22–65,*** *From Frangieh, GT, Green, WR, and Fine, SL: A histopathologic study of Best's macular dystrophy, Arch Ophthalmol 100:1115–1121, 1982.*

(Case continued on next page.)

22–66

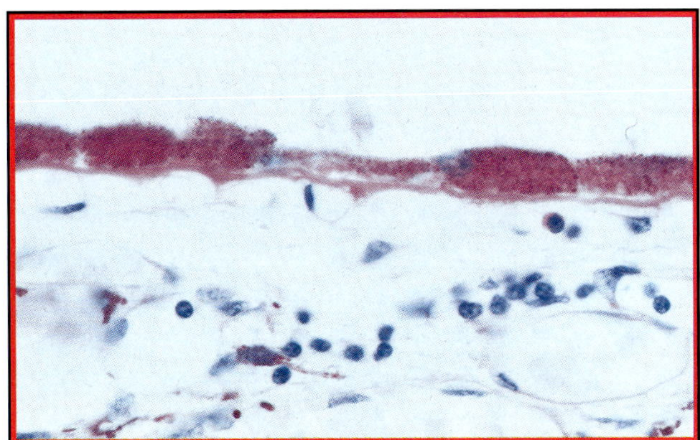

22–67

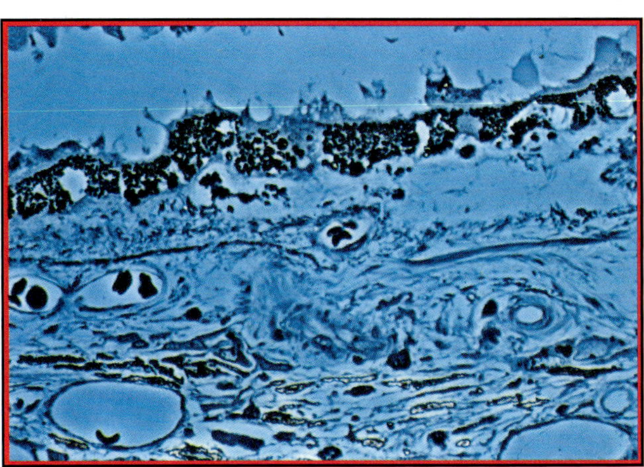

22–68

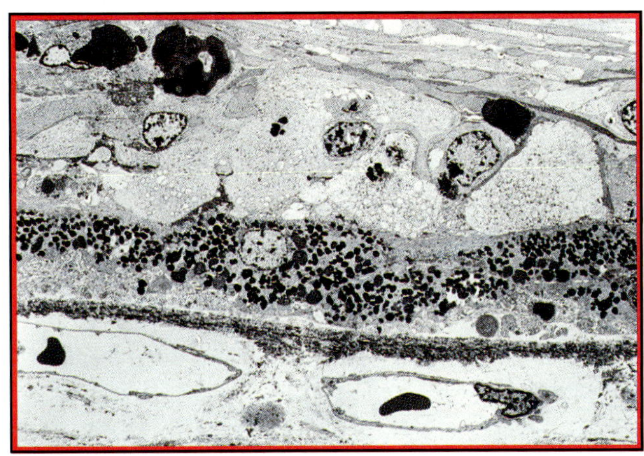

22–66 Light microscopy reveals that the retinal pigment epithelium in the macular area was intact and distended with abundant periodic acid–Schiff positive material.

22–67 The phase-contrast appearance shows distended retinal pigment epithelial cells and an area of choroidal neovascularization.

22–68 Electron microscopy shows distended RPE with lipofuscin and marked photoreceptor cell degeneration. Bruch's membrane and the choriocapillaris are intact.

22–66 *through* ***22–68,*** *From Frangieh, GT, Green, WR, and Fine, SL: A histopathologic study of Best's macular dystrophy, Arch Ophthalmol 100:1115–1121, 1982.*

22–69 PATTERN DYSTROPHIES

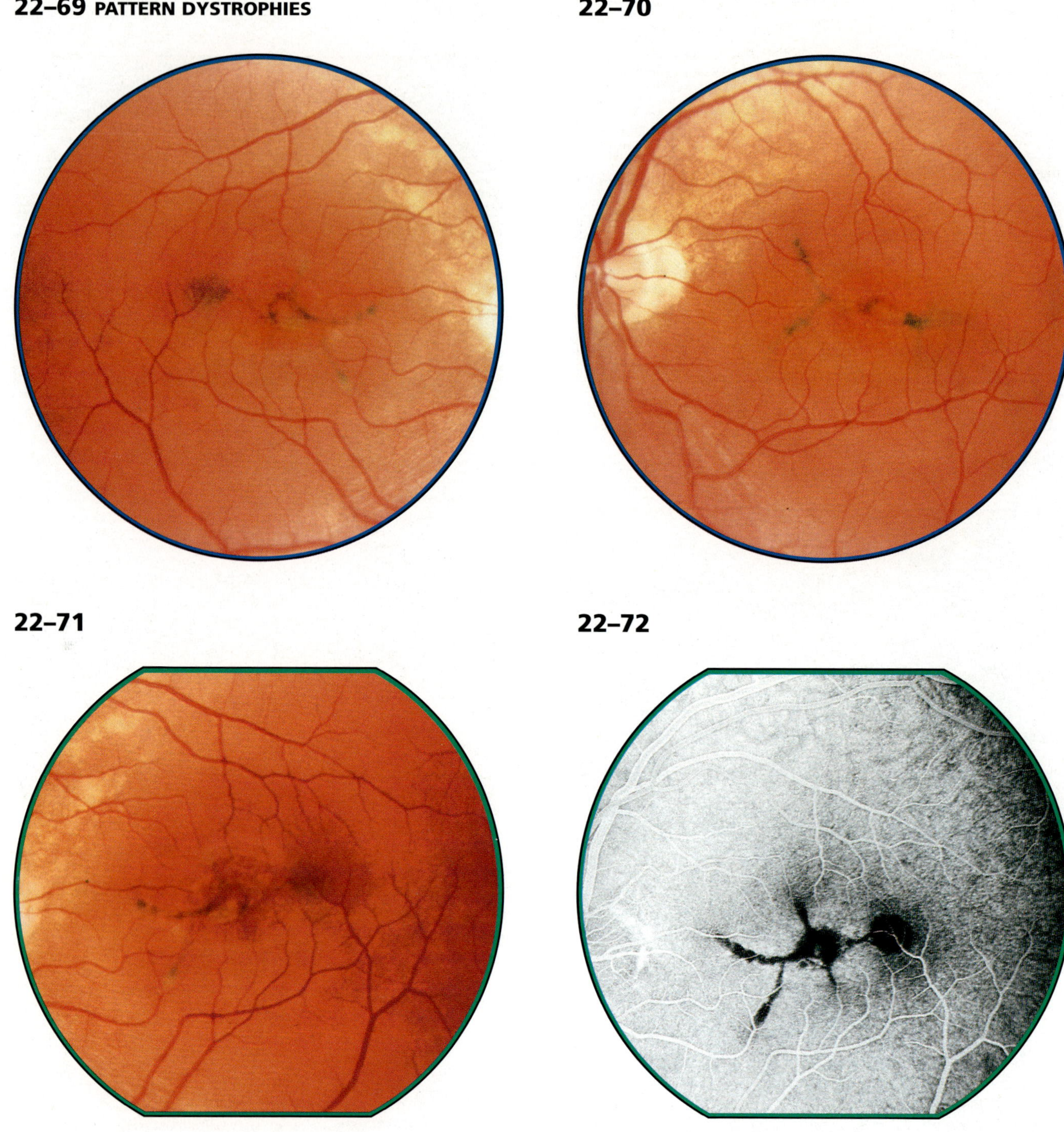

22–69 and 22–70 Pattern dystrophies are hereditary forms of macular degeneration. The bilateral symmetric pigmentary maculopathy in this patient prompted the term "butterfly-shaped pigment dystrophy." This condition is slowly progressive.

22–71 and 22–72 The butterfly-like pattern is accentuated by fluorescein angiography.

***22–69** and **22–70,** From Deutman, AF, and van Blommenstein, JDA: Butterfly-shaped pigment history of the fovea, Arch Ophthalmol 83:558–569, 1970. Courtesy of Drs. Ron Carr, Ken Noble, and August Deutman.*

22–73

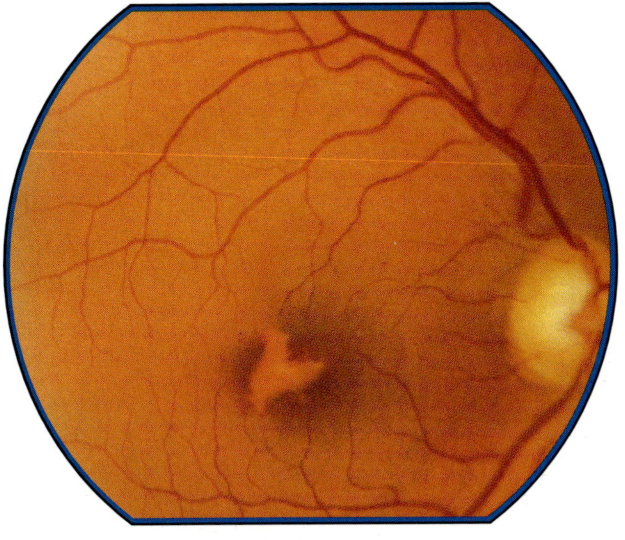

22–74

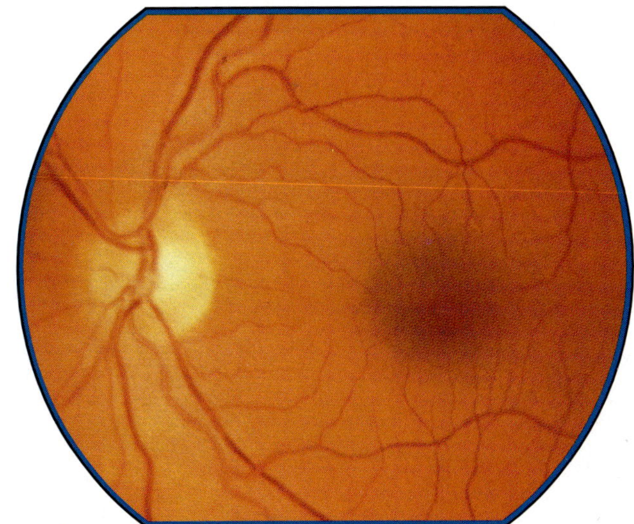

22–75

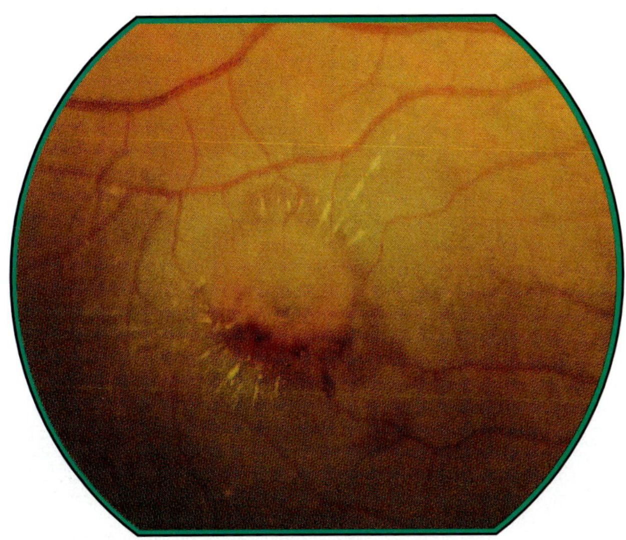

22–76

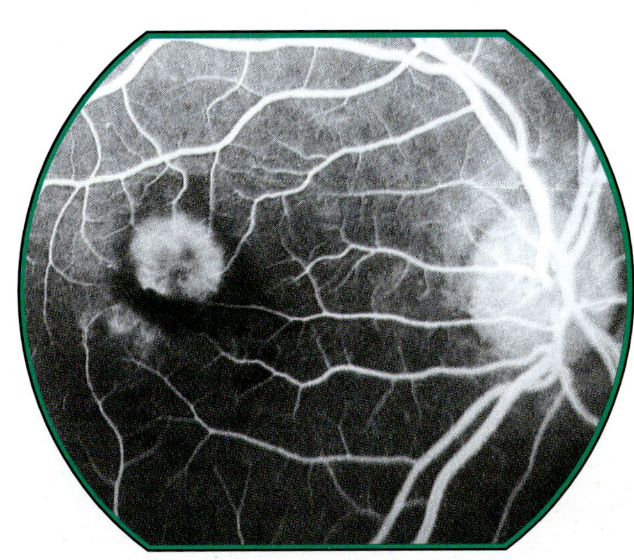

22–77

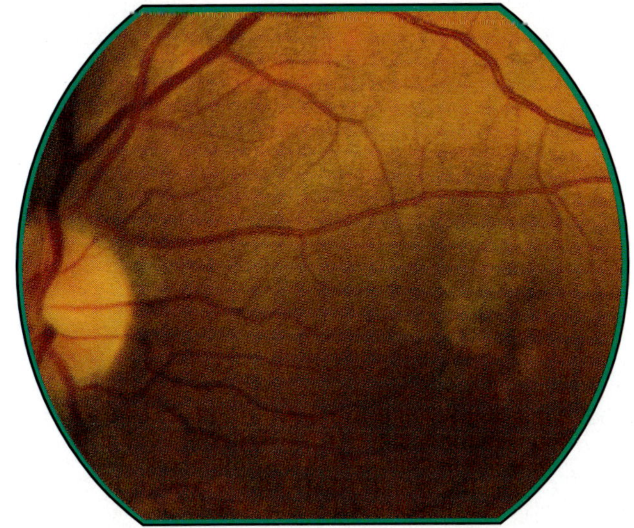

22–73 and 22–74 Rarely, pattern dystrophies can be unilateral, as demonstrated in this patient with a family history of a bilateral pattern dystrophy.

22–75 through 22–77 Choroidal neovascularization may uncommonly be associated with pattern dystrophies, as demonstrated in this patient. This young female with a pattern dystrophy has subretinal fluid, lipid, and hemorrhage secondary to choroidal neovascularization (22–75 and 22–76). The other eye showed evidence of a pattern dystrophy without neovascularization (22–77).

22–78 PATTERN DYSTROPHIES

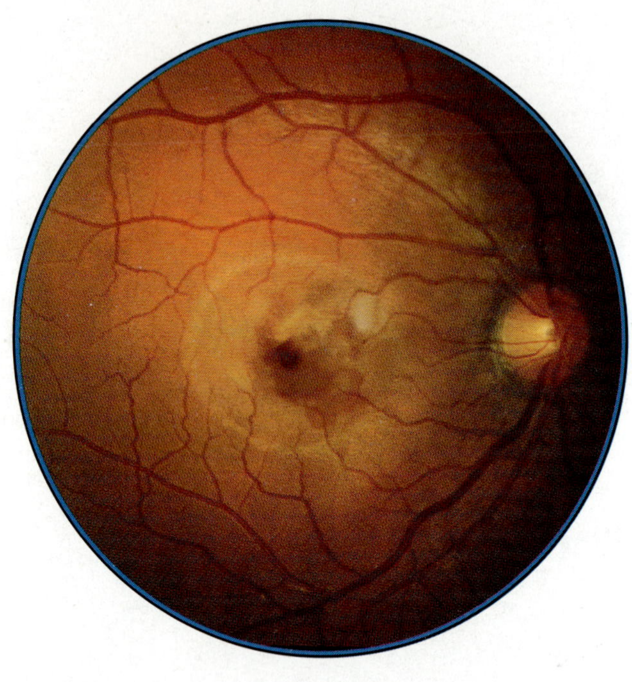

22–79

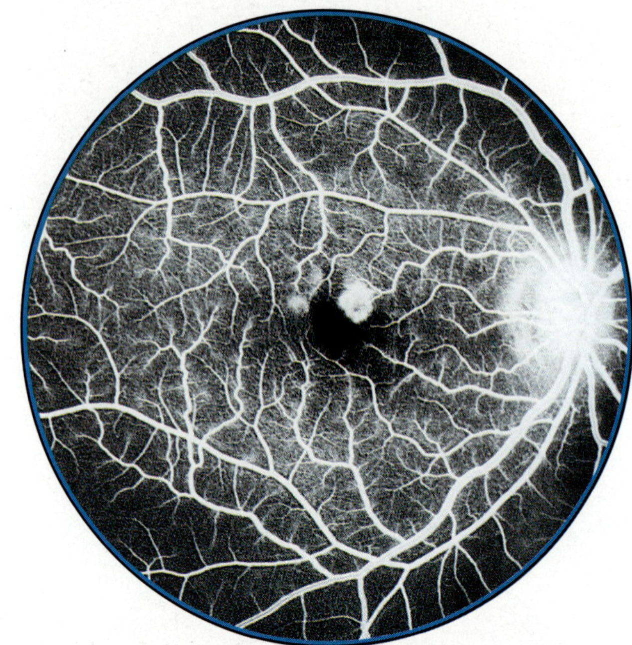

22–80

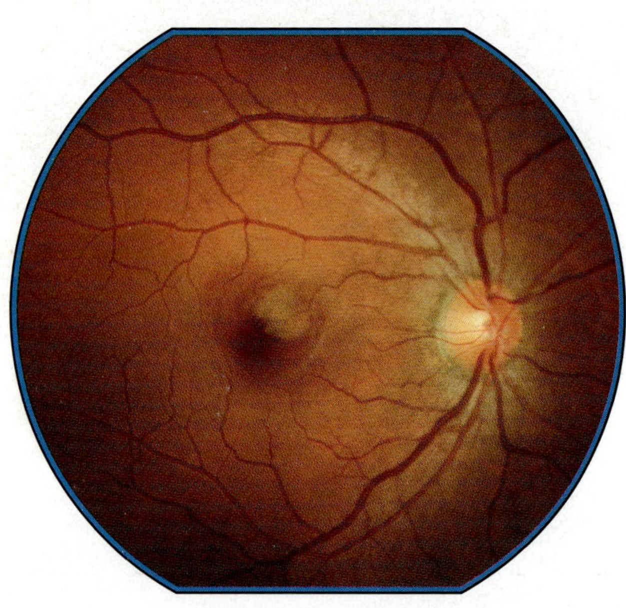

22–81

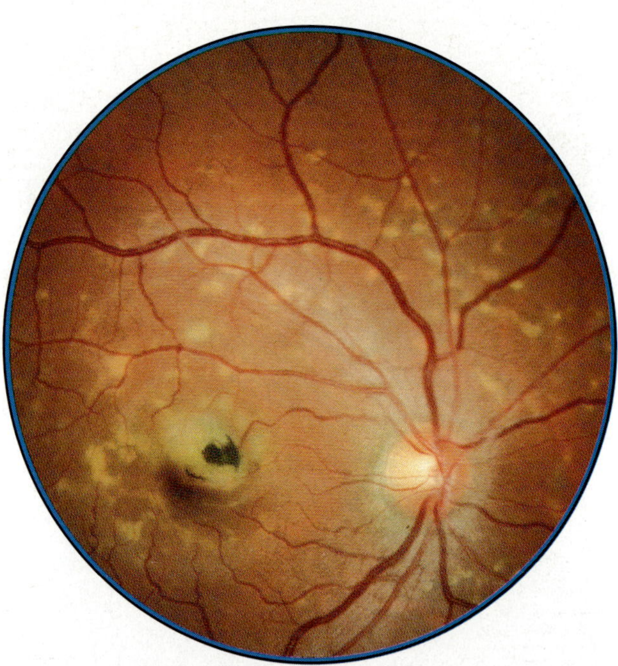

22–78 and 22–79 This 26-year-old male presented with presumed idiopathic choroidal neovascularization.

22–80 The patient was successfully treated with laser photocoagulation.

22–81 Four years later, however, multiple hypopigmented spots were seen throughout the posterior pole and peripapillary area.

(Case continued on next page.)

22–82

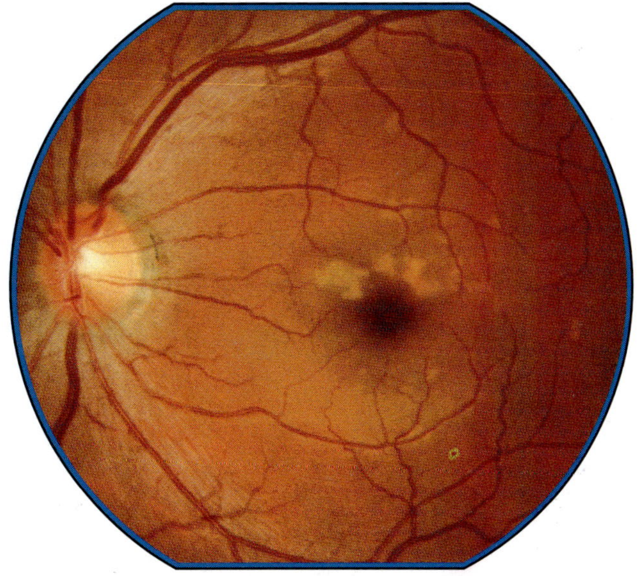

22–83

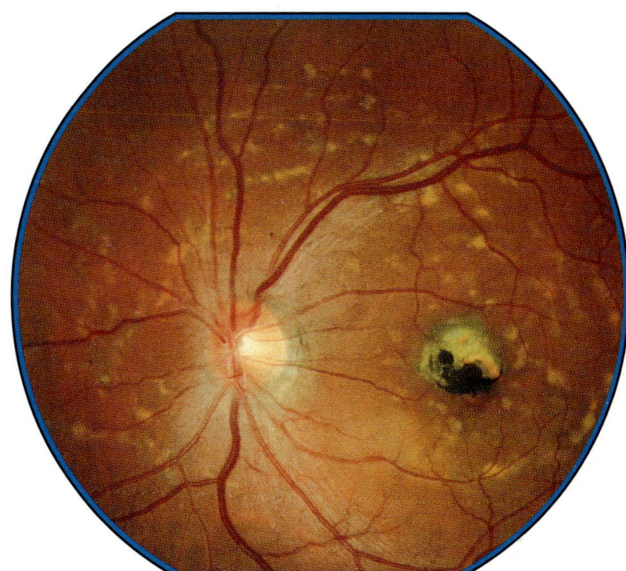

22–84 ADULT-ONSET FOVEOMACULAR DYSTROPHY

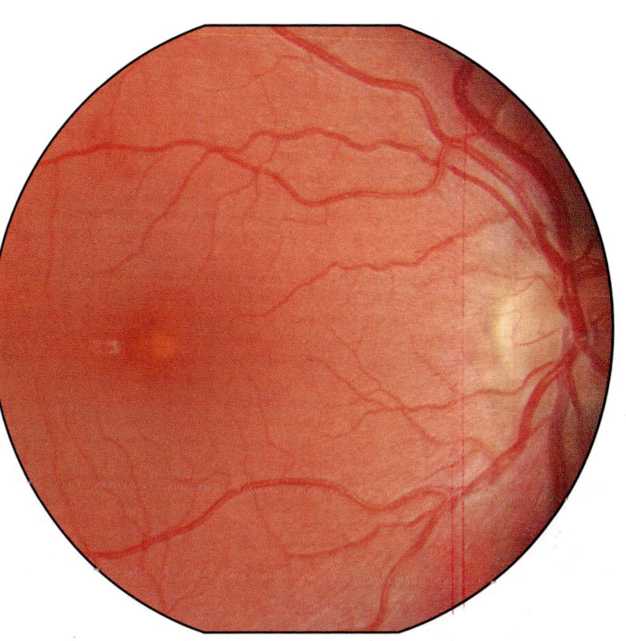

22–85

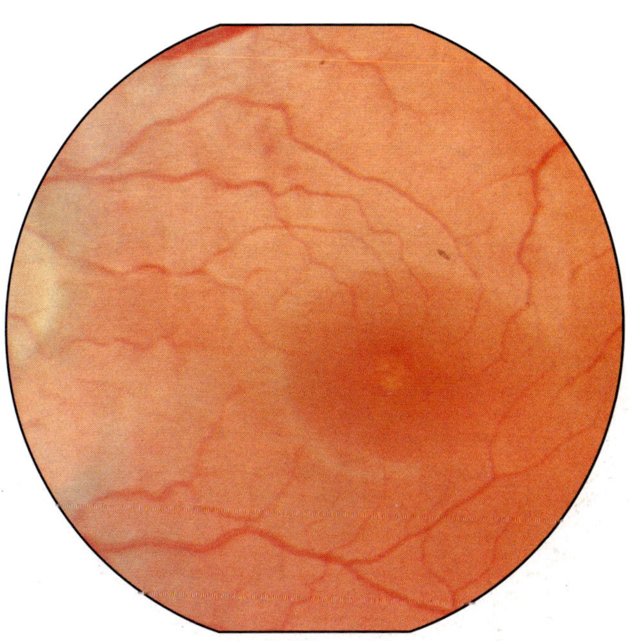

22–82 and 22–83 The other eye developed a pattern dystrophy in the macular region (22–82) and choroidal neovascularization with increasing hypopigmented spots over three years (22–83). This case is an example of a patient with presumed idiopathic choroidal neovascularization that later developed findings suggestive of a multifocal pattern dystrophy. These eyes resemble fundus flavimaculatus.

22–84 and 22–85 Pattern dystrophy is also called adult-onset foveomacular dystrophy. On this patient, a small yellowish lesion that may be confused with Best's disease is seen in this disorder. The lesion is usually smaller, and patients do not have the classic electro-oculogram findings noted in Best's disease.

22–84 *and* ***22–85,*** *Courtesy of Dr. Stuart L. Fine.*

22–86 SJÖGREN'S (RETICULAR) DYSTROPHY

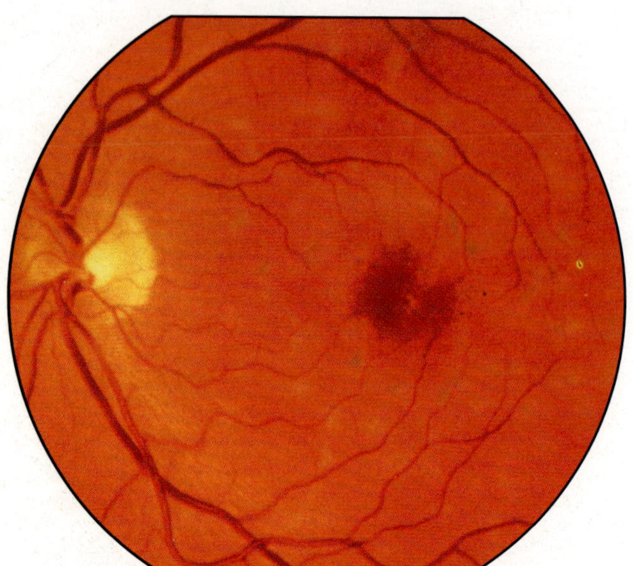

22–87

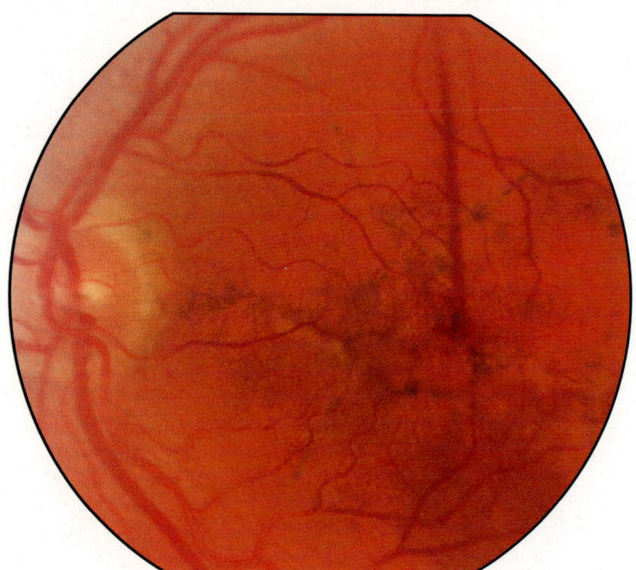

22–88

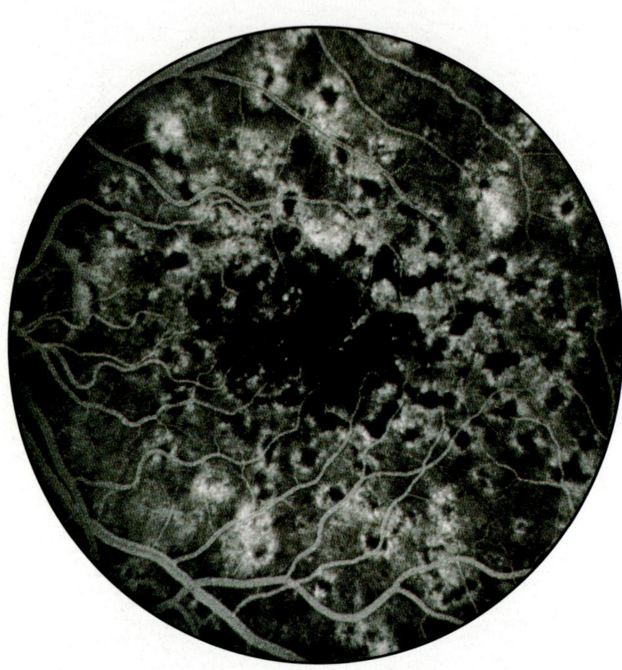

22–86 through 22–88 This rare retinal pigment epithelial dystrophy is a maculopathy with a fishnet or meshed network of pigmentation. It is probably inherited in an autosomal recessive pattern. In the early stages, a pigmentary or atrophic maculopathy is noted. A pigmentary reticular network then forms centrally.

22–87, *From Hsieh, RC, Fine, BS, and Lyons, JS: Pattern dystrophy of the retinal pigment epithelium, Arch Ophthalmol 95:1494, 1977. Courtesy of Drs. Ron Carr and Ken Noble.*

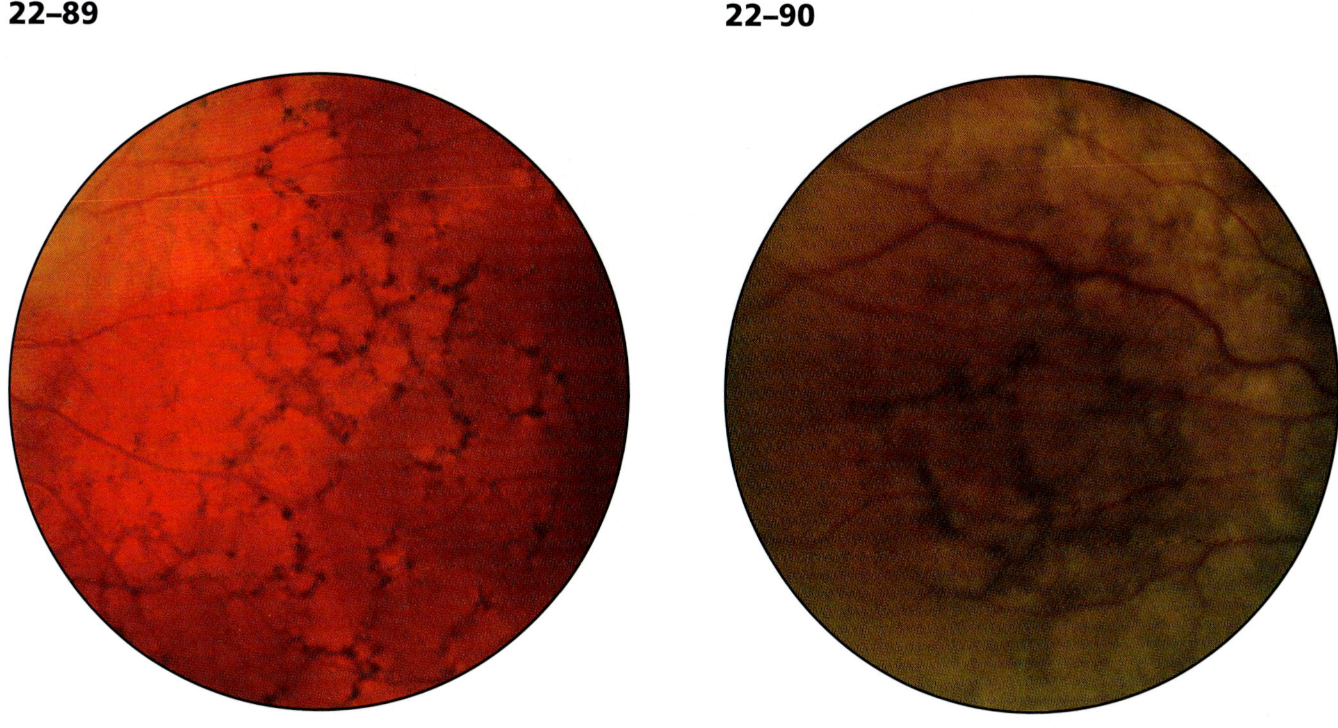

22–89 and 22–90 Later a fishnet-like peripheral pigmentary retinopathy is observed.

22–91 BENIGN CONCENTRIC ANNULAR MACULAR DYSTROPHY

22–92

22–93

22–94

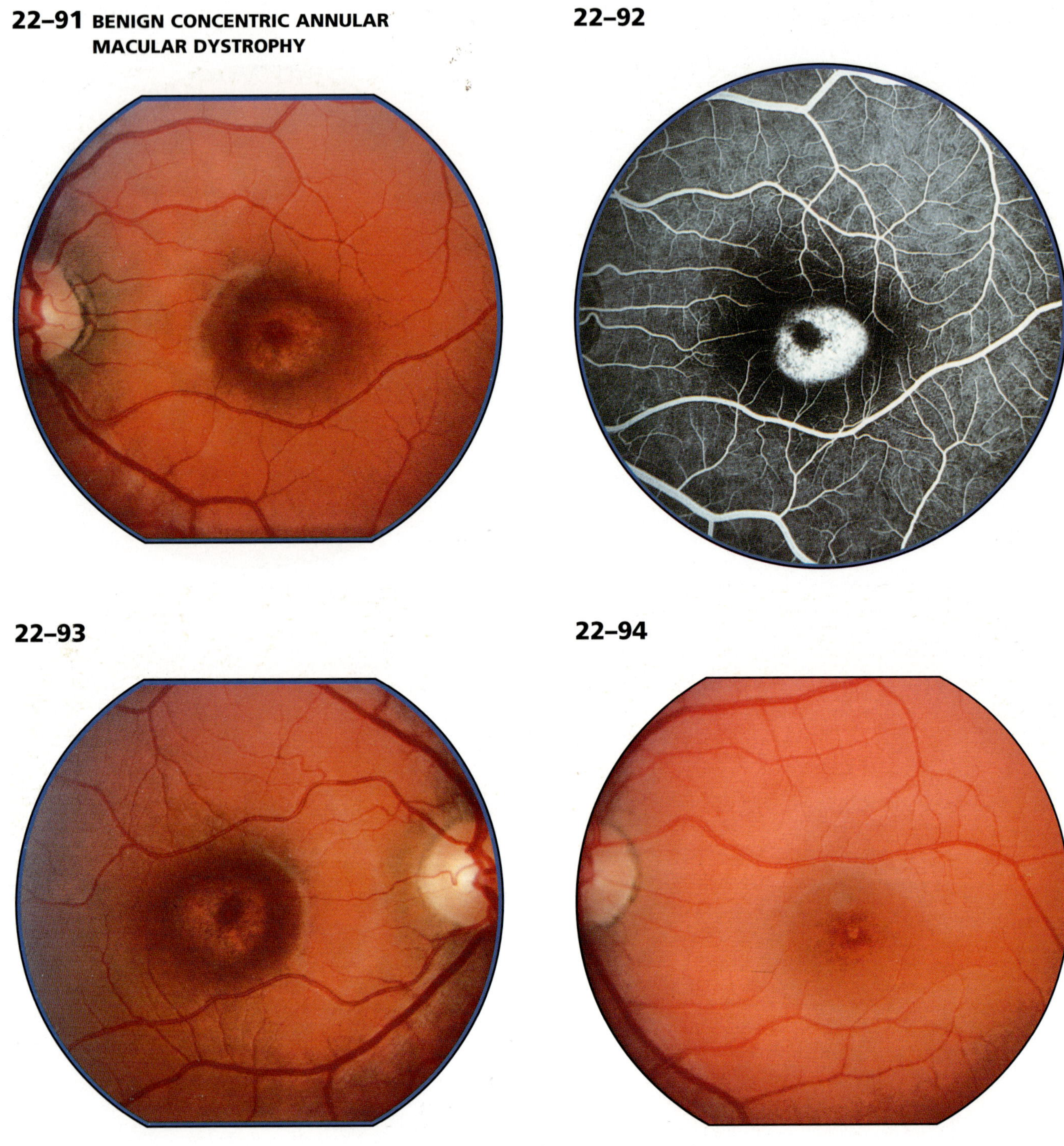

22–91 through 22–93 This autosomal dominant condition consists of a bull's eye maculopathy.

22–94 This patient's sister showed milder macular abnormalities. Initially, it was stated that these patients had a good visual prognosis. However, long-term follow-up of these patients reveals progressive visual acuity loss, macular changes, and peripheral retinal involvement.

***22–91** through **22–94,** Courtesy of Dr. Stuart L. Fine.*

22–95 DOMINANT DRUSEN

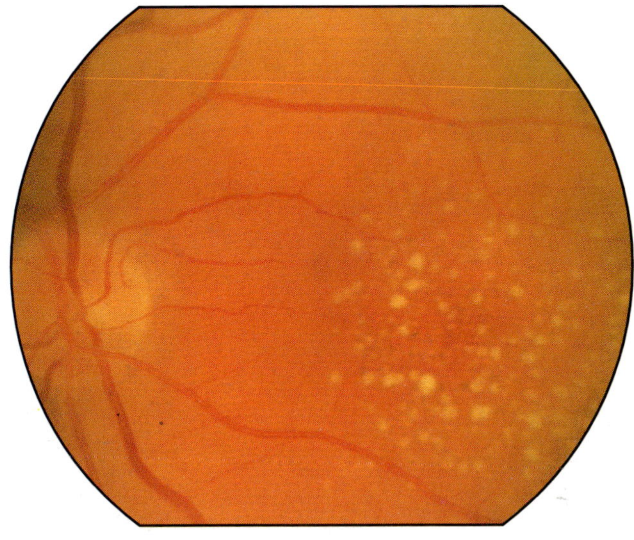

22–96

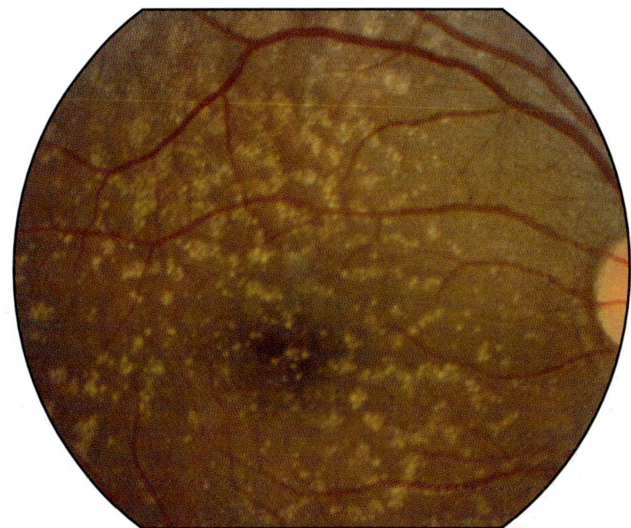

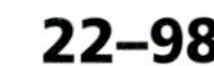

22–97

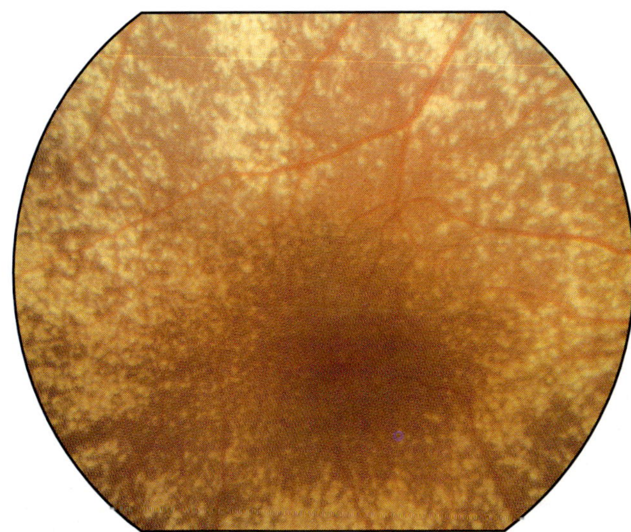

22–98

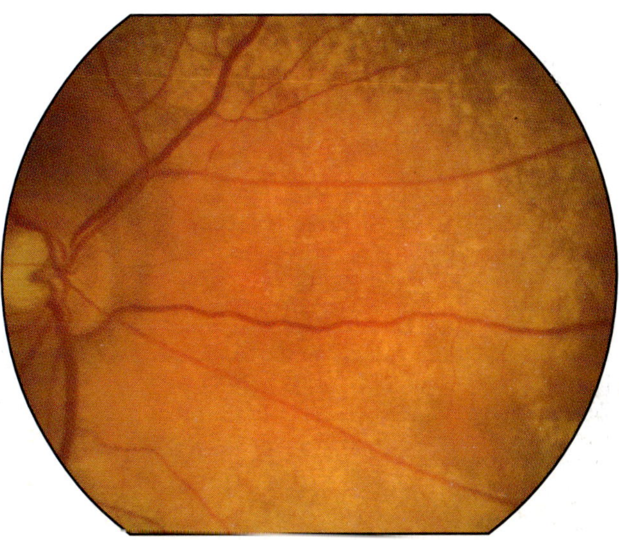

22–95 Dominant drusen is an autosomal dominant disorder, which mimics drusen seen in age-related macular degeneration. This disorder occurs in younger patients. This condition has also been termed Doyne's honeycomb dystrophy. Affected patients may later develop choroidal neovascularization. Dominant drusen may not be a separate disease entity and may simply be an early form of age-related macular degeneration. The fundus appearance and topographic distribution of dominant drusen of Bruch's membrance may vary. In this case, the drusen are confined to the macular region.

22–96 In this patient with dominant drusen, the lesions involve the entire posterior pole.

22–97 Another variation of dominant drusen shows sparing of the macular region.

22–98 The drusen may sometimes be seen only nasal to the disc.

22–95 *through* ***22–98,*** *Courtesy of Drs. Ron Carr and Ken Noble.*

22–99 SORSBY'S PSEUDOINFLAMMATORY MACULAR DYSTROPHY

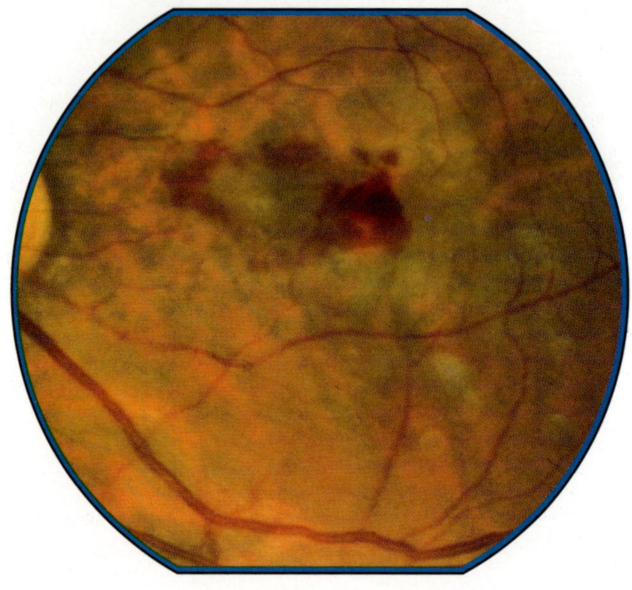

22–100

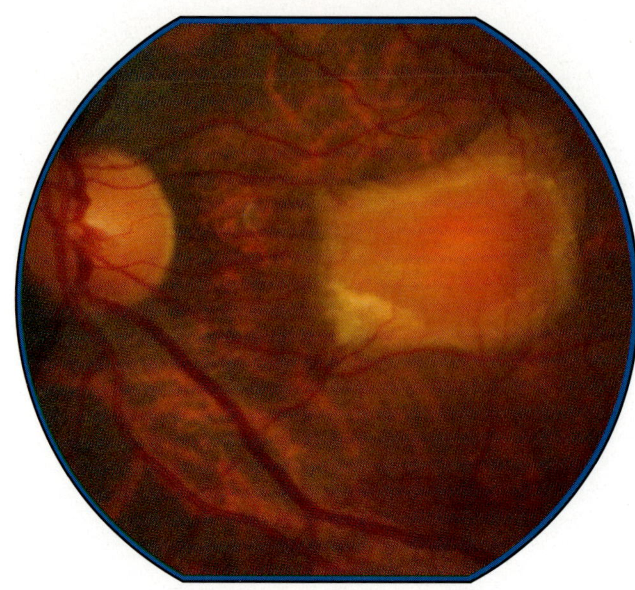

22–101

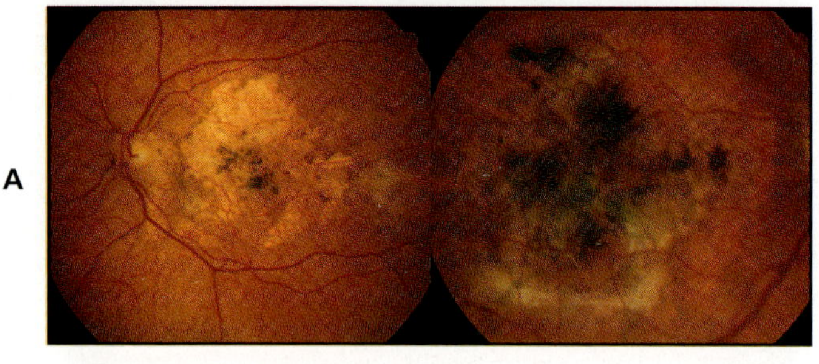

A B

22–99 This rare autosomal dominant macular dystrophy initially shows edema, hemorrhages, and exudation; scarring then occurs. This patient is a 30-year-old man from a family with this disorder. Note the hemorrhagic maculopathy associated with a subretinal neovascular membrane.

22–100 This lesion progressed to a dense glial scar in the macula, as seen in the next photograph.

22–101 This patient (A) with Sorsby's pseudo-inflammatory maculopathy developed choroidal neovascularization in her early forties. She now has an atrophic scar with subretinal fibrosis. The proband (B) developed choroidal neovascularization in her early forties. She ultimately developed widespread fibrovascular changes with hyperpigmentation. None of the family members had soft exudative drusen. No yellow deposits were seen in other family members of this dominant dystrophy.

***22–99** and **22–100,** From Carr, RE, Noble, KG, and Nasaduk, EI: Hereditary hemorrhagic macular dystrophy, Am J Ophthalmol 85:318–328, 1978. **22–101A** and **B,** Courtesy of Dr. A. Peters.*

22–102 FENESTRATED SHEEN MACULAR DYSTROPHY

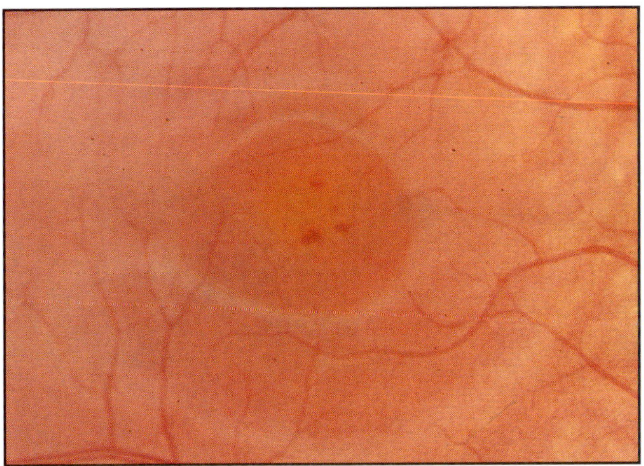

22–103

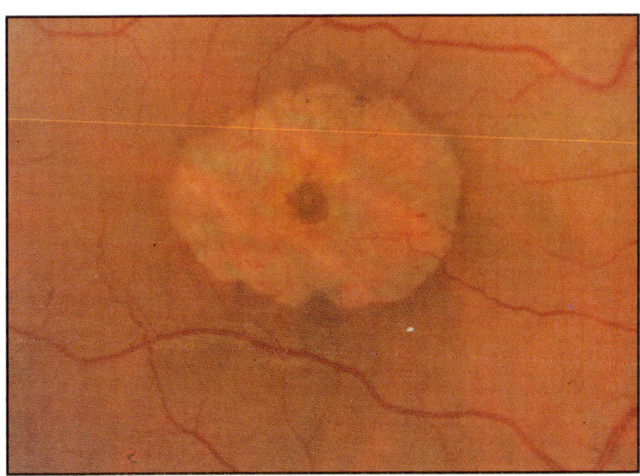

22–104 CENTRAL PIGMENTARY DYSTROPHY

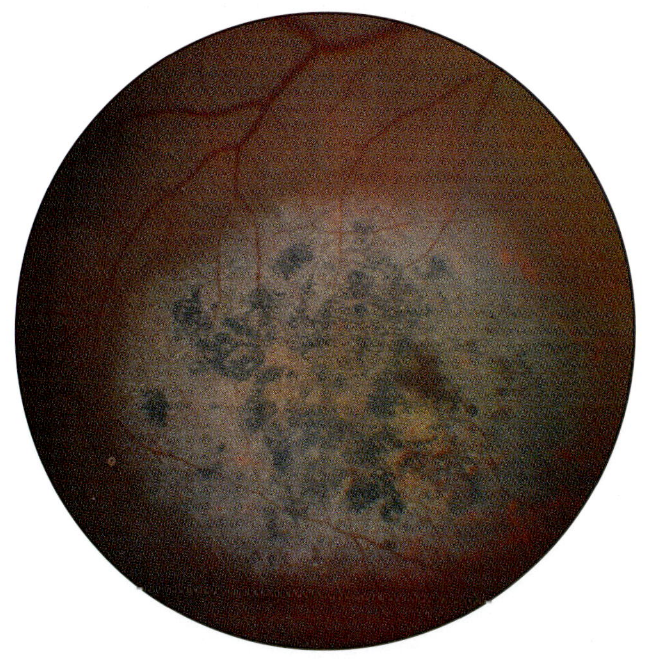

Fenestrated Sheen Macular Dystrophy

Fenestrated sheen macular dystrophy is an autosomal dominant condition, in which a yellowish refractile sheen and red fenestrations can be demonstrated in the macula. Affected patients have a relatively good prognosis.

22–102 The first patient demonstrates the early stage of the condition with several red fenestrations within an abnormal yellowish macular sheen.

22–103 The second patient exhibits the later stage of the disease with a complete ring of retinal pigment epithelium hypopigmentation surrounding a central island of preserved retinal pigment epithelium.

Central Pigmentary Dystrophy

22–104 The typical bone-spicule pigmentation and grayish metallic sheen, which is confined to the posterior pole, are seen in this patient with central pigmentary dystrophy. This dystrophy is extremely rare.

22–102 *and* ***22–103,*** *From O'Donnell, FE, and Welch, RB: Fenestrated sheen macular dystrophy, Arch Ophthalmol 97:1292–1296, 1979. Courtesy of Drs. Ron Carr and Ken Noble.* ***22–104,*** *Courtesy of Drs. Ron Carr and Ken Noble.*

22–105 NORTH CAROLINA MACULAR DYSTROPHY

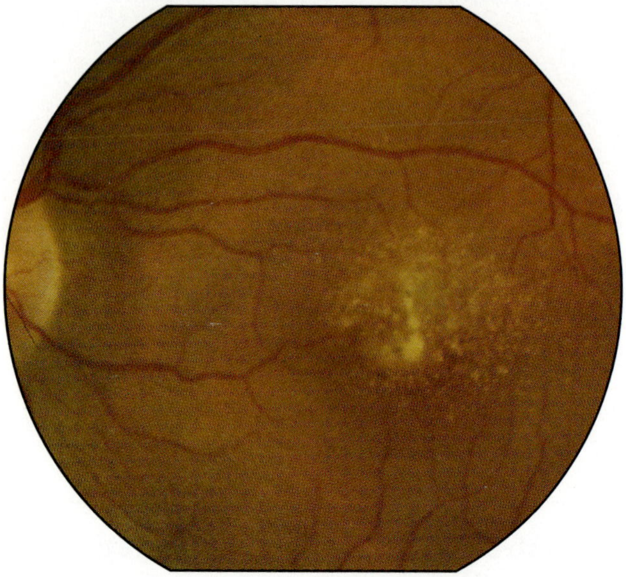

22–106

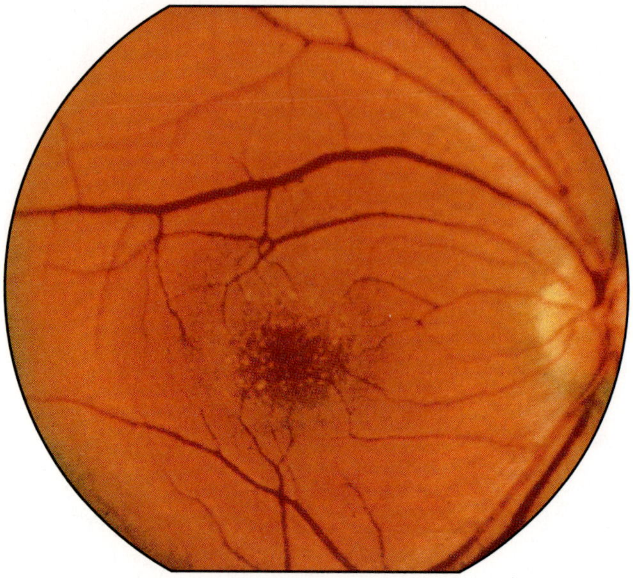

22–107

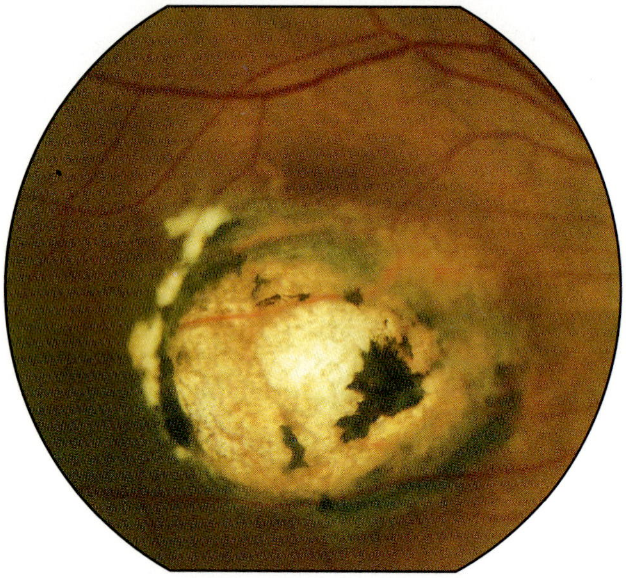

22–108

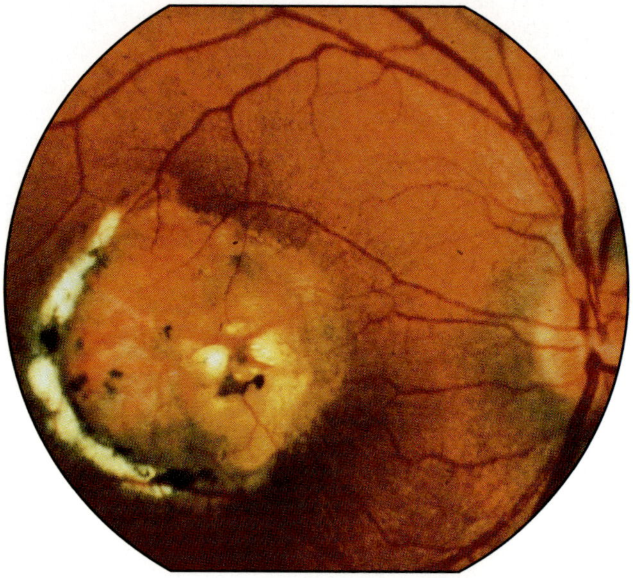

22–105 and 22–106 This dominantly inherited macular dystrophy was reported in a large pedigree from western North Carolina. Affected patients have a rapidly progressive loss of visual acuity. Loss of central vision occurs in the first few years of life and usually reaches its most severe level during the teenage years. Early in the dystrophy, drusen-like lesions with a pigmentary retinopathy are noted.

22–107 and 22–108 Progressive atrophy involving the choroid, retinal pigment epithelium, and retina may occur. These areas may resemble a staphyloma. Choroidal neovascularization has been demonstrated in such patients.

22–105 *through* ***22–108,*** *Courtesy of Dr. Kent Small.*

Suggested Readings

Blodi, FC: The pathology of central tapeto–retinal dystrophy (hereditary macular degenerations), Trans Am Acad Ophthalmol Otolaryngol 70:1047, 1966

Carr, RF: Central areolar choroidal dystrophy, Arch Ophthalmol 73:32, 1965

de Jong, PTVM, and Delleman, JW: Pigment epithelial pattern dystrophy, Arch Ophthalmol 100:1416, 1982

Deutman, AF: The hereditary dystrophies of the posterior pole of the eye, Assen, Netherlands, 1971, Van Gorcum

Frangieh, GT, Green, WR, and Fine, SL: A histopathologic study of Best's macular dystrophy, Arch Ophthalmol 100:1115, 1982

Krill, AE, and Archer, D: Classification of the choroidal atrophies, Am J Ophthalmol 72:562, 1971

Krill, AE, Deutman, AF, and Fishman, M: The cone degenerations, Doc Ophthalmol 35:1, 1973

Noble, KG, Carr, RE, and Siegel, EM: Fluorescein angiography of the hereditary choroidal dystrophies, Br J Ophthalmol 61:43, 1977

Sorsby, A, and Crick, RP: Central areolar choroidal sclerosis, Br J Ophthalmol 37:129, 1953

Weingeist, TA, Kobrin, JL, and Watzke, RC: Histopathology of Best's macular dystrophy, Arch Ophthalmol 100:1108, 1982

Yanoff, M, Rahn, EK, and Zimmerman, LE: Histopathology of juvenile retinoschisis, Arch Ophthalmol 79:49, 1968

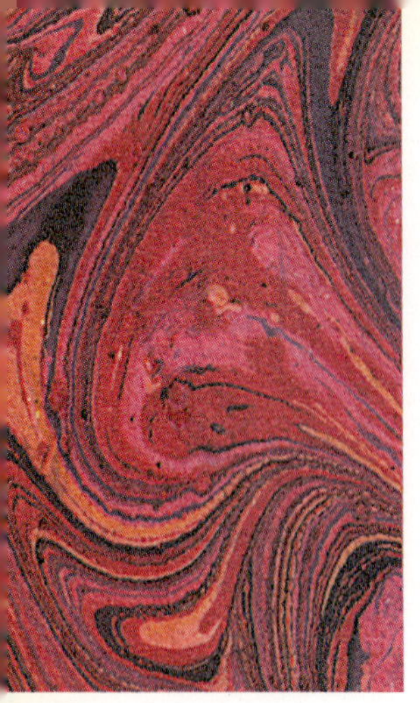

Chapter 23

Chorioretinal Folds

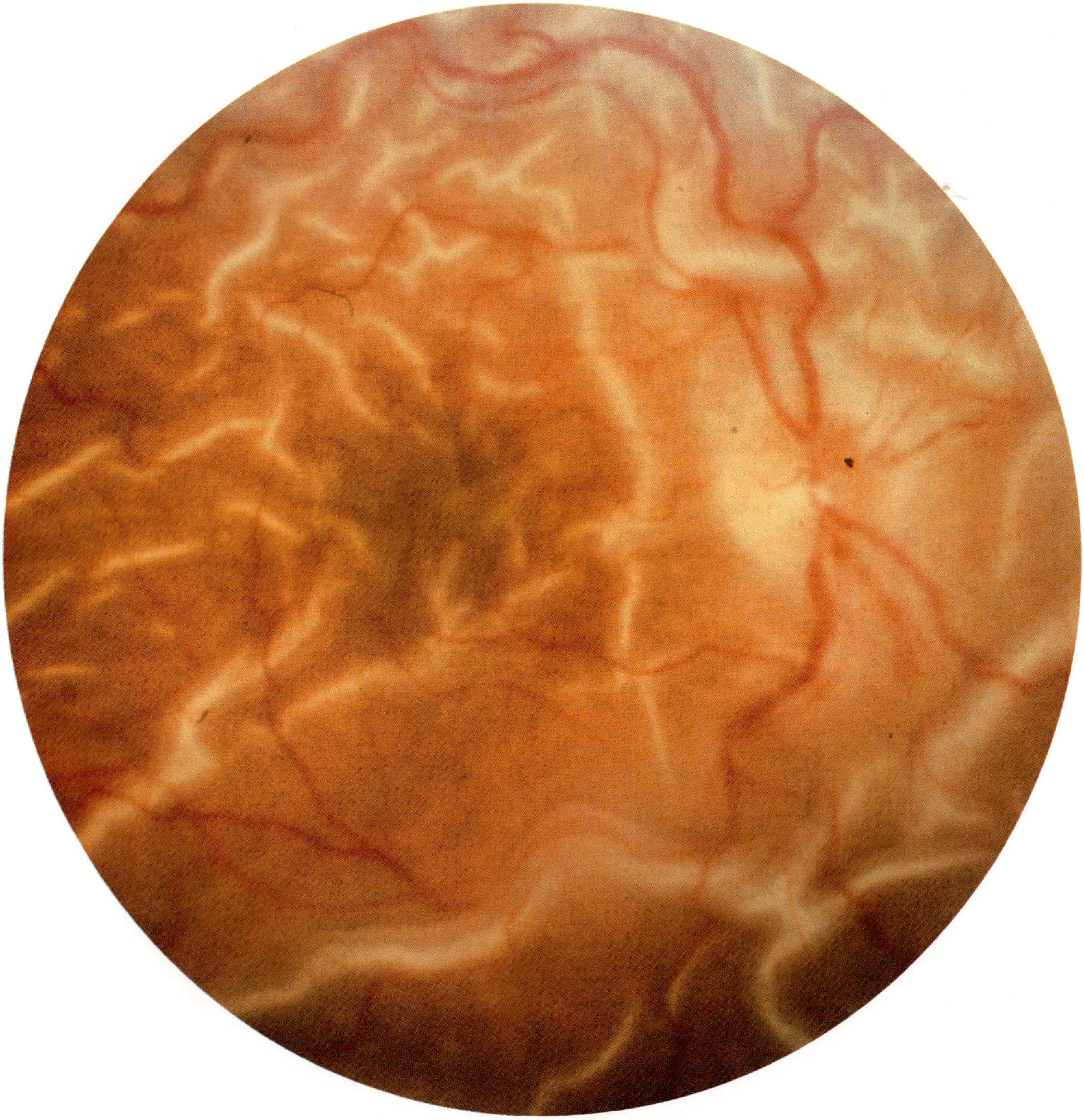

Chorioretinal folds can be seen associated with many conditions. These conditions include hyperopia, age-related macular degeneration, posterior scleritis, optic nerve head diseases, postsurgical conditions, retrobulbar tumors, hypotony, and idiopathic.

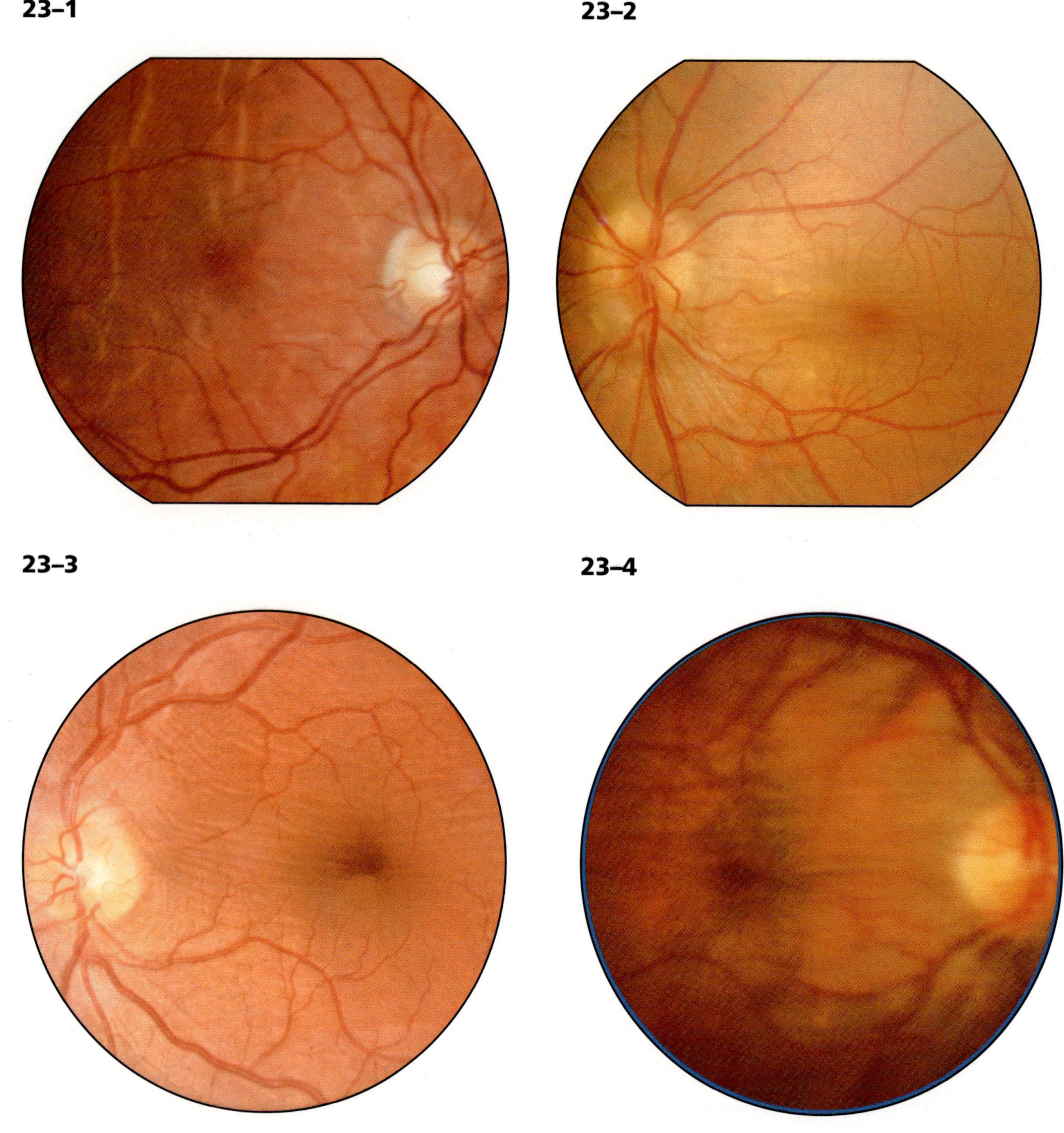

23–1 through 23–6 Chorioretinal folds may be associated with various conditions including retrobulbar or choroidal tumors (23–1, 23–2, and 23–3), hypotony (23–4, and 23–5), posterior scleritis, status postscleral buckling surgery, papilledema, pseudopapilledema, ischemic optic neuropathy, or age-related macular degeneration (23–6). Age-related macular degeneration is a common cause of chorioretinal folds, especially bilateral cases. The chorioretinal folds may also be vertical (23–1). Note the alternating black and white lines on the fluorescein study, which are characteristic of folds (23–5).

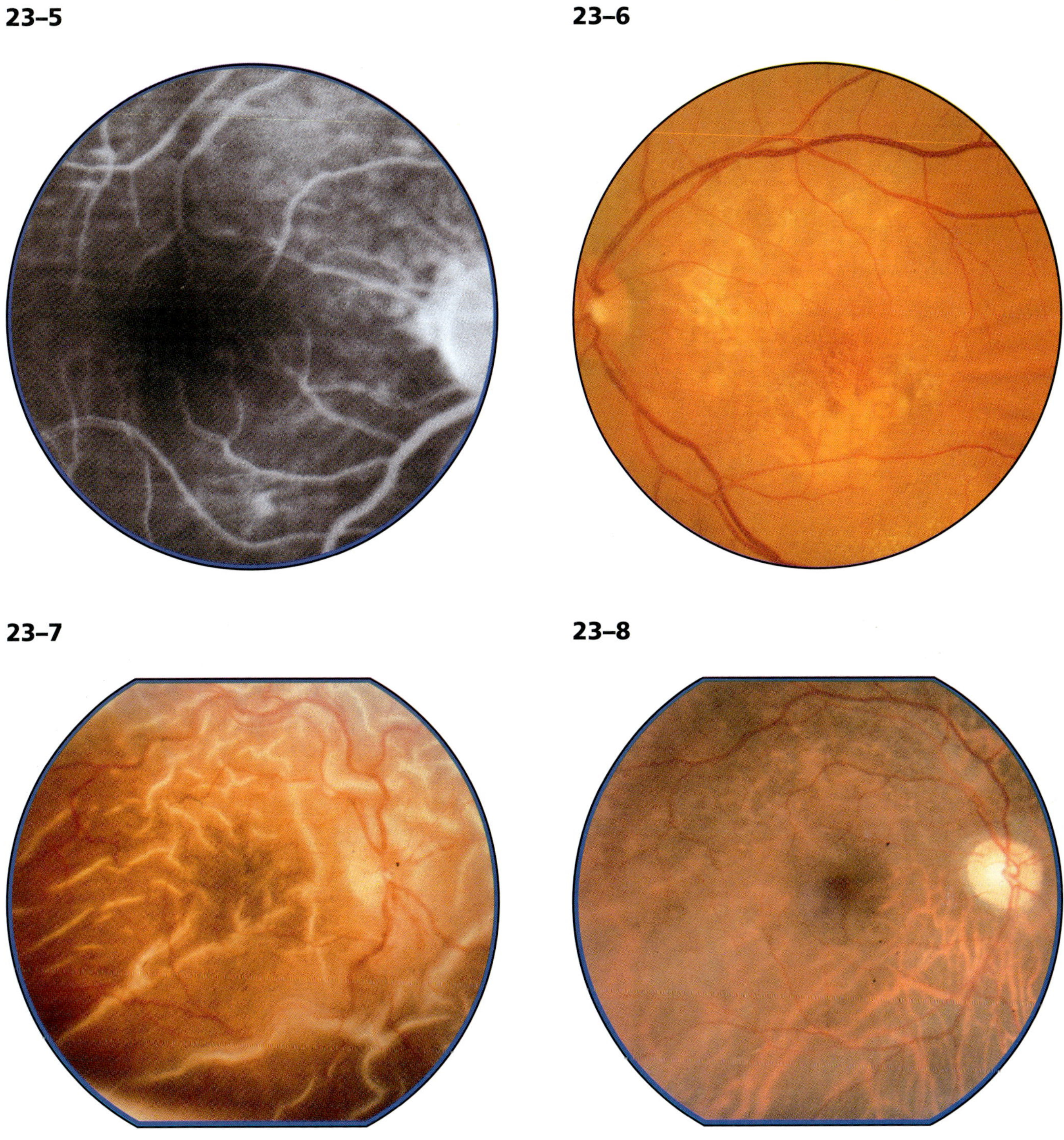

23–7 and 27–8 This patient had a trabeculectomy with mitomycin performed. The patient had a visual acuity of 20/400 and intraocular pressure of 2 mm of Mercury. Chorioretinal folds were noted.

***23–7** and **27–8,** Courtesy of Dr. Eric Suan.*

Suggested Readings

Bird, AC, and Sanders, MD: Choroidal folds in association with papilloedema, Br J Ophthalmol 57:89, 1973

Cangemi, FE, Trempe, CL, and Walsh, JB: Choroidal folds, Am J Ophthalmol 86:380, 1978

Friberg, TR, and Grove, AS, Jr: Subretinal neovascularization and choroidal folds, Ann Ophthalmol 12:245, 1980

Friberg, TR, and Grove, AS, Jr: Choroidal folds and refractive errors associated with orbital tumors: an analysis, Arch Ophthalmol 101:598, 1983

Gass, JDM: Hypotony maculopathy. In Bellows, JC, editor: Contemporary ophthalmology, honoring Sir Stewart Duke-Elder, Baltimore, 1972, Williams & Wilkins, p 343

Hyvarinen, L, and Walsh, FB: Benign chorioretinal folds, Am J Ophthalmol 70:14, 1970

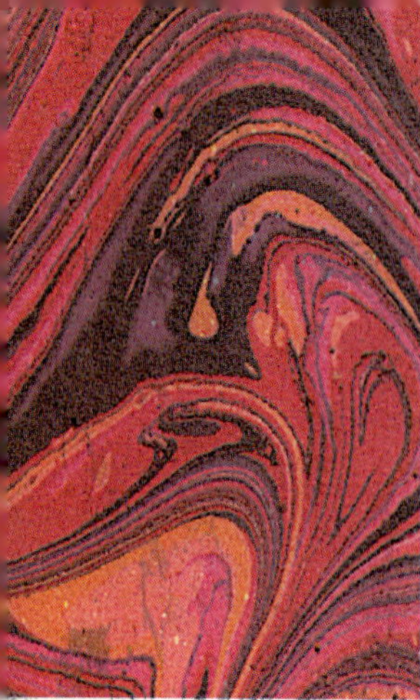

Chapter 24

Angioid Streaks

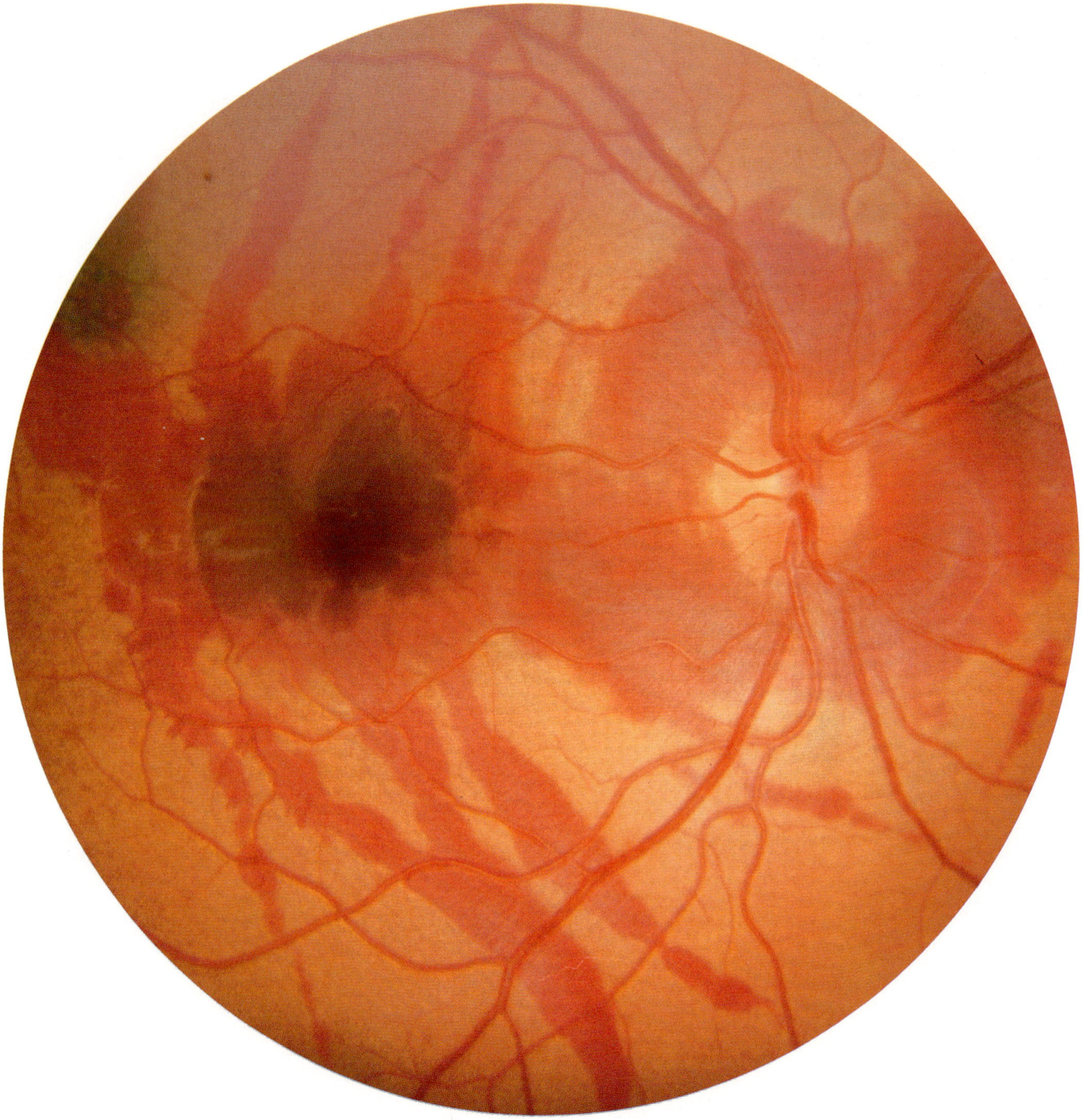

Angioid streaks are idiopathic in 50% of cases. The most commonly associated systemic finding is pseudoxanthoma elasticum. Other associated conditions include Paget's disease of bone, sickle cell anemia, and Ehlers-Danlos syndrome. These streaks, which are breaks in Bruch's membrane, may lead to choroidal neovascularization with subsequent scarring.

24–1 ANGIOID STREAKS AND CRYSTALLINE DEPOSITS 24–2

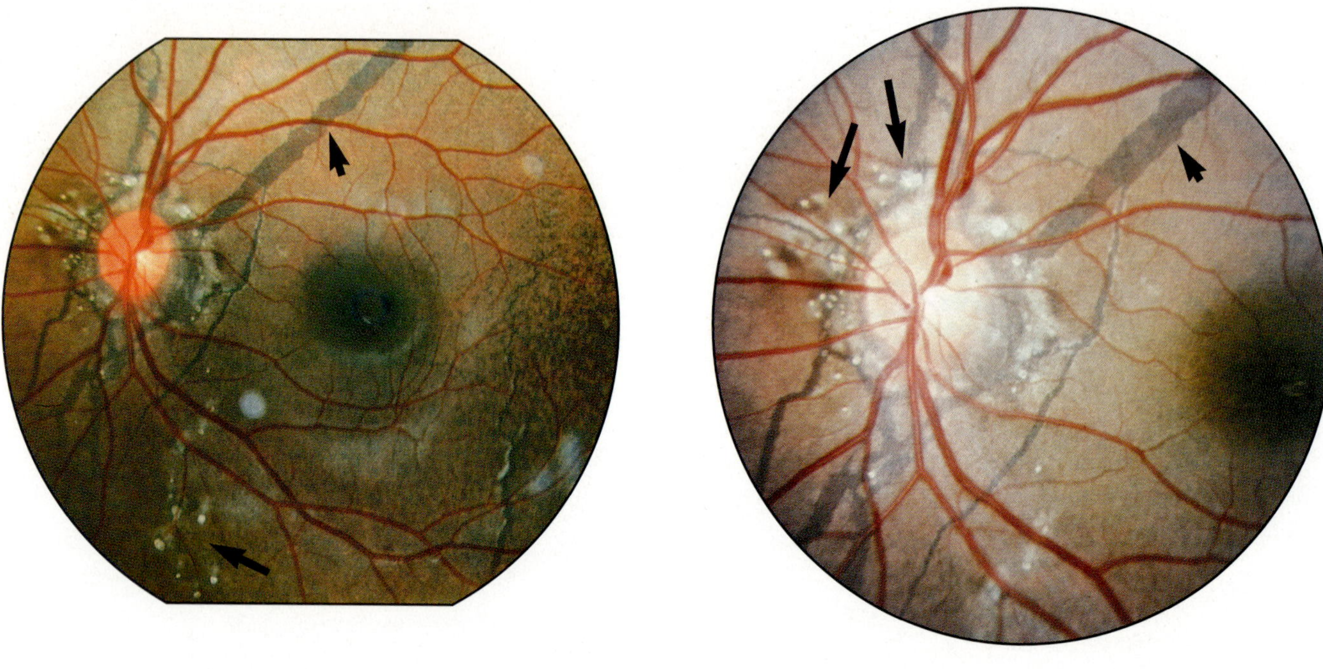

24–1 and 24–2 Angioid streaks appear as reddish-brown streaks, often in the peripapillary region *(arrowheads)*. The streaks may be red or darker brown. In some cases, subretinal crystalline deposits are noted *(arrows)*. A peau d'orange pigmentary change is also noted temporally.

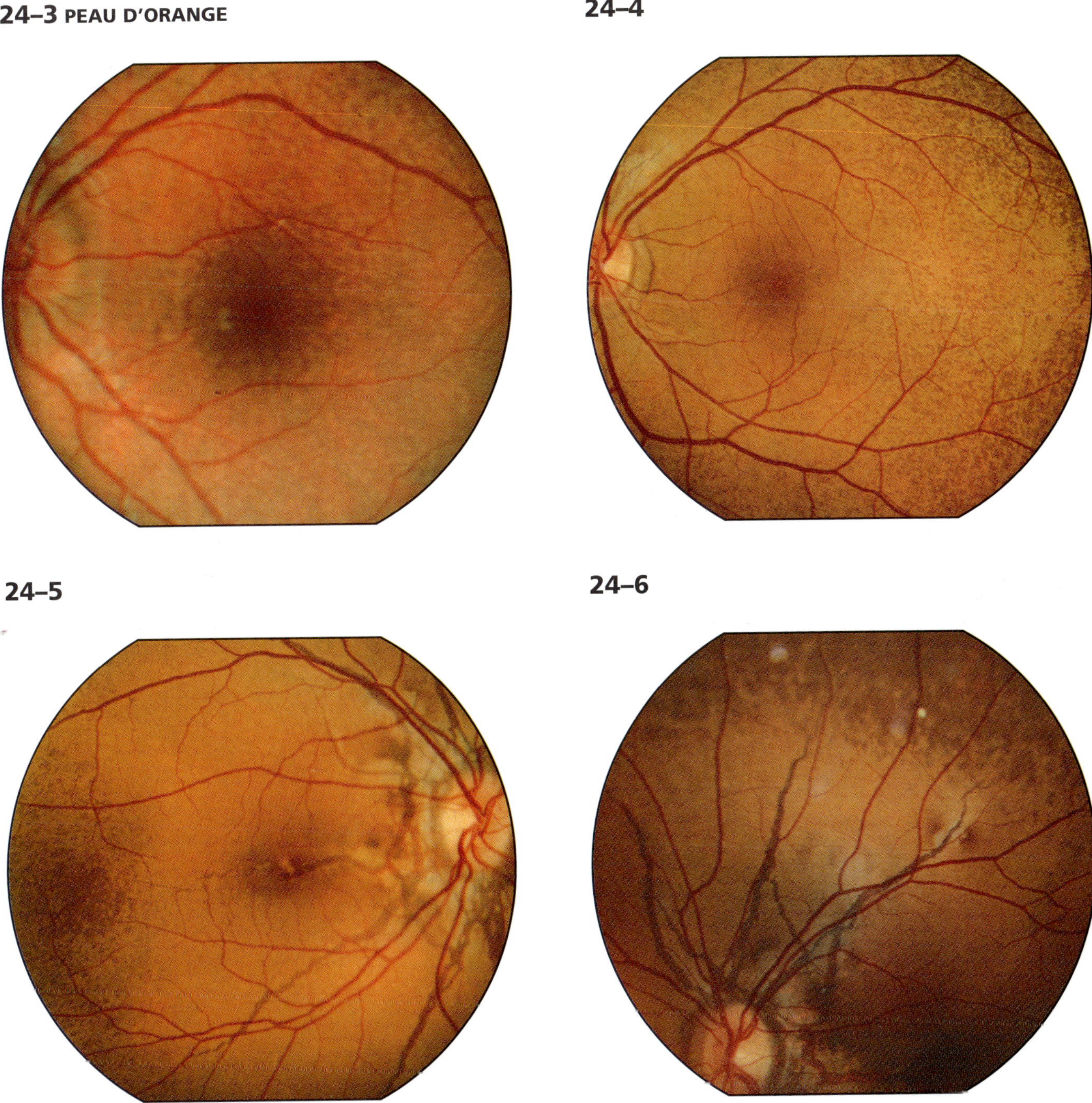

24–3 through 24–6 Peau d'orange (orange skin) or yellow mottling at the retinal pigment epithelial level first starts in the macular region (24–3) and then as atrophy ensues, the peau d'orange is noted progressively more temporally (24–4, 24–5, and 24–6). Note how progressive atrophy causes the peau d'orange to disappear with age. The lesion disappears in the macular region and with aging is only seen further anteriorly over time (24–3 through 24–6). Angioid streaks can traverse the macular region, often without a decrease in visual acuity (24–5). Choroidal neovascularization with subsequent disciform scarring may occur in these eyes, especially after age 50.

24–3, *Courtesy of Dr. Wayne Fuchs.*

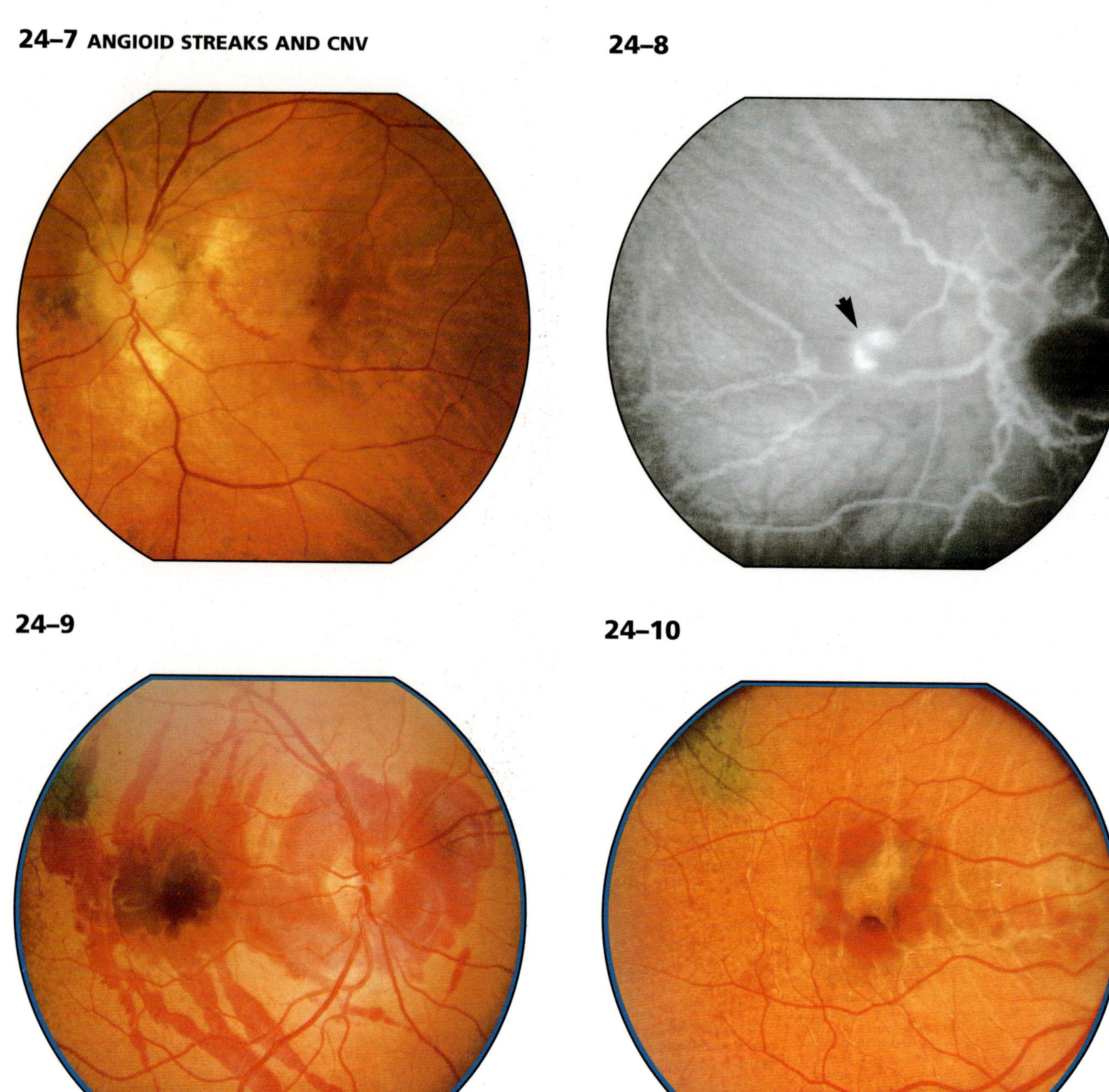

24–7 Choroidal neovascularization with subretinal hemorrhage is demonstrated in this case with angioid streaks secondary to Paget's disease.

24–8 Indocyanine-green angiography of another case may reveal multiple angioid streaks as well as active choroidal neovascularization *(arrowhead)*.

24–9 and 24–10 This patient presented with subretinal hemorrhage in the macular region and around the optic nerve. The blood spontaneously resolved and multiple angioid streaks could be noted. Note that a peau d'orange can be seen temporal to the macula but that no angioid streaks could initially be seen. The peau d'orange lesions in this patient with angioid streaks are not seen in areas of atrophy.

24–11

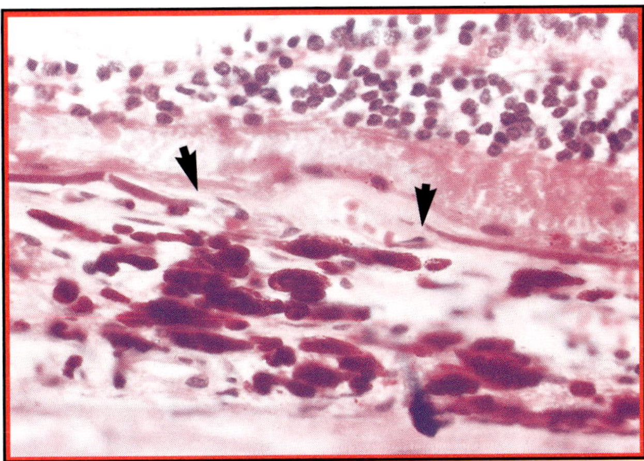

24–11A

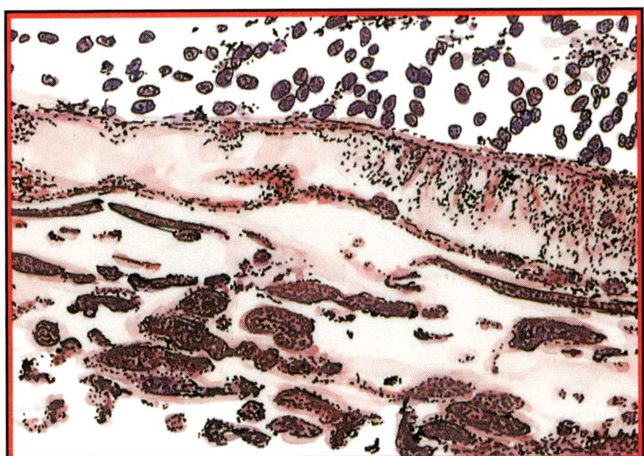

24–12

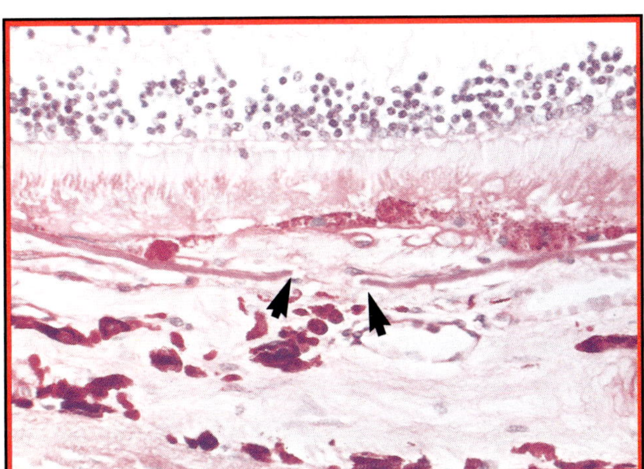

24–13

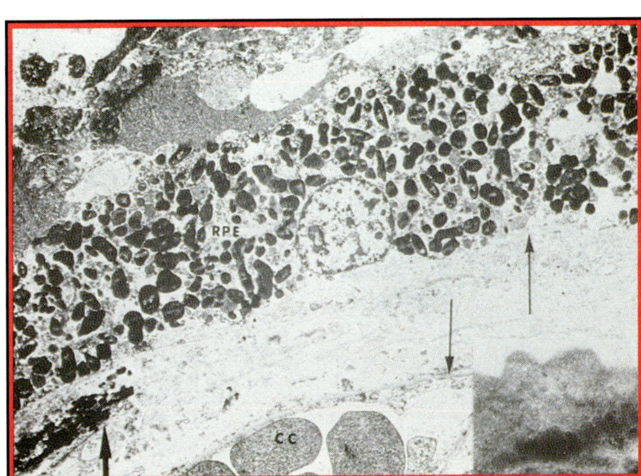

24–11, 24–11A, and 24–12 Fibrovascular tissue from the choroid extends through a defect in Bruch's membrane and between the retinal pigment epithelium and Bruch's membrane to either side of the angioid streak in these cases. Note the discontinuities in Bruch's membrane, which constitutes the streak *(arrowheads)*. Hypertrophy of the retinal pigment epithelium is present in 24–12.

24–13 Electron microscopy of an angioid streak from a patient with pseudoxanthoma elasticum shows calcium deposits in the elastic layer of Bruch's membrane *(large arrow and inset)*. The outer segments are visible. The retinal pigment epithelium and its basement membrane, as well as the basement membrane of the choriocapillaris, are intact.

***24–11, 24–12,** and **24–13,** From Dreyer, R, and Green, WR: Pathology of angioid streaks, Trans Penn Acad Ophthalmol Otolaryngol 31:158–167, 1978.*

24–14 DISCIFORM SCARRING

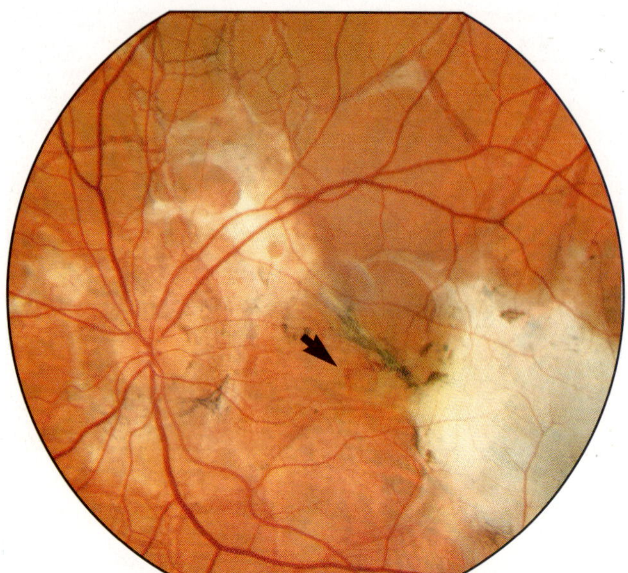

24–15

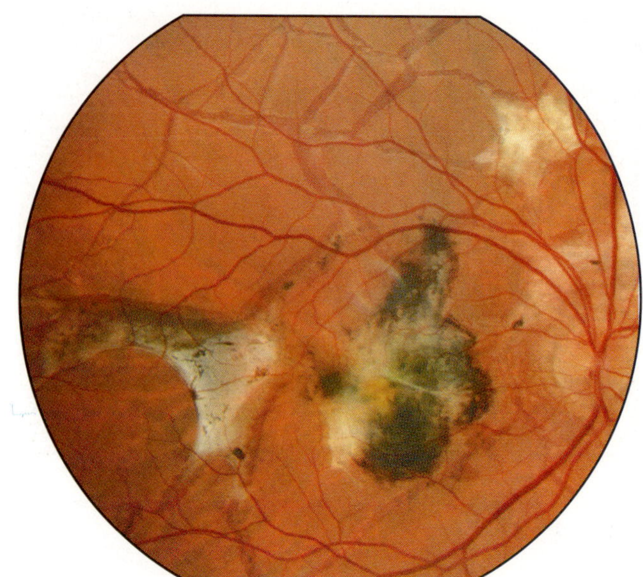

24–16 OPTIC DISC DRUSEN

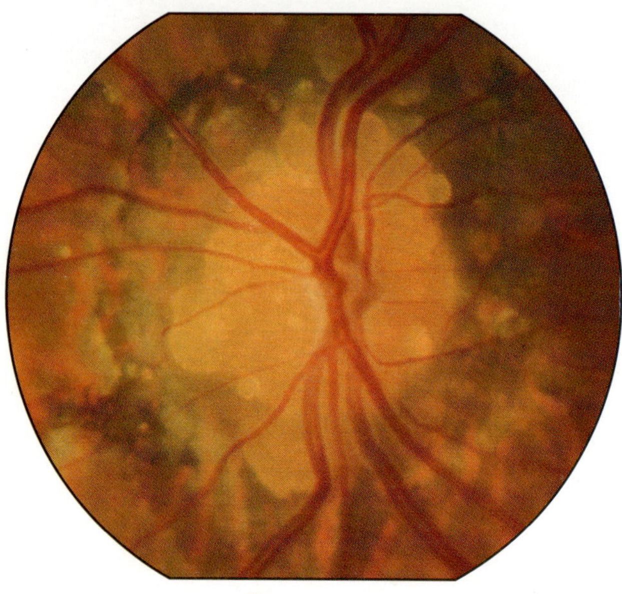

24–14 Disciform scarring may occur in eyes that develop choroidal neovascularization. This patient with multiple angioid streaks shows extensive scarring from previous choroidal neovascularization. Note that the scarring is especially fibrotic inferotemporally. In addition, a small area of active choroidal neovascularization with subretinal hemorrhage is present inferior to an island of fibrosis that connects the two larger areas of scarring *(arrowhead)*.

24–15 Another patient with angioid streaks and pseudoxanthoma elasticum developed disciform scarring.

24–16 Optic nerve head drusen may be an associated finding in patients with angioid streaks.

24–17 SYSTEMIC FINDINGS

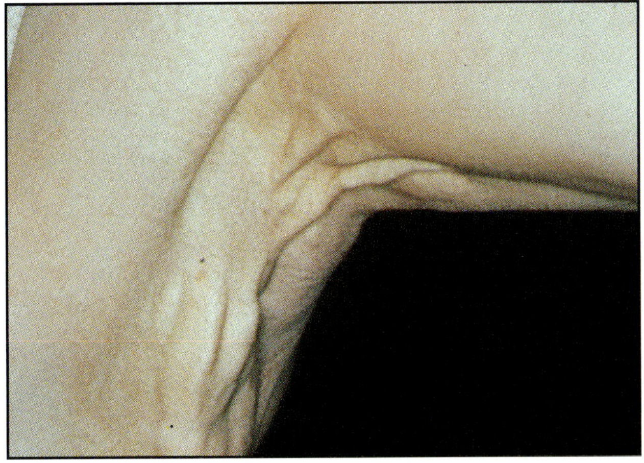

24–18

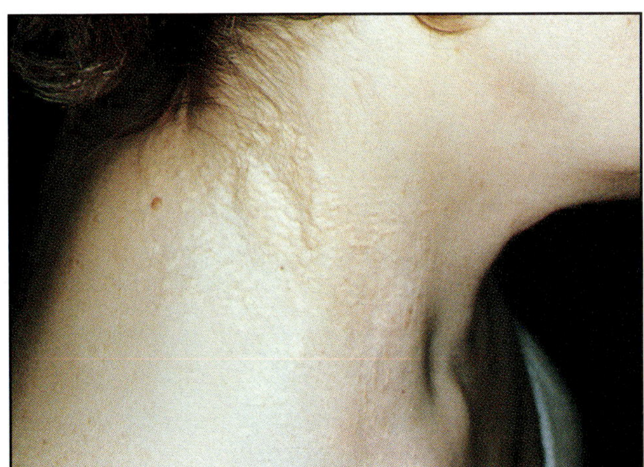

24–19

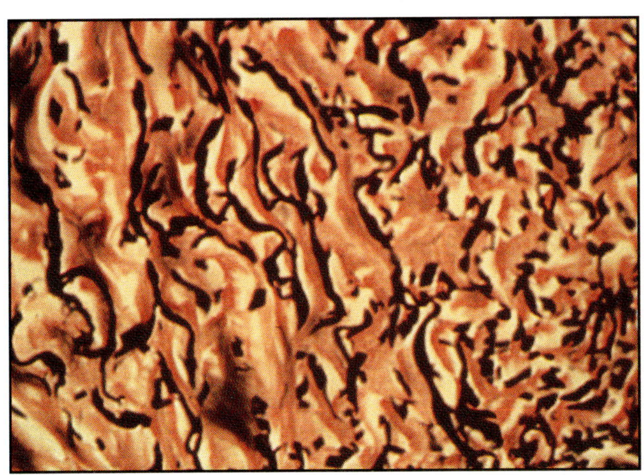

24–17 and 24–18 The characteristic systemic findings of pseudoxanthoma elasticum include skin changes (plucked chicken–like appearance). Gastrointestinal or cardiac abnormalities may also be associated with this condition.

24–19 Calcification of an increased number of enlarged elastic fibers is present in a skin biopsy.

***24–17** and **24–18,** Courtesy and copyright Dr. Mark Lebwohl.*

Suggested Readings

Clarkson, JG, and Altman, RD: Angioid streaks, Surv Ophthalmol 26:235, 1982

Connor, PJ, Jr, Juergens, JL, Perry, HO, et al: Pseudoxanthoma elasticum and angioid streaks: a review of 106 cases, Am J Med 30:537, 1961

Gass, JDM, and Clarkson, JG: Angioid streaks and disciform macular detachment in Paget's disease (osteitis deformans), Am J Ophthalmol 75:576, 1973

Green, WR, Friedman-Kien, A, and Banfield, WG: Angioid streaks in Ehlers-Danlos syndrome, Arch Ophthalmol 76:197, 1966

Nagpal, KC, Asdourian, G, Goldbaum, M, et al: Angioid streaks and sickle haemoglobinopathies, Br J Ophthalmol 60:31, 1976

Singerman, LJ, and Hatem, G: Laser treatment of choroidal neovascular membranes in angioid streaks, Retina 1:75, 1981

Woodcock, CW: Pseudoxanthoma elasticum, angioid streaks of retina and osteitis deformans, Arch Dermatol Syph 65:623, 1952

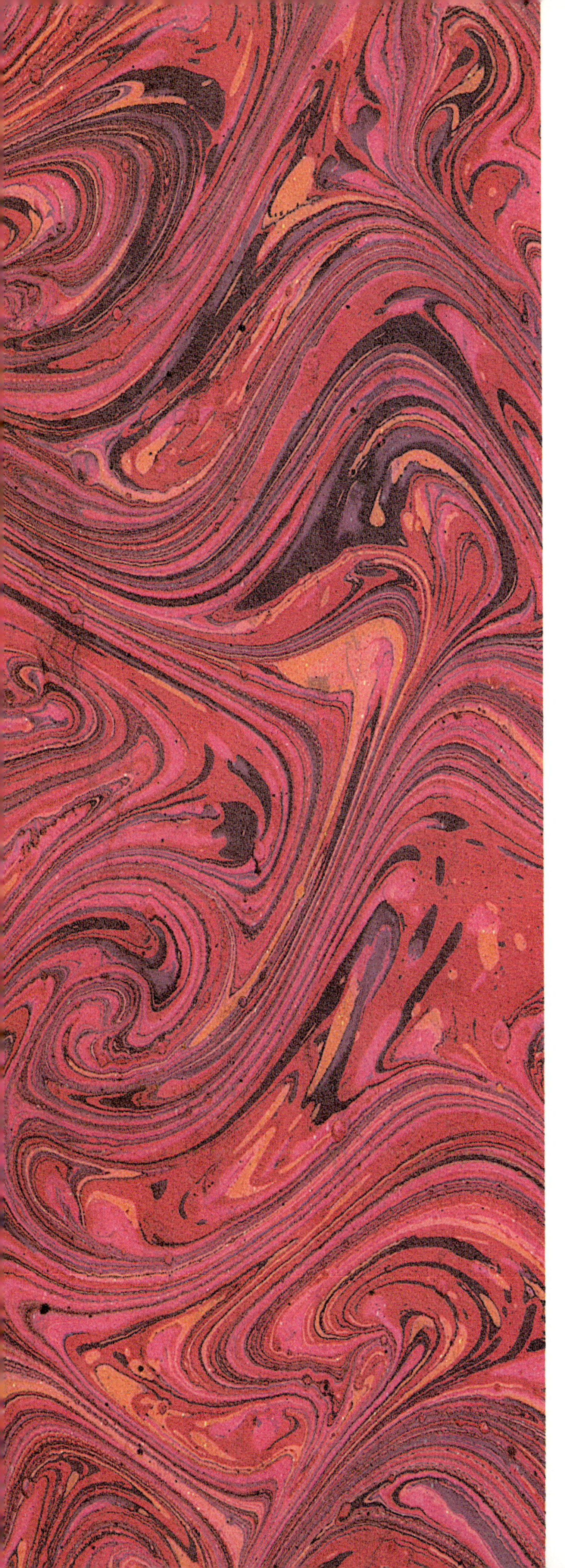

Part VII

Retinal Vascular Diseases

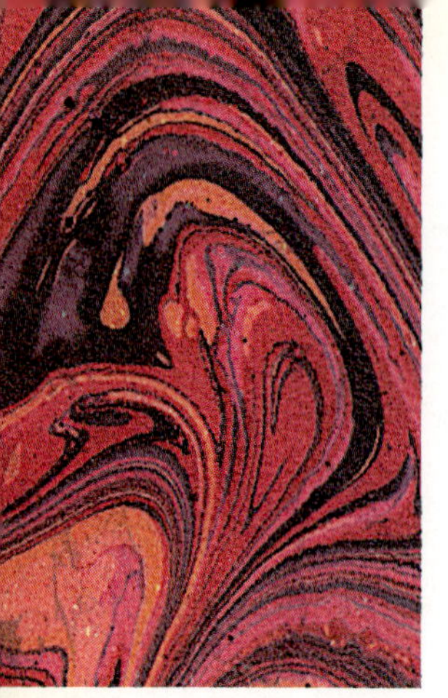

Chapter 25

Diabetic Retinopathy

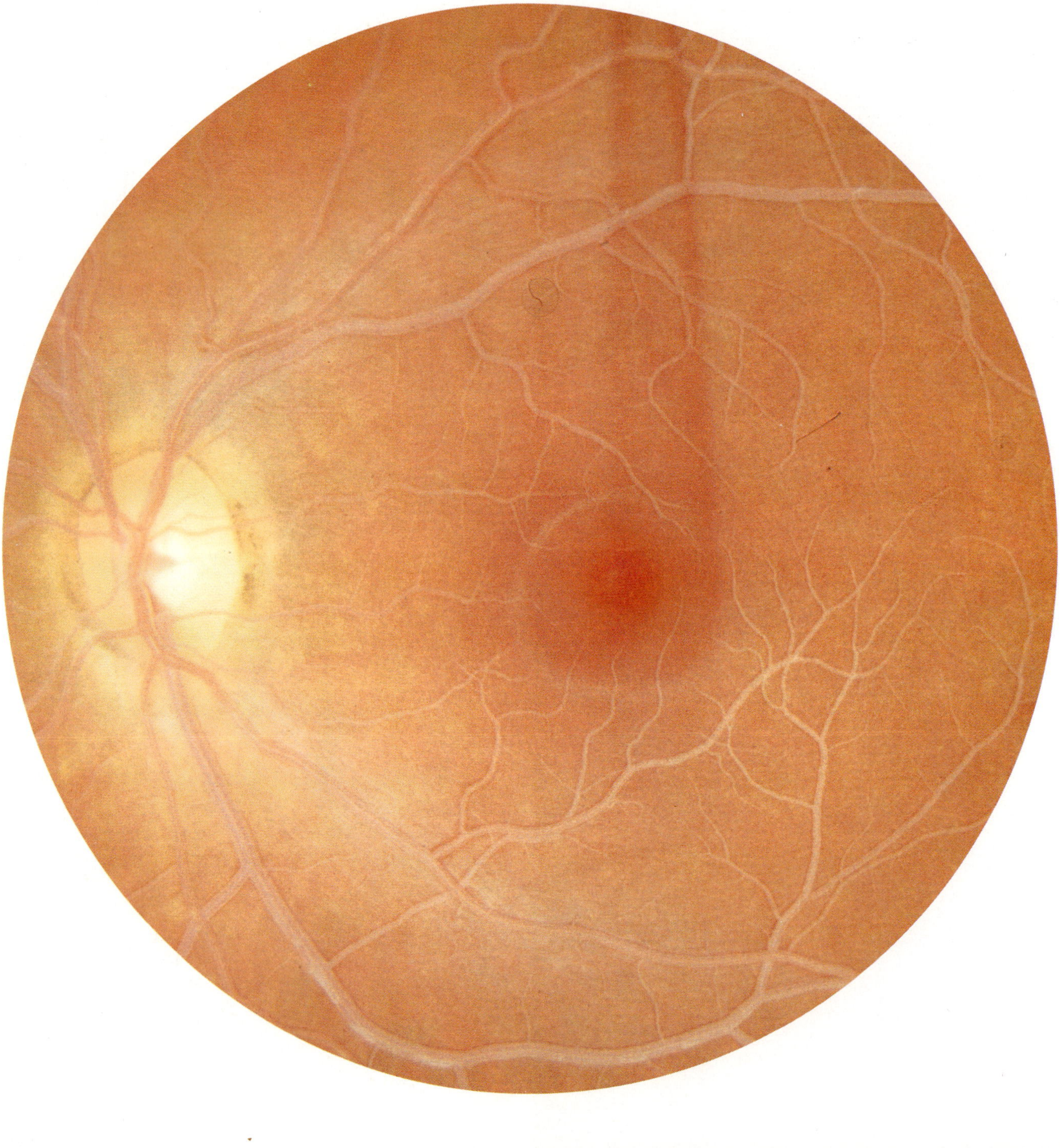

Nonproliferative diabetic retinopathy findings include intraretinal hemorrhages, microaneurysms, cotton-wool spots, macular edema, venous tortuosity and beading, and intraretinal microvascular abnormalities (IRMA). Proliferative diabetic retinopathy consists of neovascularization at the disc, neovascularization elsewhere, rubeosis irides, vitreous hemorrhage, and rhegmatogenous and/or tractional retinal detachment.

The most frequent cause of vision loss among patients with diabetic retinopathy is macular edema. The Early Treatment Diabetic Retinopathy Study has shown the beneficial role of laser photocoagulation for patients with clinically significant diabetic macular edema. Laser photocoagulation is also beneficial for patients with high-risk proliferative diabetic retinopathy. A commonly overlooked reason for decreased visual acuity in a diabetic is macular ischemia, which leads to an enlarged capillary-free zone.

25–1 NONPROLIFERATIVE DIABETIC RETINOPATHY

25–1A

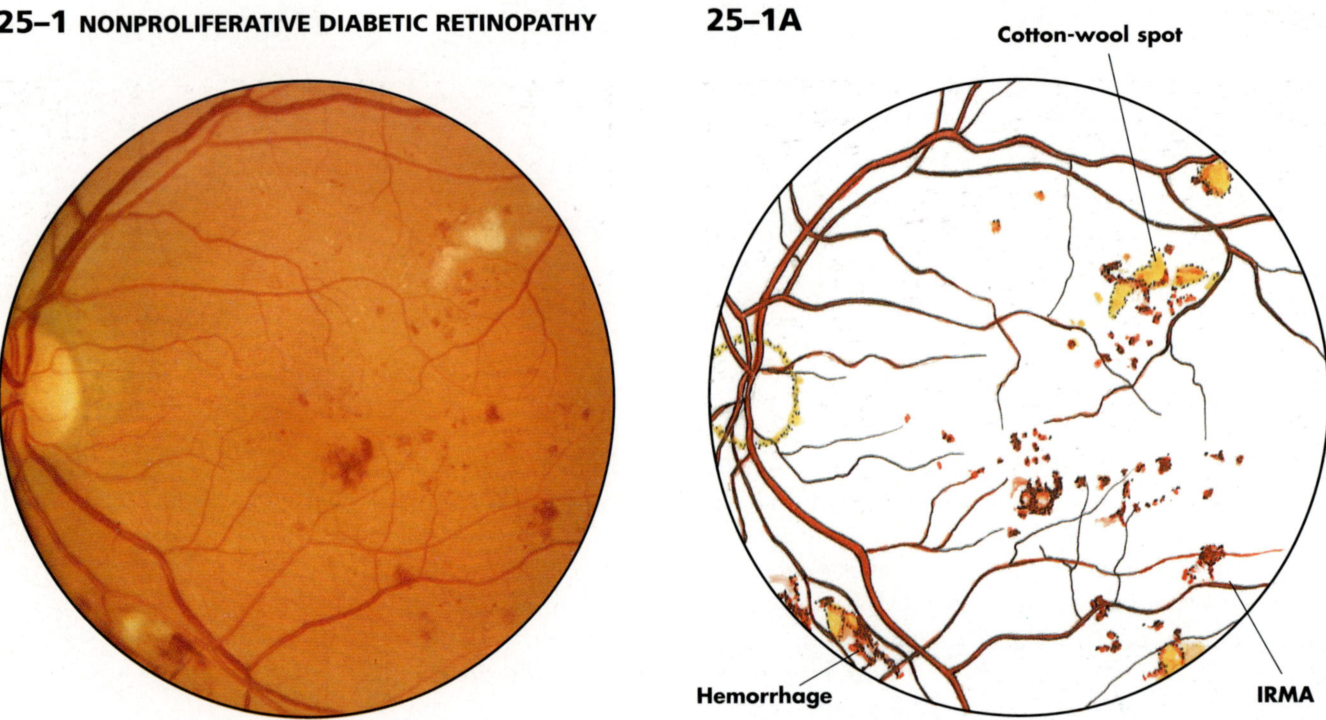

25–1 and 25–1A This patient has nonproliferative diabetic retinopathy with flame-shaped and dot-blot hemorrhages, cotton-wool spots, and microaneurysms. The patient also has intraretinal microvascular abnormalities (IRMA). This case represents moderate nonproliferative diabetic retinopathy.

25–1, *Courtesy of Drs. George Blankenship and Everett Ai and the Diabetes 2000 Program.*

25–2

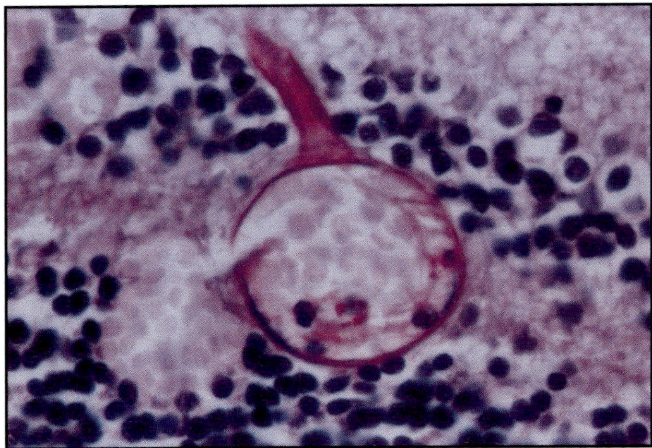

25–3

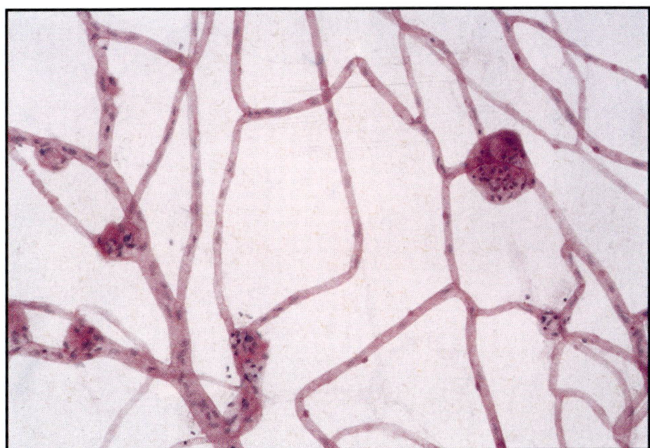

25–4

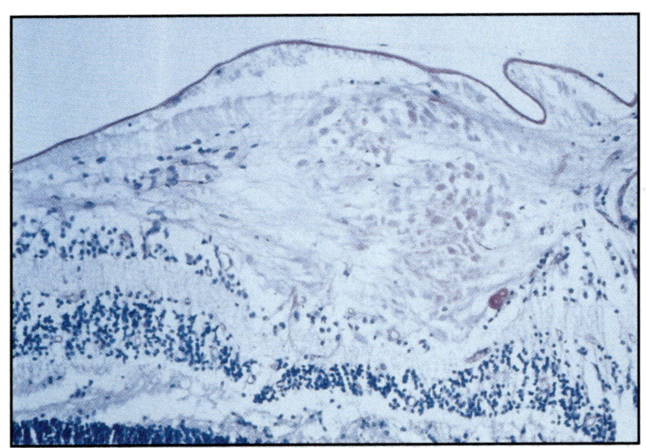

25–2 Capillary microaneurysms are a principal feature of diabetic retinopathy. Histopathologic examination shows a microaneurysm associated with an area of hemorrhage.

25–3 Trypsin digestion reveals an area of microaneurysms and absence of pericytes.

25–4 Precapillary arteriole occlusion causes microinfarction of the nerve fiber layer—a cotton-wool spot. Obstruction of axoplasm appears as swollen axons (cytoid bodies).

***25–2** through **25–4**, From Green, WR, and Wilson, DJ: Histopathology of diabetic retinopathy. In Franklin, RM, ed.: Proceedings of the symposium on retina and vitreous, New Orleans, La, 1993, New York, Kugler Publications.*

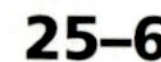

25–5 MACULAR EDEMA

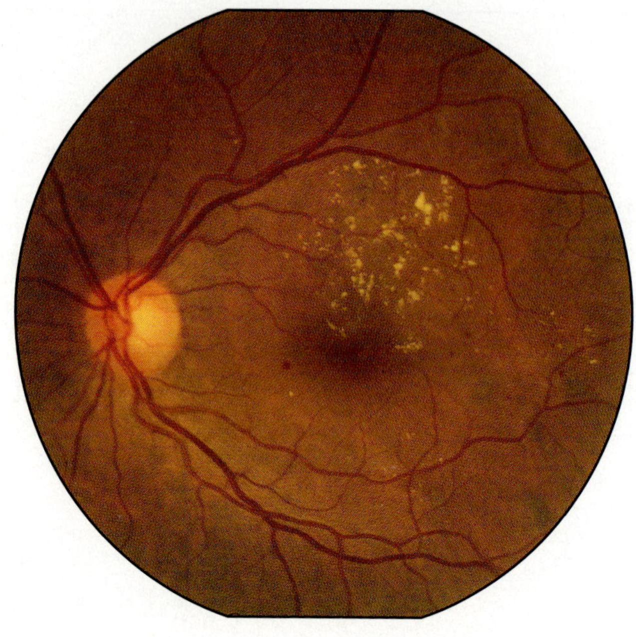

25–6

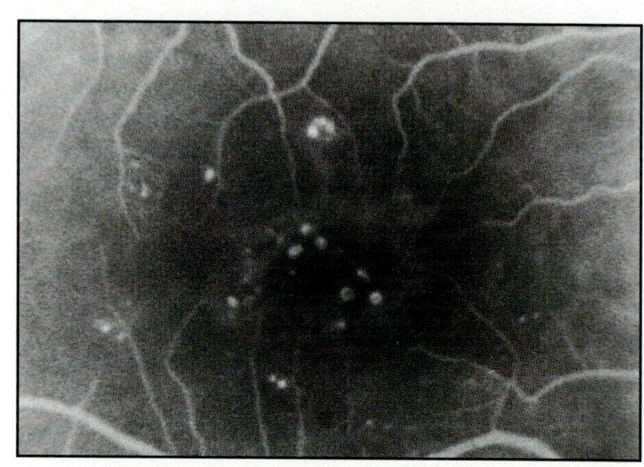

25–7

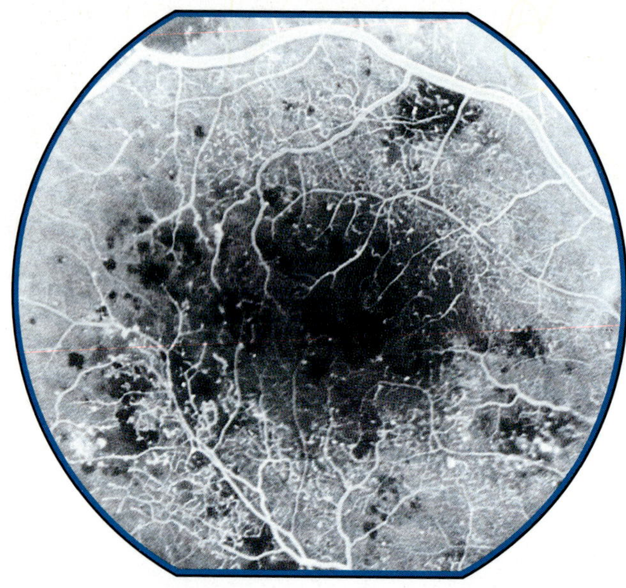

25–8

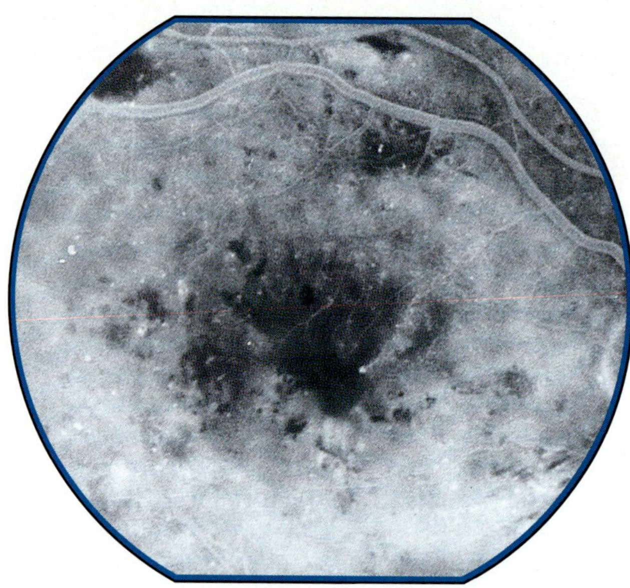

25–5 This patient has nonproliferative diabetic retinopathy with microaneurysms and clinically significant diabetic macular edema with lipid exudation.

25–6 Microaneurysms appear as focal dilatations on a fluorescein angiogram.

25–7 Early frames of the fluorescein angiogram in this patient reveal numerous microaneurysms, as well as capillary nonperfusion.

25–8 Later frames show the diffuse leakage caused by these microaneurysms.

25–9

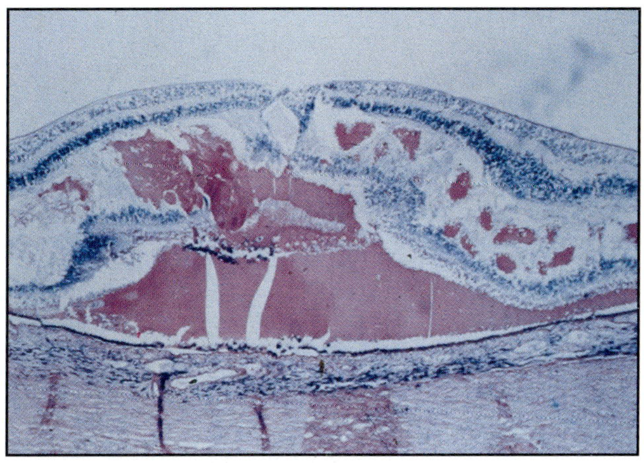

25–10

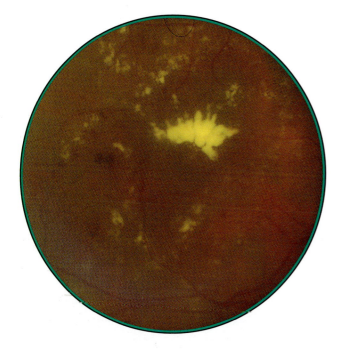

25–11

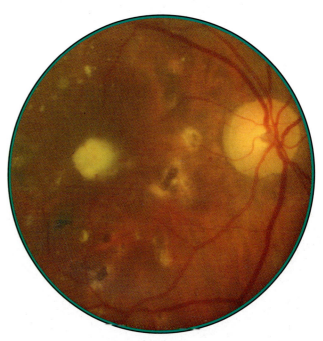

25–9 This histopathologic specimen shows marked diabetic macular edema.

25–10 and 25–11 This patient presented with marked diabetic macular edema and lipid exudation. Focal and grid laser photocoagulation was performed with resolution of the edema. However, with such severe macular edema, fibrous metaplasia or scarring often is noted, as in this case.

25–9, *From Green, WR, and Wilson, DJ: Histopathology of diabetic retinopathy. In Franklin, RM, ed: Proceedings of the symposium of retina and vitreous, New Orleans, La, 1993, New York, Kugler Publications.*

25–12 MACULAR EDEMA

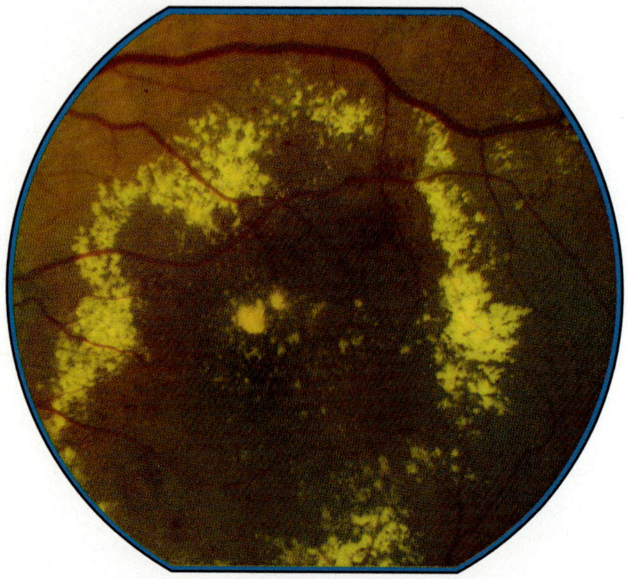

25–13

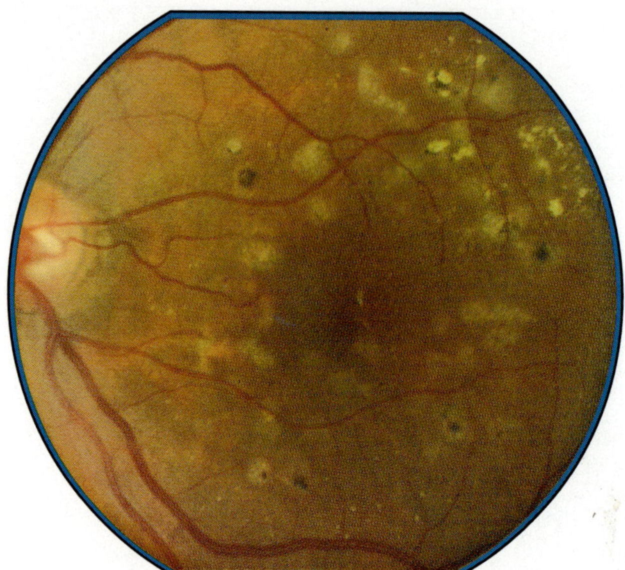

25–14

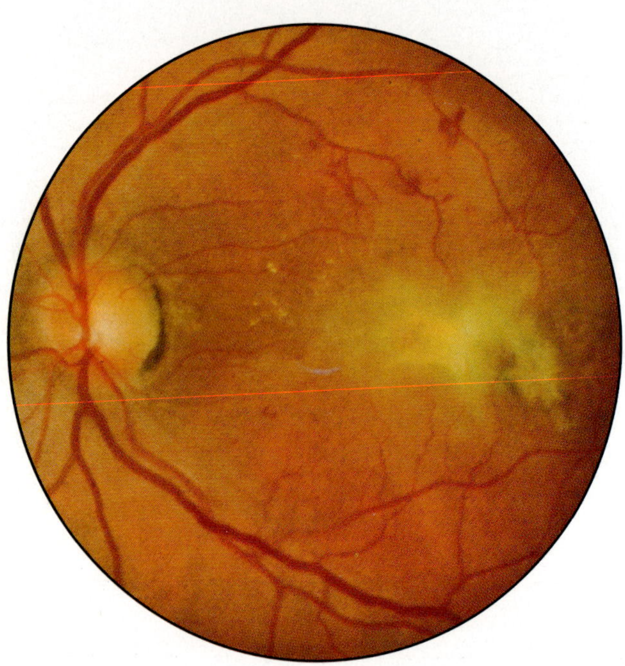

25–12 Another patient presented with massive lipid exudation in a circinate-like pattern.

25–13 Laser photocoagulation was performed in a focal and grid pattern. Note the resolution of the macular edema and lipid exudation without fibrotic change. Thus, although marked macular edema may lead to fibrosis, in some cases laser photocoagulation can cause resolution of the edema and exudation without fibrotic changes occurring.

25–14 Subretinal fibrosis may also occur secondary to untreated chronic lipid exudation.

25–15 CNV

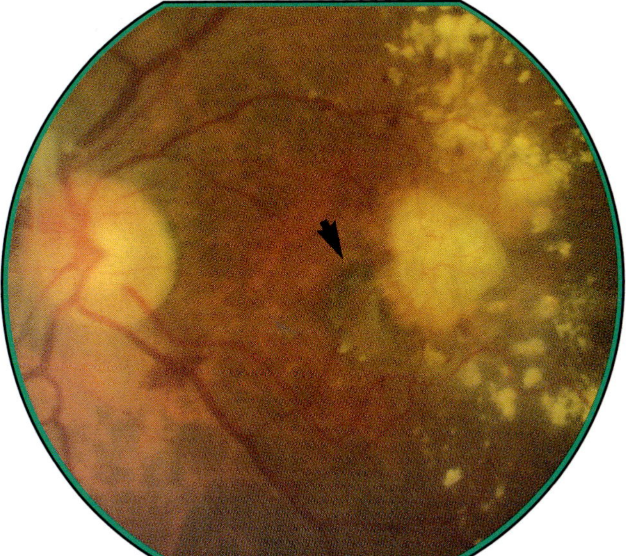

25–16

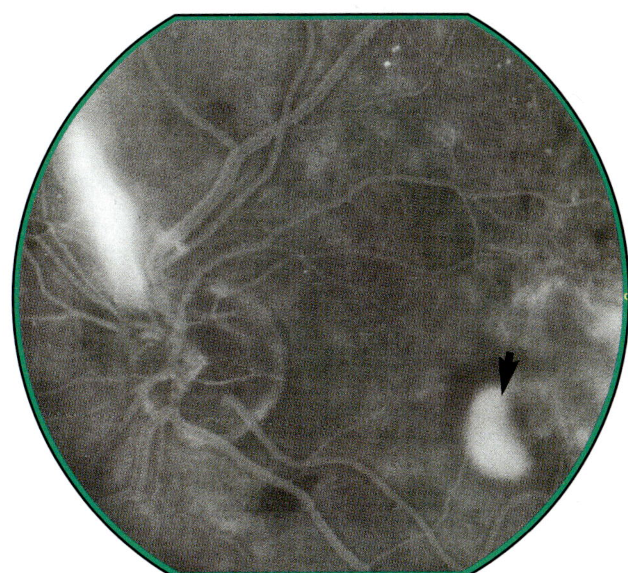

25–17 CAPILLARY NONPERFUSION

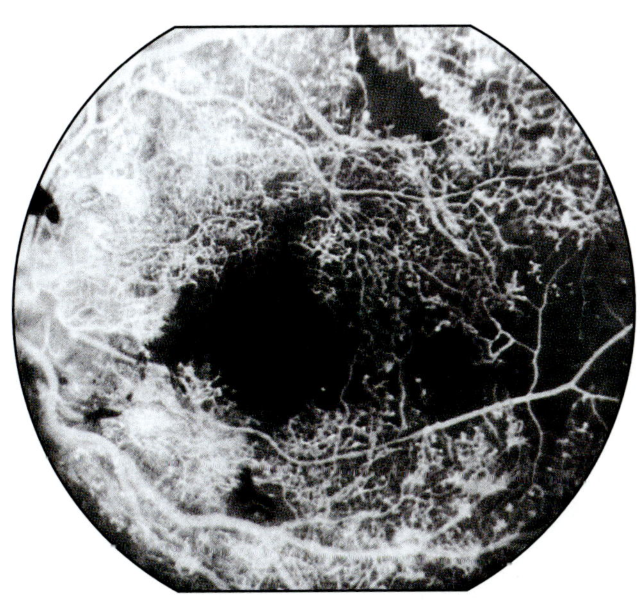

25–15 This patient had chronic exudation from diabetic macular edema, which led to fibrosis. A grayish-green choroidal neovascular membrane can be demonstrated adjacent to the fibrotic area *(arrowhead)*.

25–16 Fluorescein angiography reveals hyperfluorescence in the macular region consistent with choroidal neovascularization *(arrowhead)* and hyperfluorescence of the optic disc, consistent with proliferative diabetic retinopathy.

25–17 Fluorescein angiography may also reveal capillary nonperfusion, which is untreatable and may be the cause of severe vision loss.

25–18 SEVERE NONPROLIFERATIVE DIABETIC RETINOPATHY

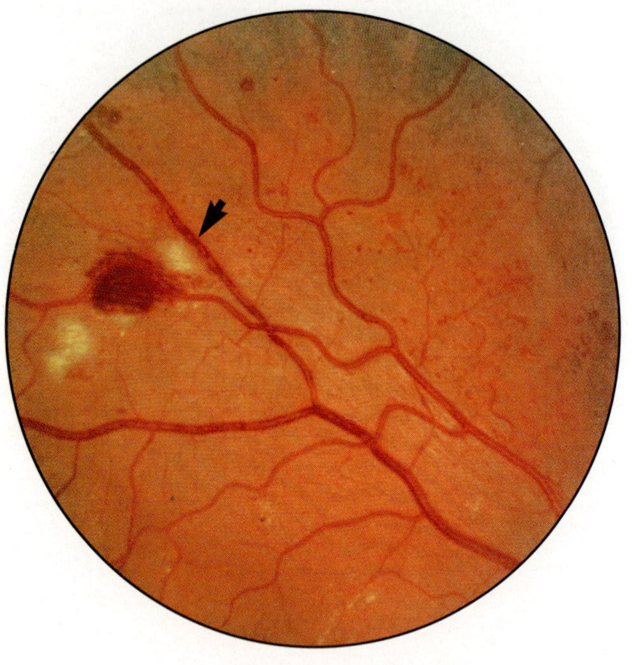

25–19 PROLIFERATIVE DIABETIC RETINOPATHY

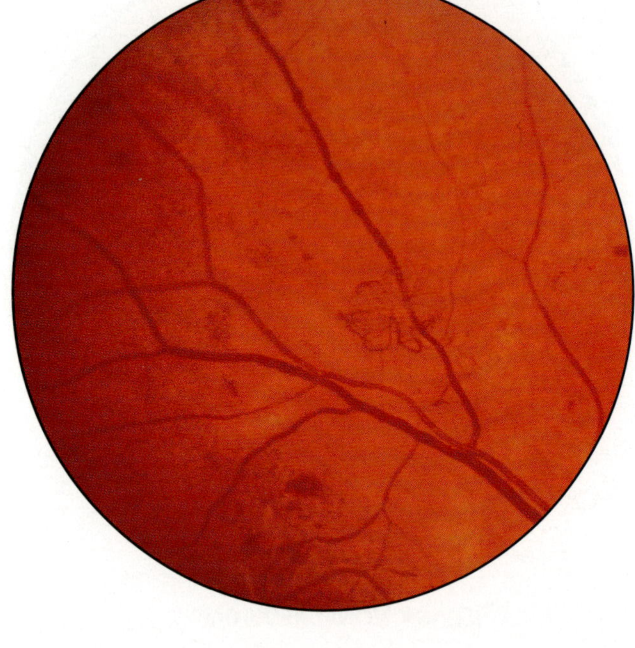

25–20

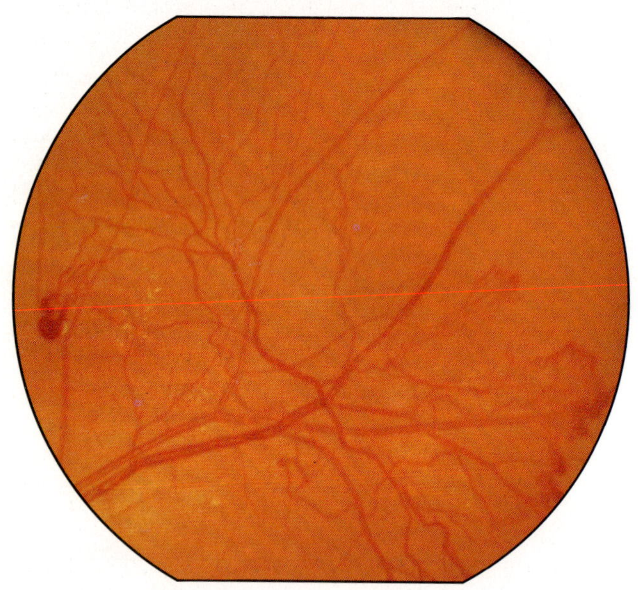

25–18 Severe nonproliferative diabetic retinopathy can be seen in this patient. On the left side of the figure are two prominent soft exudates with a large blot hemorrhage between them. Venous beading is present where the superior branch of the superior temporal vein passes by the upper exudate *(arrowhead)*. On the right side of the figure are many IRMA.

25–19 This patient has early proliferative diabetic retinopathy. New vessels form a small wheel-like network in the supertemporal quadrant with venous beading, IRMA, and blot-dot hemorrhages.

25–20 Neovascularization elsewhere (NVE) without prominent network formation is noted in this case. These vessels did not form networks over much of their course. Large aneurysmal dilatations were present at the end of a long new vessel loop on the left side of the photograph and at the circumference of a partial wheel-like network on the lower right.

25–18 *through* ***25–20,*** *Courtesy of the ETDRS Research Group. From Ryan, SJ: Retina, ed 2, St Louis, 1994, Mosby–Year Book.*

25–21 PROLIFERATIVE DIABETIC RETINOPATHY

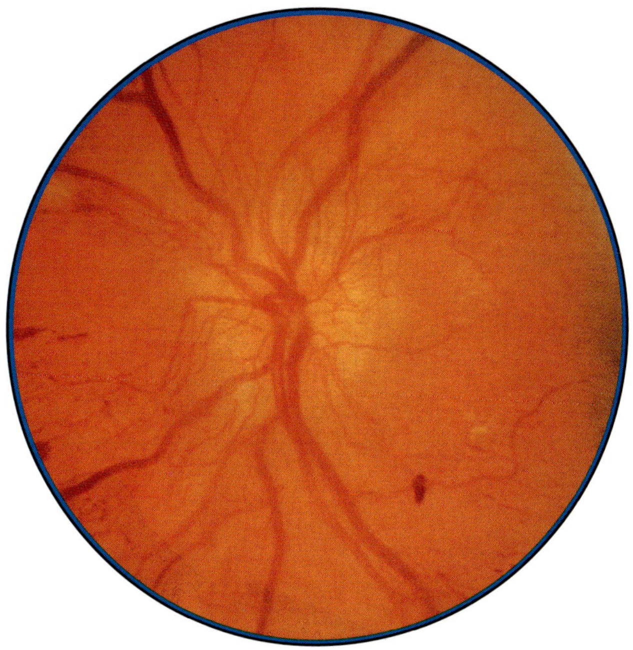

25–22

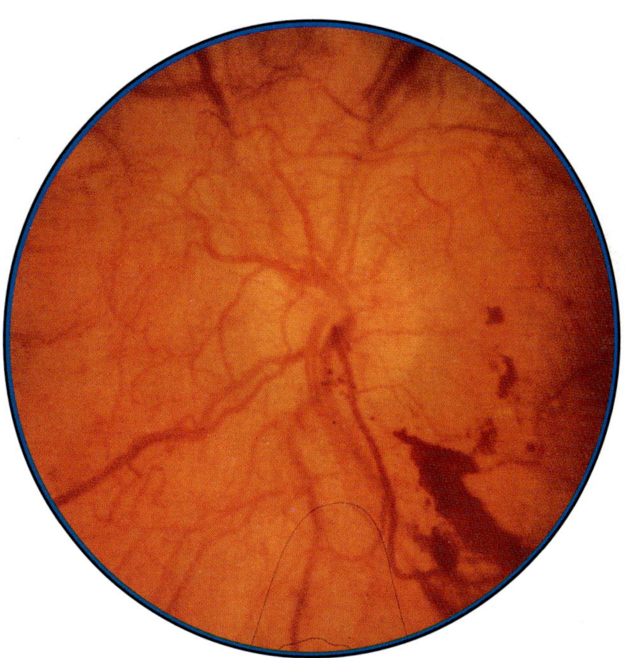

25–23

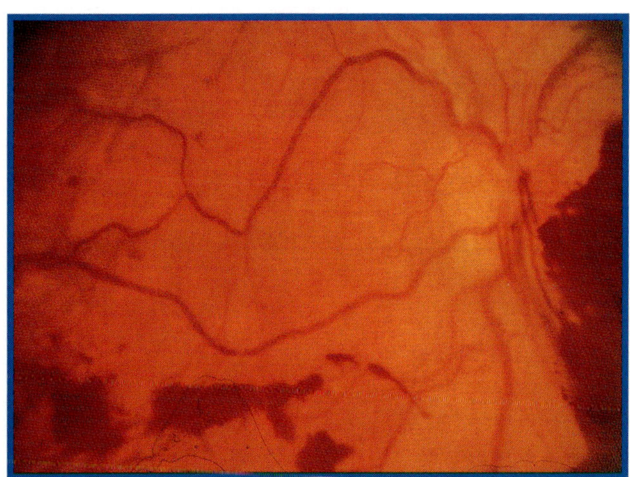

25–21 through 25–23 This case shows rapid development of large-caliber new vessels from the disc secondary to diabetic retinopathy. In the first photograph, new vessels arose on the disc and extended across its margins in all quadrants (25–21). The disc margins are blurred and there are soft and hard exudates, IRMA, and hemorrhages. The second photograph was taken 2 months later and shows that the new vessels had grown remarkably and that preretinal hemorrhage had increased (25–22). On the lower right, a large new vessel crosses the inferotemporal vessels. The third photograph shows the same patient 3 months later, when one of the new vessels had become as large as a major retinal vein and extended nasally beyond the edge of the photograph (25–23). The new vessels along and adjacent to the disc had partially regressed.

***25–21** through **25–23,** Courtesy of Dr. Matthew Davis. From Ryan, SJ: Retina, ed 2, St Louis, 1994, Mosby–Year Book.*

25–24 PROLIFERATIVE DIABETIC RETINOPATHY

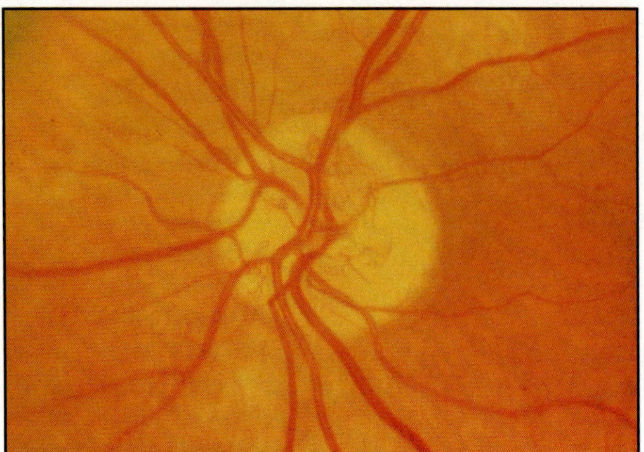

25–24A

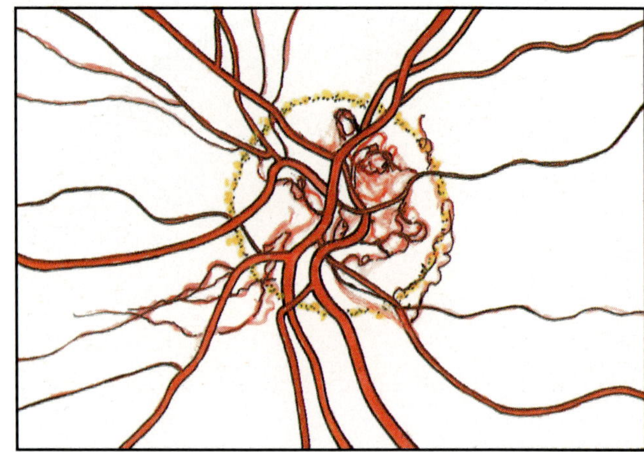

25–25

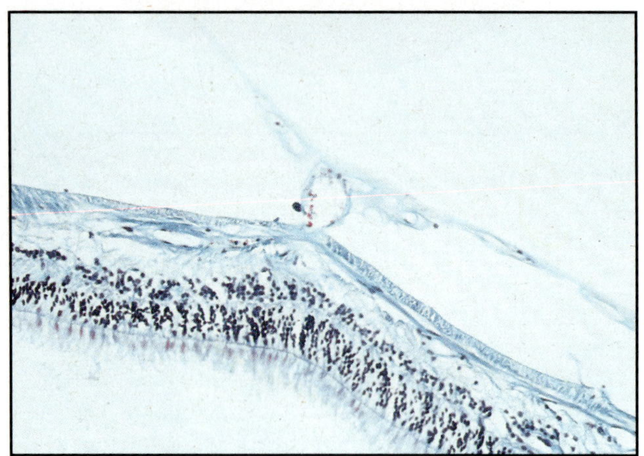

25–25A

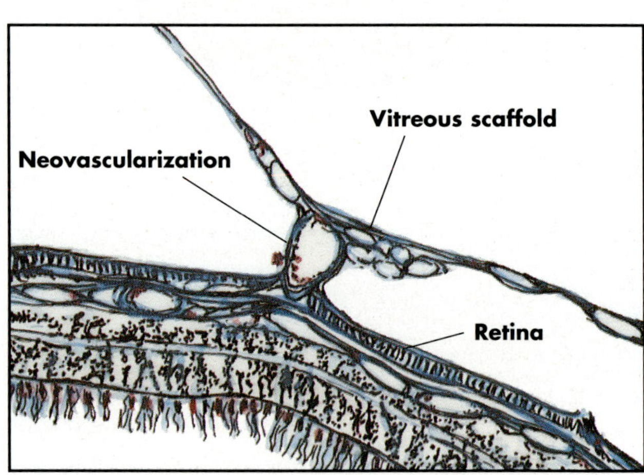

25–24 and 25–24A This is standard photograph 10a of the modified Airlie House classification, which defines a lower limit of moderate new vessels on or within 1 disc diameter of the disc (NVD). Eyes with NVD of this or greater severity have "high-risk" proliferative retinopathy and are candidates for panretinal laser photocoagulation.

25–25 and 25–25A This histopathologic specimen illustrates proliferative diabetic retinopathy with neovascularization elsewhere. The neovascular tissue extends from the retina and into the vitreous.

25–24, *Courtesy of the DRS Research Group, Invest Ophthalmol Vis Sci 21:210, 1981. From Ryan, SJ: Retina, ed 2, St Louis, 1994, Mosby–Year Book.* ***25–25,*** *From Green, WR, and Wilson, DJ: Histopathology of diabetic retinopathy. In Franklin, RM, ed: Proceedings of the symposium of retina and vitreous, New Orleans, La, 1993, New York, Kugler Publications.*

25–26

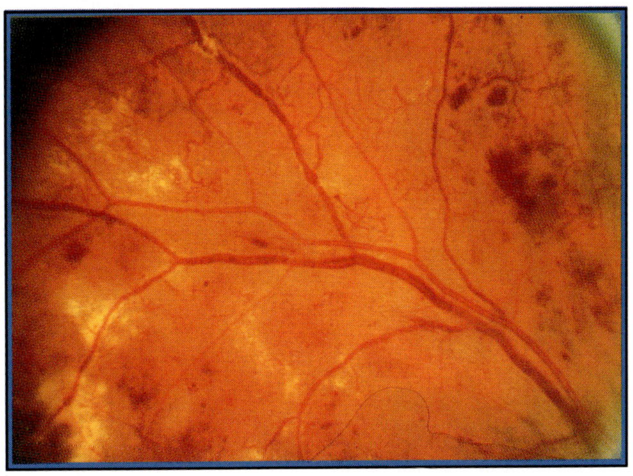

25–27

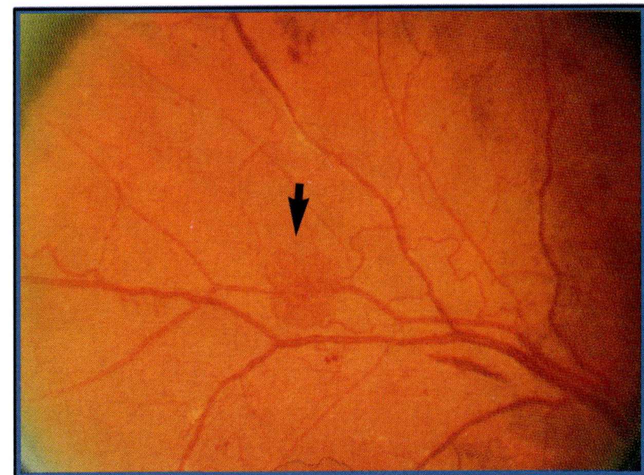

25–28

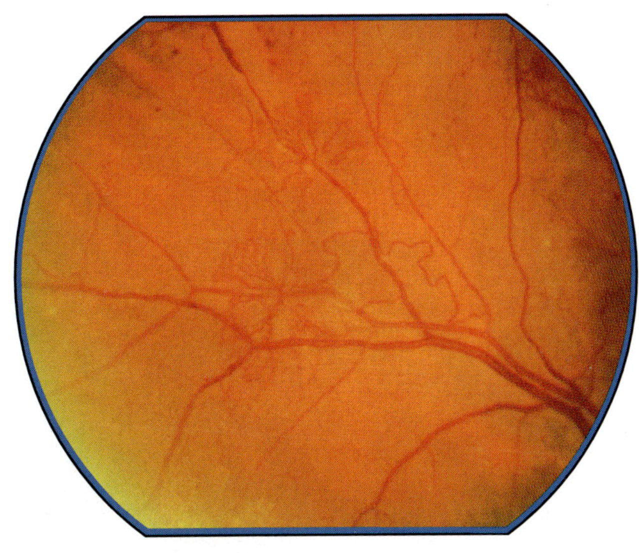

25–29

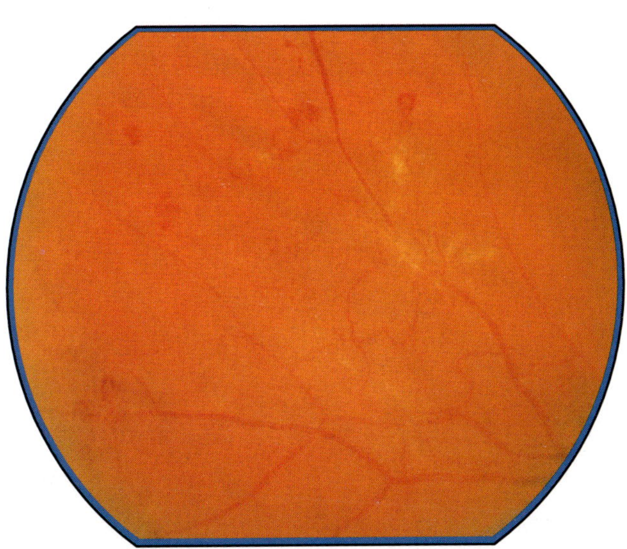

25–26 This case illustrates proliferation and regression of NVE. The first photograph shows severe nonproliferative diabetic retinopathy in a patient with newly diagnosed type II diabetes. There are many microaneurysms, hemorrhages, and hard exudates, as well as extensive edema and venous beading. Most of the tortuous small vessels appear to be within the retina (large IRMA), but some may have been on its surface (NVE).

25–27 The second photograph was taken 8 months later and shows a marked improvement in the intraretinal abnormalities, but a wheel-like network of new vessels has appeared on the surface of the retina *(arrowhead)*.

25–28 The third photograph was taken 3 months later when the new vessel patch has enlarged and a second patch has developed above it. During the next 2 years, the new vessels continued to grow slowly at the edges of the patches while regressing at their centers.

25–29 The final photograph in this series shows that 3 years after the vessels appeared, most of the new vessels had regressed, although there was still one dilated loop at the upper edge of the upper patch. No contraction of fibrous proliferation of vitreous had occurred. There has been no vitreous hemorrhage and the vision remained good.

25–26 *through* ***25–29,*** *Courtesy of Dr. Matthew Davis. From Ryan, SJ: Retina, ed 2, St Louis, 1994, Mosby–Year Book.*

25–30 PROLIFERATIVE DIABETIC RETINOPATHY

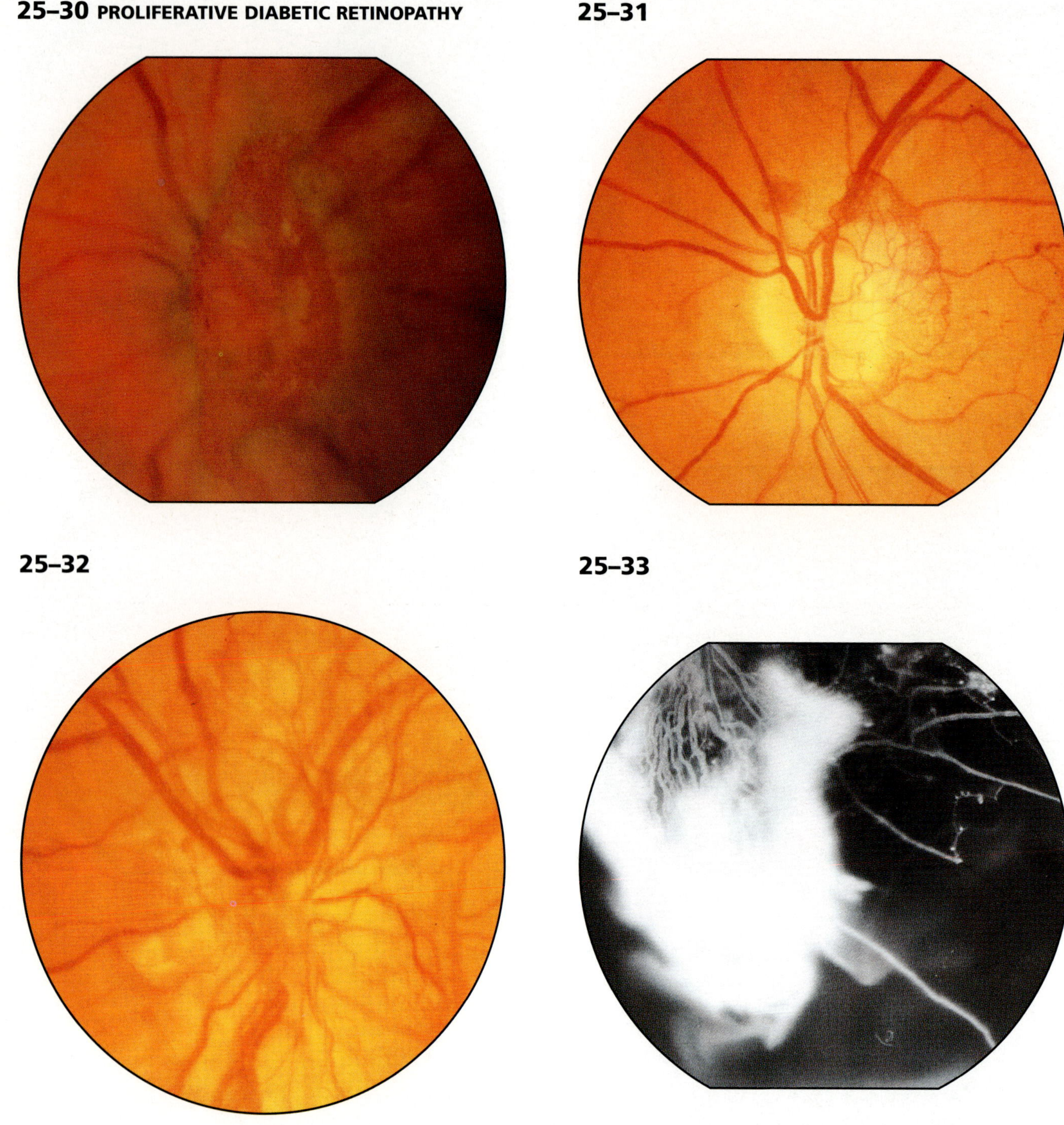

25–30 through 25–35 These photographs illustrate additional cases of diabetic retinopathy with optic disc neovascularization. Note the fluorescein angiographic appearance of the hyperfluorescence secondary to the retinal neovascularization (25–33).

25–31, *Courtesy of Dr. George Blankenship.* ***25–34,*** *Courtesy of Peter Buch, CRA.* ***25–35,*** *Courtesy of Bruce Morris, CRA.*

25–34

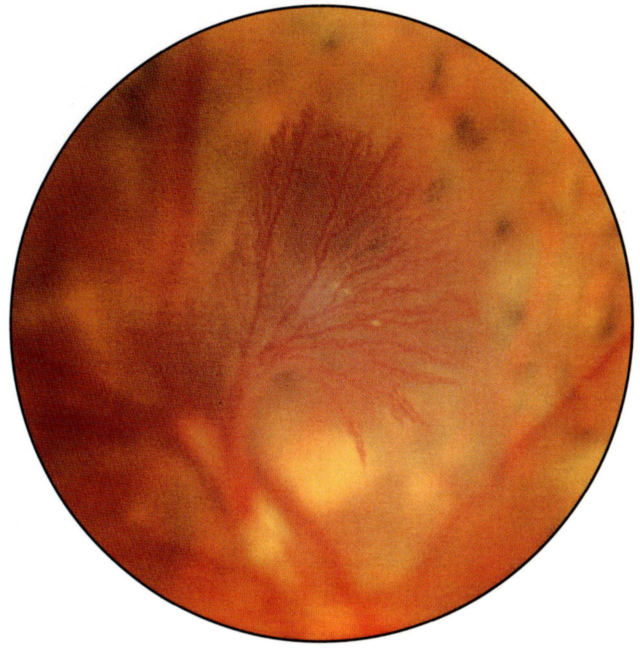

25–35

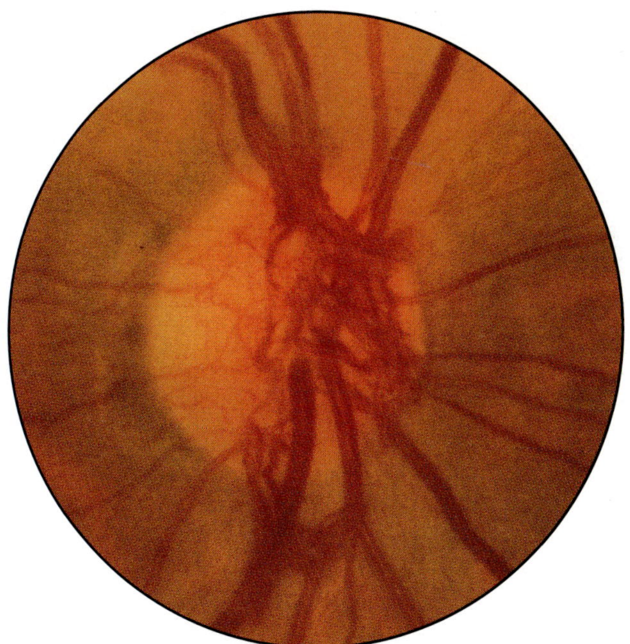

25–36 PROLIFERATIVE DIABETIC RETINOPATHY

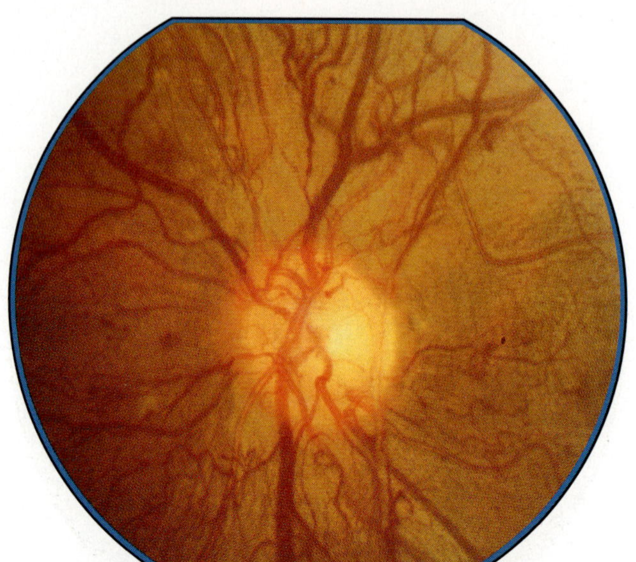

25–37

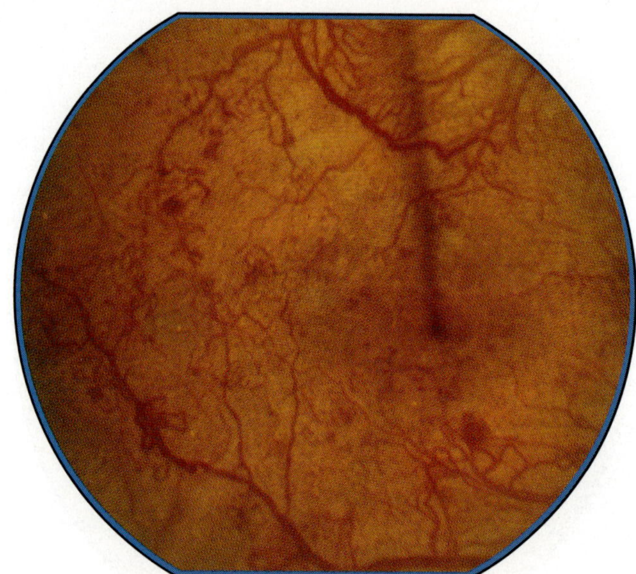

25–38

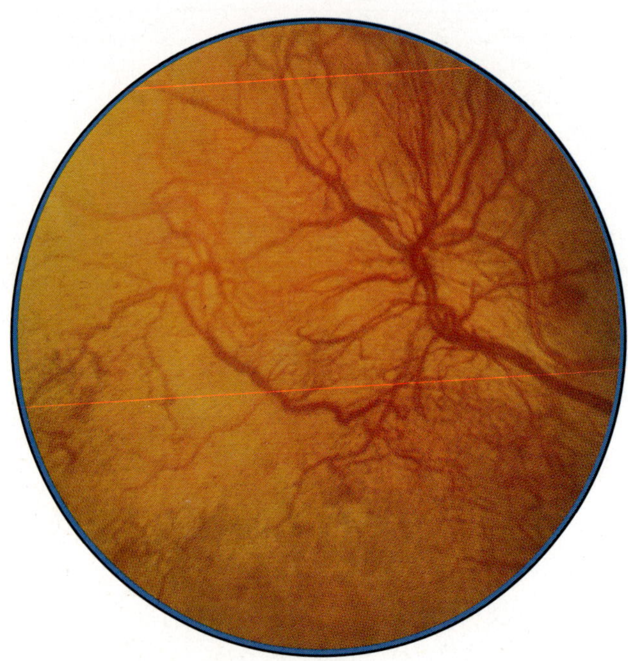

25–36 through 25–38 Florid neovascularization at the optic disc and elsewhere is demonstrated in the next patient.

25–36 *through* ***25–38,*** *Courtesy of Dr. R. N. Frank.*

25–39 LASER PHOTOCOAGULATION: PREOPERATIVE

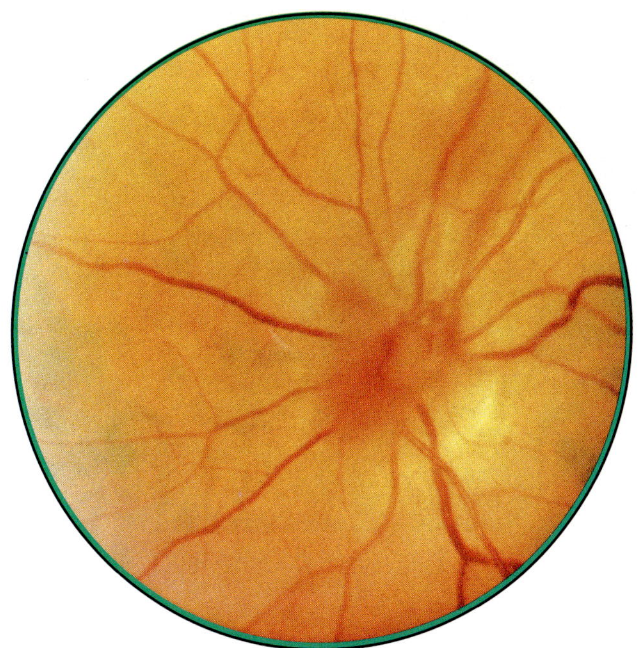

25–40 POSTOPERATIVE

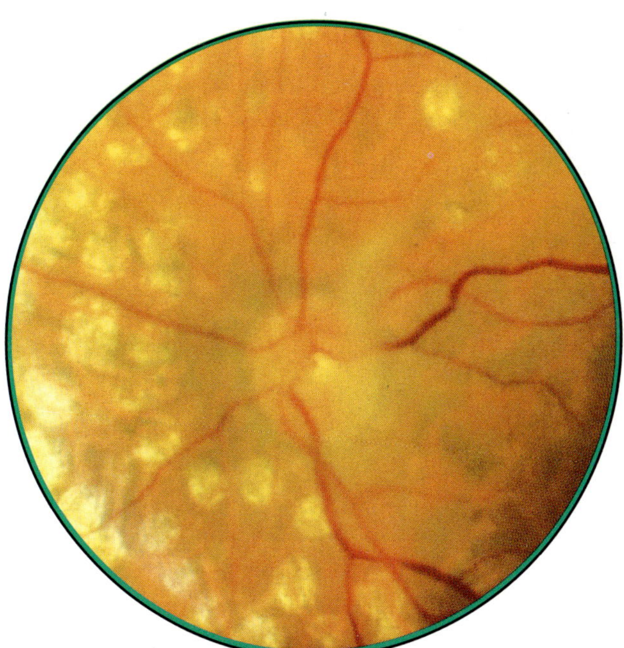

25–41 PREOPERATIVE

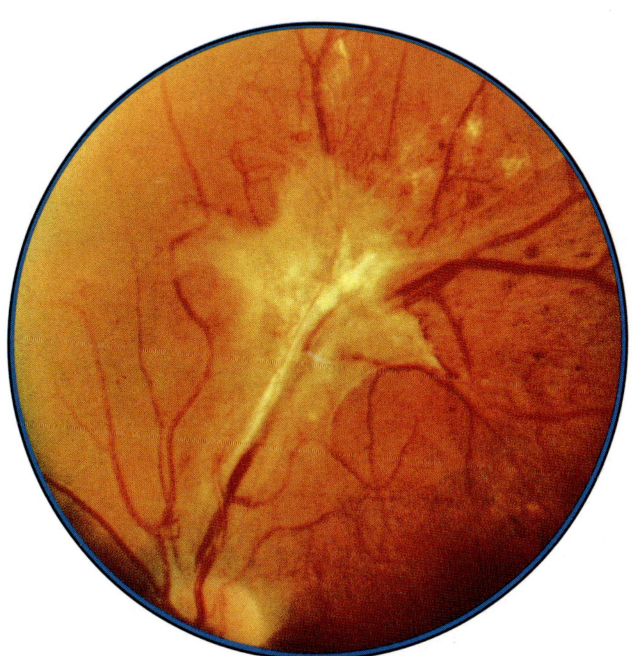

25–42 POSTOPERATIVE

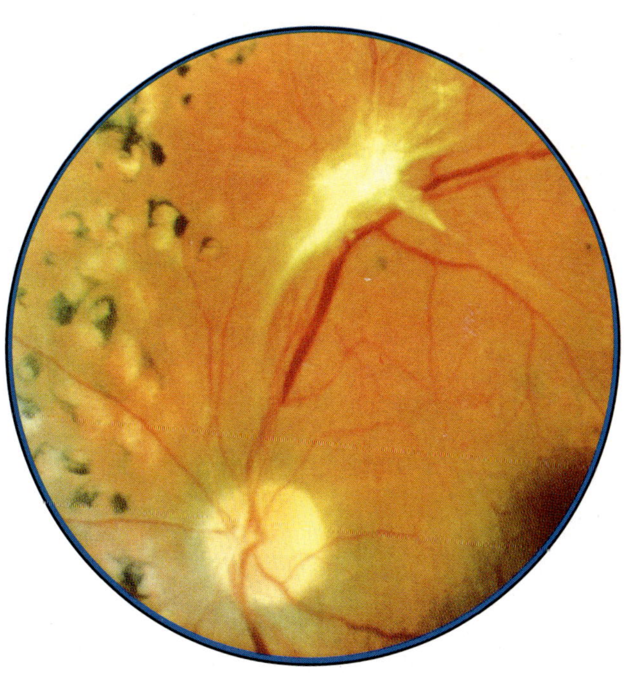

25–39 through 25–42 These photographs show preoperative (25–39 and 25–41) and postoperative (25–40 and 25–42) examples of patients treated with panretinal laser photocoagulation for proliferative diabetic retinopathy. In the first case, neovascularization at the disc is noted (25–39). On the follow-up examination, the neovascularization has regressed and laser photocoagulation scars can be appreciated (25–40). In the second photograph, neovascularization and fibrous proliferation is noted (25–41), which shows regression in the postoperative photograph (25–42). Laser photocoagulation scars are present.

25–43 FOVEAL RETINAL NEOVASCULARIZATION

25–44

25–45

25–46

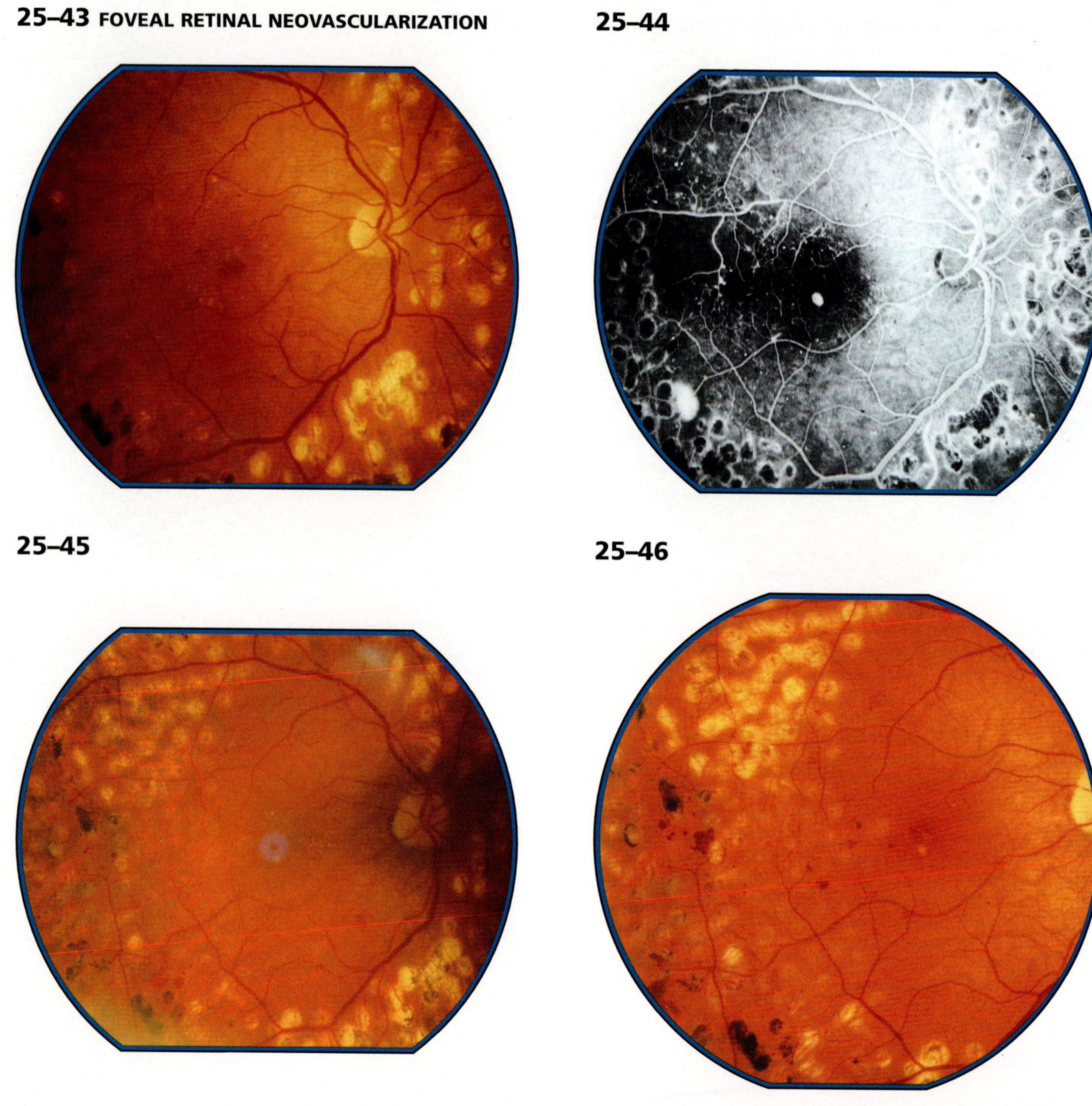

25–43 This patient presented with retinal neovascularization in the foveal region.

25–44 Fluorescein angiography confirmed the retinal neovascularization in the macular region. Note the capillary nonperfusion adjacent to the macula.

25–45 and 25–46 Laser photocoagulation was performed peripheral to the macula with resolution of the foveal retinal neovascularization.

25–47 CAPILLARY NONPERFUSION

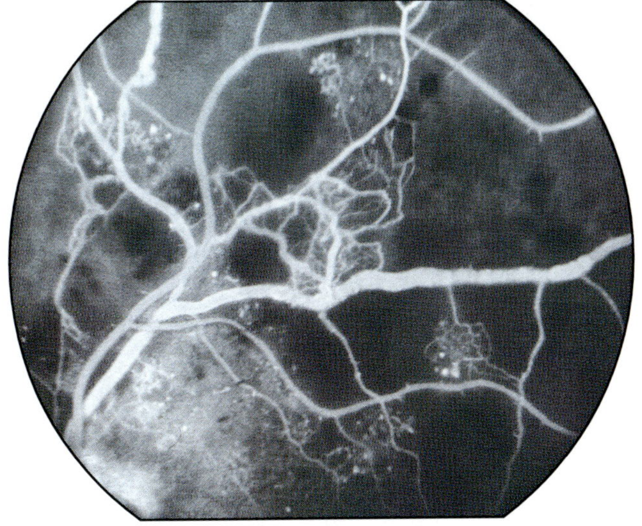

25–48

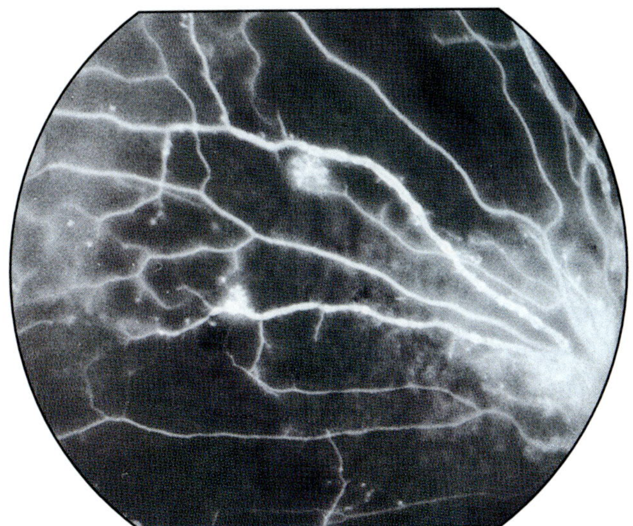

25–49 FIBROUS PROLIFERATION

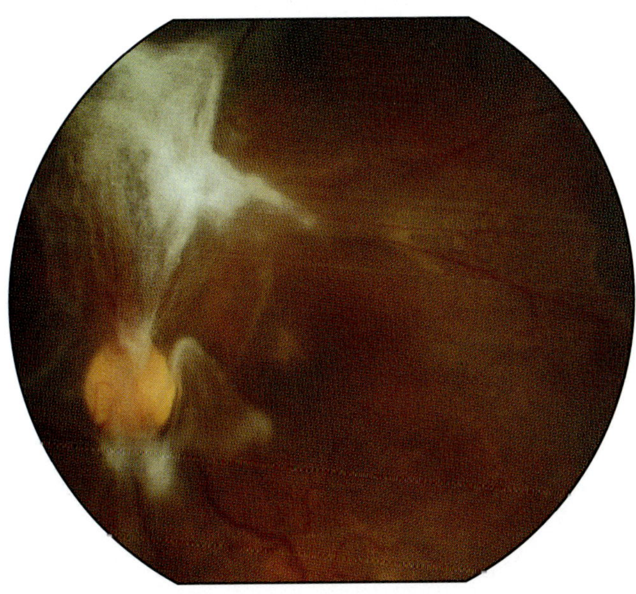

25–47 and 25–48 Extensive peripheral capillary nonperfusion may be marked in patients with advanced proliferative diabetic retinopathy.

25–49 Proliferative diabetic retinopathy can lead to extensive fibrous proliferation as seen in this patient.

25–50 TRACTIONAL RETINAL DETACHMENT

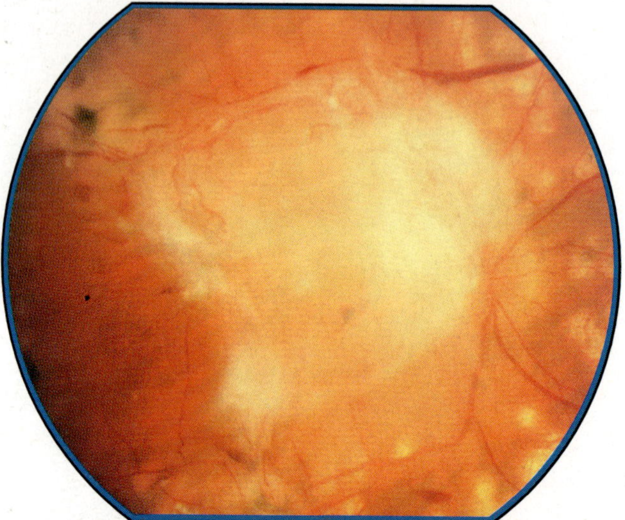

25–51

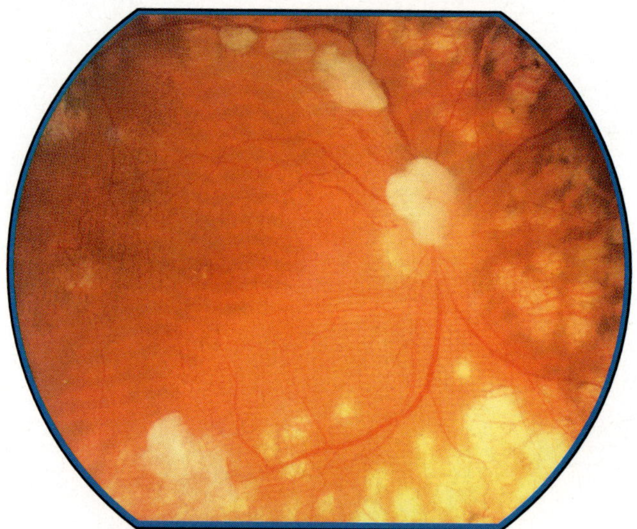

25–52

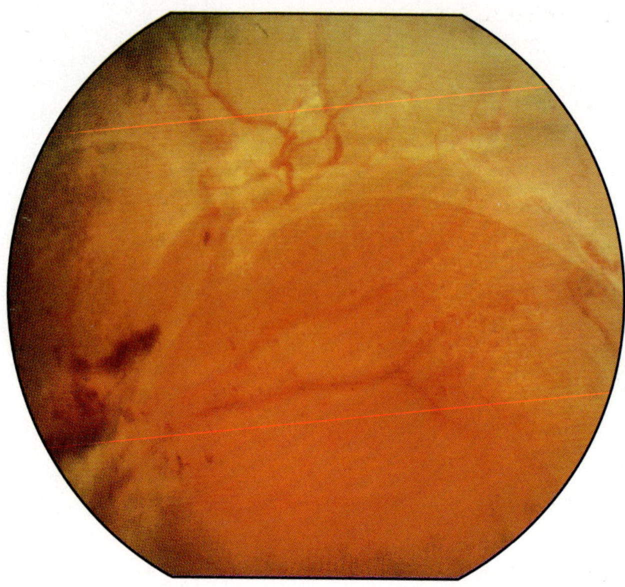

25–50 and 25–51 Tractional retinal detachment can occur from proliferative diabetic retinopathy as seen in this case. Note that the posterior pole is detached preoperatively. After vitrectomy, the posterior pole is flat.

25–52 In this eye fibrovascular proliferations are present at the optic disc and above the supertemporal vascular arcade. The posterior vitreous surface is adherent to these proliferations but is detached elsewhere. In the center of the photograph, the posterior vitreous surface is thin (visible only with slit illumination), but its position is marked by fine dots of hemorrhage deposited on it. Temporal to this area, the posterior vitreous surface has a typical Swiss cheese appearance. There are round and oval clear areas in a surface that appears as a semiopaque sheet. The same appearance is present 1–2 disc diameters above the disc, near the left edge of the photograph. The retina is attached but is blurred in part because the camera is focused on the elevated proliferations and in part because of blood in the posterior vitreous.

***25–50** and **25–51**, Courtesy of Dr. Yale Fisher.*

25–53 DRAGGING OF THE MACULA 25–54 25–55

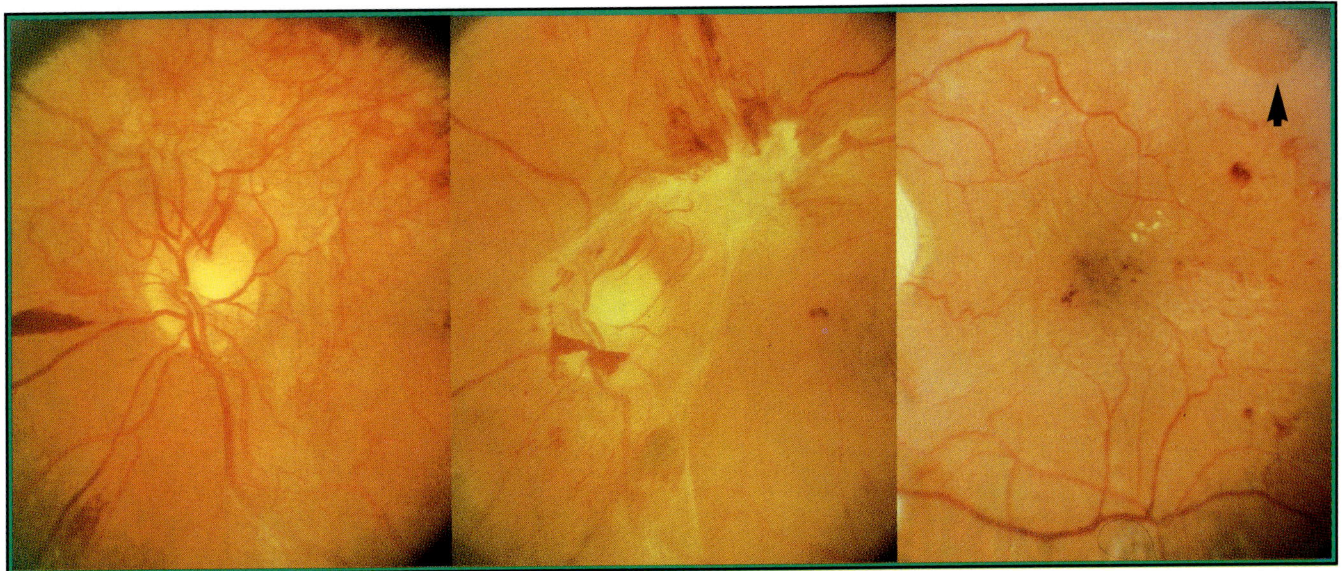

25–53 through 25–55 This case illustrates dragging of the macula. The first photograph of this 39-year-old white female shows extensive fibrovascular proliferations on and adjacent to the disc (25–53). The temporal edge of the patch of proliferation is tightly opposed to the retina, and the nasal edge is elevated about one-third of a disc diameter by localized posterior vitreous detachment, the lower edge of which was marked by preretinal hemorrhage. Visual acuity is 20/60. Panretinal photocoagulation was performed. The second photograph shows the patient 3 weeks after laser photocoagulation (25–54). The patient noted a marked decrease in visual acuity and returned for examination. There was marked regression of the new vessels. Contraction of the proliferations pulled the neurosensory macula (but not the corresponding more deeply pigmented RPE) up and nasally. Vitrectomy was performed. The third photograph shows the patient 2 months later when visual acuity had improved to 20/30 and the neurosensory macula had returned to its normal position (25–55). There appeared to be a rather large full-thickness retinal break *(arrowhead),* but this did not lead to retinal detachment during the remaining 3 years of follow-up. At the 4-year follow-up visit, vision had improved to 20/20.

***25–52** through **25–55,** Courtesy of the DRVS Research Group. From Ryan, SJ: Retina, ed 2, St Louis, 1994, Mosby–Year Book.*

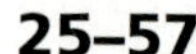

25–56 DIABETIC PAPILLOPATHY

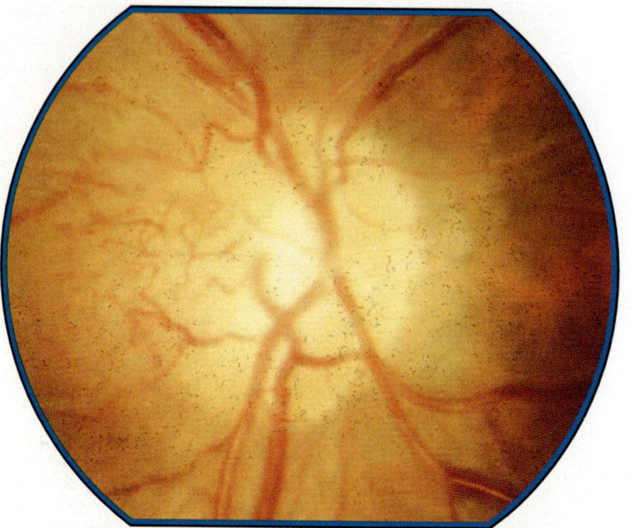

25–57

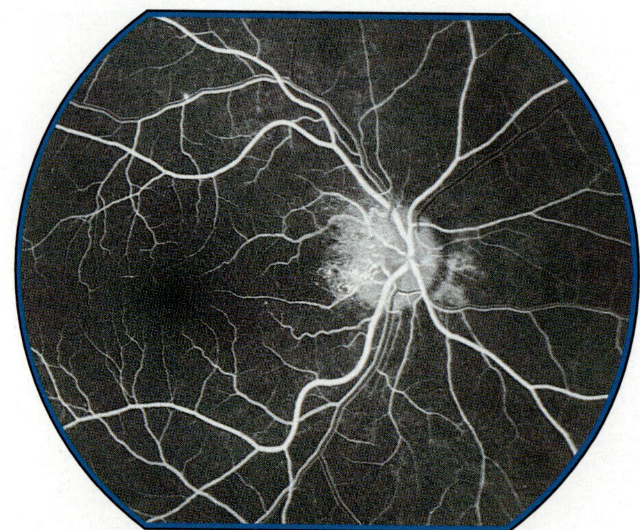

25–58

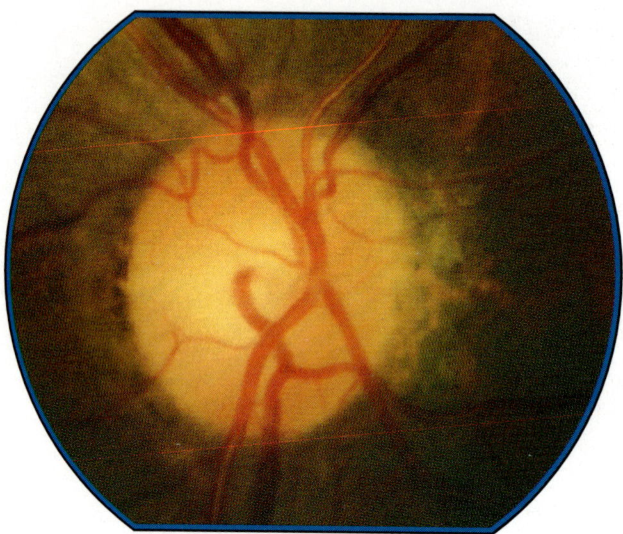

25–59

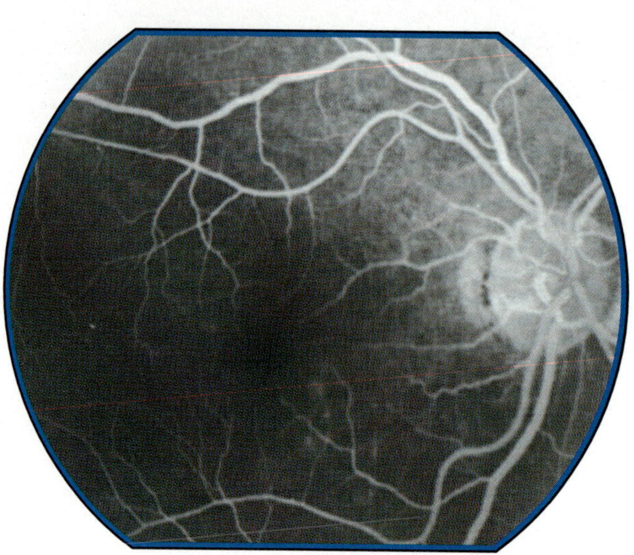

25–56 This patient has diabetic papillopathy that simulates an angioma. The patient presented with a vascular-appearing lesion at the optic nerve.

25–57 Fluorescein angiography reveals mild hyperfluorescence. It was believed by many experts that this represented an angioma of the optic nerve.

25–58 and 25–59 However, the lesion spontaneously resolved, which suggested that it was caused by diabetic papillopathy. This case shows that diabetic papillopathy may mimic an angioma.

***25–56** through **25–58,** Courtesy of Drs. Wendy Klein and Ron Carr.*

25–60 LIPEMIA RETINALIS

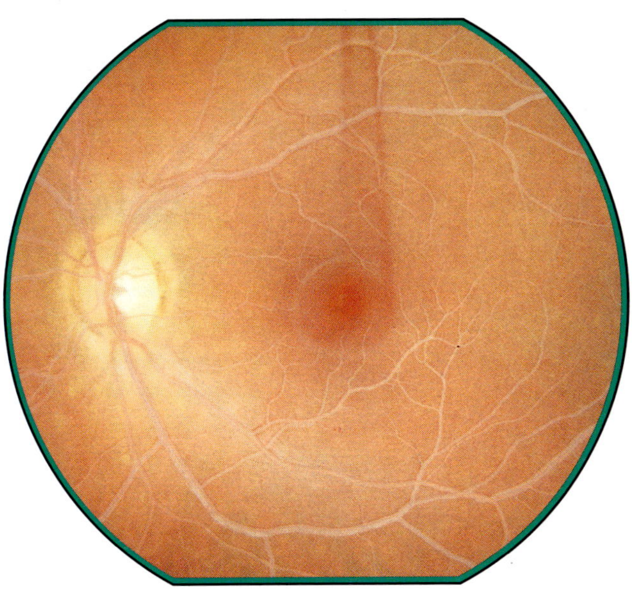

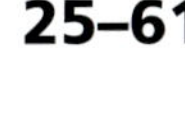

25–61

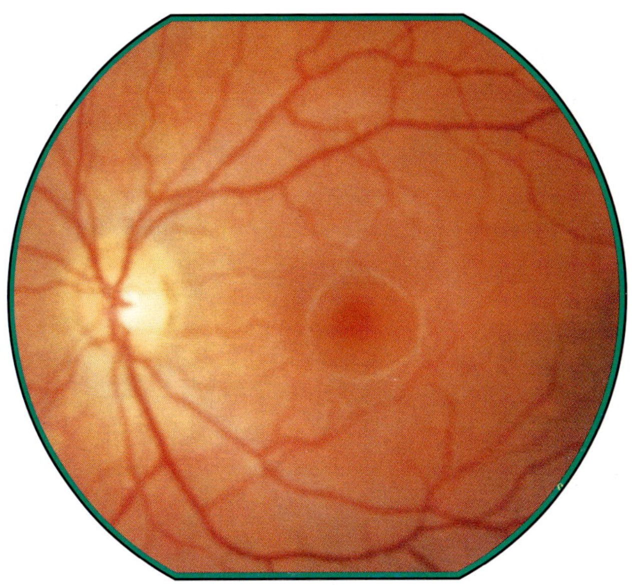

25–60 This 9-year-old female with diabetes mellitus had 20/20 vision in both eyes and creamy-white–appearing blood vessels. The background fundus appearance was also lightened. Laboratory findings revealed elevated serum cholesterol, triglycerides, low-density lipoproteins, and very-low-density lipoproteins. She was also found to have hypothyroidism.

25–61 Six weeks later after insulin therapy and thyroid supplementation, her triglyceride levels were lower and her abnormal retinal findings had resolved. This case illustrates lipemia retinalis, which is due to elevated serum triglycerides. In this case, the hypertriglyceridemia was secondary to her diabetes mellitus and hypothyroidism.

25–60 *and* ***25–61,*** *From Martinez, K, et al: Lipemia retinalis, Arch Ophthalmol 110:1171, 1992. Copyright 1992, American Medical Association.*

Suggested Readings

Aiello, LM, Rand, LI, Briones, JC, Wafai, MZ, and Sebestyen, JG: Diabetic retinopathy. In Joslin Clinic patients with adult-onset diabetes, Ophthalmology 88:619–623, 1981

Blankenship, GW: Diabetic macular edema and argon laser photocoagulation: a prospective randomized, Ophthalmology 86:69–78, 1979

Blankenship, GW: A clinical comparison of central and peripheral argon laser panretinal photocoagulation for proliferative diabetic retinopathy, Ophthalmology 95:170–177, 1988

Bresnick, GH: Diabetic maculopathy: a critical review highlighting diffuse macular edema, Ophthalmology 90:1301–1317, 1983

Bresnick, GH, de Venecia, G, Myers, FL, Harris, JA, and Davis, MD: Retinal ischemia in diabetic retinopathy, Arch Ophthalmol 93:1300–1310, 1975

Bresnick, GH, Engerman, R, Davis, MD, de Venecia, G, and Myers, FL: Patterns of ischemia in diabetic retinopathy, Trans Am Acad Ophthalmol Otolaryngol 81:694–709, 1976

Davis, MD, Norton, EWD, and Myers, FL: The Airlie classification of diabetic retinopathy. In Goldberg, MF, and Fine, SL, eds: Symposium on the treatment of diabetic retinopathy, Washington DC, 1968, US Public Health Servication Publication no. 1890

Diabetic Retinopathy Study Research group: A modification of the Airlie House classification of diabetic retinopathy, Invest, Ophthalmol Vis Sci 21:210–226, 1981

Early Treatment Diabetic Retinopathy Study Research Group: Photocoagulation for diabetic macular edema, Int Ophthalmol Clin 27:265–272, 1987

Early Treatment Diabetic Retinopathy Study Research Group: Aspirin effects on mortality and morbidity in patients with diabetes mellitus, JAMA 268:1292–1300, 1992

Ferris, FL, III, and Patz, A: Macular edema: A complication of diabetic retinopathy, Surv Ophthalmol 28:452–461, 1984

Gordon, B, Chang, S, and Yannuzzi, LA: The effects of lipid-lowering on diabetic retinopathy, Am J Ophthalmol 112:385–391, 1991

Green, WR, and Wilson, DJ: Histopathology of diabetic retinopathy. In Franklin, RM, ed: Proceedings of the Symposium on Retina and Vitreous, New Orleans Academy of Ophthalmology, New Orleans, LA, 1993, New York, Kugler Publications, pp 63–81

Guyer, DR, D'Amico, DJ, and Smith, C: Subretinal fibrosis following laser photocoagulation for diabetic macular edema, Am J Ophthalmol 113:652–656, 1992.

Henkind, P, and Wise, GN: Retinal neovascularization, collaterals, and vascular shunts, Br J Ophthalmol 58:413–422, 1974

Klein, R, Klein BEK, Moss SE, Davis, MD, and DeMets, DL: The Wisconsin Epidemiologic Study of Diabetic Retinopathy: X. Four-year incidence and progression of diabetic retinopathy when age at diagnosis is 30 years of age or more, Arch Ophthalmol 107:244–249, 1989

Kohner, EM, and Henkind, P: Correlation of fluorescein angiogram and retinal digest in diabetic retinopathy, Am J Ophthalmol 69:403–414, 1970

Kohner, EM: The natural history of diabetic retinopathy, J R Coll Physicians Lond 6:259–270, 1972

Lewis, H, Schachat, AP, Haimann, MH, Haller, JA, Quinlan, P, Von Frichen, MA, Fine, SL, and Murphy, RP: Choroidal neovascularization after laser photocoagulation for macular edema, Ophthalmology 97:503–511, 1990

McDonald, HR, and Schatz, H: Visual loss following panretinal photocoagulation for proliferative diabetic retinopathy, Ophthalmology 92:388–393, 1985

Okun, E, Johnston, GP, Boniuk, I, Arribas, NP, Escoffery, RF, and Grand, MG: Xenon arc photocoagulation of proliferative diabetic retinopathy: a review of 2688 consecutive eyes in the format of the Diabetic Retinopathy Study, Ophthalmology 91:1458–1463, 1984

Patz, A: Clinical and experimental studies on retinal neovascularization, Am J Ophthalmol 94:715–743, 1982

Patz, A, Schatz, H, Berkow, JW, Gittelsohn, AM, and Ticho, U: Macular edema—an overlooked complication of diabetic retinopathy, Trans Am Acad Ophthalmol Otolaryngol 77:34–42, 1973

Ramsay, RC, Knobloch, WH, and Cantrill, HL: Timing of vitrectomy for active proliferative diabetic retinopathy, Ophthalmology 93:283–289, 1986

Shimizu, K, Kobayashi, Y, and Muraoka, K: Midperipheral fundus involvement in diabetic retinopathy, Ophthalmology 88:601–612, 1981

Tso, MOM, Cunha-Vaz, JGF, Shih CY, and Jones, CW: A clinicopathologic study of blood-retinal barrier in experimental diabetes, Invest Ophthalmol Vis Sci 18(Suppl):169, 1979

Vine, AK: The efficacy of additional argon laser photocoagulation for persistent, severe proliferative diabetic retinopathy, Ophthalmology 92:1532–1537, 1985

Wetzig, PC, and Jepson, CN: Treatment of diabetic retinopathy by light coagulation, Am J Ophthalmol 62:459–465,1966

Yanoff, M: Diabetic retinopathy, N Engl J Med 274:1344–1349, 1966

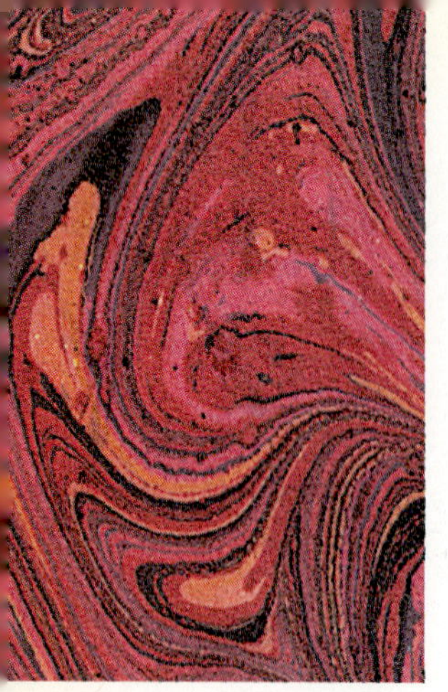

Chapter 26

Retinal Arterial Obstructive Diseases

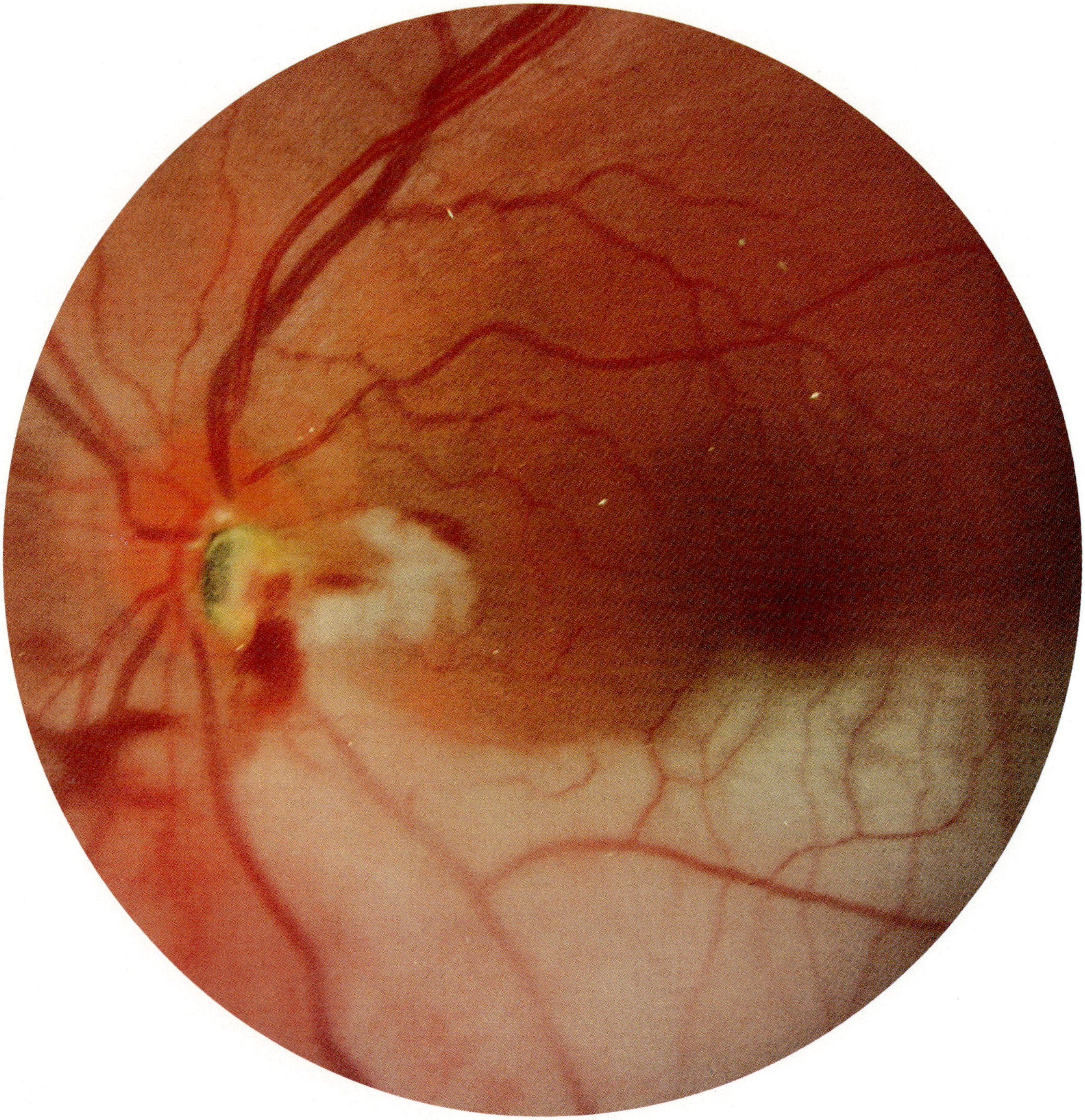

Retinal arterial obstructive diseases include ophthalmic artery obstructions, central retinal artery occlusions, branch retinal artery occlusions, cilioretinal artery occlusions, combined central retinal artery and vein obstructions, and cotton-wool spots.

Patients with an ophthalmic artery occlusion often have no light perception vision. A cherry-red spot is absent in almost half of these cases because of choroidal insufficiency. Retinal pigment epithelial changes are commonly seen after ophthalmic artery occlusion.

Central retinal artery obstructions are most commonly seen in older adults. These patients often have signs of systemic vascular disease. An afferent pupillary defect is usually noted. The superficial retina becomes opacified except for the foveola, in which a cherry-red spot is noted. The cherry-red spot occurs since the foveola is very thin, which allows visualization of the underlying retinal pigment epithelium and choroid. In more severe disease, segmentation or "box-carring" of the vasculature is seen. In approximately one-fifth of cases, an embolus is noted. The finding of an embolus is a poor prognostic factor for survival. Rubeosis may occur in 15% to 20% of cases. Various forms of treatment for an acute central retinal artery occlusion include anterior chamber paracentesis, carbogen, lowering intraocular pressure pharmacologically, and ocular massage.

A branch retinal artery obstruction has superficial retinal whitening in the distribution of a blocked branch retinal artery. The visual prognosis with branch retinal artery occlusion is relatively good. Rubeosis is extremely uncommon. A similar systemic workup is done as for patients with central retinal artery occlusion; however, since the visual prognosis is better, invasive ocular measures are usually not undertaken.

Approximately one-third of patients have a cilioretinal artery. A cilioretinal artery obstruction also has a relatively good visual prognosis.

26–1 OPHTHALMIC ARTERY OCCLUSION

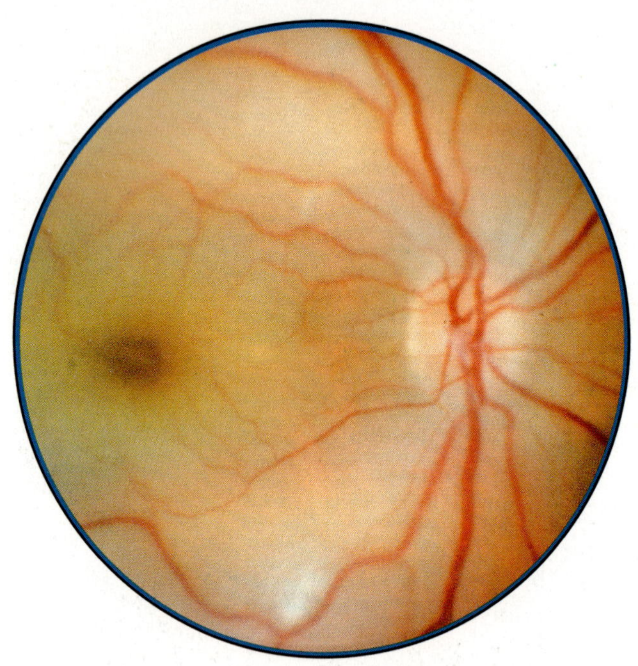

26–2

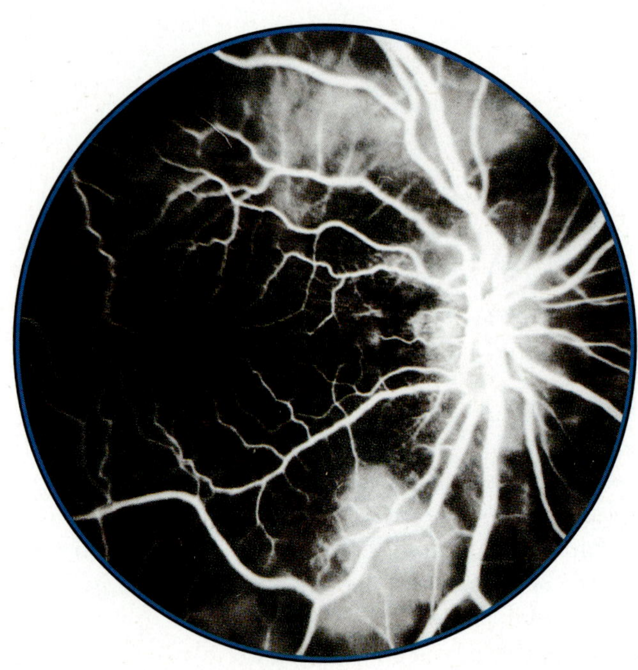

26–1 This photograph illustrates a diffuse but heterogeneous whitening of the retina corresponding to retinal as well as choroidal ischemia in a patient with an ophthalmic artery occlusion secondary to temporal arteritis.

26–2 The fluorescein study shows a marked delay in the perfusion of the choroidal circulation, which is evident in this phase of the angiogram in which the retinal circulation is already perfused.

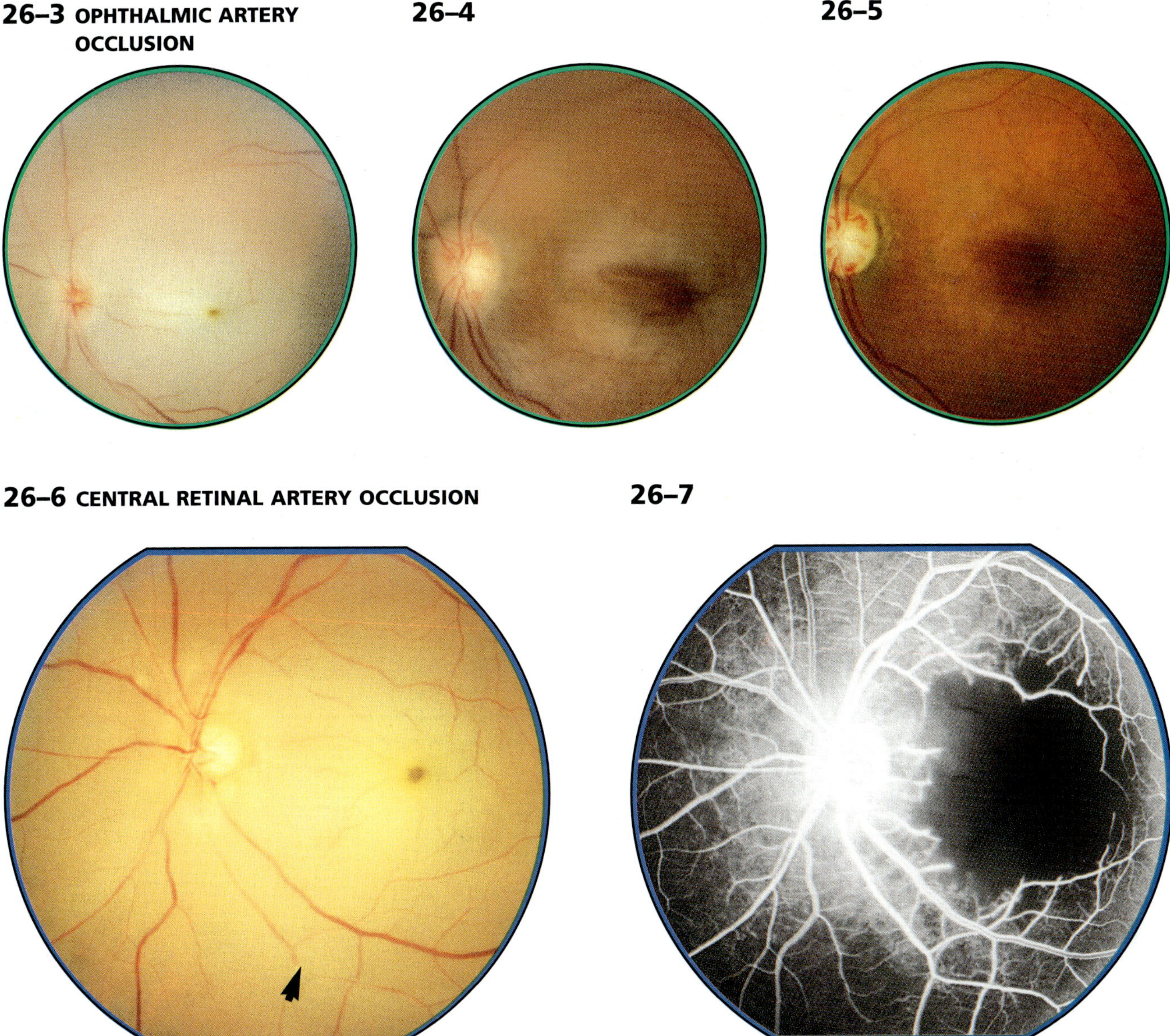

26–3 through 26–5 This patient also has had an ophthalmic artery occlusion. In the acute stages, there is diffuse whitening in the posterior fundus with a cherry-red spot. Two months later, the outer retinal ischemia has largely subsided, leaving a reddish-brown discoloration in the foveal region. There is still some perifoveal whitening of the inner retina. There are also early signs of compensatory collaterals between the retinal and choroidal circulations. The next photograph shows further resolution of the acute whitening of the retina with a diffuse granularity secondary to the choroidal ischemia, decreased retinal vascular caliber, and sheathing irregularities from the retinal arteriolar ischemia. There are also compensatory arteriole-arteriole connections between the retinal and ciliary circulations at the optic nerve head.

26–6 and 26–7 This patient has a central retinal artery occlusion. Note the plaque inferiorly *(arrowhead)*. Fluorescein angiography in this case reveals blockage secondary to the overlying edema in the macular region.

26–8 CENTRAL RETINAL ARTERY OCCLUSION

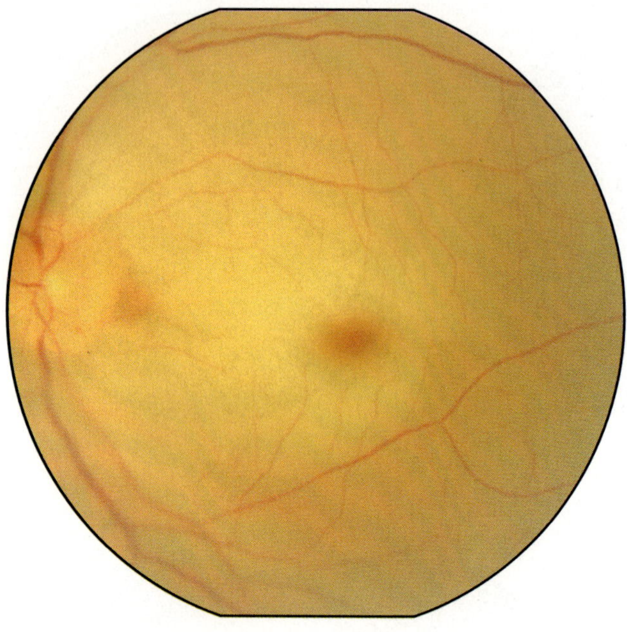

26–9

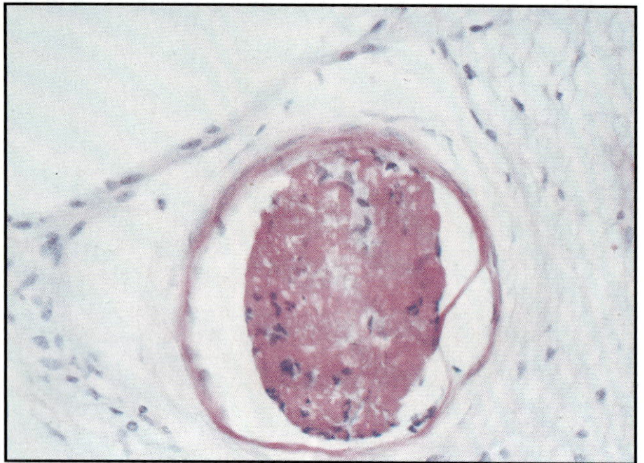

26–10

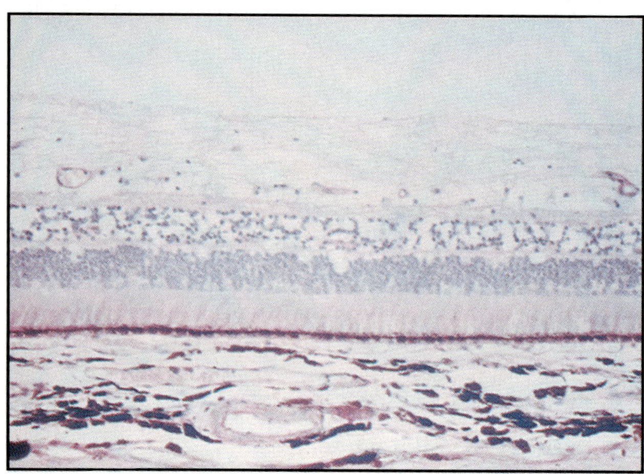

26–8 This patient also has a central retinal artery occlusion with a cherry-red spot and retinal edema. There is very minimal sparing of the peripapillary retina from perfused ciliary vessels.

26–9 and 26–10 Recent central retinal artery occlusion with a fresh thrombus and edema and pyknosis of the inner retinal layers.

26–11

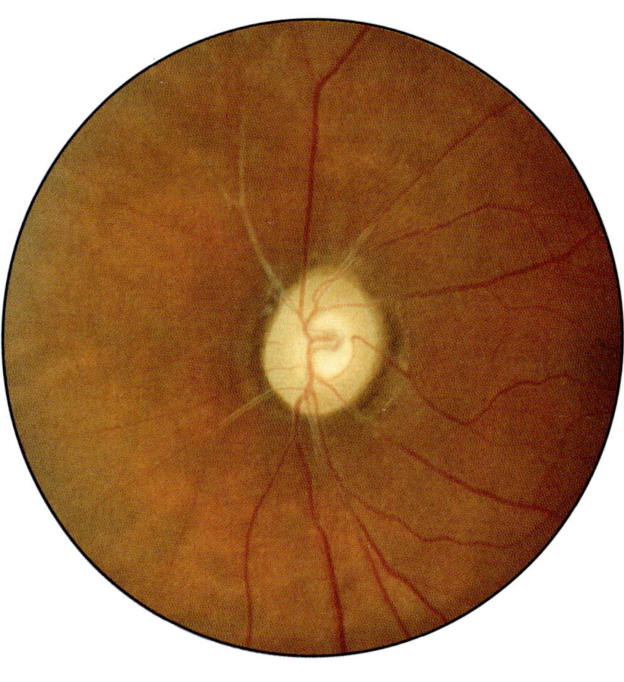

26–12 **26–13**

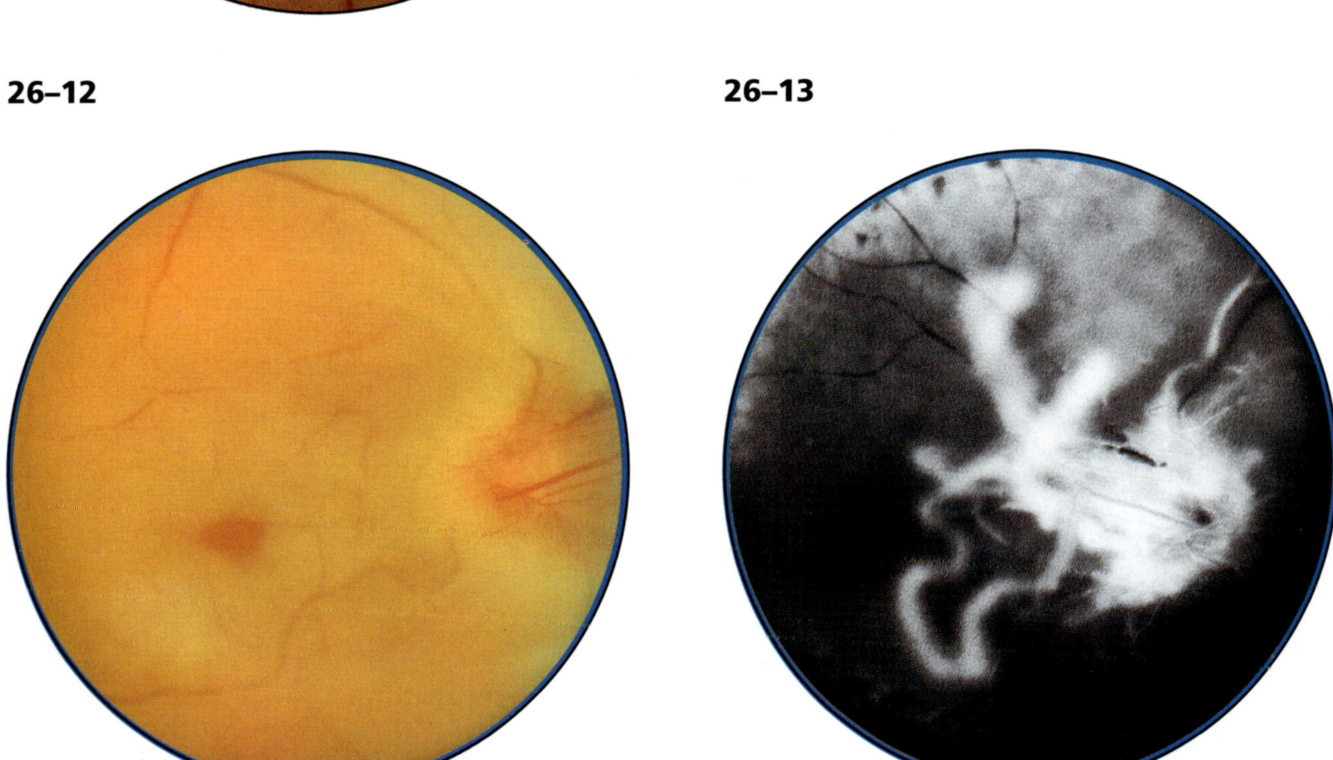

26–11 This patient has a pale optic disc and sheathed vessels from a central retinal artery occlusion secondary to a retrobulbar intrasheath hemorrhage.

26–12 and 26–13 This patient has proliferative diabetic retinopathy, optic disc neovascularization, and a central retinal artery occlusion. Note the cherry-red spot and the perfused area derived from the ciliary circulation. Note the neovascularization on the disc. The fluorescein angiogram confirms the presence of neovascularization, which originates from the patent choroidal circulation.

26–14 BRANCH RETINAL ARTERY OCCLUSION

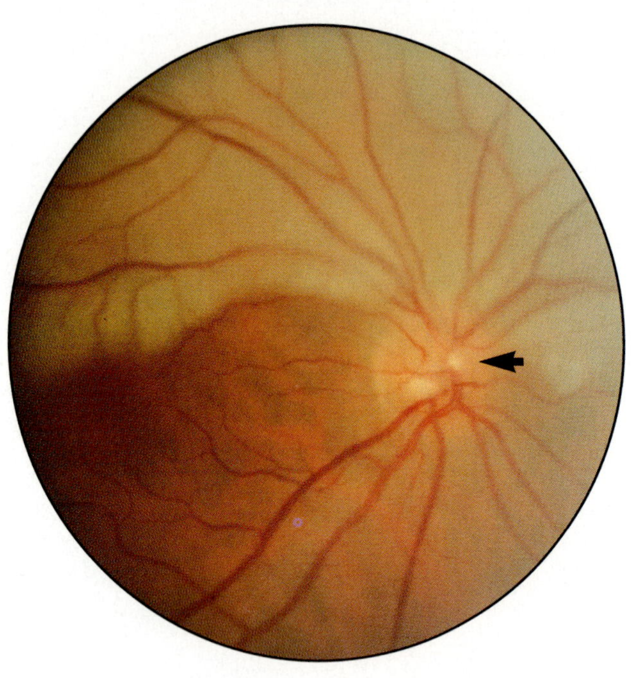

26–15

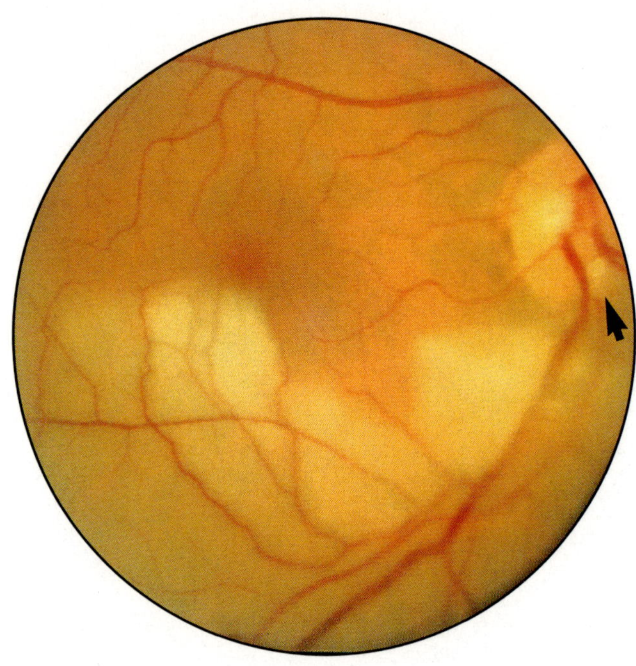

26–14 This patient has a branch retinal artery occlusion with a hemispheric whitening of the retina from the occlusion. There is a plaque on the surface of the disc within the arteriole *(arrowhead)*. This patient's embolism was secondary to mitral valve prolapse (Barlow's syndrome).

26–15 This patient has a branch retinal artery occlusion with whitening secondary to retinal edema. There is a sectorial sparing of the retina in the inferonasal macula from a patent, perfusing, ciliary retinal artery. Note the glistening plaque on the optic disc *(arrowhead)* consistent with embolic disease.

26–16

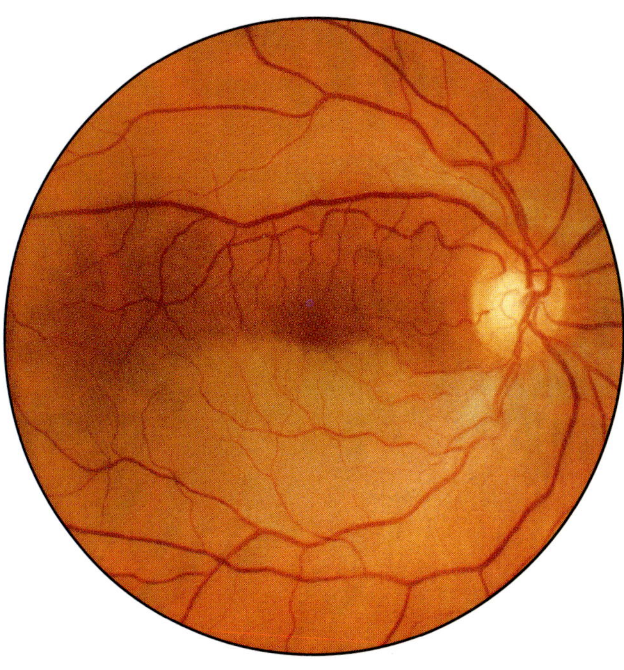

26–17

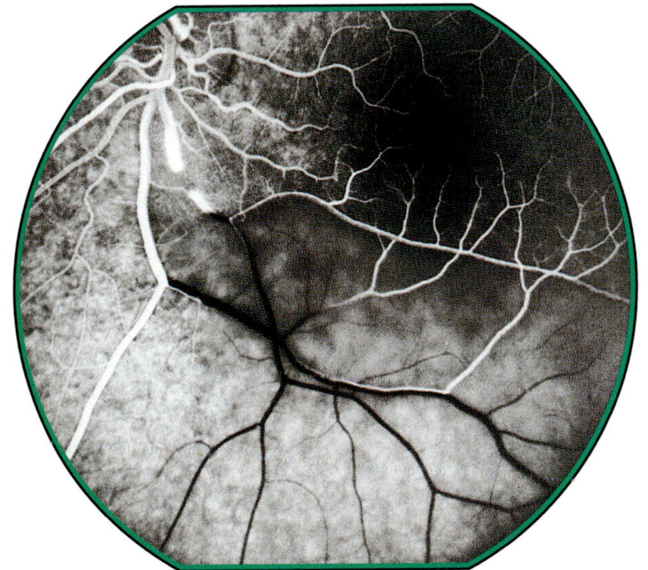

26–18

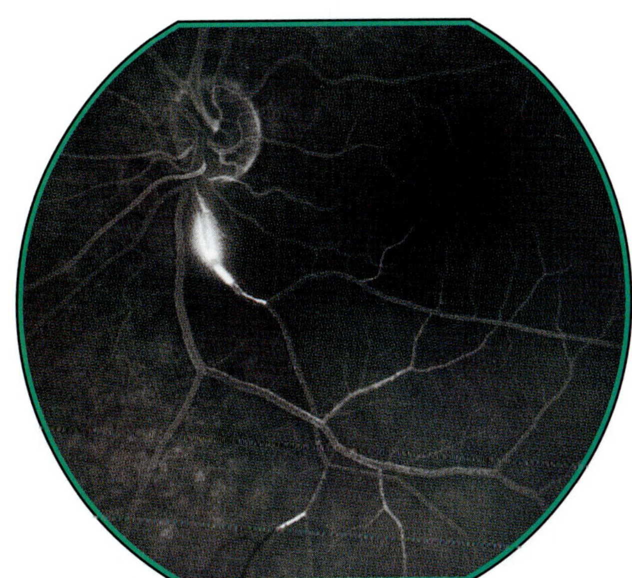

26–16 This patient shows acute whitening of the superior and inferior retina secondary to artery occlusions. There is sparing of the superior macula by a patent ciliary vessel.

26–17 and 26–18 The fluorescein angiogram in another patient with recurrent retinal branch artery occlusions shows delayed perfusion of the involved arteriole as well as the corresponding venule. The fluorescein angiogram of an additional patient with recurrent retinal branch artery occlusions shows staining at the proximal segment of acute arteriolar obstruction. There is also a more peripheral area of nonperfusion from an older branch retinal occlusion in the more peripheral distribution of the vessel.

26–19 RECURRENT BRANCH RETINAL ARTERY OCCLUSIONS

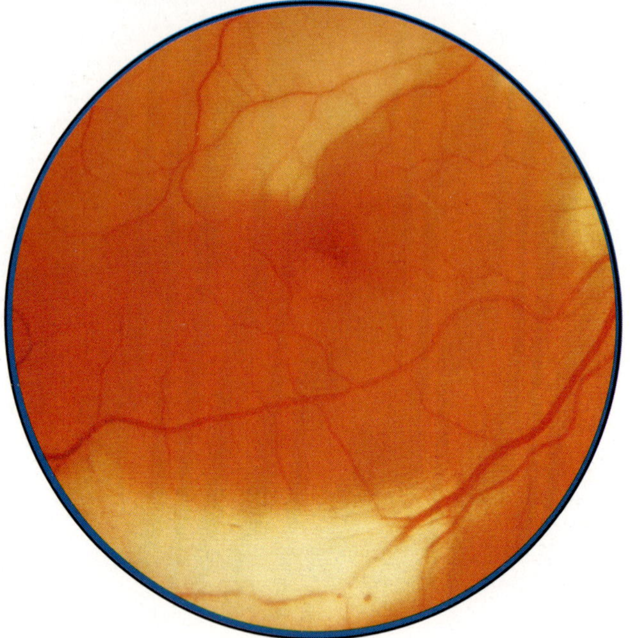

26–20

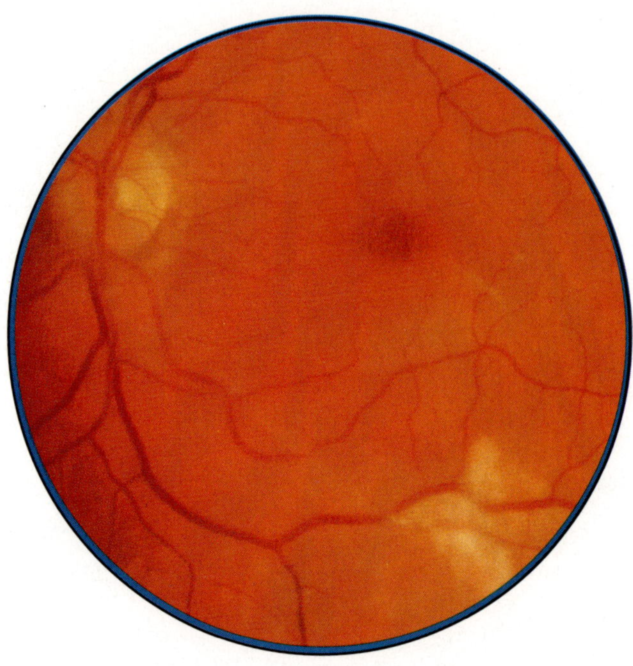

26–21

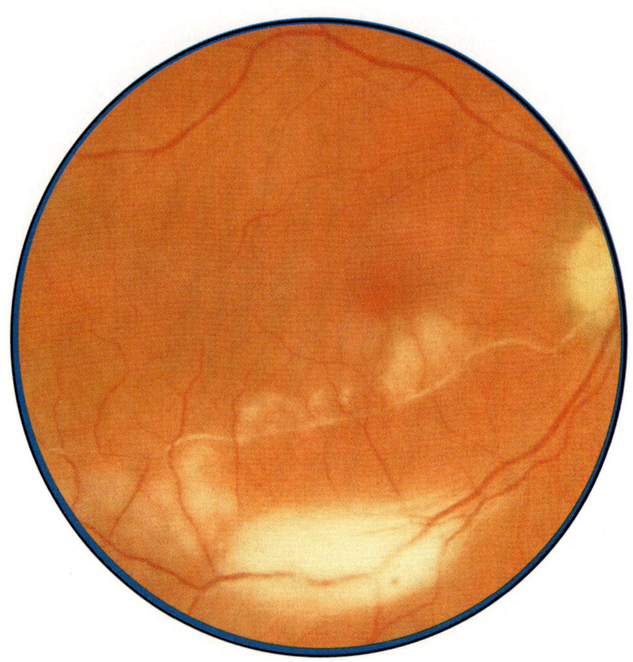

26–19 This patient had recurrent branch retinal artery occlusions. He first had a branch retinal artery occlusion in the right eye. Note the myelinated nerve fibers inferiorly.

26–20 Approximately 5 weeks later, a branch retinal artery occlusion was noted in his left eye.

26–21 Two years after the initial presentation, another branch retinal artery occlusion was noted in the right eye. This patient had incidental myelinated nerve fibers of the inferior artery and vein region, with an associated small aneurysm.

26–19 *through* ***26–21,*** *Courtesy of Dr. Len Joffe.*

26–22 SHEATHING

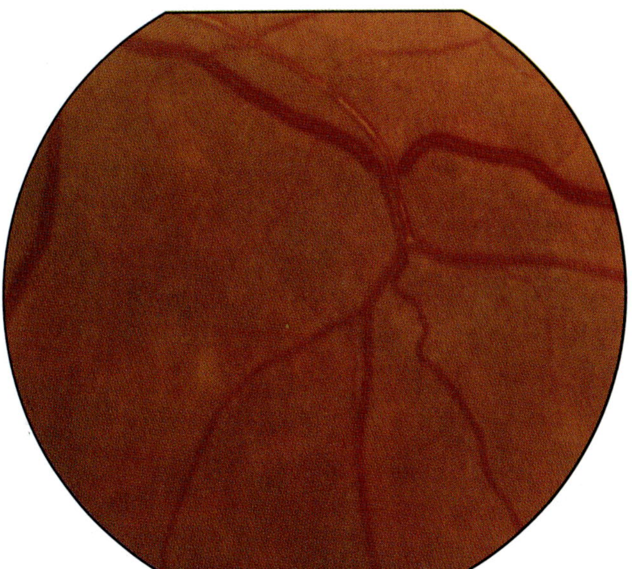

26–23 TRAUMA

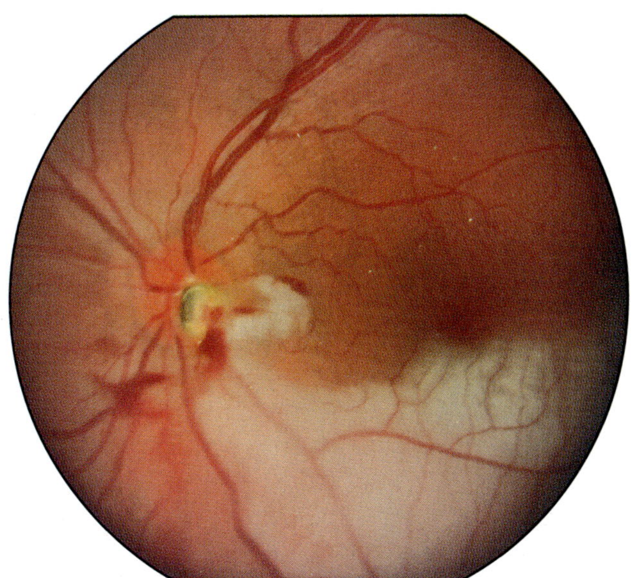

26–24 CILIORETINAL ARTERY OCCLUSION

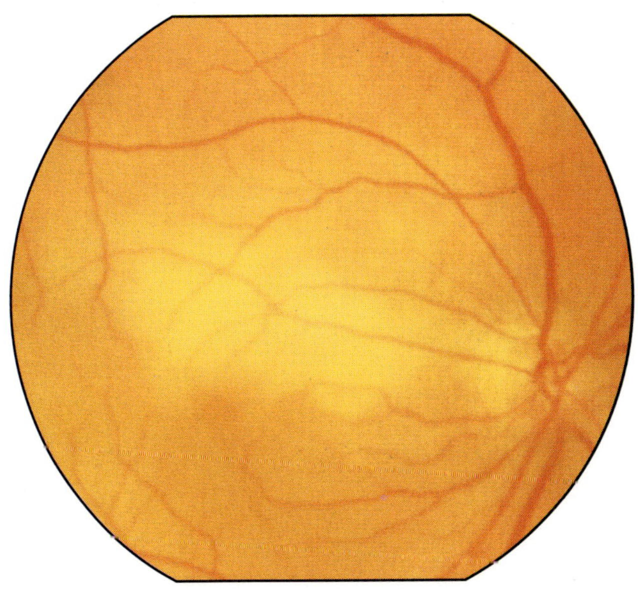

26–22 In this patient with an arterial occlusion, the sheathing extends to the bifurcation of the arteriole, which is the site of the antecedent occlusion.

26–23 This patient has a branch retinal artery occlusion with vitreous hemorrhage secondary to a metallic foreign body. He was struck with a hammer. There is also some preretinal hemorrhage induced by the impact of the foreign body on the surface of the optic nerve.

26–24 A cilioretinal artery occlusion is noted in this patient with whitening in the distribution of the cilioretinal artery.

26–22, *Courtesy of Bruce Morris, CRA.* ***26–23,*** *Courtesy of Dr. Keith Zinn.*

26–25 CHOROIDAL ISCHEMIA

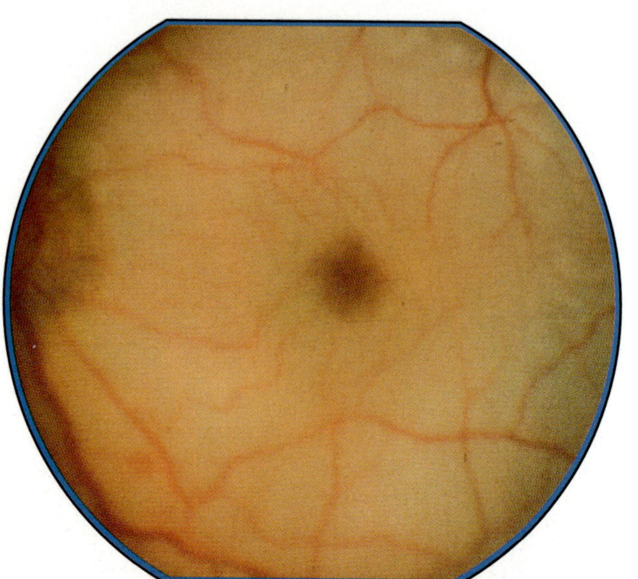

26–26

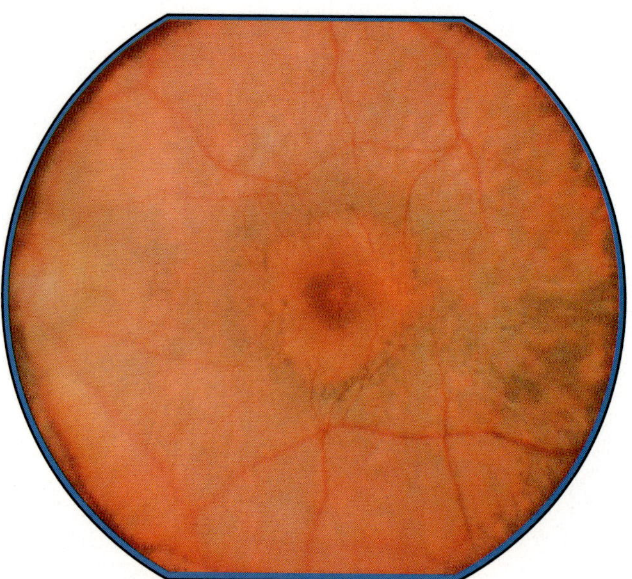

26–27

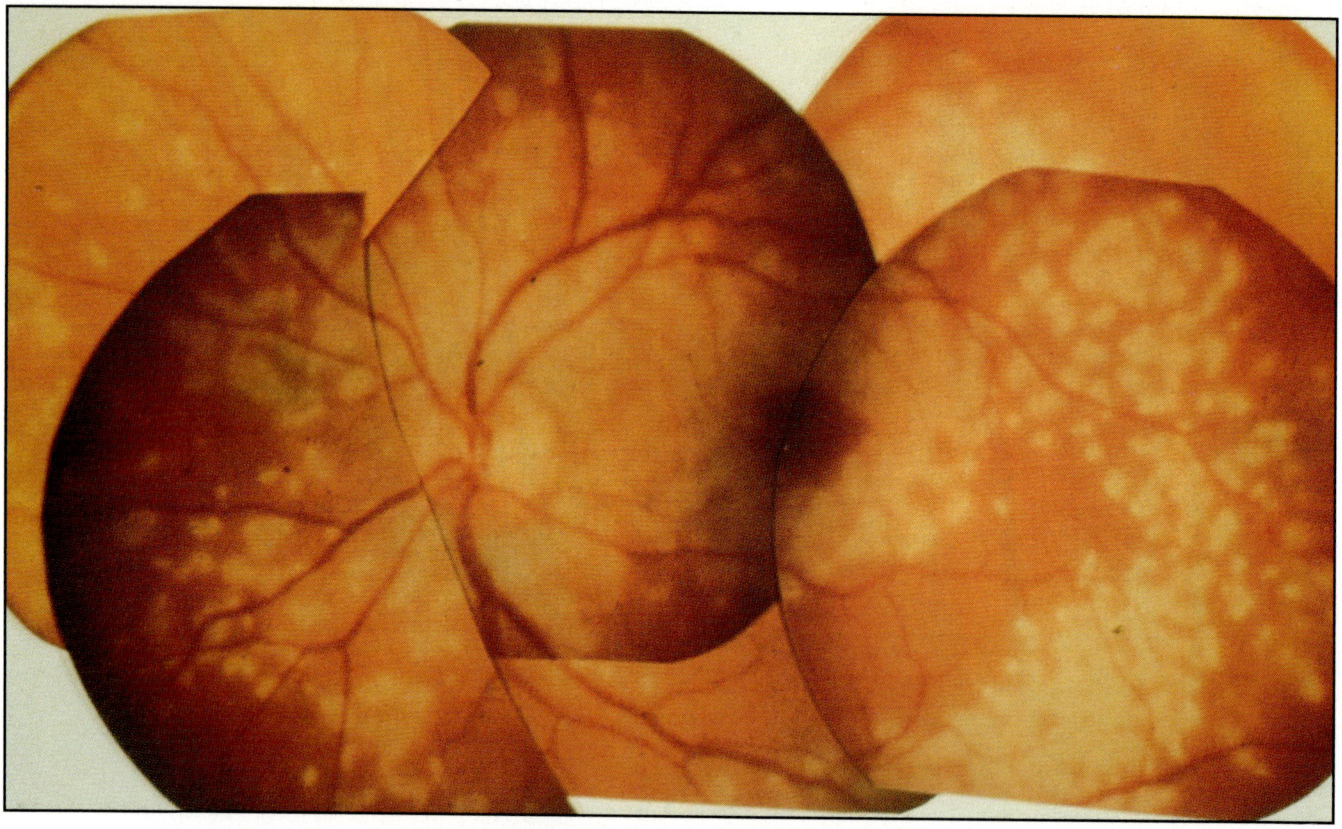

26–28

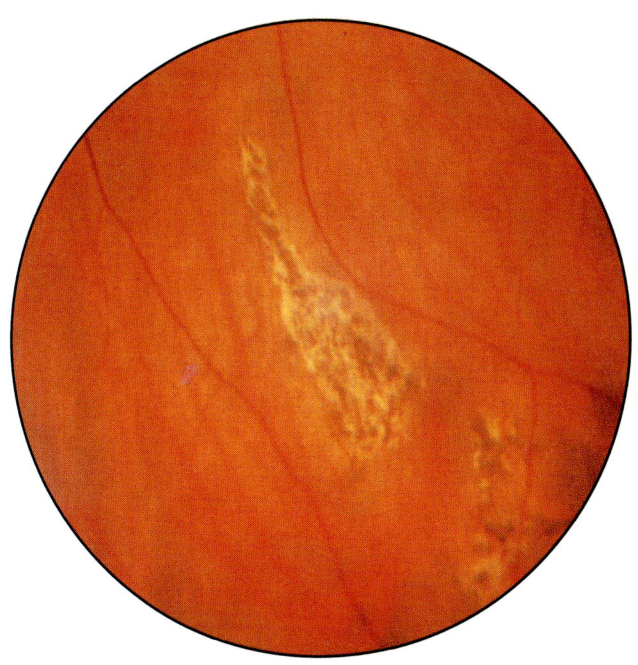

26–29

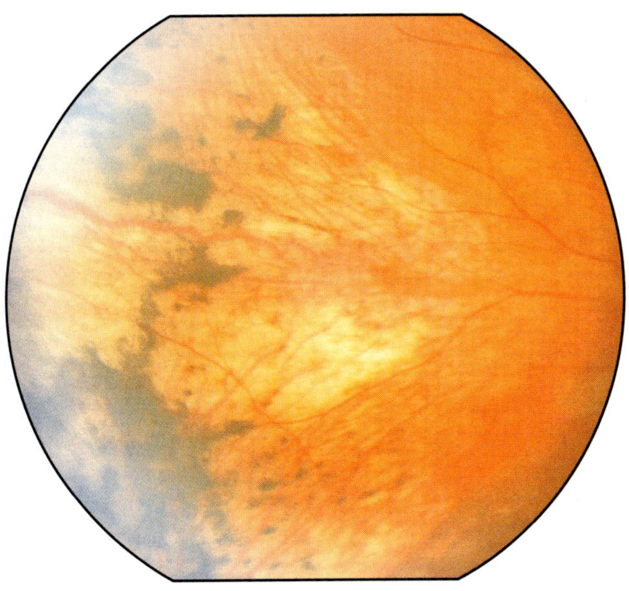

26–25 and 25–26 This patient has acute outer retinal infarction and choroidal ischemia following intraocular surgery. There is a cherry-red spot at the fovea. The optic nerve and retinal vasculature appear clinically uninvolved. The next photograph (25–26) is of the same patient following spontaneous resolution of the ischemia. Note the widespread retinal pigment epithelial atrophic and pigmentary disturbance, and the sparing of the perifoveal region. The visual acuity has returned to 20/25; however, there are areas of visual field loss corresponding to the choroidal pathology.

26–27 In this patient with choroidal ischemia following intraocular surgery, there is more diffuse ischemia. Some areas of deep or outer retinal infarction (choroidal ischemia) appear in a multifocal and variably confluent distribution. Again, there is sparing of the far periphery, fovea, optic nerve, and retinal circulation. The patchy outer choroidal ischemia may resemble a Purtscher's-like retinopathy.

26–28 There are multiple healed choroidal infarctions in this patient with embolic obstructive disease secondary to a cardiac myxoma. The tail of the larger infarction follows the course of the occluded ciliary vessel.

26–29 This larger choroidal infarct was caused by ischemia to the posterior ciliary arteries during central retinal vein decompression.

26–25 *through* ***26–27,*** *Courtesy of Dr. Ronald G. Michels.* ***26–28,*** *Courtesy of Dr. Dan Weidenthal.* ***26–29,*** *From Rodriguez, A, Rodriguez, FJ, Betancourt, F: Presumed occlusion of posterior ciliary arteries following central retinal vein decompression surgery, Arch Ophthalmol 112:54–56, 1994. Courtesy of Dr. Francisco Rodriguez.*

Suggested Readings

Augsburger, JJ, and Magargal, LE: Visual prognosis following treatment of acute central retinal artery obstruction, Br J Ophthalmol 64:913–917, 1980

Brown, GC, Brown, MM, Hiller, T, Fischer, D, Benson, WE, and Magargal, LE: Cotton-wool spots, Retina 5:206–214, 1985

Brown, GC, Magargal, LE, Augsburger, JJ, and Shields, JA: Preretinal arterial loops and retinal arterial occlusion, Am J Ophthalmol 87:646–651, 1979

Brown, GC, and Reber, R: An unusual presentation of branch retinal artery obstruction in association with ocular neovascularization, Can J Ophthalmol 21:103–106, 1986

Duker, J, and Brown, GC: Neovascularization associated with obstruction of the central retinal artery, Ophthalmology 95;1244–1249, 1988

ffytche, TJ, Bulpitt, CJ, Kohner, EM, Archer, D, and Dollery, CT: Effects of changes in intraocular pressure on the retinal microcirculation, Br J Ophthalmol 58:514–522, 1974

Gold, D: Retinal arterial occlusion, Trans Am Acad Ophthalmol Otolaryngol 83:392–408, 1977

Hayreh, SS: The cilio-retinal arteries, Br J Ophthalmol 47:71–89, 1963

Henkind, P, and Wise, GN: Retinal neovascularization, collaterals, and vascular shunts, Br J Ophthalmol 58:413–422, 1974

Jampol, Lm, Wong, AS, and Albert, DM: Atrial myxoma and central retinal artery occlusion, Am J Ophthalmol 75:242–249, 1973

Kraushar, MF, and Brown, GC: Retinal neovascularization after branch retinal arterial obstruction, Am J Ophthalmol 104:294–296, 1987

Manschot, WA, and Lee, WR: Development of retinal neovascularization in vascular occlusive disease, Trans Ophthalmol Soc UK 104:880–886, 1985

McLeod, D, Marshall, J, Kohner, EM, and Bird, AC: The role of axoplasmic transport in the pathogenesis of retinal cotton-wool spots, Br J Ophthalmol 61:177–191, 1977

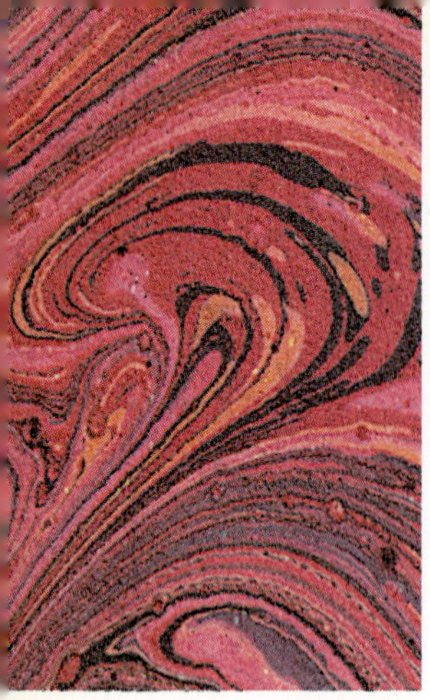

Chapter 27

Central Retinal Vein Occlusions

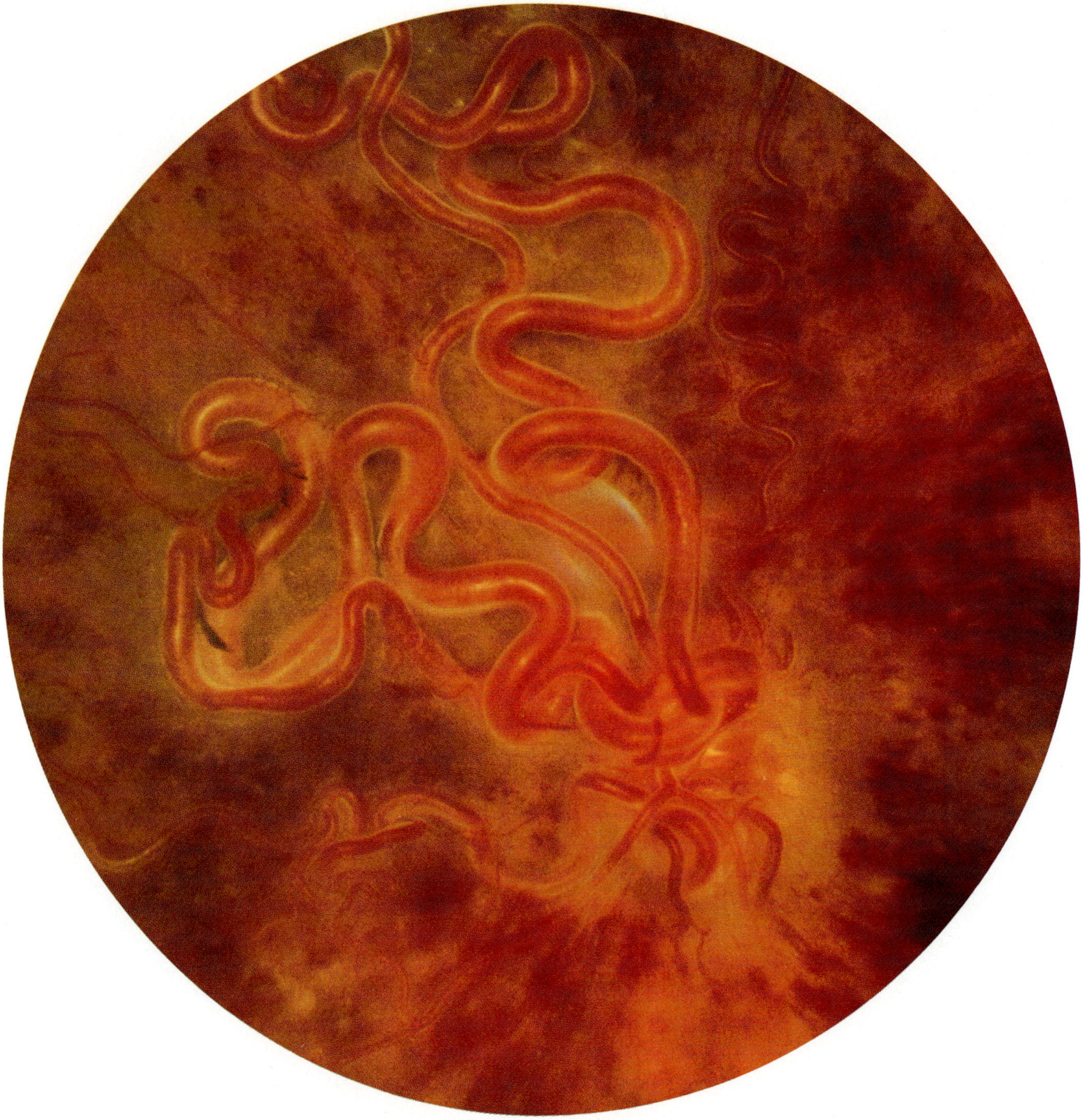

A central retinal vein occlusion is a common retinal vascular abnormality usually seen in patients over 50 years of age. Thrombosis of the central retinal vein in the area of the lamina cribrosa is commonly seen on histopathologic examination. There are two types of central retinal vein occlusions: an ischemic and a nonischemic type. An ischemic retinal vein occlusion may progress to capillary nonperfusion, retinal neovascularization, and vitreous hemorrhage. Neovascular glaucoma is a dreaded complication of an ischemic vein occlusion. Nonischemic vein occlusions have a better prognosis. Macular edema may also occur in eyes with venous occlusions.

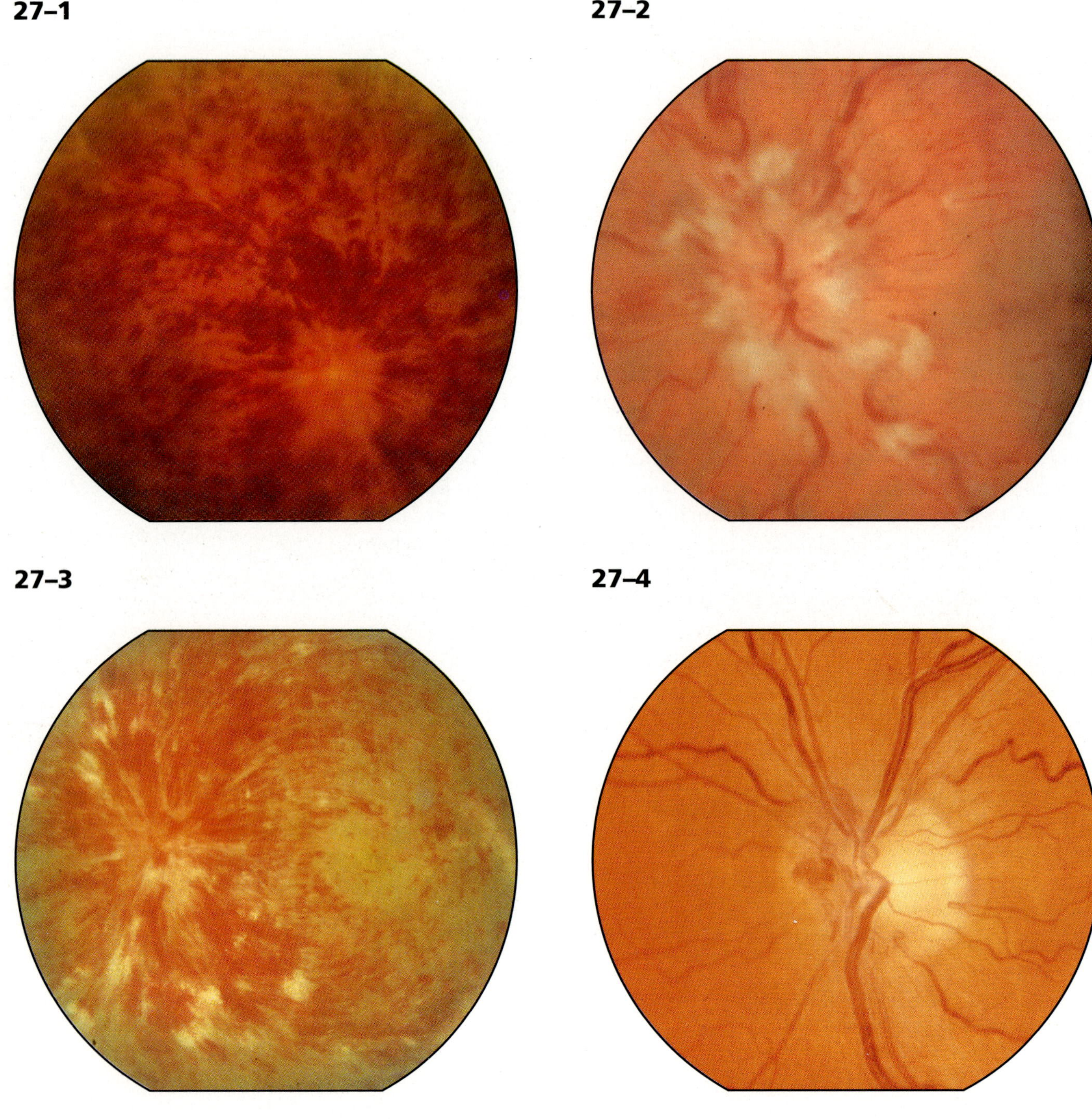

27–1 This patient has a central retinal vein occlusion with extensive intraretinal hemorrhages.

27–2 The next patient has an ischemic central retinal vein occlusion with optic disc edema and multiple cotton-wool spots, in addition to retinal hemorrhages.

27–3 This 32-year-old female with an underlying blood dyscrasia initially had a hemispheric branch retinal vein occlusion inferiorly as is evident by the tortuous, sheathed venule in that area. She subsequently developed a complete central retinal vein occlusion. There is widespread hemorrhage and axoplasmic debris as well as severe macular edema.

27–4 In this patient, compensatory collateralization evolved at the disc following a central retinal vein occlusion. These compensatory vessels are slow to perfuse, and they do not stain with fluorescein, which differentiates them from preretinal neovascularization.

27–5

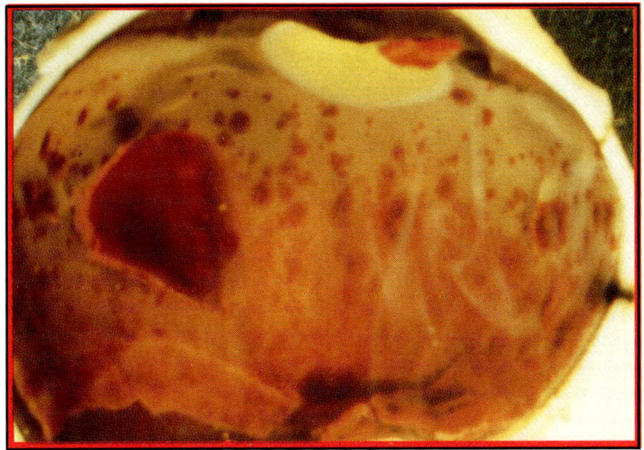

27–6

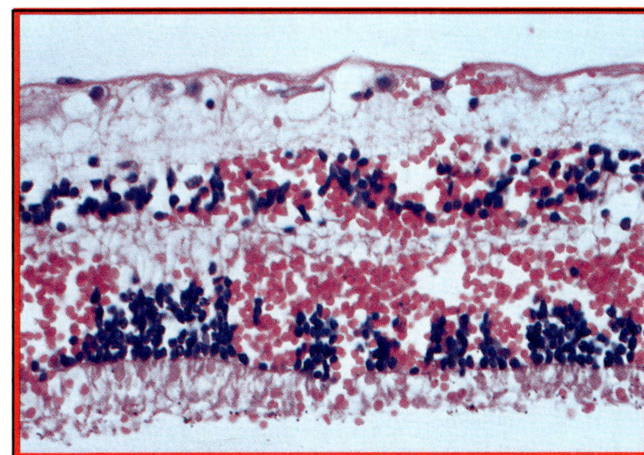

27–7

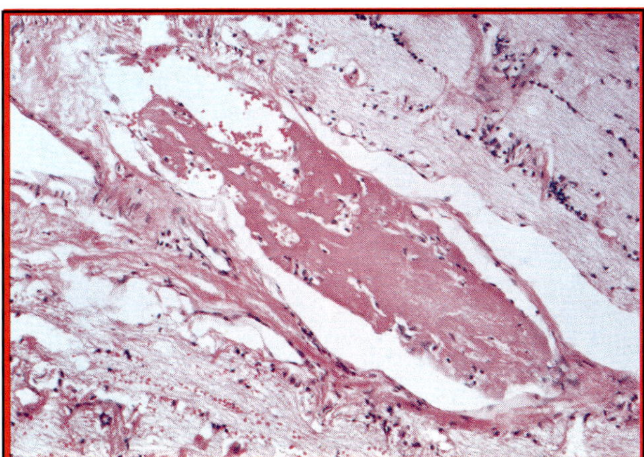

27–7A

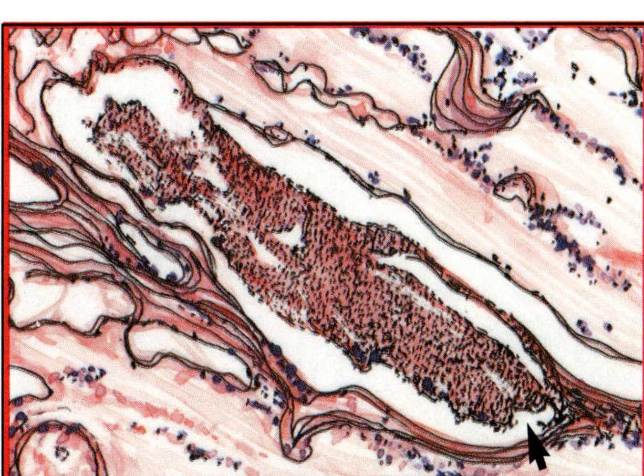

27–5 through 27–7A This is a clinicopathologic correlation of a central retinal occlusion of 24 hours duration. Extensive hemorrhage is present throughout the retina. Light microscopy shows deep retinal hemorrhage (27–6) and a fresh thrombus *(arrowhead)* in the central retinal vein at the posterior aspect of the lamina cribrosa (27–7). Hemorrhage can be seen throughout the retina.

***27–5** through **27–7,** From Green, WR, Chan, CC, Hutchins, GM, and Terry, JM: Central retinal vein occlusion: a prospective histopathologic study of 29 eyes in 28 cases, Retina 1:27–55, 1981.*

27–8 WYBURN-MASON SYNDROME

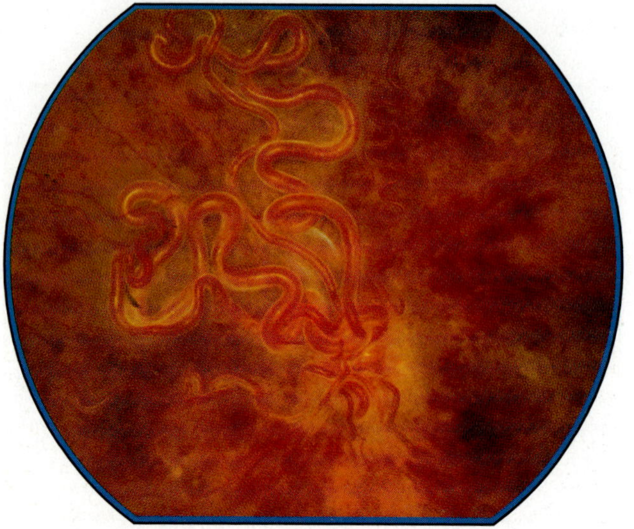

27–9

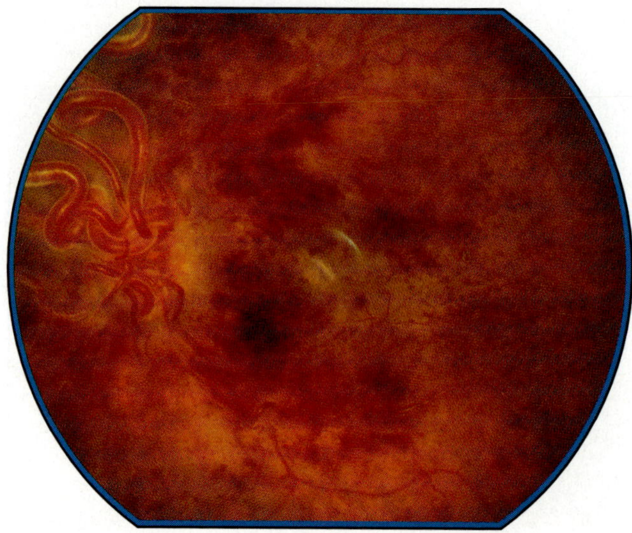

27–10

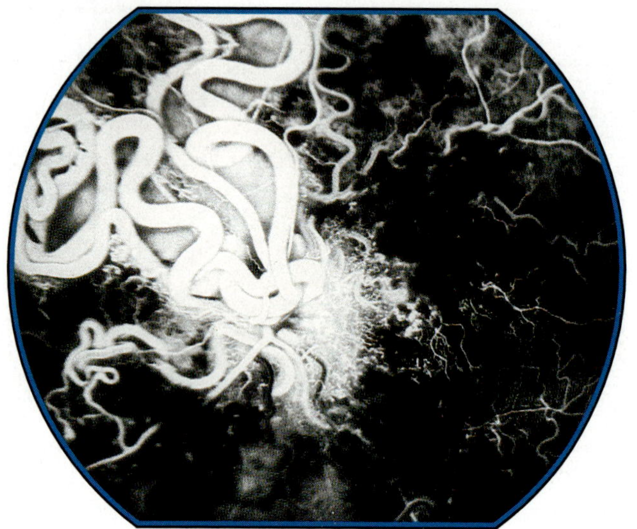

27–11

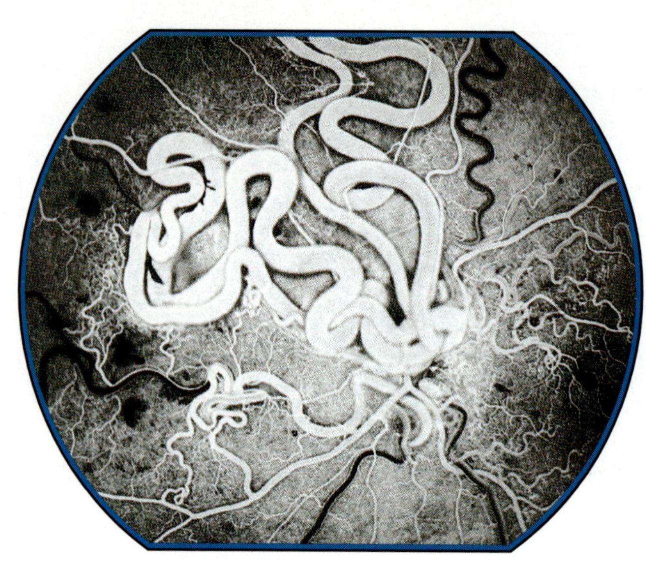

27–12

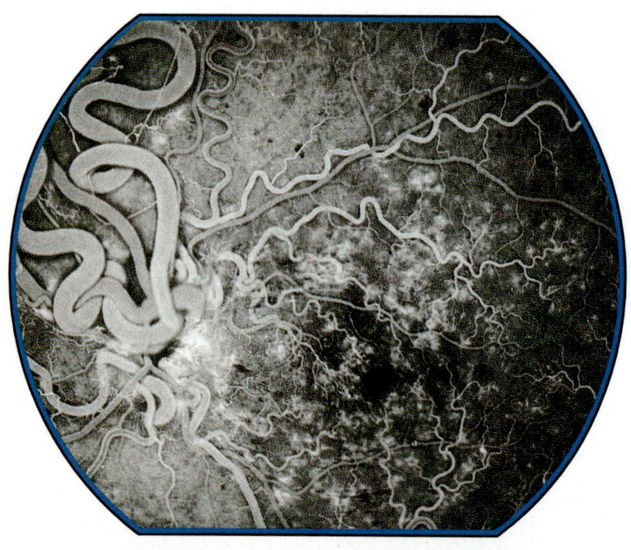

27–8 and 27–9 This patient has an arteriovenous malformation associated with the Wyburn-Mason syndrome and developed a central retinal vein occlusion.

27–10 through 27–12 Note the dilated vessels on the fluorescein angiogram. Telangiectatic vessels can be demonstrated in the macular region. Figures 27–11 and 27–12 were taken at another time than 27–10, which shows blockage secondary to the blood.

27–13 CAROTID CAVERNOUS FISTULA

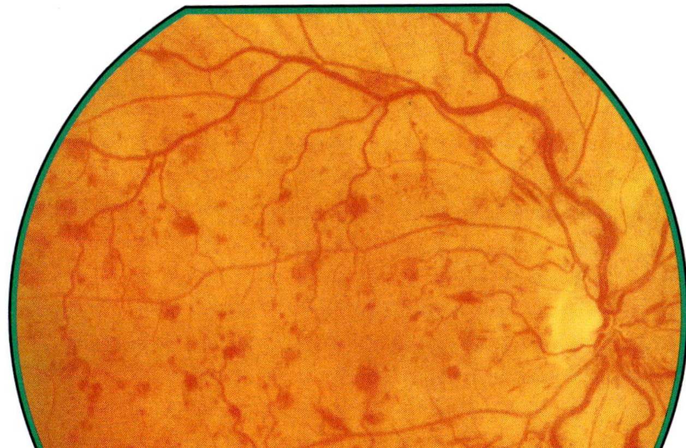

27–14

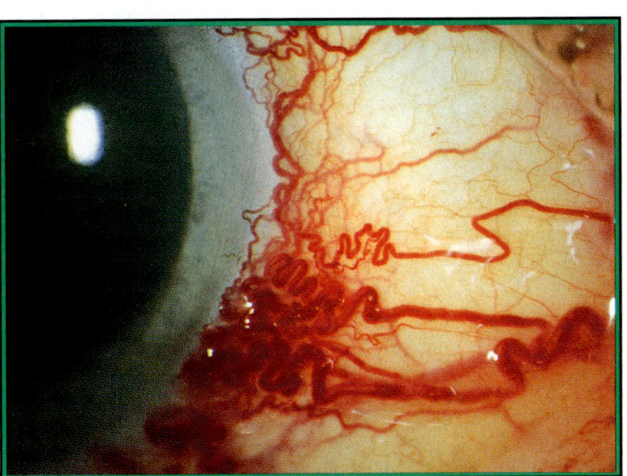

27–13 This patient has intraretinal hemorrhages and tortuous vessels.

27–14 The same patient also has dilated conjunctional vessels due to a carotid cavernous fistula. Carotid cavernous fistulas should be considered in the differential diagnosis of central retinal vein occlusions.

27–13 *and* ***27–14,*** *Courtesy of Robert Hammond.*

27–15 CRVO AND BRVO

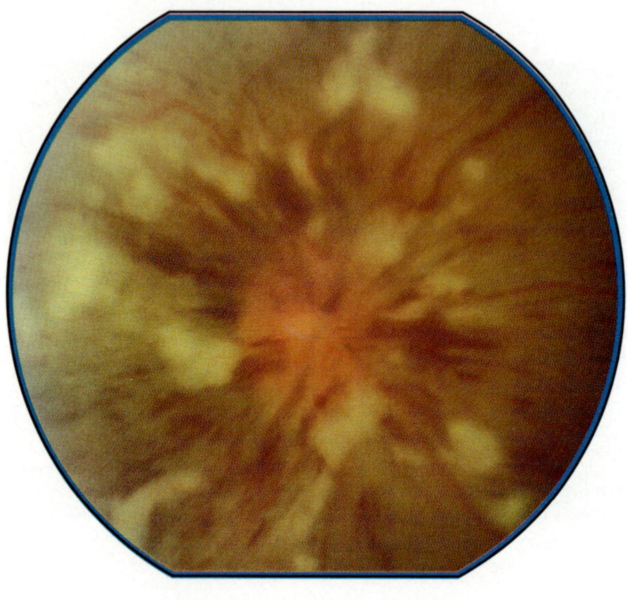

27–16

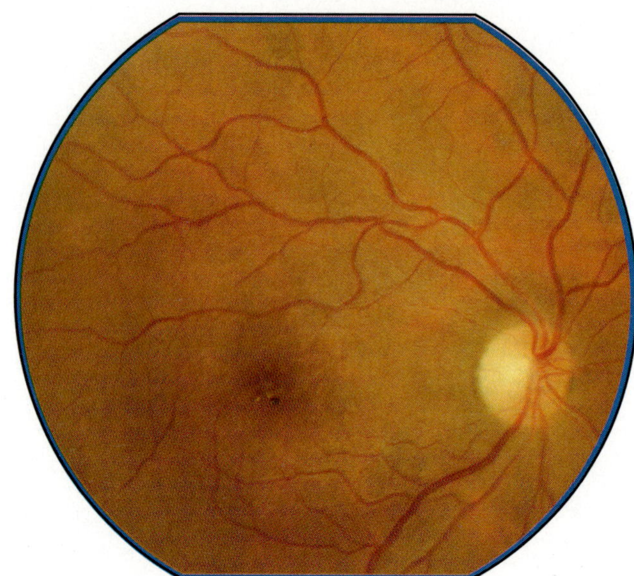

27–17

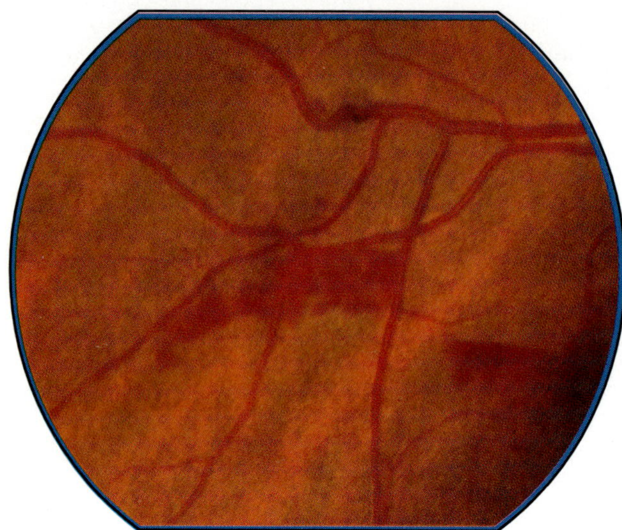

27–18

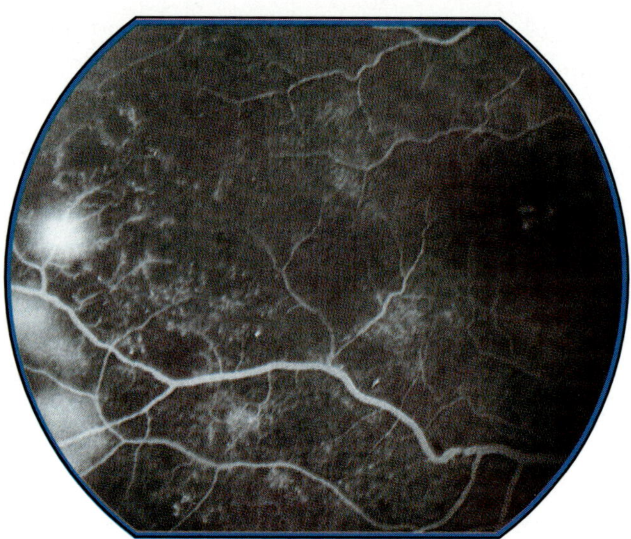

27–15 This patient has a central retinal vein occlusion with intraretinal hemorrhages and cotton-wool spots.

27–16 The central retinal vein occlusion cleared. There was residual minor pigmentary and atrophic change at the level of the retinal pigment epithelium from the antecedent edema. There was no sign of residual edema or a retinal vascular occlusive abnormality suggestive of a previous central retinal vein occlusion.

27–17 The patient subsequently presented with vitreous hemorrhage.

27–18 The fluorescein angiogram taken at this time revealed a retinal microangiopathy and preretinal neovascularization in the distribution of the inferior temporal vasculature, consistent with an independent secondary branch retinal vein occlusion. The rest of his retina did not reveal any perfusion abnormalities.

Suggested Readings

The Central Vein Occlusion Study Group: Baseline and early natural history report: the Central Vein Occlusion Study (CVOS), Arch Ophthalmol 111:1087–1095, 1993

Green, WR, Chan, CC, Hutchins, GM, and Terry, JM: Central retinal vein occlusion: a prospective histopathologic study of 29 eyes in 28 cases, Retina 1:27–55, 1981

Gutman, FA: Evaluation of a patient with central retinal vein occlusion, Ophthalmology 90:481–483, 1983

Hayreh, SS: Classification of central retinal vein occlusion, Ophthalmology 90:458–474, 1983

Hayreh, SS, Rojas, P, Podhajsky, P, Montague, P, and Woolson, RF: Ocular neovascularization with retinal vascular occlusion. III. Incidence of ocular neovascularization with retinal vein occlusion, Ophthalmology 90:488–506, 1983

Johnson, MA, and Finkelstein, D: Neovascularization and retinal sensitivity loss in patients with retinal ischemia, Invest Ophthalmol Vis Sci 27(Suppl):145, 1986

Kohner, E: Photocoagulation prevents thrombotic glaucoma in ischemic central retinal vein occlusion, Symposium on Central Vein Occlusion, 10th Annual Macula Society Meeting, June 26, 1987, Cannes, France

Laatikainen, L, Kohner, EM, Khoury, D, and Blach, RK: Panretinal photocoagulation in central retinal vein occlusion: a randomized controlled clinical study, Br J Ophthalmol 61:741–753, 1977

Magargal, LE, Brown, GC, Augsburger, JJ, and Donoso, LA: Efficacy of panretinal photocoagulation in preventing neovascular glaucoma following ischemic central retinal vein obstruction, Ophthalmology 89:780–784, 1982

Magargal, LE, Donoso, LA, and Sandborn, GE: Retinal ischemia and risk of neovascularization following central retinal vein obstruction, Ophthalmology 89:1241–1245, 1982

Sabates, R, Hirose, T, and McMeel, JW: Electroretinography in the prognosis and classification of central retinal vein occlusion, Arch Ophthalmol 101:232–235, 1983

Smith, P, Green, WR, Miller, NR, and Terry, JM: Central retinal vein occlusion in Reye's syndrome, Arch Ophthalmol 98:1256–1260, 1980

Trempe, CL: Central retinal vein occlusion: Prevention of rubeosis iridis by proper medical management, Symposium on Central Vein Occlusion, 10th Annual Macula Society Meeting, June 26, 1987, Cannes, France

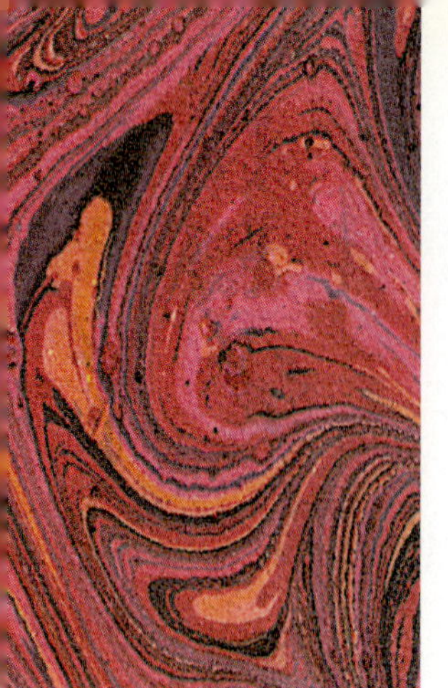

Chapter 28

Branch Retinal Vein Occlusion

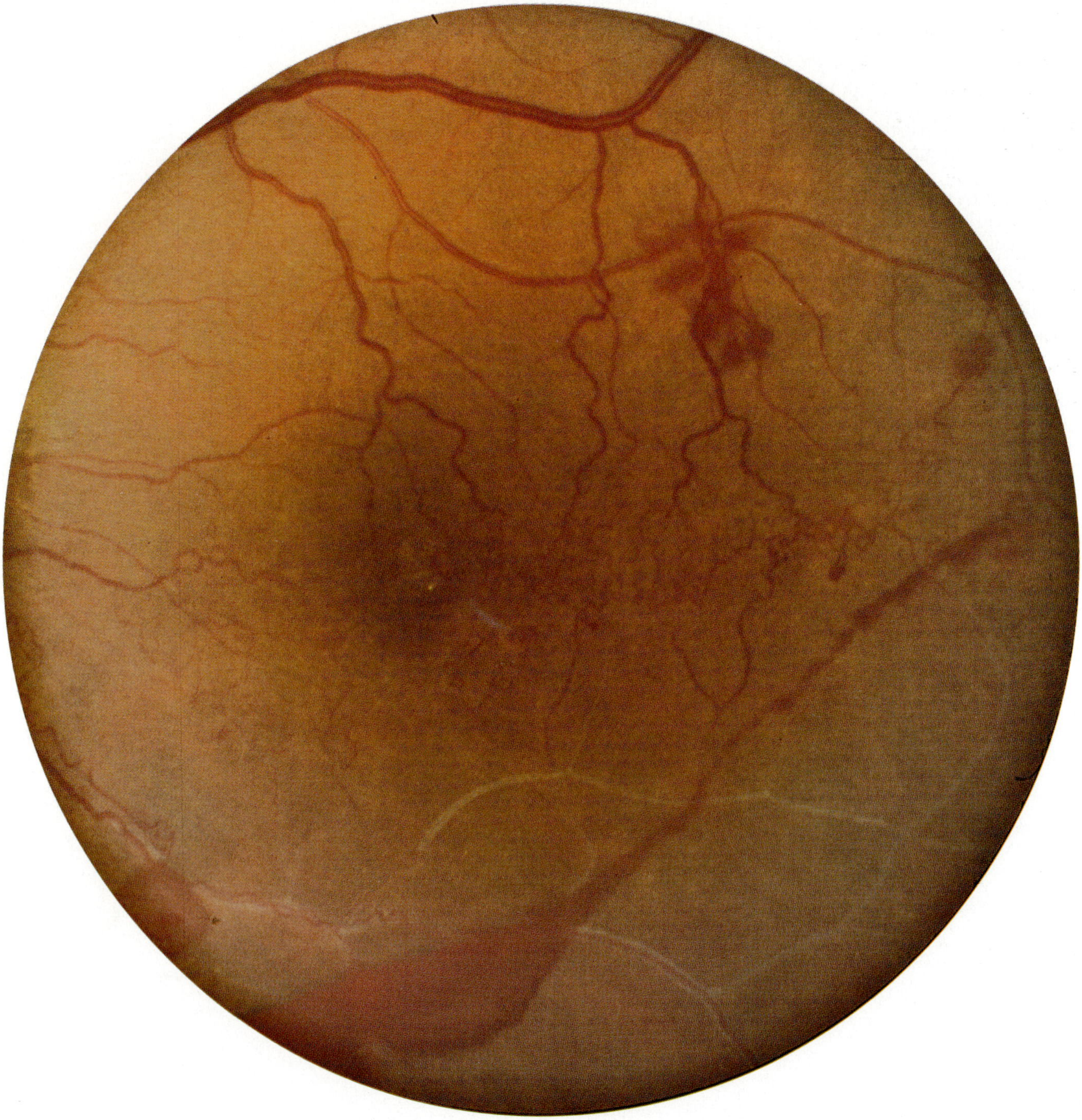

A branch retinal vein occlusion appears most frequently in elderly patients. The occlusion occurs at the site of an arteriovenous crossing. There is no conclusive evidence that any systemic disease plays an important role in the pathogenesis of this condition, although many of these patients have systemic hypertension. Complications of branch retinal vein occlusions include macular edema, capillary nonperfusion, and vitreous hemorrhage secondary to retinal neovascularization. Retinal neovascularization often occurs if a vein occlusion produces an area of capillary nonperfusion that is greater than 5 disc diameters by fluorescein angiography. Collateral formation must be distinguished from neovascularization. Fluorescein angiography will often be helpful in distinguishing these collaterals from actual neovascularization in difficult cases. The Collaborative Branch Retinal Vein Occlusion Study has described guidelines for laser photocoagulation for proliferative disease as well as for macular edema.

28–1

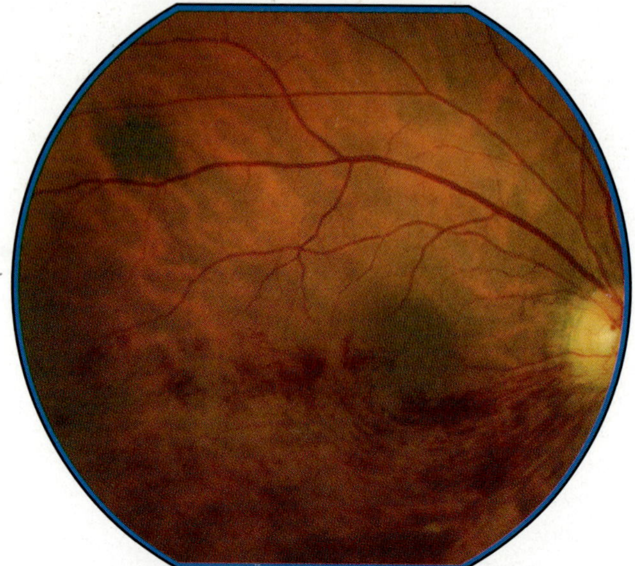

28–2

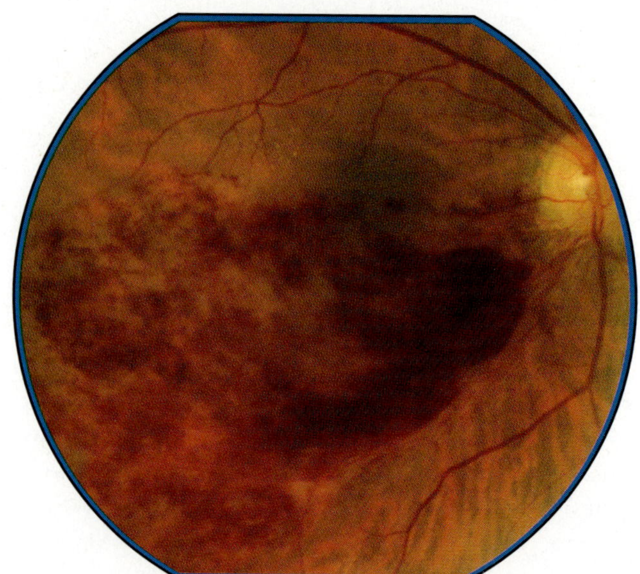

28–3

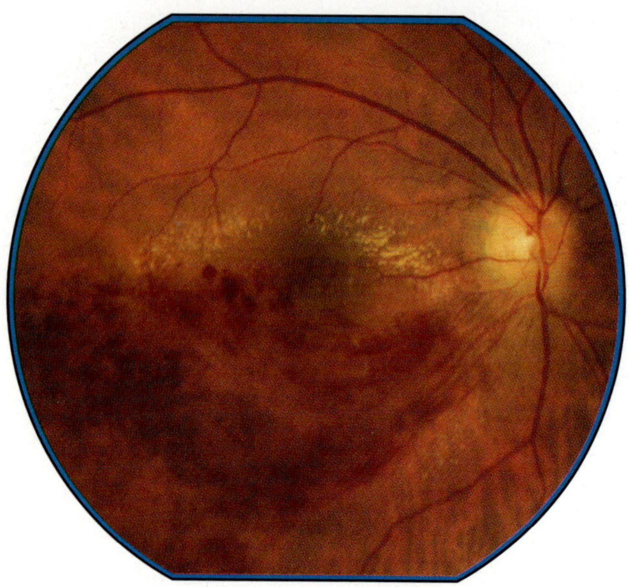

28–1 In this patient with a quadrantic branch retinal vein occlusion, there is diffuse retinal hemorrhage.

28–2 Two months later rebleeding occurred.

28–3 Three additional months later there is chronic and diffuse hemorrhage and intraretinal edema, which is fringed with lipid deposition.

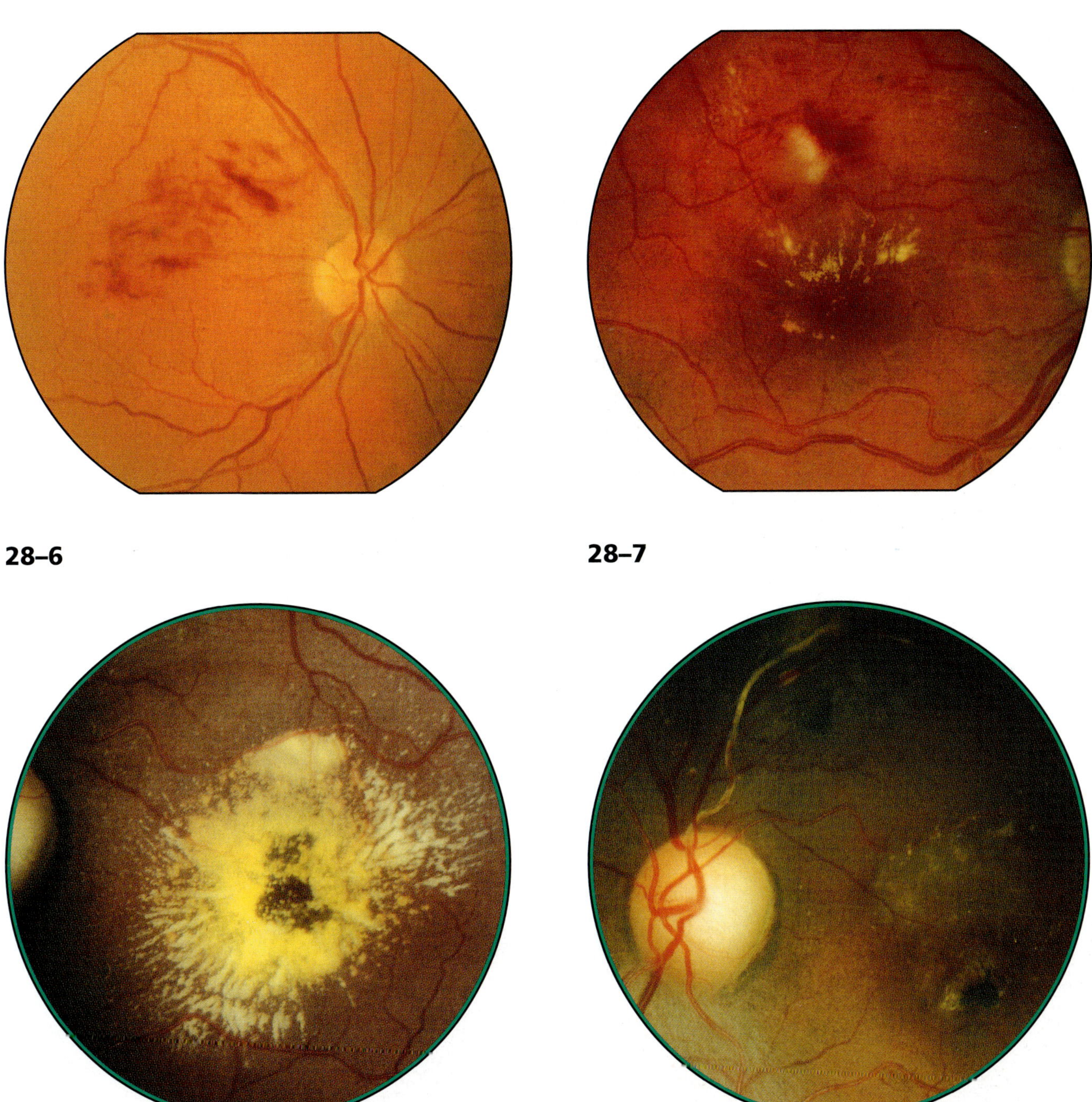

28–4 There are intraretinal hemorrhages and macular edema along the course of an occluded macular branch retinal vein in this patient. There is also more generalized arteriosclerotic vascular disease present.

28–5 This patient was referred with a diagnosis of diabetic macular edema. However, one can see that the patient actually has a superior branch retinal vein occlusion with cotton-wool spots, retinal hemorrhages, and secondary macular edema from the vein occlusion.

28–6 and 28–7 This patient with a branch retinal vein occlusion developed extensive macular edema. Following scatter laser photocoagulation there was resolution of the dense lipid. Some pigmentary degenerative change is evident along with sheathing of the involved vasculature.

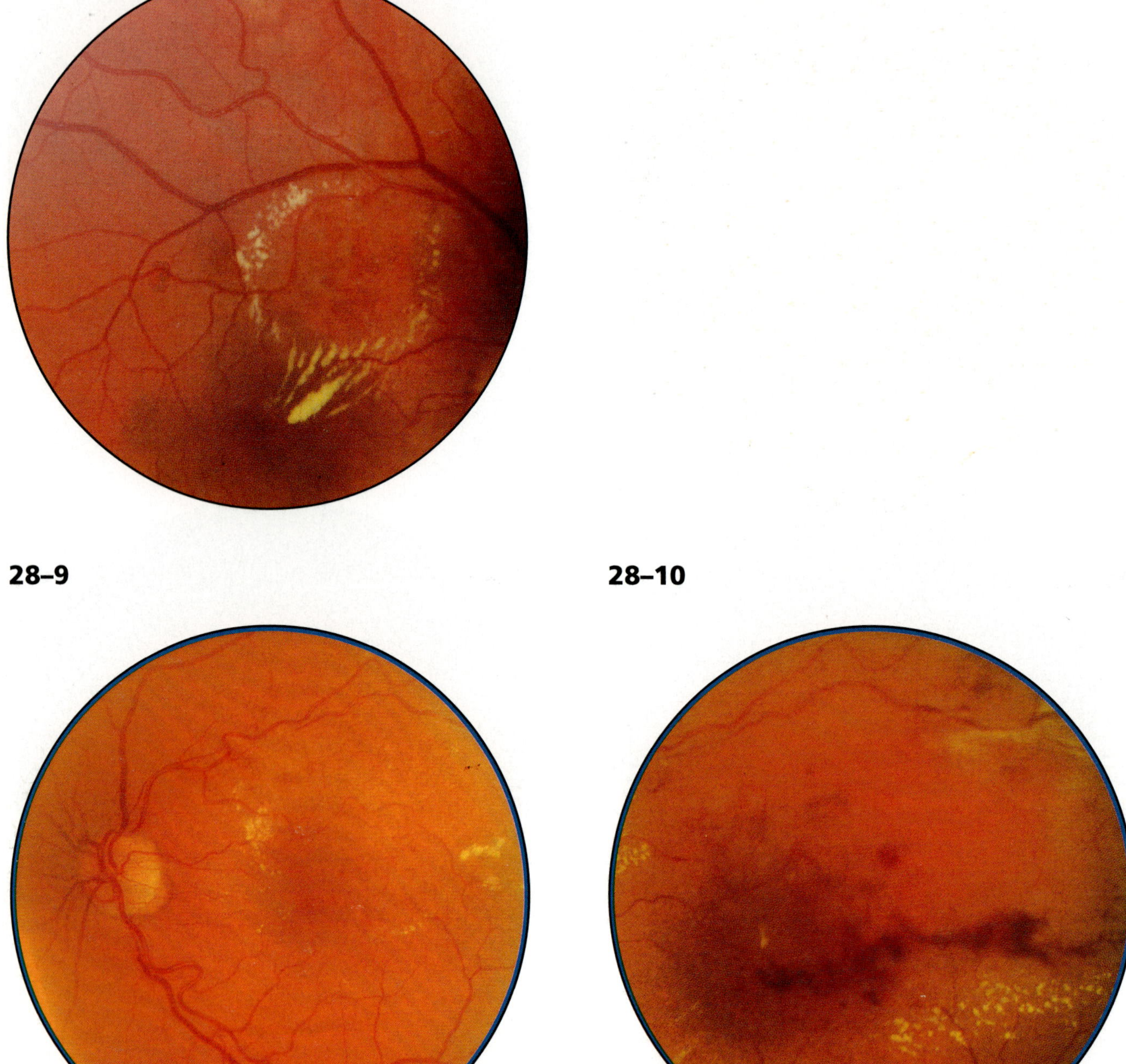

28–8 This patient has a macular branch retinal vein occlusion with a chronic microangiopathy consisting of telangiectatic and aneurysmal changes along the distribution of the vein, retinal thickening or edema, and a circinate pattern of lipid deposition with multiple wedged deposits toward the fovea.

28–9 and 28–10 This patient demonstrates a quadrantic macular vein occlusion with a chronic microangiopathy and persistent serous and lipid deposition. The patient refused laser photocoagulation treatment, and she experienced progressive exudative hemorrhagic change, epiretinal formation, and visual decline. No signs of compensatory collateralization evolved.

28–11

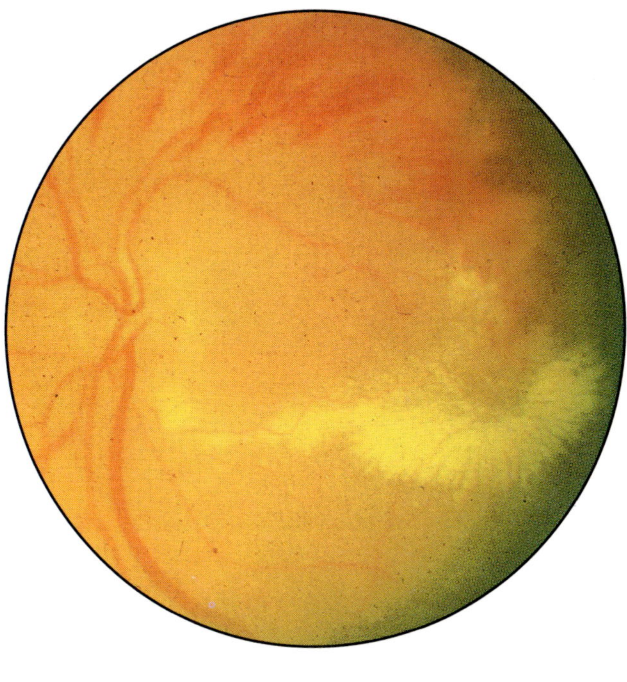

28–12

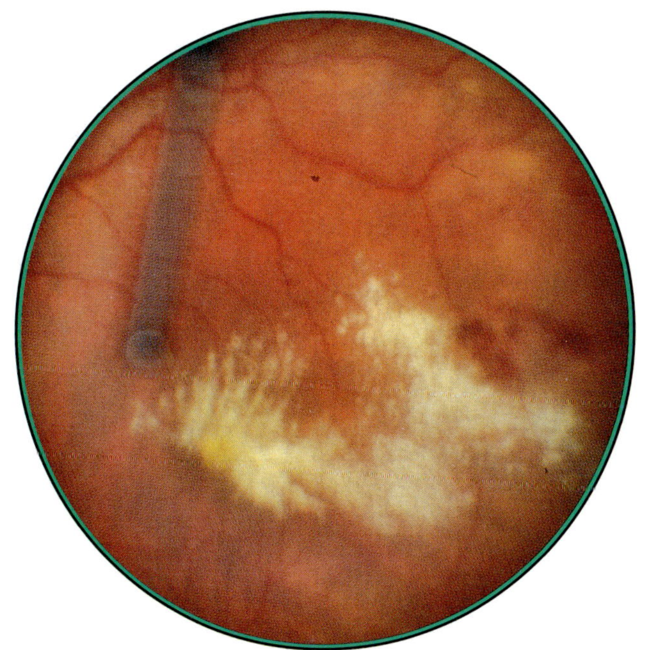

28–13

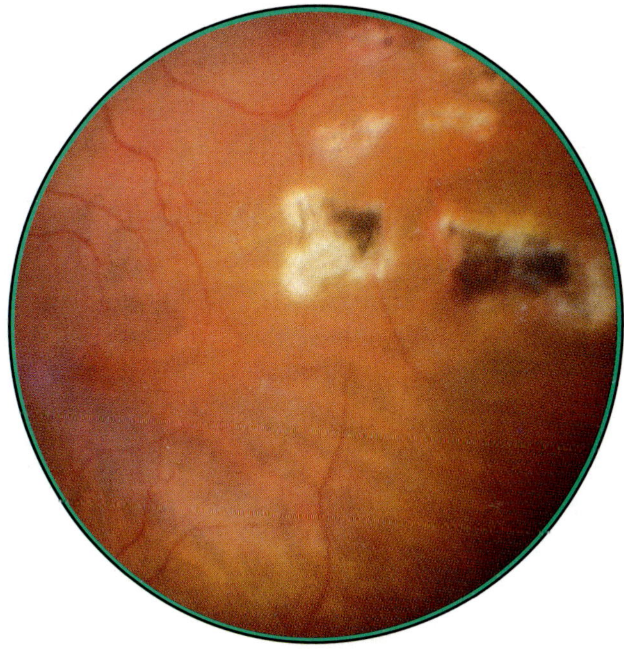

28–11 This patient demonstrates a branch retinal vein occlusion with heavy lipid deposition in the macula. There is also a neurosensory retinal detachment in the superior macula.

28–12 and 28–13 This patient has a branch retinal vein occlusion just beyond the central macula, associated with very heavy lipid deposition in the posterior pole. Laser photocoagulation treatment was carried out with minimal scattered applications in the superotemporal macula. This was associated with resolution of the exudative changes and improvement in the vision.

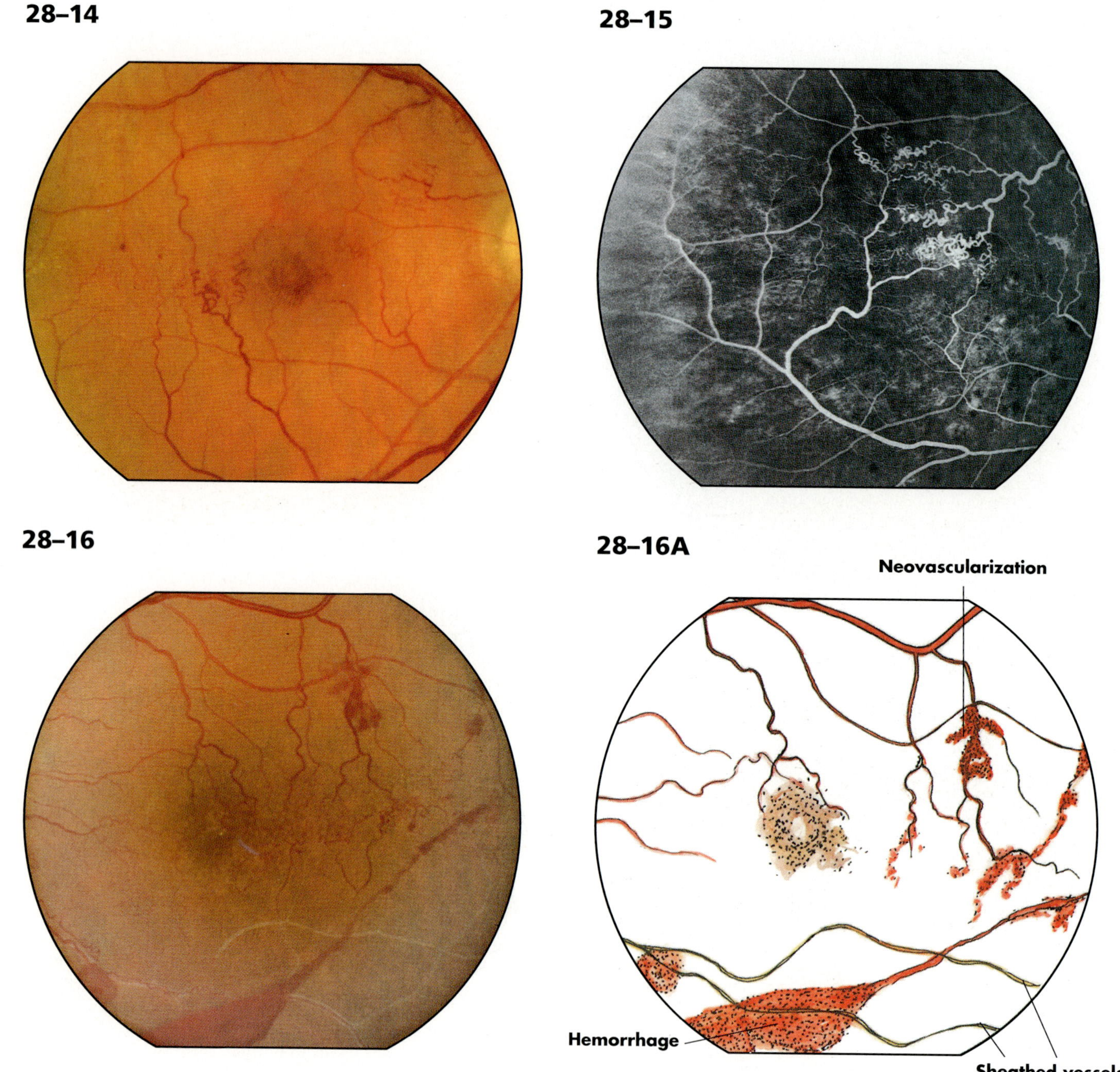

28–14 This patient experienced a branch retinal vein occlusion that evolved spontaneously with collateral formation in the papillomacular bundle as well as in the temporal macula along the course of the horizontal raphe. Some residual epiretinal membrane disturbance occurred in the perifoveal region.

28–15 In this patient with a compensating branch retinal vein occlusion, the fluorescein study confirmed the nature of the tortuous vessels as venous-venous anastomotic communications or collateralizations. Note that these vessels do not leak.

28–16 and 28–16A This patient had an inferior branch retinal vein occlusion. The occlusion resolved spontaneously, but several years later vitreous hemorrhage occurred. Note the blood in front of the retina inferiorly and the marked paucity of vessels. Vessels that are evident are irregular and sheathed. Minimal collateralization is evident along the course of the horizontal raphe, but there is also preretinal neovascularization—in this case in the superior hemisphere, which is normally perfused.

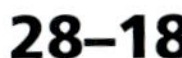

28–17

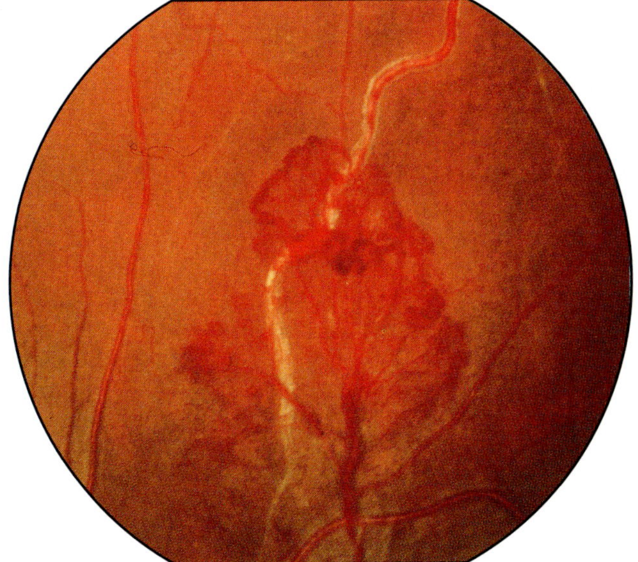

28–18

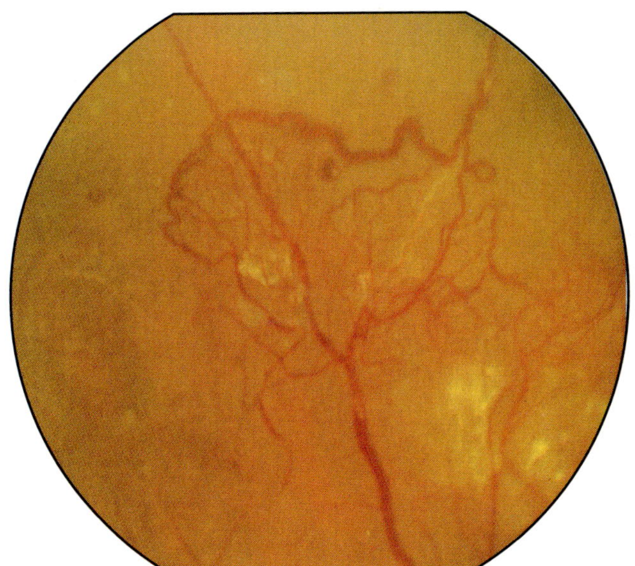

28–19

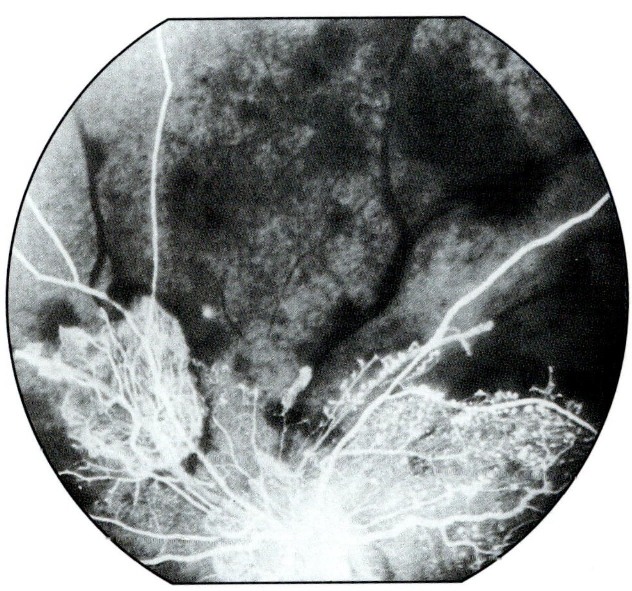

28–17 This patient with a branch retinal vein occlusion demonstrates a very prominent area of preretinal neovascularization within the ischemic area. The involved vein is markedly tortuous and sheathed. It is also located between two arterioles that are also irregular and narrowed in their vessel caliber.

28–18 This patient experienced a branch retinal vein occlusion. Peripheral neovascularization eventually evolved. Note the dilated preretinal capillaries along a broad front. Some fibrous proliferation and generalized retinal vascular ischemia also is evident.

28–19 In another patient with a branch retinal vein occlusion, the fluorescein angiogram reveals a markedly ischemic retina. The perfused area is associated with an array of microangiopathic changes including tortuosity, aneurysmal formation, larger vascular occlusions, and a patch of preretinal neovascularization.

28–20

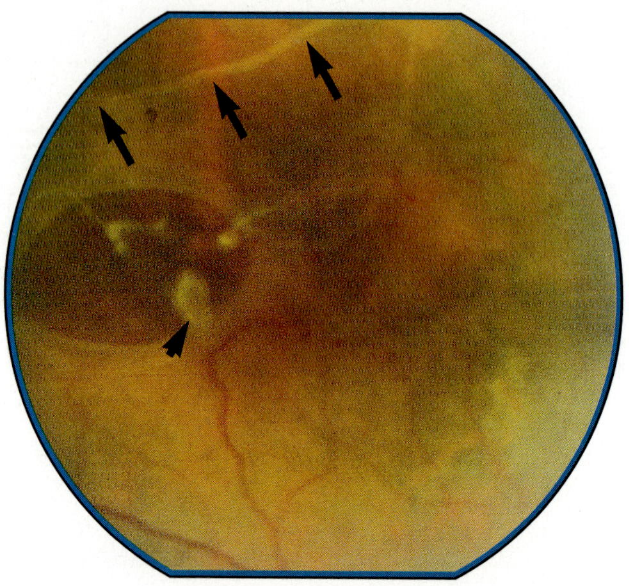

28–21 **28–21A**

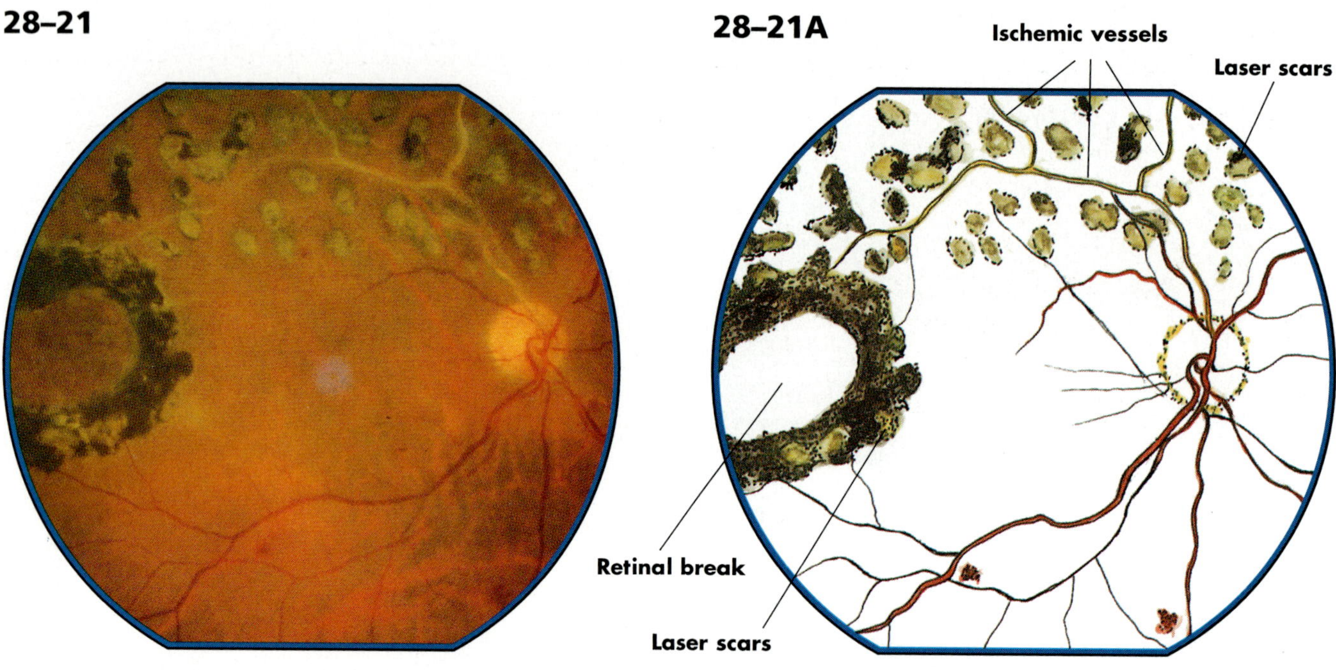

28–20 through 28–21A In this patient, the branch retinal vein occlusion is associated with a retinal break. Note the ischemic retinal vessels in the distribution of the occlusion *(arrows),* the operculum overlying an ovoid retinal hole *(arrowhead),* and a fringe of neurosensory retinal elevation at its margins. This patient was treated with laser photocoagulation by the scatter technique to the ischemic area. The retinal break was also encircled with a wreath of confluent photocoagulation. The visual acuity was surprisingly good at the level of 20/30 despite the ischemia and rhegmatogenous pathology.

28–22

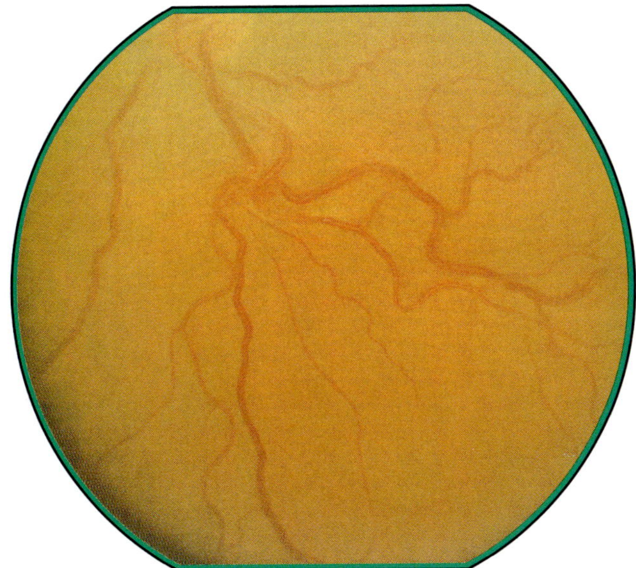

28–23

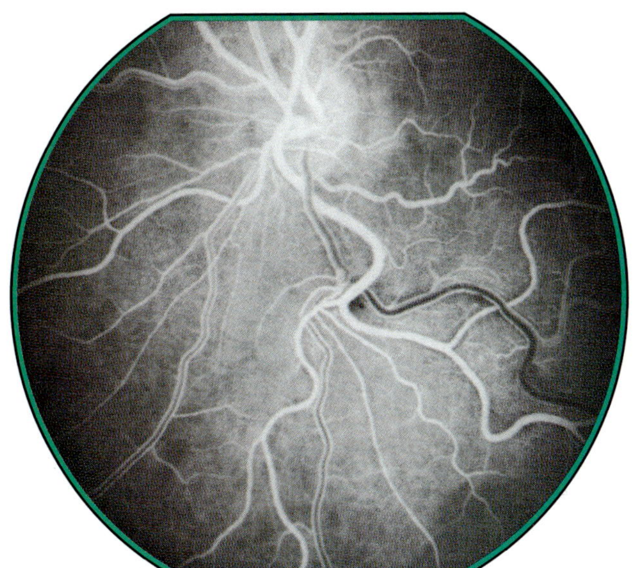

28–22 An arteriovenous crossing defect is demonstrated in this patient and is characterized by prominence of the venule at its proximal segment, a patch of subretinal hemorrhage, and obliteration of the venule at its common sheath with the crossing arteriole, as well as a trace of intraretinal edema. This constellation of findings has been referred to as the prethrombotic sign of Bonnet, since some of these patients eventually experience an acute vein occlusion.

28–23 In the same patient the fluorescein angiogram shows a localized perfusion delay in the branch of a vein from incomplete obliterative changes.

28–24

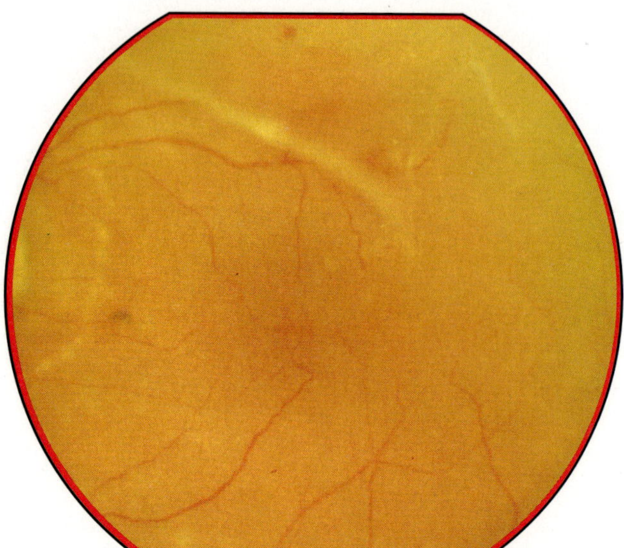

28–25

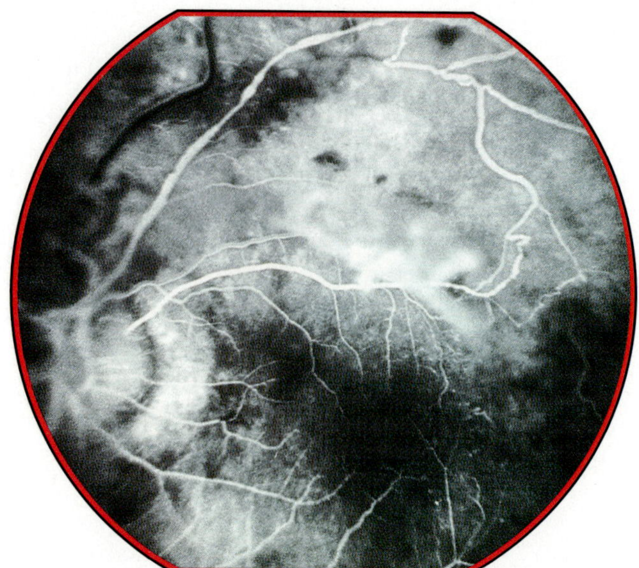

28–26

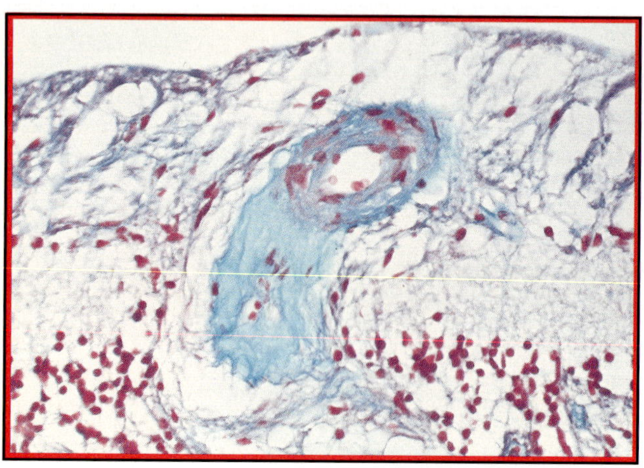

28–24 Clinicopathologic correlation of a branch retinal vein occlusion. This patient experienced a superior branch retinal vein occlusion. There are sheathed vessels, residual retinal edema, and a band of preretinal fibrosis coursing obliquely through the temporal vascular arcades.

28–25 The fluorescein angiogram reveals a superotemporal ciliary artery that is anastomosing with a branch of the superior temporal occluded vein, filling it in a retrograde fashion. The involved vein does not completely fill its distal and proximal segments in the laminar phase of the study. The corresponding arteriole appears narrowed and irregular or beaded.

28–26 Area of occlusion reveals a single channel of recanalization of the branch of the superotemporal vein as it crosses under the arteriosclerotic artery.

28–24 *through* ***28–26,*** *From Vaghefi, HA, Green, WR, Kelly, JS, Sloan, LL, Hoover, RE, and Patz, A: Correlation of clinicopathologic findings in a patient: congenital night blindness, branch retinal vein occlusion, cilioretinal artery drusen of the optic nerve head, and intraretinal pigmented lesion, Arch Ophthalmol 96:2097–2104, 1978.*

Suggested Readings

Bowers, DK, Finkelstein, D, Wolff, SM, and Green, WR: Branch retinal vein occlusion, Retina 7:252–259, 1987

Branch Vein Occlusion Study Group: Argon laser photocoagulation for macular edema in branch vein occlusion, Am J Ophthalmol 98:271–282, 1984

Branch Vein Occlusion Study Group: Argon laser scatter photocoagulation for prevention of neovascularization and vitreous hemorrhage in branch vein occlusion, Arch Ophthalmol 104:34–41, 1986

Clemett, RS, Kohner, EM, and Hamilton, AM: The visual prognosis in retinal branch vein occlusion, Trans Ophthalmol Soc UK 93:523–535, 1973

Finkelstein D: Ischemic macular edema: recognition and favorable natural history in branch vein occlusion, Arch Ophthalmol 110:1427–1434, 1992

Finkelstein, D, Clarkson, JG, and The Branch Vein Occlusion Study Group: Branch and central retinal vein occlusions. Focal points 1987: clinical modules for ophthalmologists 5(module 12), no. 3, Am Acad Ophthalmol

Frangieh, GT, Green, WR, Barraquer-Somers, E, and Finkelstein, D: Histopathologic study of nine branch retinal vein occlusions, Arch Ophthalmol 100:1132–1140, 1982

Gutman, FA: Macular edema in branch retinal vein occlusion: prognosis and management, Trans Am Acad Ophthalmol Otolaryngol 83:488–495, 1977

Gutman, FA, and Zegarra, H: The natural course of temporal retinal branch vein occlusion, Trans Am Acad Ophthalmol Otolaryngol 78:178–192, 1974

Gutman, FA, and Zegarra, H: Macular edema secondary to occlusion of the retinal veins, Surv Ophthalmol 28:462–470, 1984

Hayreh, SS, Rojas, P, Podhajsky, P, Montague, P, and Woolson, RF: Ocular neovascularization with retinal vein occlusion, Ophthalmology 90:488–506, 1983

Joffe, L, Goldberg, RE, Magargal, LE, and Annesley, WH: Macular branch vein occlusion, Ophthalmology 87:91–98, 1980

Orth, DH, and Patz, A: Retinal branch vein occlusion, Surv Ophthalmol 22:357–376, 1978

Shilling, JS, and Kohner, EM: New vessel formation in retinal branch vein occlusion, Br J Ophthalmol 60:810–815, 1976

Vanghefi, HA, Green, WR, Kelley, JS, Sloan, LL, Hoover, RE, and Patz, A: Correlation of clinicopathologic findings in a patient: congenital night blindness, branch retinal vein occlusion, drusen of optic nerve head and intraretinal pigmented lesion, Arch Ophthalmol 96:2097–2104, 1978

Wilson, DJ, Finkelstein, D, Quigley, HA, and Green, WR: Macular grid photocoagulation: an experimental study on the primate retina, Arch Ophthalmol 106:100–105, 1988

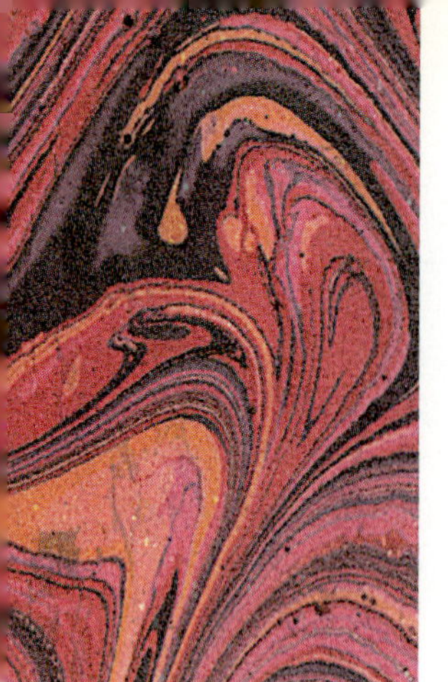

Chapter 29

Pregnancy and Retinal Disease

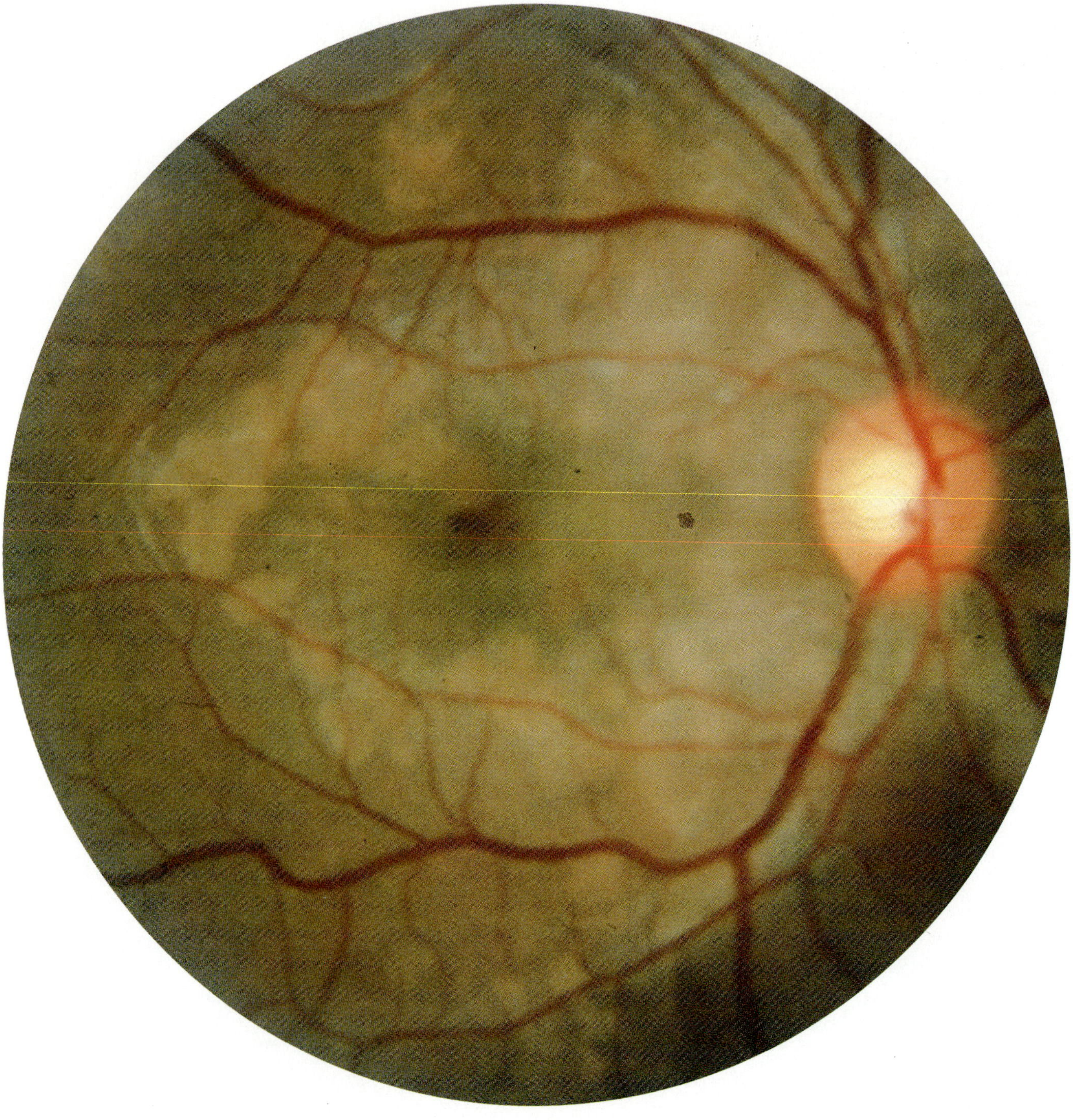

Toxemia of pregnancy refers to both preeclampsia (hypertension, edema, proteinuria) and eclampsia (the above with seizures). Retinal findings in toxemia of pregnancy include reversible focal arteriolar spasm, generalized arteriolar narrowing, hemorrhages, exudates, edema, and papilledema. Serous exudative detachments may rarely occur.

29–1

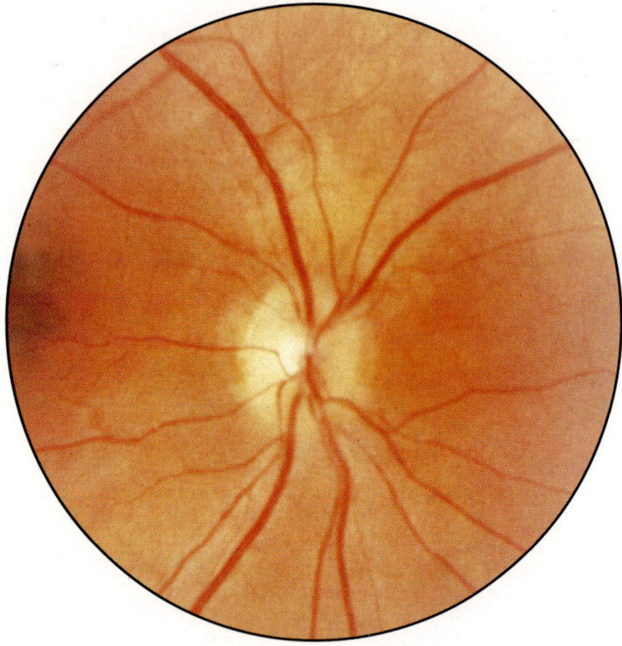

29–2

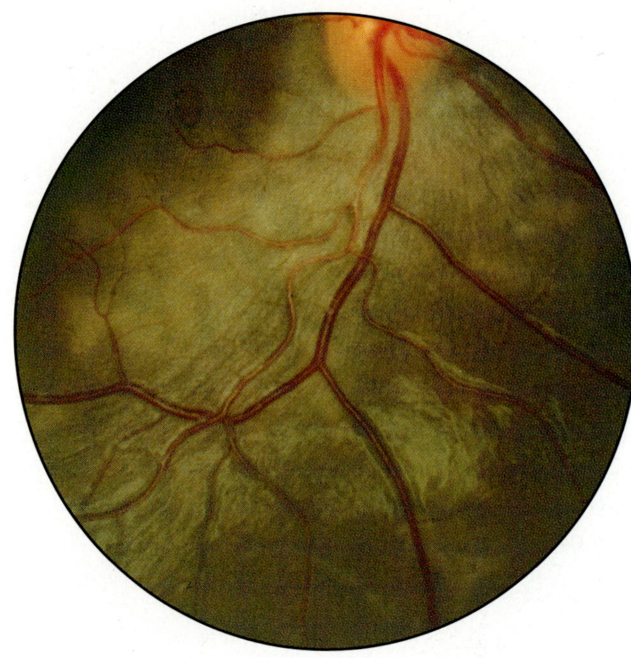

29–1 This patient with severe preeclampsia has generalized retinal arteriolar narrowing with an increased arteriole-to-vein ratio.

29–2 The next patient illustrates a neurosensory retinal elevation with Elschnig's spots.

29–1, *Courtesy of Drs. Glenn Jaffe, Howard Schatz, and Richard Ober. From Ryan, SJ: Retina, ed 2, St Louis, 1994, Mosby–Year Book.* ***29–2,*** *Courtesy of Dr. Kurt Gitter.*

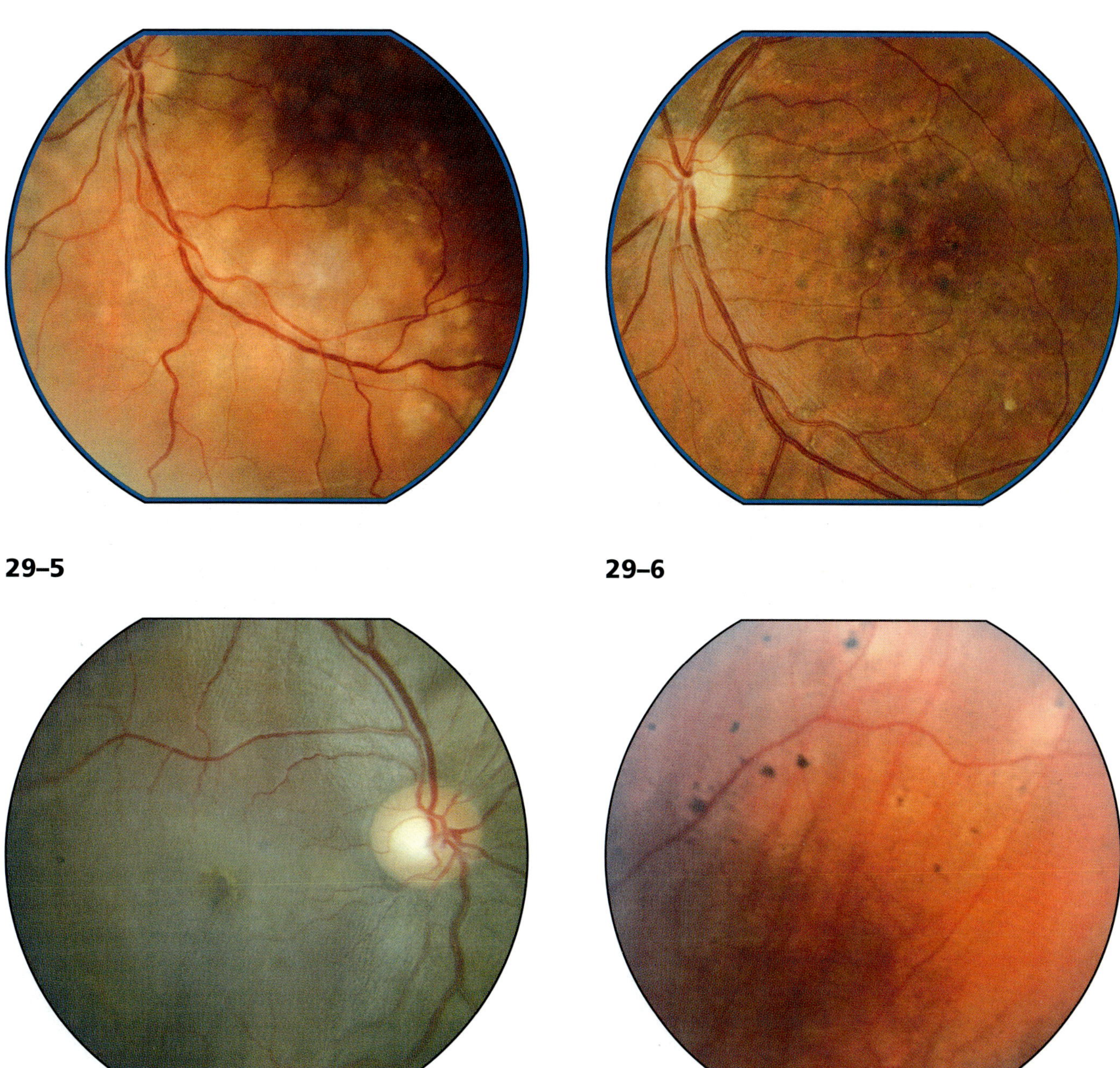

29–3 and 29–4 This preeclamptic patient was noted to have hand motions vision during pregnancy. She had bilateral deep white lesions, Elschnig's spots, an inferior detachment, and retinal striae. Her vision returned to 20/20 in the right eye and 20/30 in the left eye after delivery. Note the atrophic pigmentary changes.

29–5 In this patient with toxemia of pregnancy, there is a bullous detachment of the retina with barely evident white spots at the level of the retinal pigment epithelium.

29–6 This patient demonstrates multiple pigmentary spots that seem to have a vasculotropic orientation with regard to the choroidal circulation. These abnormalities are commonly referred to as Elschnig's spots. When associated with atrophic linear areas, they are called Siegrist's lines and are indicative of anterior choroidal ischemia, such as found in patients with toxemia of pregnancy.

***29–3** and **29–4,** Courtesy of Dr. Ken Noble. **29–5** and **29–6,** Courtesy of Dr. Lee Jampol.*

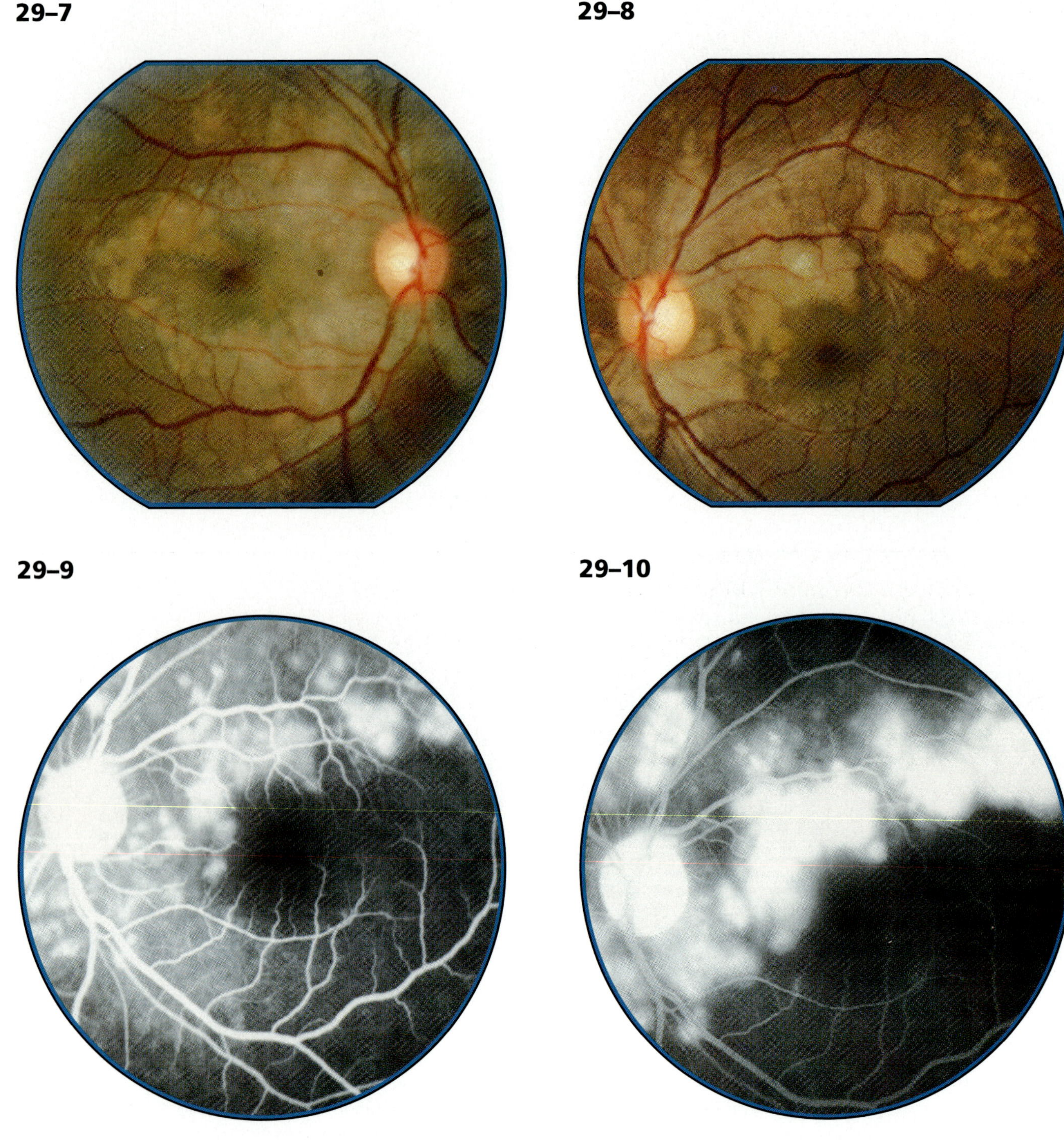

29–7 and 29–8 This patient with toxemia of pregnancy noted acute loss of vision in both eyes after delivery. Ophthalmoscopy revealed bilateral serous exudative detachments with yellow-white deposits at the level of the retinal pigment epithelium.

29–9 and 29–10 Fluorescein angiography performed after delivery illustrates the multiple serous detachments secondary to multiple retinal pigment epithelial leaks presumably due to fibrinoid necrosis.

29–7 *and* ***29–8,*** *Courtesy of Dr. Gaetano Barile.* ***29–9*** *and* ***29–10,*** *Courtesy of Dr. Gaetano Barile and Mr. José Martinez.*

29–11

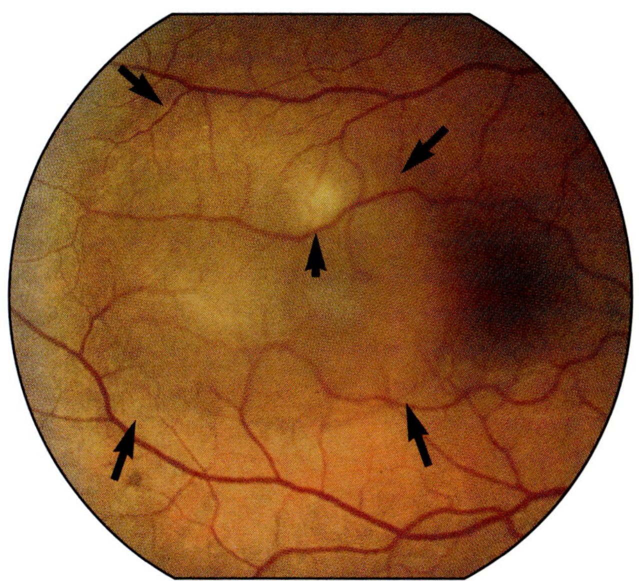

29–12

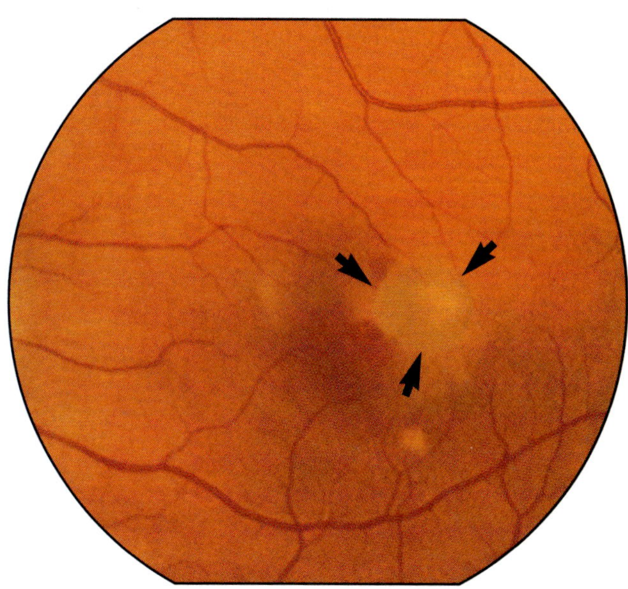

29–11 This pregnant patient developed a serous macular detachment *(arrows)* due to central serous chorioretinopathy. Note the fibrin superiorly *(arrowhead)*. The occurrence of central serous chorioretinopathy is probably related to the pregnancy.

29–12 This pregnant patient developed subretinal fluid and hemorrhage due to a choroidal neovascular membrane *(arrowheads)*. Choroidal neovascularization may simply represent a coincidental finding in pregnant patients.

Suggested Readings

Brancato, R, Menchini, U, and Bandello, F: Proliferative retinopathy and toxemia of pregnancy, Ann Ophthalmol 19:182–183, 1987

Carpenter, F Kava, HL, and Plotkin, D: The development of total blindness as a complication of pregnancy, Am J Obstet Gynecol 66:641–647, 1953

Chang, M, and Herbert, WNP: Retinal arteriolar occlusions following amniotic fluid embolism, Ophthalmology 91:1634–1637, 1984

Chumbley, LC, and Frank, RN: Central serous retinopathy and pregnancy, Am J Ophthalmol 77: 158–160, 1974

Fastenberg, DM, and Ober, RR: Central serous choroidopathy in pregnancy, Arch Ophthalmol 101:1055–1058, 1983

Gitter KA, Houser, BP, Sarin, LK, and Justice, J: Toxemia of pregnancy. An angiographic interpretation of fundus changes, Arch Ophthalmol 80:449–454, 1968

Greenber, F, and Lewis, RA: Safety of fluorescein angiography during pregnancy (letter), Am J Ophthalmol 110:323–324, 1990

Klein, BEK, and Klein, R: Gravidity and diabetic retinopathy, Am J Epidemiol 119:564–569, 1984

Laatikainen, L, Teramo, K, Heita-Heikurainen, H, Koivisto, V, and Pelkonen, R: A controlled study of the influence of continuous subcutaneous insulin infusion treatment on diabetic retinopathy during pregnancy, Acta Med Scand 221:367–376, 1987

Seddon, JM, MacLaughlin, DT, Albert, DM, et al: Uveal melanomas presenting during pregnancy and the investigation of estrogen receptors in melanomas, Br J Ophthalmol 66:695–704, 1982

Soubrane, G, Canivet, J, and Coscas, G: Influence of pregnancy on the evolution of background retinopathy: preliminary results of a prospective fluorescein angiography study. In Ryan, SJ, Dawson, AK, and Little, HL, eds: Retinal diseases, New York, 1985, Grune & Stratton, pp 15–20

Sunness, JS: The pregnant woman's eye, Surv Ophthalmol 32: 219–238, 1988

Wiebers, DO: Ischemic cerebrovascular complications of pregnancy, Arch Neurol 42:1106–1113, 1985

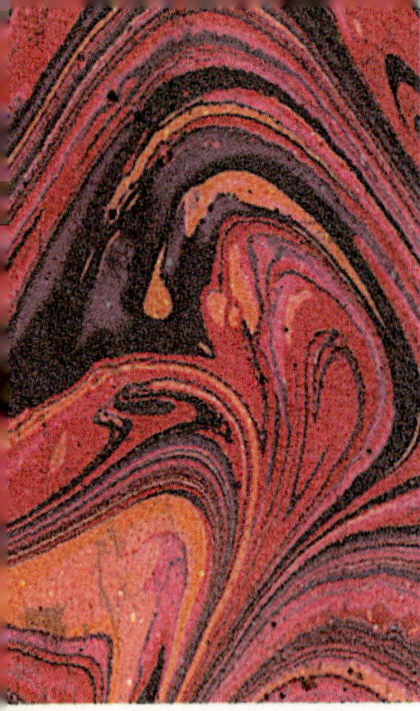

Chapter 30
Hypertension

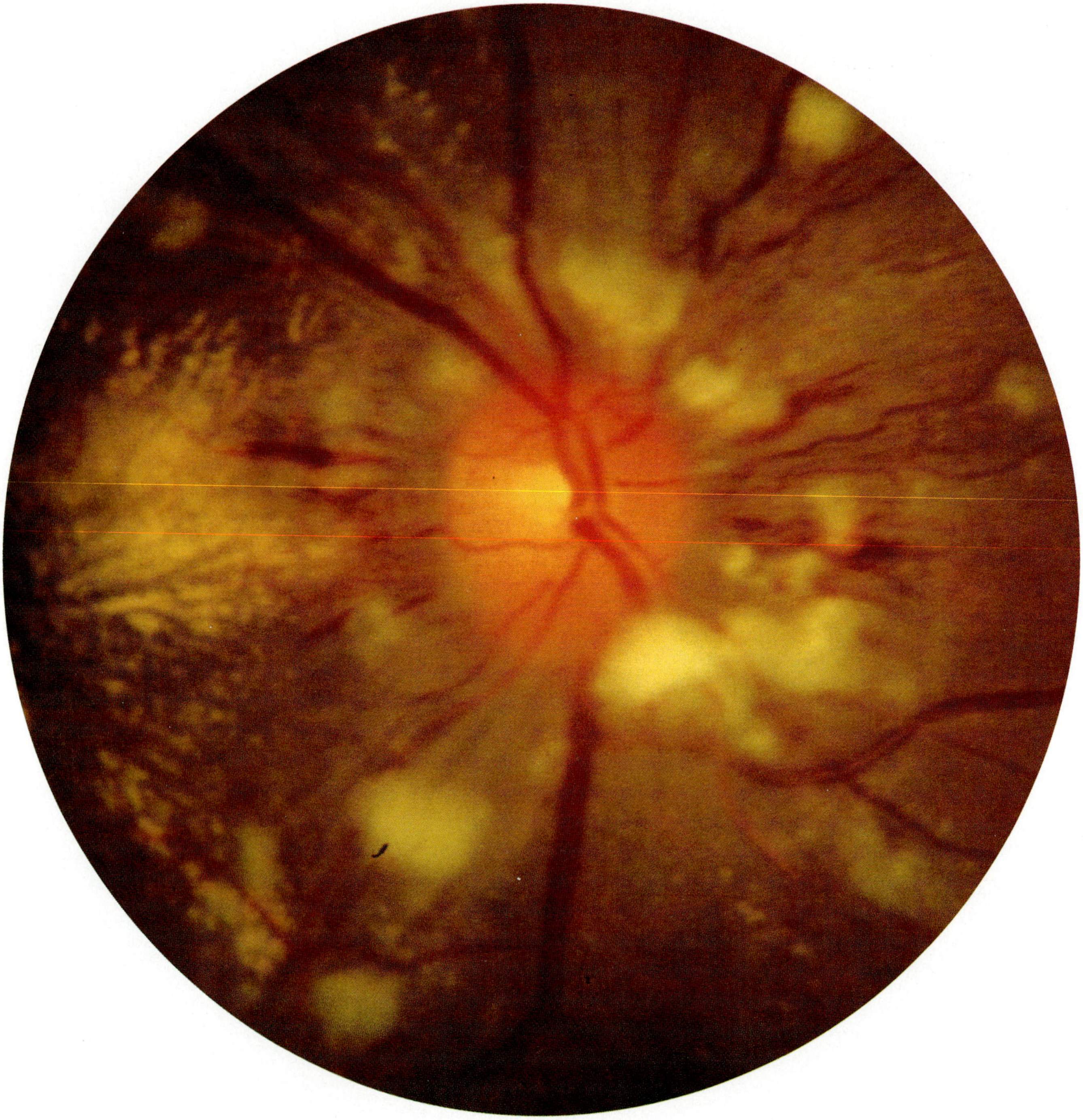

Hypertension may cause both focal and generalized constriction of the retinal arterioles. These findings are usually due to chronic disease. Acutely elevated blood pressure levels can be associated with breakdown of the blood-retinal barrier and significant exudation.

Intraretinal hemorrhages, cotton-wool spots, and macular edema may occur. Fibrinoid necrosis of the choroidal vessels can also occur as can damage to the optic nerve.

30–1

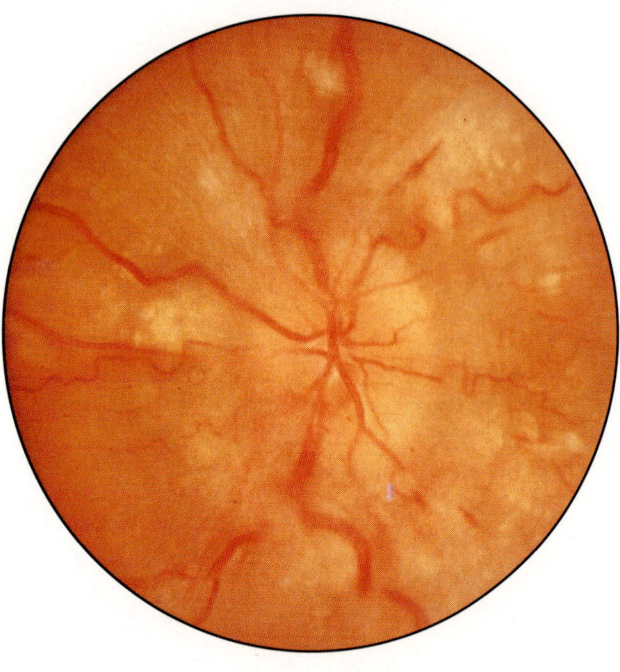

30–2

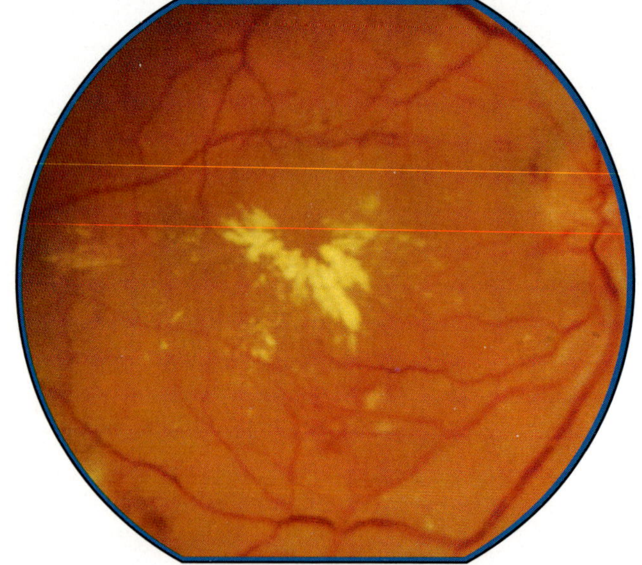

30–3

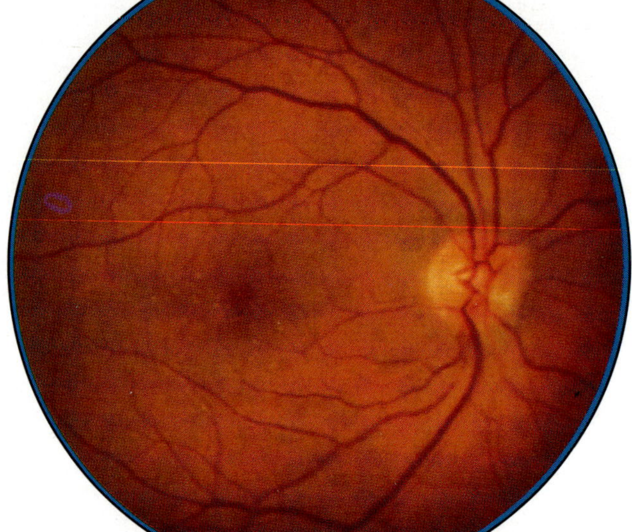

30–1 Optic disc swelling is noted in this patient secondary to hypertension.

30–2 and 30–3 This patient had acutely elevated blood pressure, which caused intraretinal hemorrhages, cotton-wool spots, lipid exudation, and macular edema. Sometimes these changes can be due to venous occlusive disease. However, in this case, it was due to a hypertensive microangiopathy, as indicated by the resolved state after the blood pressure was medically controlled.

30–1, *Courtesy of Dr. Kurt Gitter.*

30–4

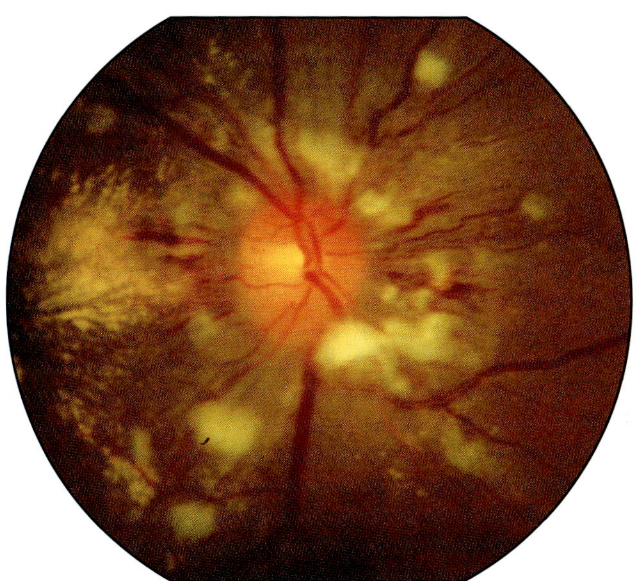

30–5

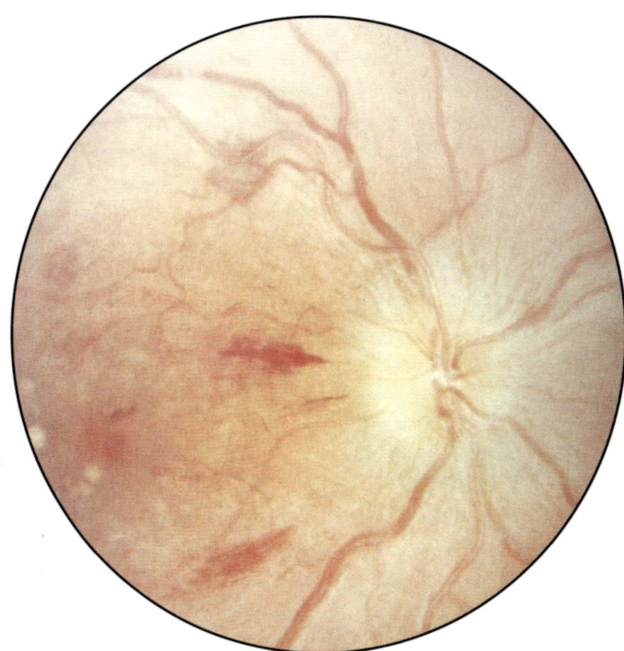

30–6

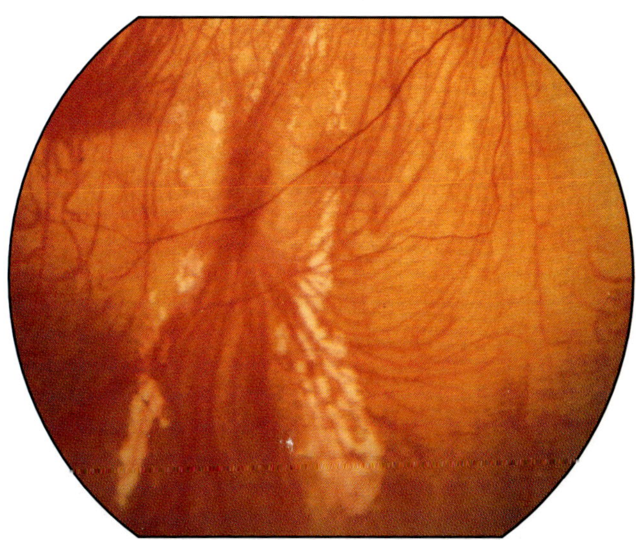

30–4 This 30-year-old male had a blood pressure of 220/170. He demonstrated multiple cotton-wool spots, intraretinal hemorrhage, and macular edema. Visual acuity was 20/100 in both eyes. The patient showed improvement after his blood pressure was lowered.

30–5 This patient has malignant hypertension with optic disc edema and intraretinal hemorrhages.

30–6 This patient developed multiple triangular infarcts of the choroid during an acute hypertensive episode.

30–4, *Courtesy of Dr. Wendell Bauman.*

30–7

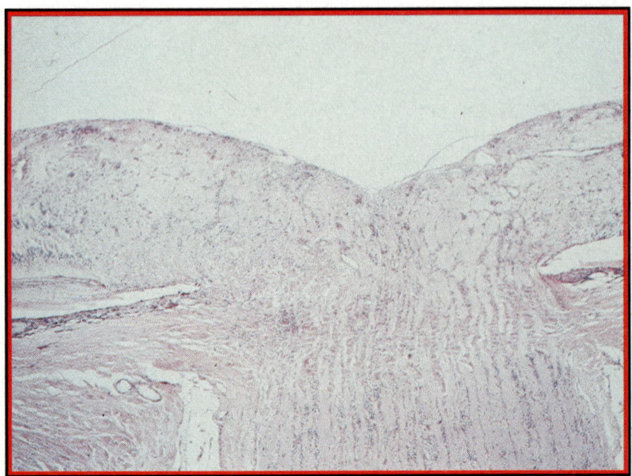

30–8

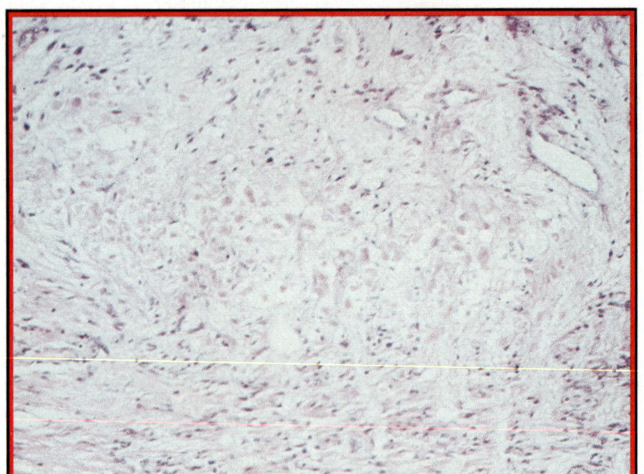

30–9

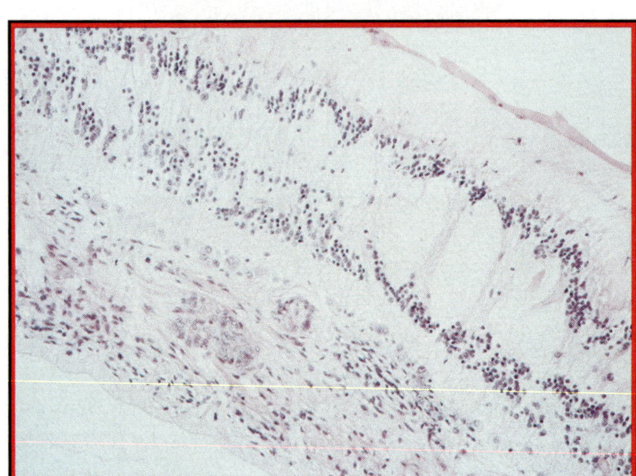

30–7 and 30–8 This case illustrates the changes in the eye of a 26-year-old male who died of malignant hypertension. This photograph demonstrates papilledema with partial obliteration of the optic cup and thickening of the optic nerve head with peripapillary crowding of the retina. The retina adjacent to the optic nerve head has been pushed to the side. A microinfarction is noted in the temporal prelaminar area of the optic nerve head. Higher magnification reveals an area of axonal swelling (cytoid bodies). Disruption of the nerve fibers can be seen in this area of infarction.

30–9 This photograph demonstrates cystoid macular edema with some fibrinous material.

30–7 *through* ***30–9,*** *From Green, WR: Retina. In Spencer, WR, ed: Ophthalmic pathology. An atlas and textbook, Philadelphia, 1985, WB Saunders.*

Suggested Readings

Ashton, N: The eye in malignant hypertension, Trans Am Acad Ophthalmol Otolaryngol 76:17–40, 1972

Ashton, N and Harry, J: The pathology of cotton wool spots and cytoid bodies in hypersensitive retinography and other diseases, Trans Ophthalmol R Soc UK 83:91–114, 1963

deVenecia, G, Wallow, I, Houser, JD, and Wahlstrom, M: The eye in accelerated hypertension. I. Elschnig's spots in nonhuman primates, Arch Ophthalmol 98:913–918, 1980

Green, WR: Systemic diseases with retinal involvement. In Spencer, WH, ed: Ophthalmic pathology: an atlas and textbook, Philadelphia, 1985, WB Saunders, pp 1034–1047

Hayreh, SS, Servais, G, and Virdi, PS: Macular lesions in malignant arterial hypertension, Ophthalmologica 198:230–246, 1989

Scheie, HG: Evaluation of ophthalmoscopic changes of hypertension and arteriolar sclerosis, Arch Ophthalmol 49:117, 1953

Tso, MOM, and Jampol, LM: Pathophysiology of hypertensive retinopathy, Ophthalmologica 89:1132, 1982

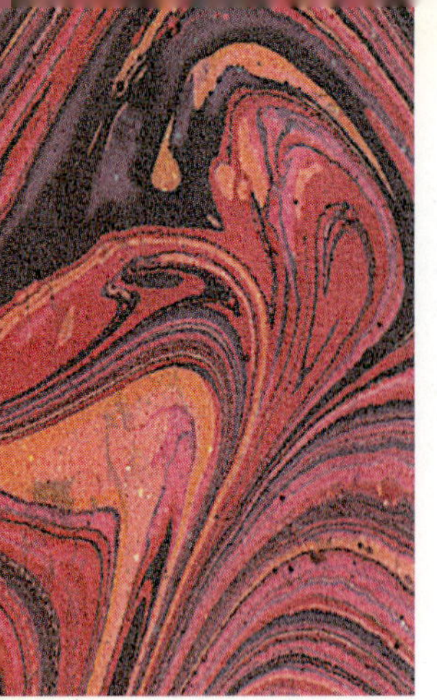

Chapter 31

The Rheumatic Diseases

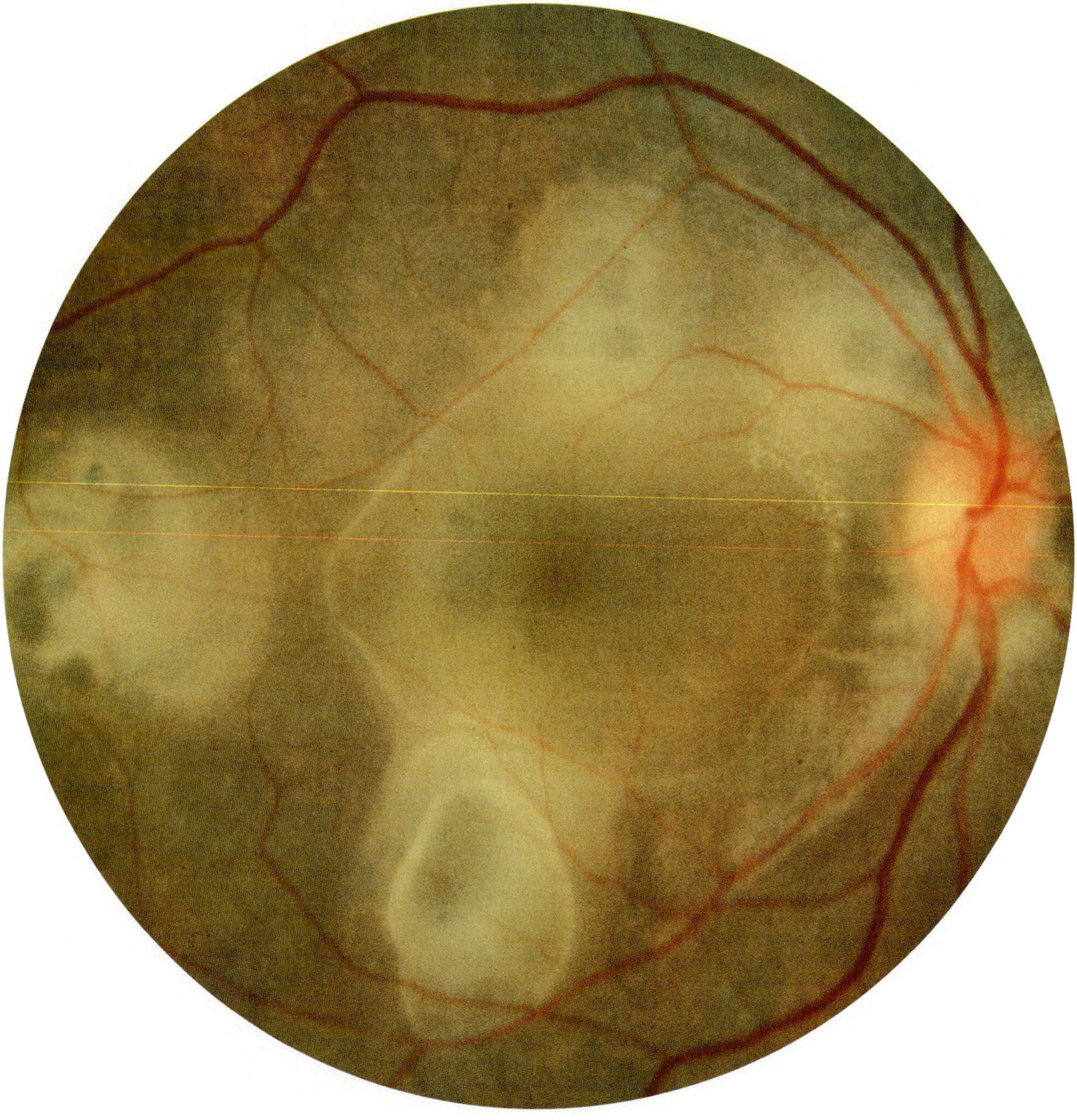

Systemic lupus erythematosus has several ocular manifestations including eyelid involvement, secondary Sjögren's syndrome, retinal vascular disease, and neuro-ophthalmic lesions. Retinal vascular involvement includes cotton-wool spots, intraretinal hemorrhages, and a Purtscher's-like picture. In addition, central retinal artery occlusions, vein occlusions, and more diffuse vaso-occlusive disease can occur. Cases of lupus choroidopathy have also been reported.

Behçet's disease is noted for the classical triad of oral ulcers, genital ulcers, and hypopyon uveitis. Ocular involvement includes iritis, hypopyon, and retinal vasculitis. Rarely, secondary neovascularization or detachment will occur. Immunosuppressive drugs have recently improved the treatment of this condition.

31–1 SYSTEMIC LUPUS ERYTHEMATOSUS

31–2

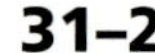

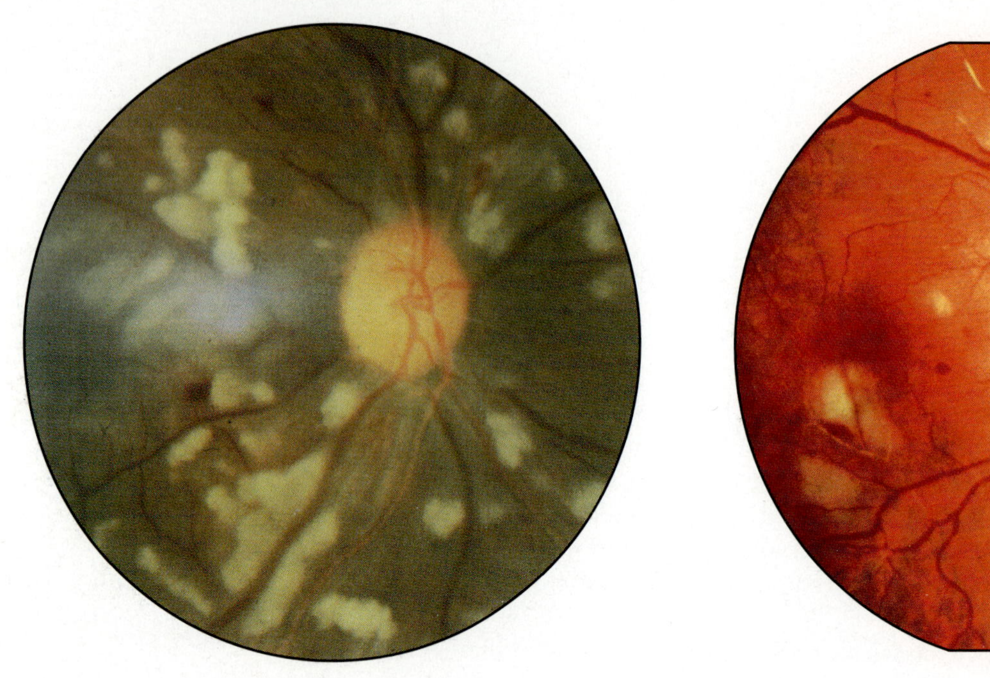

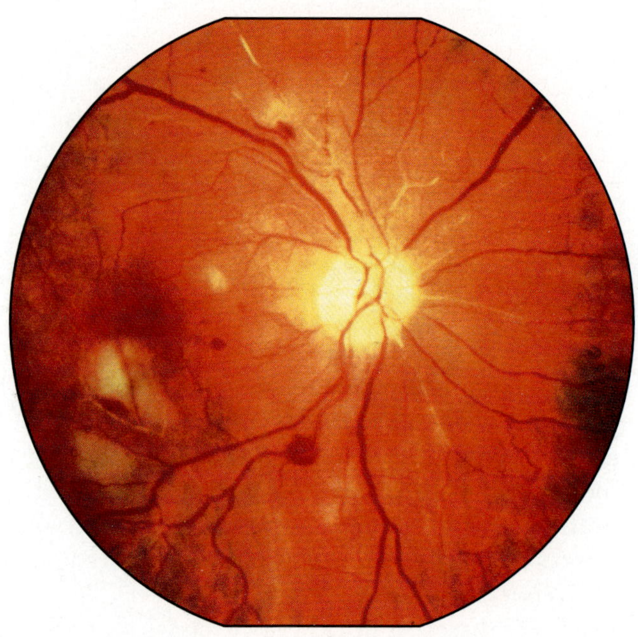

31–1 This patient with systemic lupus erythematosus has extensive cotton-wool spots. Some hemorrhages are also present.

31–2 This patient with systemic lupus erythematosus demonstrates diffuse vaso-occlusive disease with hemorrhages and zones of intraretinal whitening from capillary occlusions. Note the extensive sheathing of the retinal vessels. In this case, the patient has anticardiolipin antibodies.

31–1 *and* ***31–2,*** *From Jabs, DA, et al: Arch Ophthalmol 104:558–563, 1986. Copyright 1986 American Medical Association. From Ryan, SJ: Retina, ed 2, St. Louis, 1994, Mosby–Year Book.*

31–3

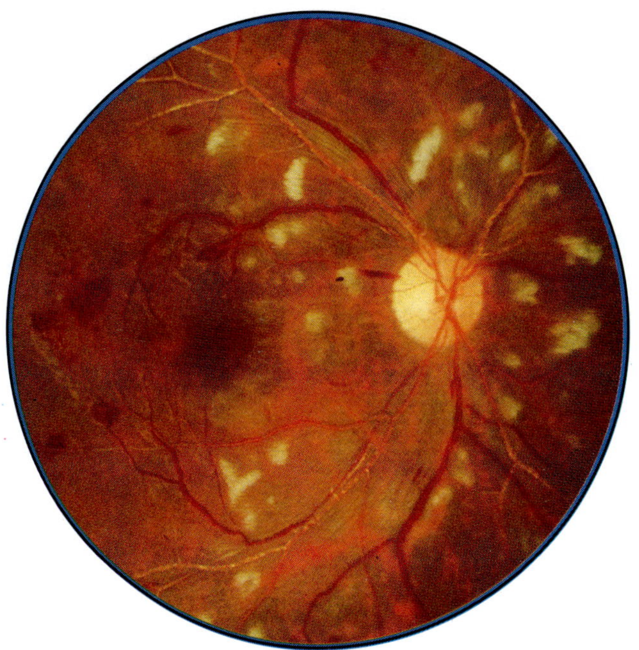

31–4

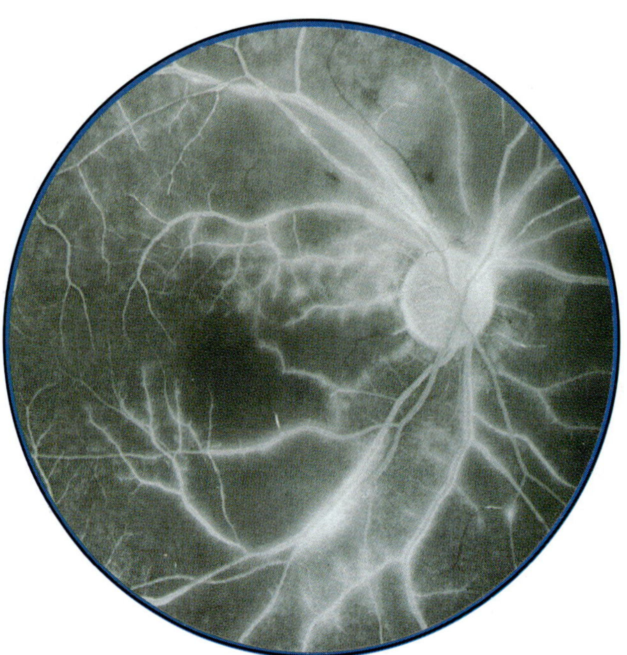

31–3 This patient with systemic lupus erythematosus has multiple cotton-wool spots, intraretinal hemorrhages, nonperfusion, and sheathed retinal vessels in a beaded appearance.

31–4 The fluorescein angiogram shows capillary nonperfusion (especially inferonasal to the optic disc), as well as staining of the vessels consistent with retinal vasculitis.

31–5 SYSTEMIC LUPUS ERYTHEMATOSUS

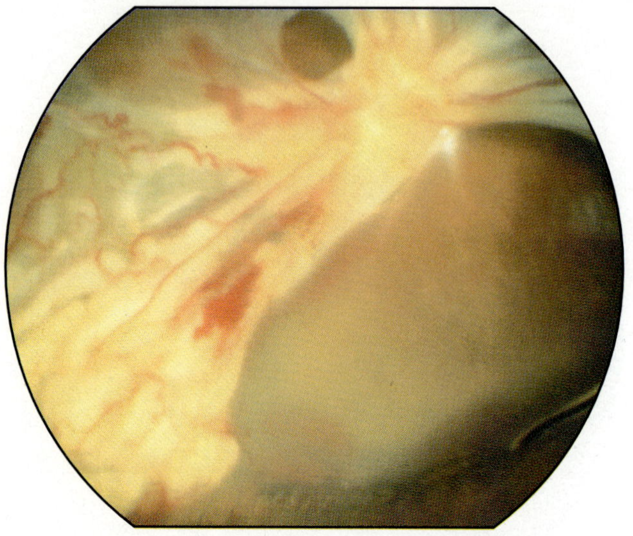

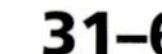

31–6

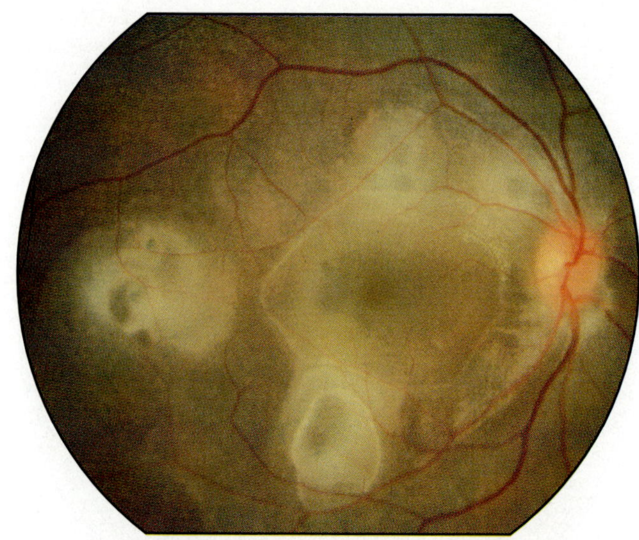

31–7

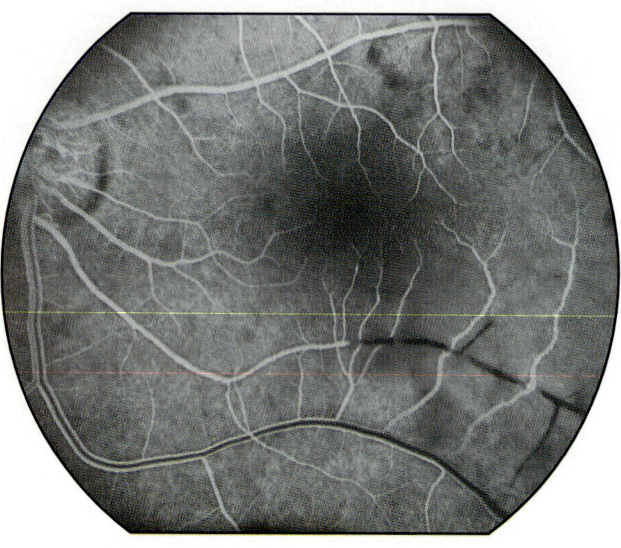

31–8

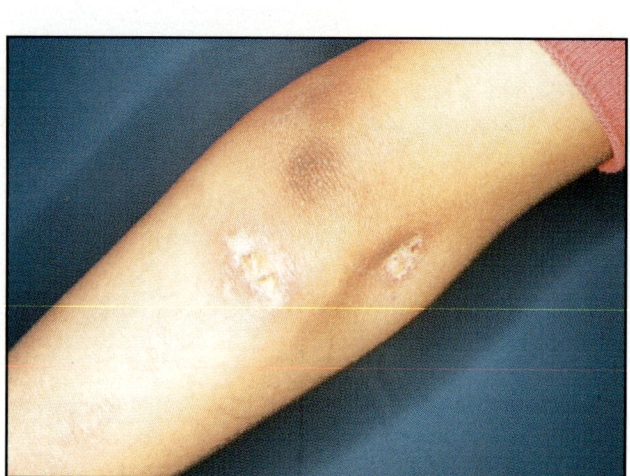

31–5 This patient with systemic lupus erythematosus has extensive fibrovascular proliferation with vitreous hemorrhage, retinal traction, and a retinal tear.

31–6 This patient has a choroidopathy with multiple detachments secondary to systemic lupus erythematosus. Fibrin is present under the retina. This condition represents a type of disseminated intravascular coagulopathy. This condition may alternatively be caused by steroid administration.

31–7 This patient with systemic lupus erythematosus has a retinal arteriole occlusion.

31–8 These skin lesions are secondary to discoid lupus erythematosus.

***31–6** and **31–7**, From Green, WR, et al: Histopathologic features of idiopathic macular holes and cysts, Ophthalmology 97:1045–1051, 1990. **31–8**, Courtesy and copyright Dr. Mark Lebwohl.*

31–9 BEHÇET'S DISEASE

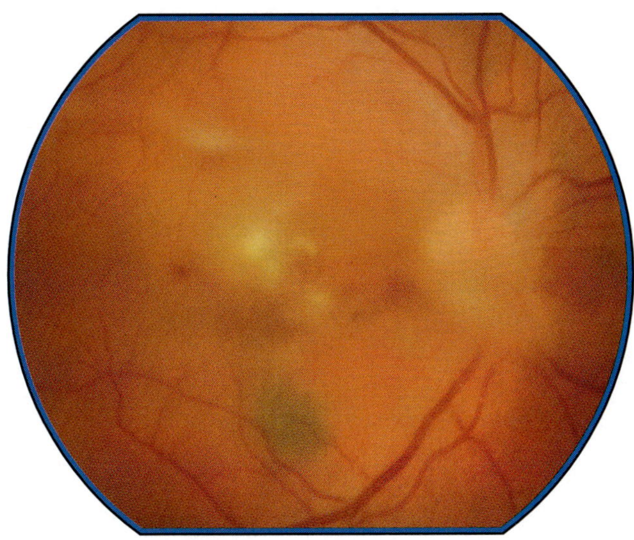

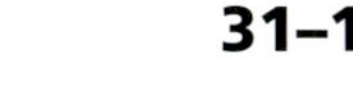

31–10

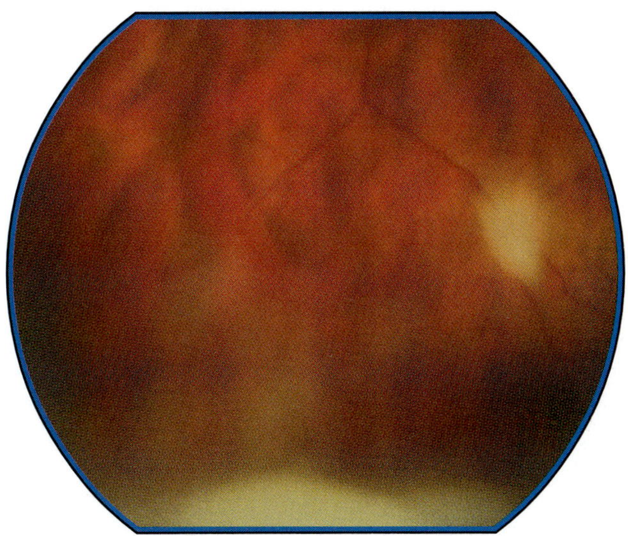

31–9 This patient with Behçet's disease has a serous detachment with lipid in the macular region. There is also vitreous opacification, especially near the optic disc.

31–10 This patient has snowbanks secondary to inflammation from Behçet's disease.

***31–9** and **31–10,** Courtesy of Dr. Richard Klein.*

31–11 BEHÇET'S DISEASE

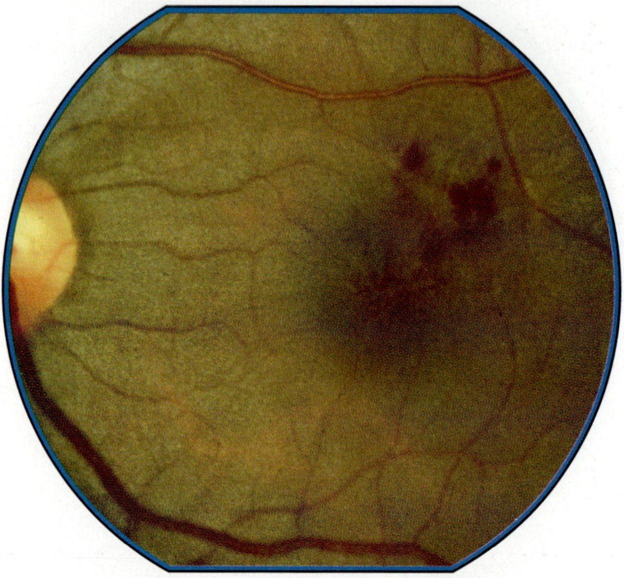

31–12

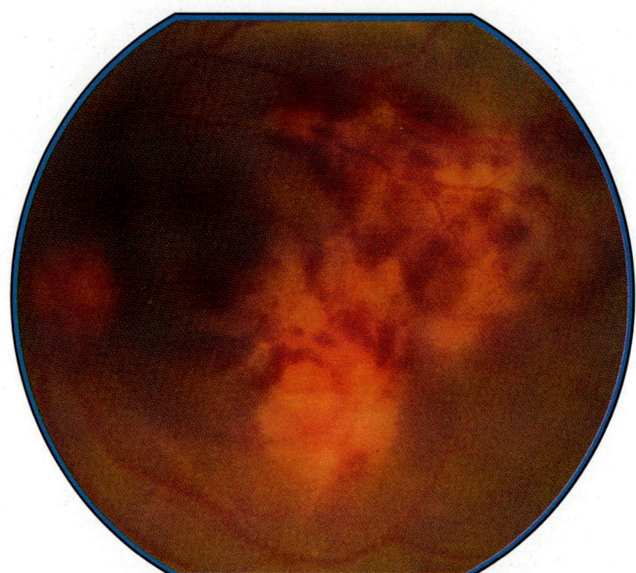

31–13

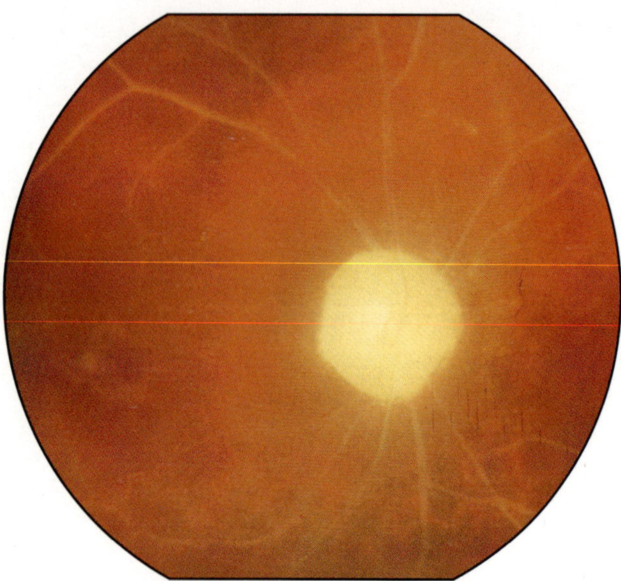

31–11 and 31–12 These fundus photographs from a patient with Behçet's disease demonstrate retinal vasculitis. The first photograph shows an early lesion. One month later, the disease had progressed. There is acute whitening within the retina and arterial as well as venular inflammatory changes. The fundus details are clouded by inflammatory and hemorrhagic cells within the vitreous.

31–13 This patient has end-stage Behçet's disease in the fundus with optic atrophy and severe sheathing of the retinal vessels.

31–11 *and* ***31–12,*** *Courtesy of Dr. Douglas A. Jabs. From Ryan, SJ: Retina, ed 2, St Louis, 1994, Mosby–Year Book.* ***31–13,*** *Courtesy of Dr. Leyla-Suna Atmaca.*

31–14 **31–15**

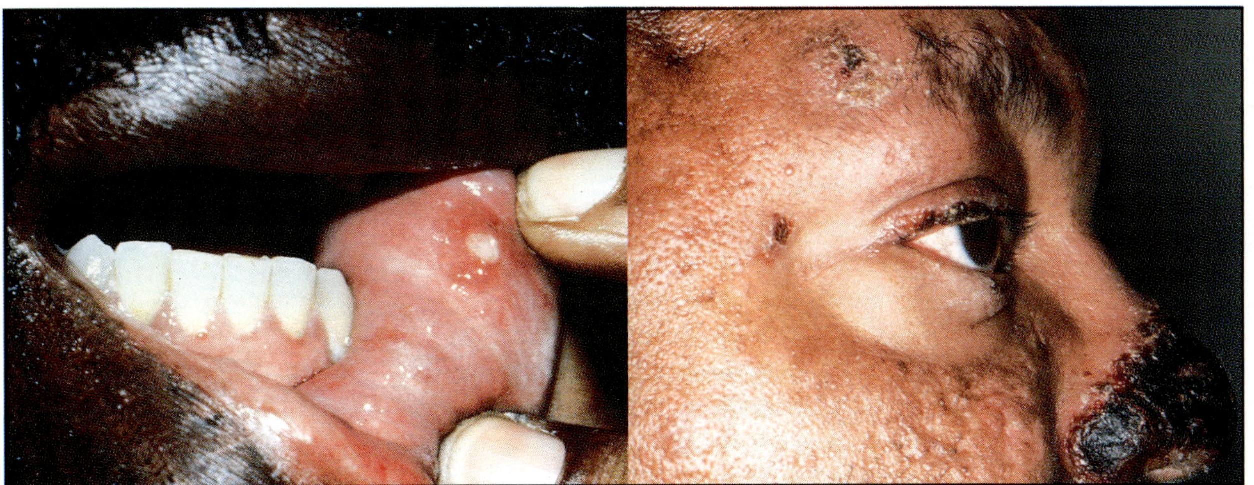

31–14 and 31–15 Behçet's disease can have numerous systemic manifestations that may involve the oral cavity (aphthous ulcer), (31–14), genitals, and/or skin (31–15).

31–14, *Courtesy of Dr. W. Culbertson.* ***31–15,*** *From Lebwohl, M: Atlas of the skin and systemic disease, New York, 1995, Churchill Livingstone.*

31–16 WEGENER'S GRANULOMATOSIS

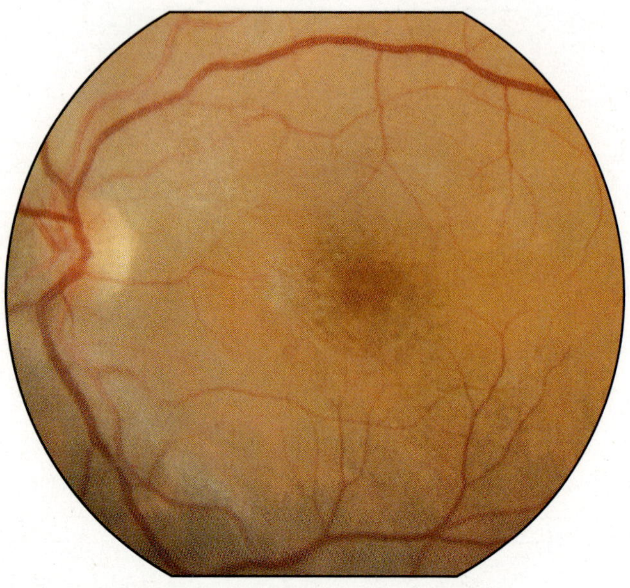

31–17 CREST SYNDROME

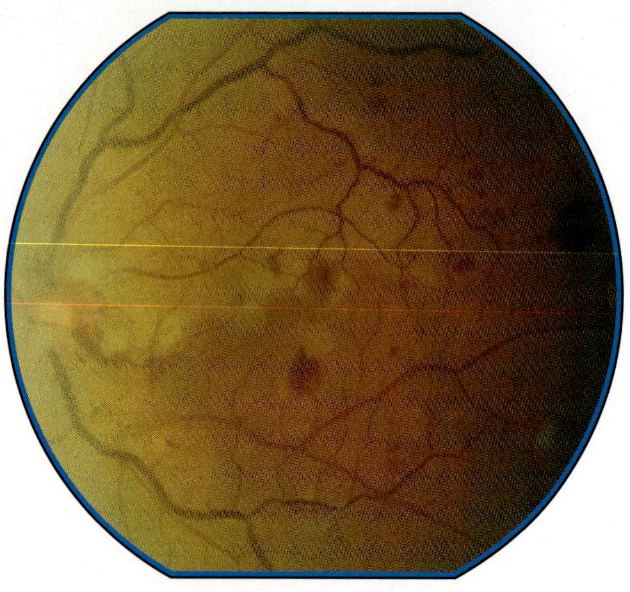

31–18

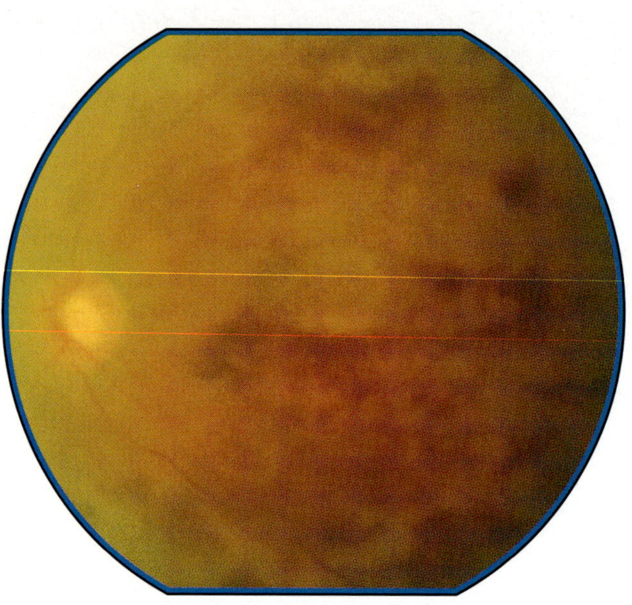

31–16 This patient with Wegener's granulomatosis has cystoid macular edema with a foveal cyst, an epiretinal membrane, and vitreous inflammation.

31–17 and 31–18 The CREST syndrome is a milder variant of scleroderma with calcinosis, Raynaud's phenomenon, esophageal, and dermatologic disease. This 60-year-old female with the CREST syndrome developed combined central retinal artery and vein occlusions.

31–17 *and* ***31–18,*** *Courtesy of Dr. John Sorenson.*

31–19 PROTEIN C DEFICIENCY

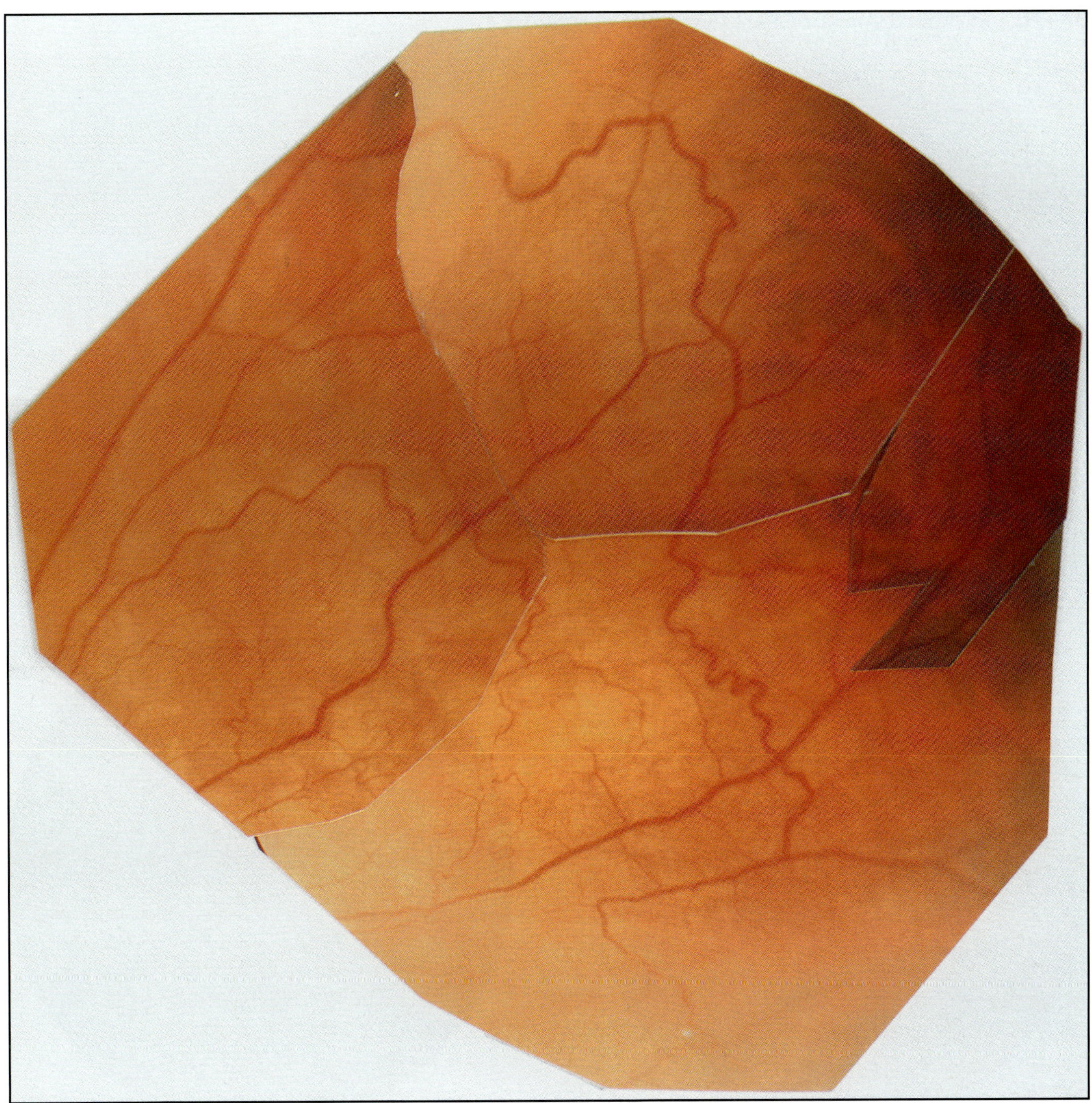

31–19 This patient with protein C deficiency illustrates arterial to arterial anastomosis following peripheral arterial occlusive disease.

Other Systemic Diseases

31–20 GASTROINTESTINAL DISEASES: REGIONAL ENTERITIS

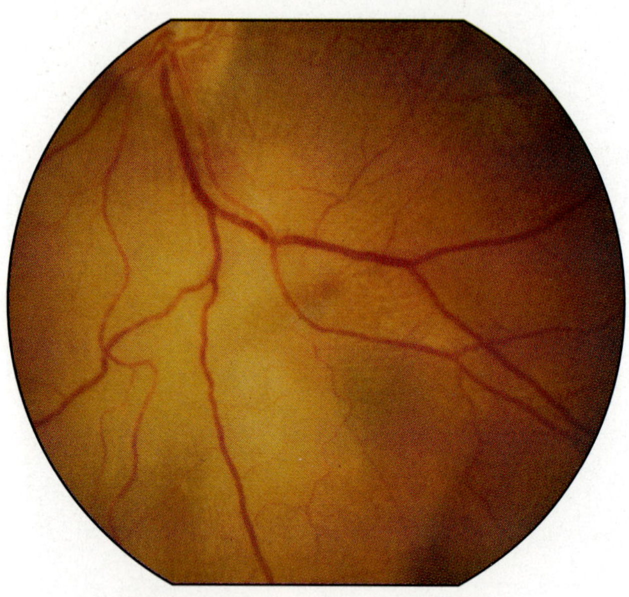

31–21 GIARDIA

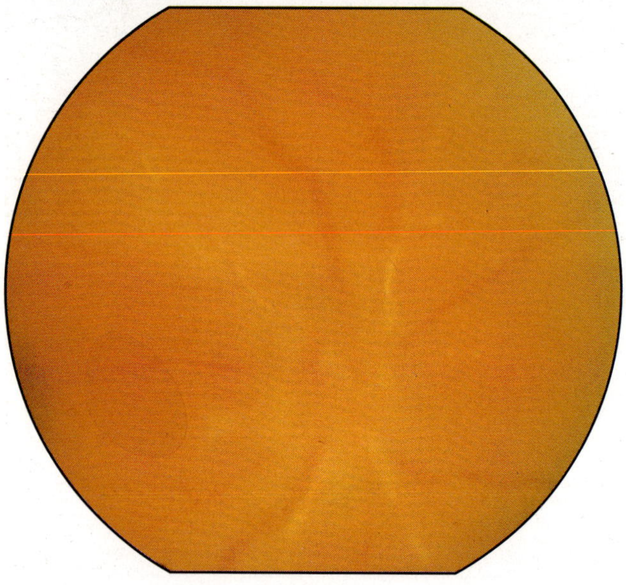

31–22

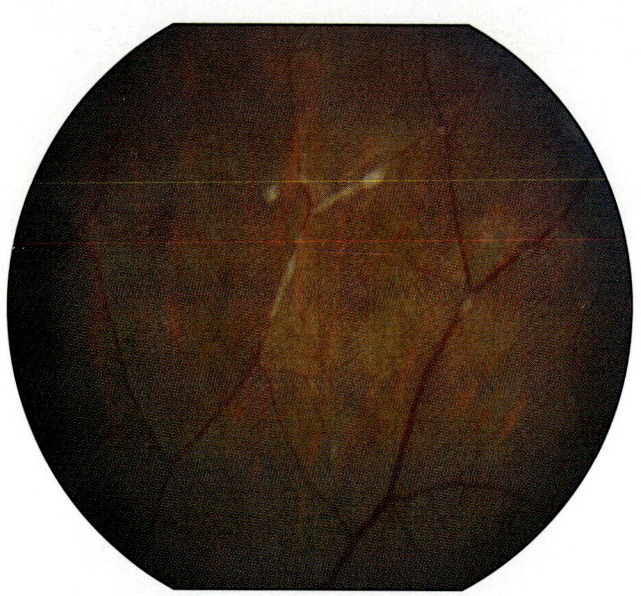

31–20 This patient with regional enteritis developed exudative retinal detachments over multifocal choroiditis.

31–21 and 31–22 Two patients have a hazy vitreous and yellow-white deposits around thickened retinal vessels with sheathing. Jejunal biopsy specimen demonstrated Giardia lamblia. Antiparasite drug treatment was followed with improvement of the ocular and systemic findings.

31–20 *Courtesy of Dr. David Knox. From Knox, DL, Schachat, AP, and Mustonen, E: Primary, secondary and coincidental ocular complications of Crohn's disease, Ophthalmology 91:163–173, 1984.* ***31–21*** *and* ***31–22,*** *Courtesy of Dr. David Knox. From Knox, DL, and King, J: Retinal arteritis, iridocyclitis, and giardiasis, Ophthalmology 89:1303–1308, 1982.*

31–23 PANCREATITIS

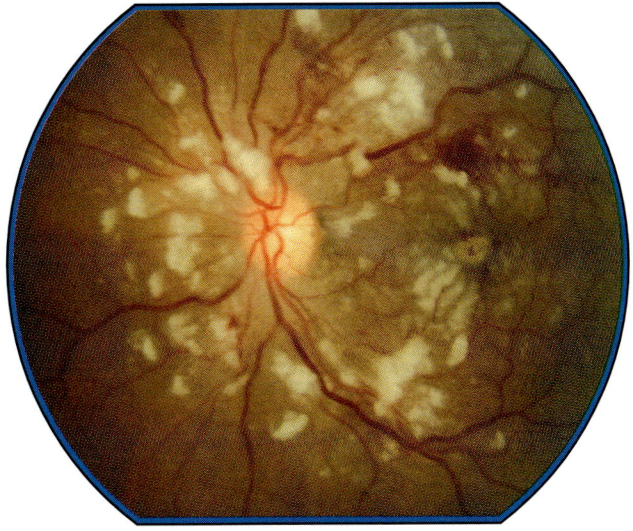

31–24

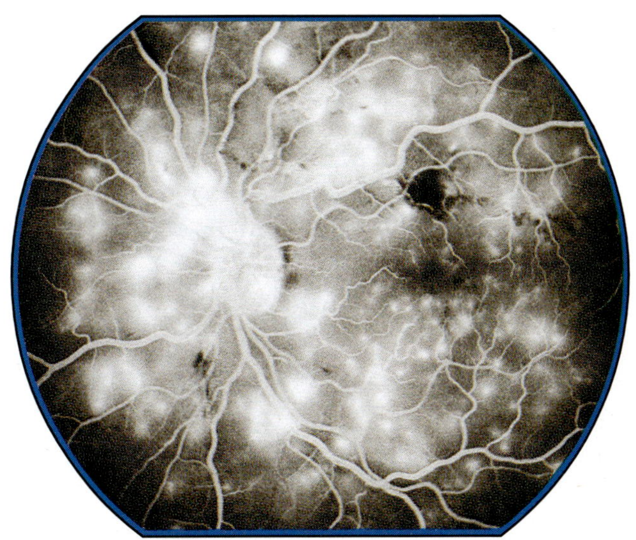

31–25 WHIPPLE'S DISEASE

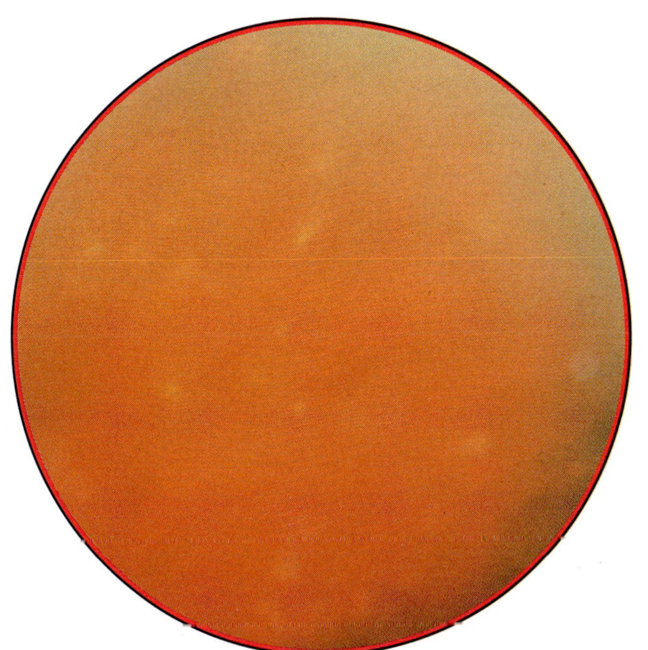

31–26 and 31–27

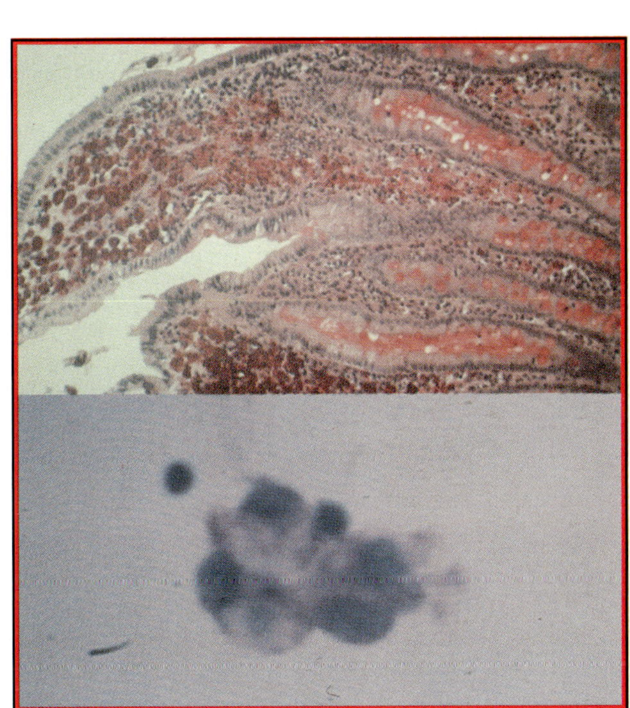

31–23 and 31–24 Acute pancreatitis may cause a Purtscher's-like retinopathy. This patient developed visual loss during trimethoprim and sulfamethoxazole (Bactrim)-induced pancreatitis. Note the multifocal inner and outer retinal infarcts. In this case, there is a disseminated intravascular coagulopathy-like picture, whereas in other cases only the inner retina may be affected. Leukoembolization has been proposed as the cause of this type of retinopathy.

31–25 through 31–27 Whitish choroidal lesions (31–25) are noted in this patient with biopsy-proven Whipple's disease (31–26 and 31–27).

31–23 and 31–24, Courtesy of Dr. Mark W. Johnson. 31–25 through 31–27, Courtesy of Dr. Alan Friedman.

31–28 WEBER-CHRISTIAN DISEASE

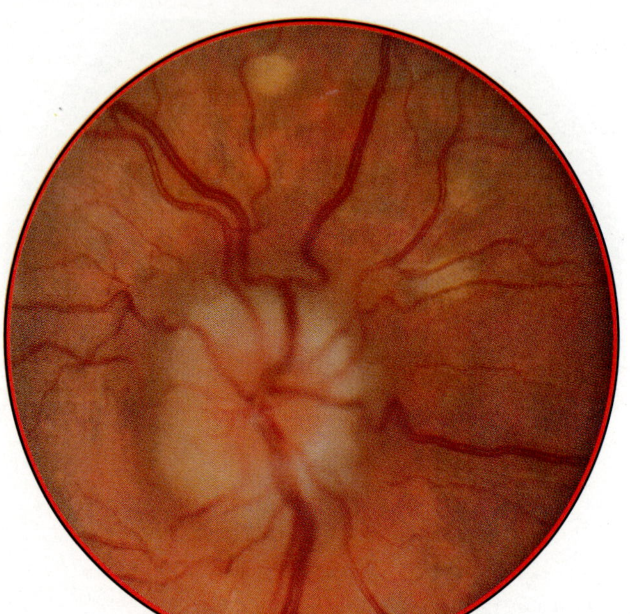

31–29

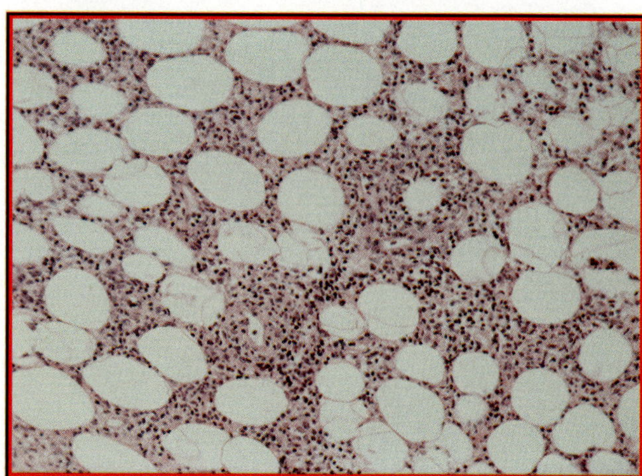

31–28 Weber-Christian disease consists of nodular panniculitis and fever. Bone marrow, pulmonary, and/or pancreatic disease may also occur. If the panniculitis occurs with acute systemic symptoms, a collagen vascular, pancreatic, or lymphomatous disease is often present. This patient with Weber-Christian disease has yellowish white subretinal lesions and optic disc edema.

31–29 Biopsy was consistent with panniculitis.

Suggested Readings

Arnett, FC, Bias, WB, and Stevens, MB: Juvenile-onset chronic arthritis: clinical and roentgenographic features of a unique HLA-B27 subset, Am J Med 69:369–376, 1980

Belmont, JB, and Michelson, JB: Vitrectomy in uveitis associated with ankylosing spondylitis, Am J Ophthalmol 94:300–304, 1982

Bohan, A, Peter, JB, Bowman, RL, and Pearson, CM: A computer assisted analysis of 153 patients with polymyositis and dermatomyositis, Medicine (Baltimore) 56:255, 1977

Bullen, CL, Liesegang, TJ, McDonald, TJ, and DeRemee, RA: Ocular complications of Wegener's granulomatosis, Ophthalmology 90:279–290, 1983

Calabro, JJ, Parrino, GR, Atchoo, PD, Marchesano, JM, and Goldberg, JS: Chronic iridocyclitis in juvenile rheumatoid arthritis, Arthritis Rheum 13:406–413, 1970

Chamberlain, MA: Behçet's syndrome in 32 patients in Yorkshire, Ann Rheum Dis 36:491–499, 1977

Cullen, JF, and Coleiro, JA: Ophthalmologic complications of giant cell arteritis, Surv Ophthalmol 20:247–260, 1976

Diddie, KR, Aronson, AJ, and Ernest, JT: Chorioretinopathy in a case of systemic lupus erythematosus, Trans Am Ophthal Soc 75:122–129, 1977

Duguid, JB: Periarteritis nodosa, Trans Ophthalmol Soc UK 74:25–40, 1954

Gold, D, Feiner, L, and Henkind, P: Retinal arterial occlusive disease in systemic lupus erythematosus, Arch Ophthalmol 95:1580–1585, 1977

Hamilton, CR, Shelley, WM, and Tumulty, PA: Giant cell arteritis: including temporal arteritis and polymyalgia rheumatica, Medicine (Baltimore) 50:1–27, 1971

Hochberg, MC, Boyd, RE, Ahearn, JM, Arnett, FC, Bis, WB, Provost, TT, and Stevens, MB: Systemic lupus erythematosus: a review of clinico-laboratory features and immunogenetic markers in 150 patients with emphasis on demographic subsets, Medicine (Baltimore) 64:285–295, 1985

Hopkins, DJ, Horan, E, Burton, IL, Clamp, SE, Dombal, FT, and Goligher, JC: Ocular disorders in a series of 332 patients with Crohn's disease, Br J Ophthalmol 58:732–737, 1974

Issak, BL, Liesegang, TJ, and Michel, CJ: Ocular and systemic findings in relapsing polychondritis, Ophthalmology 93:681–689, 1986

Michelson, JB, and Chisari, FV: Behçet's disease, Surv Ophthalmol 26:190–203, 1982

Scherbel, AL, Mackenzie, AH, Nousek, JE, and Atdjian, M: Ocular lesions in rheumatoid arthritis and related disorders with particular reference to retinopathy: a study of 741 patients treated with and without chloroquine drugs, N Engl J Med 273:360–366, 1965

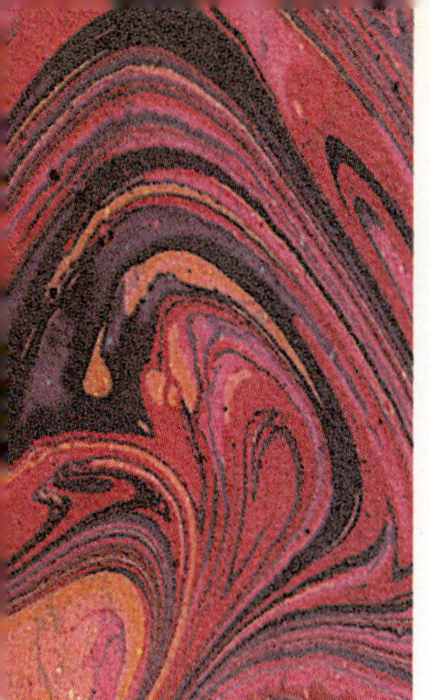

Chapter 32

Parafoveal Telangiectasis

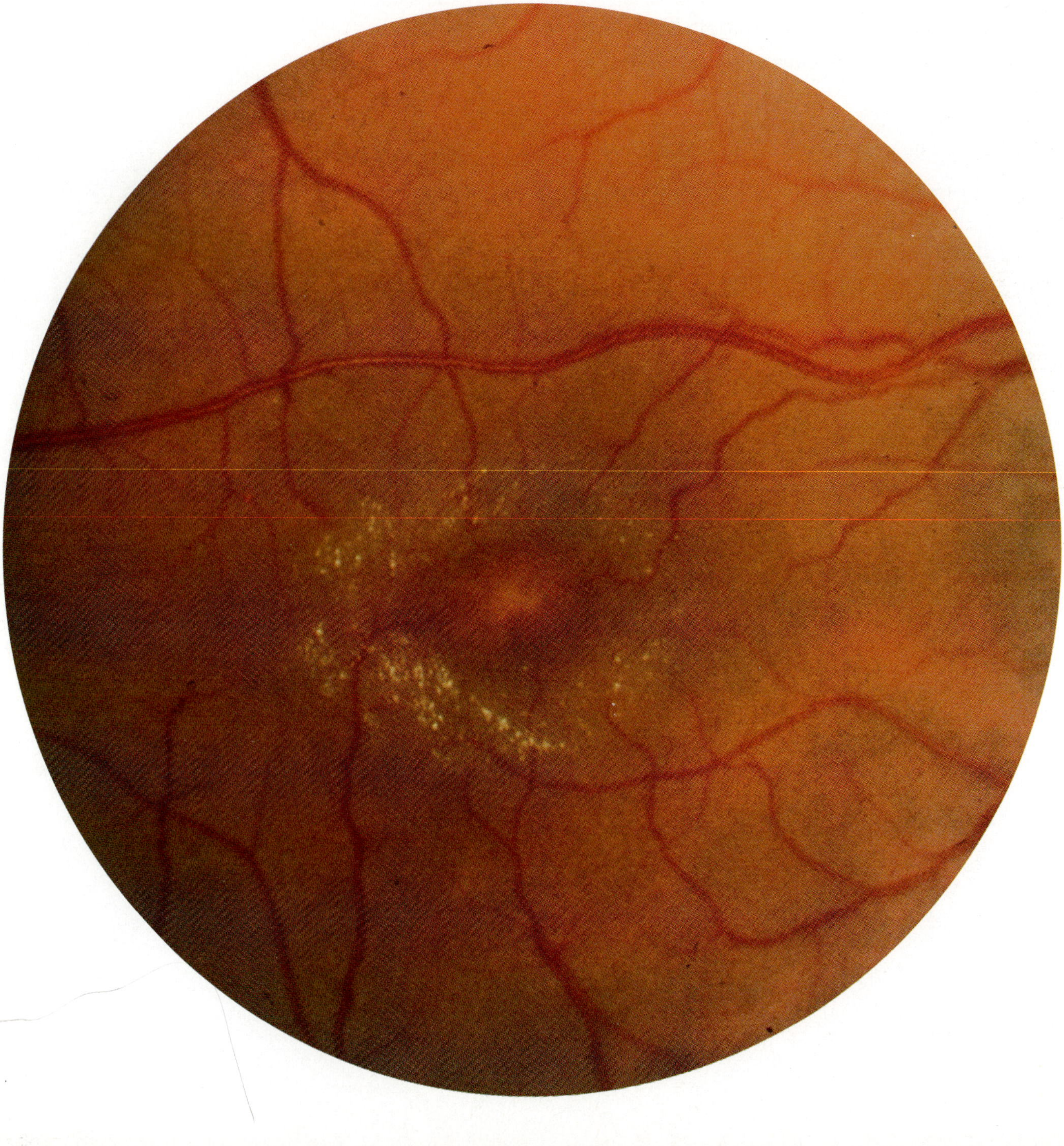

Parafoveal telangiectasis may be divided into several subgroups. Group IA consists of unilateral congenital parafoveal telangiectasis; group IB consists of unilateral idiopathic parafoveal telangiectasis, group II consists of bilateral or acquired parafoveal telangiectasis. In addition, there is a group III category of patients who have bilateral idiopathic perifoveal telangiectasis with capillary occlusion.

Patients with group IA or congenital disease have telangiectasis unilaterally in the temporal portion of the macula. Macular edema and exudation are common. Group IB or unilateral idiopathic disease is noted in middle-aged men. Hard exudates may be seen, but there is rarely leakage on fluorescein angiography. Visual acuity is usually very good. The most common group of patients have group II or bilaterally acquired parafoveal telangiectasis. These patients are usually elderly and may be of either sex. Usually telangiectasis is symmetric and bilateral and seen in the temporal area but can involve the entire capillary zone. Macular edema is commonly seen in this group. The retinal capillaries are mildly dilated. Superficial glistening crystals may be noted. These patients eventually develop retinal pigment epithelial hyperplasia along right-angled venules. Choroidal neovascularization may occur in these patients. The visual prognosis of patients who do not develop choroidal neovascularization is good. Thus, laser photocoagulation is not usually indicated for these patients. The role of abnormal glucose levels in these patients is controversial.

32–1

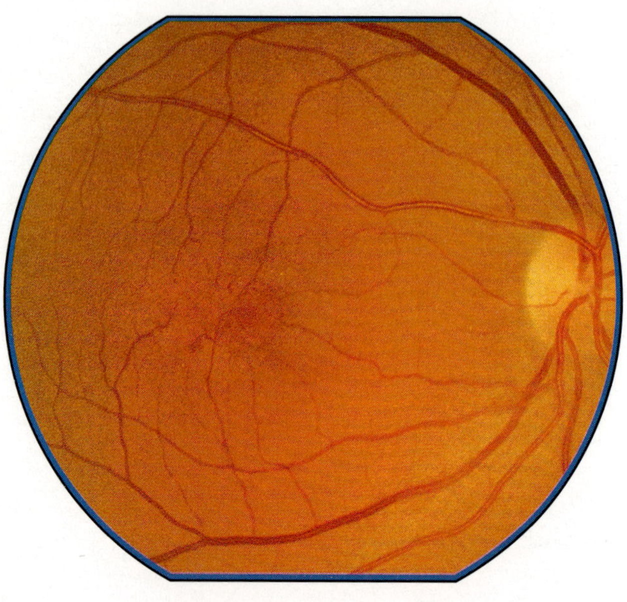

32–2

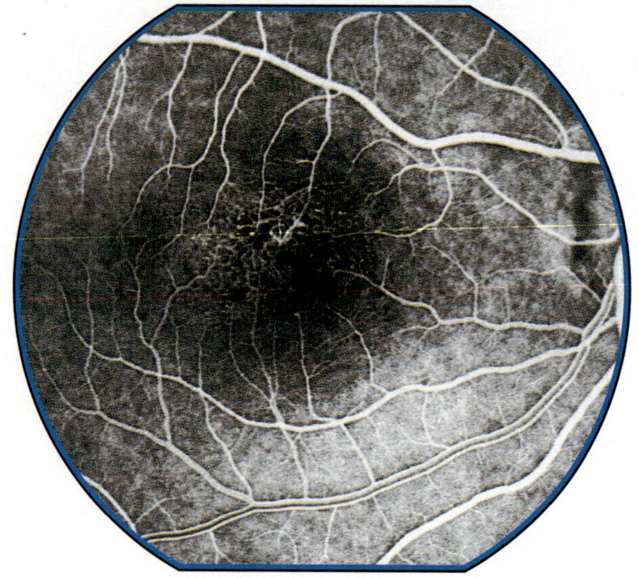

32–3

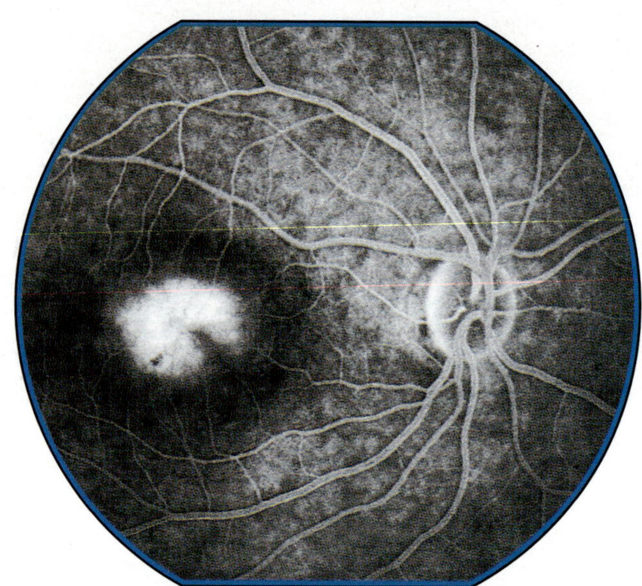

32–1 This patient has serous fluid with an area of small reddish telangiectasia noted temporally.

32–2 The early fluorescein angiogram shows telangiectatic vessels and confirms the diagnosis of parafoveal telangiectasis.

32–3 Late leakage can be demonstrated on the angiogram.

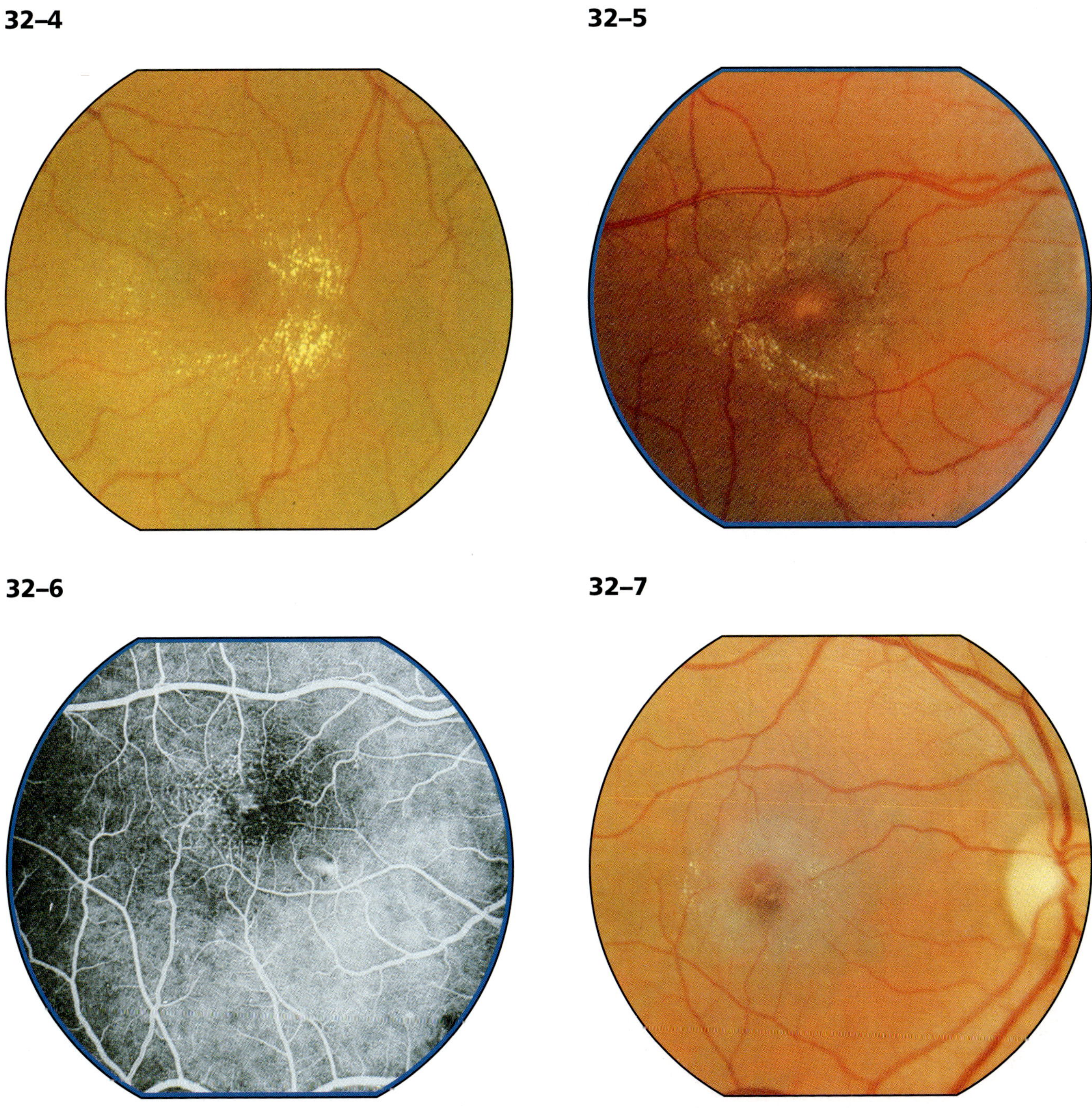

32–4 through 32–7 Crystals on the retinal surface may be seen in patients with parafoveal telangiectasis (32–4, 32–5, 32–7). Note the telangiectatic vessels, which are well illustrated on the fluorescein study (32–6). As the disease progresses, the retinal thickening and grayish discoloration encircle the parafoveal area (32–7). This patient also has some inner retinal crystalline deposits.

32–8

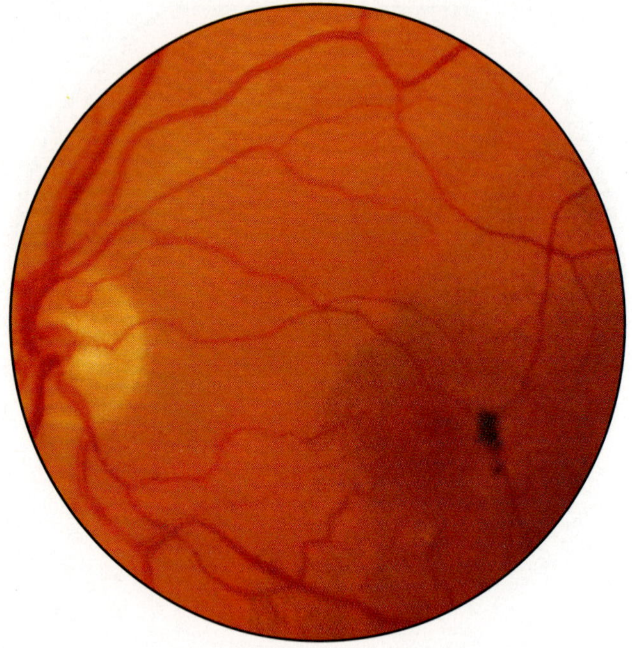

32–9

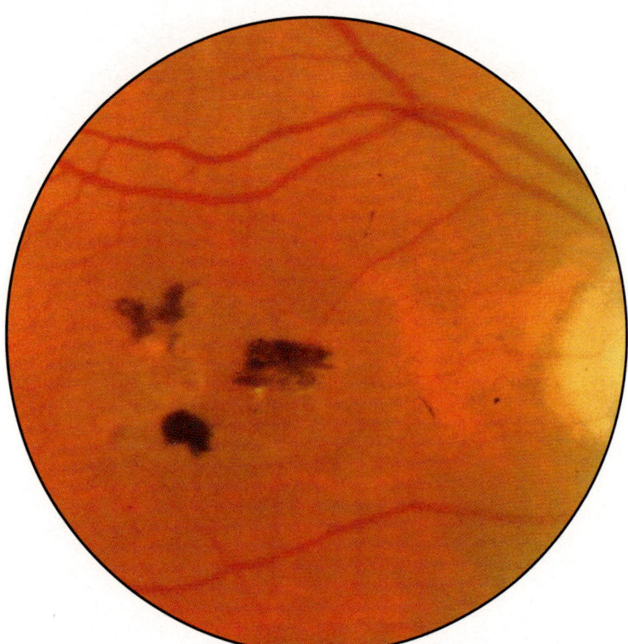

32–10

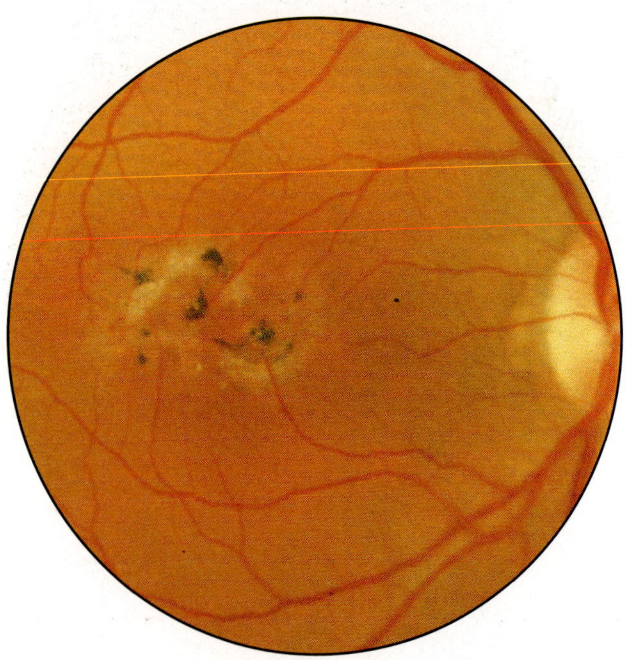

32–8 These patients may have focal areas of subretinal hyperpigmentation.

32–9 Multifocal areas of pigment epithelial hyperplasia are noted in this eye.

32–10 Later in the course of the disease, patients may experience fibrous metaplasia, as well as pigment epithelial hyperplasia, as demonstrated in this case.

32–11

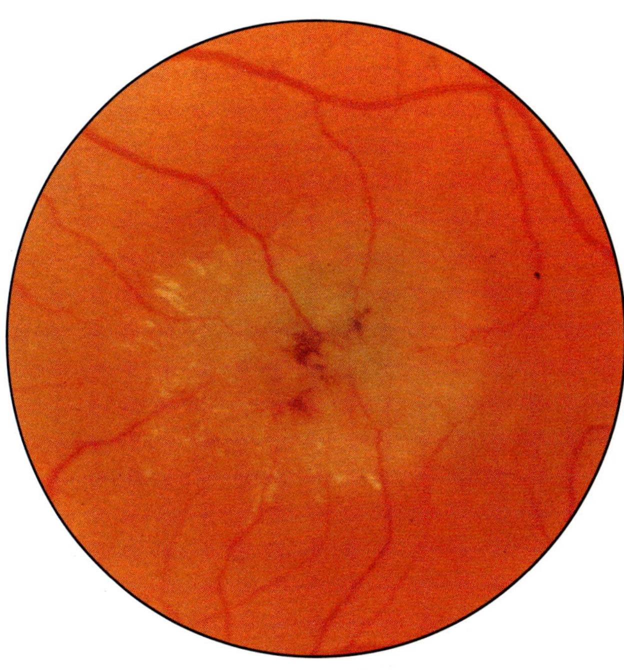

32–12

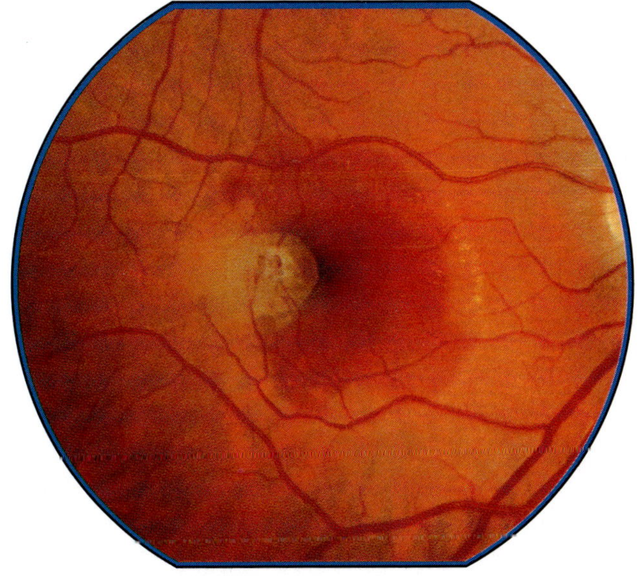

32–13

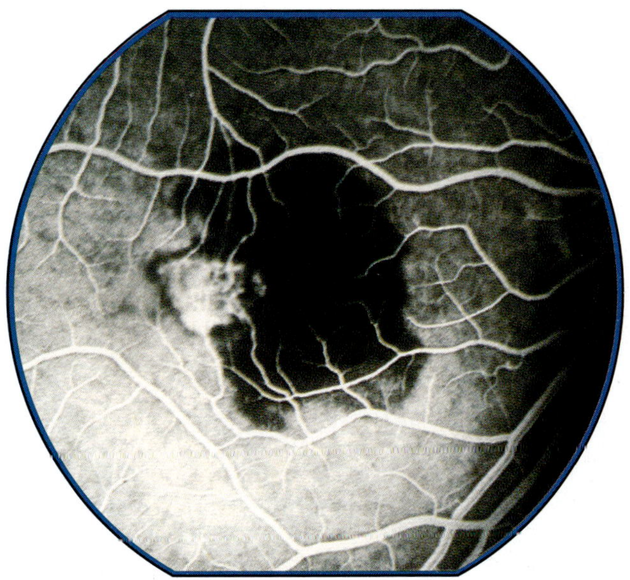

32–11 A consequence of the disturbance in the pigment epithelium may be choroidal neovascularization and its sequelae, bleeding and disciform scarring. This patient developed hemorrhage, shallow neurosensory detachment, and lipid deposition. Lipid is not characteristic of parafoveal telangiectasis unless choroidal neovascularization evolves.

32–12 and 32–13 This patient has subretinal fluid and hemorrhage secondary to choroidal neovascularization. Fluorescein angiography reveals a well-defined choroidal neovascular membrane.

(Case continued on next page.)

32–14

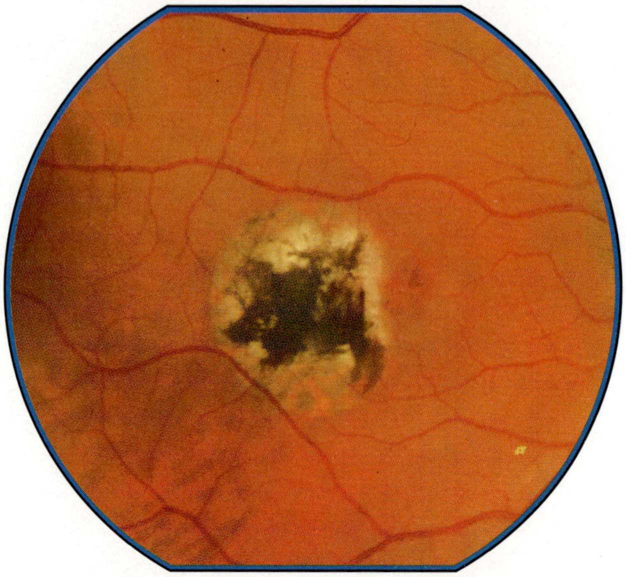

32–15

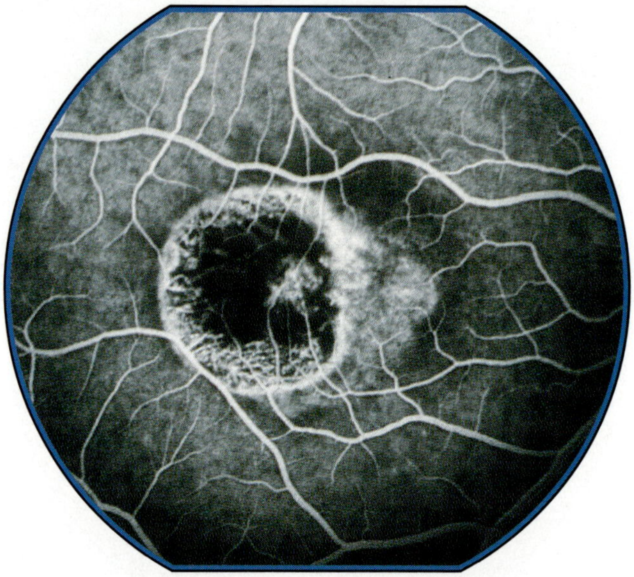

32–16

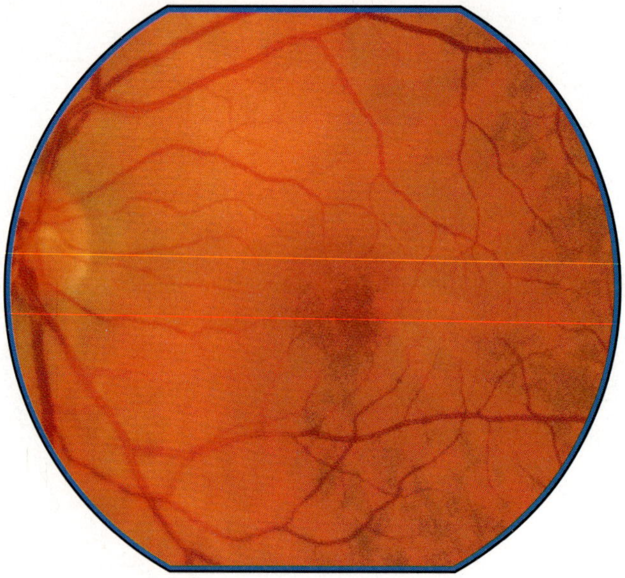

32–17

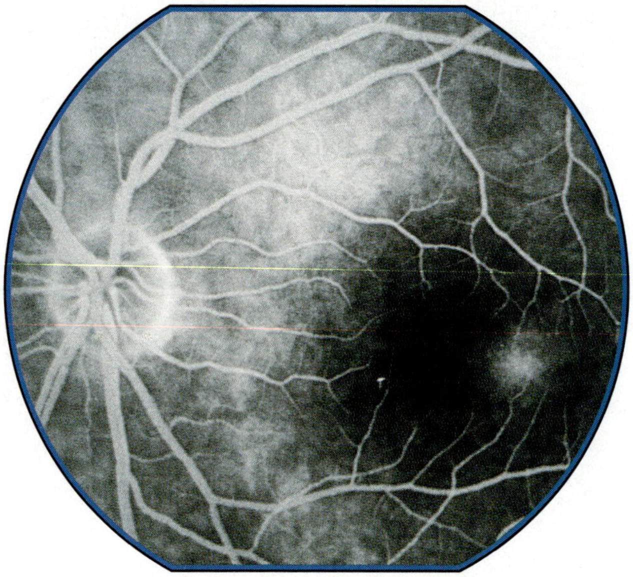

32–14 and 32–15 However, 12 years later, signs of parafoveal telangiectasis are noted. In the treated eye, telangiectatic areas are demonstrated adjacent to the laser photocoagulation scars.

32–16 and 32–17 In the other eye, which had been normal, telangiectasia can be appreciated temporally. This case also illustrates that the disease may begin unilaterally but is generally bilateral.

32–18

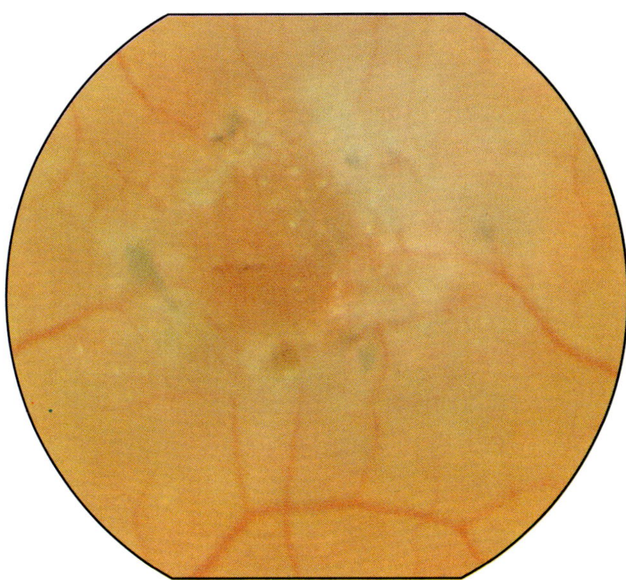

32–19

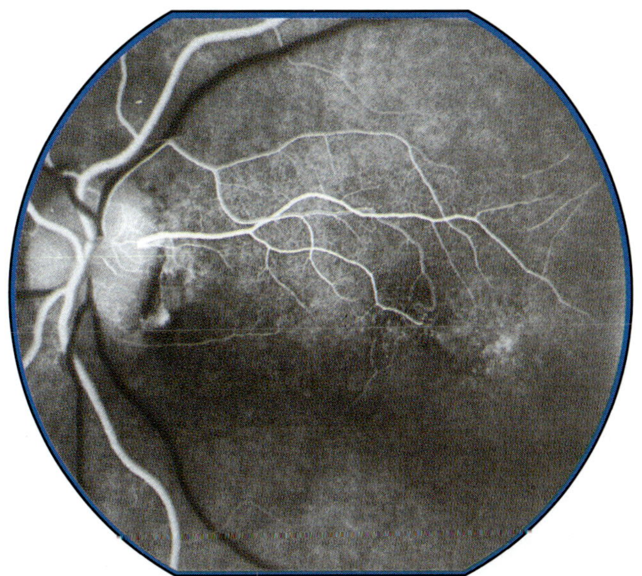

32–20

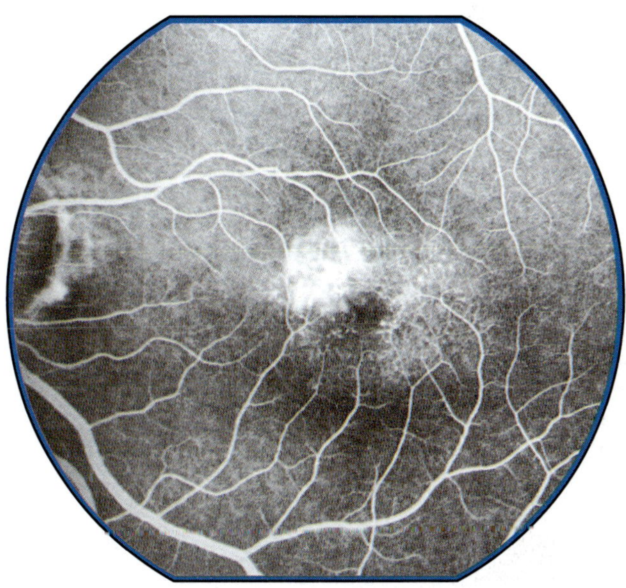

32–18 This patient has parafoveal telangiectasia with foveal atrophy. There is no lipid exudation, ischemia, aneurysmal formation, or cystoid macular edema characteristically seen in this disease. Foveal atrophy, crystallization, pigmentation, and fibrous metaplasia are characteristic of this disorder.

32–19 and 32–20 This fluorescein angiogram reveals an intraretinal arteriovenous communication as well as telangiectatic vascular changes. The anastomosis is derived from a ciliary arteriole. The later fluorescein angiogram reveals parafoveal telangiectasia with leakage.

32–21

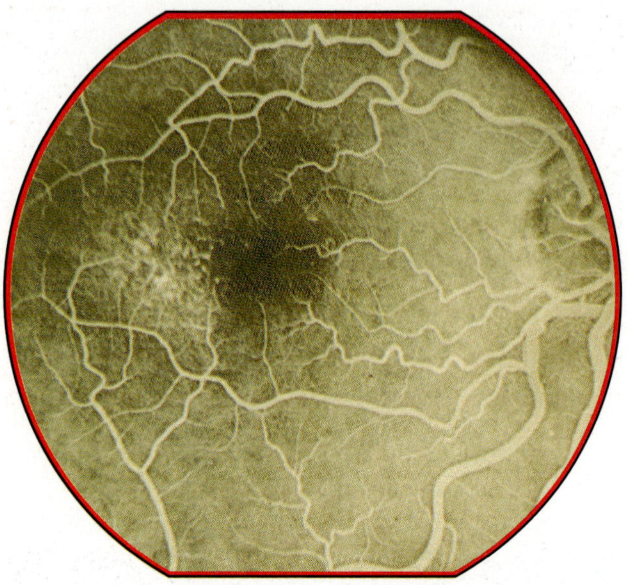

32–22

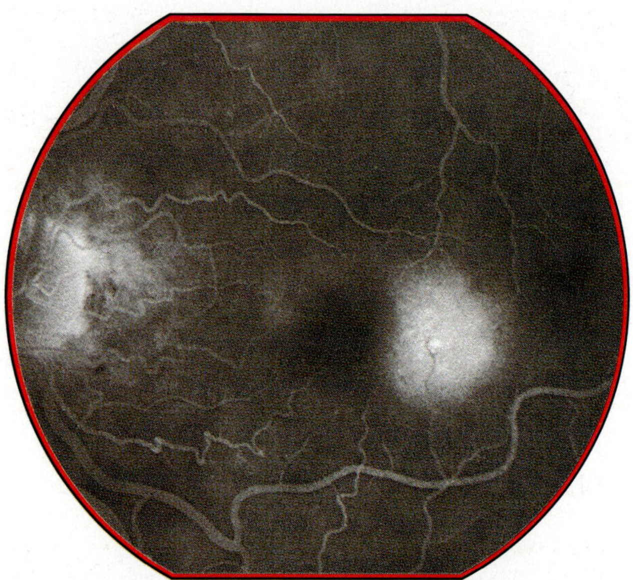

32–21 A clinicopathologic study of a patient with parafoveal telangiectasis demonstrated thickening of the capillary walls, multilamination of the basement membrane, narrowing of the capillary lumen, pericyte degeneration, lipid deposits in the capillary wall, and focal endothelial cell degeneration. No telangiectasis was noted. Although the changes were greater in the parafoveal area, similar but milder changes were noted throughout the retina. These changes were probably caused by endothelial cell degeneration and regeneration with successive basement membrane production. Secondary degeneration of pericytes also occurs.

32–22 The fluorescein angiograms of this clinicopathologic correlation reveal apparent telangiectatic vessels temporal to the fovea with late hyperfluorescence consistent with parafoveal telangiectasis.

32–21 *and* ***32–22,*** *From Green, WR, Quigley, HT, de la Cruz, Z, Cohen, B: Parafoveal retinal telangiectasia: light and electron microscopy studies, Trans Ophthalmol Soc UK 100:162–170, 1980.*

(Case continued on next page.)

32–23

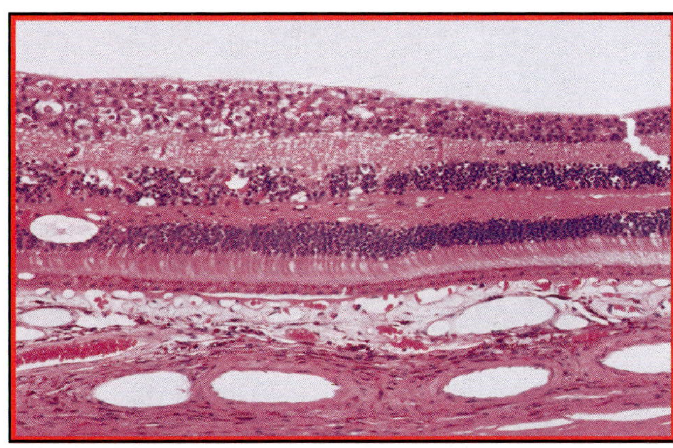

32–24

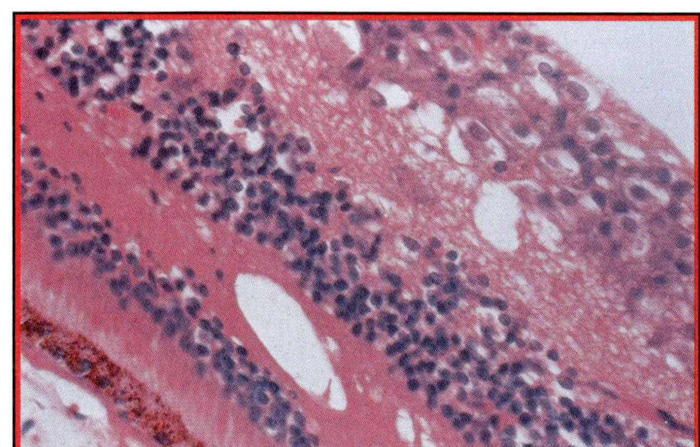

32–25

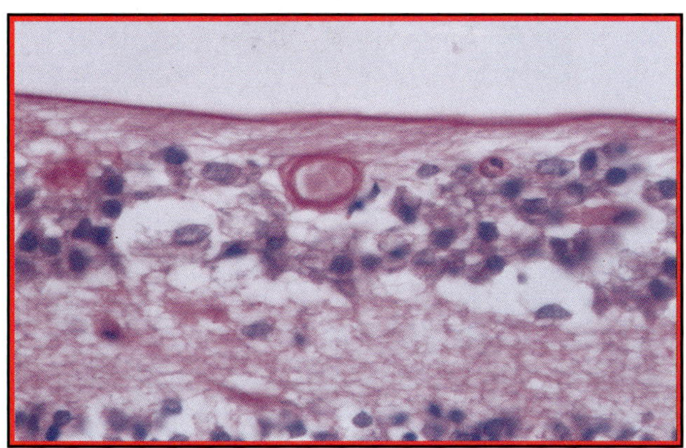

32–26

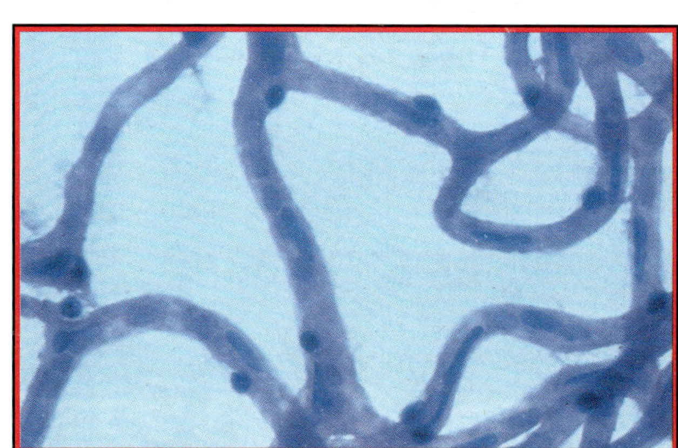

32–23 and 32–24 There is no cystoid macular edema present. Light microscopy from the temporal parafoveal area shows that the retina is thickened by edema that involves mainly the inner layers.

32–25 and 32–26 Several microcystic cavities can be appreciated. The retinal pigment epithelium is normal. Capillaries have thickened walls with multiple layers of basement membranes. No pericytes were noted in this temporal parafoveal area.

32–23 *through* ***32–26,*** *From Green, WR, Quigley, HT, de la Cruz, Z, Cohen, B: Parafoveal retinal telangiectasia: light and electron microscopy studies, Trans Ophthalmol Soc UK 100:162–170, 1980.*

(Case continued on next page.)

32–27

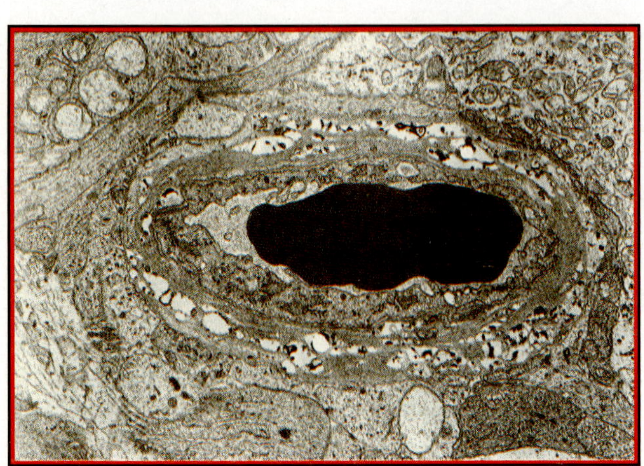

32–28

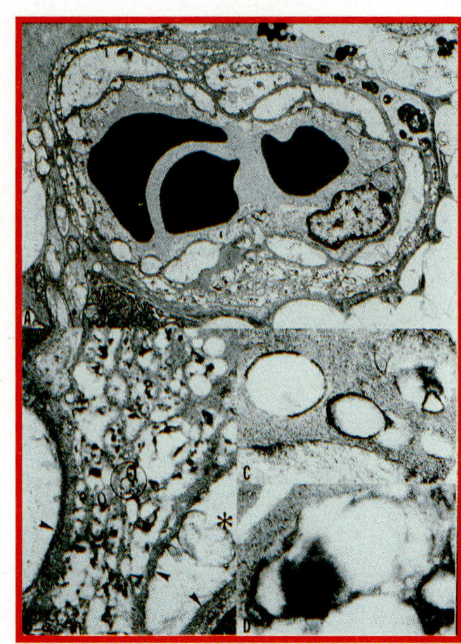

32–29

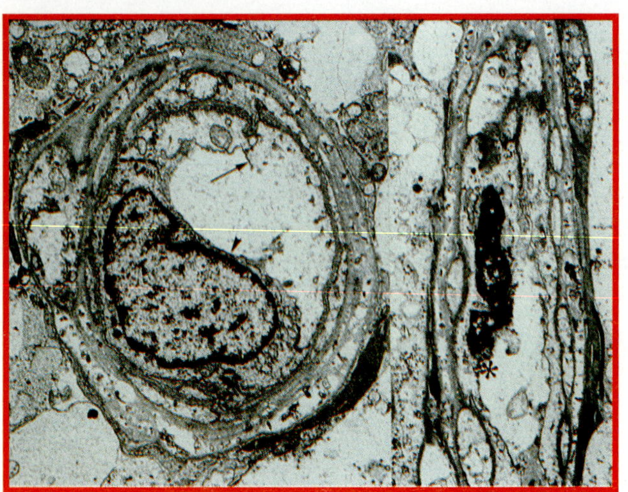

32–30

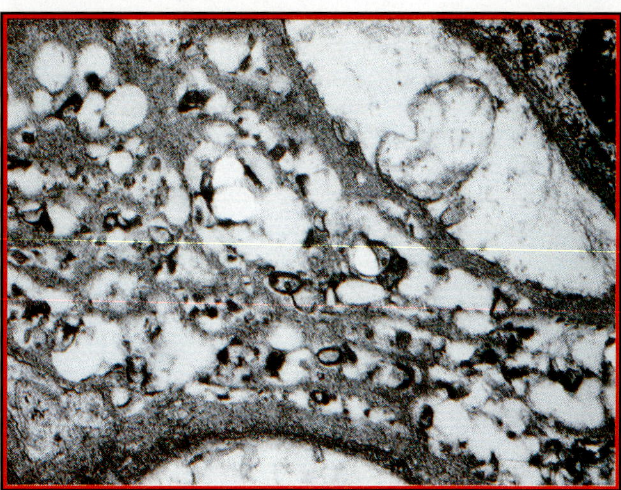

32–27 through 32–30 Electron microscopy reveals multilaminated basement membrane and deposits of lipid material in the wall of the vessels.

32–27 *through* ***32–30,*** *From Green, WR, Quigley, HT, de la Cruz, Z, Cohen, B: Parafoveal retinal telangiectasia: light and electron microscopy studies, Trans Ophthalmol Soc UK 100:162–170, 1980.*

Suggested Readings

Chew, EY, Murphy, RP, Newsome, DA, and Fine, SL: Parafoveal telangiectasis and diabetic retinopathy, Arch Ophthalmol 104:71–75, 1986

Chopdar, A: Retinal telangiectasis in adults: fluorescein angiographic findings and treatment by argon laser, Br J Ophthalmol 62:243–250, 1978

Gass, JD, and Oyakawa, RT: Idiopathic juxtafoveolar retinal telangiectasis, Arch Ophthalmol 100:769–780, 1982

Green, WR, Quigley, HA, de la Cruz, Z and Cohen, B: Parafoveal retinal telangiectasis: light and electron microscopy studies, Trans Ophthalmol Soc UK 100:162–170, 1980

Millay, RH, Klein, ML, Handelman, IL, and Watzke, RC: Abnormal glucose metabolism and parafoveal telangiectasia, Am J Ophthalmol 102:363–370, 1986

Moisseiev, J, Lewis, H, Bartov, E, Fine, SL, and Murphy, RP: Superficial retinal refractile deposits in juxtafoveal telangiectasis, Am J Ophthalmol 109:604–605, 1990

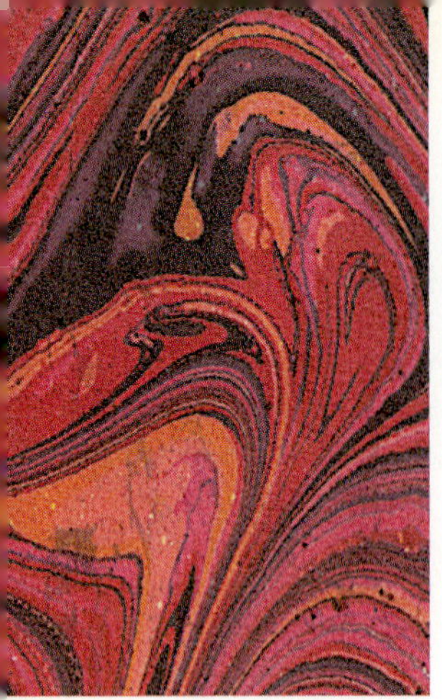

Chapter 33

Coats' Disease

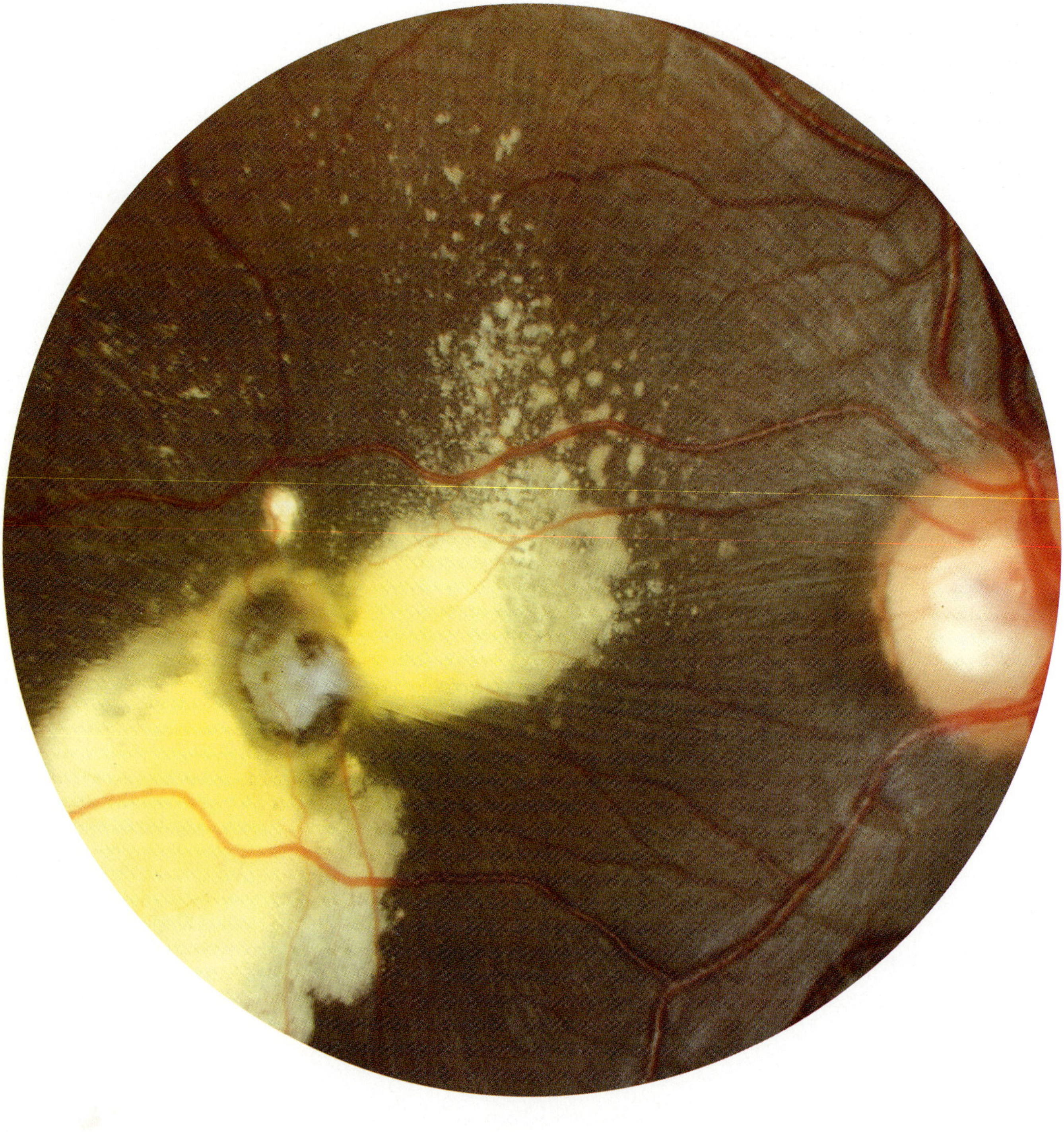

In Coats' disease, telangiectatic vessels occur and may cause exudation. Coats' disease is more common in males. It is unilateral in over 80% of cases. Leber described a disease with similar vascular abnormalities that lacked the massive subretinal exudation often seen in Coats' disease. This condition is known as Leber's multiple miliary aneurysms. This latter condition is probably simply an early or nonprogressive form of Coats' disease.

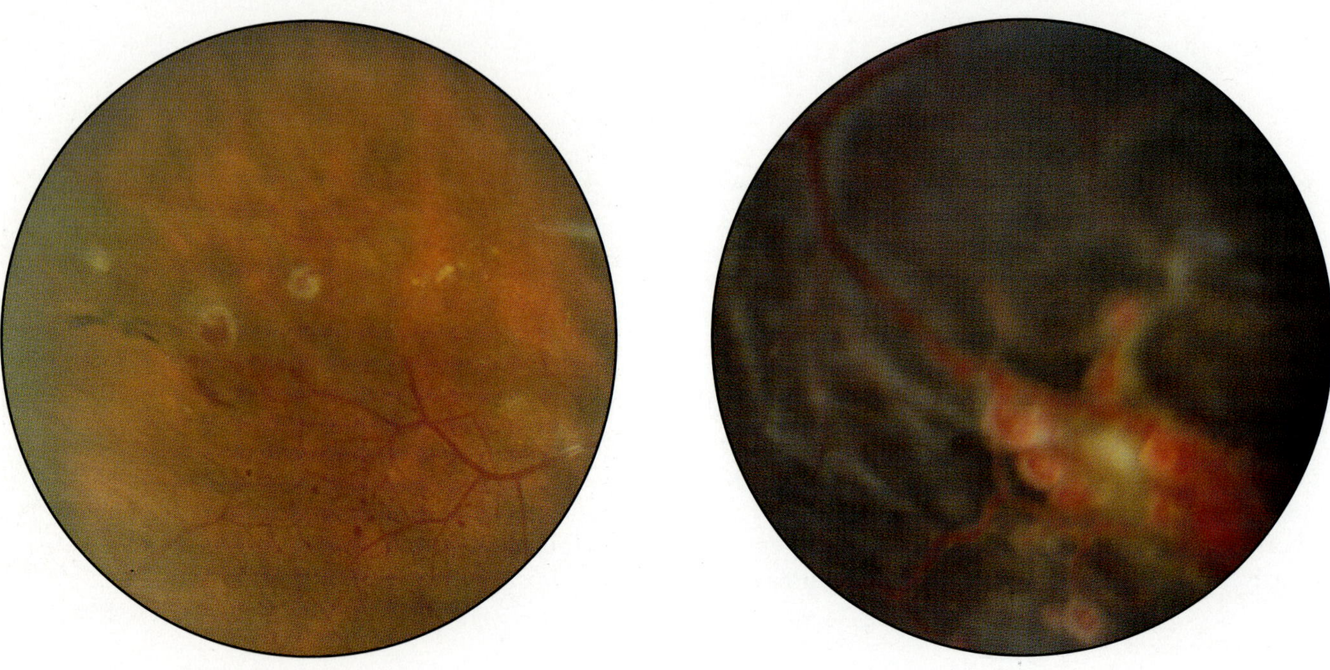

33–1 This is a patient with congenital telangiectasis and virtually no visual dysfunction. On incidental examination, dilated telangiectatic vessels were noted, associated with multiple aneurysmal changes of various size. There is sheathing of some vessels, peripheral ischemia, and a halo of exudate or fibrous proliferation around some of the larger aneurysms. In the region of the nonperfusion, there is some pigment epithelial hyperplasia presumably resulting from antecedent exudative change. Curiously, neither hemorrhage nor preretinal neovascularization is demonstrated in this patient, as is characteristic of this vasculopathy.

33–2 In Coats' disease, telangiectasis with secondary exudation is noted. This patient has peripheral telangiectasis with a secondary exudation detachment.

33–3

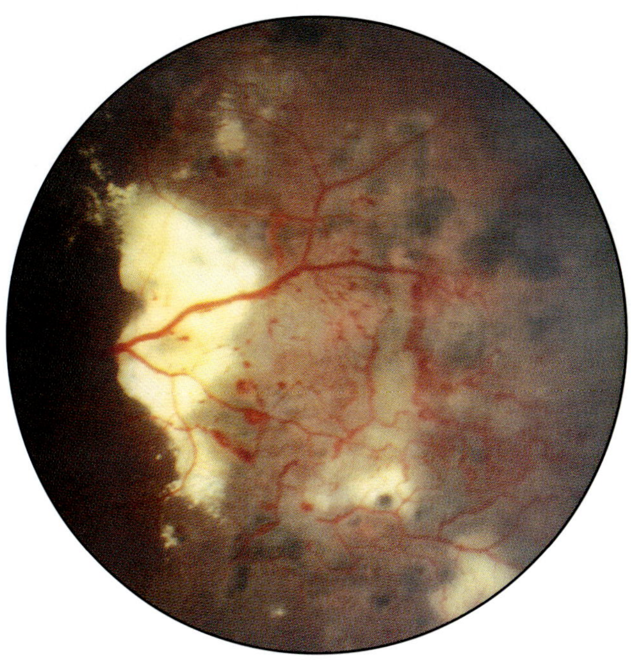

33–4

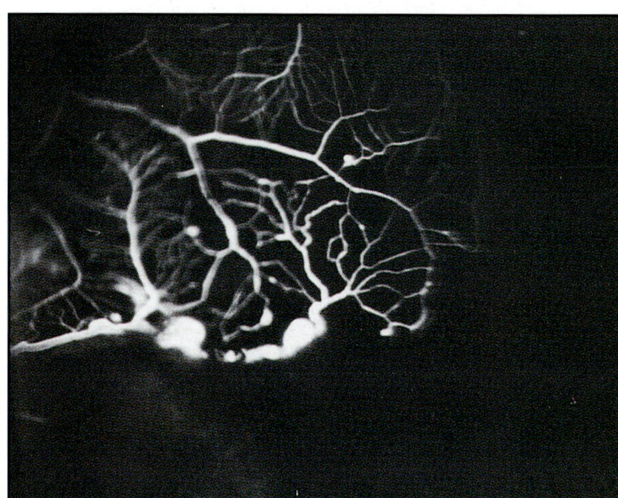

33–3 Dilated telangiectatic vessels can also be demonstrated in this case. There are scattered photocoagulation scars from previous treatment. Note the widespread aneurysmal changes on both the venous and arteriolar side of the circulation, and the extensive secondary exudation.

33–4 Fluorescein angiography of patients with Coats' disease reveals dilated vessels, as well as capillary nonperfusion.

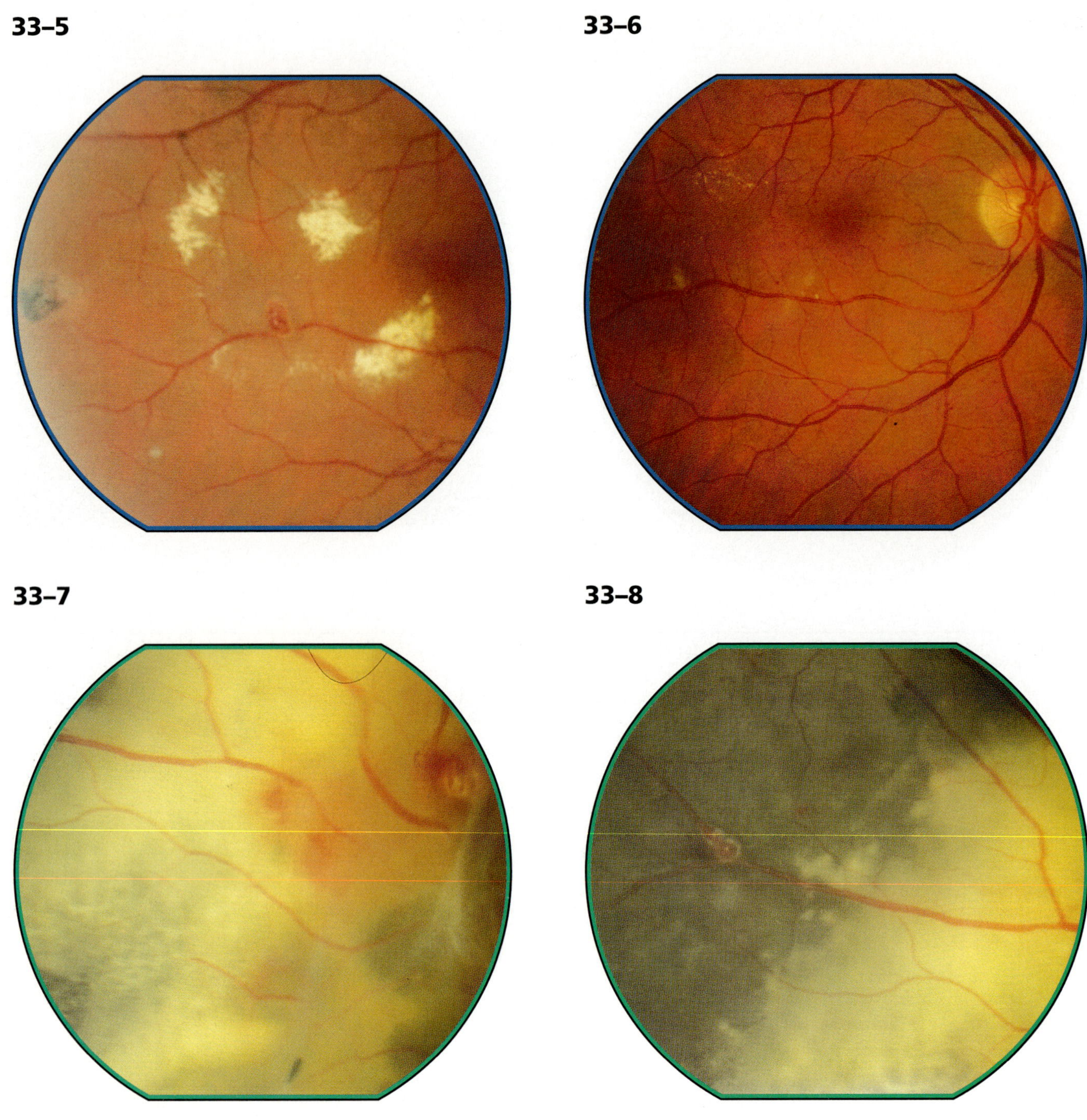

33–5 and 33–6 A localized macroaneurysmal change and dilated telangiectatic vessels are seen with secondary serous and lipid exudation in this case. This patient was treated with laser photocoagulation and showed resolution of the exudative findings.

33–7 and 33–8 This patient has congenital telangiectasis with aneurysmal changes. There is also subretinal hemorrhage, but most evident is massive lipid exudation that has diffused beneath the retina and gravitated toward the posterior pole. A secondary exudative detachment with some fibrous proliferation is also noted. In the same patient, the typical aneurysmal changes on a venule are evident where there is no extensive exudation.

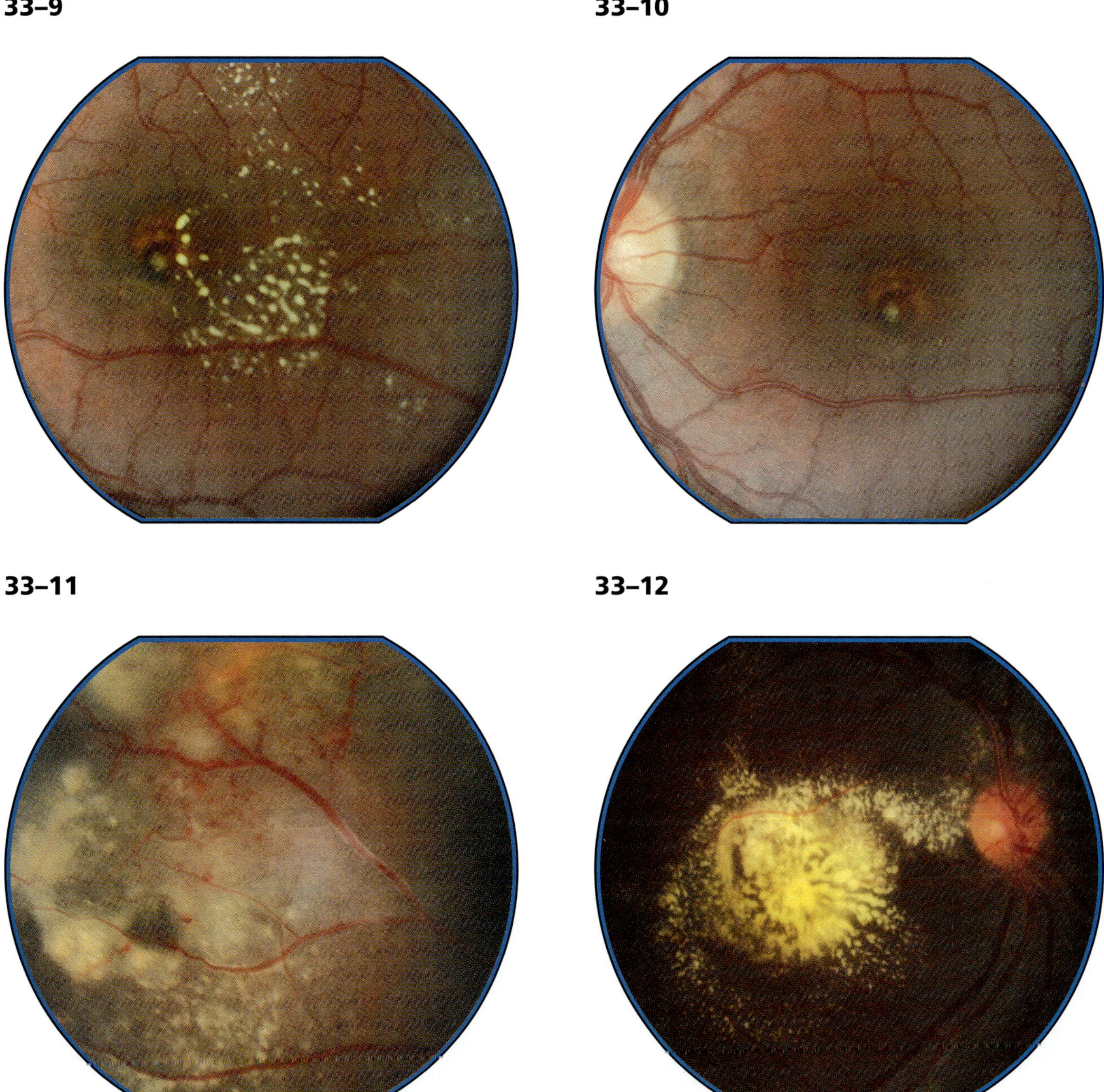

33–9 and 33–10 This patient presented with lipid deposition in the macula. There was also an atrophic pigment epithelial disturbance and a small, focal area of choroidal neovascularization in the juxtafoveal region from the exudative disturbance of the macula. Rarely is neovascularization or vitreous hemorrhage demonstrated in Coats' disease. The peripheral telangiectasis was photocoagulated with resolution of the lipid deposition in the macula.

33–11 and 33–12 This patient had extensive macular edema secondary to exudation from Coats' disease. Note the telangiectasis and exudation in the periphery (33–11) and the macular edema (33–12).

(Case continued on next page.)

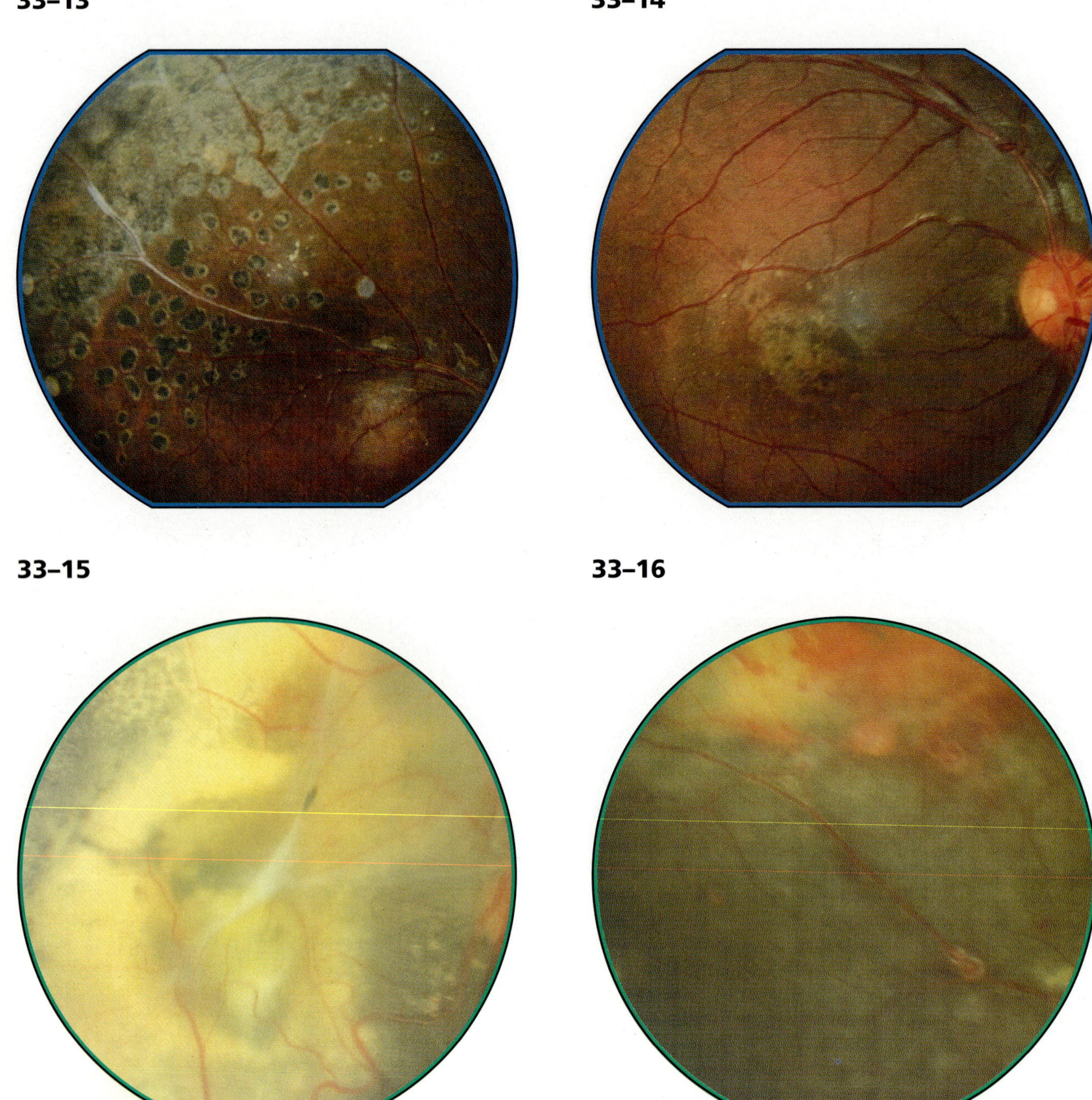

33–13 Laser photocoagulation was applied to the periphery.

33–14 This treatment caused resolution of the macular edema. Note the atrophic changes in the macula after resolution of the lipid and edema.

33–15 This patient has massive lipid exudation in the macula (a Coats' response in the macula). In addition, there is a circular area of choroidal neovascularization or disciform scarring at the fovea. Preretinal fibrosis with vitreoretinal tractional elements are also evident. A small clump of telangiectatic vessels is seen in the superior macula.

33–16 In the same patient, the retinal vascular aneurysmal, telangiectatic, exudative, and hemorrhage changes characteristic of Coats' disease may be seen.

33–17

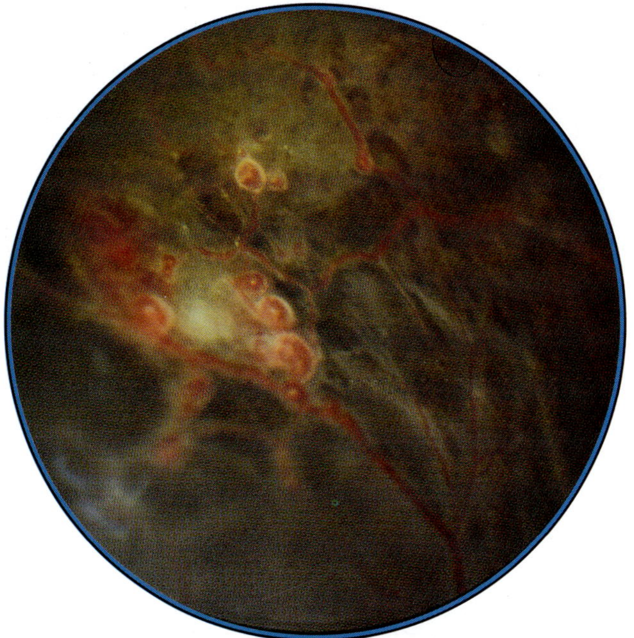

33–18

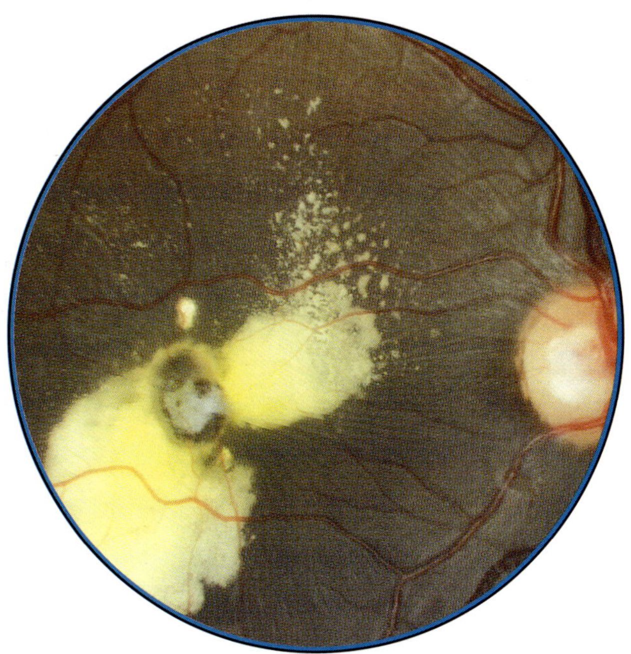

33–19

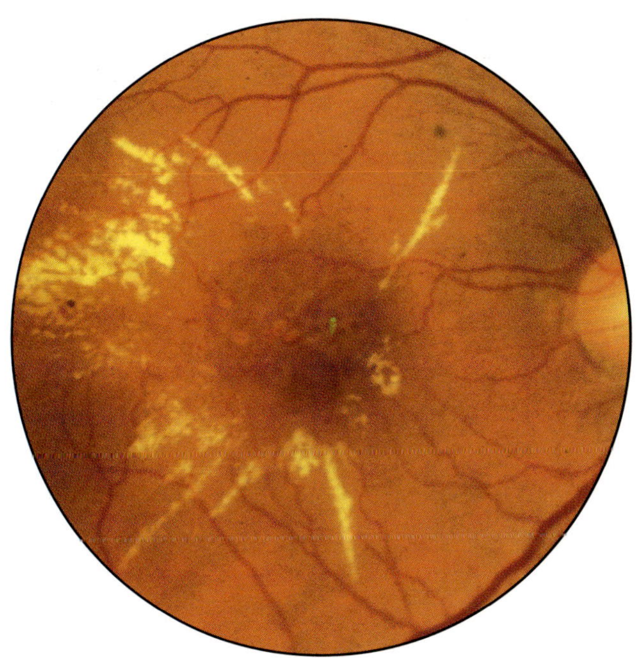

33–17 and 33–18 This patient with Coats' disease had extensive telangiectasis in the periphery. Note the halo around the multiple telangiectatic vessels. The patient had a Coats'-like response with massive lipid exudation in the macular region. Note the striae and secondary choroidal neovascularization with disciform scarring.

33–19 Leber's miliary aneurysms with secondary lipid exudation can be seen in this case in which there are prominent aneurysms with encircling whitish halos in the macula. Cystoid macular edema and lipid exudation are noted. In general, the greater the aneurysmal involvement, the more the exudation is associated with lipid deposition.

33–20

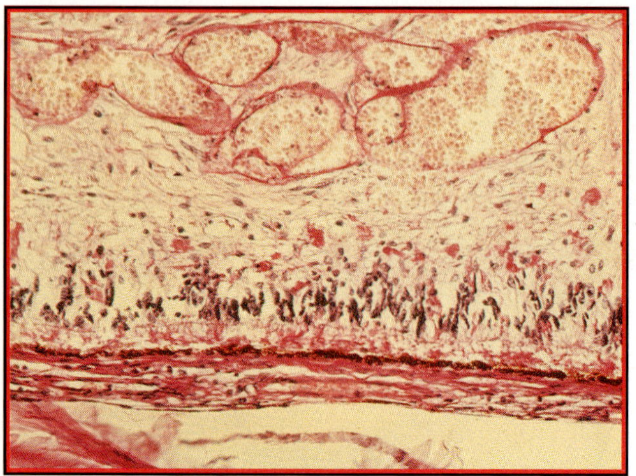

33–20A

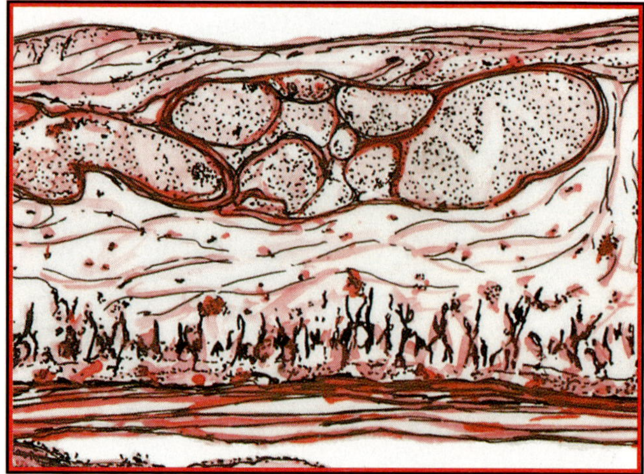

33–21

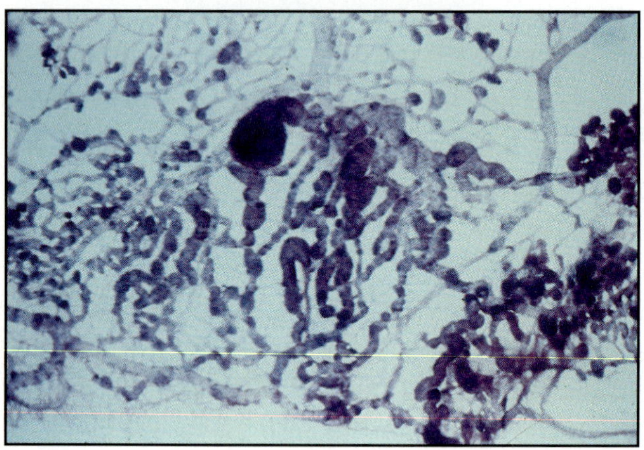

33–22

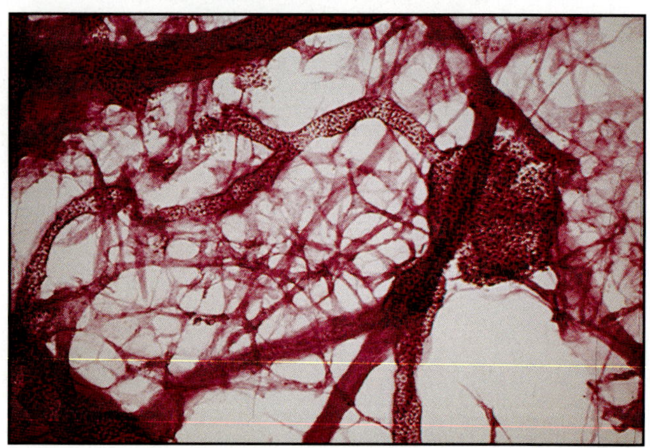

33–23

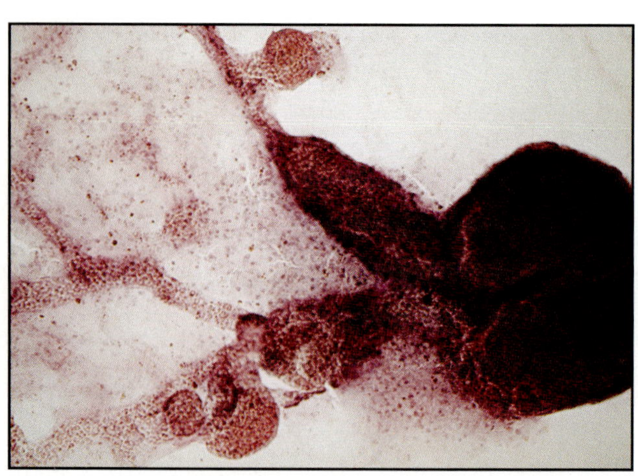

33–20 and 33–20A This histopathologic photograph shows the thin-walled telangiectatic retinal vessels in Coats' disease.

33–21 through 33–23 Trypsin digest preparations of the retina in Coats' disease reveal dilated capillaries with numerous small microaneurysms. The first of these trypsin preparations shows large aneurysms with sausage-like beading of the vessels. Note the bulbous distension of the vessels.

33–20, *From Green, WR: Bilateral Coats' disease, Arch Ophthalmol 77:378–385, 1967.* ***33–21,*** *From Egbert, PR, Chang, CC, and Winter, FC: Flat preparations of the retinal vessels in Coats' disease, J Pediatr Ophthalmol Strabismus 14:336–339, 1977.*

Suggested Readings

Bonnet M: Le syndrome de Coats, J Fr Ophthalmol 3:57, 1980

Deutsch, TA, Rabb, MF, and Jampol, LM: Spontaneous regression of retinal lesions in Coats' disease, Can J Ophthalmol 17:169, 1982

Green, WR: Bilateral Coats' disease, Arch Ophthalmol 77:378, 1967

Manschot, WA, DeBruijn, WC: Coats' disease: definition and pathogenesis, Br J Ophthalmol 51:145, 1967

Schatz, H, Burton, TC, Yanuzzi, LA, et al: Abnormal retinal and disc vessels and retinal leak. In Schatz, H, ed: Interpretation of fundus fluorescein angiography, St Louis, 1978, Mosby–Year Book, Inc, pp 408–418, 612–613

Shields, JA, Parsons, HM, Shields, CL, and Shah, P: Lesions simulating retinoblastoma, J Pediatr Ophthalmol Strabismus 28:338–340, 1991

Sugar, HS: Coats' disease: telangiectatic or multiple vascular origin, Am J Ophthalmol 45:508, 1958

Theodossiadis, GP: Some clinical, fluorescein-angiographic, and therapeutic aspects of Coats' disease, J Pediatr Ophthalmol Strabismus 16:257, 1979

Wise, GN: Coats' disease, Arch Ophthalmol 58:735, 1957

Yannuzzi, LA, Gitter, KA, and Schatz, H: The macula: a comprehensive text and atlas. Baltimore, 1979, Williams & Wilkins, pp 118–126

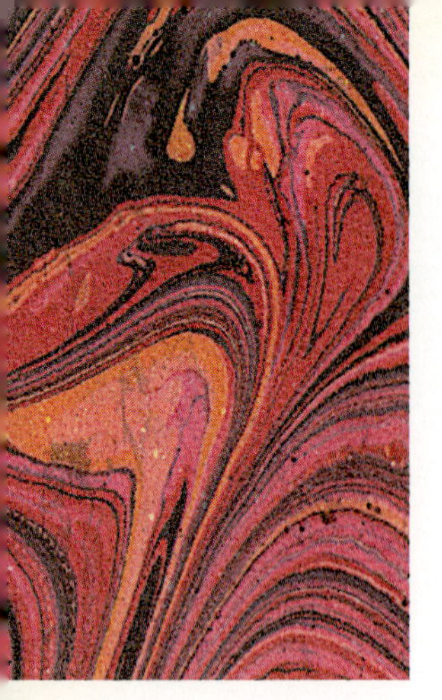

Chapter 34

Disseminated Intravascular Coagulopathy and Related Vasculopathies

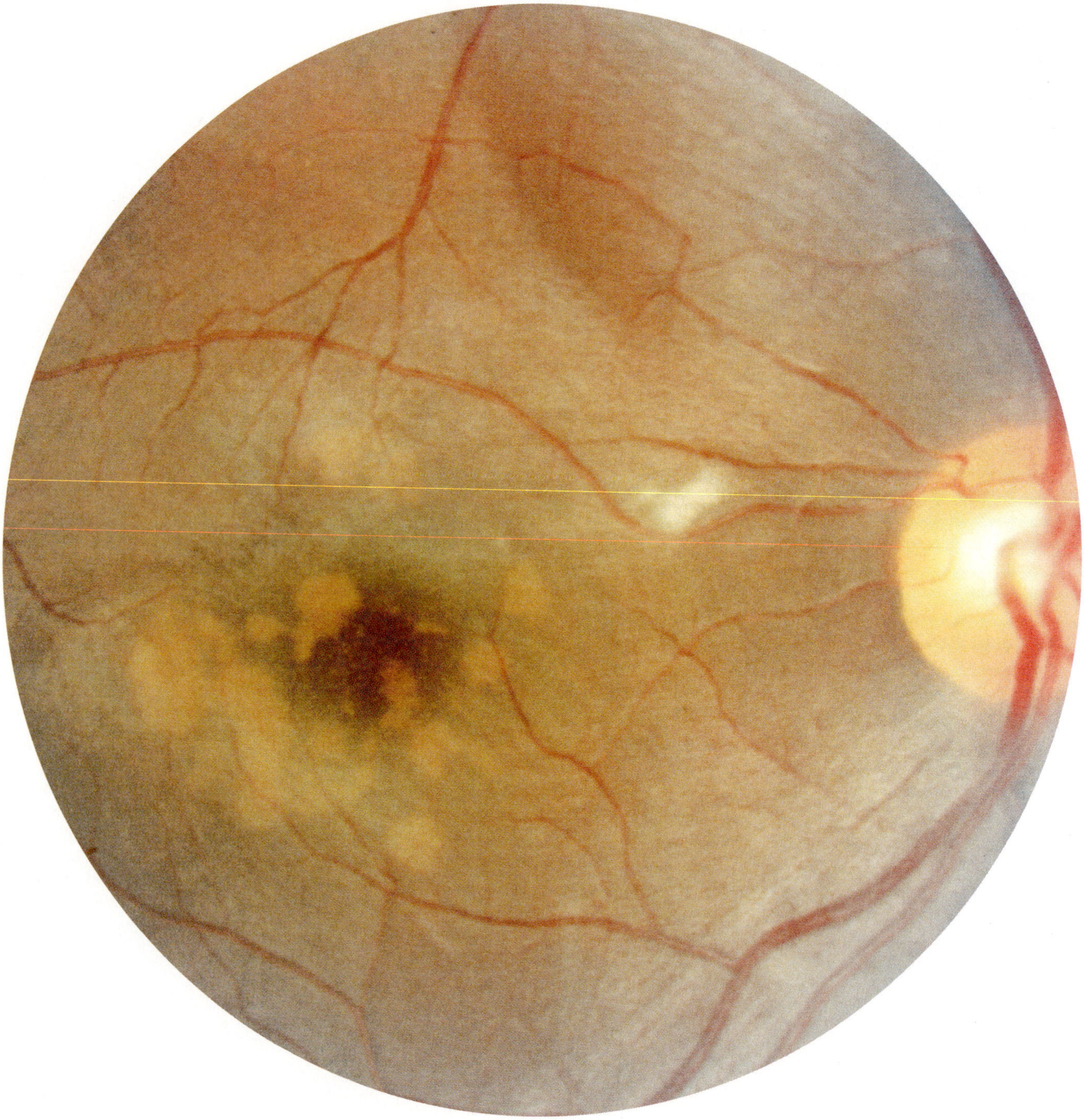

Disseminated intravascular coagulopathy (DIC) is due to the formation of fibrin clots or thrombi in small blood vessels secondary to many systemic disorders. It may be seen in hypercoagulable conditions such as abruptio placentae, trauma, carcinoma, post–organ transplantation, lupus erythematosis, leukemia, after burns, gram-negative sepsis, drug reactions, and hypertension. Thrombotic thrombocytopenic purpura (TTP) is considered an idiopathic form of DIC. Idiopathic thrombocytopenic purpura (ITP) is an autoimmune platelet disease and is less severe than DIC or TTP.

34–1

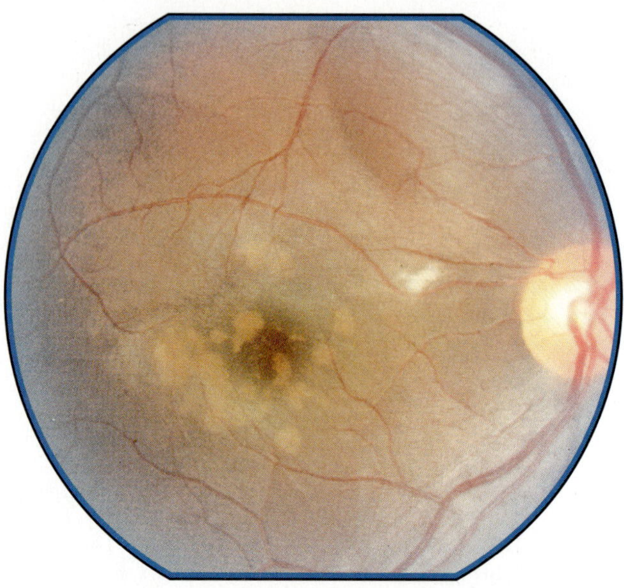

34–2

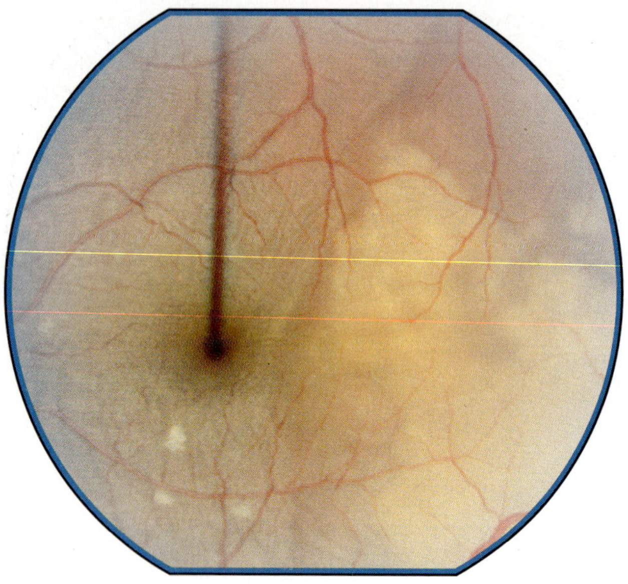

34–3

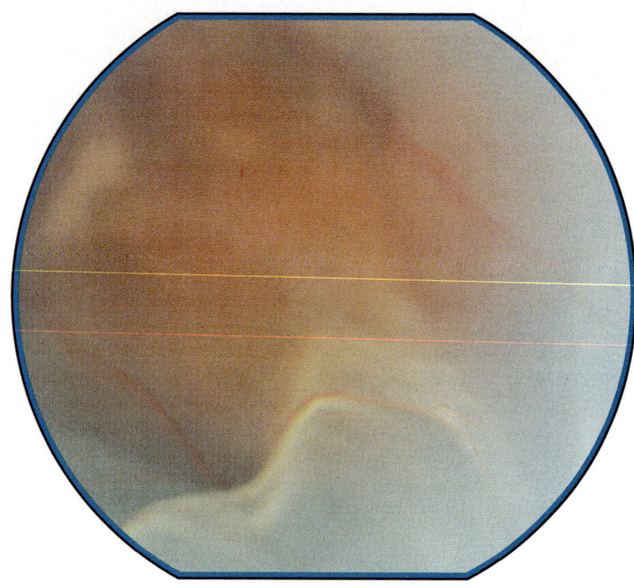

34–1 This 32-year-old male had a history of fatigue, palpitations, hematemesis, fainting, disorientation, and decreased vision. A diagnosis of TTP was established. Note the irregular discoloration in the subretinal area.

34–2 The fellow eye also has an exudative detachment. In addition, there is a greater concentration of subretinal debris.

34–3 Inferiorly, undulating folds of a secondary exudative detachment are evident.

34–1 *through* ***34–3,*** *Courtesy of Dr. Richard Spaide.*

(Case continued on next page.)

34–4

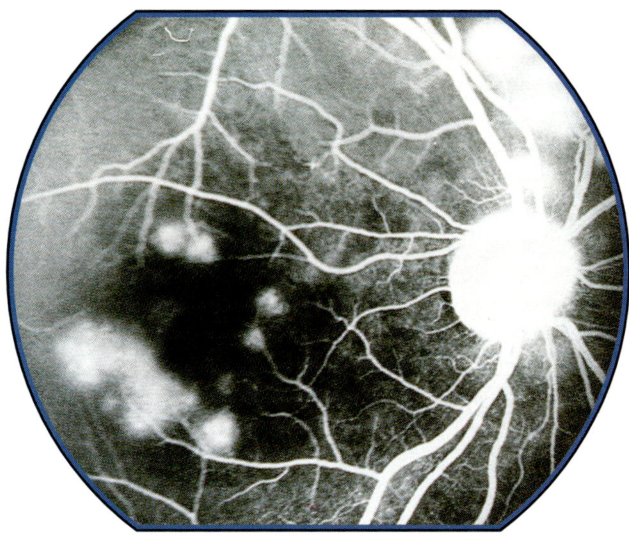

34–5

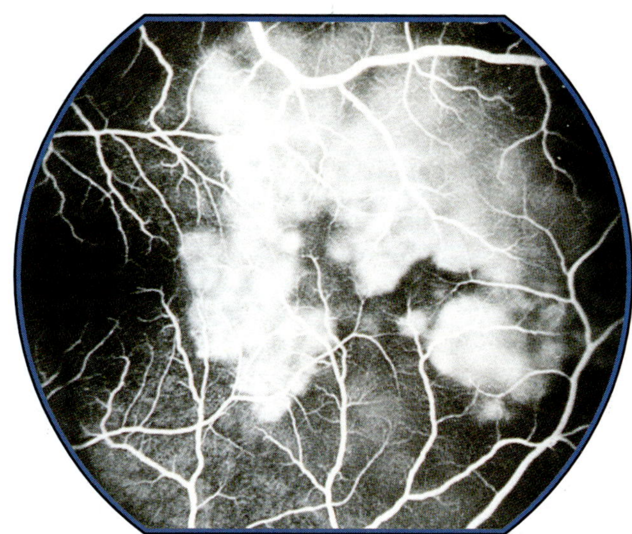

34–6

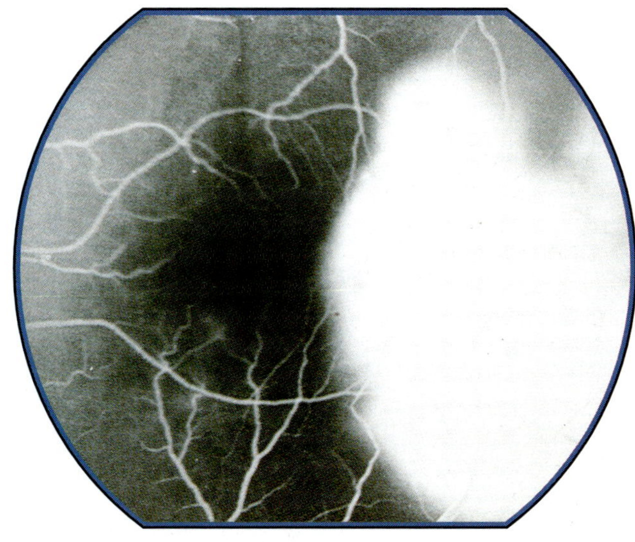

34–7

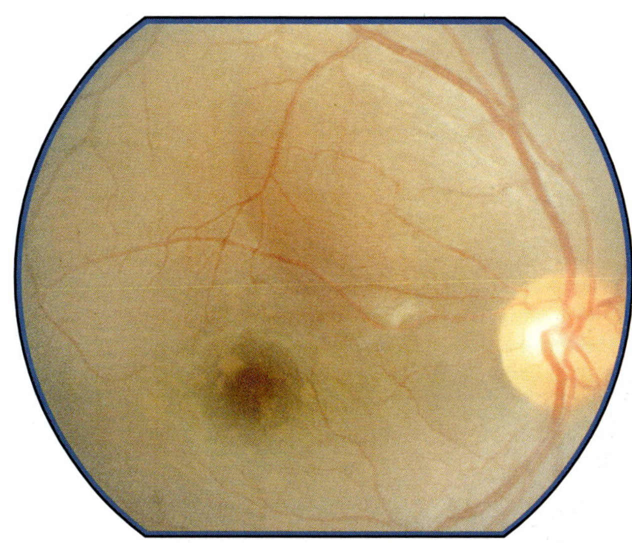

34–4 The fluorescein angiogram reveals focal leakage at the site of these blister-like elevations.

34–5 and 34–6 In the later stages of the study, the discolored areas stain confluently and ultimately begin to fill the neurosensory retinal space.

34–7 Improvement of the orange discoloration at the level of the retinal pigment epithelium is noted following treatment of the patient's TTP. There is still persistence of the exudative detachment. Presumably, fibrinoid necrosis with alterations of the retinal pigment epithelium—leading to a breakdown in the posterior blood retinal barrier—results in the orange-colored lesions at the level of the retinal pigment epithelium. It is also associated with leakage into the subneurosensory retinal space and a secondary overlying exudative detachment. This process is very similar to the case presented earlier involving toxemia of pregnancy.

***34–4** through **34–7**, Courtesy of Dr. Richard Spaide.*

34–8

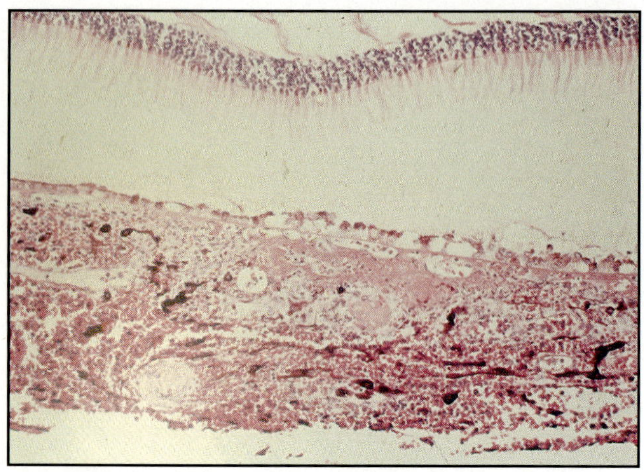

34–9

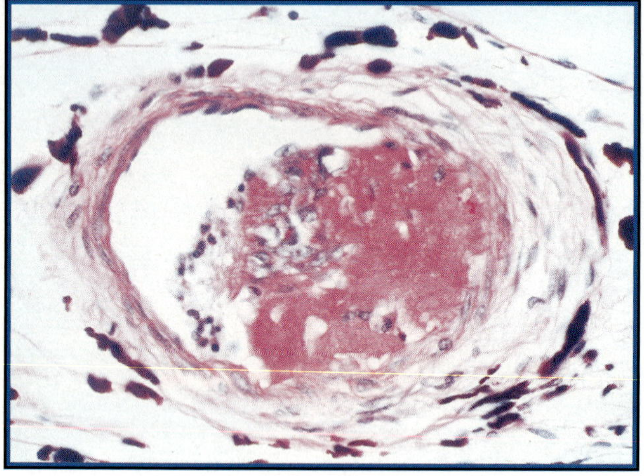

34–10

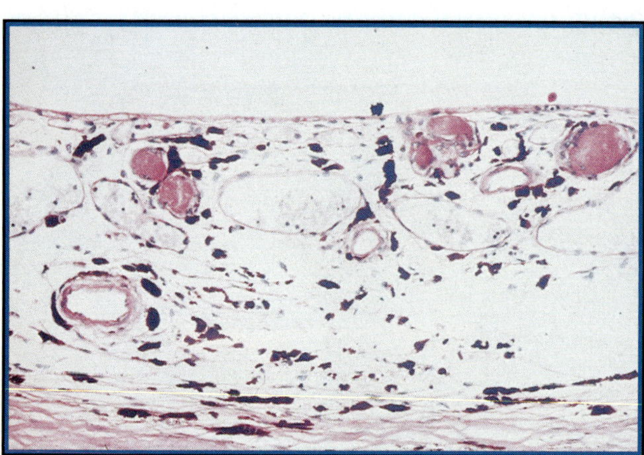

34–8 This patient shows thrombotic occlusions of the choriocapillaris and adjacent choroidal vessels and necrosis with vacuolization of the retinal pigment epithelium.

34–9 and 34–10 Patients with ITP develop anemia, thrombocytopenia, and neurologic abnormalities due to thrombotic occlusions of the blood vessels. The choriocapillaris and larger choroidal vessels may be occluded.

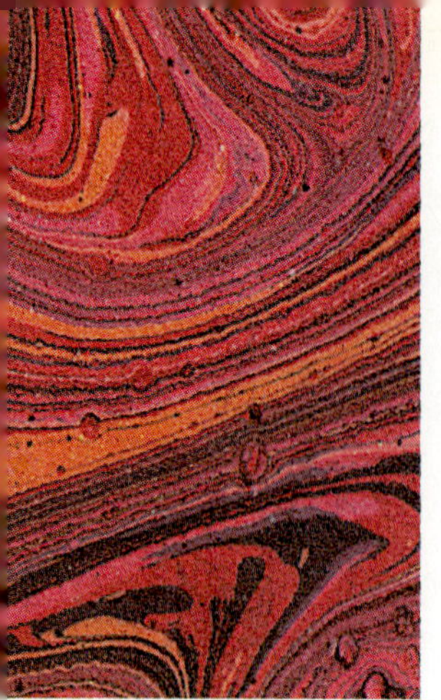

Chapter 35

Hemoglobinopathies

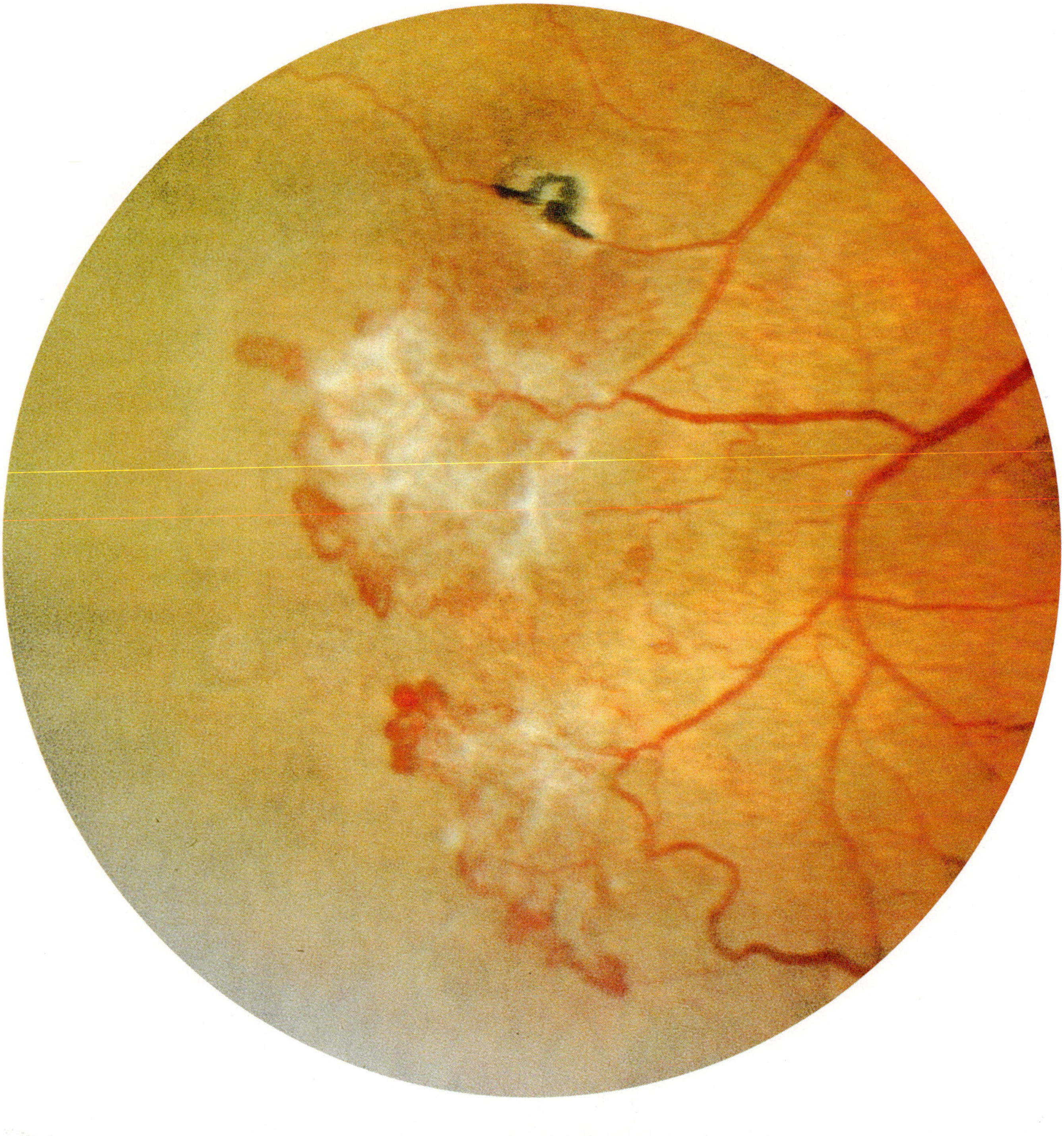

Ophthalmic manifestations of sickle cell disorders occur most frequently in sickle cell and sickle cell-thalassemia diseases. Sickling of the conjunctiva may be noted, which produces comma-shaped capillaries. Iris atrophy or synechia may occur. The sickle disc sign occurs when tiny red spots are noted on the optic disc. Nonproliferative sickle cell retinopathy findings include salmon patch hemorrhages, iridescent spots, and black sunbursts. A salmon patch is a roundish or ovalish hemorrhage of the neurosensory retina. These hemorrhages can involve the area between the neurosensory retina and the retinal pigment epithelium. Initially, these hemorrhages are reddish and then they turn salmon colored. An iridescent spot occurs when a salmon patch hemorrhage resorbs. A small cavity is left behind which contains macrophages. The black sunburst sign is a darkish chorioretinal scar that histopathologically represents retinal pigment epithelial hyperplasia and hypertrophy with migration. The origin of the black sunburst is probably an intraretinal hemorrhage. Proliferative sickle cell retinopathy usually occurs in the peripheral retina. Characteristic sea fans are areas of retinal neovascularization noted in areas between perfused and nonperfused retina. They may bleed and cause a vitreous hemorrhage, which can cause a tractional and/or rhegmatogenous retinal detachment.

Goldberg has proposed a staging criteria for the ophthalmic manifestations of sickle cell disease. Stage I or background lesions include salmon patches, iridescent spots, black sunbursts, and occluded peripheral vessels. Arteriovenular anastomoses occur in stage II disease. Neovascularization often with sea fan formation is noted in stage III disease. Vitreous hemorrhage occurs in stage IV and retinal detachment in stage V. Laser photocoagulation may be useful in preventing the progression of proliferative sickle retinopathy.

35–1 NON-PROLIFERATIVE SICKLE CELL RETINOPATHY: HEMORRHAGES

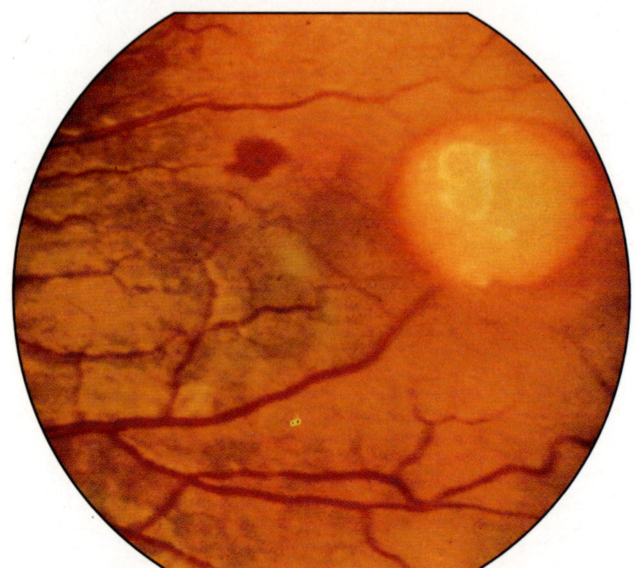

35–2

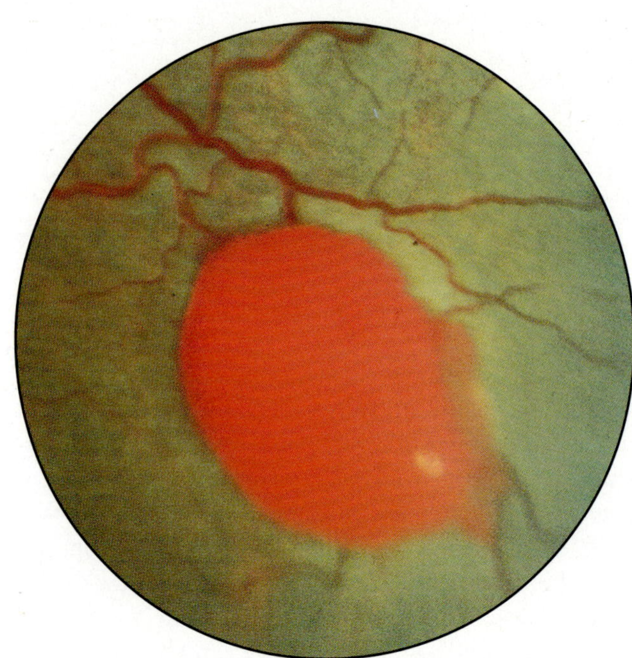

35–3

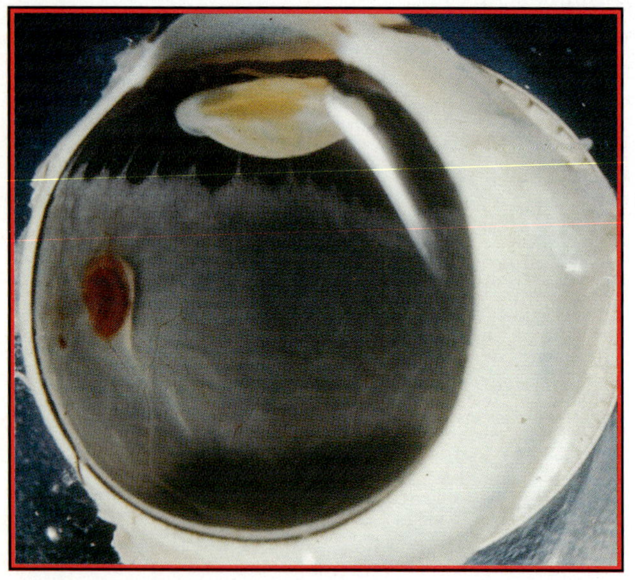

35–4

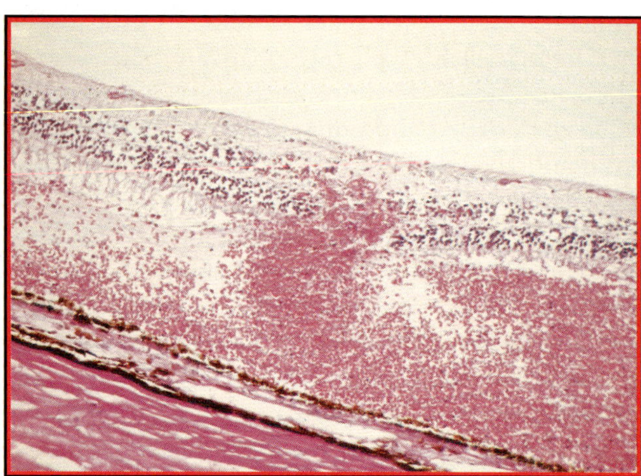

35–1 through 35–12 Findings of non-proliferative sickle cell retinopathy include retinal and preretinal hemorrhages (35–2), salmon patches (35–1, 35–3, and 35–4), iridescent spots (35–5, 35–6, and 35–7), and pigmented fundus lesions called black sunbursts (35–8 through 35–12).

35–3 and 35–4 Salmon patches are due to hemorrhage in the deep retinal and subretinal space.

***35–3** and **35–4**, From Romayananda, N, Goldberg, MF, and Green, WR: Histopathology of sickle cell retinopathy, Trans Am Ophthalmol Soc 77:652–676, 1973.*

35–5 IRIDESCENT SPOTS

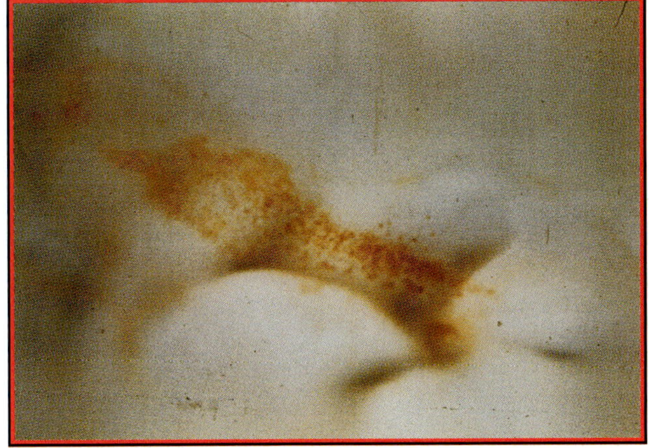

35–6

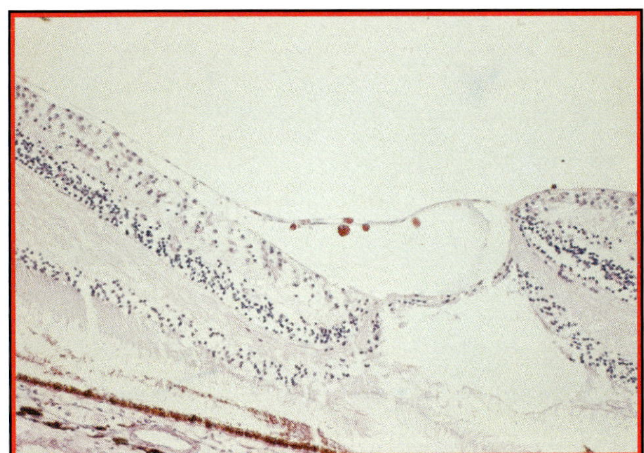

35–7

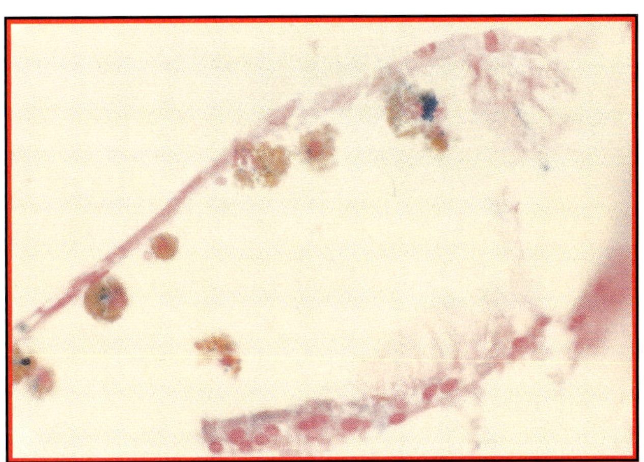

35–5 Iridescent spots are old resorbed subinternal limiting membrane hemorrhages with hemosiderin deposition. An iridescent spot in the macular region is noted in this gross photograph.

35–6 and 35–7 Light microscopy reveals an iridescent spot and schisis in the macular region (35–6) with hemosiderin deposits (35–7).

__35–5__ through __35–7,__ From Romayananda, N, Goldberg, MF, and Green, WR: Histopathology of sickle cell retinopathy, Trans Am Ophthalmol Soc 77:652–676, 1973.

35–8 BLACK SUNBURSTS

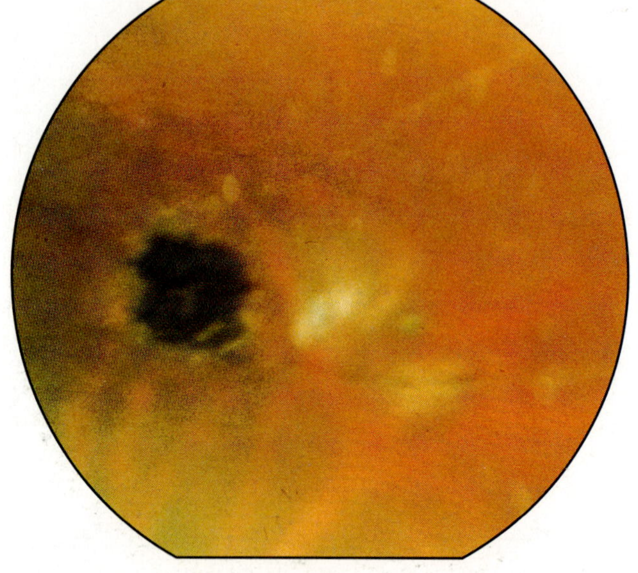

35–9

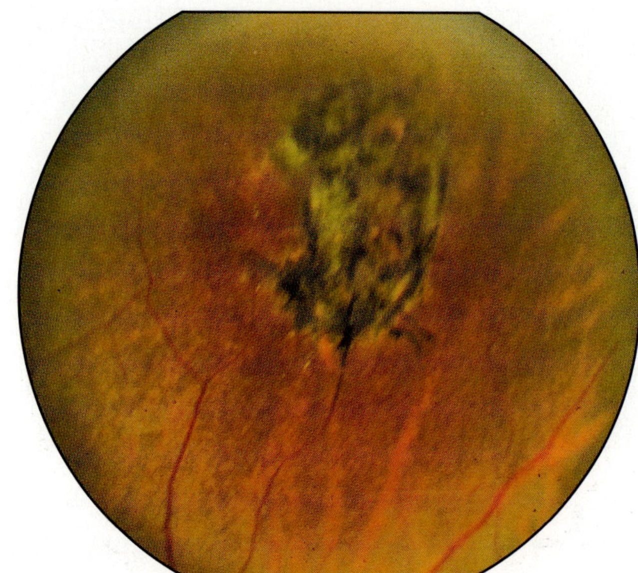

35–10

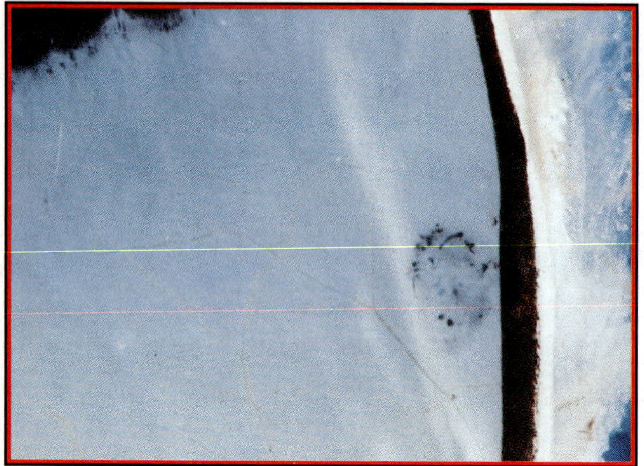

35–11

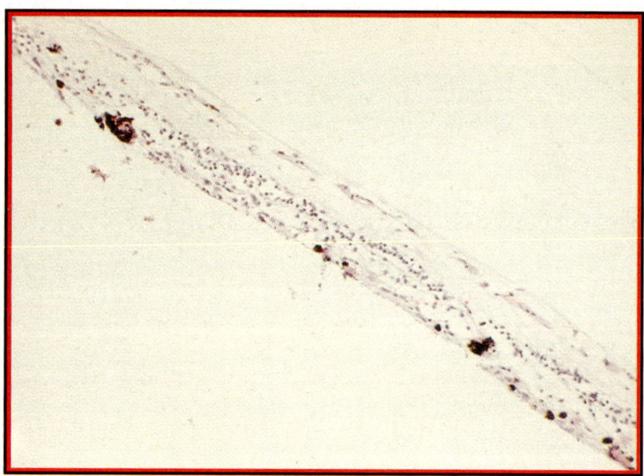

35–12

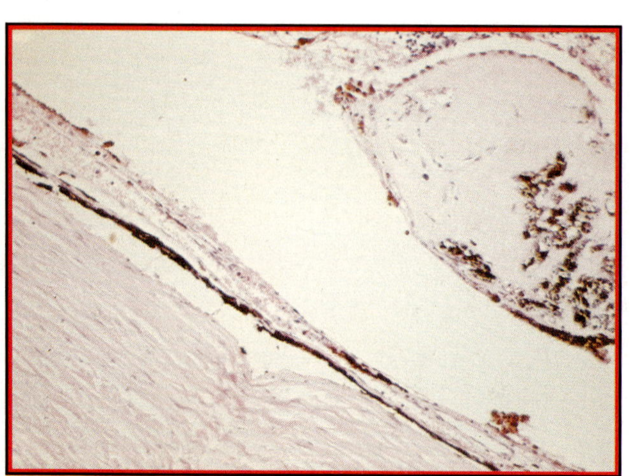

35–8 through 35–10 Black sunburst lesions are resorbed subretinal hemorrhages with secondary retinal pigment epithelial hypertrophy and hyperplasia.

35–11 and 35–12 Migration into the retina in a perivascular distribution with hemosiderin deposition is also noted. The outer nuclear layer is lost.

35–10 *through* ***35–12,*** *From Romayananda, N, Goldberg, MF, and Green, WR: Histopathology of sickle cell retinopathy, Trans Am Ophthalmol Soc 77:652–676, 1973.*

35–13 PROLIFERATIVE SICKLE CELL RETINOPATHY

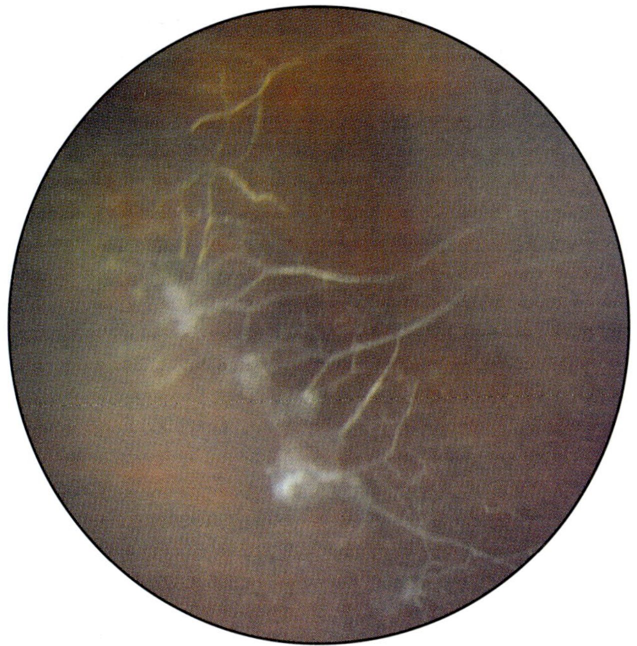

35–14

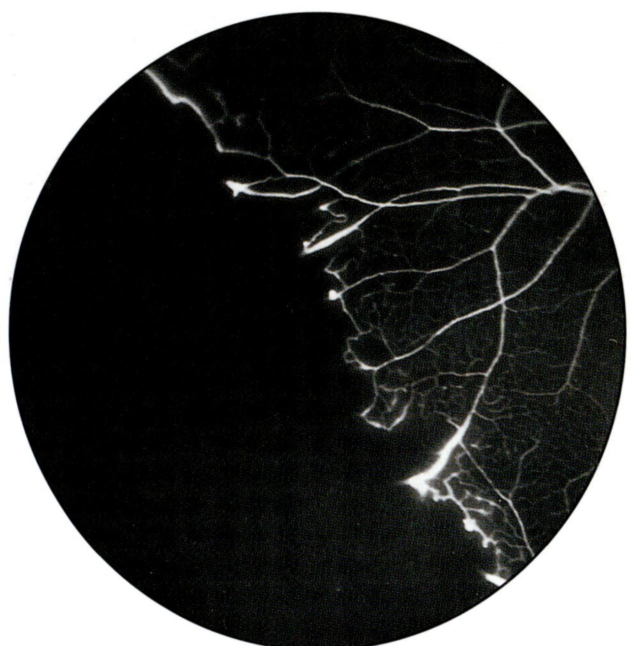

35–15 OCCLUSIVE DISEASE

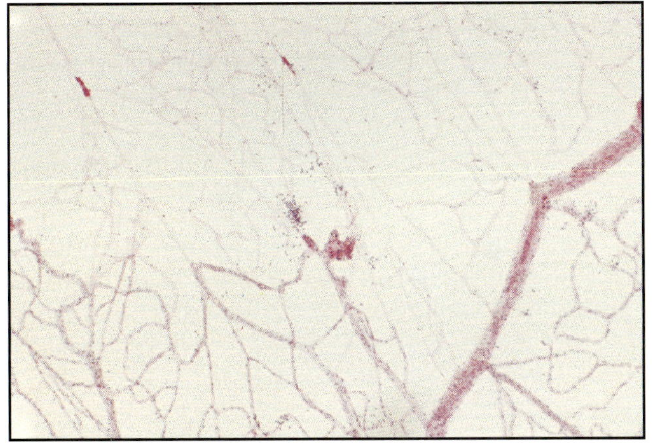

35–16

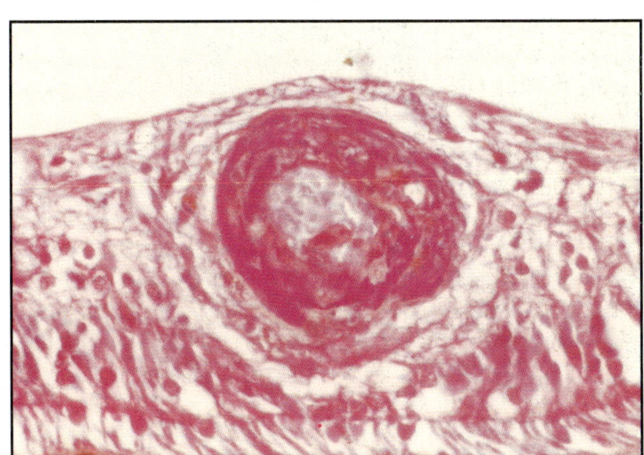

35–13 Proliferative sickle cell retinopathy consists of peripheral capillary nonperfusion and retinal neovascularization, which may be associated with vitreous hemorrhage or retinal detachment.

35–14 Peripheral capillary nonperfusion is demonstrated on the accompanying fluorescein angiogram.

35–15 Trypsin digest preparations show peripheral acellular vessels with arteriovenular looping and beading following arteriolar occlusion.

35–16 Fibrin thrombus obstructs this arteriole tertiary branch of the central retinal artery.

***35–15** and **35–16,** From Romayananda, N, Goldberg, MF, and Green, WR: Histopathology of sickle cell retinopathy, Trans Am Ophthalmol Soc 77:652–676, 1973.*

35–17 PROLIFERATIVE SICKLE CELL RETINOPATHY

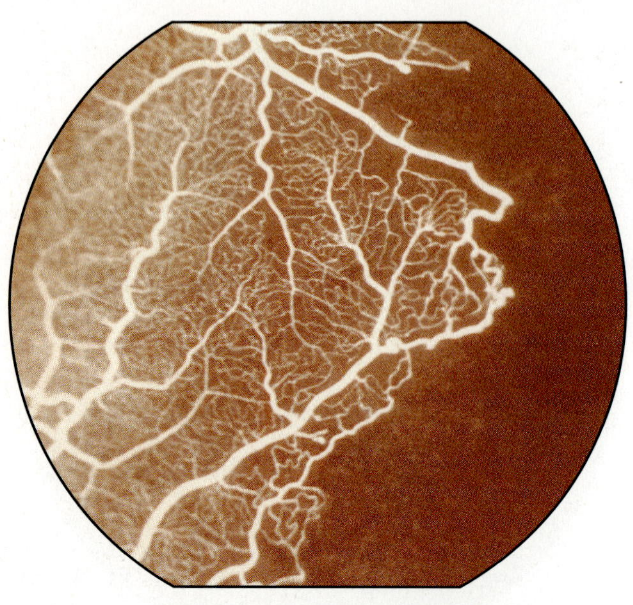

35–18

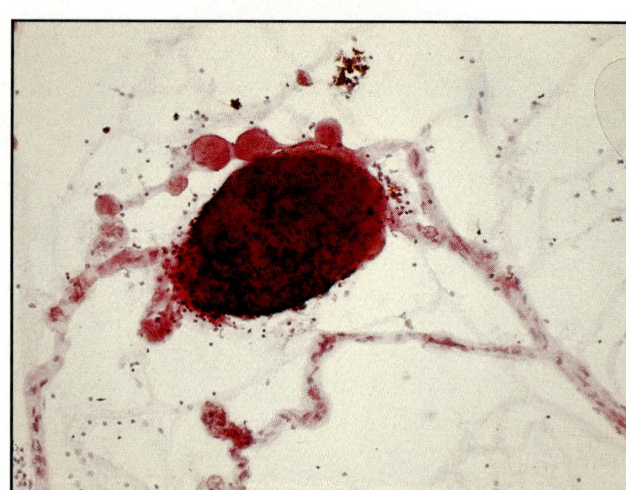

35–17 This fluorescein angiogram shows an arteriovenous anastomosis.

35–18 Looping and beading, as seen in this specimen, occurs at the margin of perfused and nonperfused retina.

35–18, *From Romayananda, N, Goldberg, MF, and Green, WR: Histopathology of sickle cell retinopathy, Trans Am Ophthalmol Soc 77:652–676, 1973.*

35–19

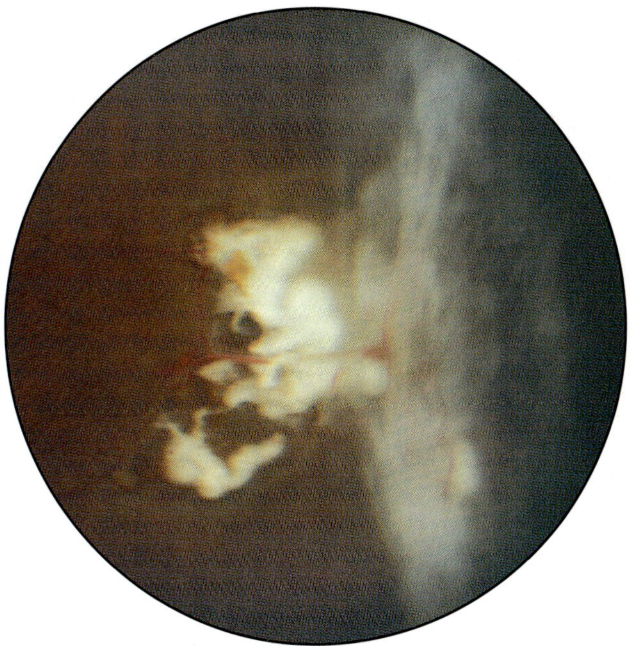

35–20

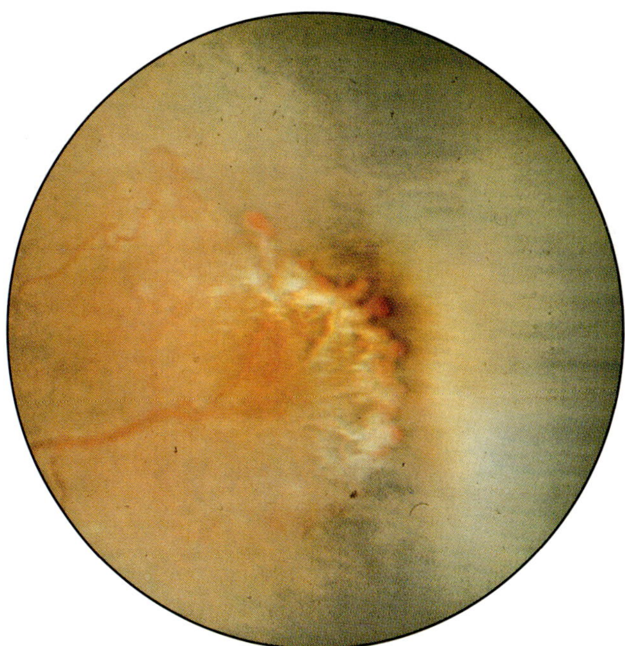

35–21

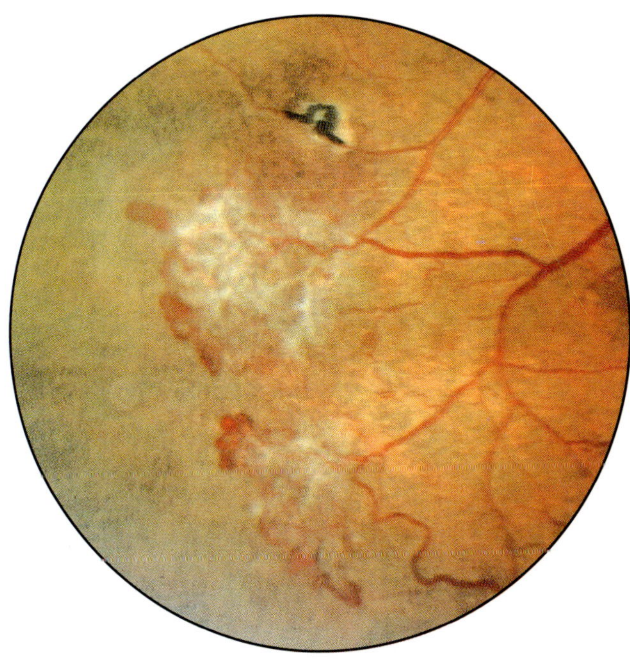

35–19 through 35–21 Sea fan formation is observed in the next photographs. Arterioles may close and form AV communications at the junction of perfused and nonperfused retina. Areas of preretinal neovascularization may occur. In these eyes, the ischemic peripheral retina is devoid of vessels, or sheathed nonperfused casts may remain as the only clinical evidence remnant of the preoccluded circulation. Fibrous proliferation and tractional elements may evolve.

35–22 PROLIFERATIVE SICKLE CELL RETINOPATHY

35–23

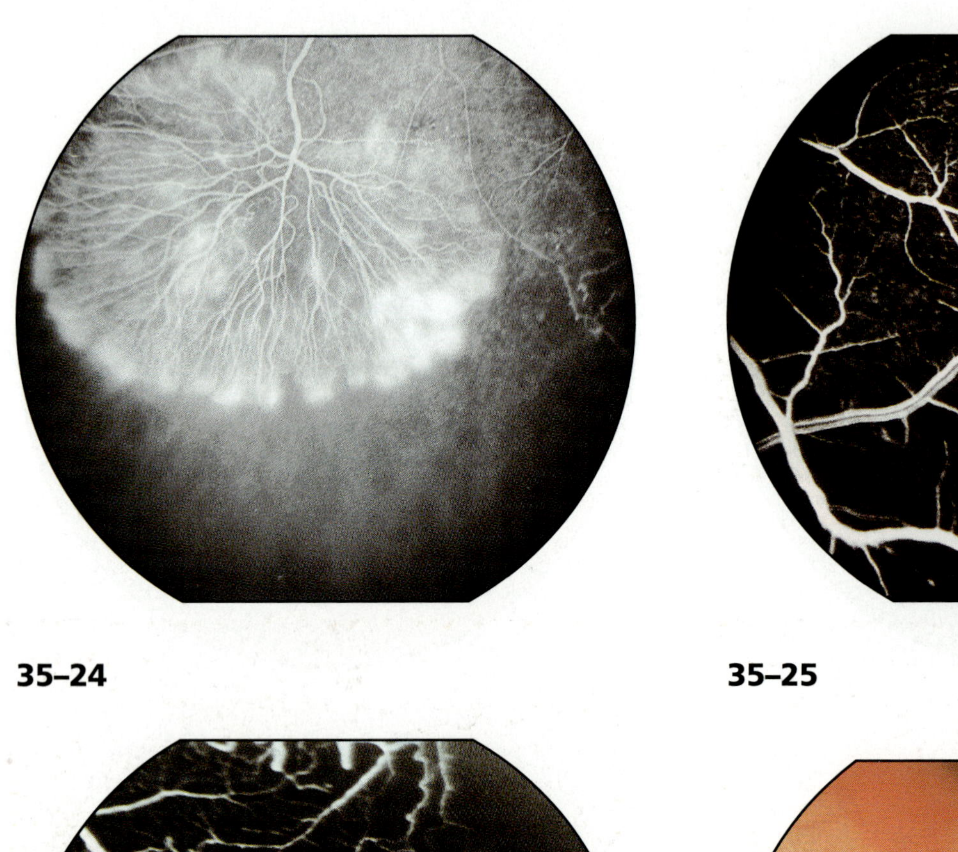

35–24

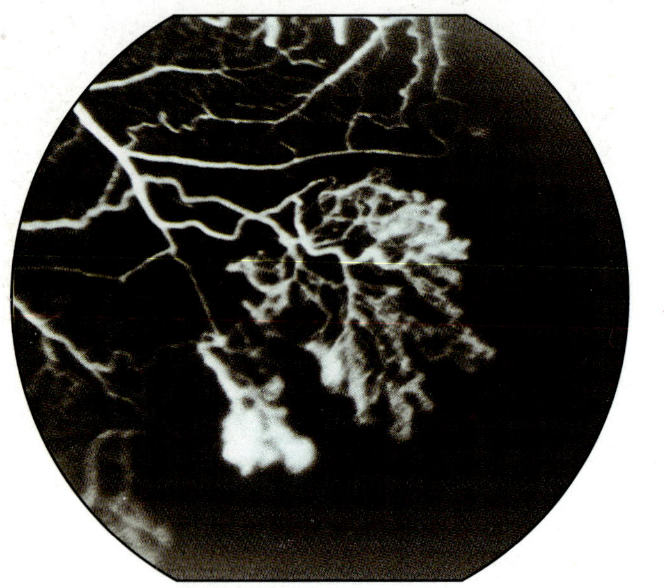

35–25

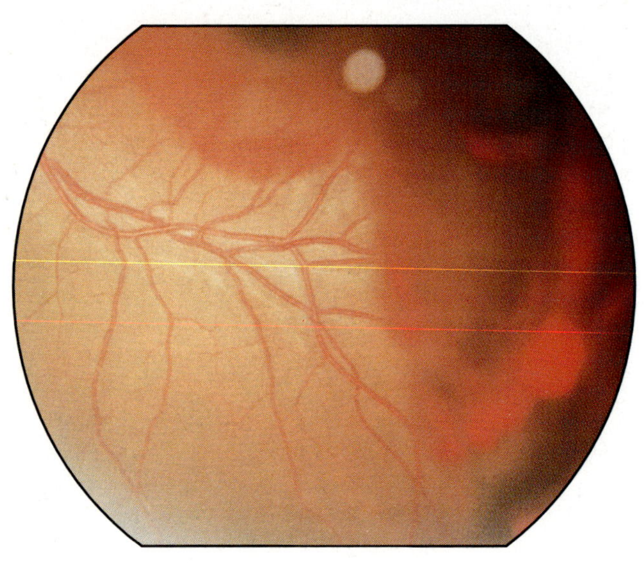

35–22 through 35–24 The fluorescein study shows a variation in the morphology of the preretinal neovascularization with early vascular, lacelike vessels that leak into the overlying vitreous in the late stages of the study. These vessels appear generally at a discrete junction between perfused and nonperfused retina. Although the nonischemic area appears very dark, no evidence of choroidal ischemia is known to occur in these patients to account for this finding. Presumably, the pigment in the fundus of those susceptible to the disease, as well as artifactual aberrations associated with peripheral photography, contribute to this effect.

35–25 Secondary vitreous hemorrhage may ensue.

35–26

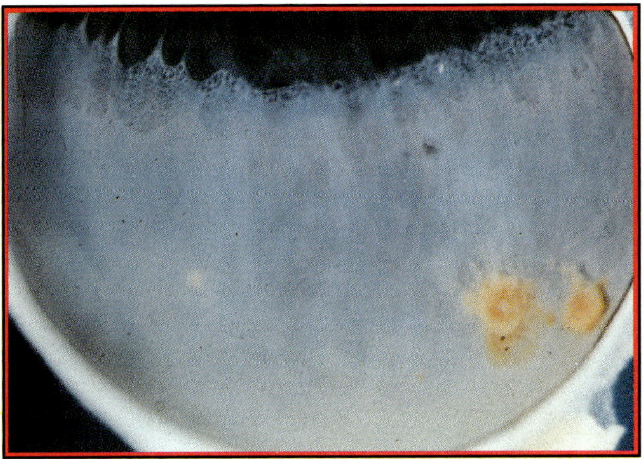

35–27

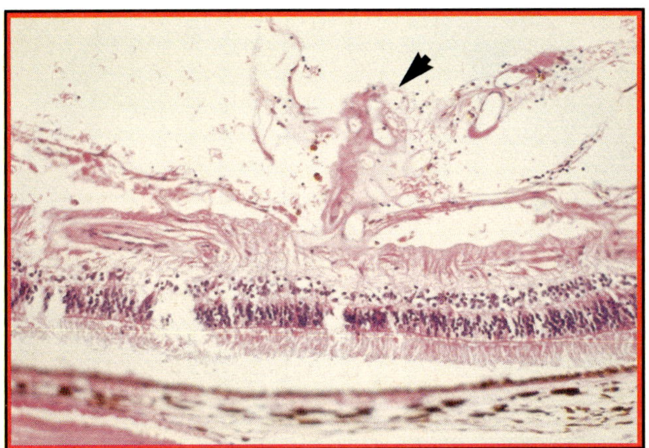

35–27A

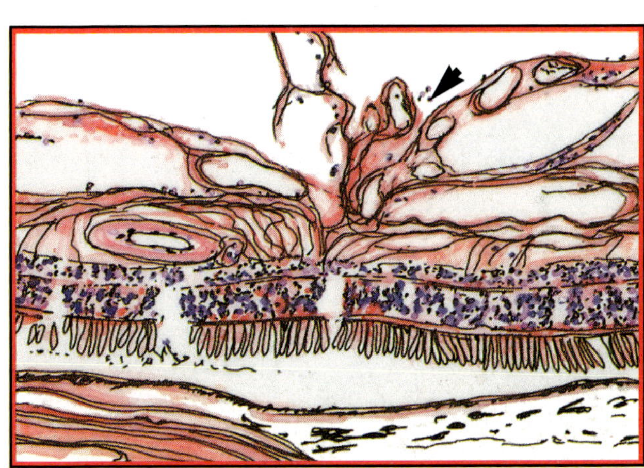

35–26, 35–27 and 35–27A Localized retinal neovascularization is also demonstrated in this patient with proliferative sickle cell retinopathy in which gross examination reveals two sea fans with surrounding hemorrhage. A section of one of these sea fans shows an area where vessels extend into the vitreous from the retina (retinal neovascularization) *(arrowhead)*. There is a discontinuity of the internal limiting membrane of the retina through which the vessels extend into the vitreous. Fibroglial tissue, a few lymphocytes, and numerous erythrocytes, which are sickled, are present near the sea fans.

***35–26** and **35–27**, From Romayananda, N, Goldberg, MF, and Green, WR: Histopathology of sickle cell retinopathy, Trans Am Ophthalmol Soc 77:652–676, 1973.*

35–28 PROLIFERATIVE SICKLE CELL RETINOPATHY

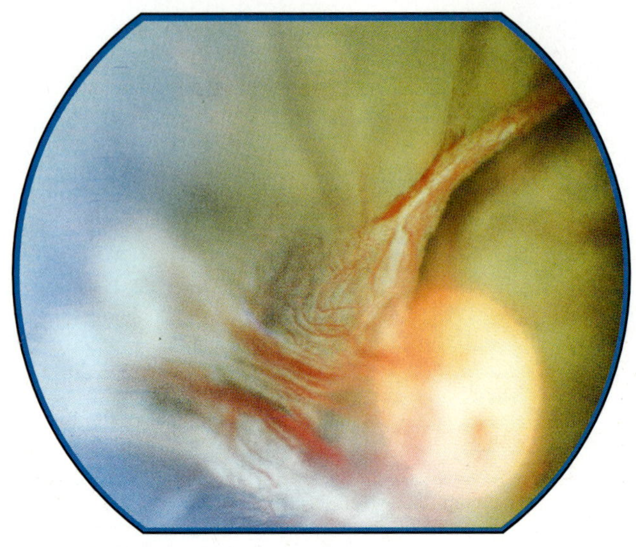

35–29

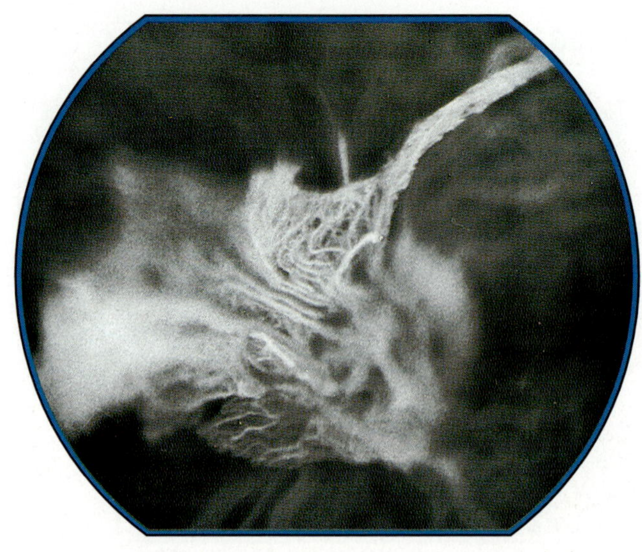

35–30 TORTUOUS VESSELS

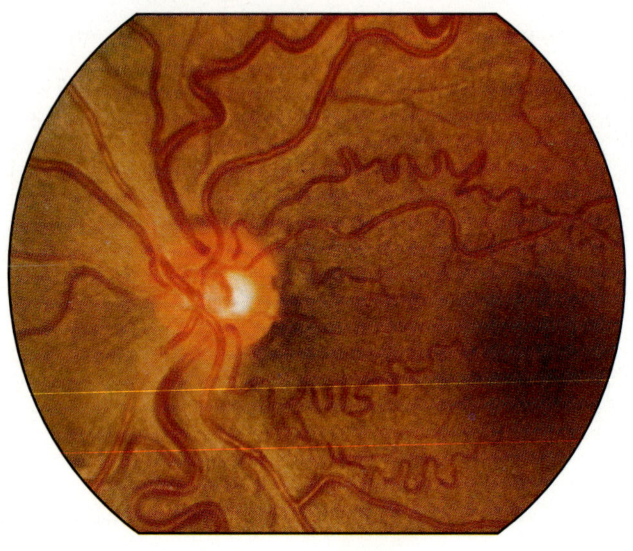

35–31 CENTRAL RETINAL ARTERY OCCLUSION

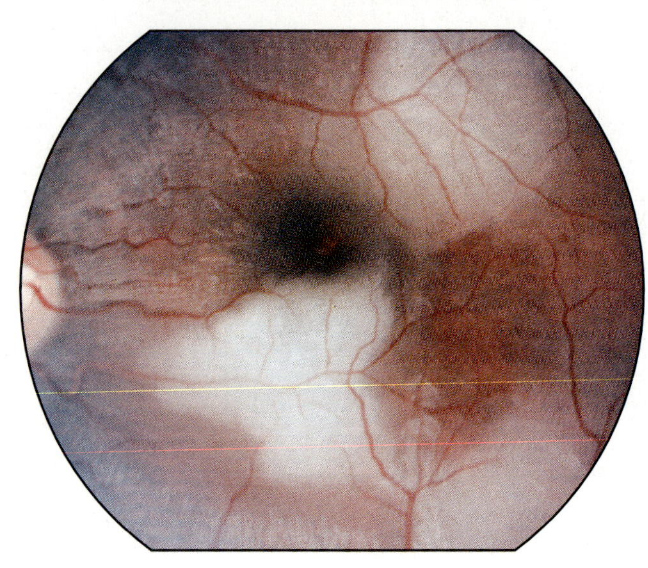

35–32 NONPERFUSION-BLUNTING OF PERIFOVEAL CAPILLARIES

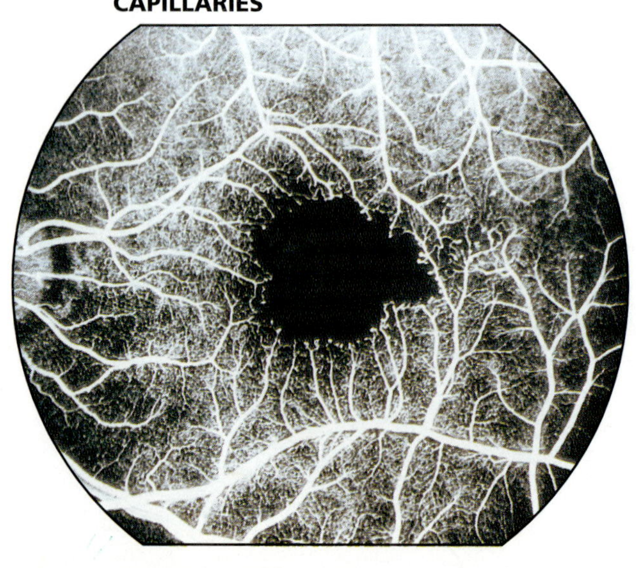

35–33 ANGIOID STREAKS

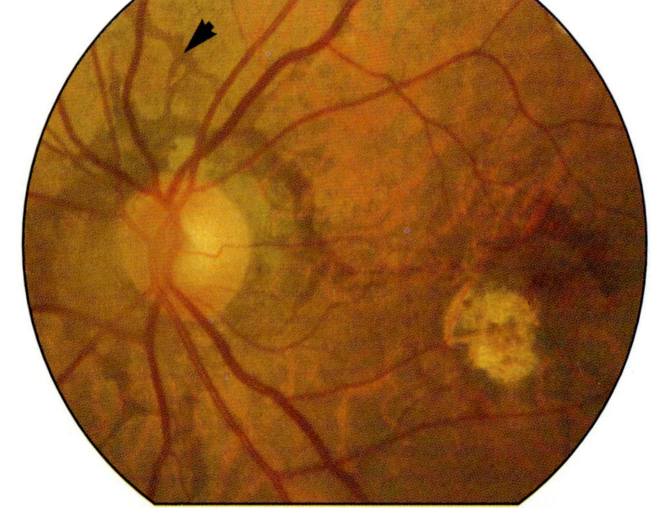

35–34 HYPEREOSINOPHILIC SYNDROME

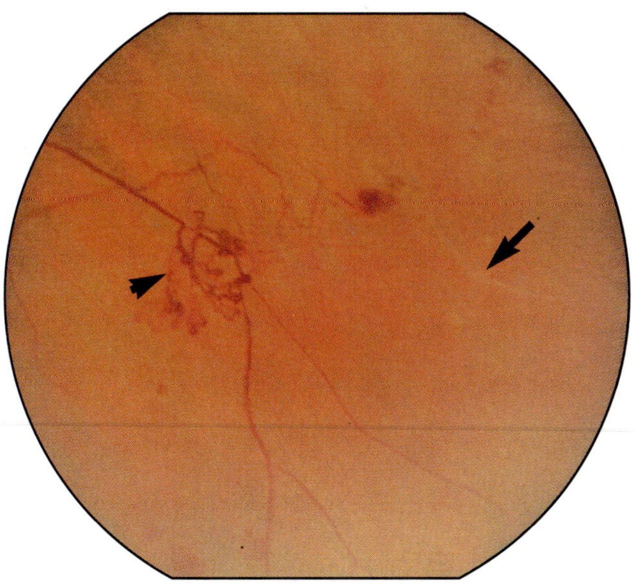

35–35 WALDENSTRÖM'S DISEASE

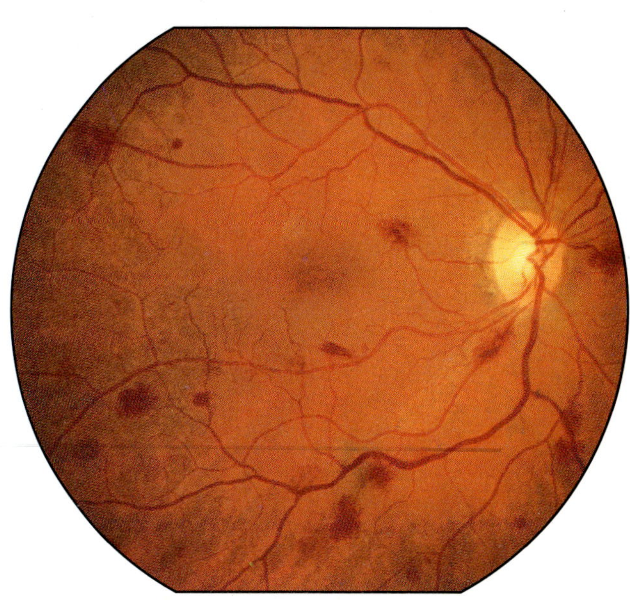

35–28 and 35–29 Neovascular proliferation at the optic disc is demonstrated in this patient.

35–30 through 35–32 Tortuous vessels may occur with sickle cell retinopathy (35–30). A central retinal artery occlusion is noted in a patient with sickle cell thalassemia (35–31). Following these occlusions, there is often thinning of the retina, termed the macular depression sign of Goldbaum. Other findings of sickle cell retinopathy include nonperfusion with blunting of the perifoveal capillaries (35–32).

35–33 Angioid streaks *(arrowhead)* may also be seen in patients with sickle cell retinopathy.

35–34 Patients with the hypereosinophilic syndrome may show intraretinal hemorrhages and neovascularization elsewhere *(arrowhead)*. There is also a sheathed vessel present in the upper right-hand corner *(arrow)*.

35–35 This patient has multiple intraretinal hemorrhages secondary to Waldenström's disease.

35–34, *Courtesy of Dr. Richard Chenoweth.*

35–36 HIGH-ALTITUDE RETINOPATHY

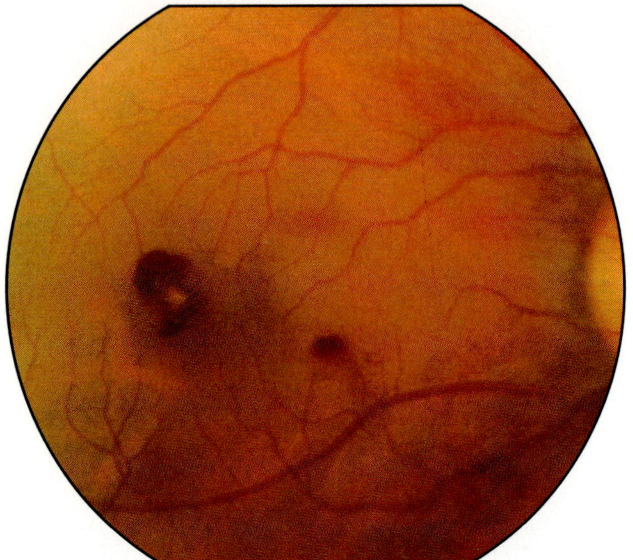

35–37

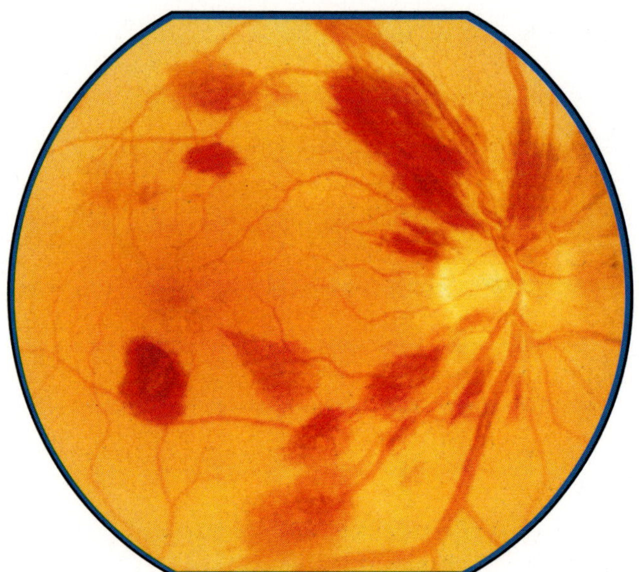

35–38

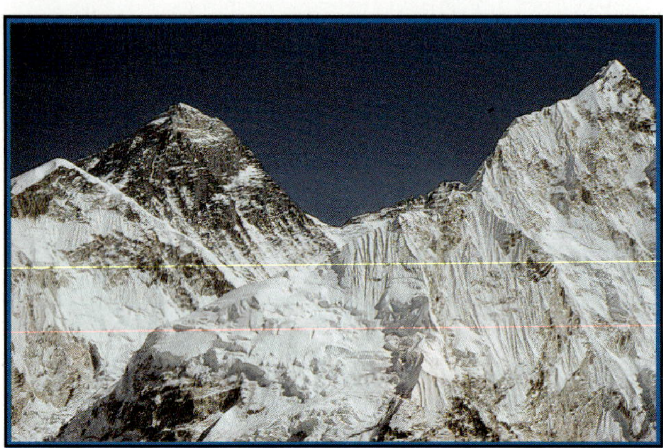

35–36 Intraretinal hemorrhages are noted in this patient with high-altitude retinopathy, at only 13,000 feet, skiing, and, in 35–37 and 35–38, climbing Mt Everest.

35–37 and 35–38 Another patient demonstrates high-altitude retinopathy with intraretinal hemorrhages (35–37) after climbing on Mt. Everest (35–38).

__35–36__ through __35–38,__ Courtesy of Dr. Michael Wiedman. __35–37,__ From Wiedman, M: High altitude retinal hemorrhage, Arch Opthalmol 93:401–403, 1975.

Suggested Readings

Asdourian, GK, Nagpal, KC, Busse, B, Goldbaum, M, Patrianakos, D, Rabb, MF, and Goldberg, MF: Macular and perimacular vascular remodeling in sickle haemoglobinopathies, Br J Ophthalmol 60:431–453, 1976

Bunn, HF: Disorders of hemoglobin structure, function, and synthesis. In Isselbacher, KJ, Adams, RD, Braunwald, E, Petersdorf, RG, and Wilson, JD, ed: Harrison's principles of internal medicine, ed 9, New York, 1980, McGraw-Hill, pp 1546–1554

Cohen, SB, Goldberg, MF, Fletcher, ME, and Jednock, NJ: Diagnosis and management of ocular complications of sickle hemoglobinopathies, part II, Ophthalmic Surg 17:110–116, 1986

Cohen, SB, Goldberg, MF, Fletcher, ME, and Jednock, NJ: Diagnosis and management of ocular complications of sickle hemoglobinopathies, part V, Ophthalmic Surg 17:369–374, 1986

Goldbaum, MH: Retinal depression sign indicating a small retinal infarct, Am J Ophthalmol 86:45–55, 1978

Goldberg, MF: Classification and pathogenesis of proliferative sickle cell retinopathy, Am J Ophthalmol 71:649–665, 1971

Goldberg, MF: Sickle cell retinopathy. In Duane, TD, and Jaeger, EA, eds: Clinical ophthalmology, vol 3, Philadelphia, 1979, Harper & Row Publishers

Jampol, LM: New techniques in treating proliferative sickle cell retinopathy. In Fine, S, and Owens, SL, eds: Management of retinal vascular and macular disorders, Baltimore, 1983, Williams & Wilkins, pp 218–224

Jampol, LM, Condon, P, Farber, M, Rabb, M, Ford, S, and Serjeant, G: A randomized clinical trial of feeder vessel photocoagulation of proliferative sickle cell retinopathy. I. Preliminary results, Ophthalmology 90:540–545, 1983

Jampol, LM, Green, Jr, Goldberg, MF, and Peyman, GA: An update on vitrectomy surgery and retinal detachment repair in sickle cell disease, Arch Ophthalmol 100:591–593, 1982

Paton, D: The conjunctival sign of sickle-cell disease, Arch Ophthalmol 66:90–94, 1961

Ryan, SJ, and Goldberg, MF: Anterior segment ischemia following scleral buckling in sickle cell hemoglobinopathy, Am J Ophthalmol 72:35–50, 1971

Welch, RB, and Goldberg, MF: Sickle-cell hemoglobin and its relation to fundus abnormality, Arch Ophthalmol 75:353–362, 1966

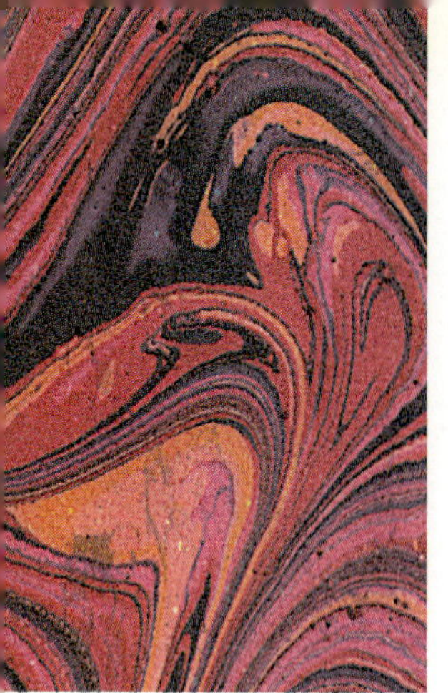

Chapter 36

Retinopathy of Prematurity

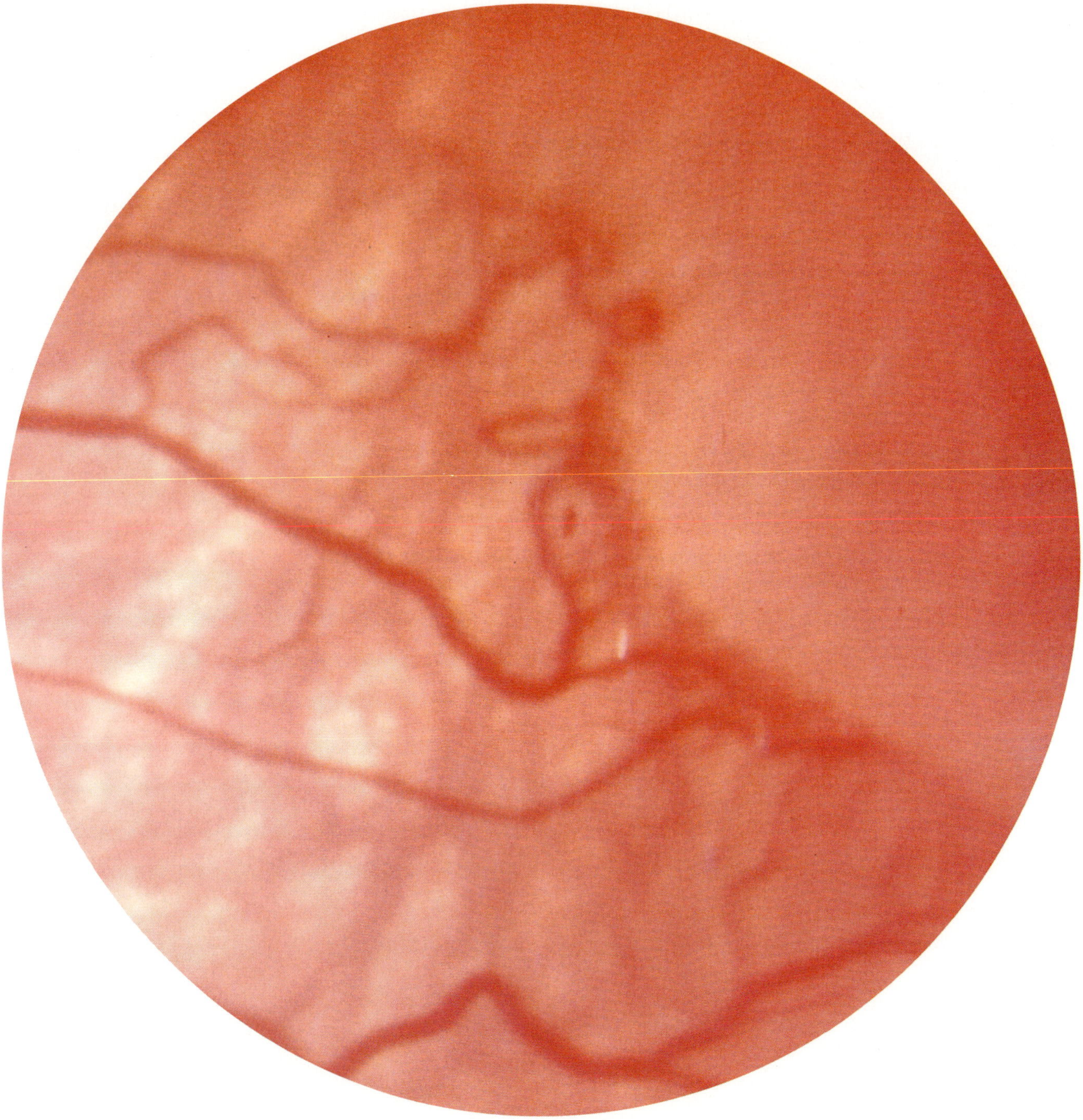

Retinopathy of prematurity may lead to retinal neovascularization. These cases can result in total retinal detachment. Cryotherapy and diode laser photocoagulation are useful in preventing the progression of this disorder.

36–1 STAGE I

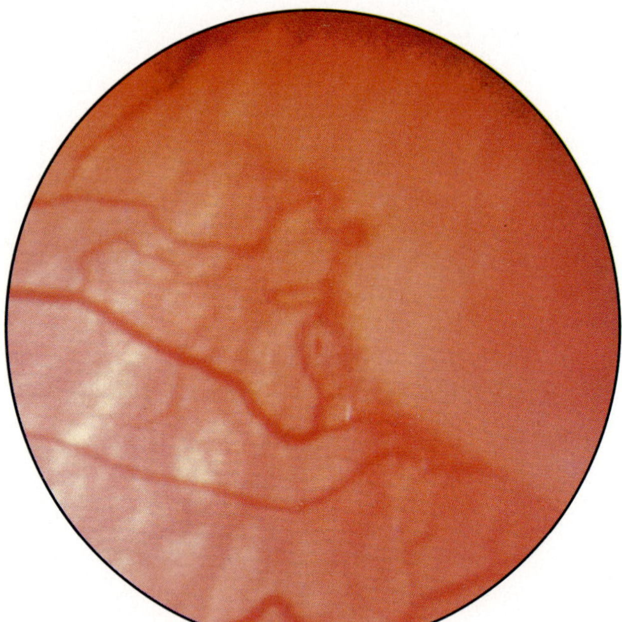

36–2 STAGE II

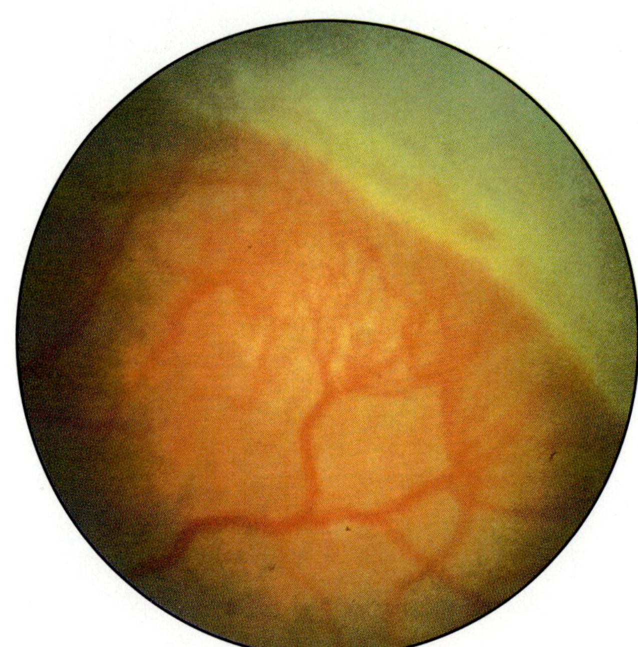

36–3 STAGE III

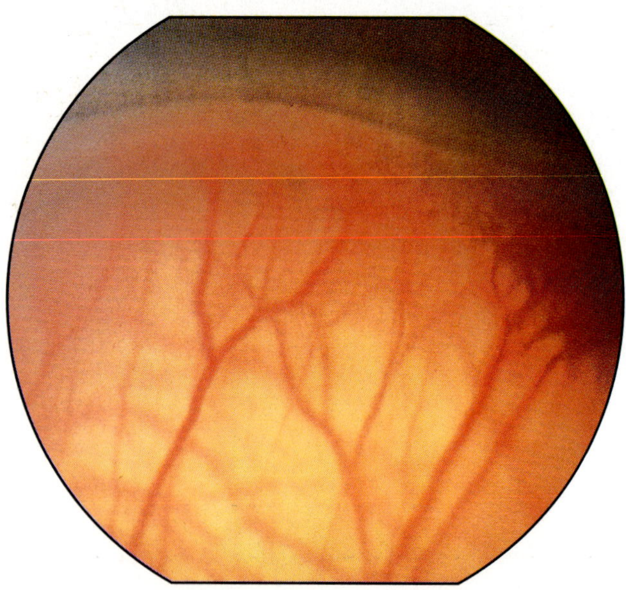

36–1 through 36–6 The international classification of retinopathy of prematurity is as follows stage I—demarcation line (36–1); stage II—a ridge (36–2); stage III—a ridge with extraretinal fibrovascular proliferation (36–3); and stage IV—retinal detachment. Stage IVA disease consists of extrafoveal subtotal retinal detachment (36–4) and stage IVB disease (36–5 and 36–6) consists of retinal detachment involving the fovea. Stage IVB detachments can be effusive (36–5) or tractional (36–6).

36–1, *Courtesy of Earl A. Palmer, Casey Eye Institute.* ***36–2*** *through* ***36–4,*** *Courtesy of Dr. Michael Trese.* ***36–5*** *and* ***36–6,*** *Courtesy of Dr. Michael Trese. From Trese, MT: Scleral buckling for retinopathy of prematurity, Ophthalmology 101:23–26, 1994.*

36–4 STAGE IVA

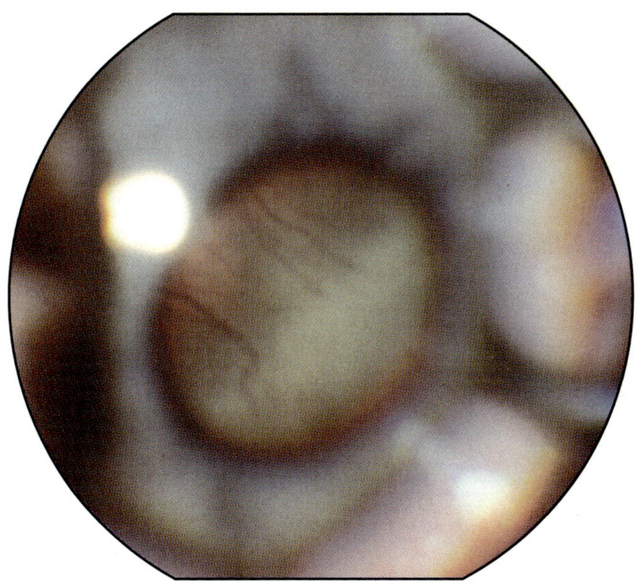

36–5 STAGE IVB

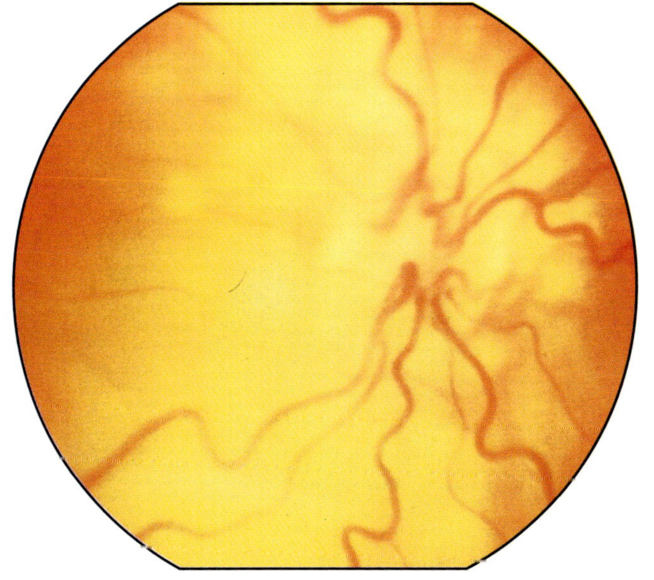

36–6

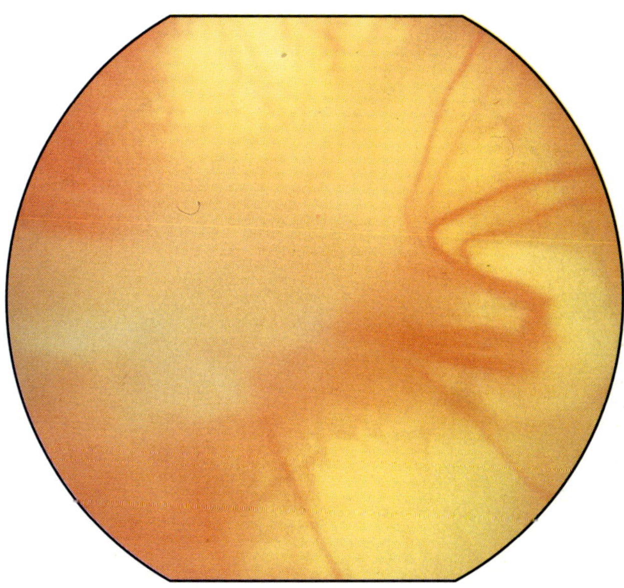

36–7 STAGE V

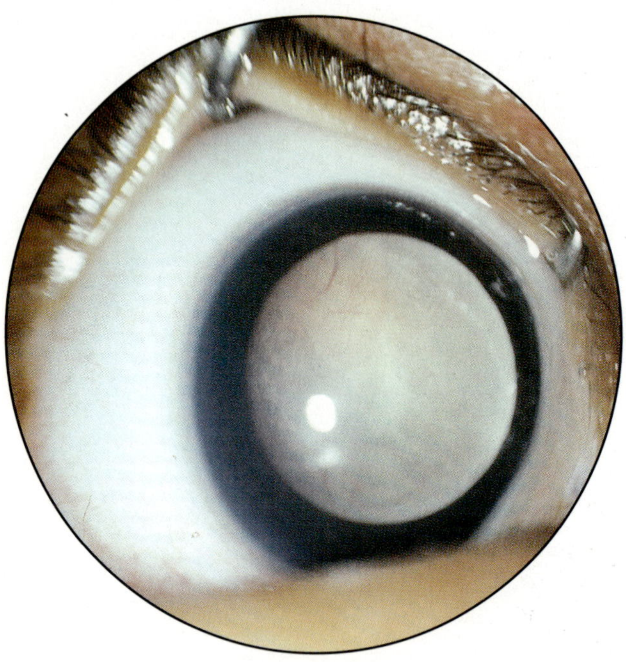

36–8

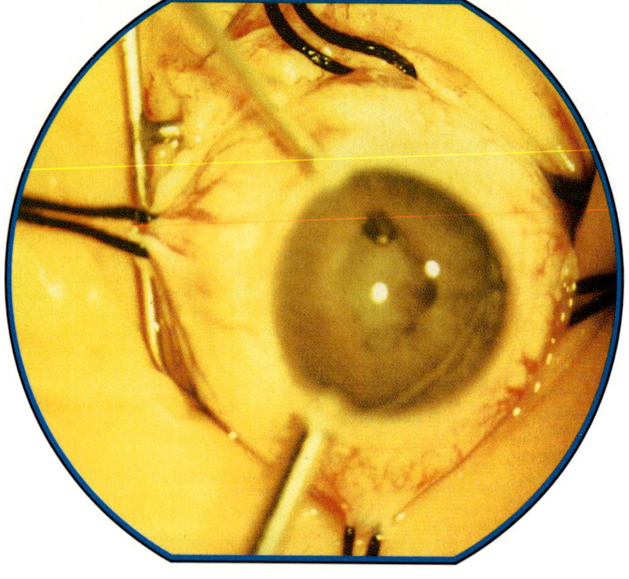

36–9

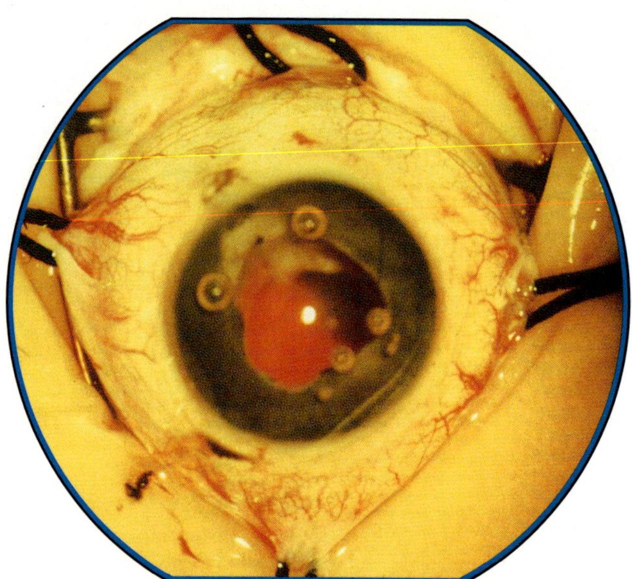

36–7 Stage V disease consists of a total retinal detachment.

36–8 and 36–9 Preoperative (36–8) and postoperative (36–9) appearance of a patient with stage V disease.

36–7 *through* ***36–9,*** *Courtesy of Dr. Michael Trese.*

36–10

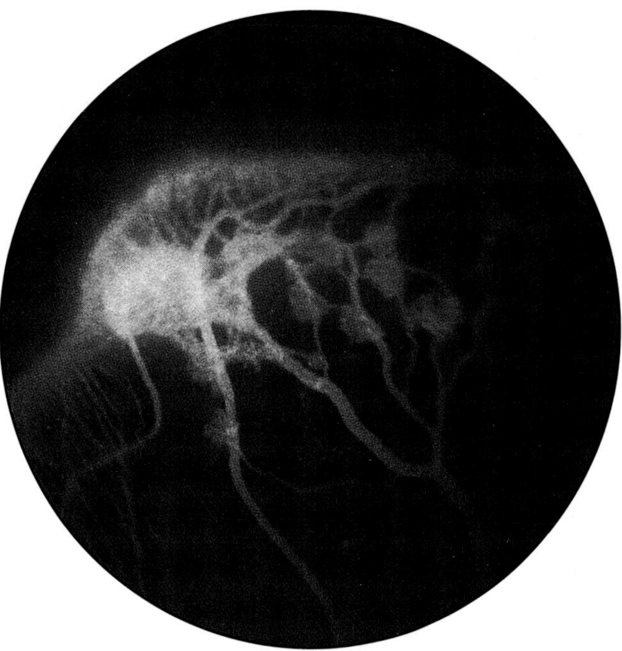

36–10 Peripheral retinal neovascularization and capillary nonperfusion are noted in this angiogram.

36–11

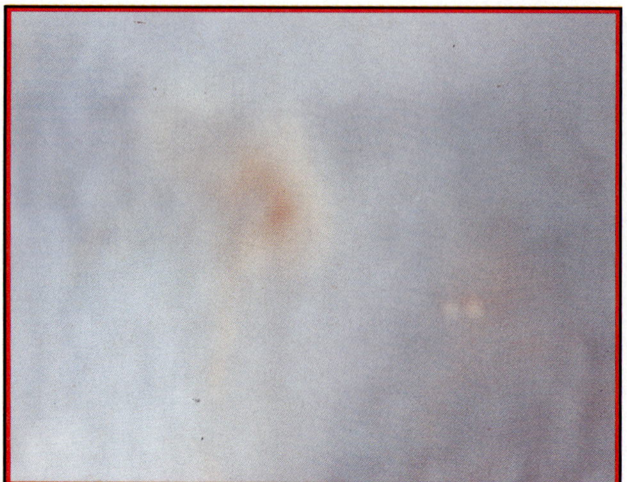

36–12

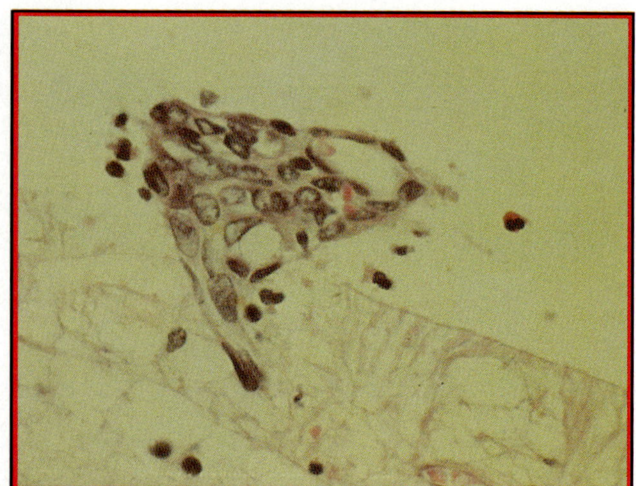

36–13

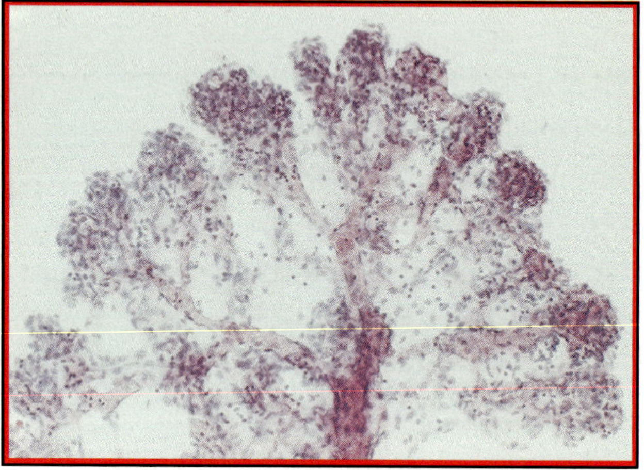

36–14

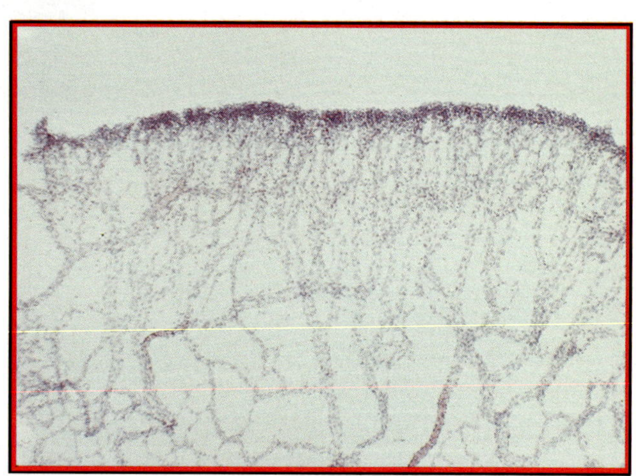

36–11 Gross appearance of the peripheral ring of retinal neovascularization and two small areas of localized retinal neovascularization that extend into the vitreous in an eye with retinopathy of prematurity.

36–12 An area of neovascularization extends through the internal limiting membrane into the vitreous.

36–13 Intraretinal neovascularization is noted, which has a sea fan–like configuration.

36–14 Increasing arborization of the retinal vessels in the peripheral region blends with a band of active neovascularization.

36–11 *through* ***36–14,*** *From Chui, HC, Green, WR: Acute retrolental fibroplasia: a clinicopathological correlation, MD Med J, 26:71–74, 1977.*

36–15

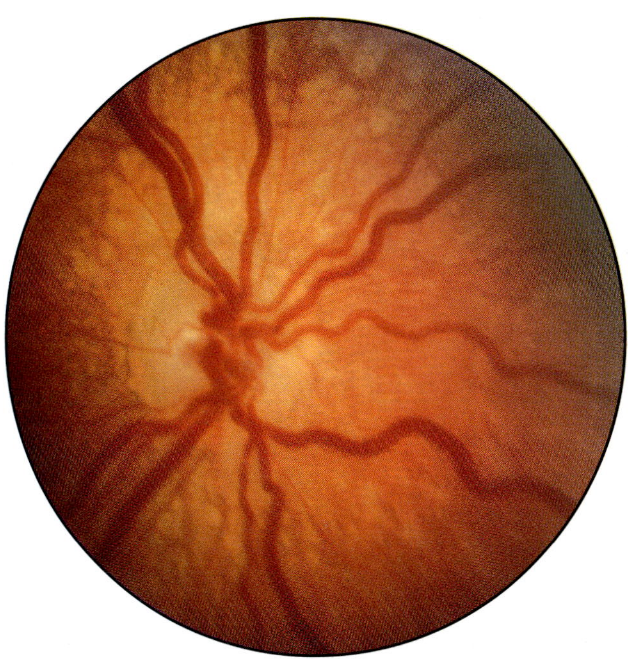

36–16

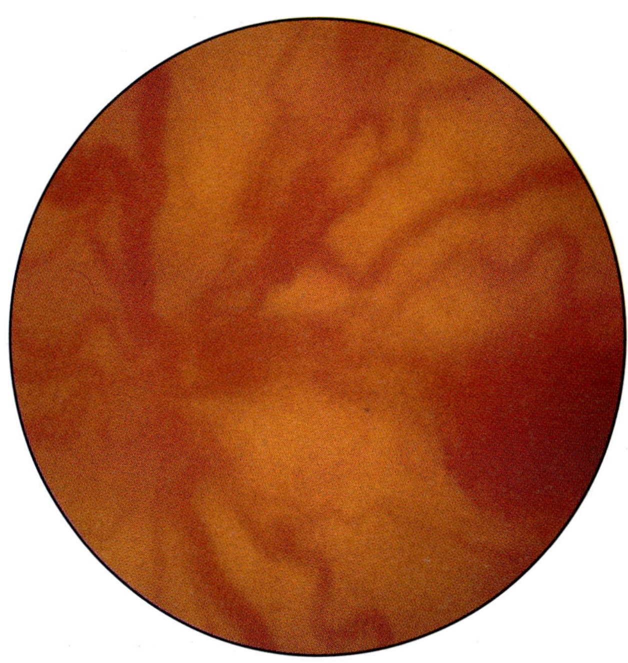

36–15 "Plus" disease is an extremely aggressive form of retinopathy of prematurity in which there is increasing dilatation and tortuosity of the retinal vessels with iris engorgement and vitreous haze.

36–16 This fundus photograph shows the appearance of an extremely severe degree of posterior pole plus disease in an eye that soon developed a total retinal detachment.

36–15, *Courtesy of Dr. Michael Trese.* ***36–16,*** *Courtesy of the Ophthalmic Photography Health Science Center. From Ryan, SJ: Retina, ed 2, St Louis, 1994, Mosby–Year Book.*

36–17 INCONTINENTIA PIGMENTI

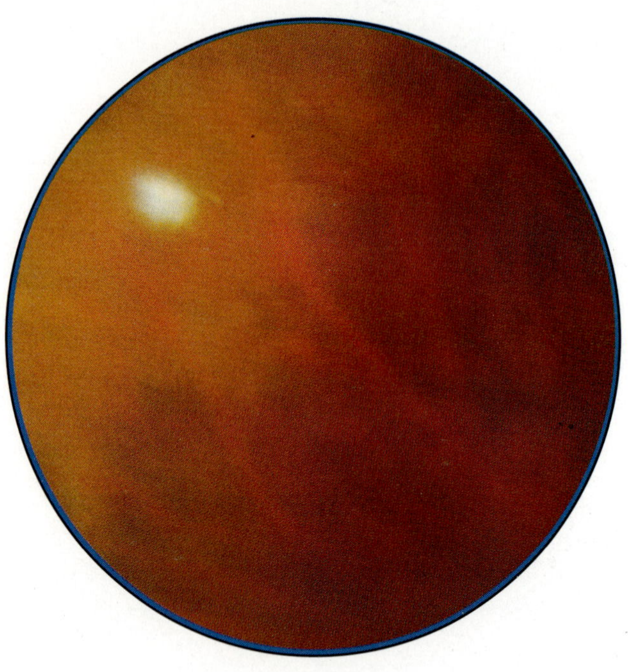

36–18

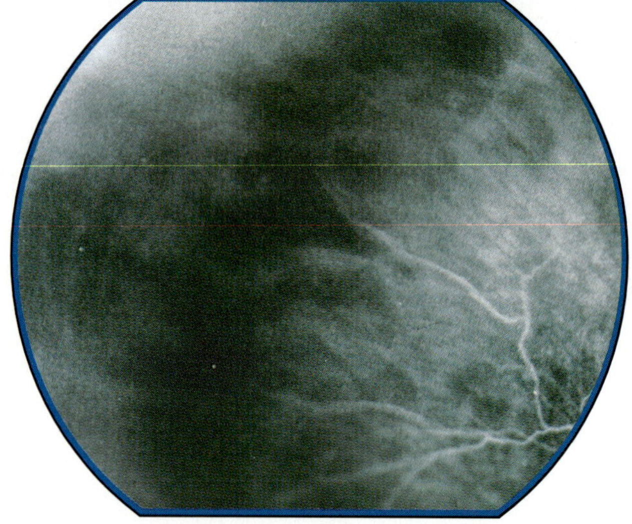

36–19

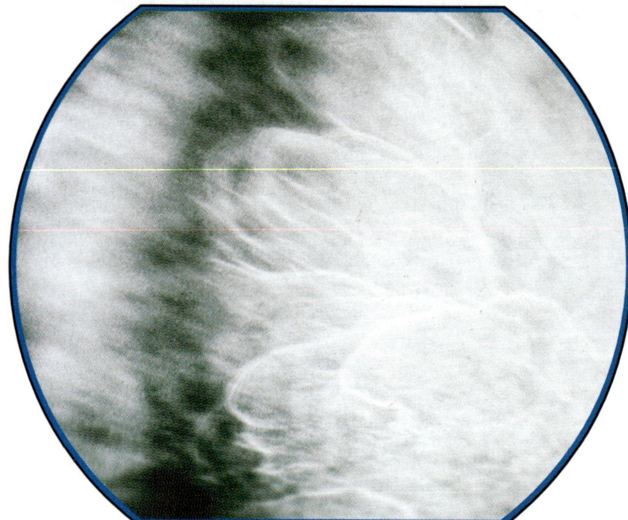

36–17 Another cause of peripheral capillary nonperfusion and retinal neovascularization is incontinentia pigmenti. This patient with incontinentia pigmenti demonstrates peripheral nonperfusion with a whitish fibrotic spot.

36–18 and 36–19 Note the transition zone between perfused and nonperfused retina.

36–17 *through* ***36–19,*** *From Wald, KJ, Hirose, T, and Topilow, H: Ectodermal dysplasia, ectrodactyly, and clefting syndrome and bilateral detachment, Arch Ophthalmol 111:734, 1993.*

Suggested Readings

Biglan, AW, Brown, DR, Reynolds, JD, and Milley, JR: Risk factors associated with retrolental fibroplasia, Ophthalmology 91:1504–1511, 1984

Cryotherapy for Retinopathy of Prematurity Cooperative Group: Manual of procedures, archived at the National Technical Information Service, Springfield, VA, US Department of Commerce, NTIS Accession No PB88–16350, 1988

Cryotherapy for Retinopathy of Prematurity Cooperative Group: Multicenter trial of cryotherapy for retinopathy of prematurity, one year outcome—structure and function, Arch Ophthalmol 108:950–955, 1990

Flower, RW: A new perspective on the pathogenesis of retrolental fibroplasia: the influence of elevated arterial CO_2, Retinopathy of Prematurity Conference, Dec 4–6, 1981

Flynn, JT, Cassady, J, Essner, D, Zeskind, J, Merritt, J, Flynn, R, and Williams, MJ: Fluorescein angiography in retrolental fibroplasia: experience from 1969–1977, Ophthalmology 86:1700–1723, 1979

Gibson, DL, Sheps, SB, Hong, Uh S, Schechter, MT, and McCormick, AQ: Retinopathy of prematurity-induced blindness: birth weight-specific survival and the new epidemic, Pediatrics 86:405–412, 1990

Keith, CG: Visual outcome and effect of treatment in stage III developing retrolental fibroplasia, Br J Ophthalmol 66:446–449, 1982

Kingham, JD: Acute retrolental fibroplasia, Arch Ophthalmol 95:39–47, 1977

Machemer, R: Description and pathogenesis of late stages of retinopathy of prematurity, Ophthalmology 92:1000–1004, 1985

O'Grady, GE, Flynn, JT, and Herrera, JA: The clinical course of retrolental fibroplasia in premature infants, South Med J 65:655–658, 1972

Payne, JW, and Patz, A: Current status of retrolental fibroplasia: the retinopathy of prematurity, Ann Clin Res 11:205–221, 1979

Seiberth, V, Linderkamp, O, Knorz, MC, and Liesenhoff, H: The effect of bright light on the incidence of acute retinopathy of prematurity: a controlled clinical trial, Ophthalmology (Suppl):120–121, 1991

Tasman, W: Vitreoretinal changes in cicatricial retrolental fibroplasia, Trans Am Ophthalmol Soc 68:548–594, 1970

Tasman, W, Brown, GC, Schaffer, DB, Quinn, G, Naidoff, M, Benson, WE, and Diamond, G: Cryotherapy for active retinopathy of prematurity, Ophthalmology 93:580–585, 1986

Yamashita Y: Studies on retinopathy of prematurity. III. Cryocautery for retinopathy of prematurity, Rinsho Ganka 26:385–393, 1972

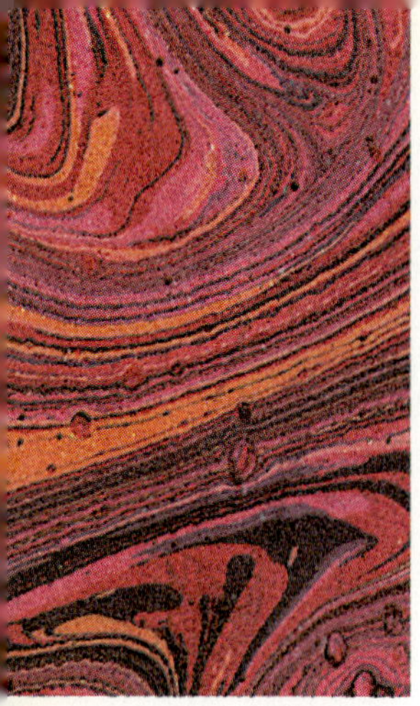

Chapter 37

Acquired Retinal Macroaneurysms

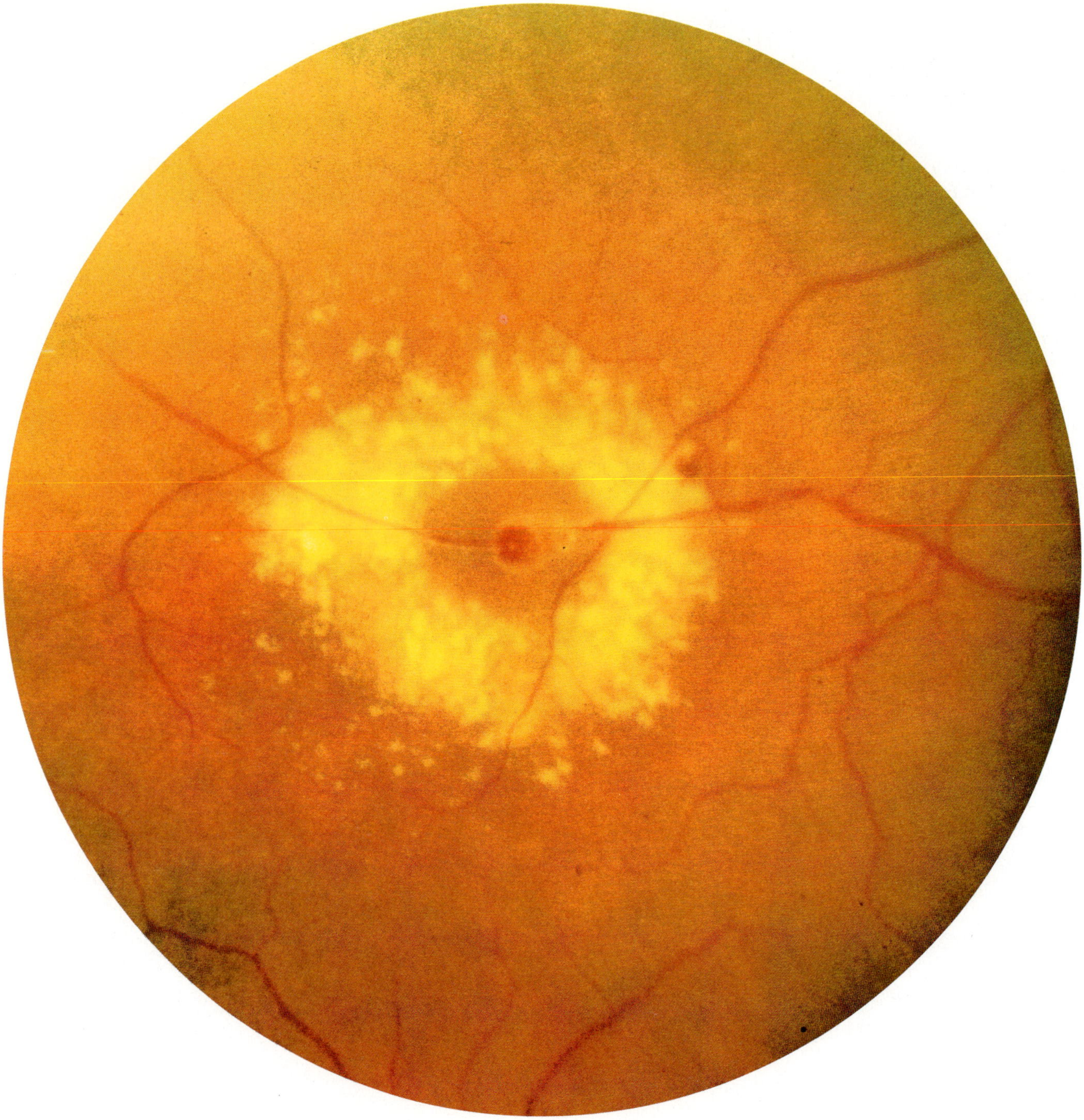

Retinal macroaneurysms consist of dilatations of the retinal arterioles. Secondary subretinal exudation and hemorrhage may occur. Systemic hypertension is often noted in these patients, which are usually women.

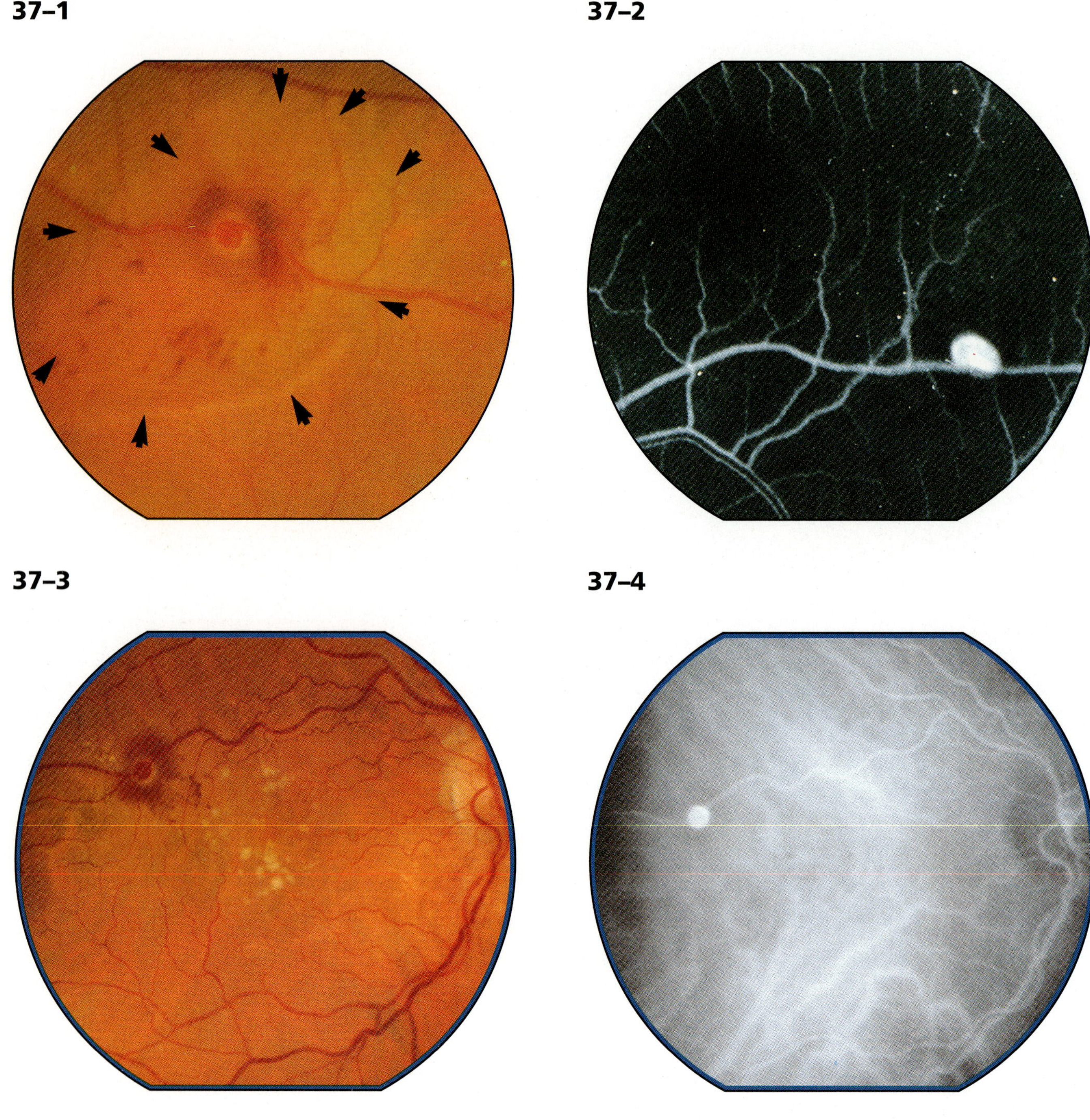

37–1 This patient has a macroaneurysm along the course of an irregular, beaded arteriole. An irregular halo of yellowish exudate surrounds the aneurysm, and in turn, there is a ring of subretinal hemorrhage. The aneurysm is also associated with an exudative detachment of the neurosensory retina *(arrowheads)*. A very faint fringe of lipoidal change is demonstrated at its inferior aspect. There are also dilated telangiectatic vessels within the detached area, possibly some attempt to compensate for slow perfusion through the aneurysm.

37–2 through 37–4 Fluorescein angiography helps to delineate a macroaneurysm (37–2) as a late intense lightbulb area of staining or a ring of staining by indocyanine-green (ICG) angiography (37–3 and 37–4).

37–5

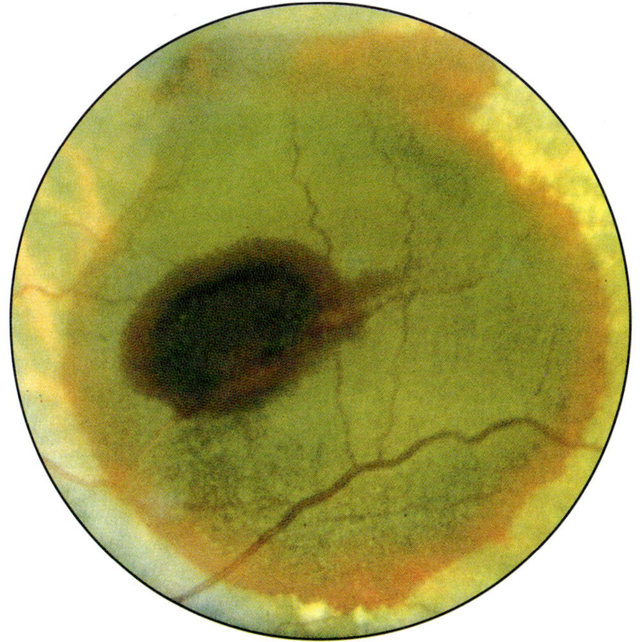

37–6

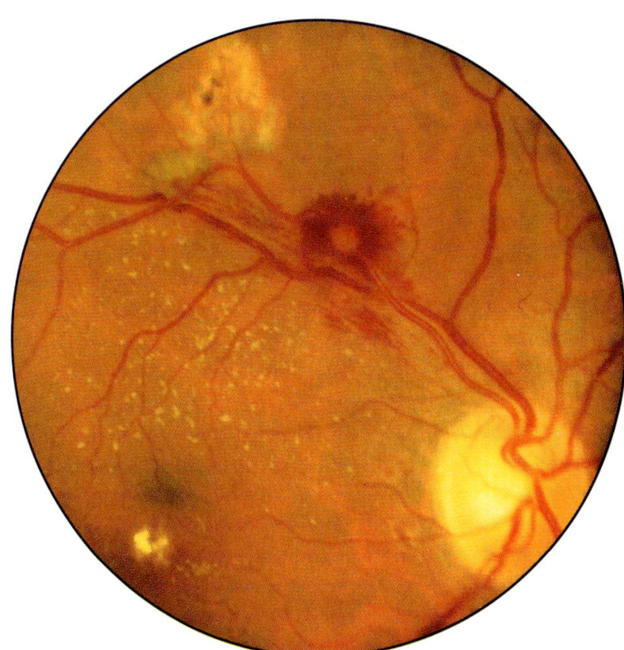

37–7

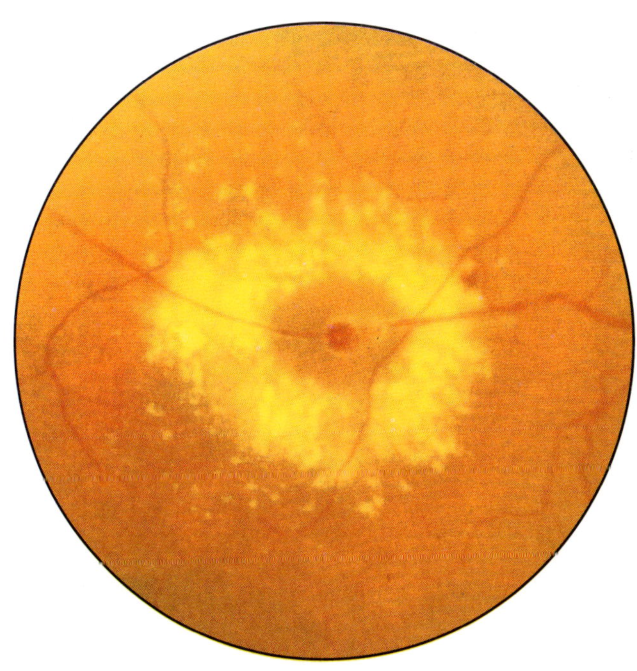

37–5 A macroaneurysm may bleed in front or behind the retina, or in some instances in both directions, forming an asymmetric, hourglass configuration of blood. When it bleeds in front of the retina, it may obscure the aneurysm itself, as demonstrated in this case.

37–6 The next patient demonstrates that macroaneurysms may be multiple and recurrent. An acute macroaneurysm is seen along the course of the superior temporal arteriole with a surrounding area of hemorrhage. Previously, the patient had experienced a macroaneurysm at the next order of bifurcation. It was photocoagulated, and now there is an atrophic scar and narrowing of the involved vessel. The patchy lipid deposition in the central macula, which is resolving, was the result of the first aneurysm.

37–7 The following patient has a macroaneurysm associated with lipid exudation.

37–8

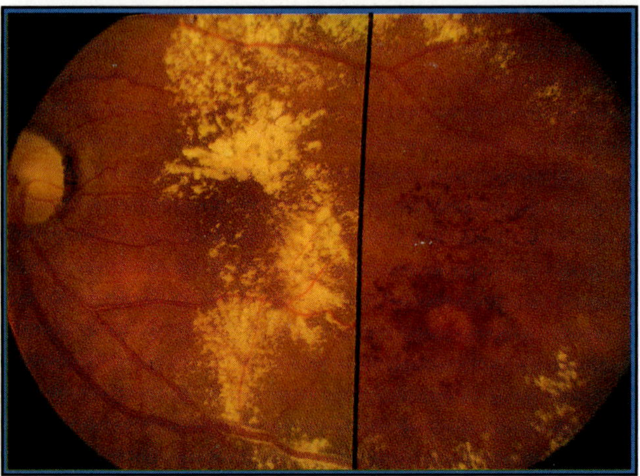

37–9

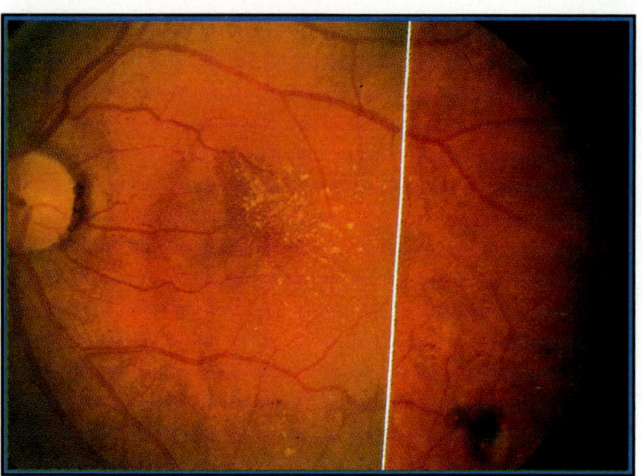

37–10

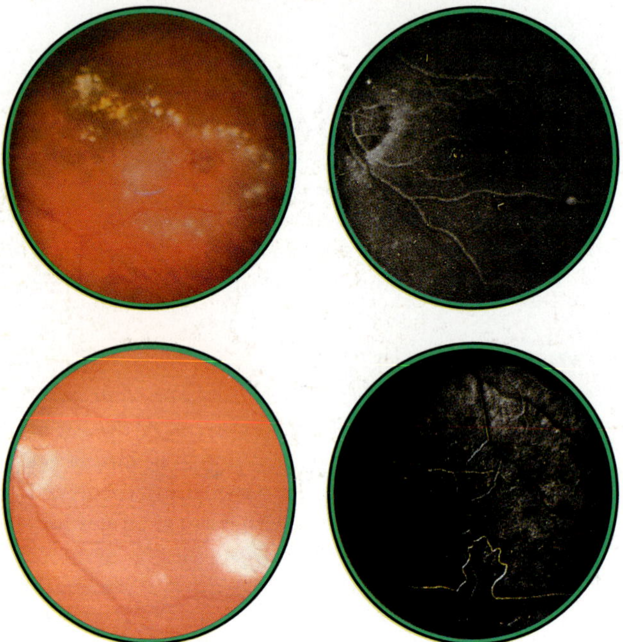

37–8 and 37–9 In this patient, there is a bilobed macroaneurysm. The distal segment of the involved arteriole is very thin, suggesting an interruption in the normal flow through that vessel. There is surrounding hemorrhage and a massive exudative response including neurosensory retinal detachment, and extensive lipid coursing in its typical fashion toward the macula. The patient had laser photocoagulation and several months after treatment there is resolving lipid deposition. In affected patients, the serous component of the exudative response tends to resolve in a matter of several days to weeks; whereas the lipid exudation takes weeks or months to be dissolved and debrided through a cellular mediated process rather than diffusion directly into one of the two circulations. The heavy concentration of lipid may have a degenerative as well as hyperplastic effect on the retinal pigment epithelium and neurosensory retina, leading to irreversible structural change and limited visual improvement potential.

37–10 Lipid deposition was noted in the macular region of this patient following cataract surgery. The lipid emanated from the inferior temporal arcade, where a "ghostlike" aneurysmal dilatation was evident clinically. The fluorescein study confirmed the presence of a macroaneurysm. Following photocoagulation, there was an atrophic scar at the site of the aneurysm, and a hairpin, arteriole-arteriole anastomosis shunting blood through the obliterated treatment site was noted. There was resolution of the exudation in the macula and improvement in the vision.

37–11

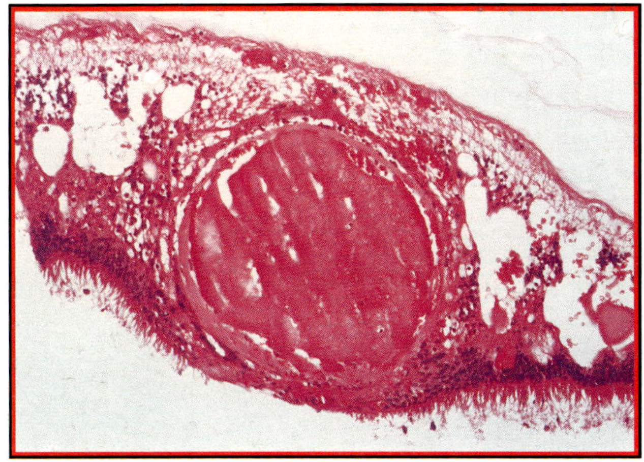

37–12 **37–12A**

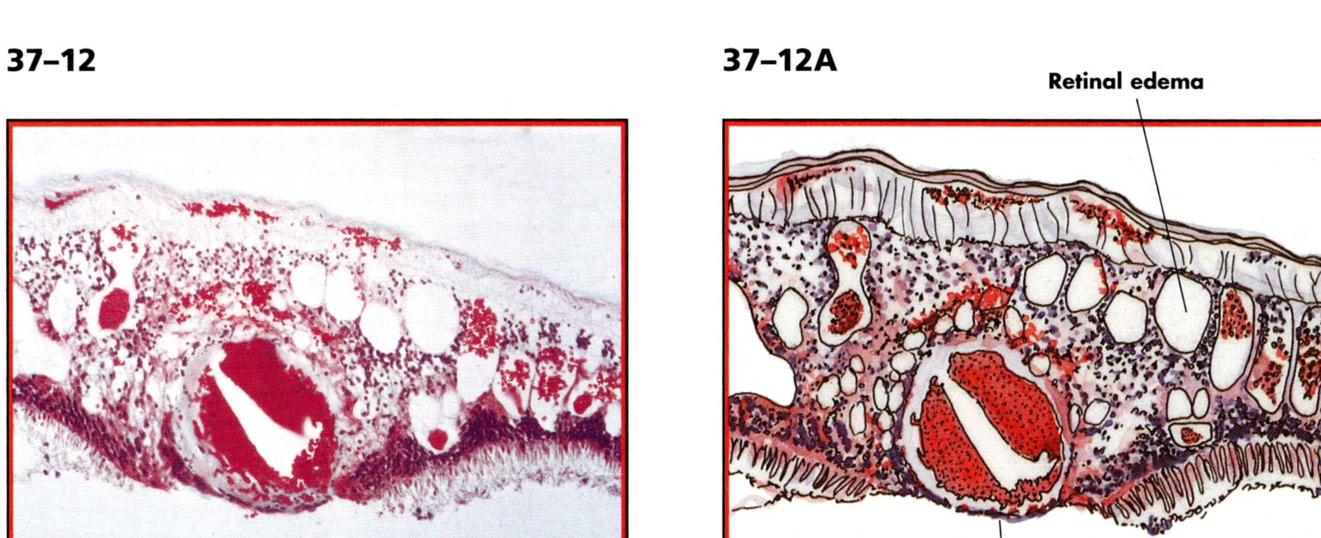

37–11, 37–12, and 37–12A These histopathologic correlates demonstrate the various features of macroaneurysms. Thrombosed retinal arterial macroaneurysms are noted with retinal hemorrhages and cystic edema.

37–13

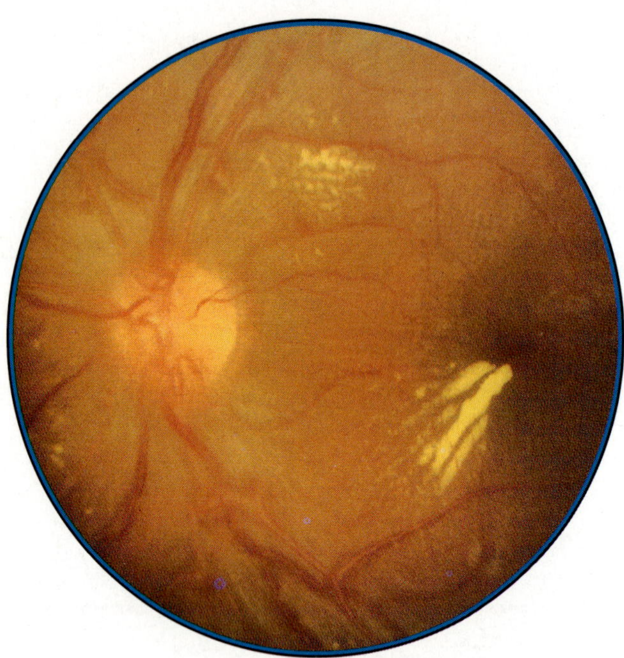

37–14

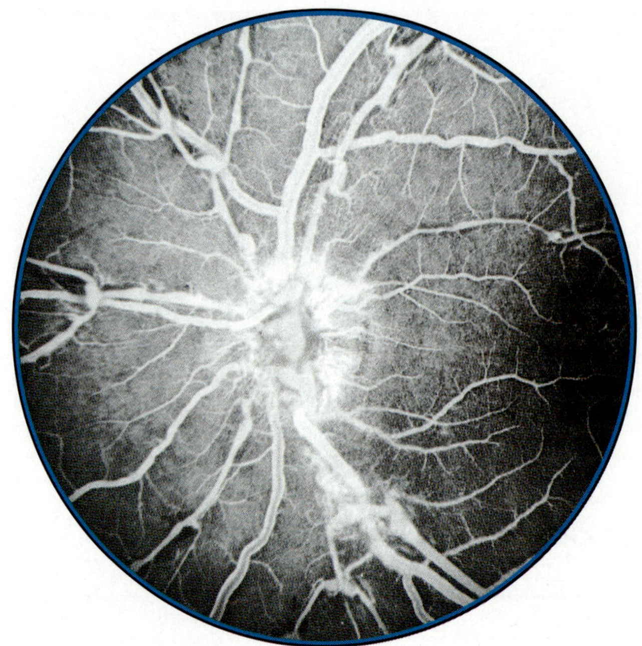

37–13 and 37–14 This healthy patient has lipid exudation and tortuous vessels secondary to a peculiar rare syndrome termed bilateral multiple retinal arterial macroaneurysms due to an idiopathic retinal vasculitis. Note how well the fluorescein angiogram delineates the multiple macroaneurysms. The findings were similar in both eyes.

37–13 *and* ***37–14,*** *Courtesy of Johnny Justice.*

Suggested Readings

Abdel-Khalek, MN, and Richardson, J: Retinal macroaneurysm: natural history and guidelines for treatment, Br J Ophthalmol 70:2–11, 1986

Cleary, PE, Kohner, EM, Hamilton, AM, and Bird, AC: Retinal macroaneurysms, Br J Ophthalmol 59:355–361, 1975

Cousins, SW, Flynn, HE, Jr, and Clarkson, JG: Macroaneurysms associated with retinal branch vein occlusion, Am J Ophthalmol 109:567–570, 1990

Green, WR: Retinal ischemia: vascular and circulatory conditions and diseases. In Spencer, WH, ed: Ophthalmic pathology, Philadelphia, 1985, WB Saunders

Joondeph, BC, Joondeph, HC, and Blair, NP: Retinal macroaneurysms treated with the yellow dye laser, Retina 9:187–192, 1989

Lewis, RA, Norton, EWD, and Gass, JDM: Acquired arterial macroaneurysms of the retina, Br J Ophthalmol 60:21–30, 1976

Mainster, MA, Whitacre, MM: Dye yellow photocoagulation of retinal arterial macroaneurysms, Am J Ophthalmol 105:97–98, 1988

Nadel, AJ, and Gupta, KK: Macroaneurysms of the retinal arteries, Arch Ophthalmol 94:1092–1096, 1976

Palestine, AG, Robertson, DM, and Goldstein, BG: Macroaneurysms of the retinal arteries, Am J Ophthalmol 93:164–171, 1982

Perry, HD, Zimmerman, LE, and Benson, WE: Hemorrhage from isolated aneurysm of a retinal artery: report of two cases simulating malignant melanoma, Arch Ophthalmol 95:281, 1977

Rabb, MF, Gaglioano, DA, and Teske, MP: Retinal arterial macroaneurysms, Surv Ophthalmol 33:73–96, 1988

Robertson, DM: Macroaneurysms of the retinal arteries, Trans Am Acad Opthalmol Otolaryngol 77:55–67, 1973

Russell, SR, and Folk, JC: Branch retinal artery occlusion after dye yellow photocoagulation of an arterial macroaneurysm, Am J Ophthalmol 104:186–187, 1987

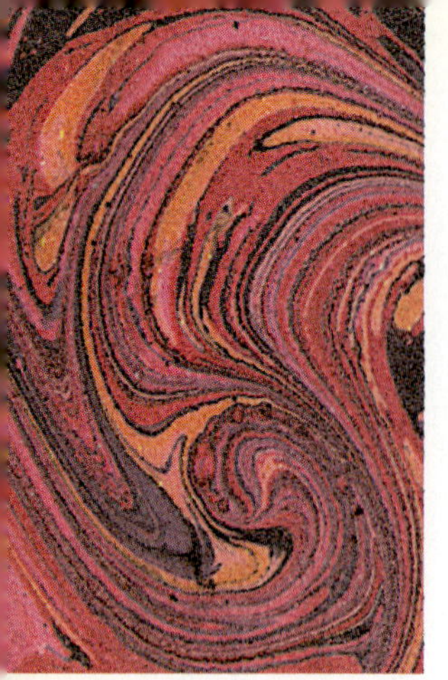

Chapter 38

Eales' Disease

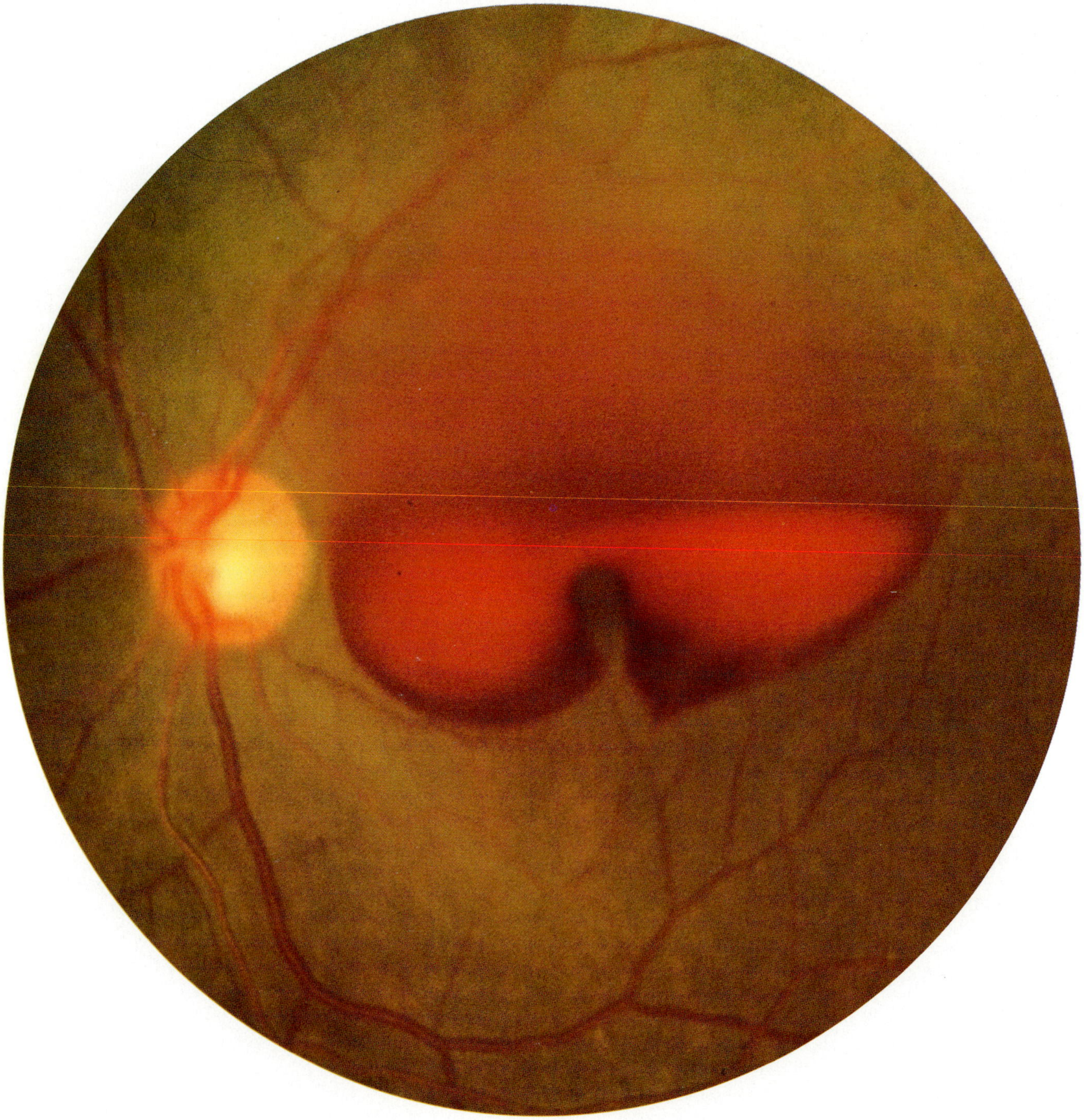

Eales' disease, or peripheral idiopathic retinal vascular occlusive disease, is usually seen in healthy young males. Vascular sheathing, intraretinal hemorrhages, and retinal phlebitis may occur without any known causes. Macular edema may also be noted. Peripheral retinal nonperfusion is very common in this condition. Up to 80% of patients with Eales' disease have retinal neovascularization. Rubeosis may also occur. Vasoproliferation may lead to retinal detachment.

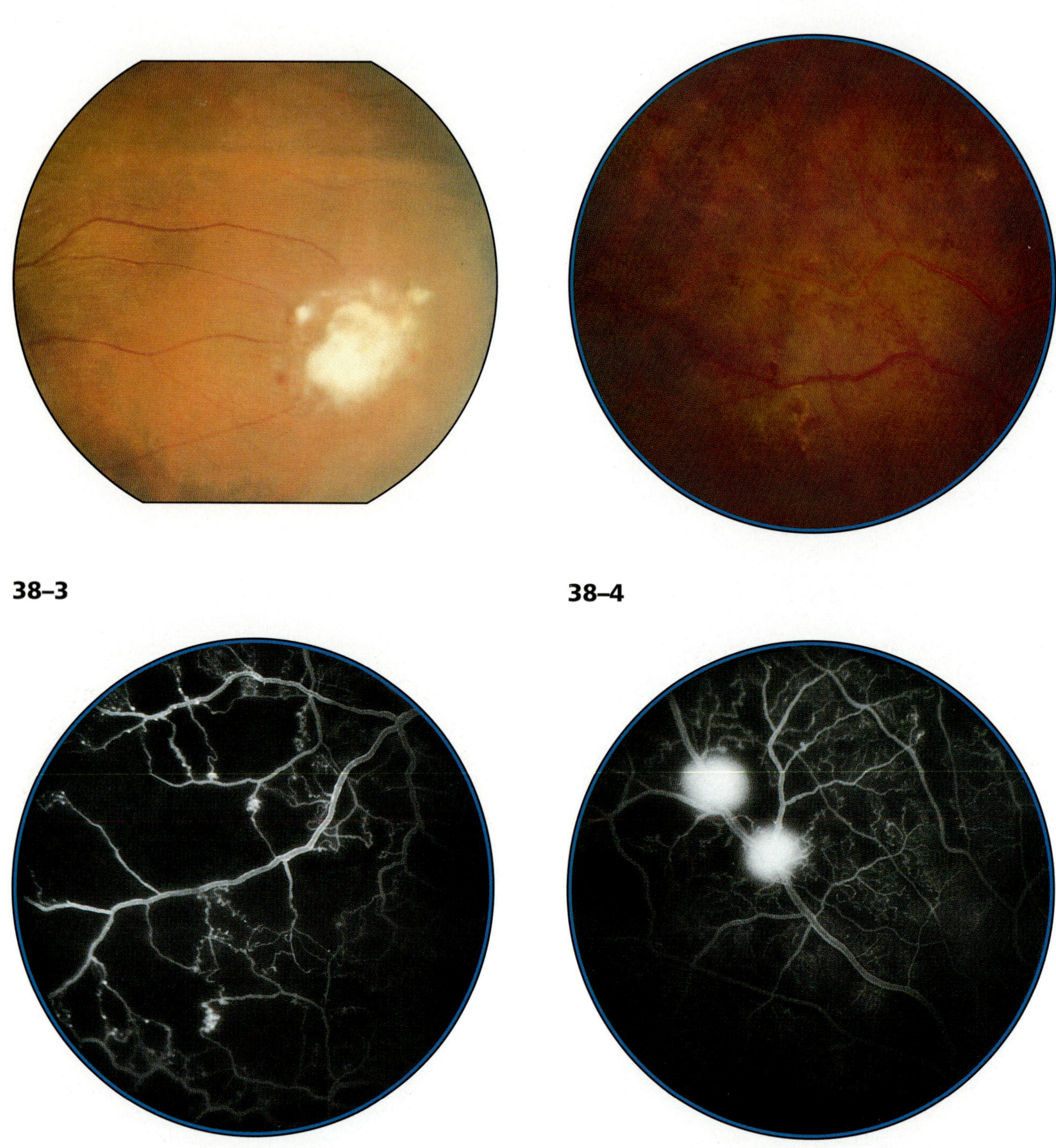

38–1 This patient with Eales' disease, who has been followed for 17 years, demonstrates fibrosis and telangiectasis that has not progressed.

38–2 through 38–4 This patient also has Eales' disease with capillary nonperfusion and retinal neovascularization demonstrated on the fluorescein angiogram (38–3). The early proliferative changes begin along the arteriovenous shunt, but there is no junction between perfused and nonperfused retina, as seen in sickle cell retinopathy (38–4).

38–5

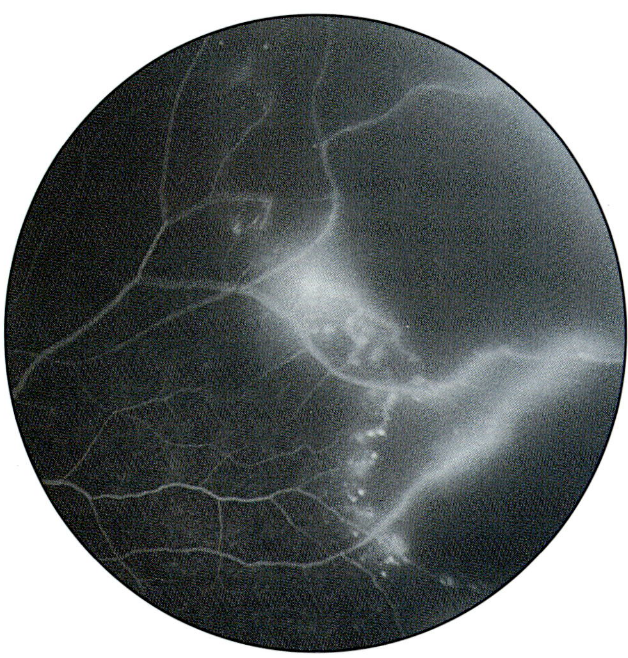

38–6

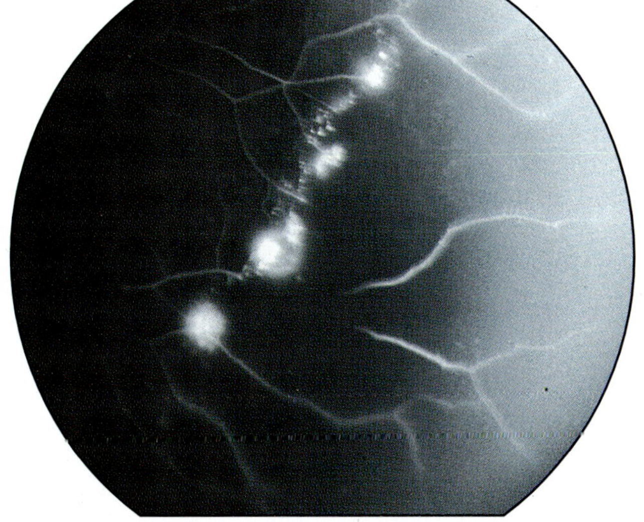

38–7

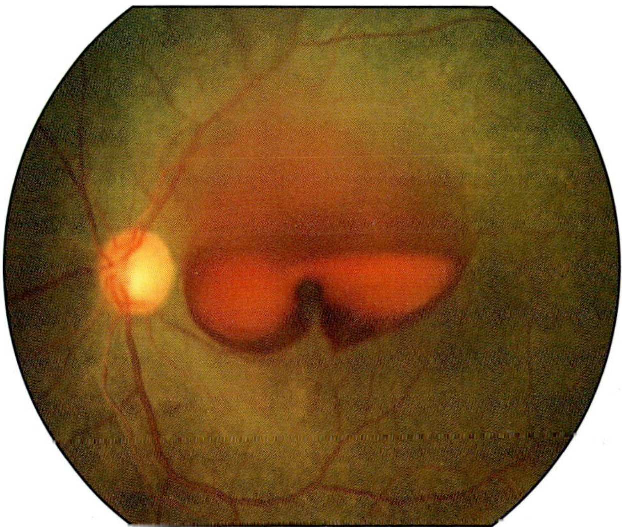

38–5 The late-stage angiogram in this patient with Eales' disease reveals leakage at the site of early proliferative change, but also staining of vessels characteristic of this disease—which is not seen in other hemoglobinopathies such as sickle cell retinopathy. This change, however, may be demonstrated in proliferative vascular disease secondary to granulomatous systemic diseases such as sarcoidosis.

38–6 Another patient with Eales' disease demonstrates retinal neovascularization.

38–7 Macular manifestations include retinal vascular leakage, cystoid macular edema, and disc neovascularization. This patient had subhyaloid hemorrhage in the macular region in addition to peripheral changes consistent with Eales' disease.

Suggested Readings

Elliot, AJ: Thirty-year observation of patients with Eales' disease, Am J Ophthalmol 80:404–408, 1975

Elliot, AJ, and Harris, GS: The present status of the diagnosis and treatment of periphlebitis retinae (Eales' disease), Can J Ophthalmol 4:117–122, 1969

Murphy, RP, Renie, WA, Proctor, LR, Shimizu, H, Lippman, SM, Anderson, KC, Fine, SL, Patz, A, and McKusick, VA: A survey of patients with Eales' disease. In Fine, SL, and Owens, SL, eds: Management of retinal vascular and macular disorders, Baltimore, Md, 1983, Williams & Wilkins

Renie, WA, Murphy, RP, Anderson, KC, Lippman, SM, McKusick, VA, Proctor, LR, Shimizu, H, Patz, A, and Fine, SL: The evaluation of patients with Eales' disease, Retina 3:243–248, 1983

Spitznas, M, Meyer-Schwickerath, GT, and Stephan, B: The clinical picture of Eales' disease, Graefes Arch Clin Exp Ophthalmol 194:73–85, 1975

Spitznas, M, Meyer-Schwickerath, G, and Stephan, B: Treatment of Eales' disease with photocoagulation, Graefes Arch Clin Exp Ophthalmol 194:193–198, 1975

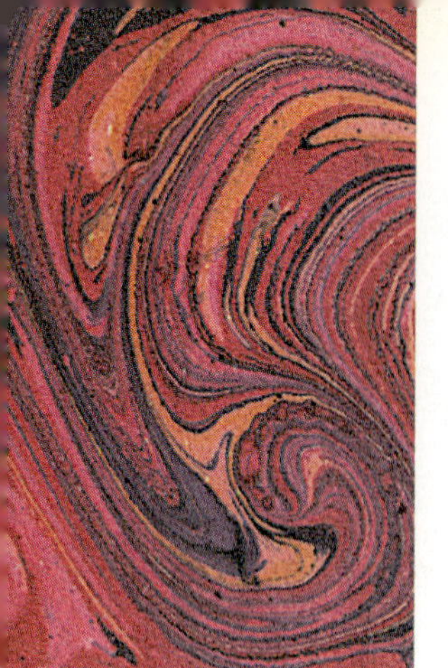

Chapter 39

Radiation Retinopathy

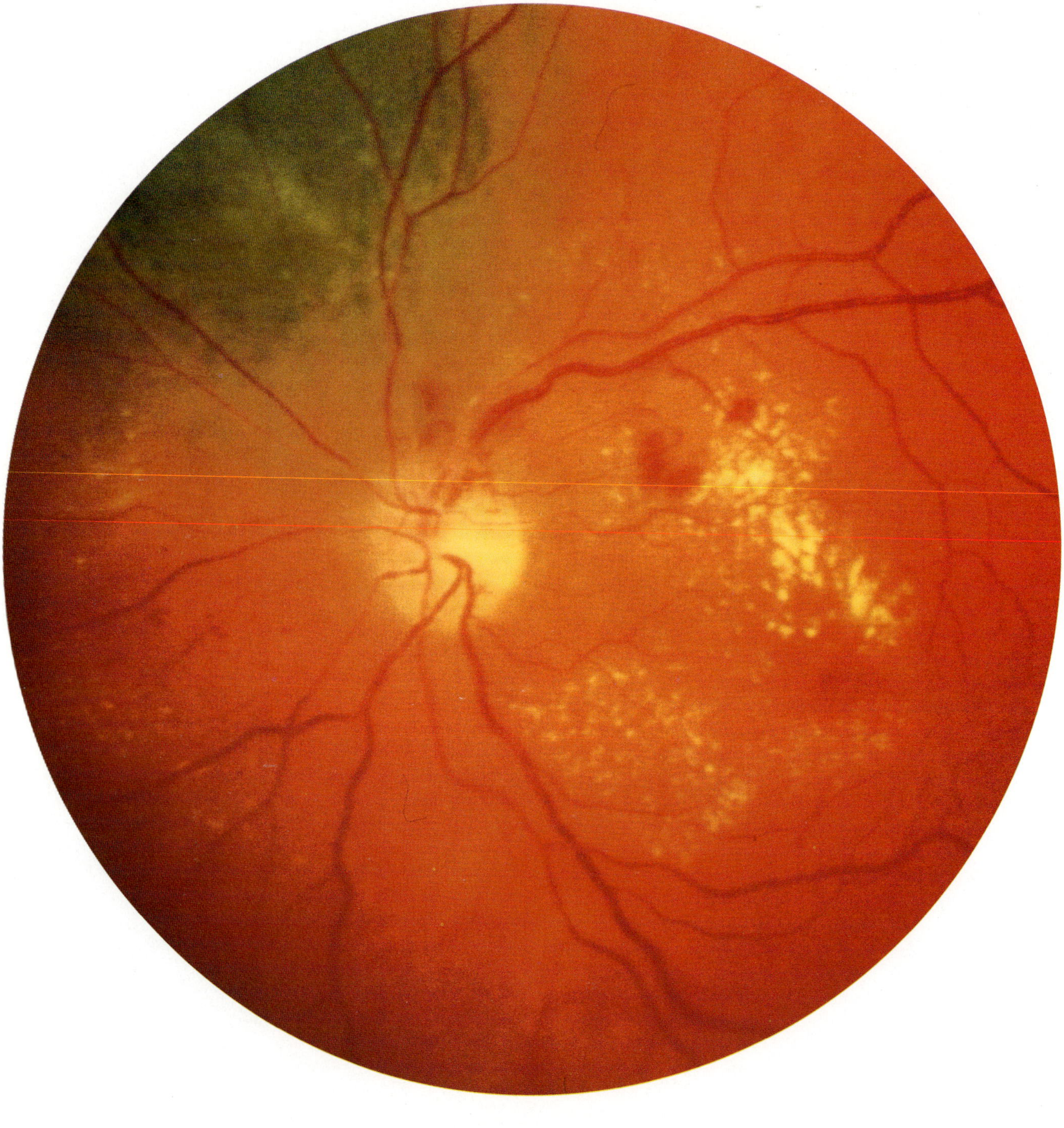

Radiation retinopathy is commonly seen following radiotherapy of various neoplasms. Intraretinal hemorrhages, cotton-wool spots, capillary nonperfusion, telangiectasis, and macular edema are common. Macular edema is demonstrated in the majority of affected patients and is the most common retinal finding.

39–1 RADIATION RETINOPATHY

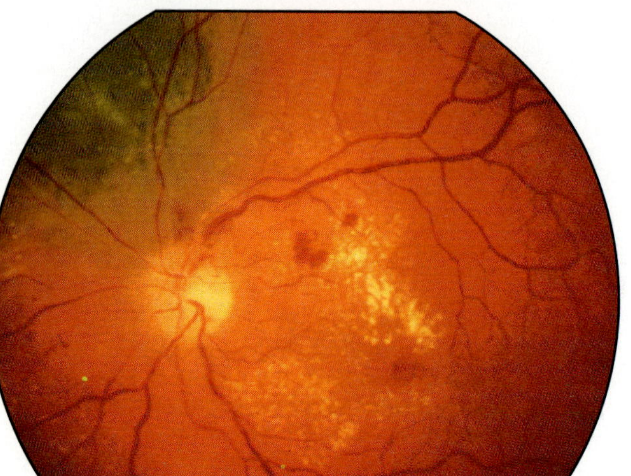

39–2

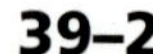

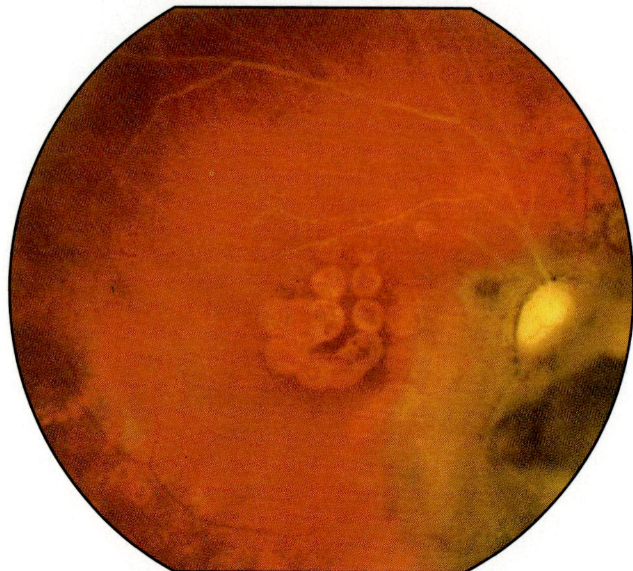

39–3

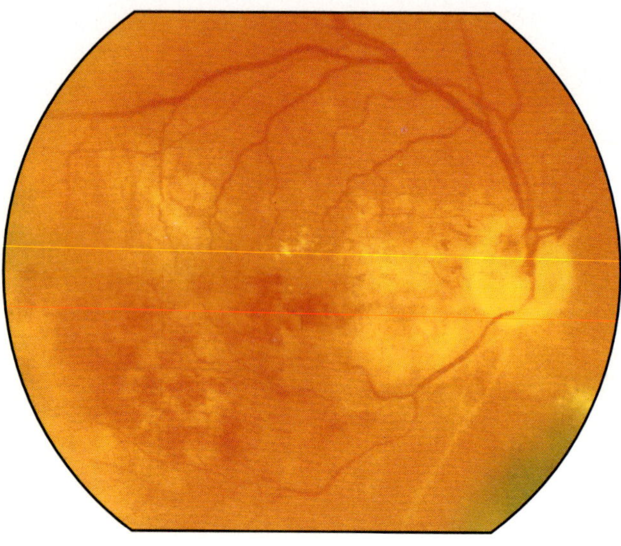

39–4

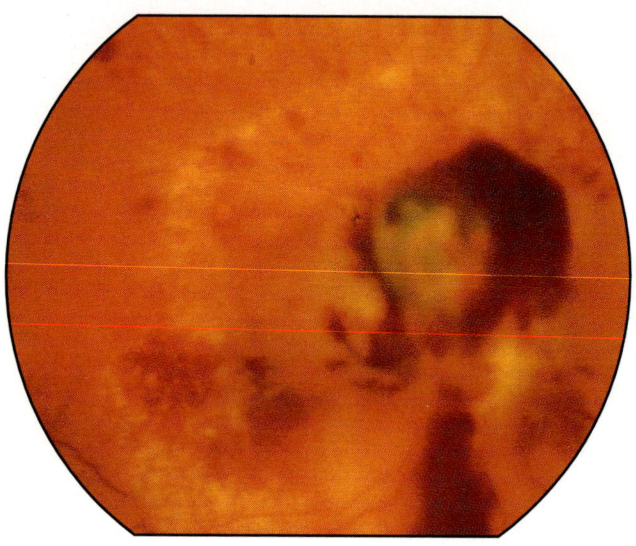

39–1 This patient had proton beam irradiation for a choroidal melanoma. Radiation retinopathy with intraretinal hemorrhages, lipid exudation, and macular edema are present. Note the irradiated choroidal melanoma superiornasal to the optic disc.

39–2 This patient also had proton beam irradiation for a choroidal melanoma. Note the vascular sheathing secondary to radiation retinopathy.

39–3 This patient developed a pale optic disc, intraretinal hemorrhages, and macular edema following proton beam irradiation for a choroidal melanoma. Note the sheathed vessel inferiorly near the irradiated choroidal melanoma.

39–4 This patient developed a papillopathy following proton beam irradiation for a choroidal melanoma.

39–1, 39–2, *and* ***39–4,*** *Courtesy of Dr. Evangelos Gragoudas.* ***39–3,*** *Gragoudas, E, et al: Radiation maculopathy after proton beam irradiation for choroidal melanoma, Ophthalmology 99:1278–1285, 1992.*

39–5 BONE MARROW TRANSPLANTATION RETINOPATHY 39–6

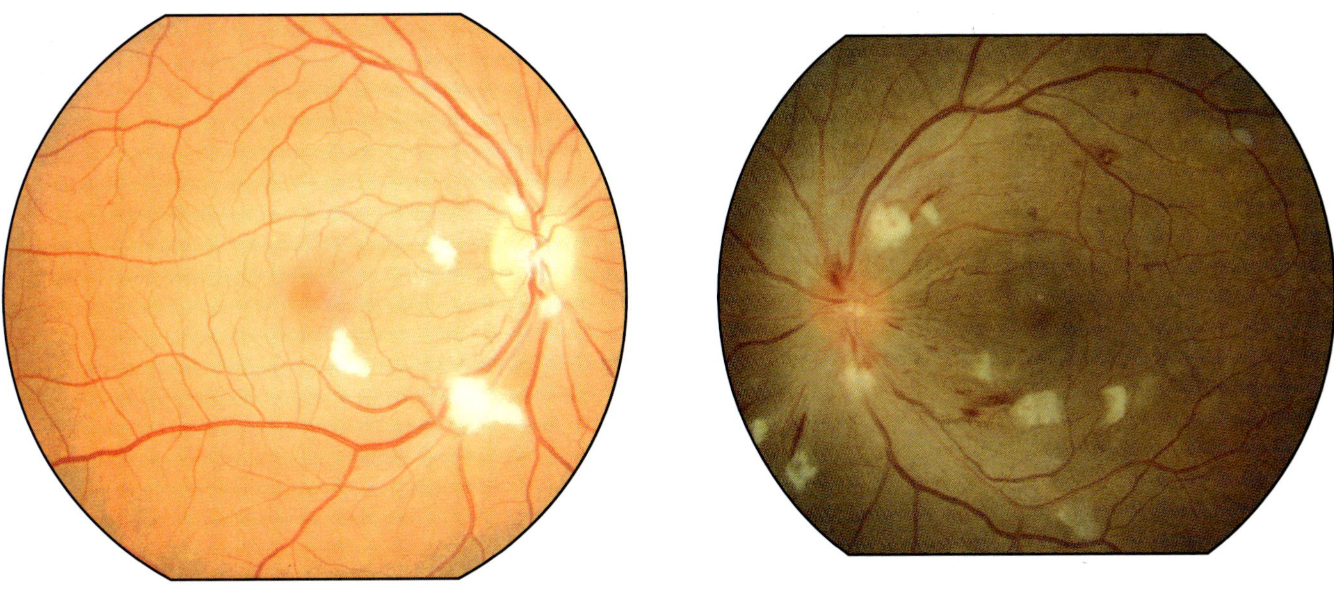

39–5 and 39–6 These two patients developed intraretinal hemorrhages and/or cotton-wool spots following bone marrow transplantation. Both patients had received autologous bone marrow transplants with high-dose chemotherapy, consisting of BCNU, cyclophosphamide, and cisplatin. The retinopathy developed approximately two months after chemotherapy. These patients may also develop progressive ischemic disease, preretinal neovascularization, and all of their sequelae.

***39–5** and **39–6,** Courtesy of Dr. Glenn Jaffe.*

Suggested Readings

Amoaku, WMK, and Archer, DB: Cephalic radiation and retinal vasculopathy, Eye 4:195–203, 1990

Amoaku, WMK, and Archer, DB: Fluorescein angiographic features, natural course and treatment of radiation retinopathy, Eye 4:657–667, 1990

Archer, DB, Amoaku, WMK, and Gardner, TA: Radiation retinopathy—clinical, histopathological, ultrastructural and experimental correlations, Eye 5:239–251, 1991

Boozalis, GT, Schachat, AP, and Green, WR: Subretinal neovascularization from the retina in radiation retinopathy, Retina 7:156–161, 1987

Brown, GC, Shields, JA, Sanborn G, Augsburger, JJ, Savino, PJ, and Schatz, NJ: Radiation retinopathy, Ophthalmology 89:1494–1501, 1982

Chaudhuri, PR, Austin, DJ, and Rosenthal, AR: Treatment of radiation retinopathy, Br J Ophthalmol 65:623–625, 1981

Chee, PHY: Radiation retinopathy, Am J Ophthalmol 66:860–865, 1968

Guyer, DR, Mukai S, Egan, KM, Seddon, JM, Walsh, SM, and Gragoudas, ES: Radiation maculopathy following proton beam irradiation for choroidal melanoma, Ophthalmology 99:1278–1285, 1992

Haye, C, Desjardins, L, Bouder, P, et al: Maculopathies par radiations chez les patients traités pour mélanomes choroidiens, Ophthalmologie 1990; 229–231

Hayreh, SS: Post-radiation retinopathy: A fluorescence fundus angiographic study, Br J Ophthalmol 54:705–714, 1970

Kinyoun, JL, Kalina, RE, and Brower, SA: Radiation retinopathy after orbital irradiation for Graves' ophthalmopathy, Arch Ophthalmol 102:1473–1476, 1984

Kinyoun, JL, and Orcutt, JC: Radiation retinopathy, JAMA, 258:610–611, 1987

Lopez, PF, Sternberg, P, Dabbs, CK, Vogler, WR, Crocker, I, and Kain, NS: Bone marrow transplant retinopathy, Am J Ophthalmol 112:635–646, 1991

Nakissa, N, Rubin, P, Strohl, R, and Keys, H: Ocular and orbital complications following radiation therapy of paranasal sinus malignancies and review of literature, Cancer 51:980–986, 1983

Ross, HS, Rosenberg, S, and Friedman, AH: Delayed radiation necrosis of the optic nerve, Am J Ophthalmol 76:683–686, 1973

Shukovsky, LJ, and Fletcher, GH: Retinal and optic nerve complications in a high dose irradiation technique of ethmoid sinus and nasal cavity, Radiology 104:629–634, 1972

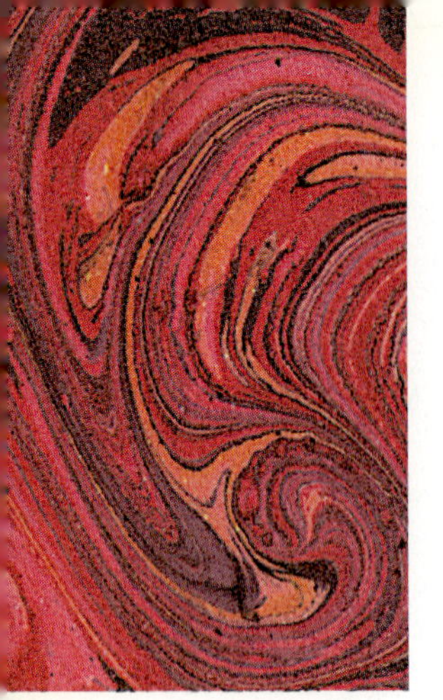

Chapter 40

Ocular Ischemic Syndrome

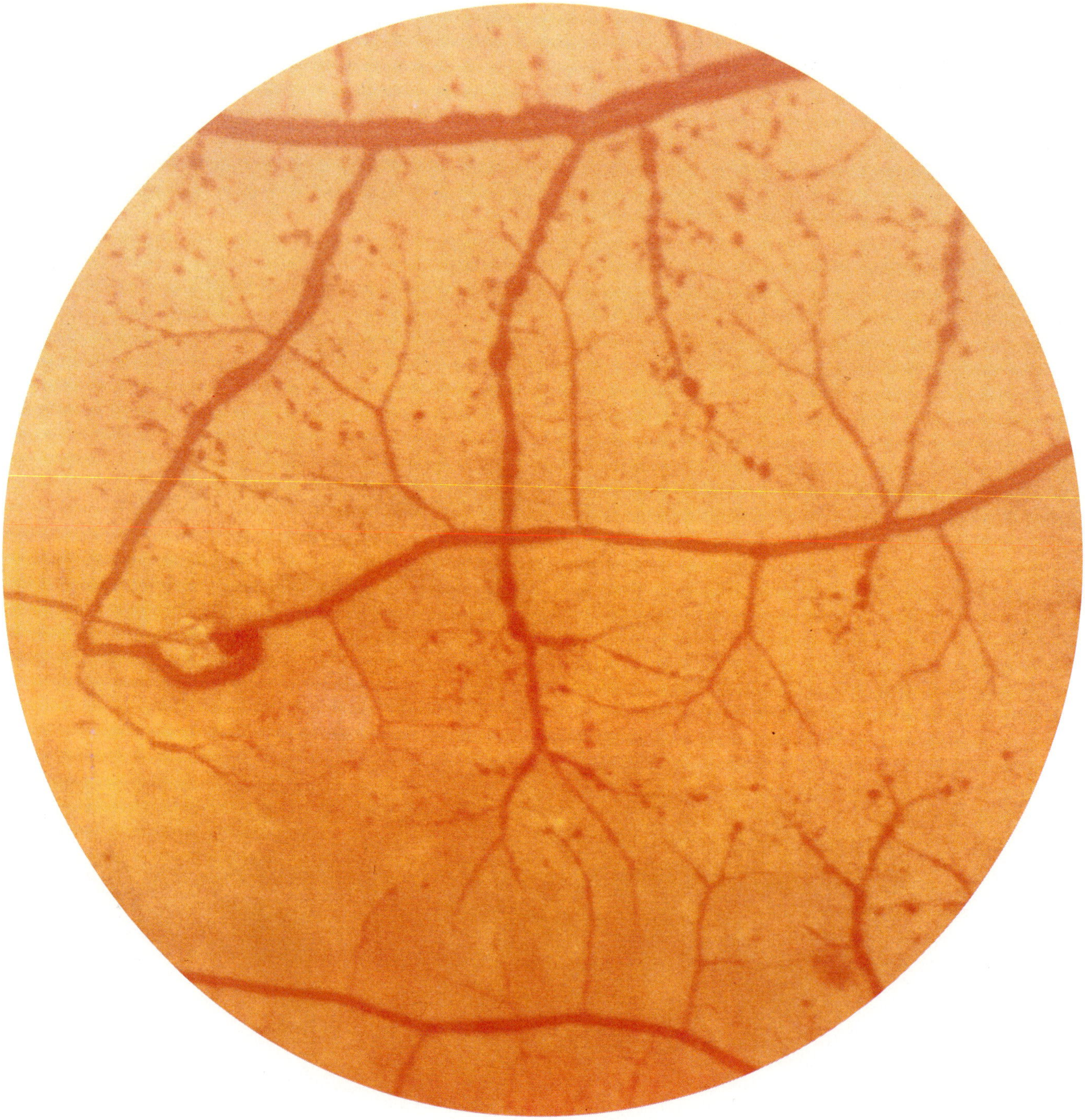

Carotid insufficiency findings in the posterior segment include midperipheral retinal hemorrhages, cotton-wool spots, dilated vessels, arteriovenous (AV) communications, microaneurysms, venous beading, retinal neovascularization, and vitreous hemorrhage.

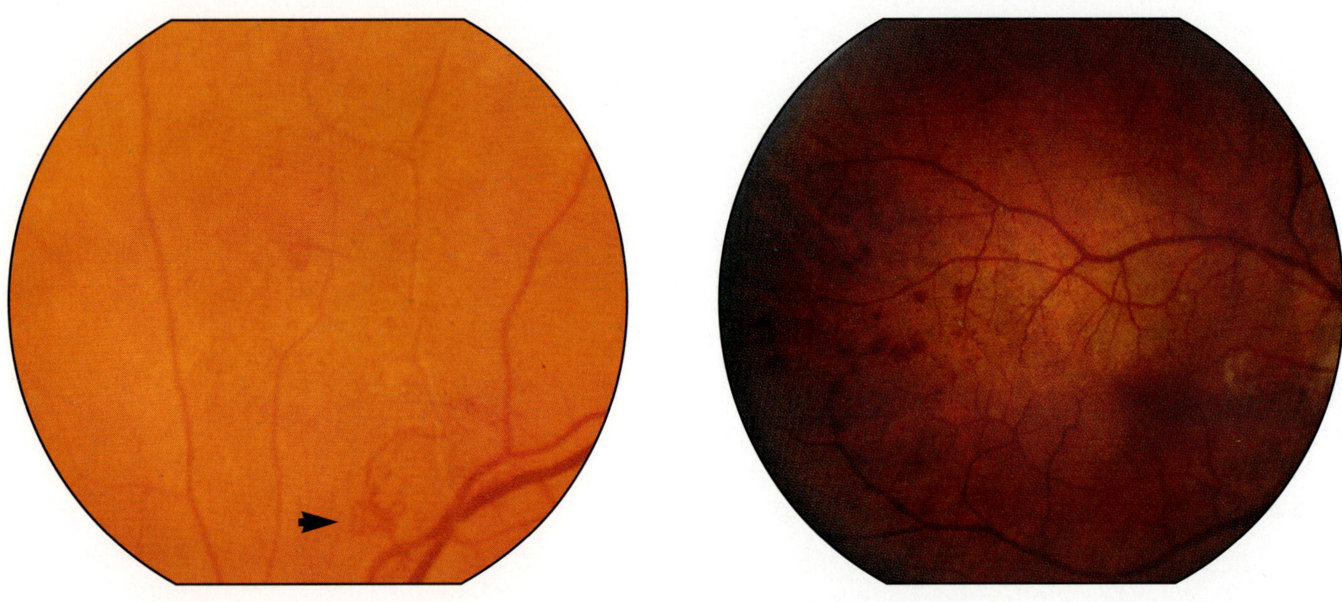

40–1 This patient has carotid artery obstructive disease with secondary ocular ischemic changes. The peripheral retina reveals irregular, narrowed, sheathed, and even obliterated vessels. Some of the smaller branches are not evident clinically or are "pruned." The clinically evident vessels have been referred to as "preferential vascular channels." There also may be secondary dotlike aneurysmal changes and preretinal neovascularization *(arrowhead),* which is demonstrated in this patient.

40–2 Dot and blot hemorrhages without venous dilation and tortuosity differentiates the ocular ischemic syndrome from venous occlusive disease and may also be seen in the posterior pole.

40–2, *Courtesy of Dr. Gary Brown.*

40–3

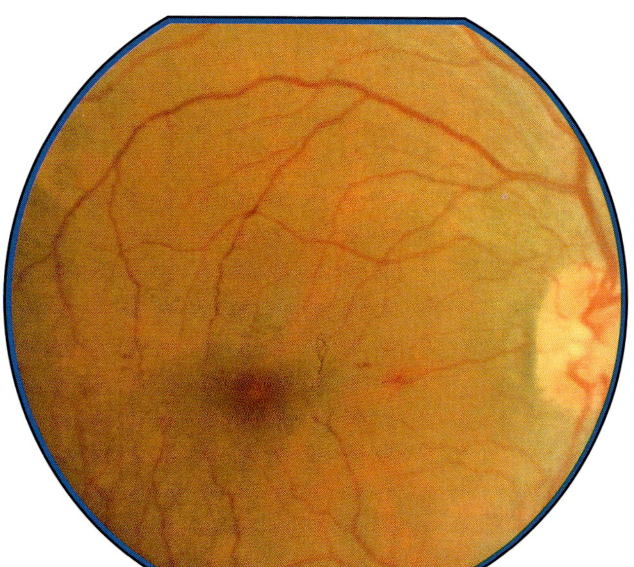

40–4

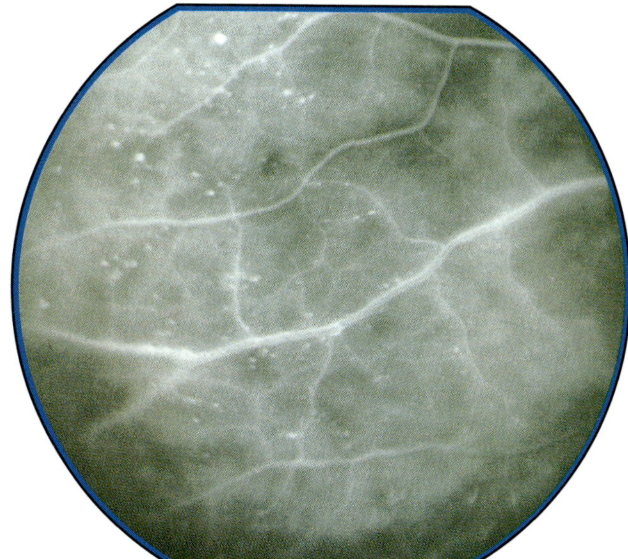

40–5

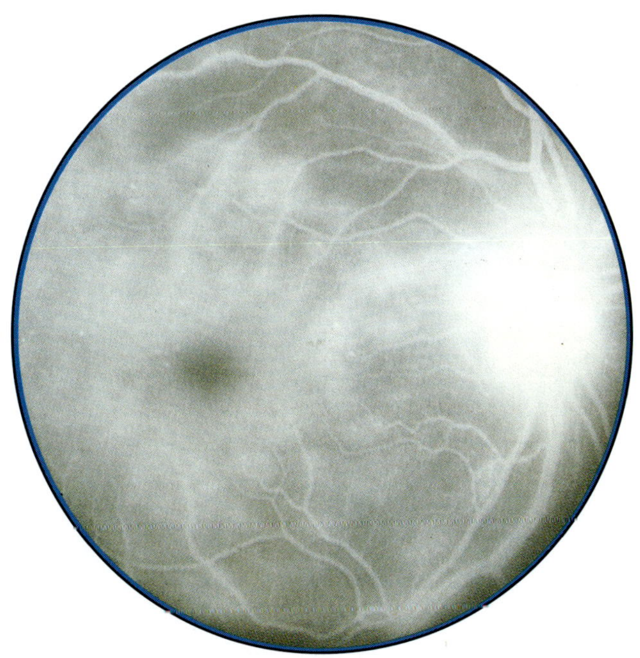

40–3 and 40–4 This 62-year-old female had a 100% left internal carotid artery obstruction and a visual acuity of 20/40. Numerous microaneurysms are demonstrated in the posterior pole (40–3) and periphery (40–4). A foveal cyst is also noted (40–3).

40–5 The late phase of the angiogram demonstrates staining of the blood vessels in the periphery and marked macular edema. The retinal veins are somewhat dilated.

__40–3__ through __40–5,__ Courtesy of Dr. Gary Brown. From Brown, G, et al: Am J Ophthalmol 102:442–448, 1986.

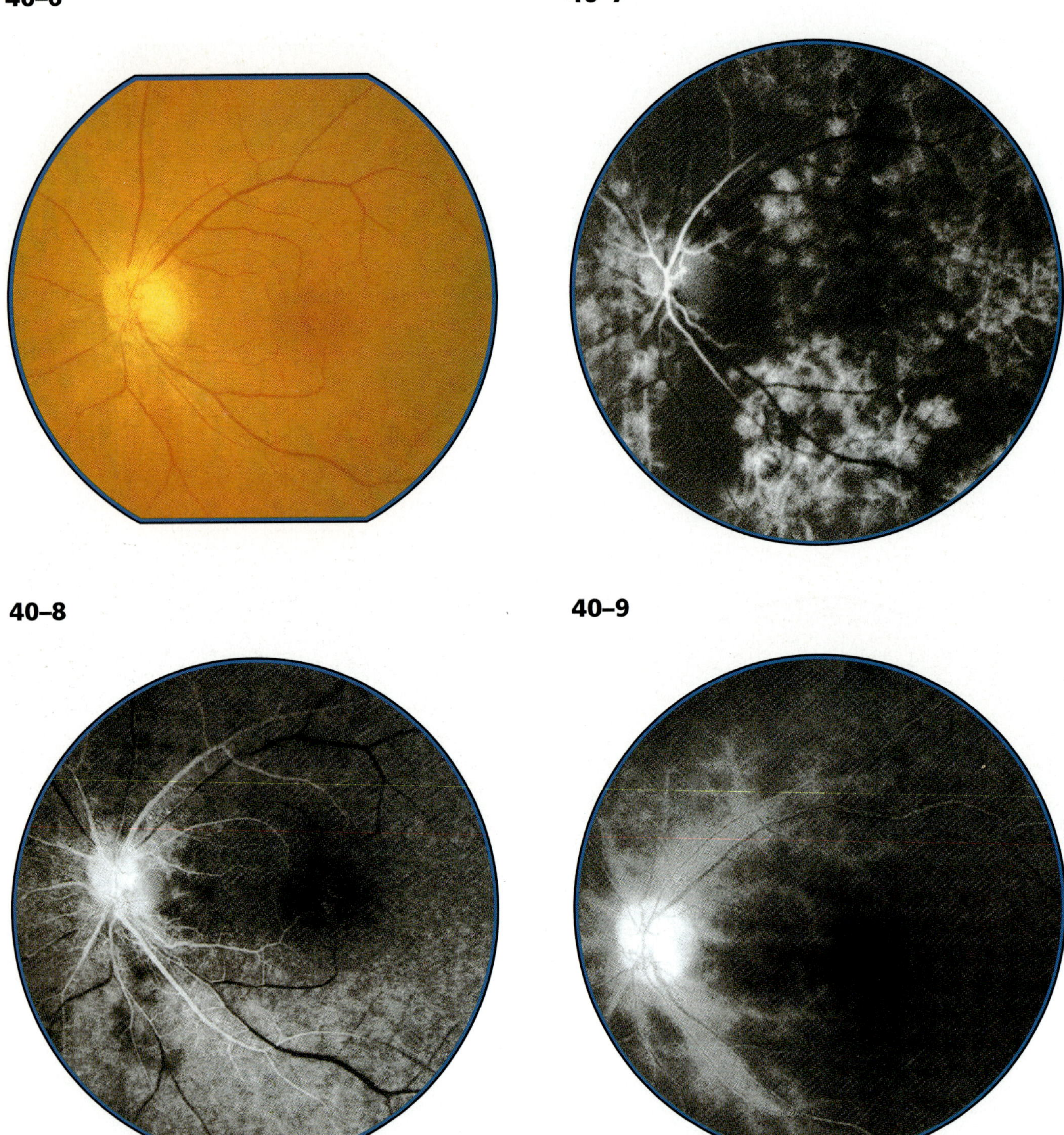

40–6 This 59-year-old male had severe carotid artery obstruction. He has generalized narrowed retinal arteries and optic disc pallor.

40–7 and 40–8 There is marked delay in his choroidal filling.

40–9 The late-stage angiogram reveals marked staining of the retinal vessels, especially the arteries. This finding is seen in over 80% of patients with the ocular ischemic syndrome. Neovascularization of the optic disc is also noted in this case.

40–6 *through* ***40–9,*** *Courtesy of Dr. Gary Brown.*

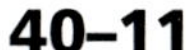

40–10

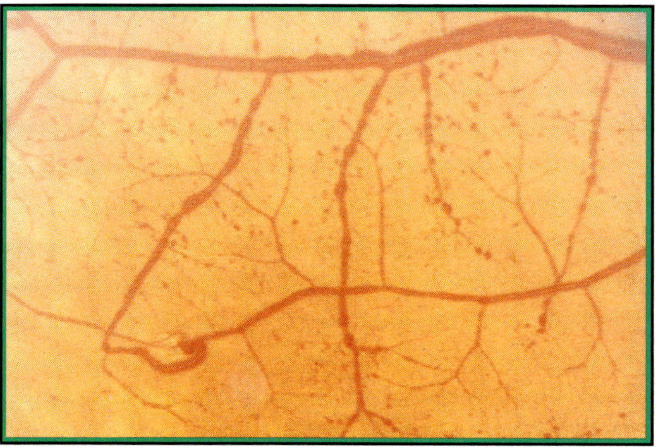

40–11

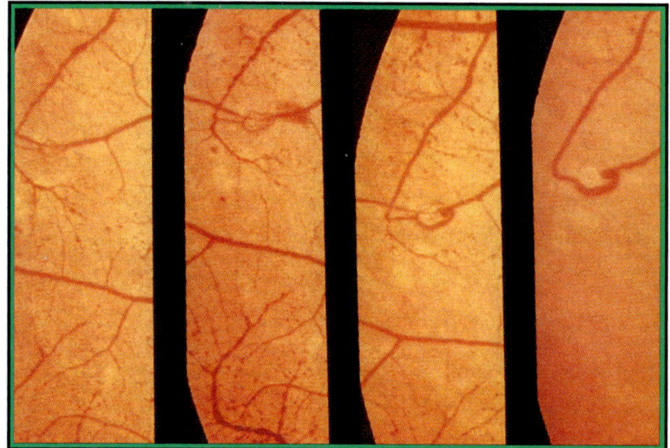

40–12

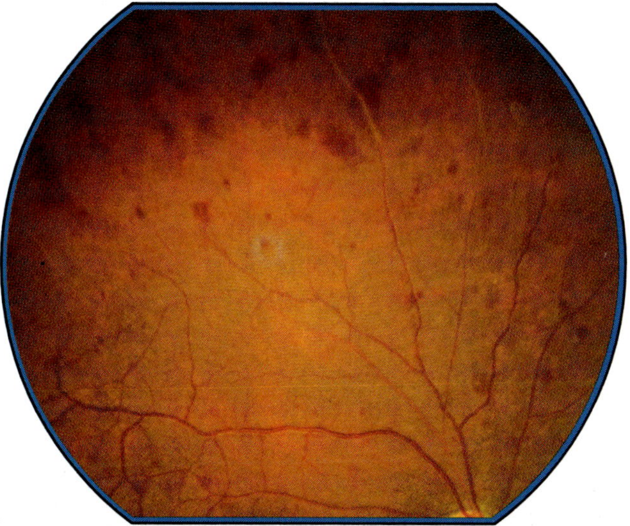

40–13

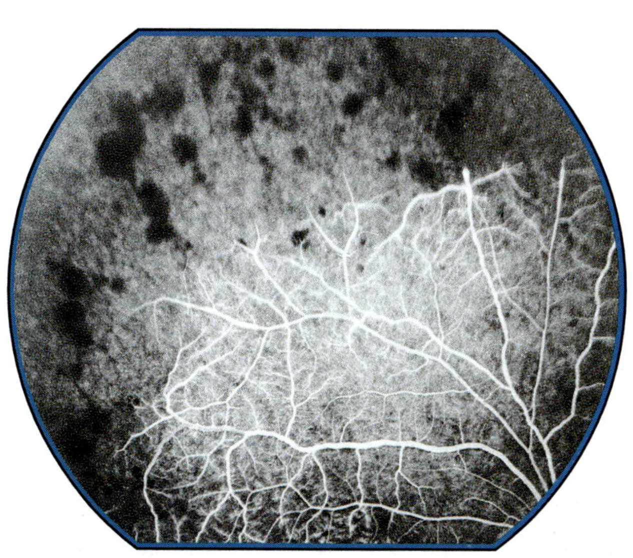

40–10 and 40–11 This patient has retinal vascular caliber irregularities including narrowing, dilation, and beading. Multiple aneurysmal changes, areas of capillary nonperfusion, and vascular shunting within and between the arterial and venular circulations are seen. A prominent arteriovenous shunt is demonstrated. Note the function of this shunt over time.

40–12 and 40–13 This patient has severe carotid artery disease. Note the multiple areas of hemorrhage and capillary nonperfusion. The presence of the hemorrhages in the ischemic area implies antecedent capillary perfusion. The extensive area of capillary nonperfusion is demonstrated on the flurorescein angiogram.

***40–10** and **40–11**, From Buethner, H and Bollins, JP: Retinal arteriovenous communications in carotid occlusive disease. In: Excerpta media: current aspects of ophthalmology, Amsterdam, 1992, Elsevier.*

Suggested Readings

Brown, GC: Anterior ischemic optic neuropathy occurring in association with carotid artery obstruction, J Clin Neurol Ophthalmol 6:39–42, 1986

Brown, GC: Macular edema in association with severe carotid artery obstructiuon, Am J Ophthalmol 102:442–448, 1986

Campo, RV, and Reeser, FH: Retinal telangiectasia secondary to bilateral carotid artery occlusion, Arch Ophthalmol 101:1211–1213, 1983

Eggleston, TF, Bohling, CA, Eggleston, HC, and Hershey, FB: Photocoagulation for ocular ischemia associated with carotid artery occlusion, Ann Ophthalmol 12:84–87, 1980

Hayreh, SS: So-called "central retinal vein occlusion." II. Venous stasis retinopathy, Ophthalmologica 172:14–37, 1976

Kearns, TP: Differential diagnosis of central retinal vein obstruction, Ophthalmology 90:475–480, 1983

Kearns, TP, Younge, BR, and Peipgras, DG: Resolution of venous stasis retinopathy after carotid artery bypass surgery, Mayo Clin Proc 55:342–346, 1980

Kobayashi, S, Hollenhorst, RW, and Sundt, TM, Jr: Retinal arterial pressure before and after surgery for carotid artery stenosis, Stroke 2:569–575, 1971

Madsen, PH: Venous-stasis retinopathy insufficiency of the ophthalmic artery, Acta Ophthalmol (Copenh) 44:940–947

Magargal, LE, Sanborn, GE, and Zimmerman, A: Venous stasis retinopathy associated with embolic obstruction of the central retinal artery, J Clin Neurol Ophthalmol 2:113–118, 1982

Sturrock, GD, and Mueller, HR: Chronic ocular ischaemia, Br J Ophthalmol 68:716–723, 1984

Young, LHY, and Appen, RE: Ischemic oculopathy: a manifestation of carotid artery disease, Arch Neurol 38:358–361, 1981

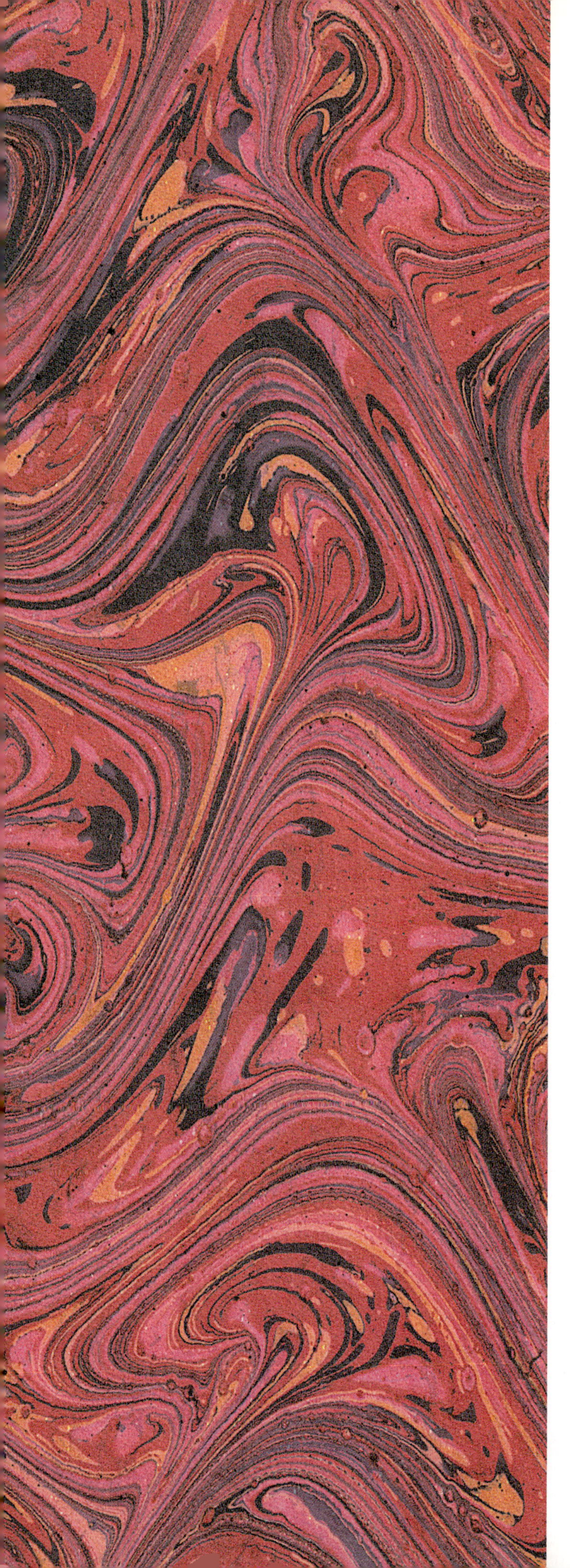

Part VIII

Inflammatory Diseases

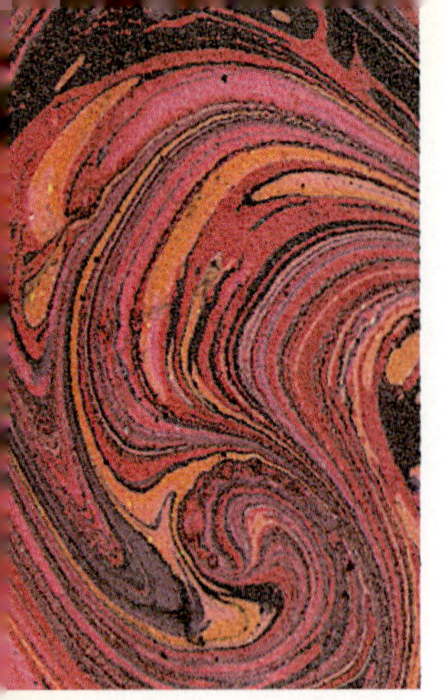

Chapter 41

Toxoplasmosis

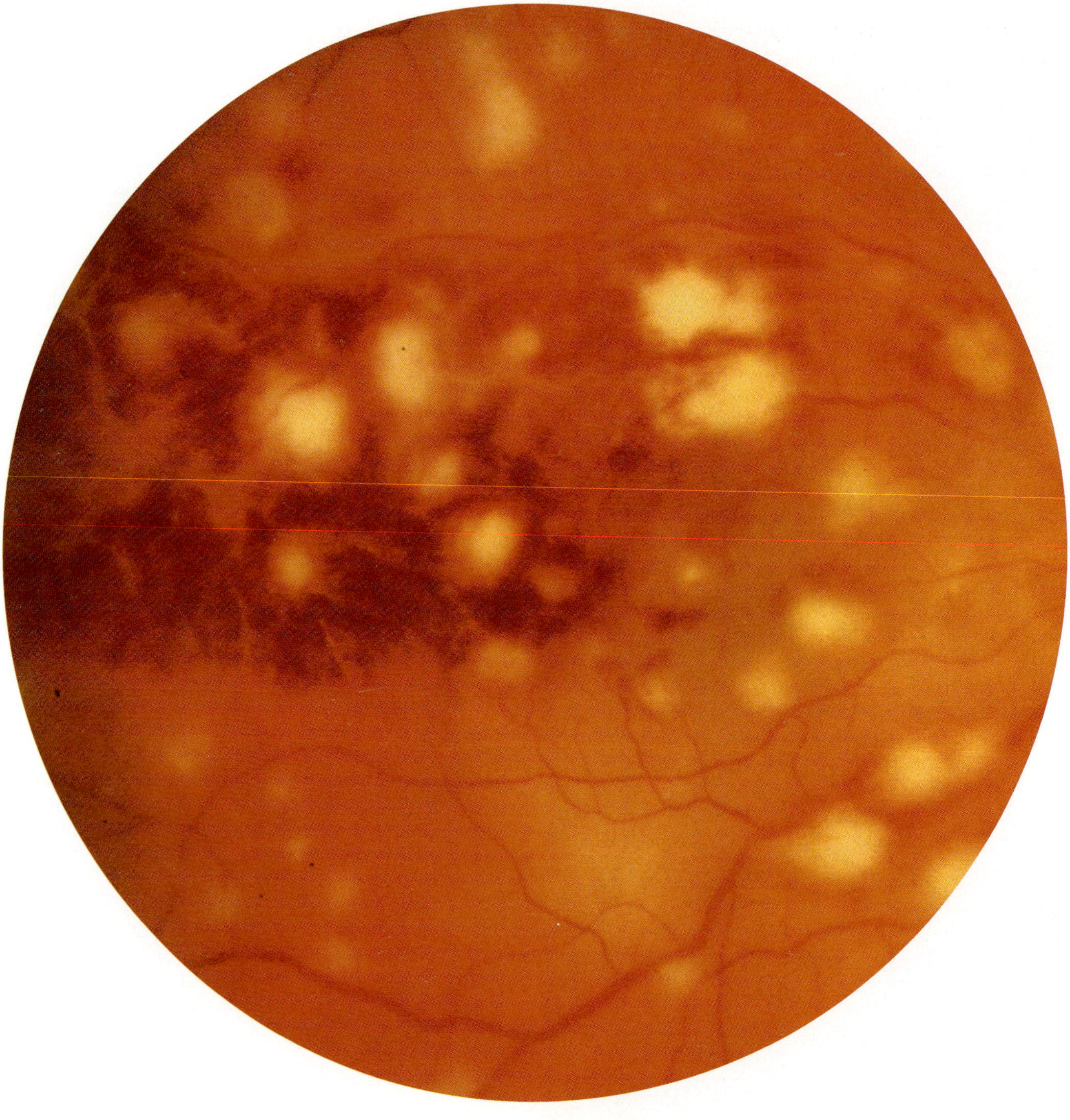

Toxoplasma gondii is an obligate intracellular parasite. A focal necrotizing retinitis is most commonly seen in ocular toxoplasmosis. Vitritis and anterior uveitis is often also noted. The inner retina is usually involved. A whitish fluffy-like lesion is seen with overlying edema. Although the retina is the primary site of infection, the choroid may also be involved. These active lesion are often noted adjacent to old chorioretinal scars. Other variants include a punctate outer or deep retinal lesion, as well as a large destructive-type lesion. The outer retinal lesions are characterized by multifocal gray-white punctate lesions at the level of the deep retina or retinal pigment epithelium. There is little or no vitritis. The large destructive lesion is common and severe.

Choroidal neovascularization may occur later in the disease. The treatment of ocular toxoplasmosis includes pyrimethamine, sulfadiazine, prednisone, clindamycin, and folinic acid.

41–1 41–1A

41–2 41–3

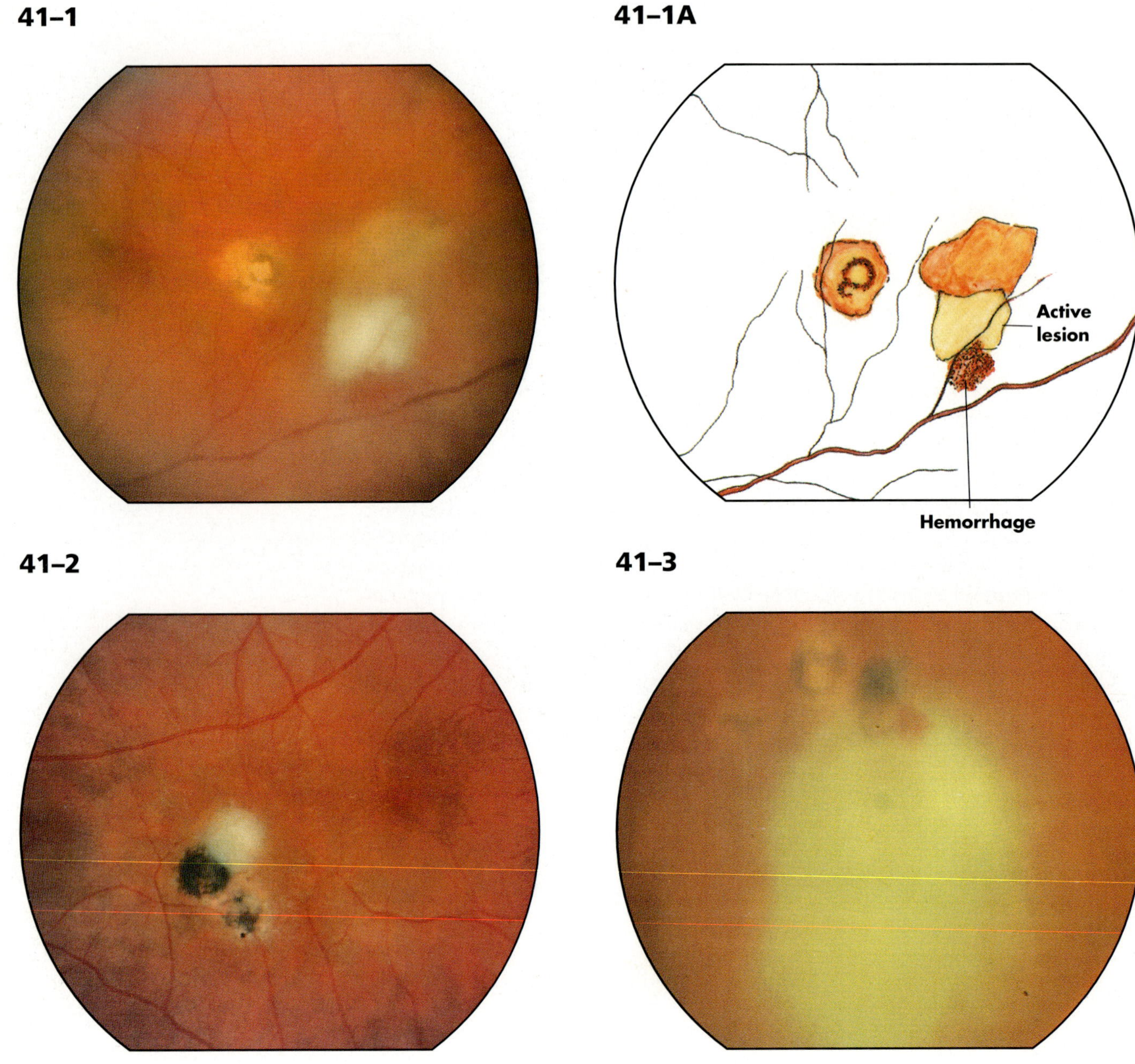

41–1 and 41–1A Active toxoplasmosis lesions have a fluffy whitish appearance. This patient has a fluffy white active toxoplasmosis lesion next to a chorioretinal scar from a previous *Toxoplasma* infection. There is also an overlying vitritis, hemorrhage, and some retinal vascular ischemic changes at the site of infection. Note the beaded arteriole secondary to an associated perivasculitis. This may lead to periarterial plaque deposition following resolution of the acute infection.

41–2 This patient has active chorioretinitis secondary to toxoplasmosis. Note the adjacent small inactive *Toxoplasma* scars.

41–3 This patient has a large destructive lesion that is also due to toxoplasmosis.

41–3, *Courtesy of Dr. Douglas A. Jabs. From Ryan, SJ: Retina, ed 2, St Louis, 1994, Mosby–Year Book.*

41–4

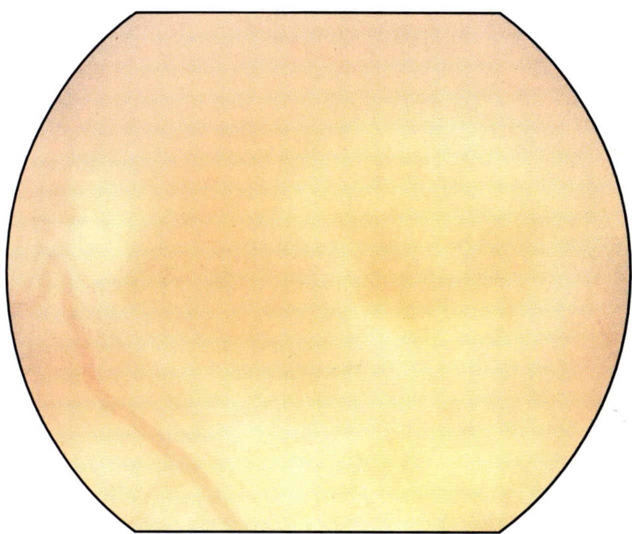

41–5

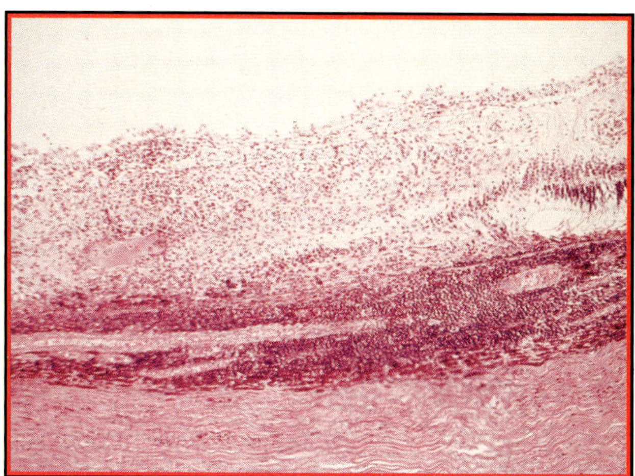

41–6

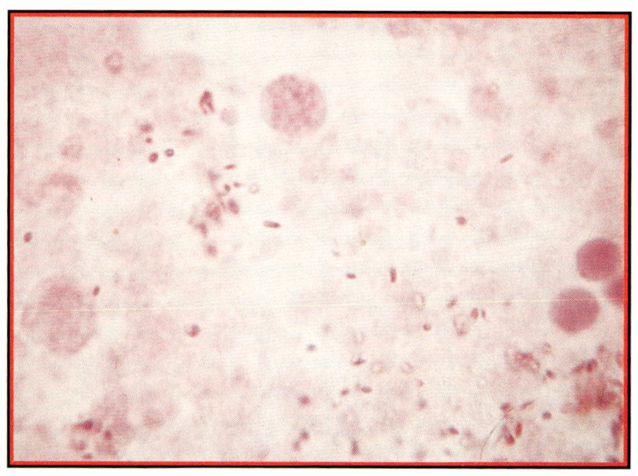

41–7

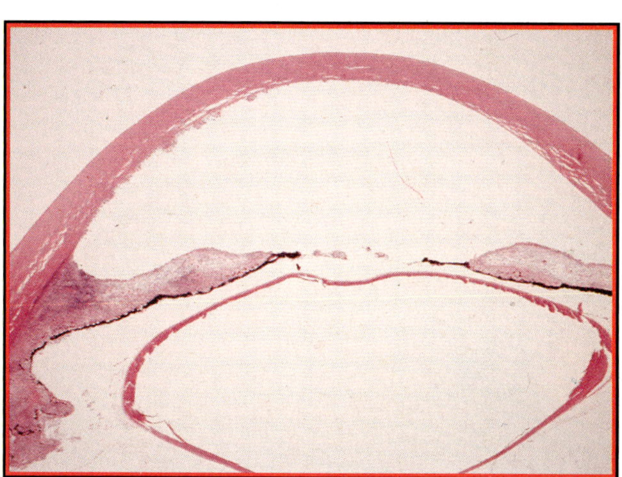

41–4 Occasionally toxoplasmosis will present with a completely obscured fundus on clinical examination secondary to massive cellular infiltration in the vitreous, a so-called "headlight in a fog." In this patient, acute retinitis in the posterior pole is associated with optic nerve as well as retinal vascular inflammation. This patient also has the acquired immune deficiency syndrome, and toxoplasmic choroiditis is commonly seen today in these patients (see Chapter 45).

41–5 through 41–7 Histopathologic correlate illustrates acute retinal necrosis with intense inflammatory cell infiltration in the subjacent choroid. Toxoplasmic cysts are present in necrotic retina. A secondary inflammatory reaction in the anterior segment with iridocyclitis, inflammatory cells in the inferior angle, an inflammatory pupillary membrane, and keratic precipitates are noted.

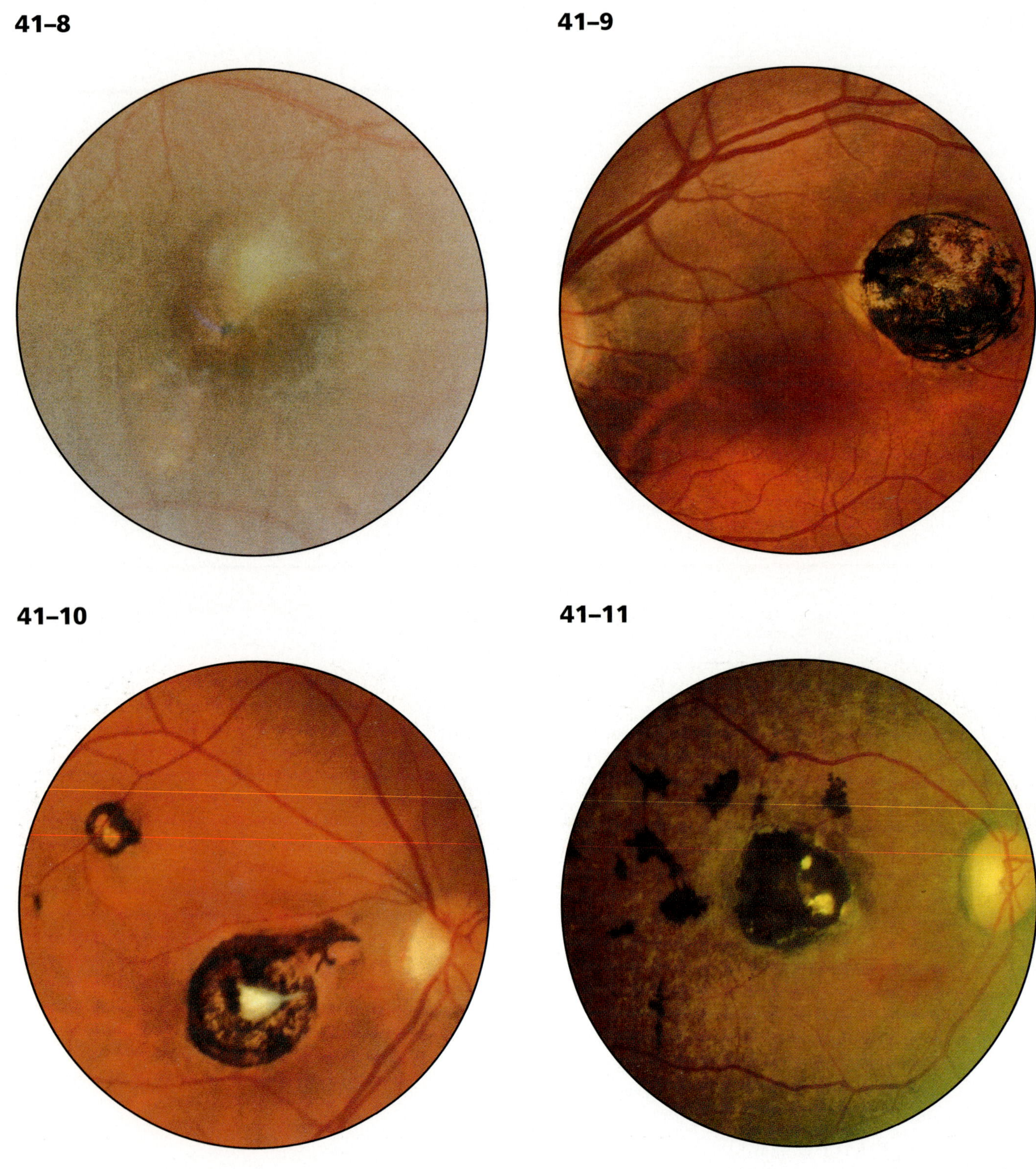

41–8 This patient has an outer retinitis in the macular region secondary to toxoplasmosis.

41–9 through 41–11 Toxoplasmosis scars may be multiple and/or associated with fibrous metaplasia, retinal vascular changes, and temporal pallor of the optic nerve.

41–12

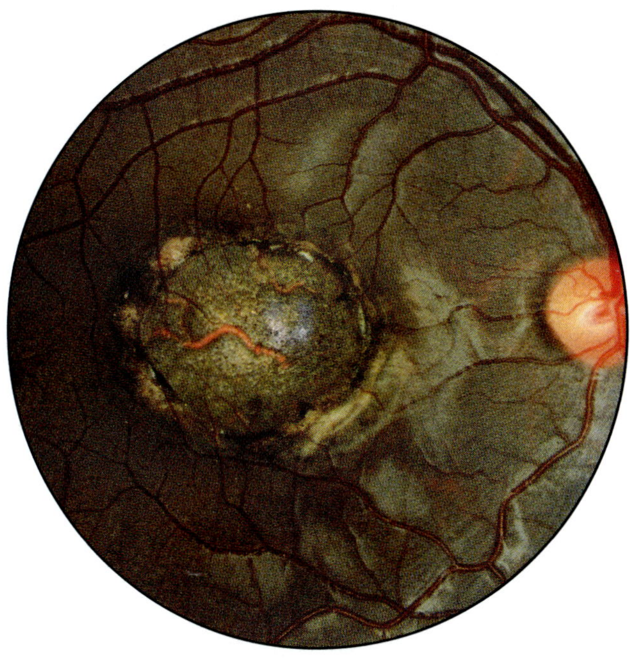

41–13

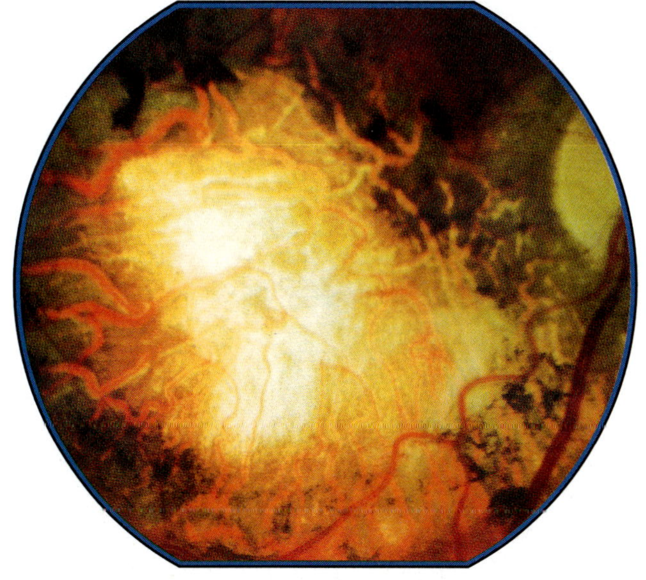

41–14

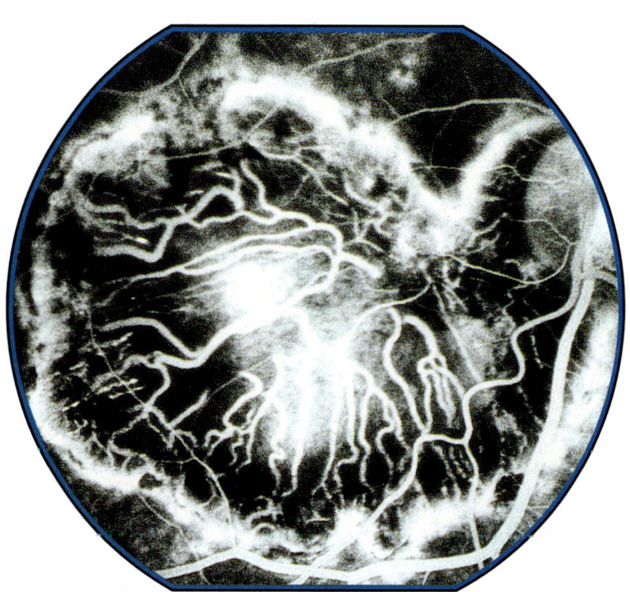

41–12 Toxoplasmosis scars show varying degrees of hyperpigmentation and atrophy.

41–13 and 41–14 Congenital toxoplasmosis may also occur at the macula.

41–12, *Courtesy of Alan Campbell, CRA.*

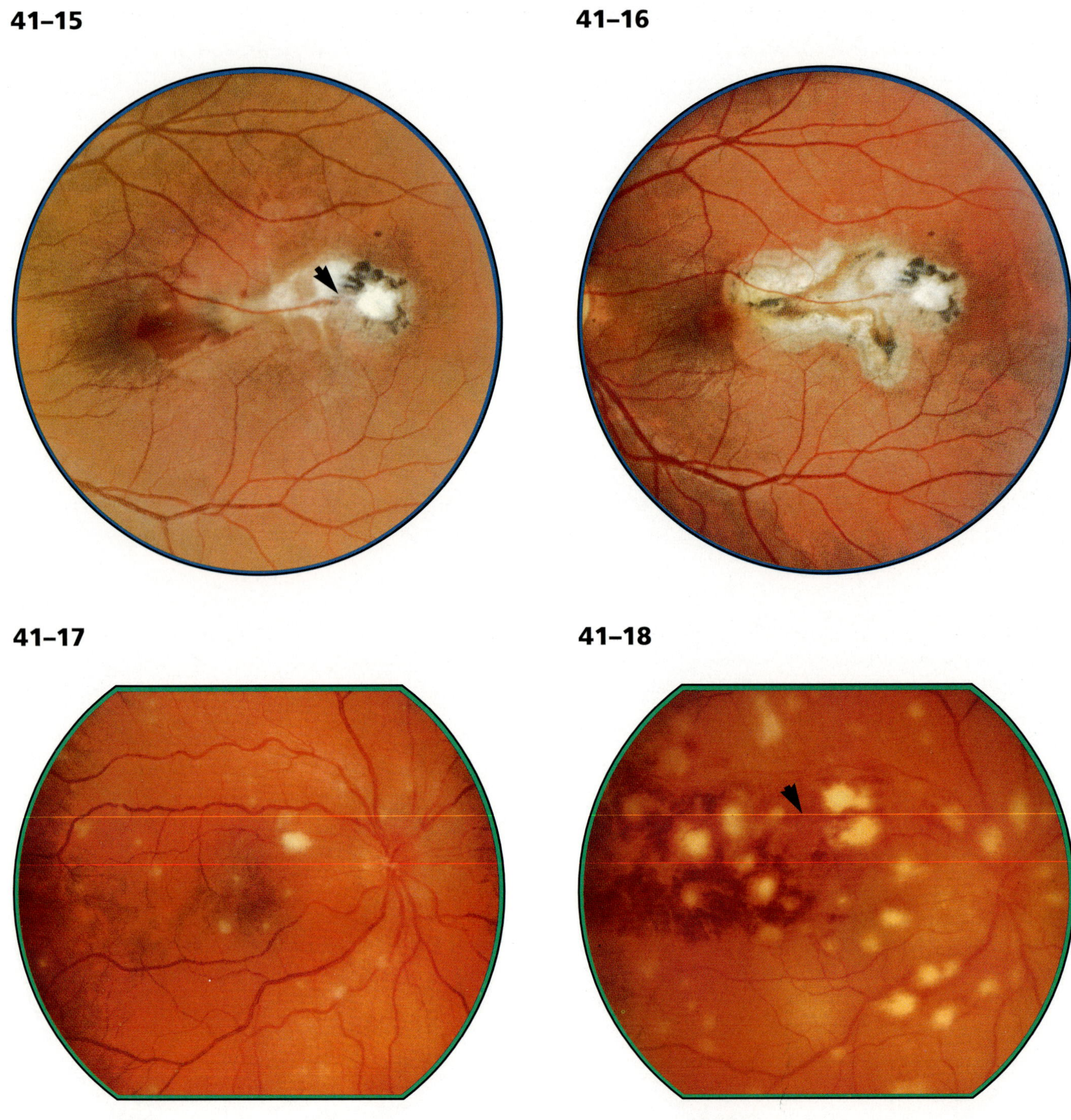

41–15 and 41–16 This patient has subretinal hemorrhage secondary to choroidal neovascularization from toxoplasmosis. The new vessels proliferated from the foveal margin of the old scar. Note the retinal choroidal anastomosis *(arrowhead)* and the ischemia temporal to the scar. After laser treatment, a scar is noted.

41–17 and 41–18 This patient had miliary toxoplasmosis. Note the multiple whitish-yellow spots. Hemorrhage was noted 5 weeks later from venous occlusive disease. Note the obstructed vessel *(arrowhead)*.

41–17 *and* ***41–18,*** *Courtesy of Dr. William Freeman.*

Suggested Readings

Akstein, RB, Wilson, LA, and Teutsch, SM: Acquired toxoplasmosis, Ophthalmology 89:1299–1301, 1982

Beverley, JKA: A rational approach to the treatment of toxoplasmic uveitis, Trans Ophthal Soc UK 78:109–116, 1958

Braunstein, RA, and Gass, JDM: Branch artery obstruction caused by acute toxoplasmosis, Arch Ophthalmol 98:512–513, 1980

Cohen, SN: Toxoplasmosis in patients receiving immunosuppressive therapy, JAMA 211:657–660, 1970

Culbertson, WW, Tabbara, KF, and O'Connor, GR: Experimental ocular toxoplasmosis in primates, Arch Ophthalmol 100:321–323, 1982

Doft, BH, and Gass, JDM: Punctate outer retinal toxoplasmosis, Arch Ophthalmol 103:1332–1336, 1985

Fine, SL, Owens, SL, Haller, JA, Knox, DL, and Patz, A: Choroidal neovascularization as a late complication of ocular toxoplasmosis, Am J Ophthalmol 91:318–322, 1981

Folk, JC, and Lobes, LA: Presumed toxoplasmic papillitis, Ophthalmology 91:64–67, 1984

Friedmann, CT, and Knox, DL: Variations in recurrent active toxoplasmic retinochoroiditis, Arch Ophthalmol 81:481–493, 1969

Nozik, RA, and O'Connor, GR: Studies on experimental ocular toxoplasmosis in the rabbit. II. Attempts to stimulate recurrences by local trauma, epinephrine, and corticosteroids, Arch Ophthalmol 84:788–791, 1970

Schwartz, PL: Segmental retinal periarteritis as a complication of toxoplasmosis, Ann Ophthalmol 9:157–162, 1977

Tabbara, KF, and O'Connor, GR: Treatment of ocular toxoplasmosis with clindamycin and sulfadiazine, Ophthalmology 87:129–134, 1980

Weiss, A, Margo, CE, Ledford, DK, Lockey, RF, and Brinser, JH: Toxoplasmic retinochoroiditis as an initial manifestation of the acquired immune deficiency syndrome, Am J Ophthalmol 101:248–249, 1986

Wilder, HC: *Toxoplasma* chorioretinitis in adults, Arch Opthalmol 48:127–136, 1952

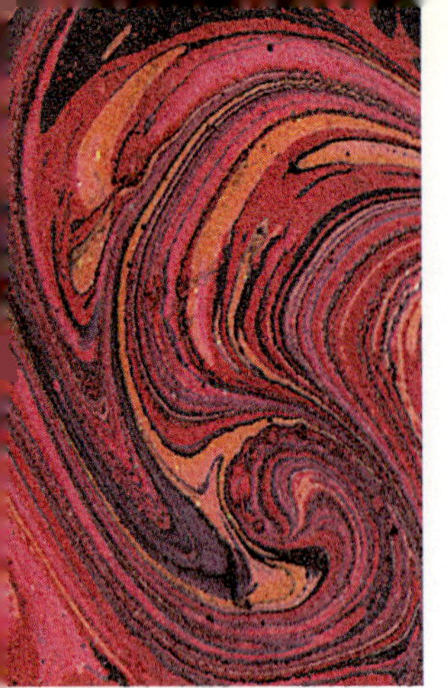

Chapter 42

Ocular Toxocariasis

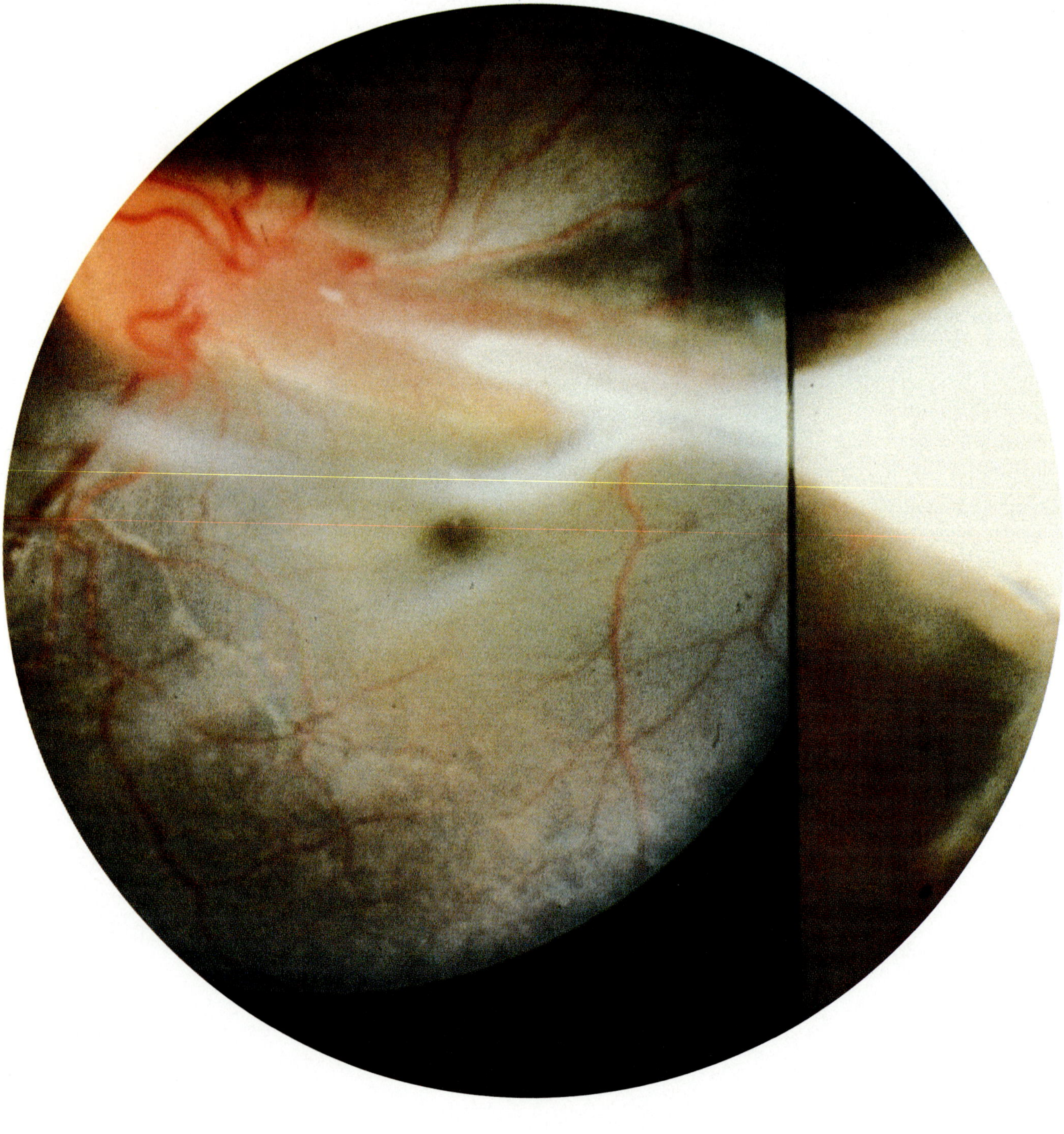

Ocular toxocariasis is caused by a roundworm and affects young children. Toxocariasis may present as a chronic endophthalmitis, posterior pole granuloma, or peripheral granulomatous type inflammatory mass.

42–1

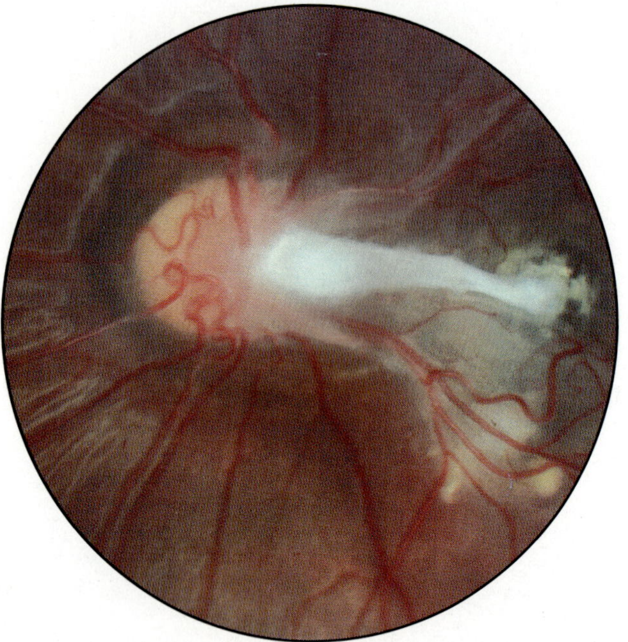

42–2

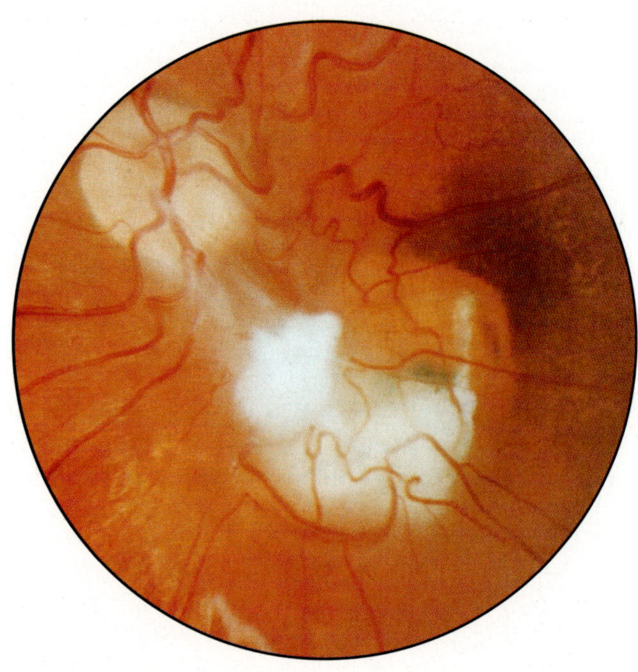

42–3

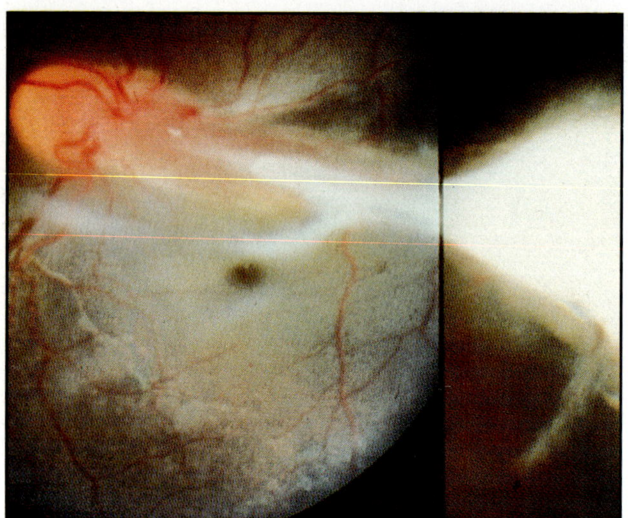

42–1 This young boy developed an inflammatory reaction secondary to presumed toxocariasis. Note the fibrous band emanating from the optic disc.

42–2 and 42–3 In these two clinical cases, whitish-yellow fibrous scar tissue can be noted connected to the optic disc.

42–3, *Courtesy of Dr. Jerry Shields.*

42–4

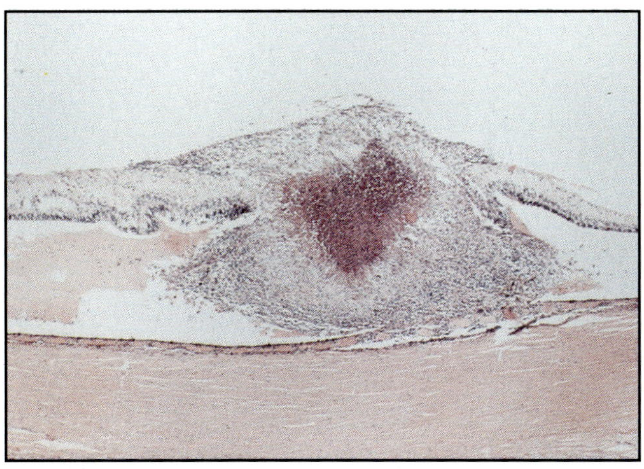

42–5 **42–5A**

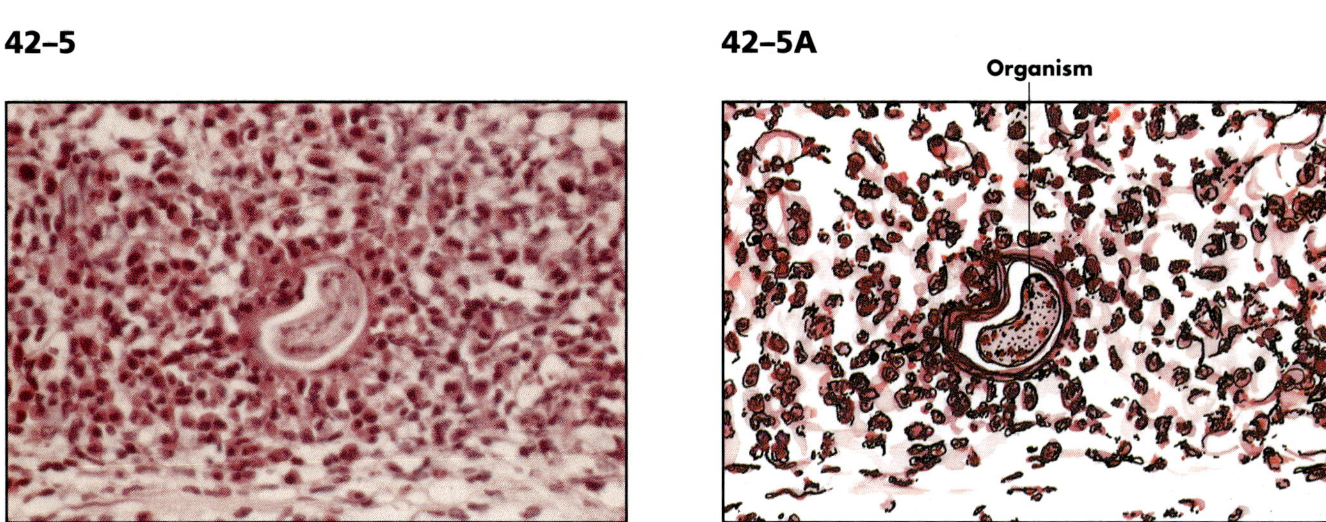

42–4, 42–5, and 42–5A Histopathologic examination of such cases at an earlier stage reveals an eosinophilic abscess (42–4) in which the second-stage larva of the organism may be present (42–5).

42–6

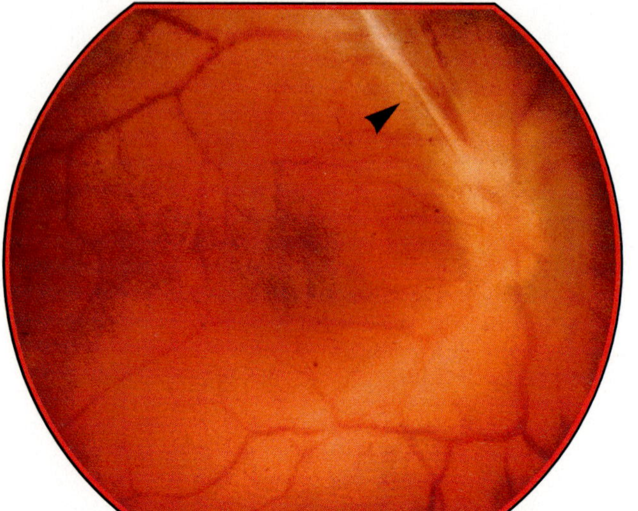

42–7

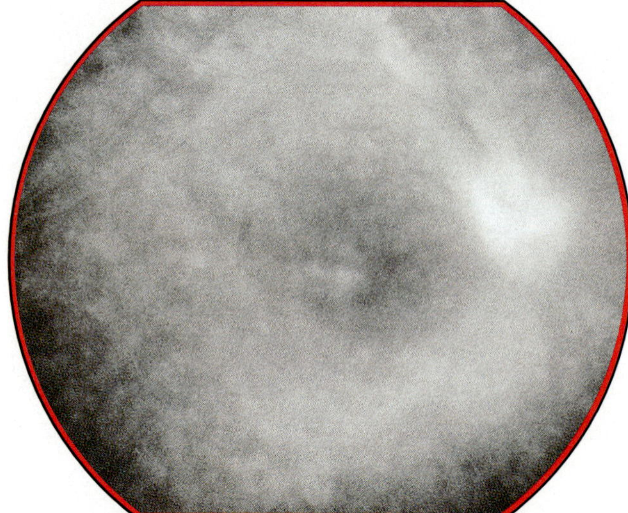

42–8

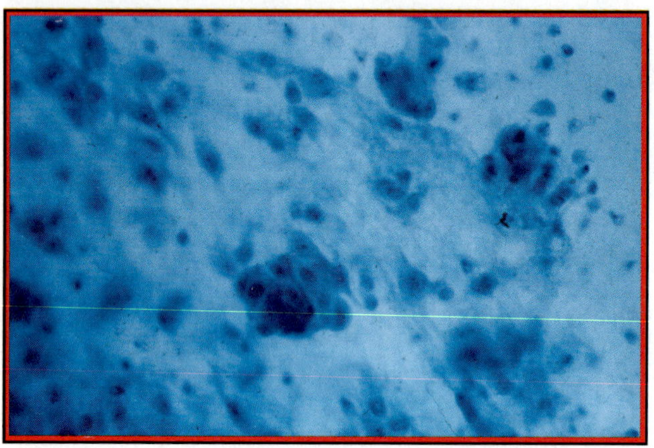

42–9

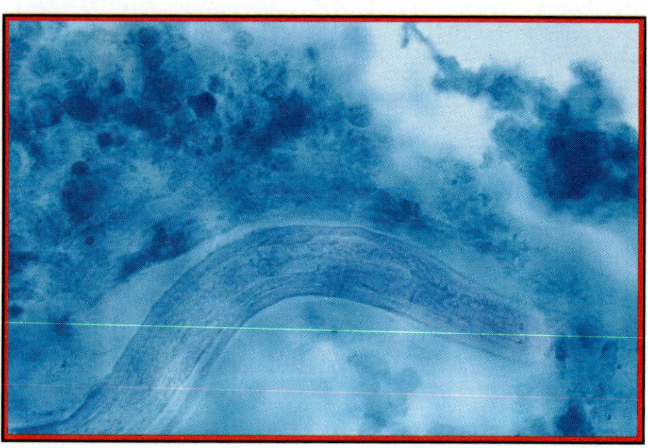

42–10

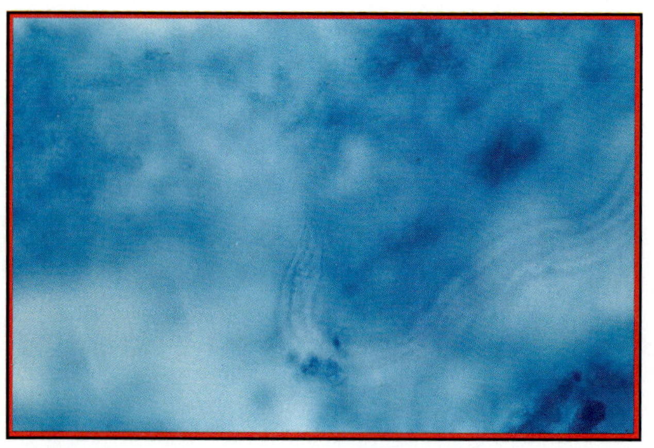

42–6 This clinicopathologic correlation describes a case in which a vitrectomy for vitreopapillary traction revealed an intact *Toxocara canis* organism. A vitreopapillary traction band from an equatorial toxocaral granuloma located in the 11-o'clock meridian is demonstrated *(arrowhead)*.

42–7 Fluorescein angiography reveals mild macular edema and late optic disc leakage.

42–8 Inflammatory infiltrate with neutrophilis, epithelioid cells, and multinucleated giant cells are present.

42–9 and 42–10 Note the rounded cephalic end (42–9) and the tapered caudal end of the parasite (42–10).

42–6 *through* ***42–10,*** *From Maguire, AM, Green, WR, Michels, RG, and Erozan, YS: Recovery of intraocular* Toxocara canis *by pars plana vitrectomy, Ophthalmology 97:675–680, 1990.*

Suggested Readings

Bass, JL, Mehta, KA, Glickman, LT, and Eppes, BM: Clinically inapparent *Toxocara* infection in children, N Engl J Med 308:723–724, 1983

Glickman, LT, and Schantz, PM: Epidemiology and pathogenesis of zoonotic toxocariasis, Epidemiol Rev 3:230–250, 1981

Maguire, AM, Green, WR, Michels, RG, and Erozan, YS: Recovery of intraocular *Toxocara canis* by pars plana vitrectomy, Ophthalmology 97:675–680, 1990

Schantz, PM, Weis, PE, Pollard, ZF, and White, MC: Risk factors for toxocaral ocular larva migrans: a case-control study, Am J Public Health 70:1269–1272, 1980

Shields, JA: Ocular toxocariasis: a review, Surv Ophthalmol 28:361–381, 1984

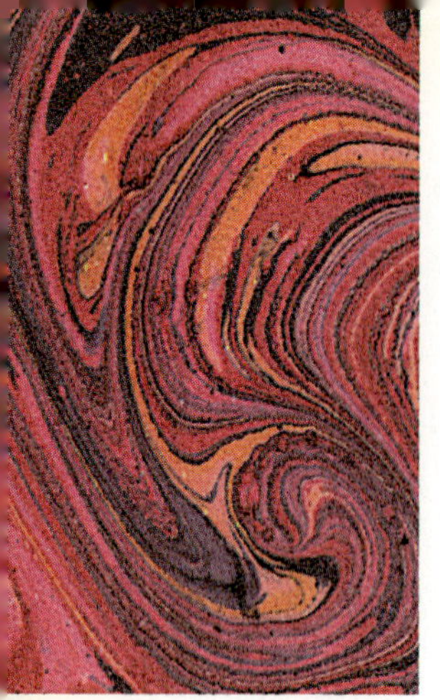

Chapter 43
Ocular Cysticercosis

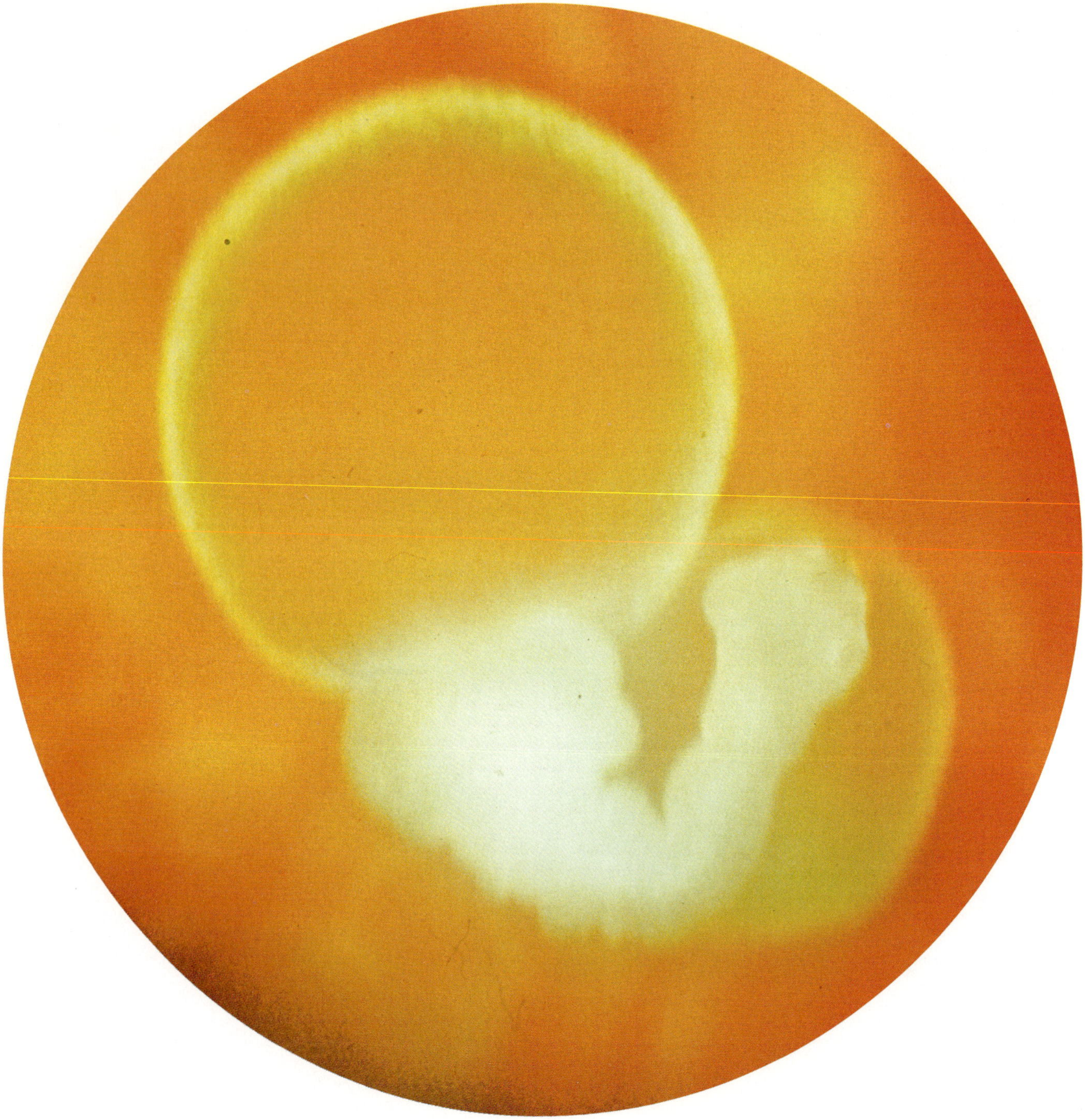

Cysticercus cellulosae is the larval form of the pork tapeworm *Taenia solium.* The organism may be noted intravitreally with a cyst and scolex. The scolex contains suckers and hooks. The organism may also be present in the subretinal space. The prognosis in untreated cases is very poor. Surgical excision is sometimes an effective treatment.

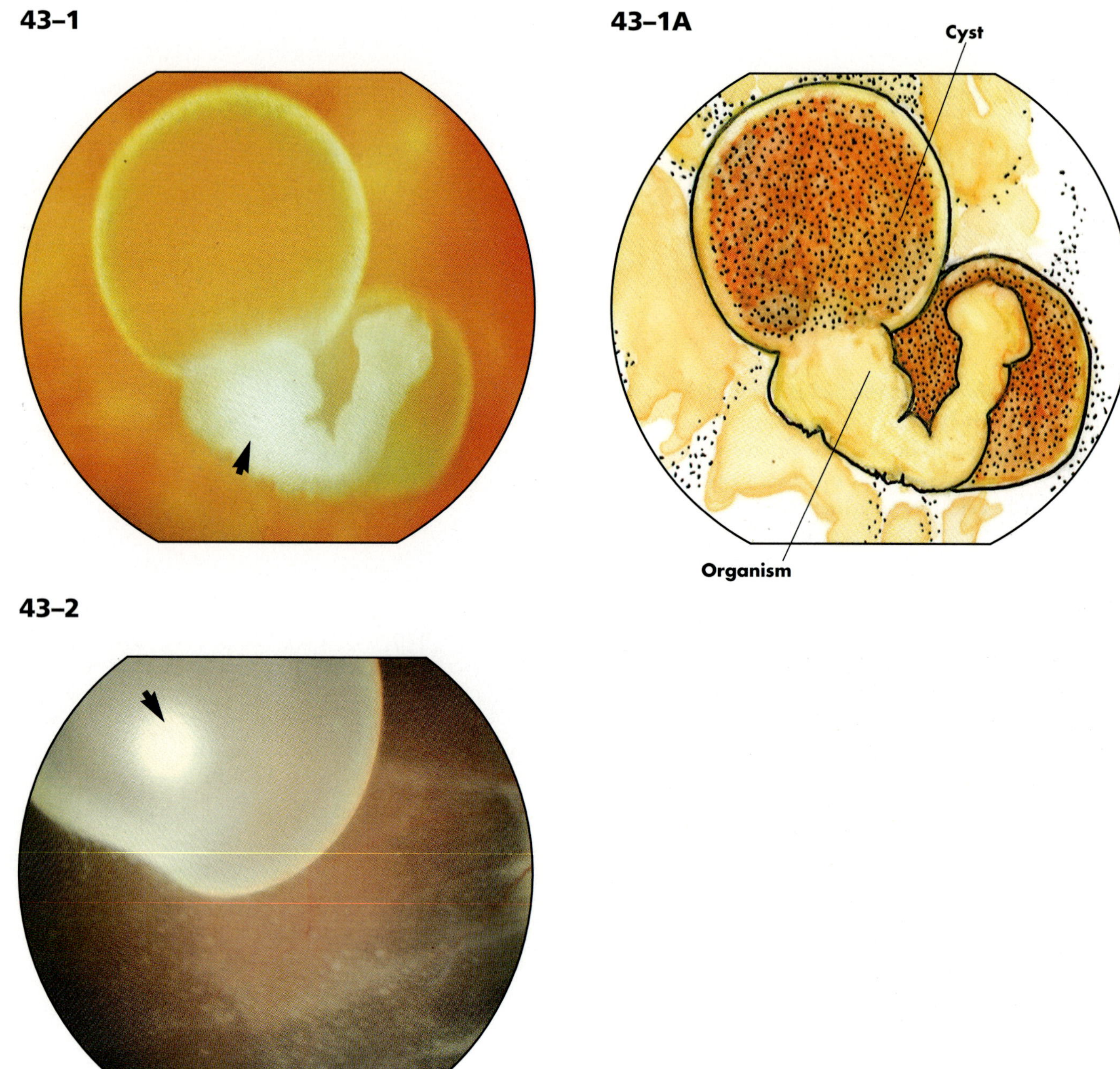

43–1, 43–1A, and 43–2 Ocular cysticercosis can be seen extending into the vitreous cavity. Note the organism *(arrowhead)* and cyst.

43–1, *Courtesy of Drs. Keith Zinn, Allen Friedman, and Katherine Burke. Reprinted from Friedman, AH, Pokorny, KS, Suhan, J, Ritch, R, and Zinn, KM: Electron microscopic observations of intravitreal* Cysticercus cellulosae (Taenia solium), *Ophthalmologica 180:267–273, 1980.* ***43–2,*** *Courtesy of Dr. Miriam Cano. Reprinted from Ryan, SJ: Retina, ed 2, St Louis, 1994, Mosby–Year Book.*

43–3

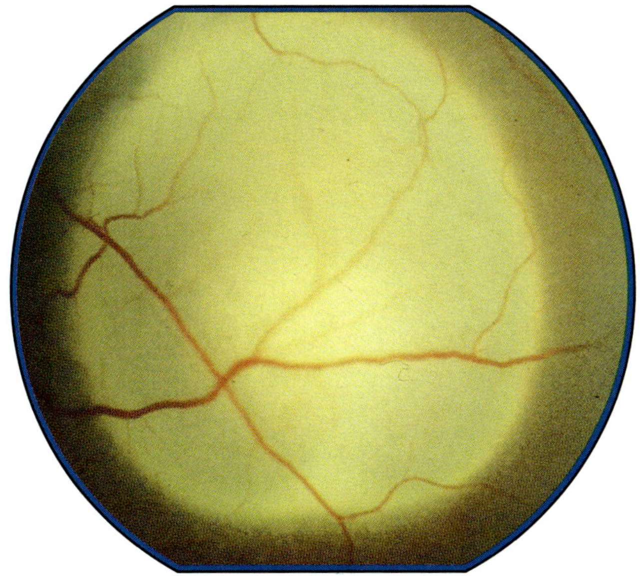

43–4

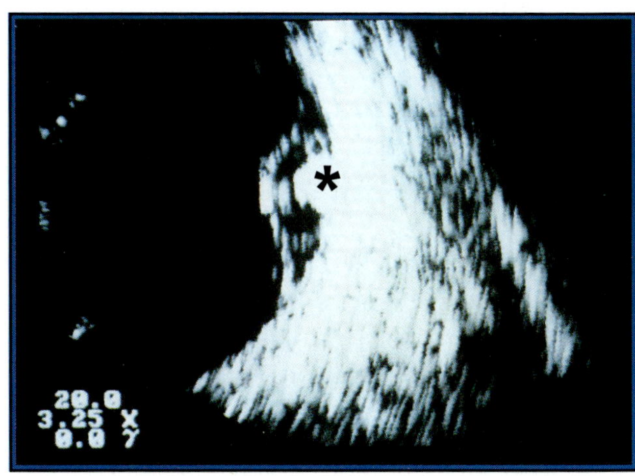

43–5

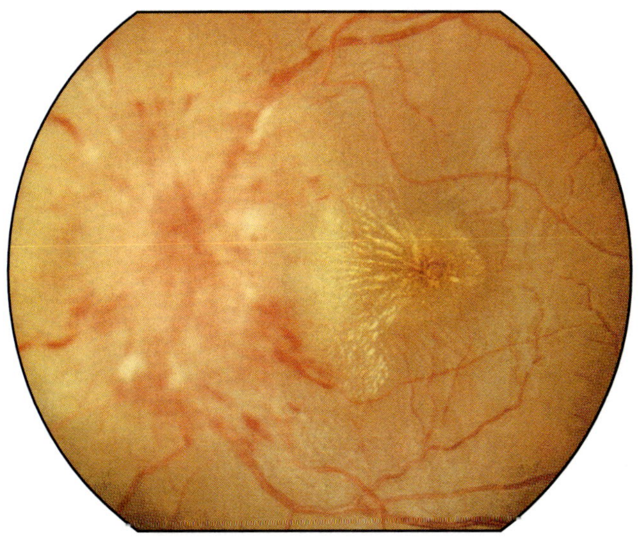

43–3 Ocular cysticercosis can be demonstrated in the subretinal space. A cystic structure can be noted with an invaginated scolex *(whitish area)*.

43–4 Ultrasonography also reveals a cystic structure with a scolex *(asterisk)*.

43–5 This 29-year-old female has massive optic disc swelling with a macular star secondary to neural cysticercosis.

***43–3** and **43–4,** Photographs courtesy of Dr. Yossi Sidikaro. **43–5,** Courtesy of Rachelle Benner.*

43–6

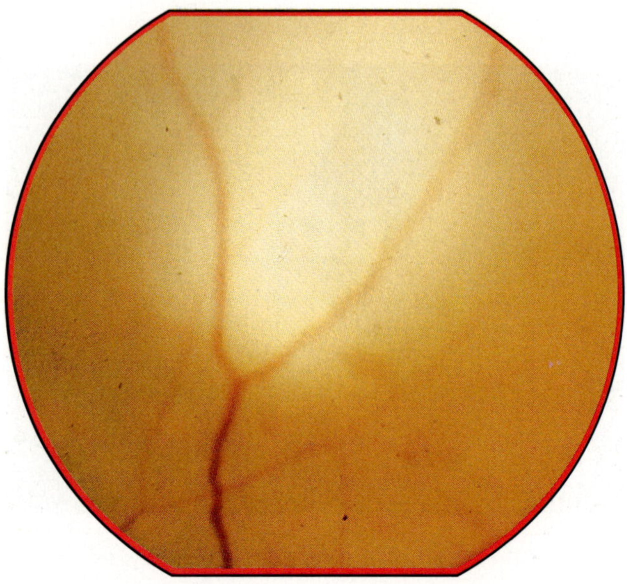

43-7

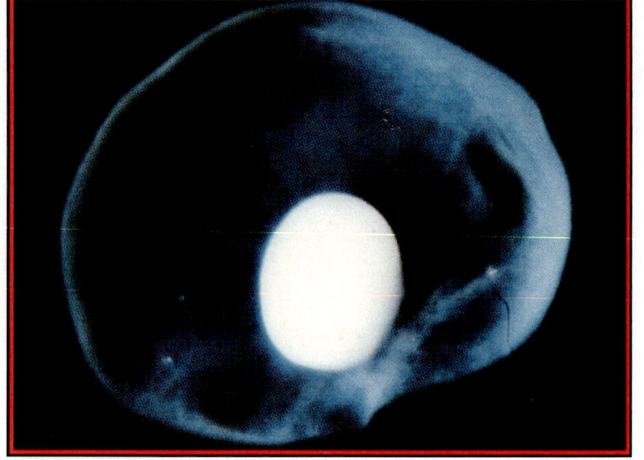

43–8

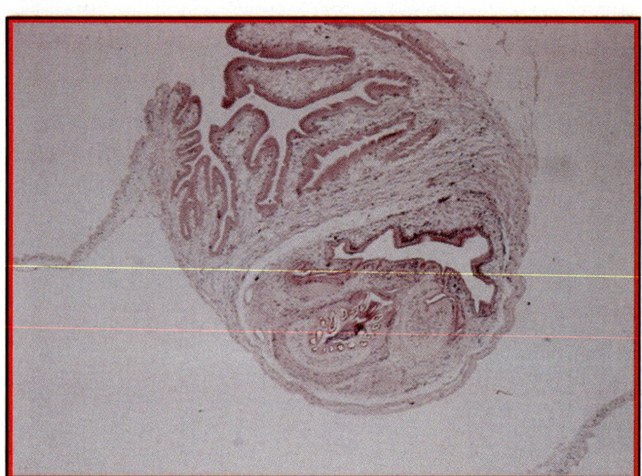

43–6 through 43–8 This patient had subretinal cysticercosis (43–6), which was successfully removed surgically (43–7) by Dr. Victor Curtin. Light microscopy reveals the intact cyst with an opening, as well as the integument and the scolex (43–8).

43–6 *through* ***43–8,*** *From Spencer, W: Ophthalmic pathology: an atlas and textbook, vol 2, ed 3, Philadelphia, 1993, WB Saunders, p 774. Case presented at the Verhoff Society, Washington, DC, April 1970. Courtesy of Dr. Victor Curtin.*

43–9

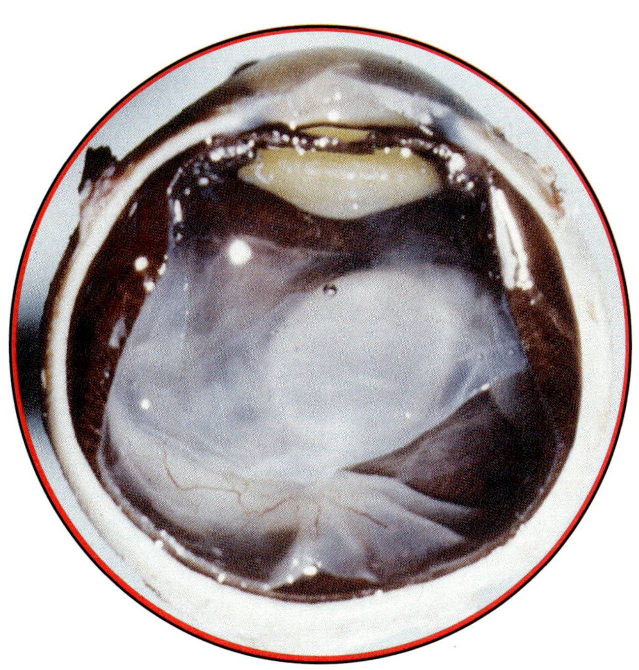

43–10

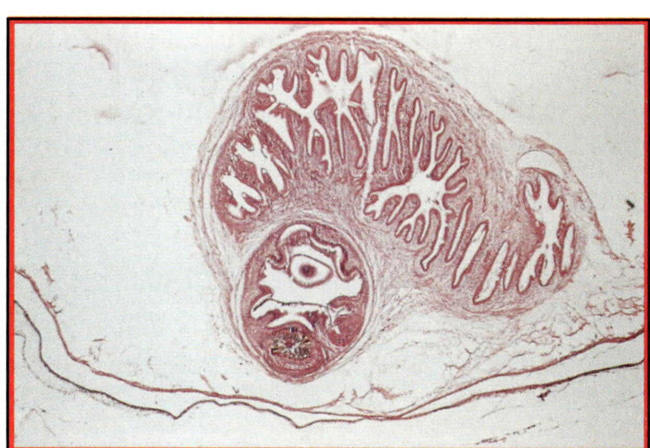

43–9 Gross appearance of *Cysticercus* in the vitreous of a 42-year-old male.

43–10 Histopathologic sectioning of the organism shows the cyst wall, scolex, body, and approximately 22 hooklets.

43–9 *and* ***43–10,*** *From Spencer, W: Ophthalmic pathology: an atlas and textbook, vol 2, ed 3, Philadelphia, 1993, WB Saunders, p 774.*

Suggested Readings

Aracena, T, and Perez-Roca, F: Macular and peripheral subretinal cysticercosis, Ann Ophthalmol 13:1265–1267, 1981

Balakrishnan, E: Bilateral intra-ocular cysticerci, Br J Ophthalmol 45:150–151, 1961

Danis, P: Intraocular cysticercus, Arch Ophthalmol 91:238–239, 1974

Hutton, WL, Vaiser, A, and Snyder, WB: Pars plana vitrectomy for removal of intravitreal cysticercus, Am J Ophthalmol 81:571–573, 1976

Kruger-Leite, E, Jalkh, AE, Quiroz, H, and Schepens, CL: Intraocular cysticercosis, Am J Ophthalmol 99:252–257, 1985

Sotelo, J, Escobedo, F, Rodriguez-Carbajal, J, Torres, B, and Rubio-Donnadieu, F: Therapy of parenchymal brain cysticercosis with praziquantel, N Engl J Med 310:1001–1007, 1984

Zinn, KM, Guillory, SL, and Friedman, AH: Removal of intravitreous cysticerci from the surface of the optic nervehead: a pars plana approach, Arch Ophthalmol 98:714–716, 1980

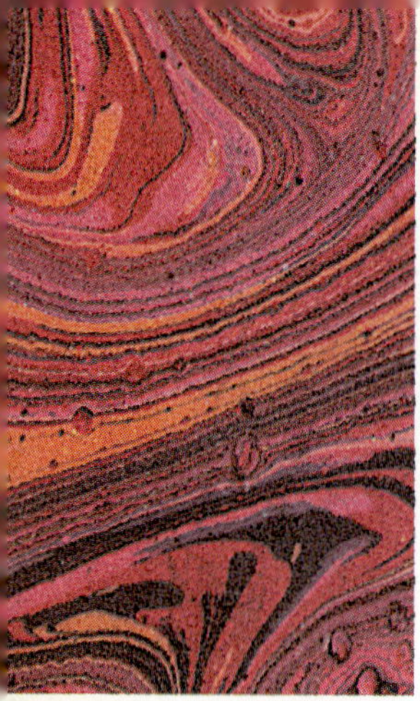

Chapter 44

Cytomegalovirus Infections of the Retina

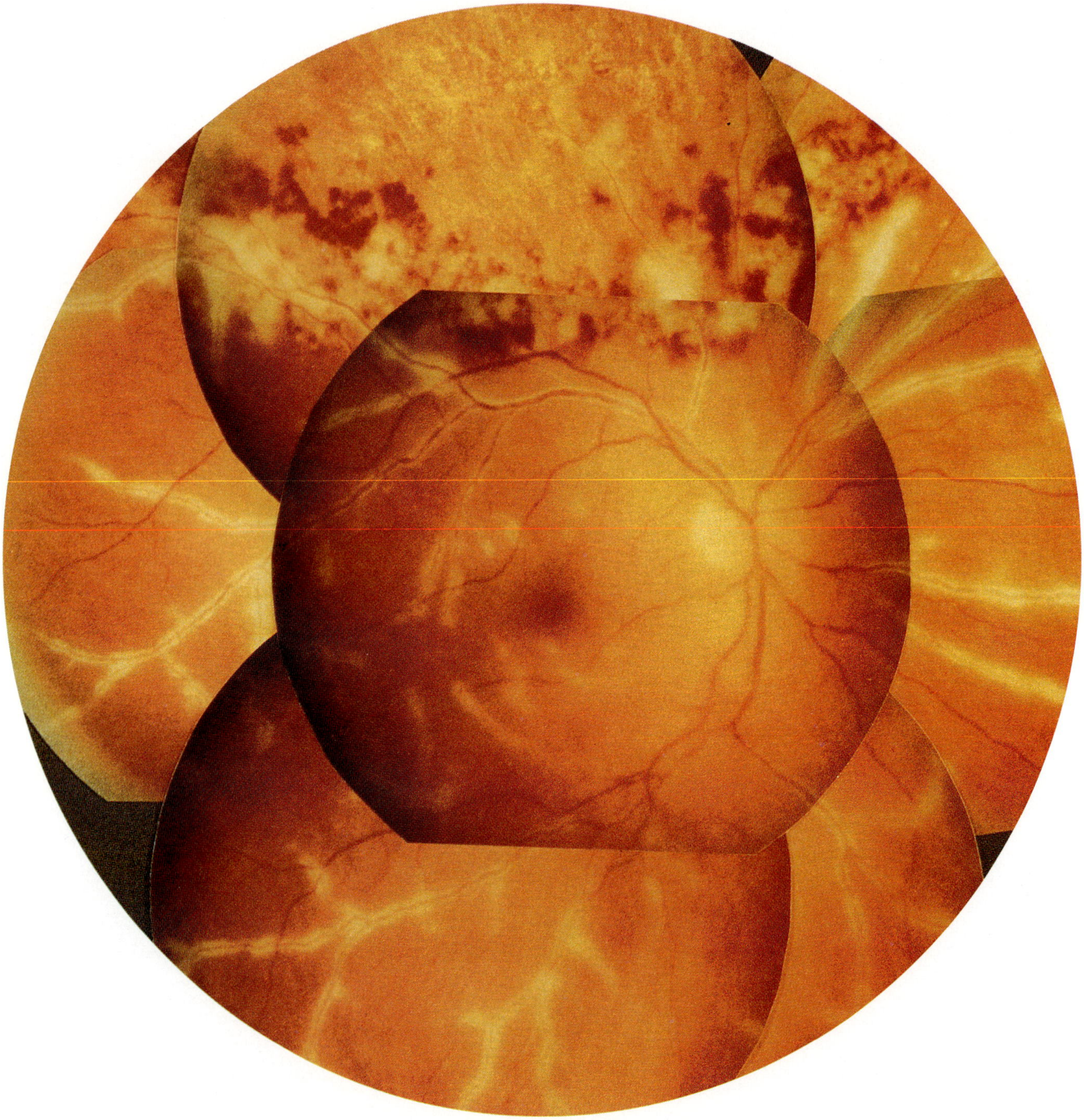

Cytomegalovirus (CMV) retinitis is common in immunocompromised patients, such as those with the acquired immune deficiency syndrome (AIDS). It is the most common infectious disease associated with AIDS. The infection first appears in a perivascular distribution and is whitish. A hemorrhagic retinal necrosis then occurs.

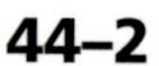

44–1

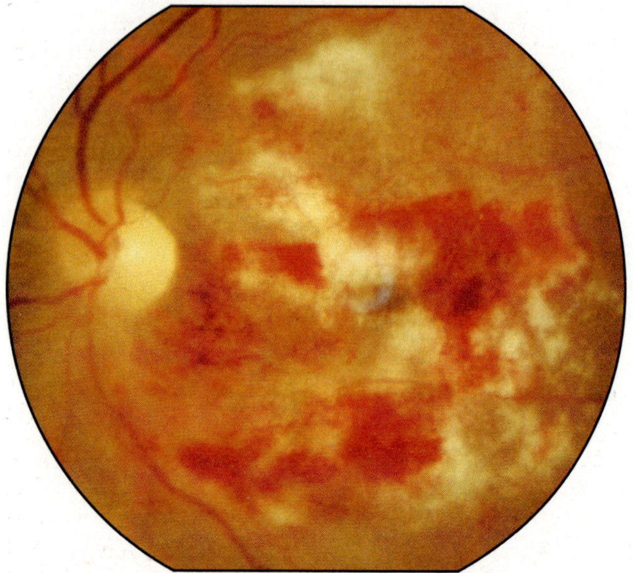

44–2

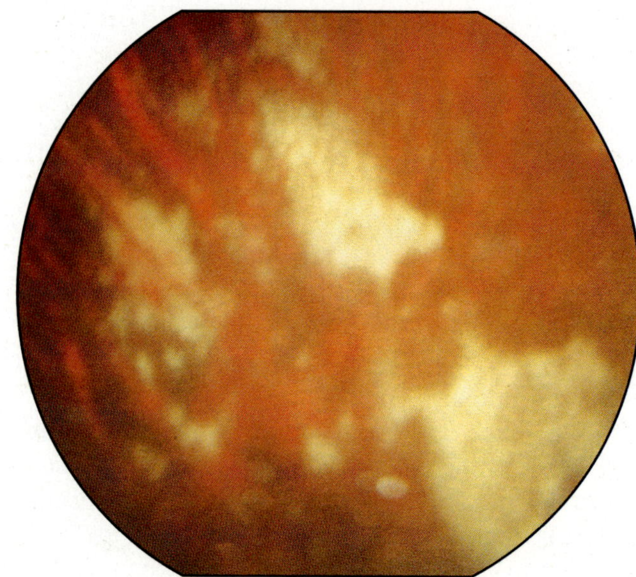

44–3

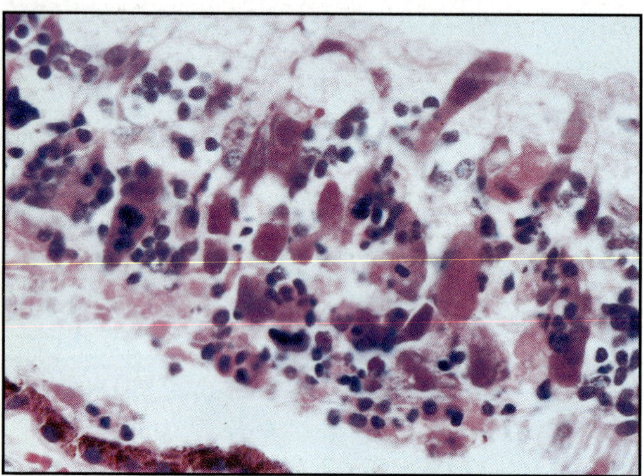

44–1 This case shows the classic hemorrhagic retinitis from CMV.

44–2 Regression of the retinitis can be demonstrated after treatment.

44–3 Light microscopy of a case of acute necrotizing retinitis due to cytomegalovirus. Large cells (neurons) containing eosinophilic intranuclear or intracytoplasmic inclusions can be noted.

44–4 through 44–6 These patients have frosted branch angiitis secondary to CMV retinitis. Note the frosted branch appearance of the vessels. Active and inactive areas of CMV retinitis are noted in these patients.

44–4

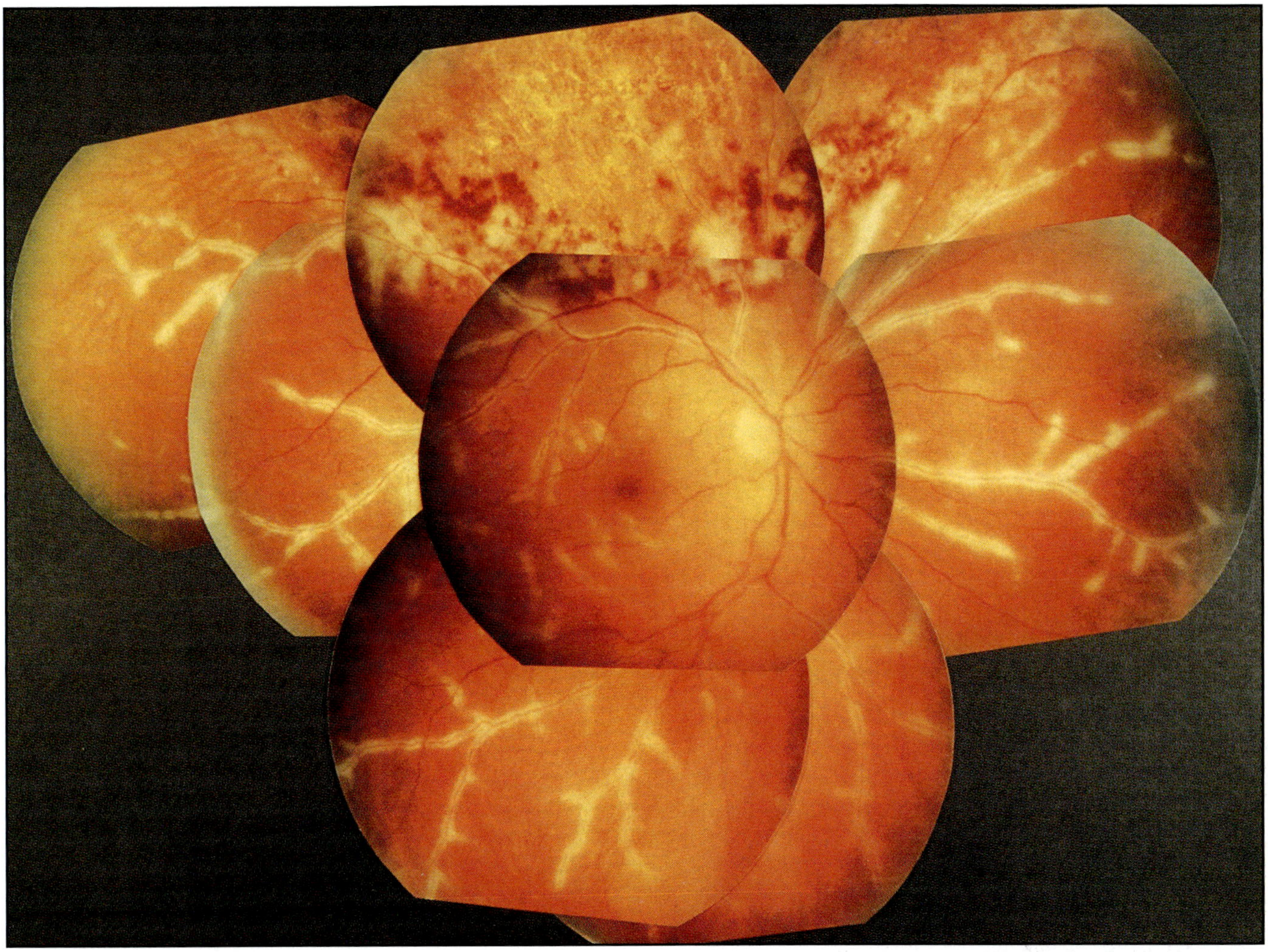

44–5

44–6

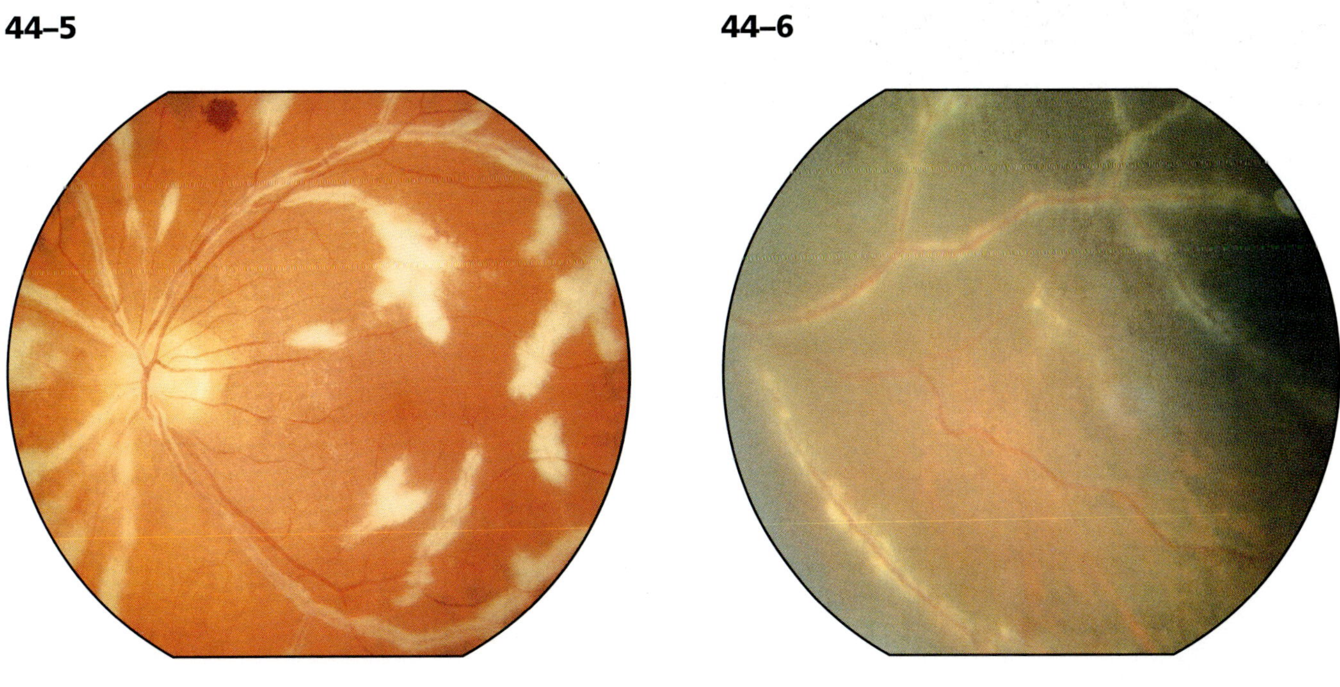

44–7 IDIOPATHIC FROSTED BRANCH ANGIITIS

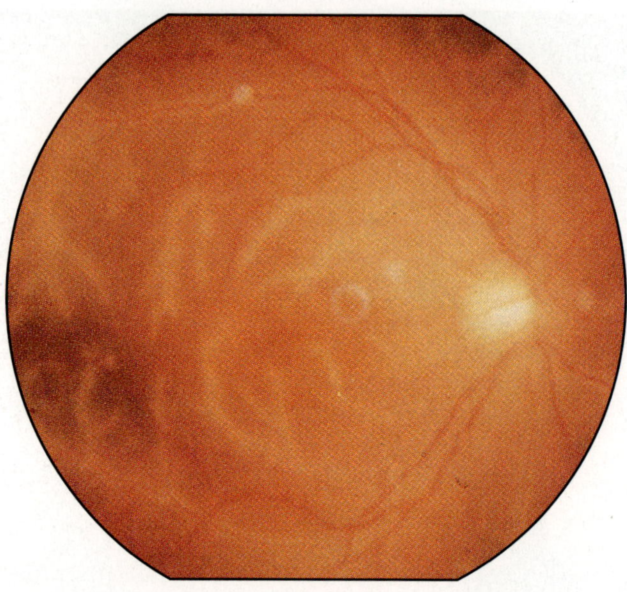

44–7 Frosted branch angiitis can also be demonstrated in patients without AIDS. This patient with idiopathic frosted branch angiitis shows a similar pattern of whitening of the vessels.

Suggested Readings

Cochereau-Massin, I, Lehoang, P, Lautier-Frau, M, Zazoun, L, Marcel, P, Robinet, M, Matheron, S, Katlama, C, Gharakhanian, S, Rozenbaum, W, Ingrand, D, and Gentilini, M: Efficacy and tolerance of intravitreal ganciclovir in cytomegalovirus retinitis in acquired immune deficiency syndrome, Ophthalmology 98:1348, 1991

D'Amico, DJ, Skdnik, PR, Kosloff, BR, Pinkston, P, Hirsch, MS, and Schooley, RT: Resolution of cytomegalovirus retinitis with zidovudine therapy, Arch Ophthalmol 106:1168, 1988

Freeman, WR, Henderly, DE, Wan, WI, Causey, D, Trousdale, MD, Green, RL, and Rao, NA: Prevalence, pathophysiology, and treatment of rhegmatogenous retinal detachment in treated cytomegalovirus retinitis, Am J Ophthalmol 103:527–536, 1987

Frenkel, LD, Keys, MP, Rola-Pleszczynski, M, and Bellanti, JA: Unusual eye abnormalities associated with congenital cytomegalovirus infection, Pediatrics 66:763–766, 1980

Guyer, DR, Jabs, DA, Brant, AM, Beschorner, WE, and Green, WR: Regression of cytomegalovirus retinitis with zidovudine: a clinicopathologic correlation, Arch Ophthalmol 107:868, 1989

Henry, K, Cantrill, H, Fletcher, C, Chinnock, BJ, and Balfour, HH, Jr: Use of intravitreal ganciclovir (dihydroxy propoxymethyl guanine) for cytomegalovirus retinitis in a patient with AIDS, Am J Ophthalmol 103:17–23, 1987

Holland, GN, and Shuler, JD: Progression rates of cytomegalovirus retinopathy in ganciclovir-treated and untreated patients, Arch Ophthalmol 110:1435–1442, 1992

Jabs, DA, Enger, C, and Bartlett, JG: Cytomegalovirus retinitis and acquired immunodeficiency syndrome, Arch Ophthalmol 107:75–80, 1989

Kinney, JS, Onorato, IM, Stewart, JA, Pass, RF, Stagno, S, Cheeseman, SH, Chin, J, Kumar, ML, Yaeger, AS, Herrmann, KL, Hurwitz, ES, and Schonberger, LB: Cytomegalovirus infection and disease, J Infect Dis 151:772–774, 1985

Palestine, AG, Rodrigues, MM, Macher, AM, Chan, CC, Lane, HC, Fauci, AS, Masur, H, Longo, D, Reichert, CM, Steis, R, Rook, AH, and Nussenblatt, RB: Ophthalmic involvement in acquired immunodeficiency syndrome, Ophthalmology 91:1092–1099, 1984

Palestine, AG, Stevens, G, Jr, Lane, HC, Masur, H, Fujikawa, LS, Nussenblatt, RB, Rook, AH, Manischewitz, J, Baird, B, Megill, M, Quinnan, G, Gelmann, E, and Fauci, AS: Treatment of cytomegalovirus retinitis with dihydroxy propoxymethyl guanine, Am J Ophthalmol 101:95–101, 1986

Pepose, JS, Holland, GN, Nestor, MS, Cochran, AJ, and Foos, RY: Acquired immune deficiency syndrome: pathogenic mechanisms of ocular disease, Ophthalmology 92:472–484, 1985

Sanborn, GE, Anand, R, Torti, RE, Nightingale, SD, Cal, SX, Yatec, B, Ashton, P, and Smith, T: Sustained-release ganciclovir therapy for treatment of cytomegalovirus retinitis: use of an intravitreal device, Arch Ophthalmol 110:188, 1992

Studies of Ocular Complications of AIDS (SOCA) Research Group in Collaboration with the AIDS Clinical Trials Group (ACTG): Studies of ocular complications of AIDS (SOCA) foscarnet-ganciclovir cytomegalovirus retinitis trial: 1. Rationale, design, and methods, Controlled Clin Trials 13:22, 1992

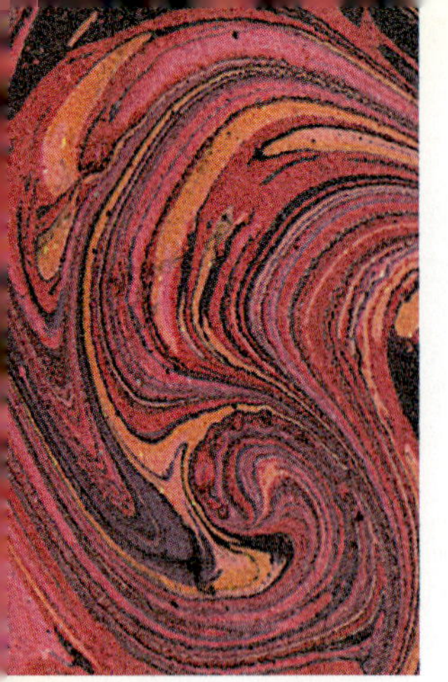

Chapter 45

Retinal Disease in the HIV-Infected Patient

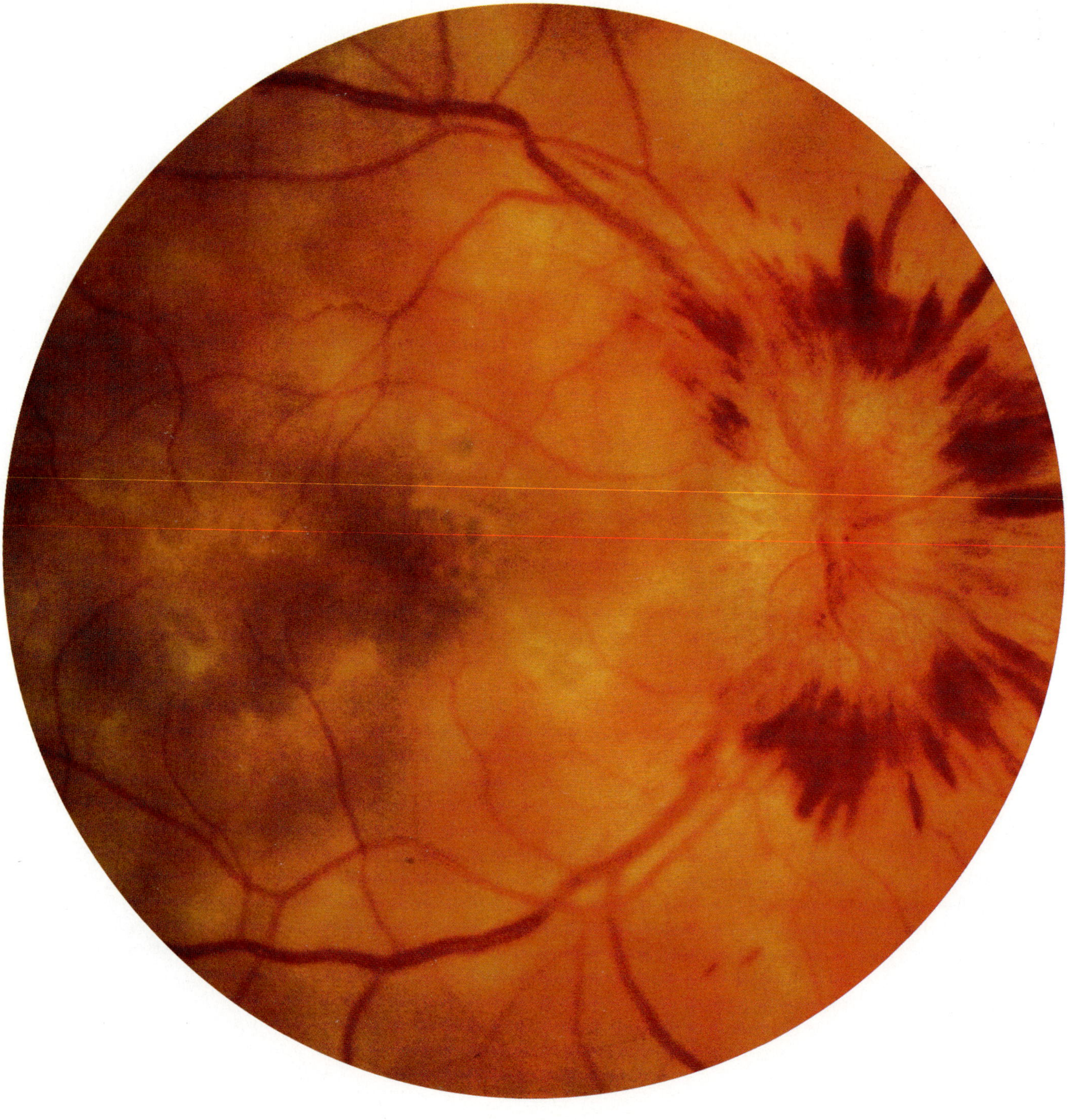

Retinal findings in the acquired immune deficiency syndrome (AIDS) include cotton-wool spots, retinal hemorrhages, microvascular abnormalities, cytomegalovirus (CMV) retinitis, and other opportunistic infections including *Cryptococcus* infection. Cotton-wool spots are the most common ophthalmic lesion noted in AIDS patients, and CMV retinitis is the most common opportunisitic infection in these patients.

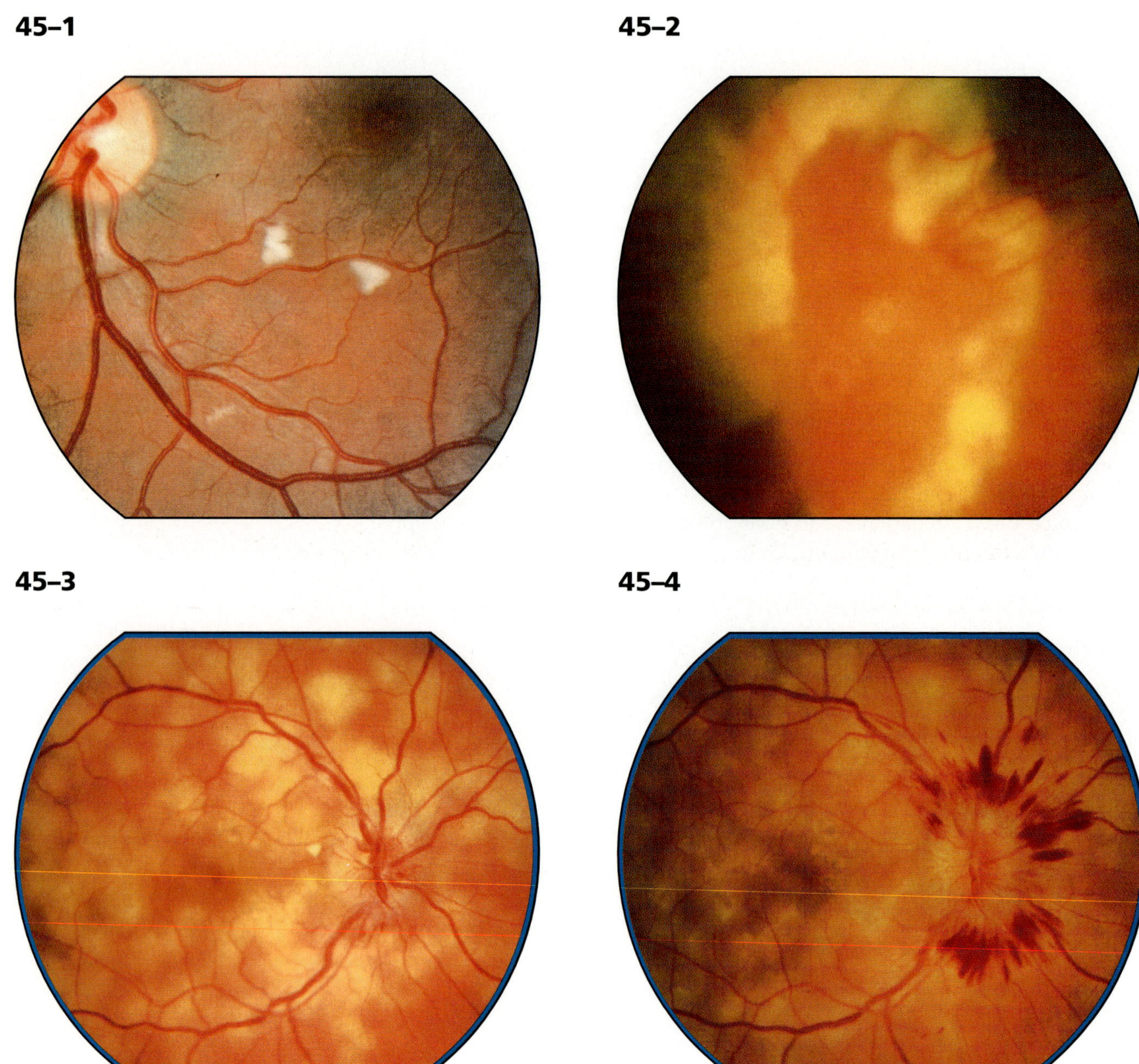

45–1 Multiple cotton-wool spots are demonstrated in this fundus photograph from an AIDS patient and may antecede foci of CMV retinitis.

45–2 This inflammatory choroidal lesion was noted in a patient who subsequently developed AIDS. Choroidal biopsy demonstrated gram-positive cocci. Cultures grew *Staphylococcus epidermidis.*

45–3 and 45–4 This patient with AIDS developed *Pneumocystis* choroiditis. The patient was a 24-year-old male with the human immunodeficiency virus (HIV) and *Pneumocystis* pneumonia. Notice the white choroidal lesions. Six weeks later, the patient developed optic disc edema with hemorrhage. Cryptococcal infection was diagnosed at this time.

45–1, *Courtesy of Dr. Jay Pepose.* ***45–2,*** *Courtesy of Dr. William Freeman. From Ryan, SJ: Retina, ed 2, St Louis, 1994, Mosby–Year Book.* ***45–3*** *and* ***45–4,*** *Courtesy of Dr. Maria Berrocal.*

45–5

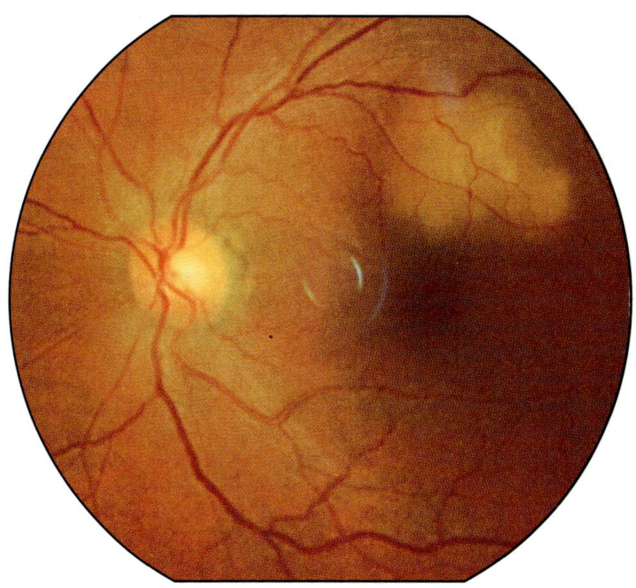

45–6

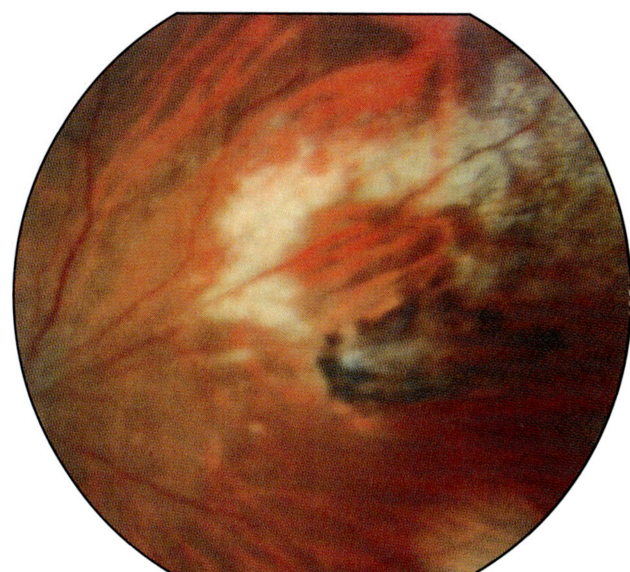

45–5 This patient has *Pneumocystis* choroiditis and HIV with multiple foci forming a confluent, solitary lesion in the fundus.

45–6 This patient with HIV has both CMV and toxoplasmosis retinitis. Note superiorly the whitish lesion secondary to CMV, and inferiorly the more hyperpigmented lesion secondary to toxoplasmosis.

***45–5** and **45–6**, Courtesy of Dr. Murk-Hein Heinemann.*

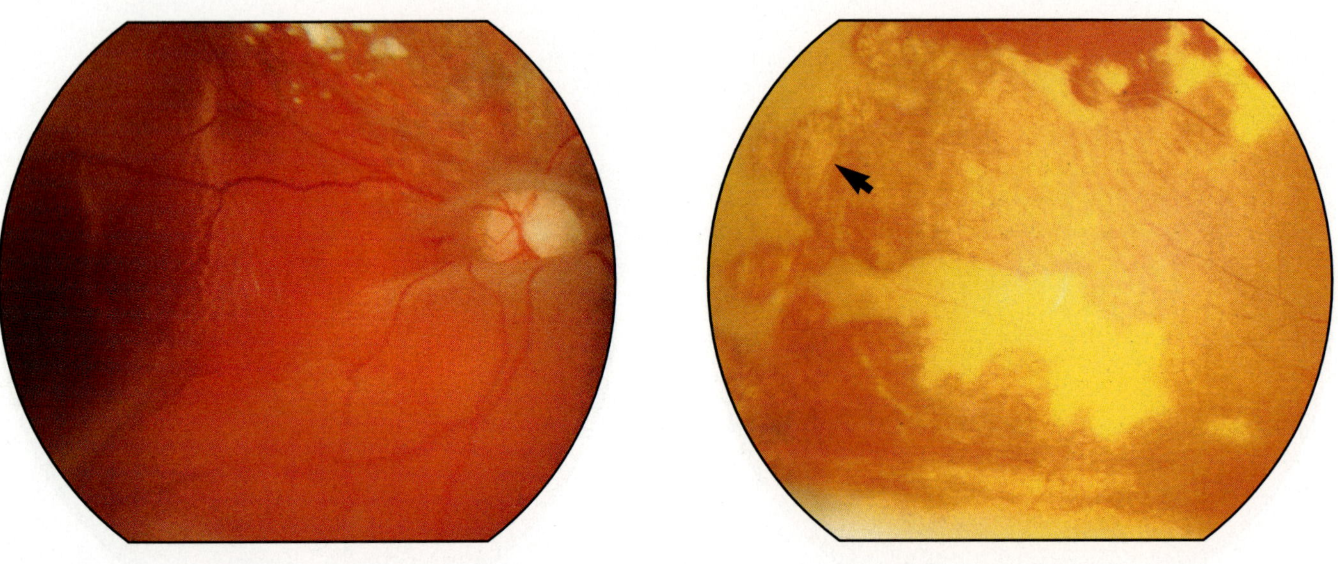

45–7 This patient had CMV retinitis which led to a retinal detachment.

45–8 AIDS patients are prone to secondary conditions such as the acute retinal necrosis syndrome, tuberculosis, cryptococcosis, toxoplasmosis, and other opportunistic infections. Acute retinal necrosis syndrome in a patient with AIDS. Some areas are resolving as evident by the presence of pigment epithelial atrophy *(arrowhead);* whereas other areas show geographic zones of retinal whitening.

45–7, *Courtesy of Dr. Murk-Hein Heinemann.*

Suggested Readings

Birch, CJ, Tachedjian, G, Doherty, RR, Hayes, K, and Gust, ID: Altered sensitivity to antiviral drugs of herpes simplex virus isolates from a patient with the acquired immunodeficiency syndrome, J Infect Dis 162:731–734, 1990

Biron, KK, Stanat, SC, Sorrell, JB, Fyfe, JA, Keller, PM, Lambe, CU, and Nelson, DJ: Metabolic activation of the nucleoside analog 9-{{2-hydroxy-1-(hydroxymethyl) ethoxy} methyl} guanine in human diploid fibroblasts infected with human cytomegalovirus, Proc Natl Acad Sci USA 82:2473–2477, 1985

Collaborative DHPG Treatment Study Group: Treatment of serious cytomegalovirus infections with 9-(1,3-dihydroxy-2-propoxymethyl) guanine in patients with AIDS and other immunodeficiencies, N Engl J Med 314:801–805, 1986

D'Amico, DJ, Skolnik, PR, Kosloff, BR, Pinkston, P, Hirsch, MS, and Schooley, RT: Resolution of cytomegalovirus retinitis with zidovudine therapy, Arch Ophthalmol 106:1168–1169, 1988

Fish, DG, Ampel, NM, Galgiani, JN, Dols, CL, Kelly, PC, Johnson, CH, Pappagianis, D, Edwards, JE, Wasserman, RB, and Clark, RJ: Coccidioidomycosis during human immunodeficiency virus infection: a review of 77 patients, Medicine (Baltimore) 69:384–391, 1990

Freeman, WR, Gross, JG, Labelle, J, Oteken, K, Katz, B, and Wiley, CA: *Pneumocystis carinii* choroidopathy: a new clinical entity, Arch Ophthalmol 107:863–867, 1989

Freeman, WR, Quiceno, JI, Crapotta, JA, Listhaus, A, Munguia, D, and Aguilar, MF: Surgical repair of rhegmatogenous retinal detachment in immunosuppressed patients with cytomegalovirus retinitis, Ophthalmology 99:466–474, 1992

Guyer, DR, Jabs, DA, Brant, AM, Beschorner, WE, and Green, WR: Regression of cytomegalovirus retinitis with zidovudine: a clinicopathologic correlation, Arch Ophthalmol 107:868–874, 1989

Heinemann, MH, Gold, JMW, and Maisel, J: Bilateral toxoplasma retinochoroiditis in a patient with acquired immune deficiency syndrome, Retina 6:224, 1986

Holland, GN, Gottlief, MS, and Foos, RY: Retinal cotton-wool patches in acquired immunodeficiency syndrome, N Engl J Med 307:1702, 1982

Kennedy, PGE, Newsome, DA, Hess, J, Narayan, O, Suresch, DL, Green, WR, Gallo, RC, and Polk, BF: Cytomegalovirus but not human T lymphotropic virus typeIII/lymphadenopathy associated virus detected by in-situ hybridization in retinal lesions in patients with the acquired immune deficiency syndrome, Br Med J 293:162–164, 1986

Palestine, AG, Rodrigues, MM, Macher, AM, Chan, C-C, Lane, HC, Fauci, AS, Masur, H, Longo, D, Reichert, CM, Stein, R, Rook, AH, and Nussenblatt, RB: Ophthalmic involvement in acquired immune deficiency syndrome, Ophthalmology 91:1092–1099, 1984

Schuman, JS, and Friedman, AH: Retinal manifestations of the acquired immune deficiency syndrome (AIDS): Cytomegalovirus, *Candida albicans*, cryptococcus, toxoplasmosis and *Pneumocystis carinii*, Trans Ophthalmol Soc UK 103:177, 1983

Studies of Ocular Complications of AIDS Research Group, in Collaboration with the AIDS Clinical Trials Group: Mortality in patients with the acquired immunodeficiency syndrome treated with either foscarnet or ganciclovir for cytomegalovirus retinitis, N Engl J Med 326:213–220, 1992

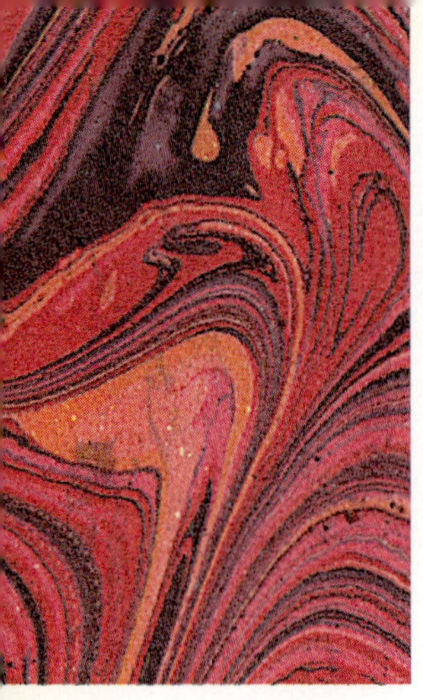

Chapter 46

Acute Retinal Necrosis Syndrome

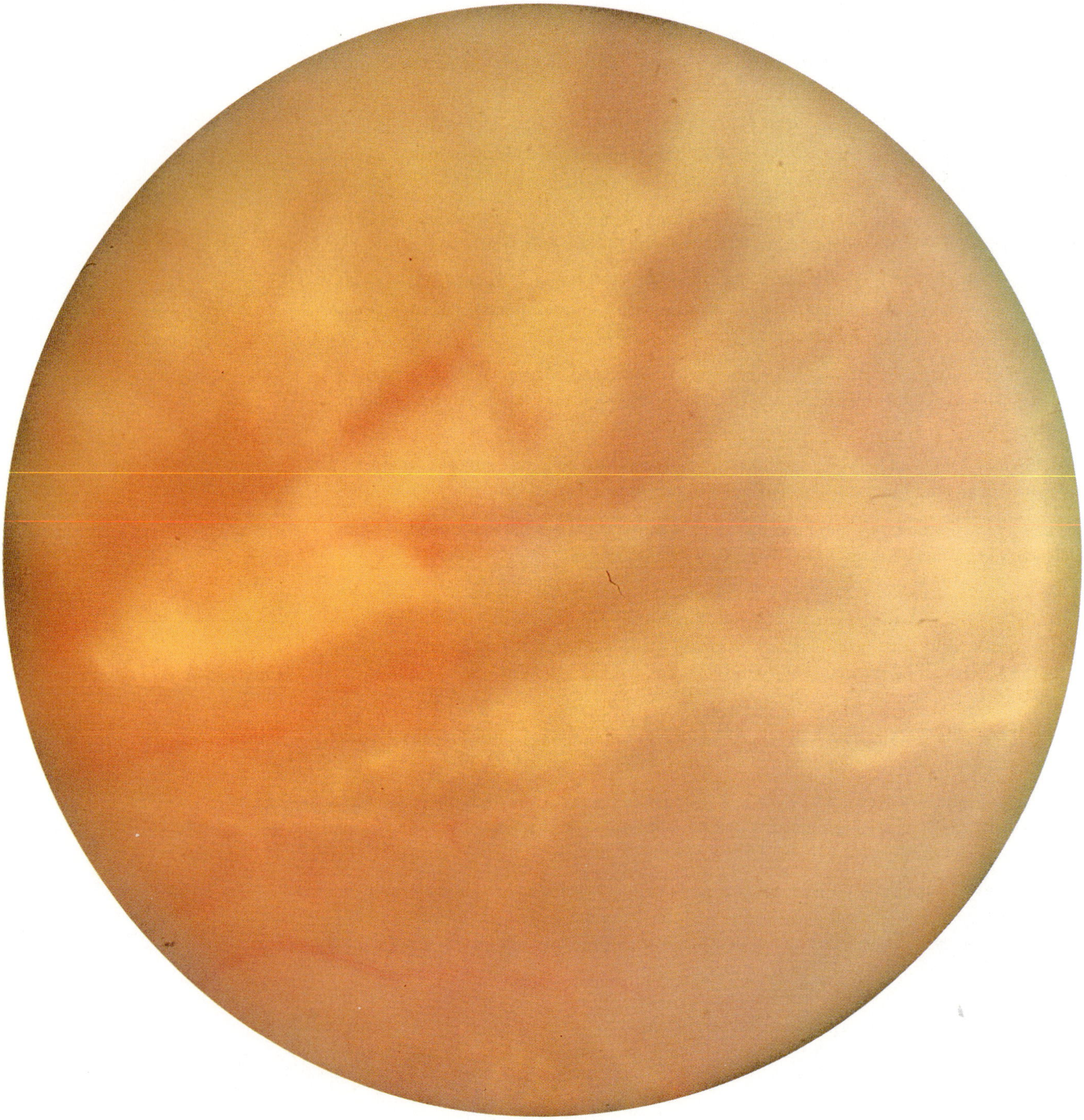

Ocular manifestations of the acute retinal necrosis syndrome include episcleritis, iritis, periorbital pain, vitreous opacification, and a necrotizing retinitis. Multifocal yellow-whitish lesions are demonstrated in patients with retinitis, which begins in the peripheral retina. Often the macula is spared. Hemorrhagic vasculitis with sheathing and obliteration of the vessels is noted; exudative retinal detachment may occur. Retinal breaks may occur at the junction of normal and necrotic retina, which may lead to a rhegmatogenous retinal detachment. Approximately three-quarters of eyes will develop such a retinal detachment within approximately 6 weeks after the start of the disease. The acute retinal necrosis syndrome occurs in otherwise healthy patients who are not immunocompromised. Herpes virus appears to be responsible for many of the cases. The fellow eye becomes involved in approximately one third of patients within 6 weeks. Acyclovir and prophylactic laser photocoagulation may be effective treatments in some cases.

46–1

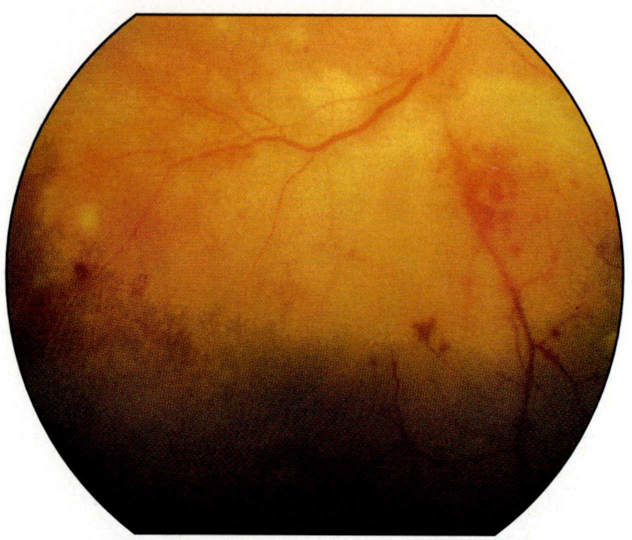

46–2

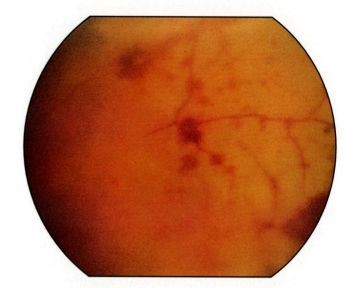

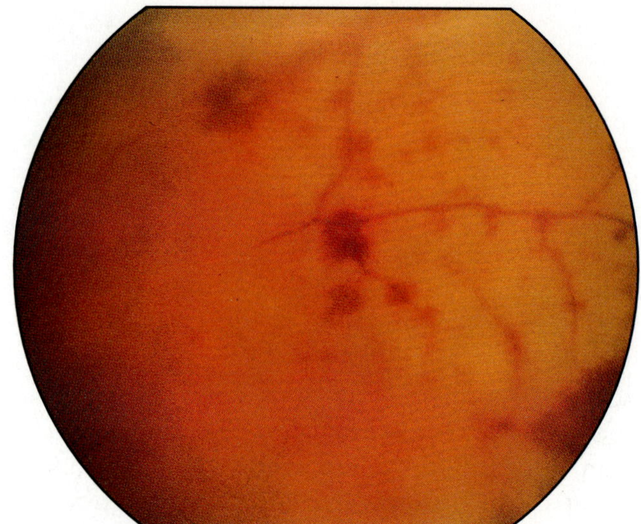

46–3

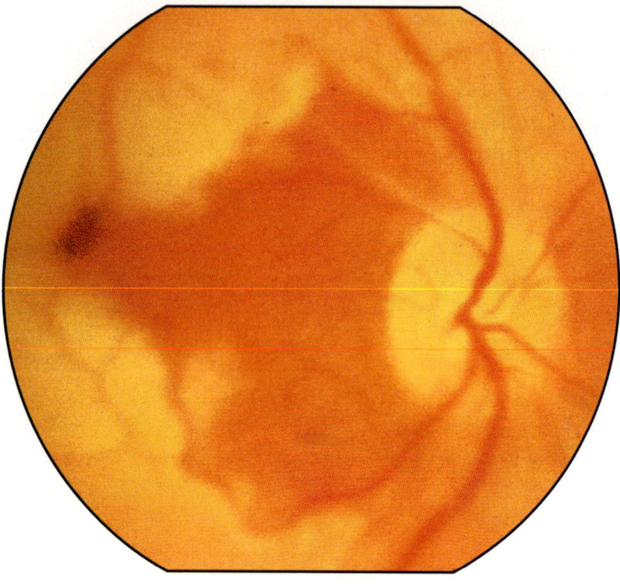

46–1 An obliterative retinal angiopathy with necrosis and vitritis can be seen in patients with the acute retinal necrosis syndrome. Note the narrowed and sheathed vessels within the retinal whitening and scattered hemorrhages.

46–2 Similar manifestations are demonstrated in this patient with marked inflammatory and hemorrhagic debris obscuring fundus details.

46–3 The necrosis may extend into the posterior pole.

46–4 **46–5**

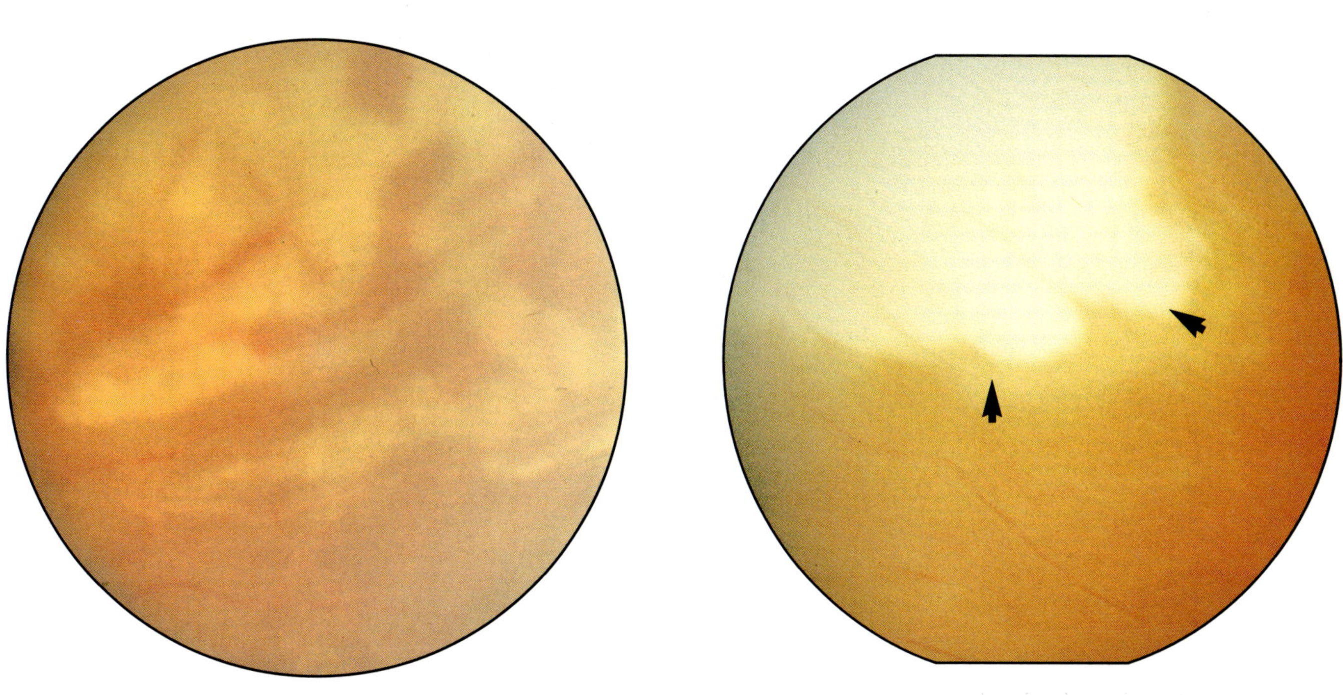

46–4 In some patients, there is a spared zone, free of necrosis, along the course of the retinal vessels. This distribution forms a geographic pattern consisting of involved and uninvolved retina.

46–5 As the process subsides, pigment epithelial stippling and atrophy evolve—which is apparent at the posterior edge of this patient who has acute retinal necrosis *(arrowheads)*.

46–5, *From Fisher, JP, Lewis, ML, Blumenkranz, M, Culbertson, WW, et al: Acute retinal necrosis syndrome. Part 1. Clinical manifest, Ophthalmology 89:1309–1316, 1982.*

46–6

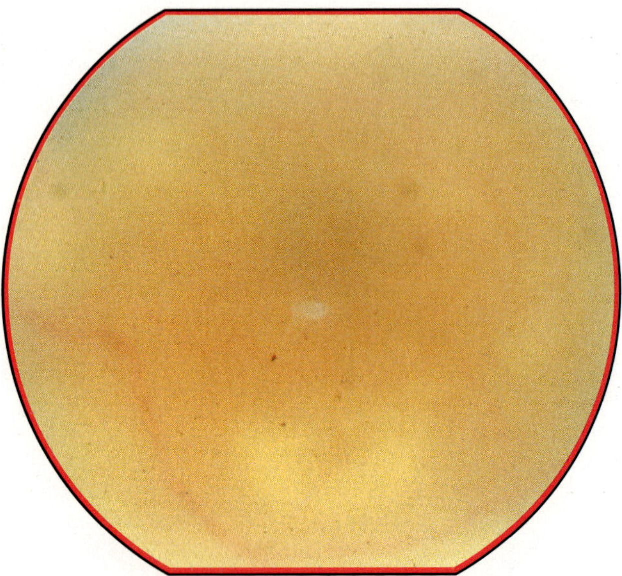

46–7

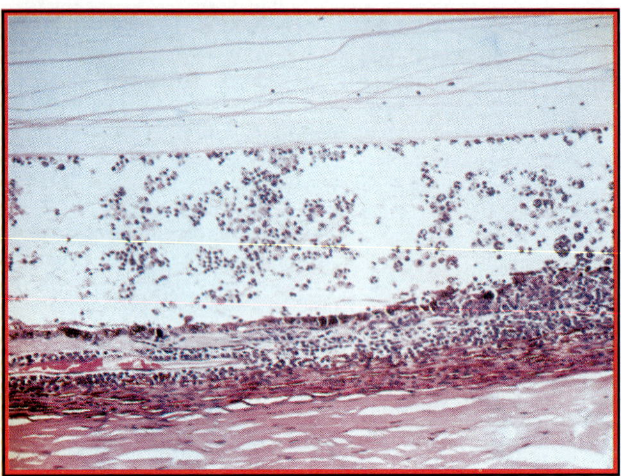

46–8

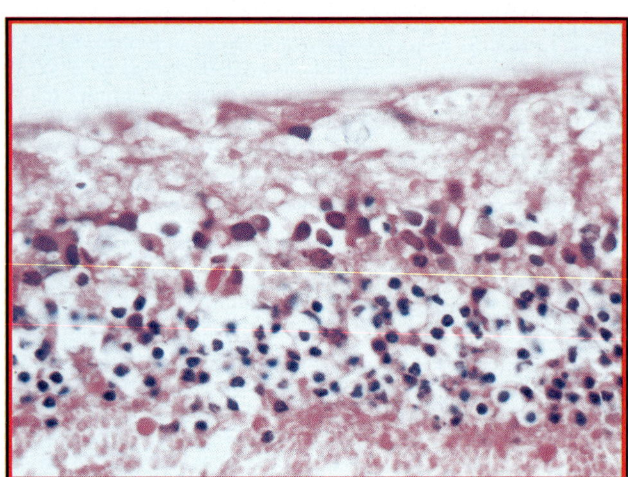

46–6 This clinicopathologic correlate of a patient with the bilateral acute retinal necrosis syndrome shows yellow-white lesions with an overlying vitritis.

46–7 and 46–8 Light microscopy reveals an infiltrate in the choroid and a partially necrotic retina with intranuclear inclusions.

46–6 *through* ***46–8,*** *From Culbertson, et al: The acute retinal necrosis syndrome, Ophthalmology 89:1317–1325, 1982.*

46–9

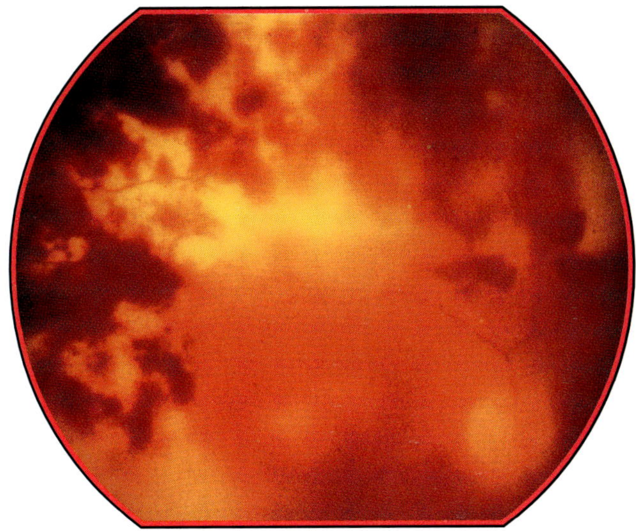

46–10

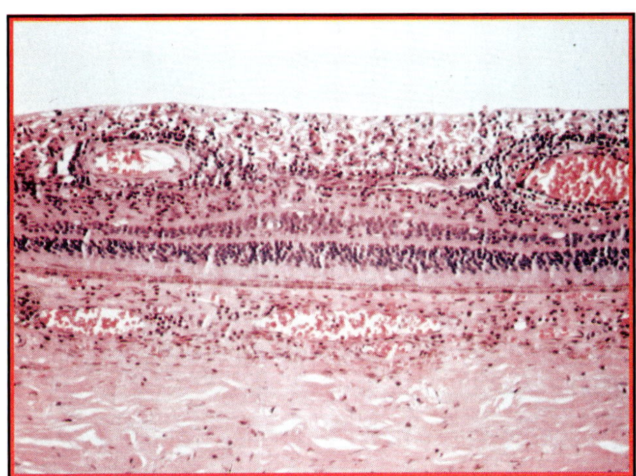

46–11

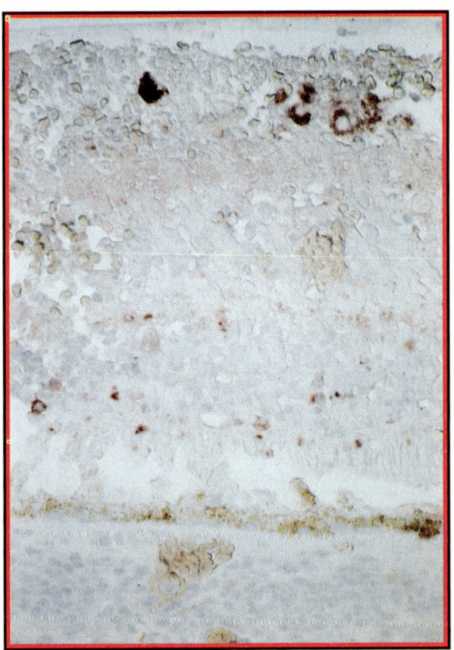

46–12

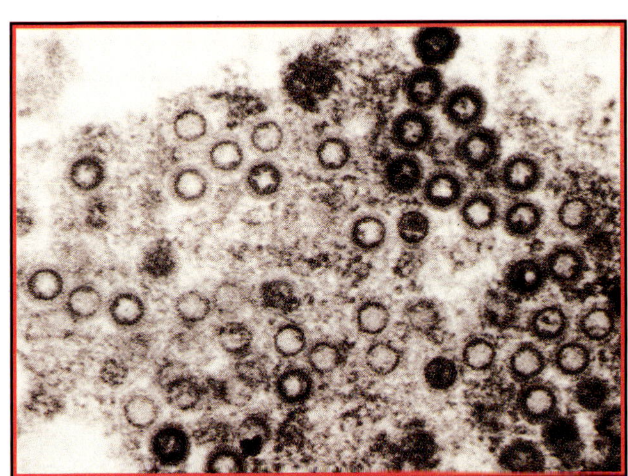

46–9 Another clinicopathologic correlation illustrates a patient that had a hemorrhagic chorioretinitis with vitritis.

46–10 Light microscopy reveals partially necrotic retina, inflammatory cells in the retina and choroid, and retinal vasculitis.

46–11 Immunoperoxidase staining was positive for herpes zoster.

46–12 Electron microscopy confirms that the virus particles had the characteristic of herpes virus.

46–9 *through* ***46–12,*** *Courtesy of Drs. Victor Curtin and Jay Pepose. Reprinted from Pepose, JS, et al: Herpes virus antibody levels in the etiologic diagnosis of the acute retinal necrosis syndrome, Am J Ophthalmol 113:248–256, 1992.*

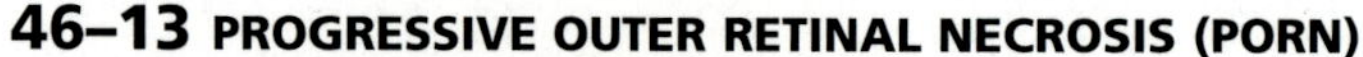

46–13 PROGRESSIVE OUTER RETINAL NECROSIS (PORN)

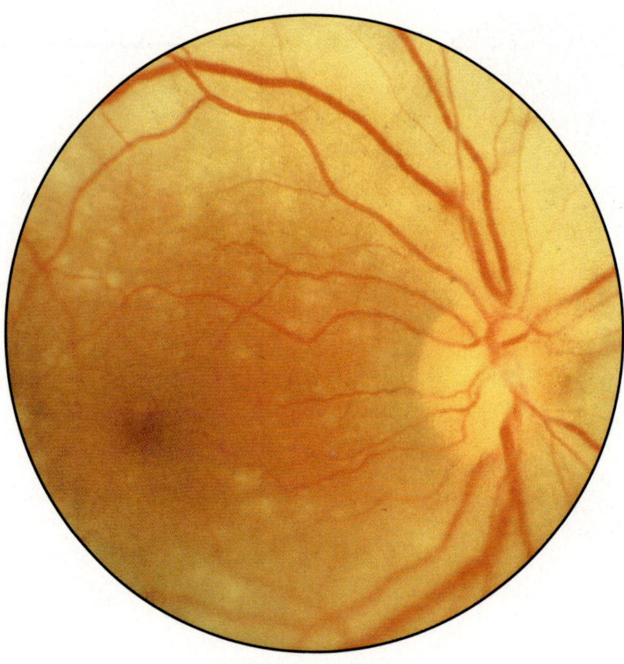

46–13 This patient with progressive outer retinal necrosis (PORN) demonstrates deep whitish-yellow lesions in the outer retina and an inferior retinal detachment.

46–13, *Courtesy of Dr. Richard Spaide.*

Suggested Readings

Blumenkranz, MS, Clarkson, JG, and Culbertson, WW: Visual results and complications after retinal reattachment in the acute retinal necrosis syndrome, Retina 9:170–174, 1989

Carney, MD, Peyman, GA, and Goldberg, MF: Acute retinal necrosis, Retina 6:85–94, 1986

Culbertson, WW, Blumenkranz, MS, Haines, H, Gass, JDM, Mitchell, KB, and Norton, EWD: The acute retinal necrosis syndrome. II. Histopathology and etiology, Ophthalmology 89:1317–1325, 1982.

Culbertson, WW, Blumenkranz, MS, Pepose, JS, Stewart, JA, and Curtin, VT: Varicella zoster virus is a cause of the acute retinal necrosis syndrome, Ophthalmology 93:559–569, 1986

Duker, JS, Nielsen, J, Eagle, RC: Rapidly progressive, acute retinal necrosis (ARN) secondary to herpes simplex virus, type 1, Ophthalmology 97:1638–1643, 1990

Freeman, WR, Thomas, EL, Rao, NA, Pepose, JS, Trousdale, MD, Howes, EL, Nadel, AJ, Mines, JA, and Bowe, B: Demonstration of herpes group virus in acute retinal necrosis syndrome, Am J Ophthalmol 102:701–709, 1986

Gorman, BD, Nadel, AJ, and Coles RS: Acute retinal necrosis, Ophthalmology 89:809–814, 1982

Holland, GN, Cornell, PJ, and Park, MS: An association between acute retinal necrosis syndrome and HLA-DQW7 and phenotype BW62, DR4, Am J Ophthalmol 108:370–374, 1989

Margolis, TP, Lowder, CY, Holland, GN, Spaide, RF, Logans, AG, Weissman, SS, Irvine, AR, Josephberg, R, Meisler, CM, and O'Donnell, JJ: Varicella-zoster virus retinitis in patients with the acquired immunodeficiency syndrome, Am J Ophthalmol 112:119–131, 1991

Matsuo, T, Date, S, Tsuji, T, Koyama, M, Nakayama, T, Koyama, T, Matsuo, N, and Koide, N: Immune complex containing herpesvirus antigen in a patient with acute retinal necrosis, Am J Ophthalmol 101:368–371, 1986

Pepose, JS, Flowers, B, Stewart, JA, Grose, C, Levy, DS, Culbertson, WW, and Kreiger, AE: Herpesvirus antibody levels in the etiologic diagnosis of the acute retinal necrosis syndrome, Am J Ophthalmol 113:248–256, 1992

Sergott, RC, Belmont, JB, and Savino, PJ: Optic nerve involvement in the acute retinal necrosis, Arch Ophthalmol 103:1160–1162, 1985

Severin, M, and Neubauer, H: Bilateral acute retinal necrosis, Ophthalmologica 192:199–203, 1981

Urayama, A, Yamada, N, Sasaki, T, Nishiyama, Y, Watanabe, H, Wakusawa, S, Satoh, Y, Takahashi, K, and Takei, Y: Unilateral acute uveitis with retinal periarteritis and detachment, Jpn J Clin Ophthalmol 25:607–619, 1971

Willerson, D, Jr, Aaberg, TM, and Reeser, FH: Necrotizing vaso-occlusive retinitis, Am J Ophthalmol 84:209–217, 1977

Young, NJA, and Bird, AC: Bilateral acute retinal necrosis, Br J Ophthalmol 62:581–590, 1978

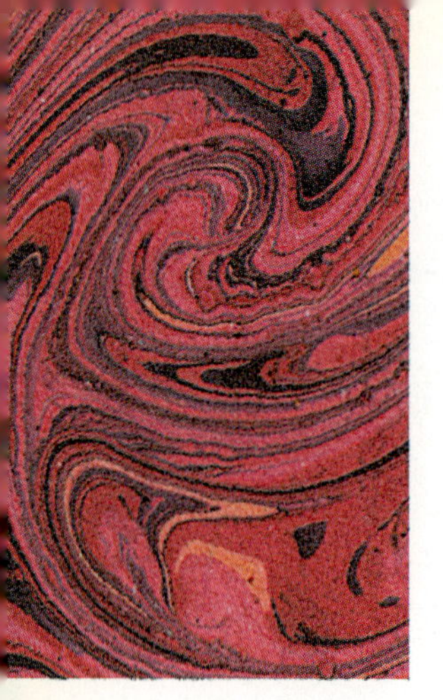

Chapter 47

Endogenous Fungal Infections of the Retina and Choroid

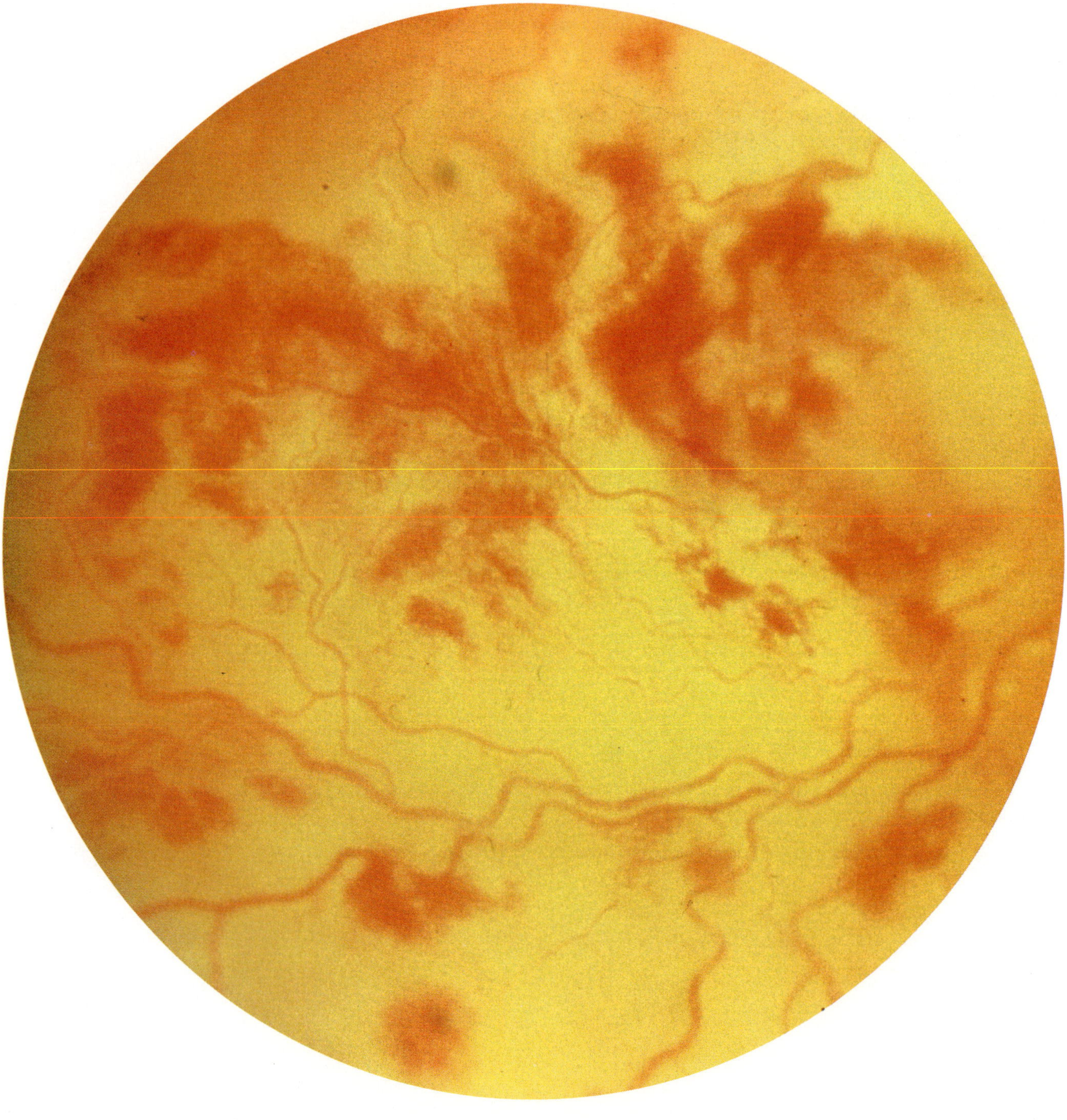

Candida is a yeast that may cause chorioretinitis especially in immunocompromised patients. A white lesion with an overlying vitritis is often noted. Histopathologic examination reveals that the *Candida* organisms are budding yeast with a pseudohyphate appearance. This infection is often seen in intravenous drug abusers. *Aspergillus, Cryptococcus, Coccidioides, Blastomyces,* and *Sporothrix* are other common fungi that may affect the retina or choroid. *Histoplasma capsulatum* is a major cause of choroidal neovascularization in patients living in the Ohio Mississippi River Valley. This condition is discussed in a separate section.

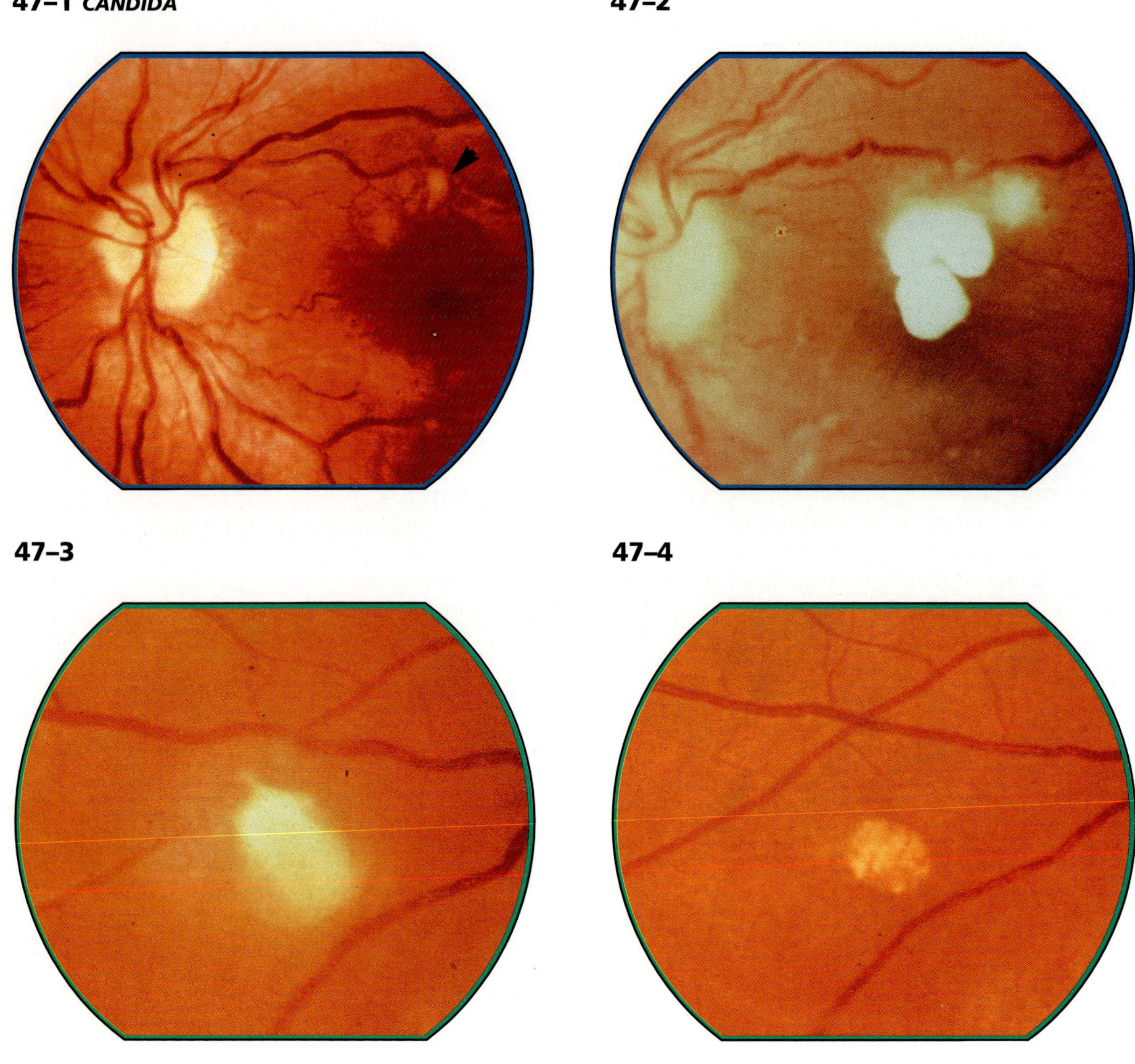

47–1 and 47–2 An early focus of *Candida* chorioretinitis in the superior macula of the left eye *(arrowhead)* is demonstrated in a patient with bacterial septicemia after abdominal surgery. The same eye 1 month later shows expansion of the lesion with vitreous invasion and multiple foci of infection. Retinal vascular tortuosity with evidence of a periphlebitis and optic disc pallor are also noted. Perivascular inflammatory plaques were present. The patient had received antifungal therapy.

47–3 and 47–4 A focus of early *Candida* chorioretinitis is also noted in this next case. The same eye can be seen after successful treatment with intravenous amphotericin B. Note the hypopigmented scar.

47–1 *and* ***47–2,*** *Courtesy of Dr. Gary Holland. From Griffin, JR, Pettit, TH, Fishman, LS, and Foss, RY: Blood-borne* Candida *endophthalmitis: a clinical and pathologic study of 21 cases, Arch Ophthalmol 89:450–456, 1973. Copyright 1973 American Medical Association.* ***47–3*** *and* ***47–4,*** *Courtesy of Drs. Gary Holland, J. Robert Griffin, and Thomas H. Pettit. From Holland, G: Endogenous fungal of the retina and choroid. In Ryan, SJ: Retina, ed 2, St Louis, 1994, Mosby–Year Book.*

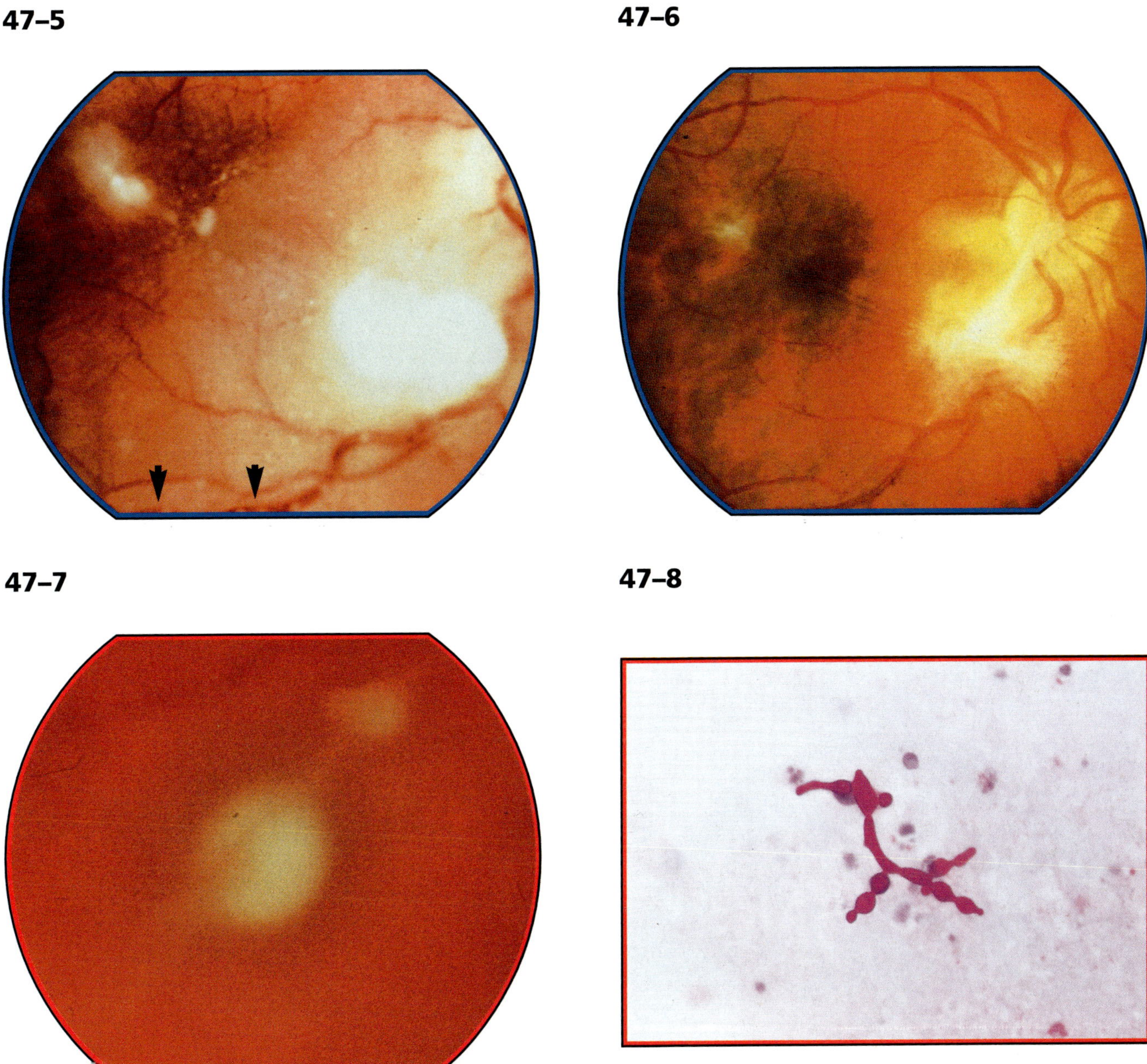

47–5 and 47–6 A large *Candida* chorioretinitis lesion with vitreous invasion is noted inferotemporal to the optic nerve head in the right eye. Note the perivascular plaques (Kyrieleis arteriolitis) inferiorly *(arrowheads)*. The same eye can be seen after successful treatment with amphotericin B. In this case, the perivascular plaques disappeared. In some eyes, especially eyes with acute toxoplasmosis, the plaques may persist. Note also that the healed lesion is associated with residual preretinal fibrosis with inner retinal striae traversing across the macula toward a small focal area of fibrosis.

47–7 and 47–8 This 27-year-old intravenous drug abuser developed *Candida* endophthalmitis. Fluffy white vitreous opacities are adjacent to and continuous with the retina. Pars plana vitrectomy was performed. Light microscopy reveals pseudohyphae and budding blastophores, which are characteristic of *Candida*.

***47–5** and **47–6,** Courtesy of Drs. Gary Holland, J. Robert Griffin, and Thomas H. Pettit. From Holland, G: Endogenous fungal of the retina and choroid. In Ryan, SJ: Retina, ed 2, St Louis, 1994, Mosby–Year Book. **47–7** and **47–8,** From Snip, RC, and Michels, RG: Pars plana vitrectomy in the management of endogenous* Candida *endophthalmitis, Am J Ophthalmol 82:699–704, 1976.*

47–9 *ASPERGILLUS*

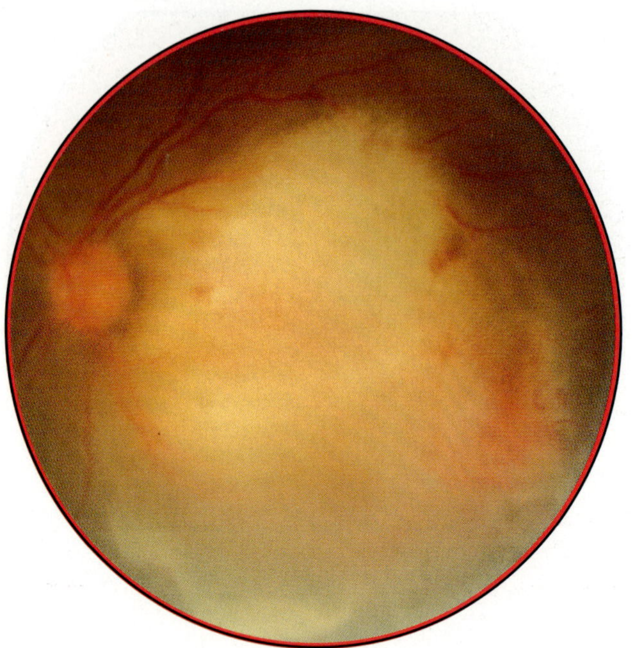

47–10

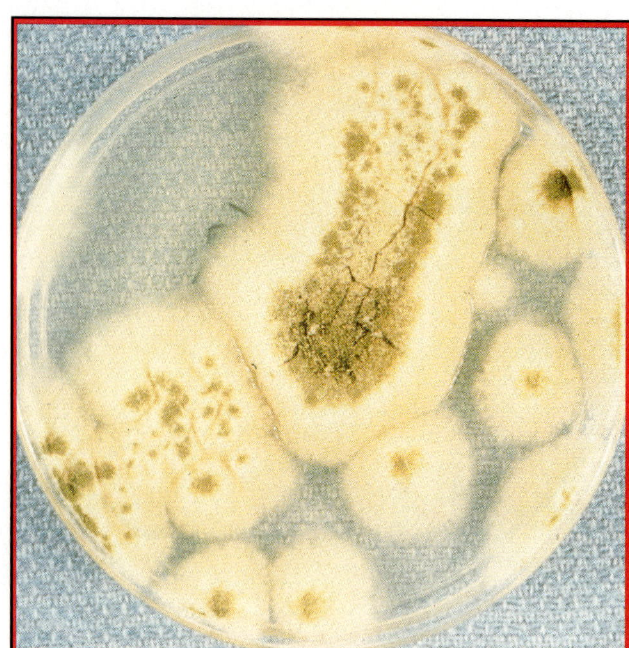

47–11

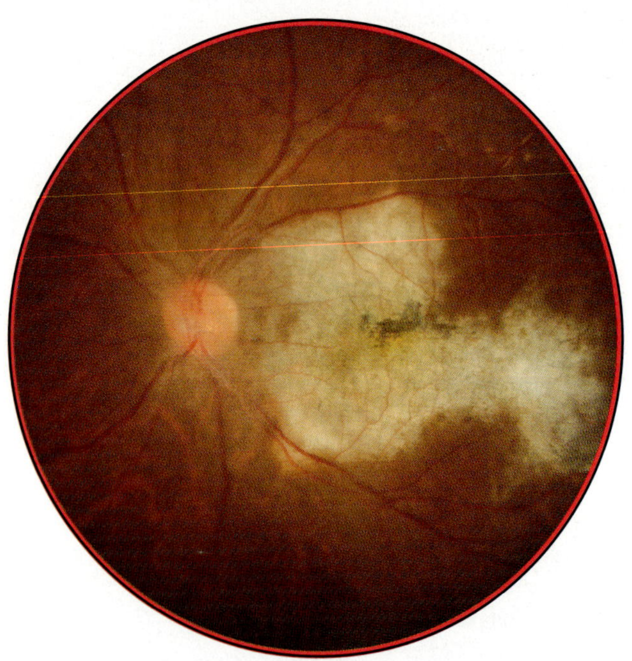

47–9 and 47–10 This patient had an endophthalmitis due to *Aspergillus.* Note the organisms in culture.

47–11 After vitrectomy an atrophic lesion is noted.

***47–9** through **47–11,** Courtesy of Dr. Charles Barr.*

47–12

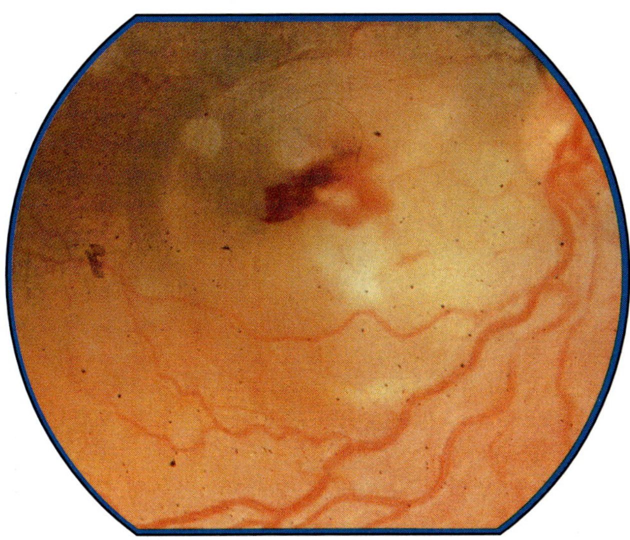

47–13

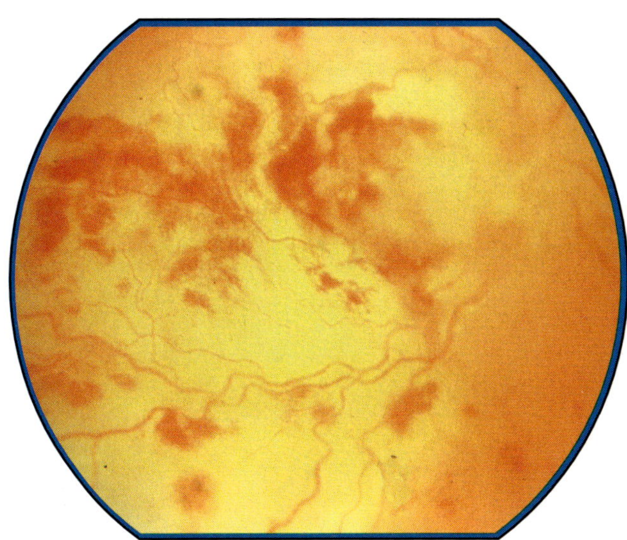

47–12 and 47–13 This patient also has *Aspergillus* infection. Note the juxtapapillary inflammation and hemorrhage. Four days later, the patient's condition progressed extensively with widespread retinal hemorrhage and infection. This case illustrates the potentially virulent nature of this pathogen.

47–12 *and* ***47–13,*** *Courtesy of Dr. Douglas A. Jabs. From Coskuncan, NM, Jabs, DA, Dunn, JP, Haller, JA, Green, WR, Vogelsang, G, Santos, GW: The eye in bone marrow transplantation: VI. Retinal complications, Arch Ophthalmol 112:372–379, 1994. Copyright American Medical Association.*

47–14 *CRYPTOCOCCUS*

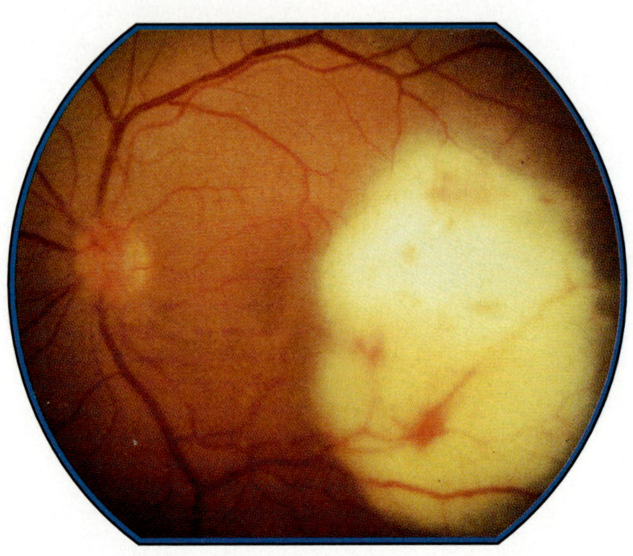

47–15

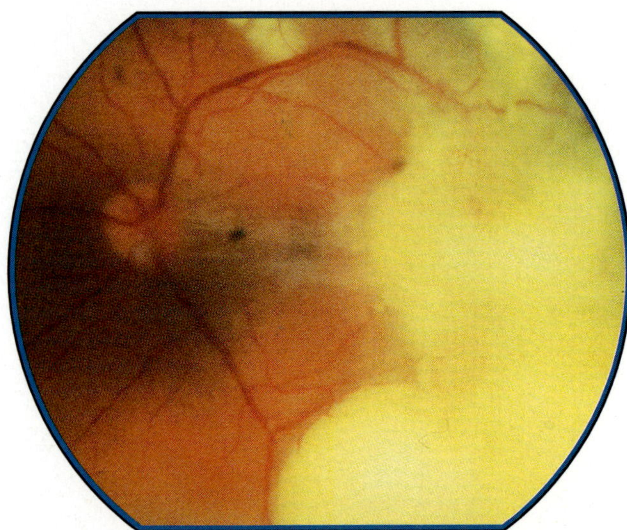

47–14 *Cryptococcus* is a fungus that primarily affects the lungs. Ocular involvement is rare and usually associated with disseminated disease. This 33-year-old male was treated with systemic steroids for a retinal inflammatory lesion before the diagnosis of cryptococcal retinitis and meningitis was suspected.

47–15 His lesion progressed. Note the extension of the mass in the macula with overlying vitreous reaction and invasion of the retina. He was eventually treated with antifungal medication but died from central nervous system complications. Histopathologic studies demonstrated ocular and disseminated systemic infection of *Cryptococcus* neoformans.

47–14 *and* ***47–15,*** *Courtesy of Dr. Joel Schulman. From Schulman, JA, Leveque, C, et al: Fatal disseminated cryptococcoses following intraocular involvement, Br J Ophthalmol 72:171–175, 1988.*

47–16

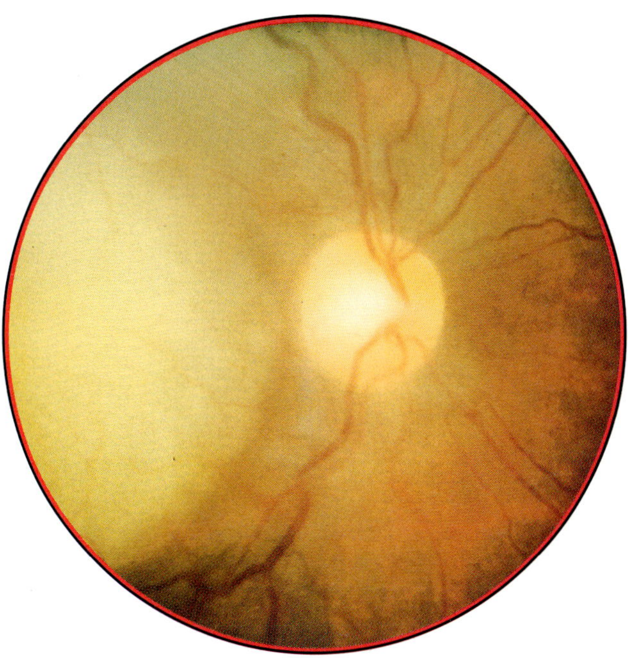

47–17

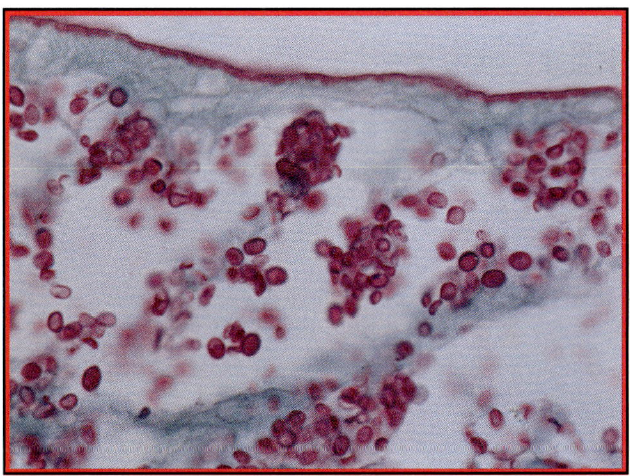

47–18

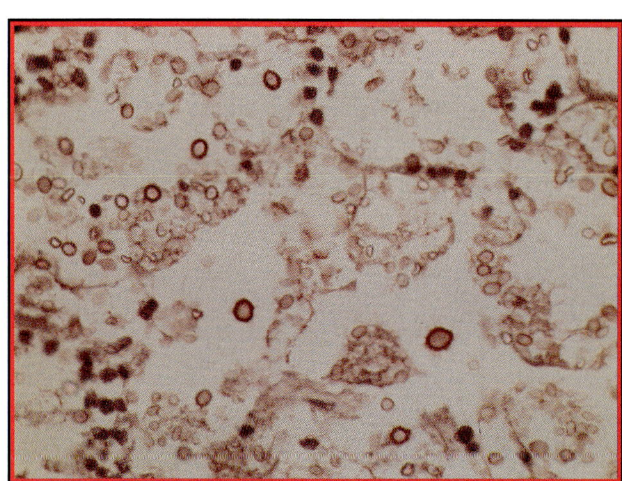

47–16 This 36-year-old female had a medical history of pulmonary tuberculosis, syphilis, and pelvic inflammatory disease. Ophthalmoscopy reveals a yellowish-white lesion.

47–17 and 47–18 Light microscopy reveals the cryptococcal organisms with their characteristic mucopolysaccharide capsule.

***47–16, 47–17,** and **47–18,** From Khodadoust, AA, and Payne, JW: Cryptococcal "torular" retinitis: a clinicopathologic case report, Am J Ophthalmol 67:745–750, 1969.*

47–19 COCCIDIOIDOMYCOSIS

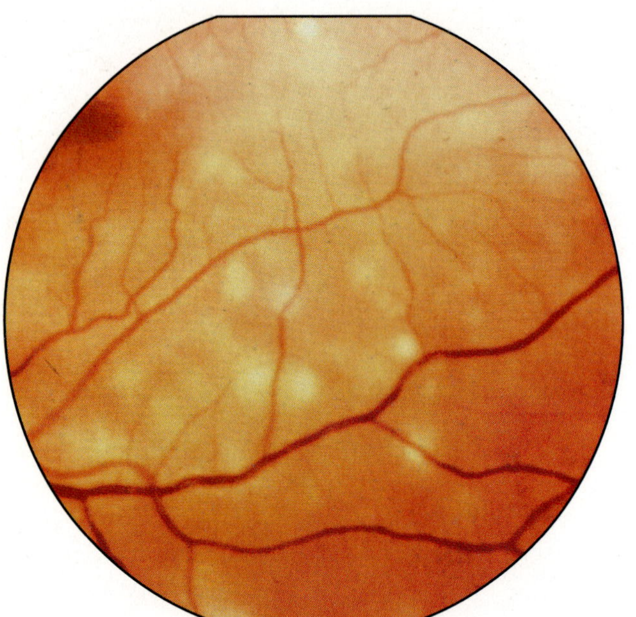

47–20

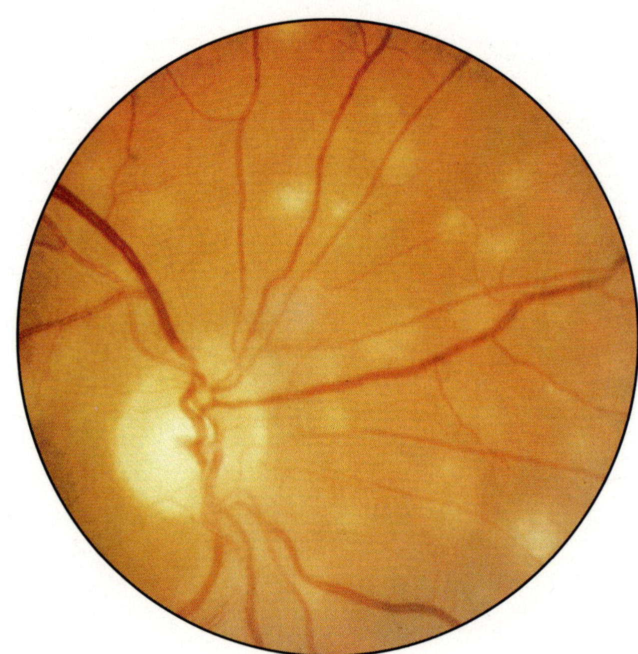

47–21

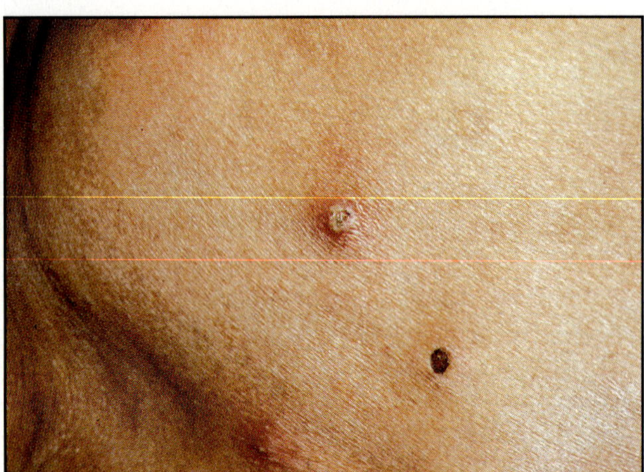

47–19 Multifocal choroidal lesions of intraocular coccidioidomycosis are noted in this eye.

47–20 This patient also has end-stage disseminated coccidioidomycosis. Note the multifocal lesions.

47–21 This patient had a cutaneous eruption secondary to coccidiodomycosis.

47–19, *Courtesy of Dr. Gary Holland. From Zakka, KA, et al: Intraocular coccidioidomycosis, Surv Ophthalmol 22:313–321, 1978.* ***47–20,*** *Courtesy of Drs. Mark Blumenkranz and Hunter Little. From Rainin, EA, and Little, HL: Ocular coccidioidomycosis: a clinical pathologic case report, Trans Am Acad Ophthalmol 76:645–651, 1972.* ***47–21,*** *Courtesy of Dr. Mark Blumenkranz.*

47–22 BLASTOMYCOSIS

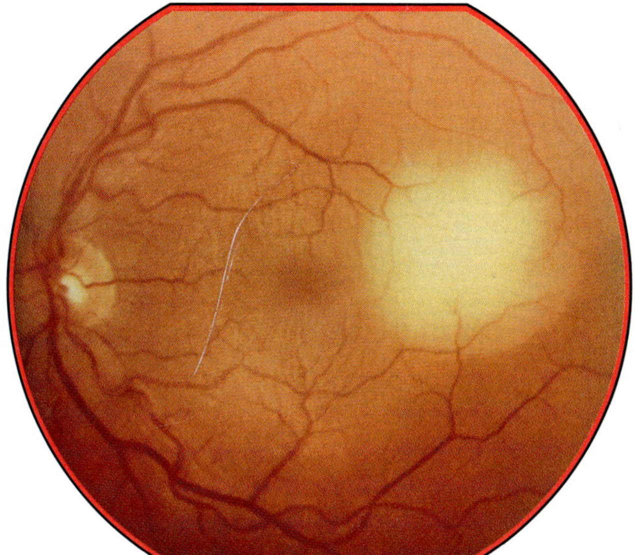

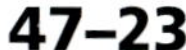

47–23

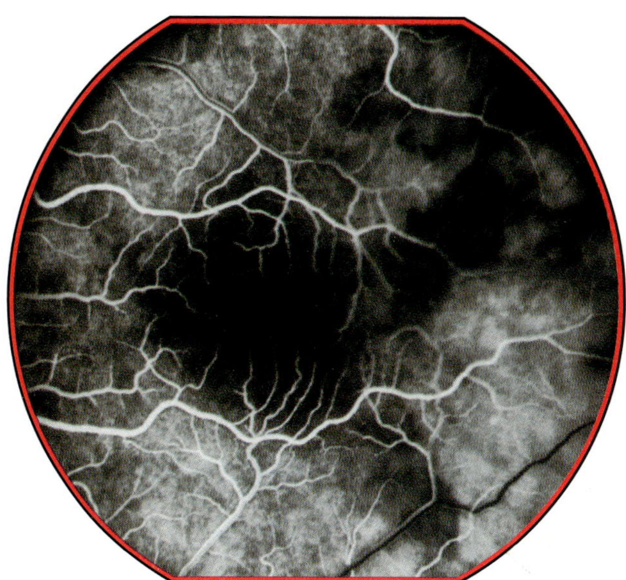

47–24

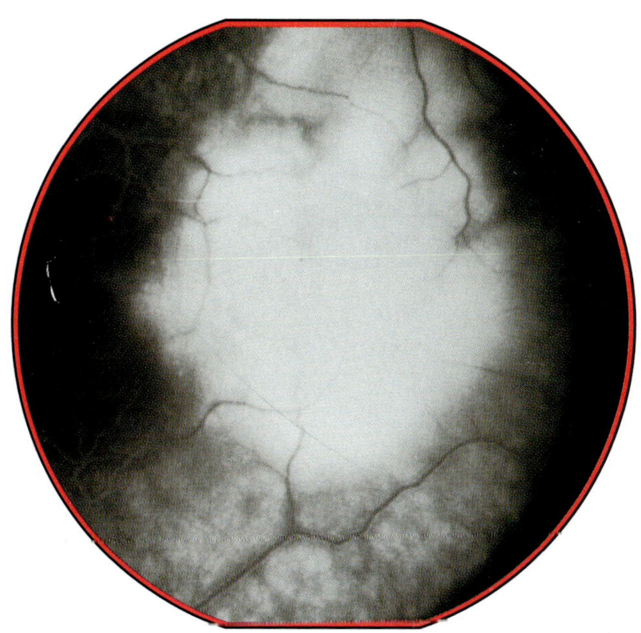

47–22 through 47–24 *Blastomyces dermatitidis* is a saprophytic fungus. Cutaneous lesions may occur from trauma, and rarely disseminated disease may follow. Blastomycosis is also a chronic granulomatous disorder. Anterior segment inflammation may occur. Choroidal involvement may occur with latent disseminated blastomycosis. Note the fluffy yellowish-white choroidal lesion (47–22), which shows early blockage with late hyperfluorescence on fluorescein angiography (47–23 and 47–24).

***47–22** through **47–24,** Courtesy of Dr. Hilel Lewis. From Lewis, H, Aaberg, TM, Fary, DRB, and Stevens, TS: Latent disseminated blastomycosis with choroidal involvement, Arch Ophthalmol 106:527–530, 1988.*

(Case continued on next page.)

47–25 BLASTOMYCOSIS

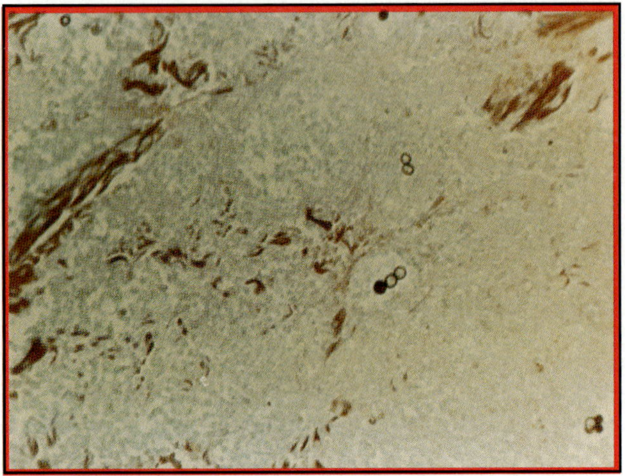

47–26

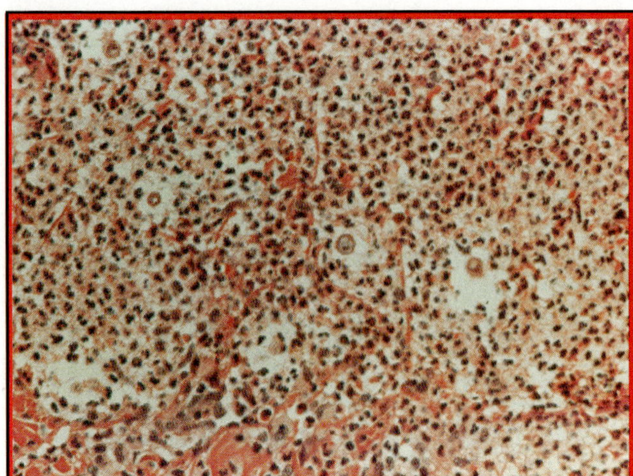

47–27

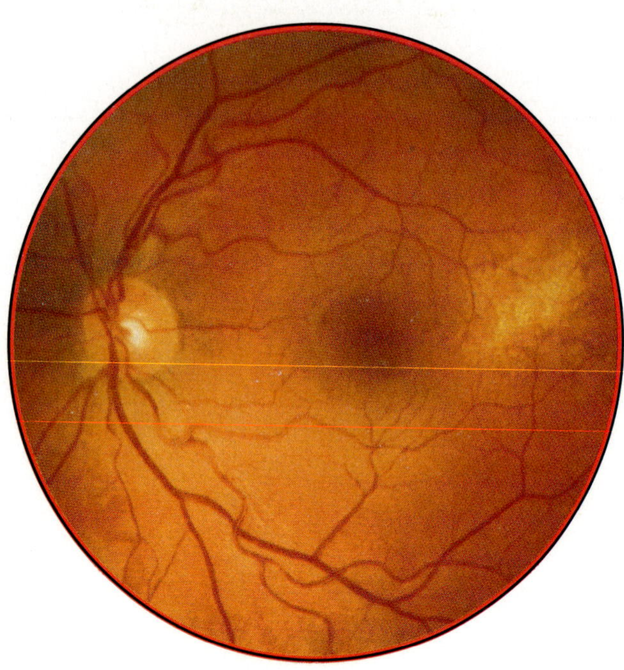

47–25 through 47–27 Blastomycosis was confirmed by histopathologic examination (47–25 and 47–26). Antifungal therapy caused resolution of the lesion (47–27).

***47–25** through **47–27,** Courtesy of Dr. Hilel Lewis. From Lewis, H, Aaberg, TM, Fary, DRB, and Stevens, TS: Latent disseminated blastomycosis with choroidal involvement, Arch Ophthalmol 106:527–530, 1988.*

47–28 BLASTOMYCOSIS

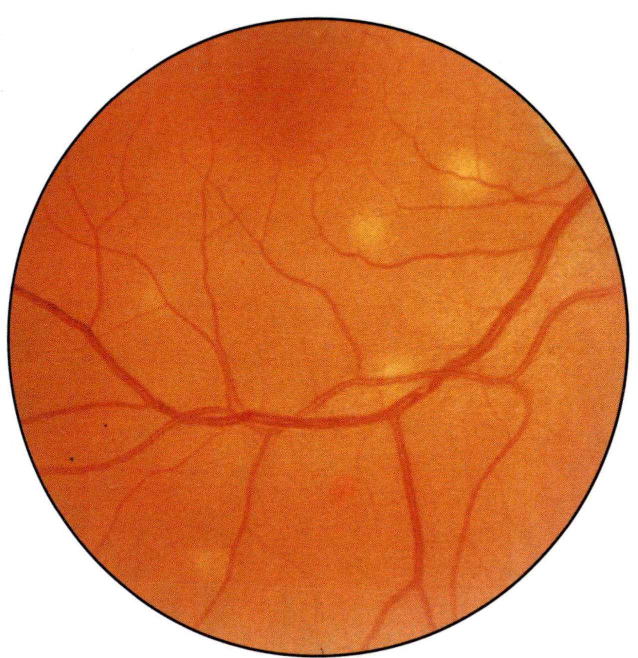

47–29 *PNEUMOCYSTIS*

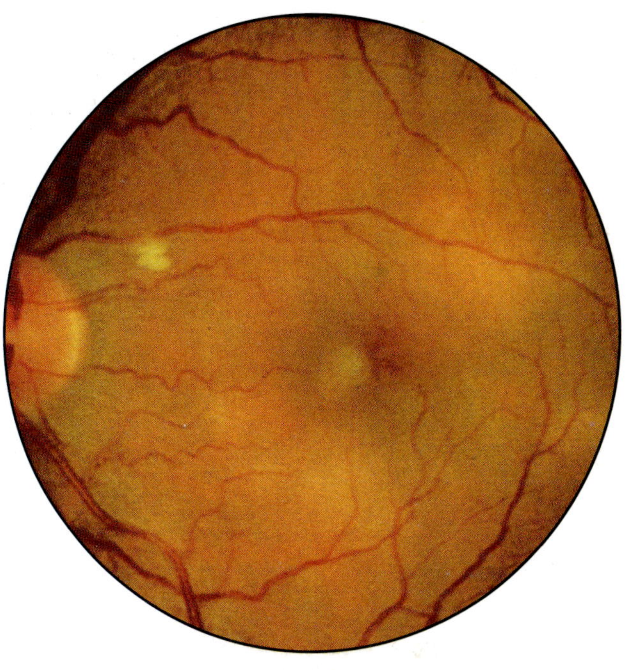

47–28 This patient had high fevers, severe headaches, a maculopapular rash, and cough. Chest X-rays revealed miliary reticular nodular infiltrates. Vision was 20/40 in the right eye and 20/30 in the left eye. Ophthalmoscopy revealed multiple small yellowish raised choroidal lesions in both eyes. The patient underwent an open-lung biopsy and *Blastomyces dermatitidis* was identified. The patient's condition improved when given intravenous amphotericin B.

47–28, *Courtesy of Dr. Froncie Gutman.*

Pneumocystis

47–29 This patient has *Pneumocystis* choroiditis. Note the deep choroidal lesions. There is also a cotton-wool spot seen in this patient with AIDS.

Suggested Readings

Blumenkranz, MS, and Stevens, DA: Endogenous coccidioidal endophthalmitis, Ophthalmology 87:974–984, 1980

Blumenkranz, MS, and Stevens, DA: Therapy of endogenous fungal endophthalmitis: miconazole or amphotericin B for coccidioidal and candidal infection, Arch Ophthalmol 98:1216–1220, 1980

Brod, RD, Clarkson, JG, Flynn, HW, Jr, and Green, WR: Endogenous fungal endophthalmitis. In: Tasman, W, and Jaeger, EA, eds: Duane's clinical ophthalmology, vol 3, 1990, pp 1–139

Cantrill, HL, Rodman, WP, Ramsay, RC, and Knobloch, WH: Postpartum *Candida* endophthalmitis, JAMA 243:1163–1165, 1980

Demicco, DD, Reichman, RC, Violette, EJ, Winn, WC, Jr: Disseminated aspergillosis presenting with endophthalmitis: a case report and a review of the literature, Cancer 53:1995–2001, 1984

Edwards, JE, Jr, Montgomerie, JZ, Ishida, K, Morrison, JO, and Guze, LB: Experimental hematogenous endophthalmitis due to *Candida*: species variation in ocular pathogenicity, J Infect Dis 135:294–297, 1977

Font, RL, Spaulding, AG, and Green, WR: Endogenous mycotic panophthalmitis caused by *Blastomyces dermatitidis*: report of a case and a review of the literature, Arch Ophthalmol 77:217–222, 1967

Jampol, LM, Dyckman, S, Maniates, V, Tso, M, Daily, M, and O'Grady, R: Retinal and choroidal infarction from *Aspergillus*: clinical diagnosis and clinicopathologic correlations, Trans Am Ophthalmol Soc 86:422–437, 1988

Klintworth, GK, Hollingsworth, AS, Lusman, PA, and Bradford, WD: Granulomatous choroiditis in a case of disseminated histoplasmosis, Arch Ophthalmol 90:45–48, 1973

McDonnell, PJ, and Green, WR: Endophthalmitis. In: Mandell, GL, Douglas, RG, Jr, Bennett, JE, eds: Principles and practice of infectious diseases, ed 3, New York, Churchill Livingstone, 1990, pp 987–995

McDonnell, PJ, McDonnell, JM, Brown, RH, and Green, WR: Ocular involvement in patients with fungal infections, Ophthalmology 92:706–709, 1985

Naidoff, MA, and Green, WR: Endogenous *Aspergillus* endophthalmitis occurring after kidney transplant, Am J Ophthalmol 79:502–509, 1975

Rodenbiker, HT, and Ganley, JP: Ocular coccidioidomycosis, Surv Ophthalmol 24:263–290, 1980

Snip, RC, and Michels, RG: Pars plana vitrectomy in the management of endogenous *Candida* endophthalmitis, Am J Opthalmol 82:699–704, 1976

Zakka, KA, Foos, RY, and Brown, WJ: Intra-ocular coccidioidomycosis, Surv Ophthalmol 22:313–321, 1978

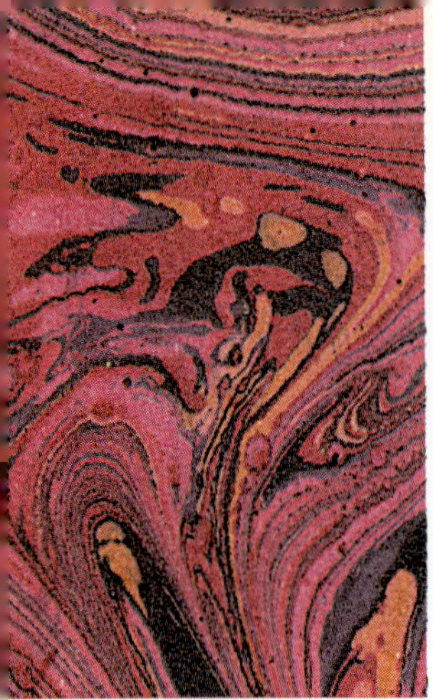

Chapter 48

Pars Planitis

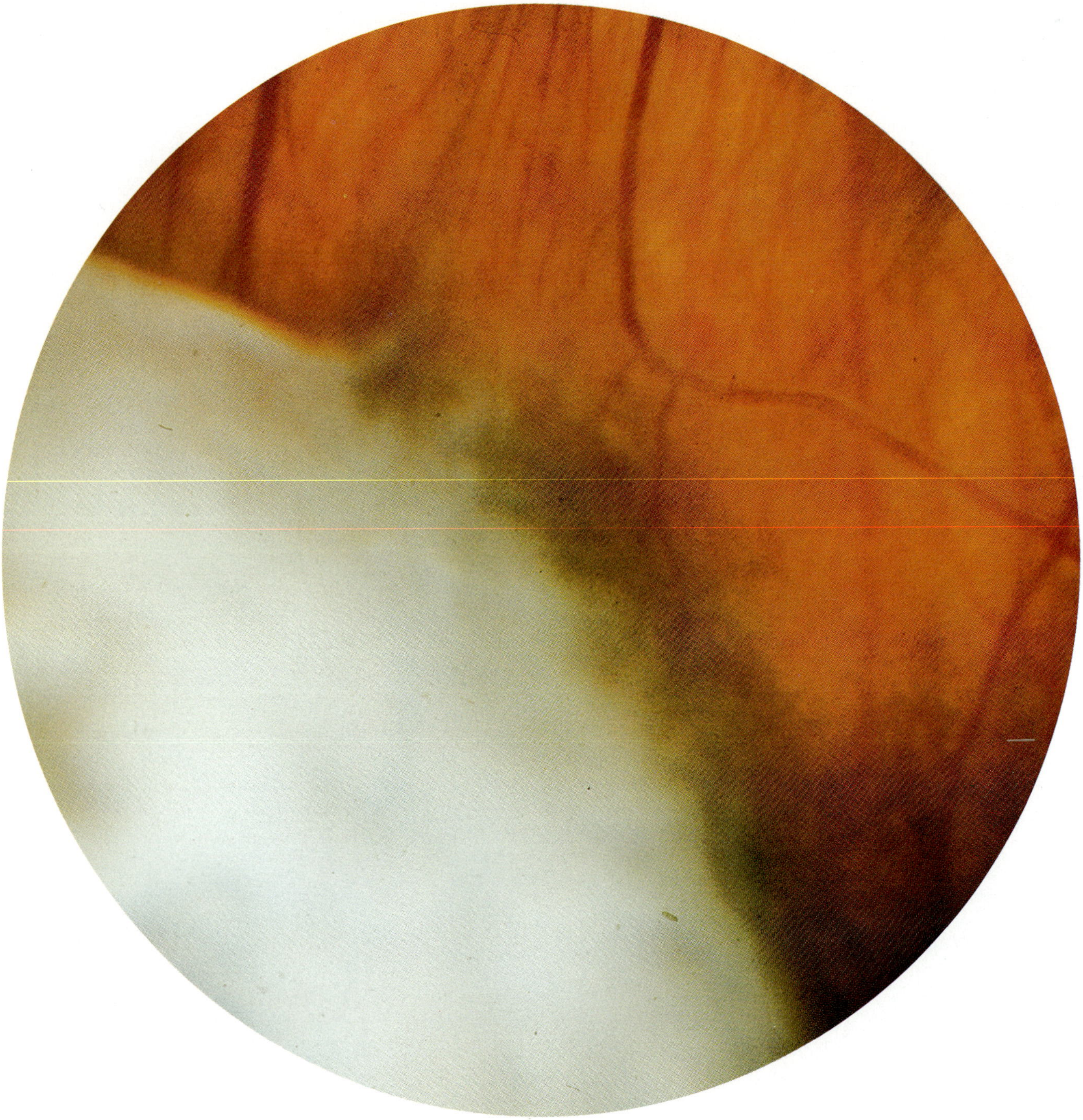

Pars planitis is seen in young adults and children. Bilateral disease is noted eventually in almost 80% of affected patients. Pars plana exudates, vitritis, snowballs, retinal periphlebitis, and cystoid macular edema may be noted. Cystoid macular edema is the most common cause of decreased vision in this disease. The characteristic lesion is the snowbank on the pars plana. The etiology of the disease is unknown. Some patients with pars planitis will have a mild form of the condition, often with a favorable prognosis.

48–1

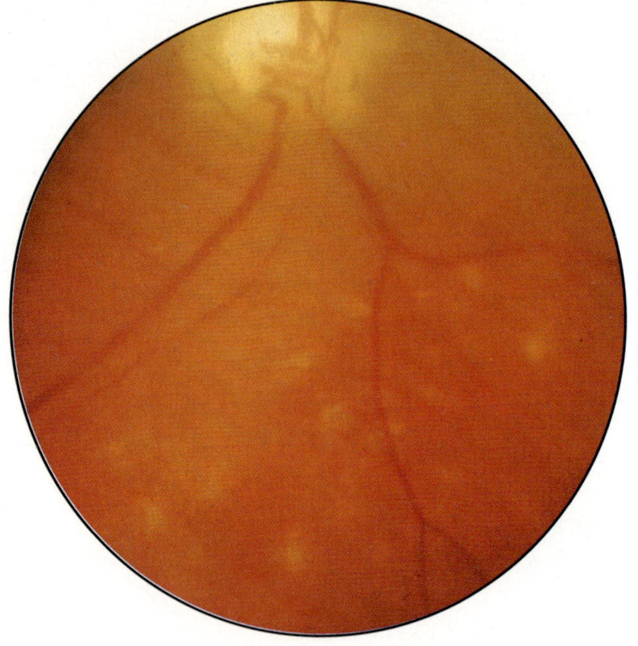

48–2

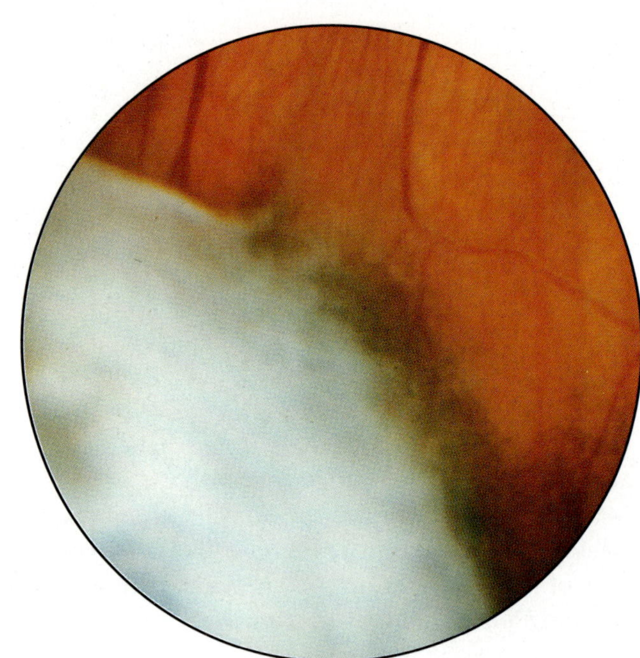

48–3

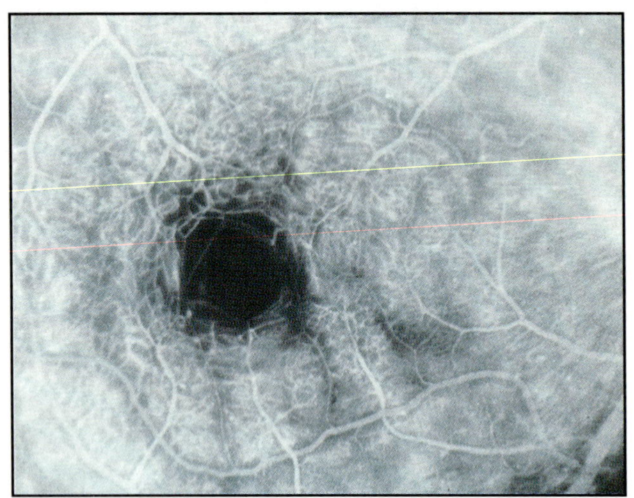

48–4

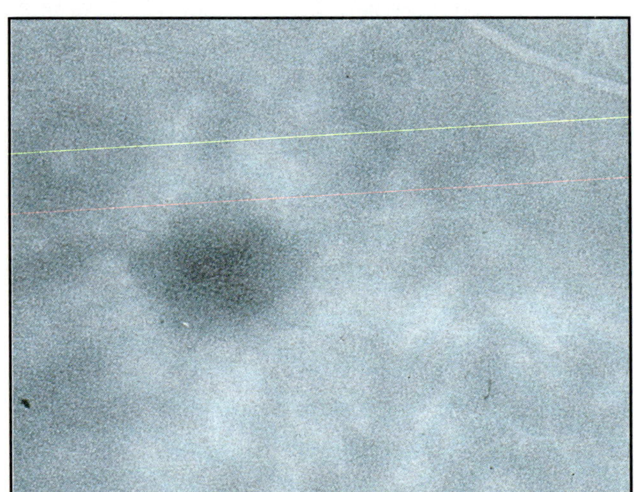

48–1 Whitish preretinal lesions can be demonstrated in patients with pars planitis. Note also the disc edema.

48–2 This patient with pars planitis has a large white snowbank lesion.

48–3 and 48–4 Fluorescein angiography reveals a more prominent foveal capillary network and cystoid macular edema in these patients.

48–1, *Courtesy of Dr. A. Edward Maumenee.*

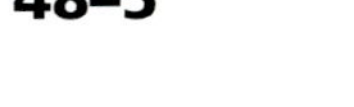

48–5

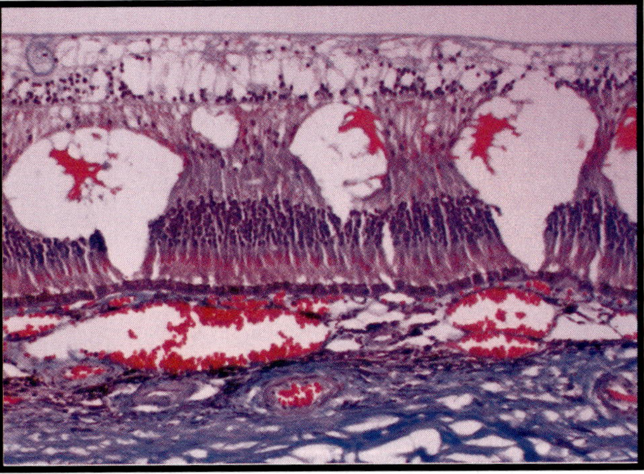

48–6

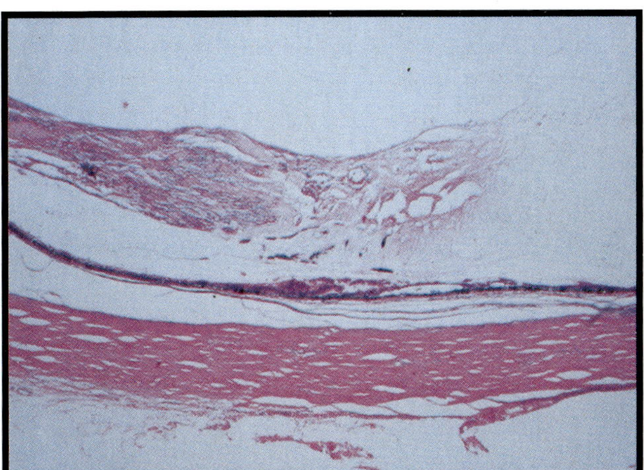

48–5 Histopathologic examination of this eye with pars planitis reveals cystoid macular edema with retinal phlebitis.

48–6 A snowbank is composed of collapsed and condensed vitreous with glial cell proliferation and neovascularization from the retina, new collagen, and minor ciliary epithelial hyperplasia.

Suggested Reading

Capone, A, Jr., Aaberg, TM: Intermediate principles and practice of ophthalmology. In Robinson, NL, ed: Clinical practice, vol 1, Philadelphia, 1994, WB Saunders, 423–442.

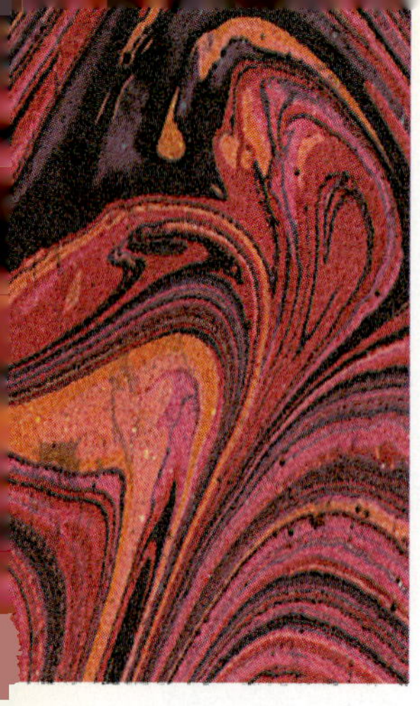

Chapter 49

Syphilis, Tuberculosis, and Other Infections

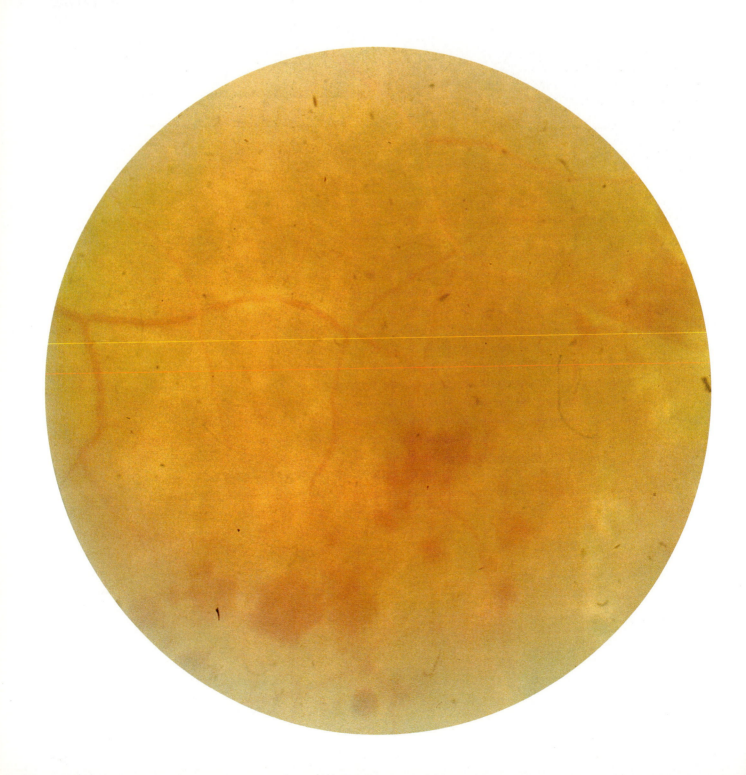

Ophthalmic manifestations of syphilis and tuberculosis are rare but important to diagnose due to the systemic consequences. Congenital syphilis is associated with a pigmentary retinopathy. A patchy, diffuse neuroretinitis is more commonly seen with acquired syphilis. Hemorrhages may be present. Patches of chorioretinal infiltrates may be seen next to pigmented scars in some cases. Two patterns may be seen: a diffuse irregular pigmentation along the major vessels, and a slowly progressive mixed atrophic and pigmentary retinopathy. Papillitis is rare but may be seen with secondary syphilis as well. Placoid choroidal involvement also may be seen with secondary syphilis.

Ophthalmic findings in tuberculosis include chronic iridocyclitis, periphlebitis, tuberculous focal choroiditis, hemorrhage, and multifocal choroiditis.

49–1 SYPHILIS

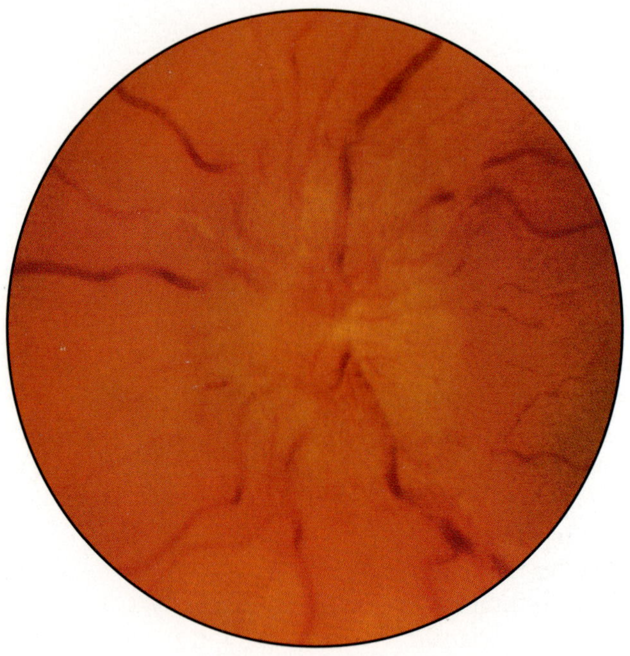

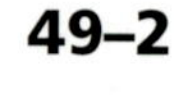

49–2

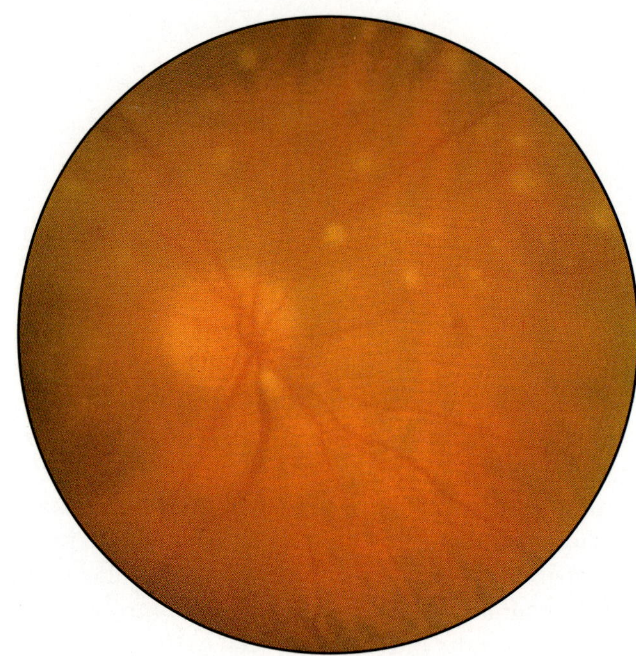

49–3

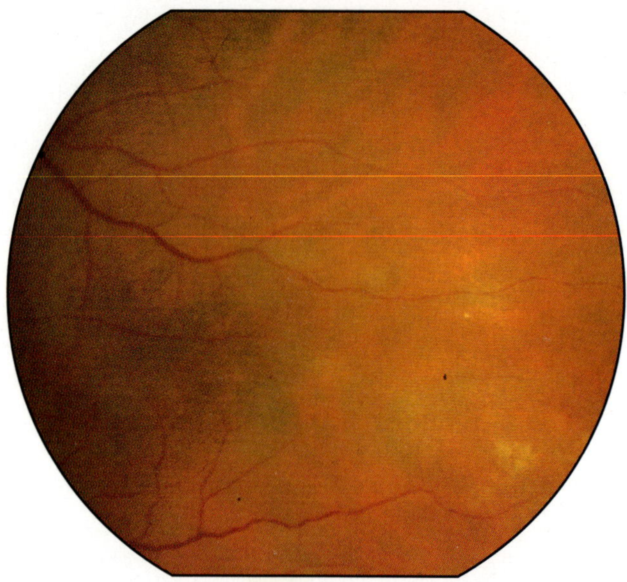

49–1 Syphilis can present with various different ophthalmic manifestations including optic disc edema.

49–2 Multiple yellowish-white spots may appear in the fundus associated with vitreous inflammatory changes.

49–3 Some patients present with a mild vasculitis, as demonstrated in this patient with vasculature narrowing, perivascular inflammation and sheathing in the peripheral fundus.

__49–1__ and __49–3__, From Folk, JF, et al: Syphilitic neuroretinitis, Am J Ophthalmol 95:480–485, 1983. Published with permission of the American Journal of Ophthalmology. Copyright by the Ophthalmic Publishing Company.

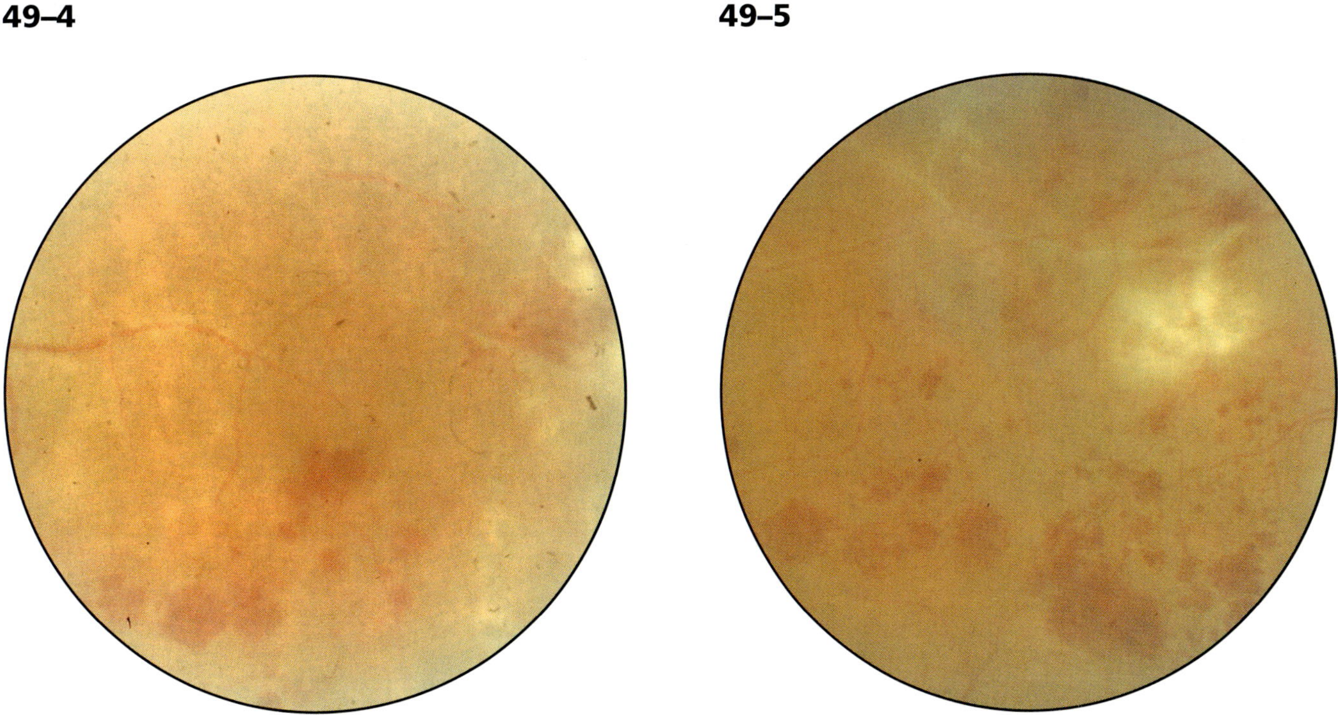

49–4 In this patient, the retinal vascular changes are associated with scattered hemorrhages and multifocal areas of whitening from infection within the retina.

49–5 The findings are similar in this patient, but more severe. Note the retinal vascular narrowing, sheathing, and whitening. There is a focal area of retinal infection and scattered hemorrhages, which are in the geographic distribution of at least two adjacent venules. These hemorrhages are often due to venous occlusive disease, as the inflammatory process within the retina obstructs the vessel.

***49–4** and **49–5,** Courtesy of Dr. David Knox.*

49–6 SYPHILIS

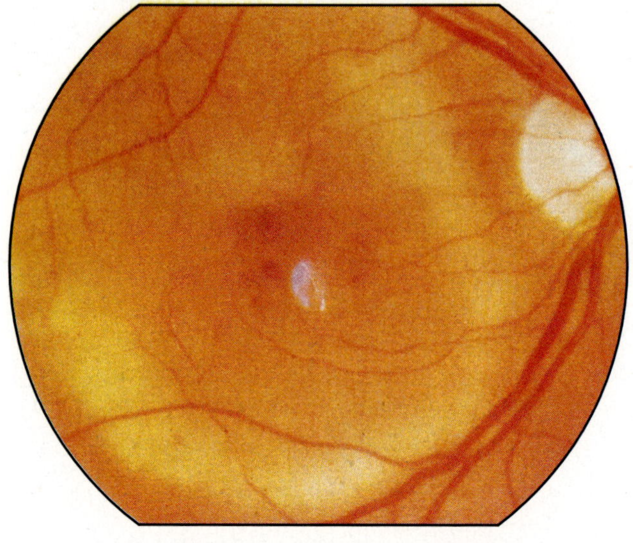

49–7

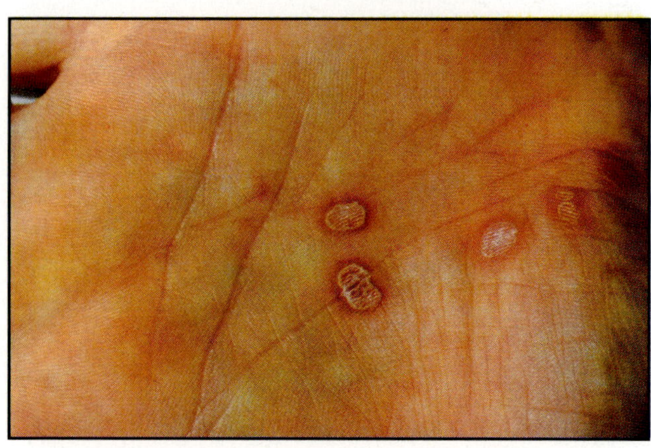

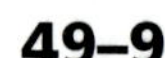

49–8

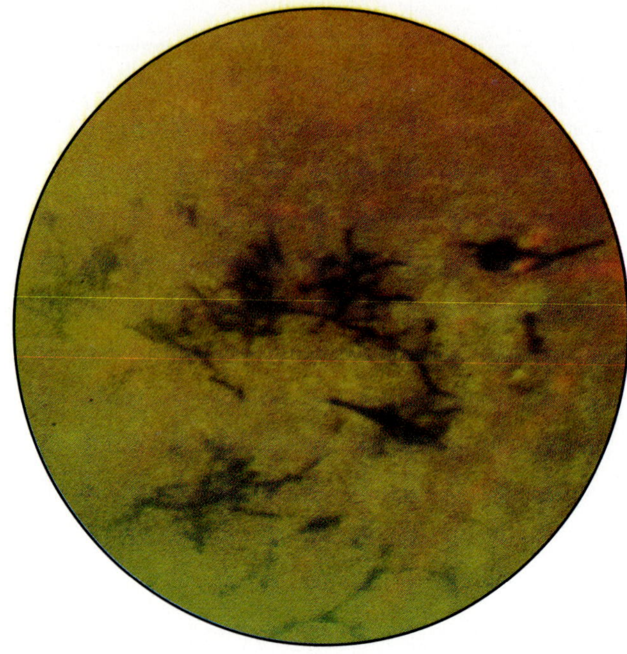

49–9

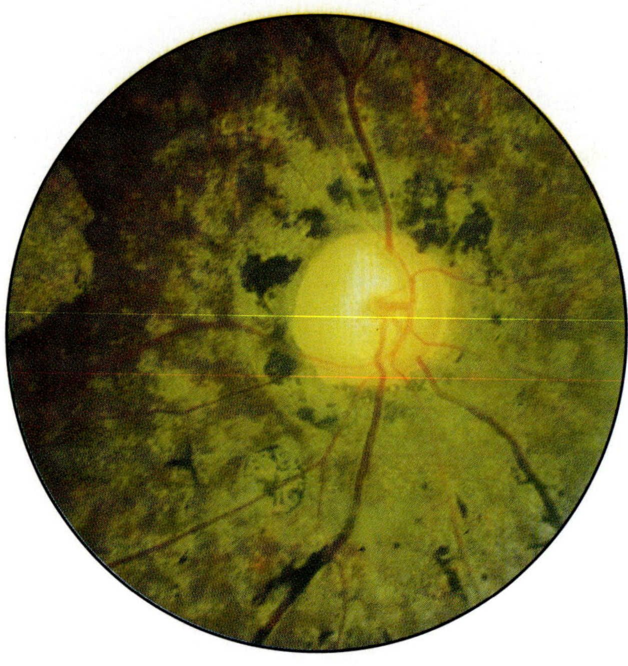

49–6 Some patients will demonstrate zonular areas of outer retinal whitening from a placoid type of chorioretinal infection which is seen with secondary syphilis. An incomplete ring of outer retinal whitening is noted in this patient with syphilitic placoid chorioretinitis. There is a cluster of hemorrhages in the central macula. As this acute reaction subsides, it reveals a corresponding area of pigment epithelial atrophy and stippling.

49–7 Chancres may occur in secondary syphilis.

49–8 and 49–9 In congenital syphilis, a retinitis pigmentosa–like presentation can occur. Note the optic disc pallor (49–9).

49–6, *From deSouza, J, et al: Am J Ophthalmol 105:271–276, 1988. Published with permission of the American Journal of Ophthalmology. Copyright by the Ophthalmic Publishing Company.* ***49–7,*** *Courtesy of Dr. R.G. Chenoweth.* ***49–8,*** *Courtesy of Dr. Irene Maumenee.* ***49–9,*** *Courtesy of Dr. David Knox.*

49–10

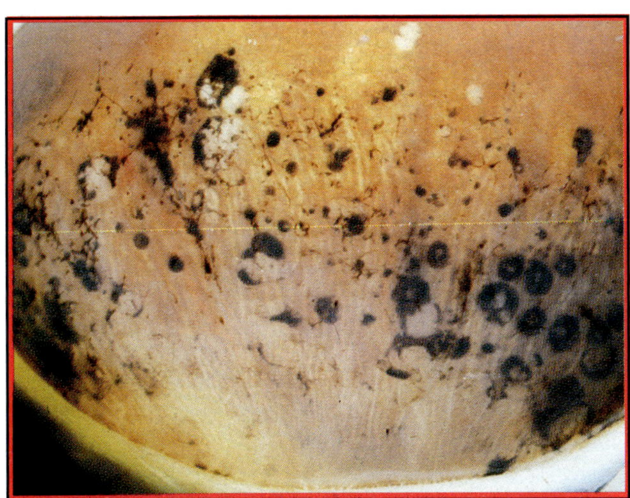

49–11

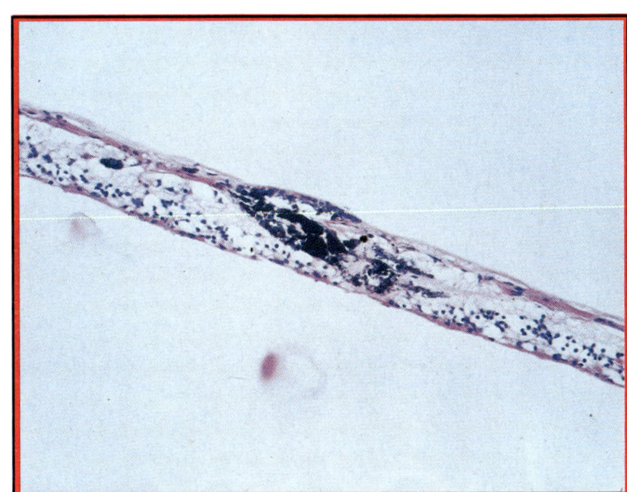

49–12

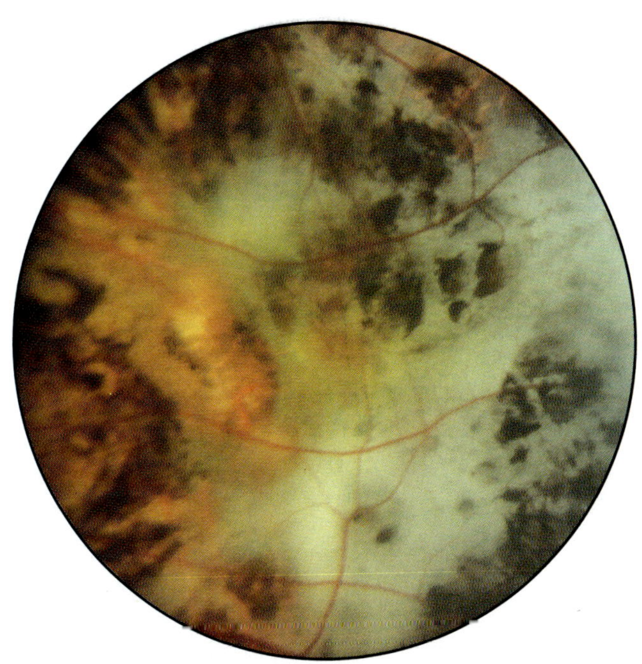

49–10 This photograph shows the bone-spicule-like appearance of such patients. This morphological picture has been termed a "salt-and-pepper" fundus.

49–11 Light microscopy reveals a loss of the photoreceptor cell layer and hyperplasia of the retinal pigment epithelium with migration into the retina in a perivascular location.

49–12 In this patient, there is massive subretinal fibrosis in addition to pigment epithelial atrophy and hyperplasia.

49–10, *Courtesy of Dr. David Knox.*

49–13 TUBERCULOSIS

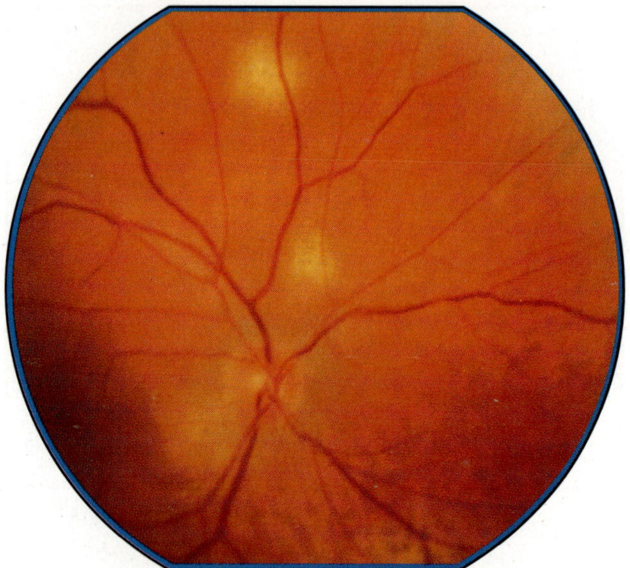

49–14

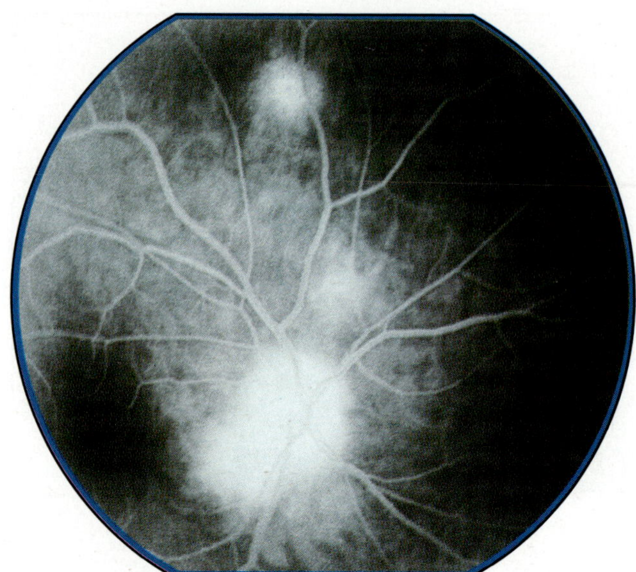

49–15

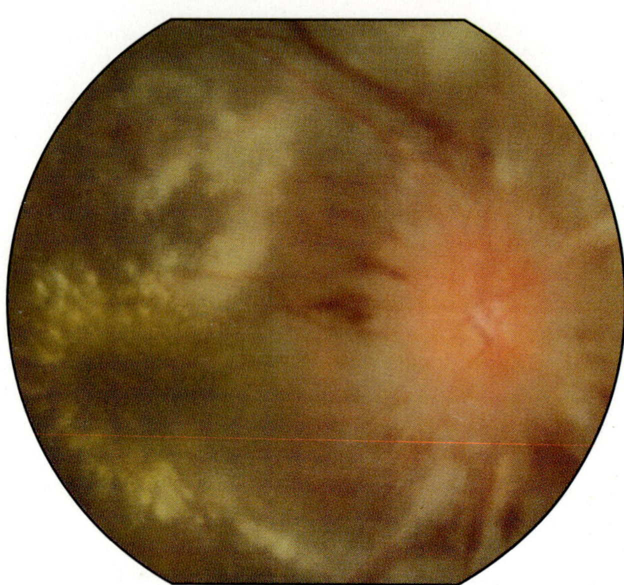

49–13 and 49–14 Ocular findings of tuberculosis include iridocyclitis and periphlebitis of the retinal vessels. Granulomas of the choroid may also occur. A focal or more diffuse choroiditis can be seen with miliary tuberculosis. Choroidal infiltration secondary to tuberculosis was noted in this patient. Note the whitish-yellow choroidal lesions that show hyperfluorescence on the fluorescein angiogram. An open lung biopsy diagnosed the tuberculosis.

49–15 This patient has massive optic disc swelling, as well as lipid exudation secondary to a granuloma due to tuberculosis.

***49–13** and **49–14,** Courtesy of Dr. Richard Spaide.*

49–16

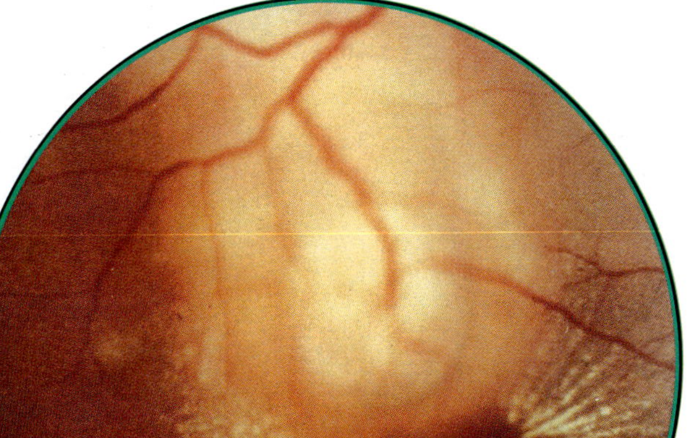

49–17

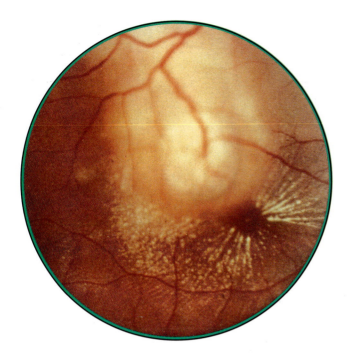

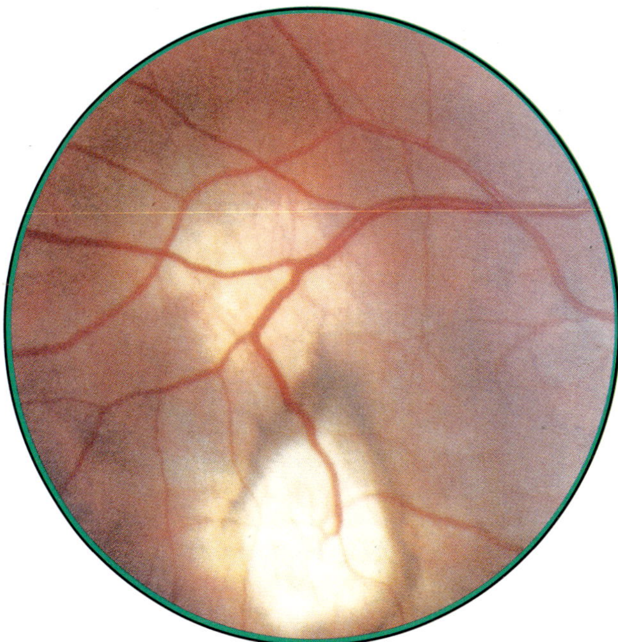

49–18

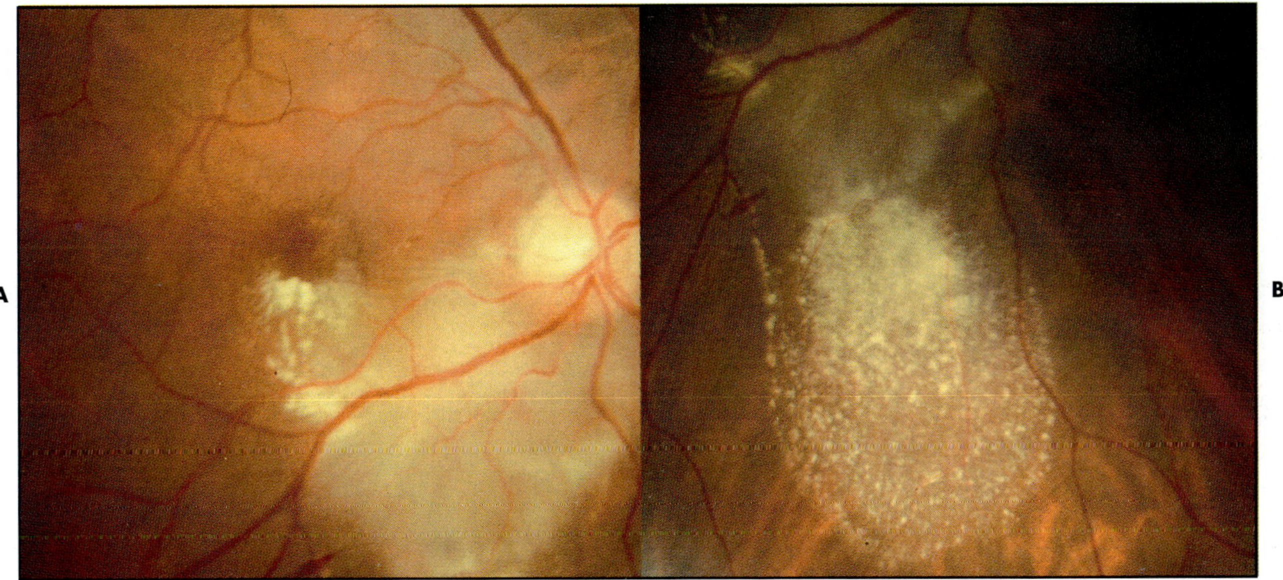

49–16 and 49–17 A chorioretinal tuberculoma with a macular star is demonstrated (49–16) that healed after antituberculosis therapy (49–17). Note the regressed scar with a retinal-choroidal anastomosis and perifoveal atrophy.

49–18 This patient with tuberculosis has a granuloma with an exudative detachment.

***49–16** and **49–17,** From Cangemi, FE, et al: Tuberculoma of the choroid, Ophthalmology 87:252–258, 1980. **49–18,** Courtesy of Dr. Scott Sneed.*

49–19 TUBERCULOSIS

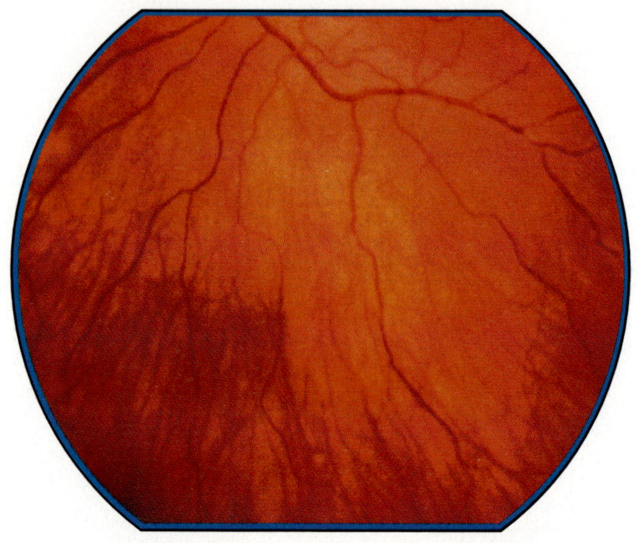

49–20

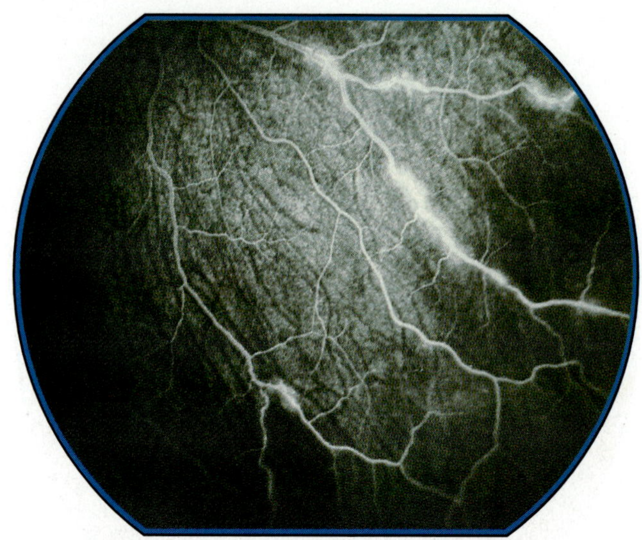

49–21

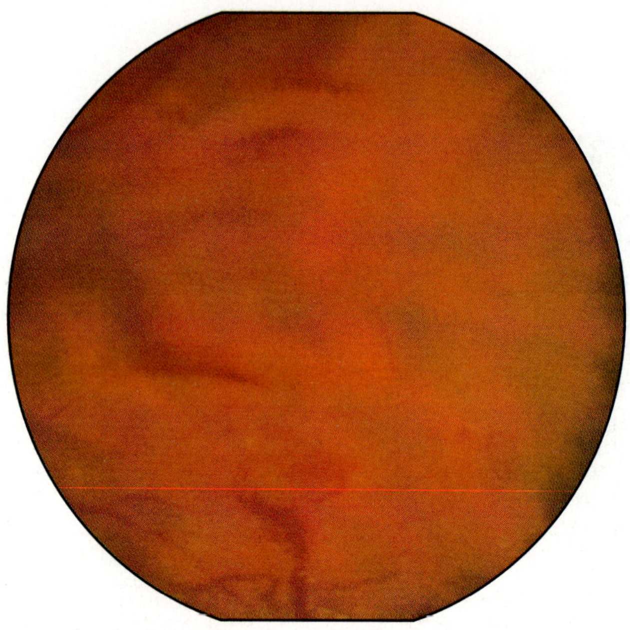

49–22

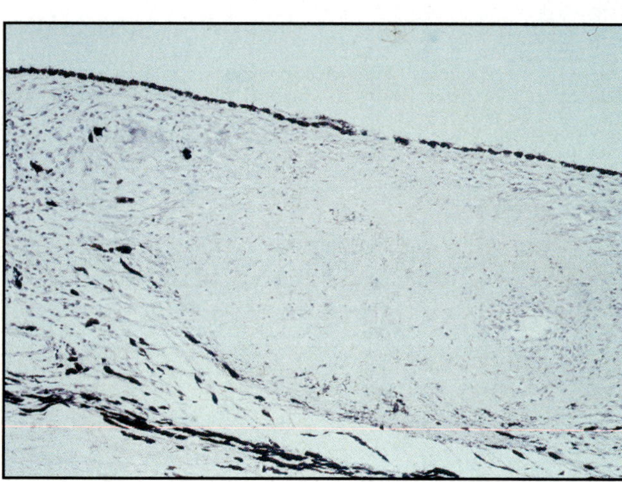

49–19 and 49–20 The color photograph of this patient with tuberculosis reveals peripheral, irregular, and dilated venules. There is swelling or periphlebitis along the course of the infratemporal vein and at a focal point along the course of a branch of an infranasal vessel. The fluorescein angiogram reveals perivascular staining.

49–21 Retinal vascular changes are more advanced in this patient with tuberculosis. There are a few aneurysmal dilatory changes, obliterated vessels, preretinal neovascularization, and vitreous hemorrhage. The later manifestation obscures some of the fundus details.

49–22 A granuloma is demonstrated in the choroid secondary to miliary tuberculosis.

49–22, *From Green, WR: Retina. In Spencer, WH, ed: Ophthalmic pathology. An atlas and textbook, vol 2, Philadelphia, 1985, WB Saunders, pp 589–1291.*

49–23 RIFT VALLEY FEVER

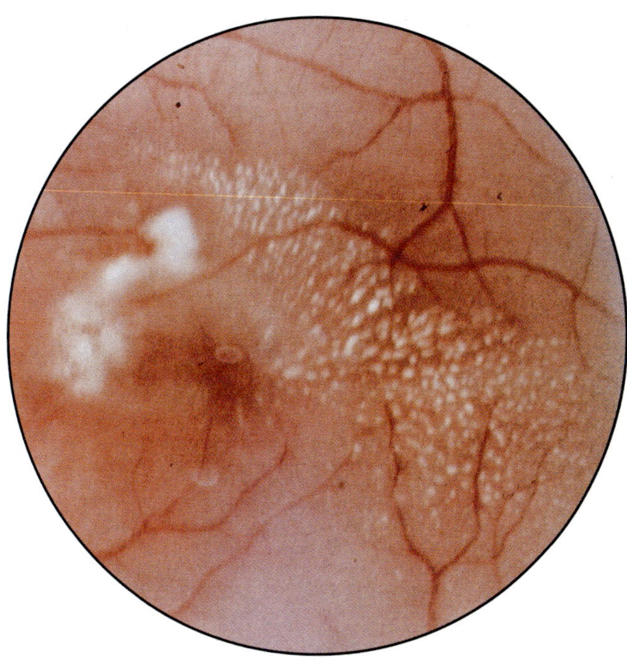

49–24 TULAREMIA

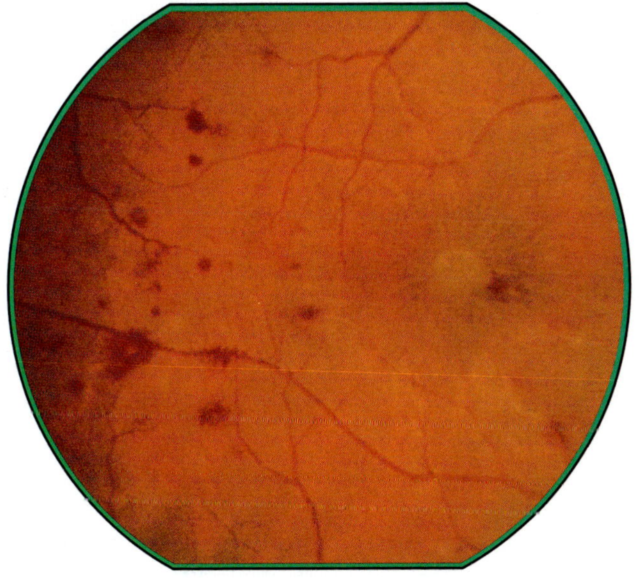

49–25

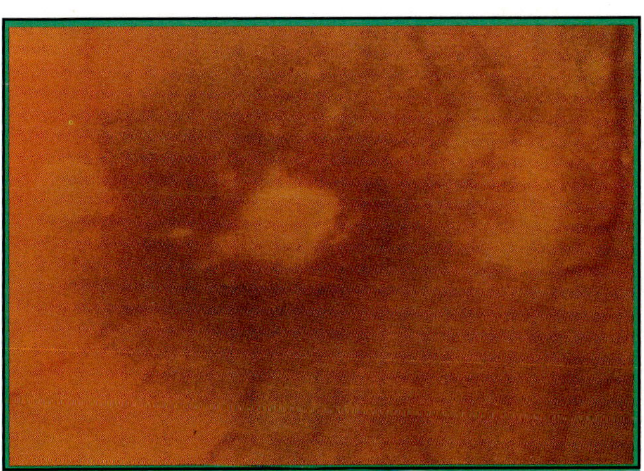

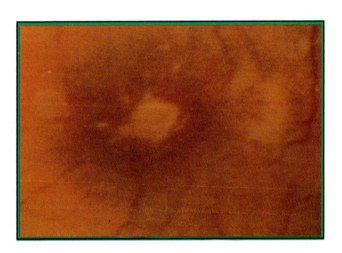

Various other infections may rarely invade the eye.

49–23 Cotton-wool spots and lipid exudation with a macular star formation is noted in this patient with Rift Valley fever.

49–24 and 49–25 Fundus appearance reveals deep retinal hemorrhages, Roth spots, superficial perivascular retinal infiltrates, and a subfoveal inflammatory focus with radiating striae secondary to tularemia.

49–23, *Courtesy of Dr. Maurice Luntz.* ***49–24*** *and* ***49–25,*** *From Marcus, DM, Frederick, AR, Hodges, T, Allan, JD, Albert, DM: Typhoidal tularemia, Arch Ophthalmol 108:118–119, 1990. Copyright 1990, American Medical Association.*

49–26 RUBELLA

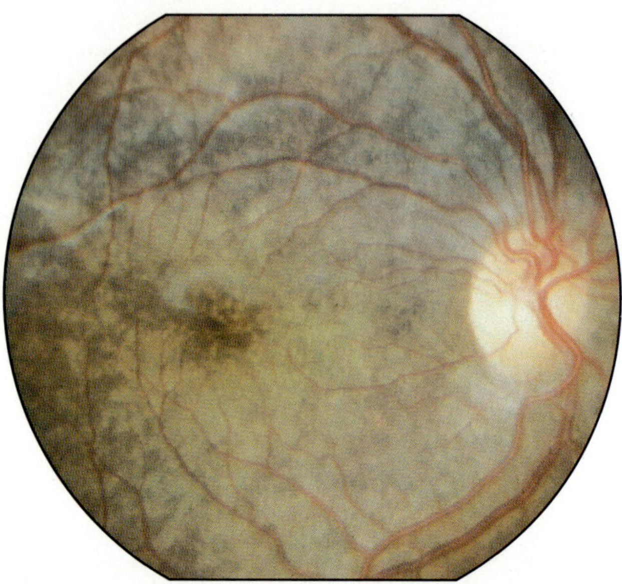

49–27

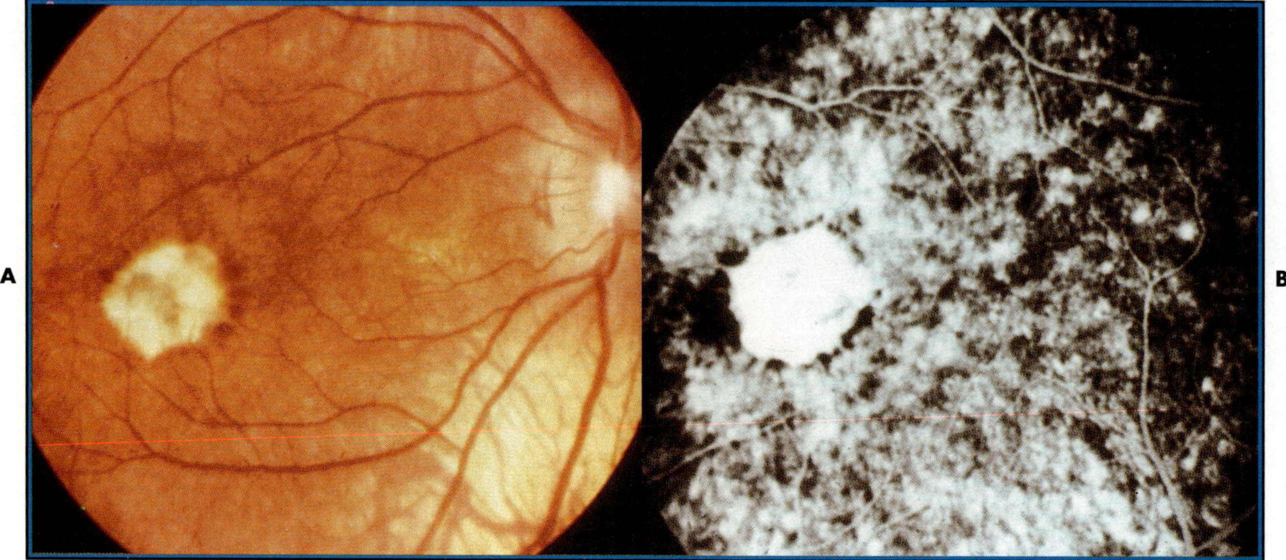

49–26 A salt-and-pepper type of retinopathy may be associated with rubella.

49–27 Rarely, choroidal neovascularization may occur in patients with rubella retinopathy.

49–28 CAT-SCRATCH FEVER

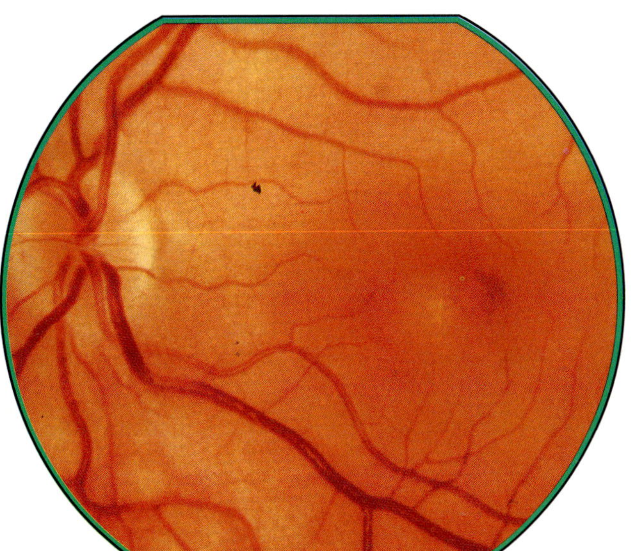

49–29

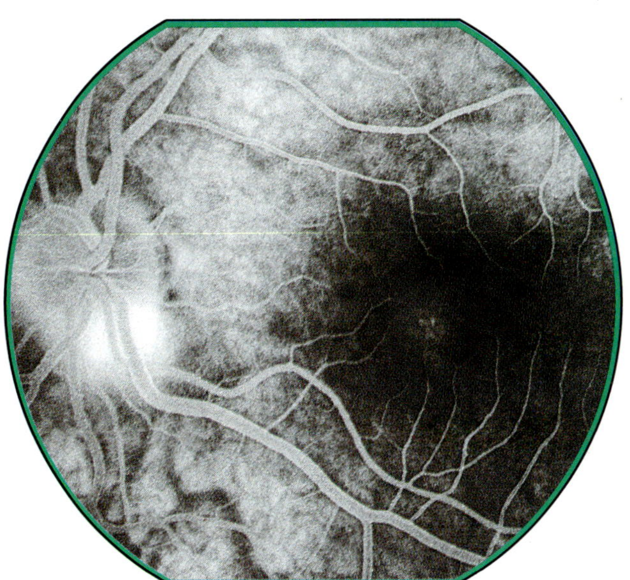

49–28 and 49–29 This 32-year-old female developed a whitish chorioretinal lesion near the macula, which showed hyperfluorescence on the fluorescein angiogram. An area of optic disc hyperfluorescence was also noted. This retinopathy was secondary to cat-scratch fever. The patient also had lymphadenopathy.

49–28 *and* ***49–29,*** *Courtesy of Dr. Thomas Aaberg.*

49–30 *NOCARDIA*

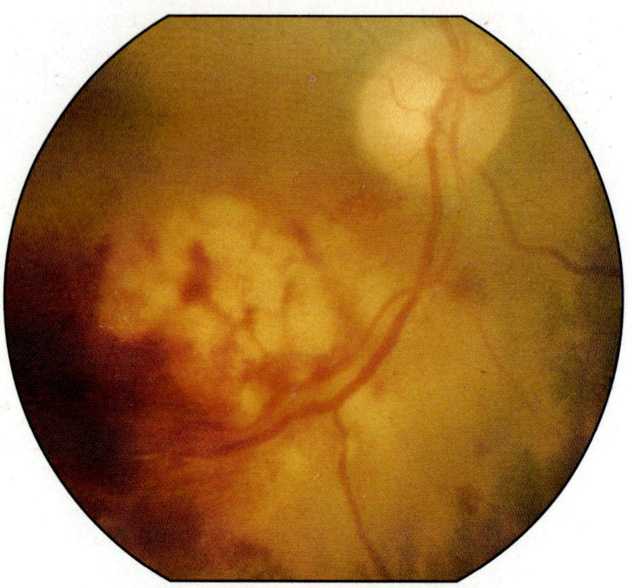

49–31

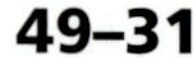

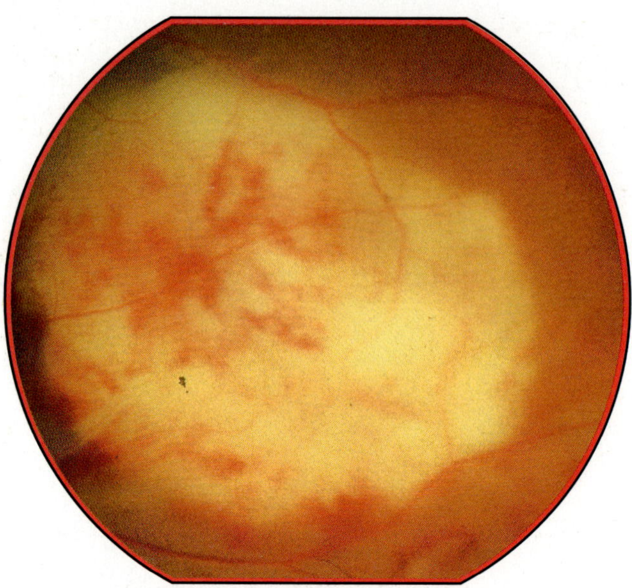

49–30 This patient has a choroiditis secondary to the bacterium *Nocardia.*

49–31 This patient has a subretinal inflammatory mass with hemorrhage and vitreous reaction secondary to the bacterium *Nocardia,* which was diagnosed by transvitreal fine-needle aspiration biopsy. There was also widespread retinal vasculitis and detachment.

49–30, *From Jampol, L, et al: Intraocular nocardiosis, Am J Ophthalmol 76:568, 1973. Published with permission of the American Journal of Ophthalmology. Copyright by the Ophthalmic Publishing Company.* ***49–31,*** *Reprinted from Gregor, RJ, Chong, CA, Augsburger, JJ, et al: Endogenous* Nocardia asteroides *subretinal abscess diagnosed by transvitreal fine-needle aspiration biopsy, Retina 9:118–121, 1989.*

(Case continued on next page.)

49–32

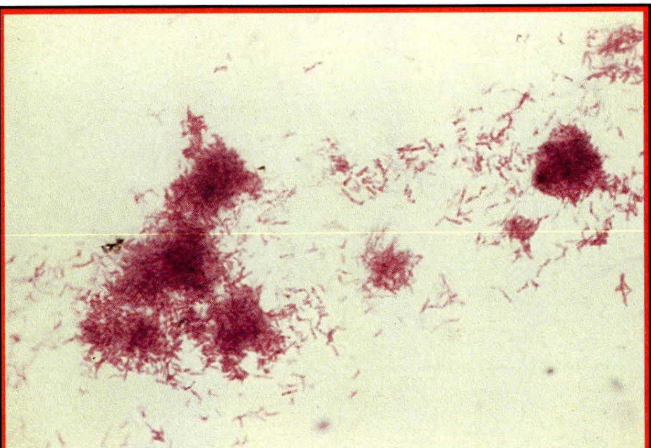

49–33

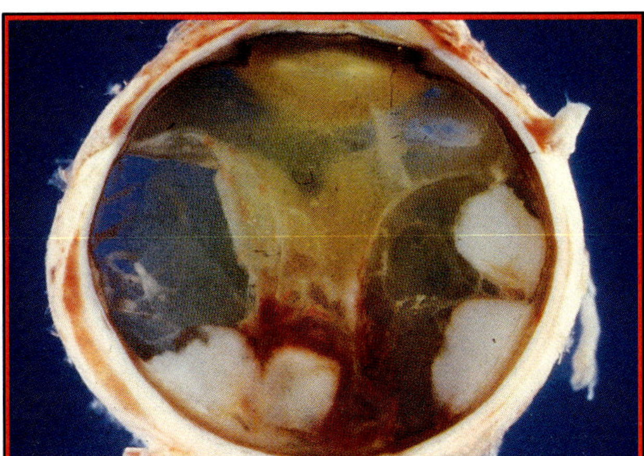

49–34

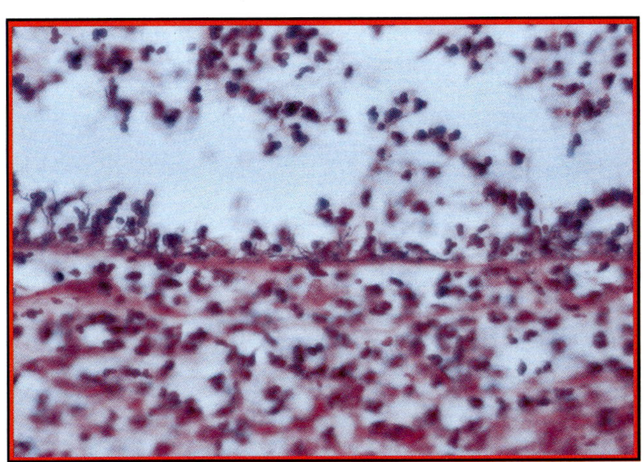

49–32 The transvitreal needle aspiration biopsy revealed *Nocardia*.

49–33 and 49–34 Histopathologic examination of another case reveals subretinal pigment epithelial whitish abscesses with organisms located along the inner aspect of Bruch's membrane.

49–32, *Reprinted from Gregor, RJ, Chong, CA, Augsburger, JJ, et al: Endogenous* Nocardia asteroides *subretinal abscess diagnosed by transvitreal fine-needle aspiration biopsy, Retina 9:118–121, 1989.* ***49–33*** *and* ***49–34,*** *Courtesy of Dr. Ramon L. Font.*

Suggested Readings

Clark, EG, and Danbolt, N: The Oslo study of the natural course of untreated syphilis, an epidemiologic investigation based on a re-study of the Boeck-Bruusgaard material, Clin North Am 48:613–623, 1964

Daley, CL, Small, PM, Schecter, GF, Schoolnik, GK, McAdam, RA, Jacobs, WR, Jr, and Hopewell, PC: An outbreak of tuberculosis with accelerated progression among persons infected with the human immunodeficiency virus, N Engl J Med 326:231–235, 1992

Darrell, RW: Acute tuberculous panophthalmitis, Arch Ophthalmol 78:51–54, 1967

Fountain, JA, and Werner, RB: Tuberculous retinal vasculitis, Retina 4:48–50, 1984

Levy, JH, Liss, RA, and Maguire, AM: Neurosyphilis and ocular syphilis in patients with concurrent human immunodeficiency virus infection, Retina 9:175–180, 1989

Mascola, L, Pelosi, R, Blount, JH, Binkin, NJ, Alexander, CE, and Cates, W, Jr: Congenital syphilis: why is it still occurring? JAMA 252:1719–1722, 1984

Ryan, SJ, Jr, Nell, EE, and Hardy, PH: A study of aqueous humor for the presence of spirochetes, Am J Ophthalmol 73:250–257, 1972

Theobald, GD: Acute tuberculous endophthalmitis, Trans Am Ophthalmol Soc 55:325, 1957

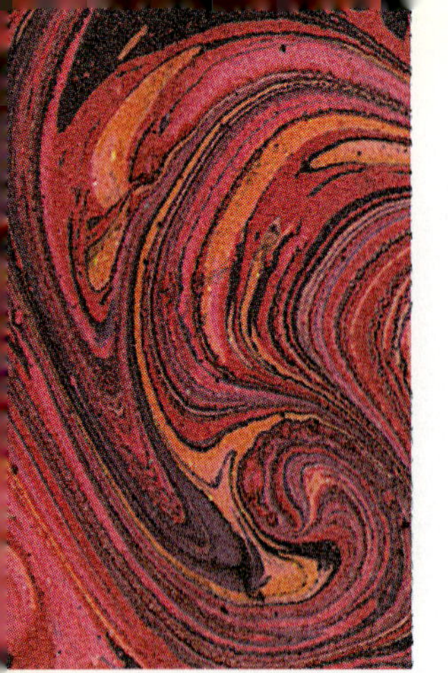

Chapter 50

Myiasis and Diffuse Unilateral Subacute Neuroretinitis

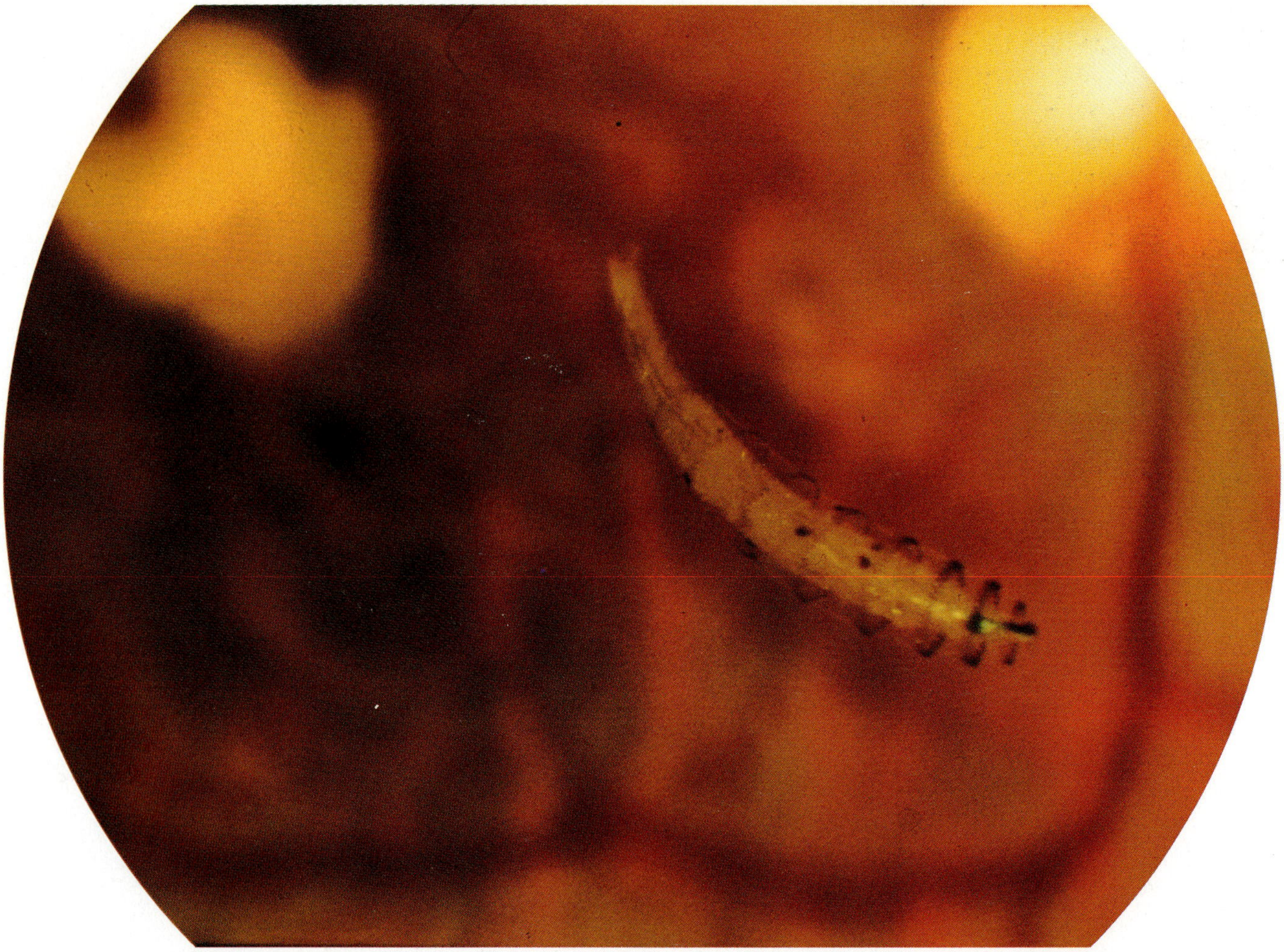

Various worms may invade the eye. This chapter presents a survey of such intraocular worms as well as illustrations of the diffuse unilateral subacute neuroretinitis syndrome (DUSN). DUSN is an infectious disease caused by a nematode. It has been previously called the unilateral wipe-out syndrome because of the profound unilateral vision loss that may occur with this condition. In the United States, DUSN is especially seen in the southeast as well as the midwest. It appears that two different nematodes are seen in the various geographic regions. Active gray-white outer retinal lesions are often noted. The nematode may also be seen in some cases.

50–1 MYIASIS

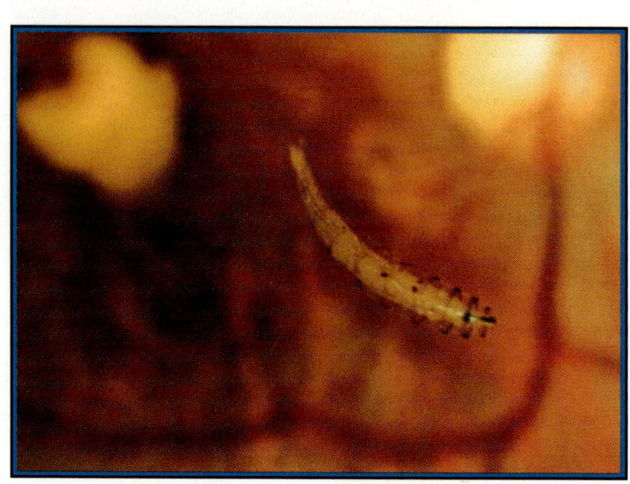

50–2

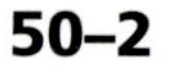

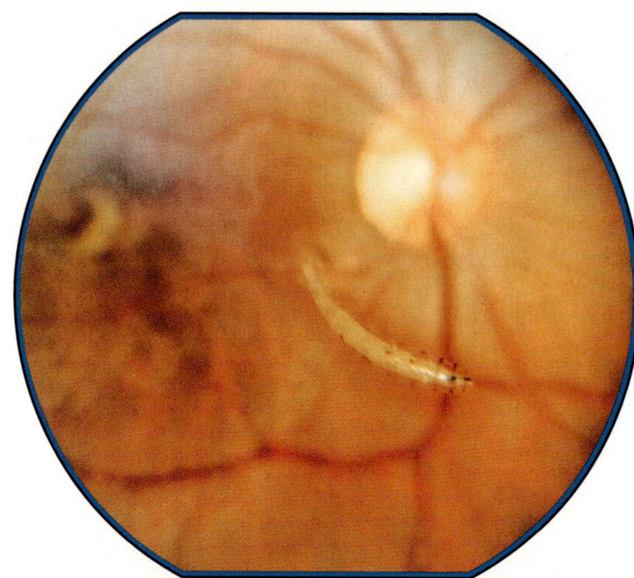

50–3

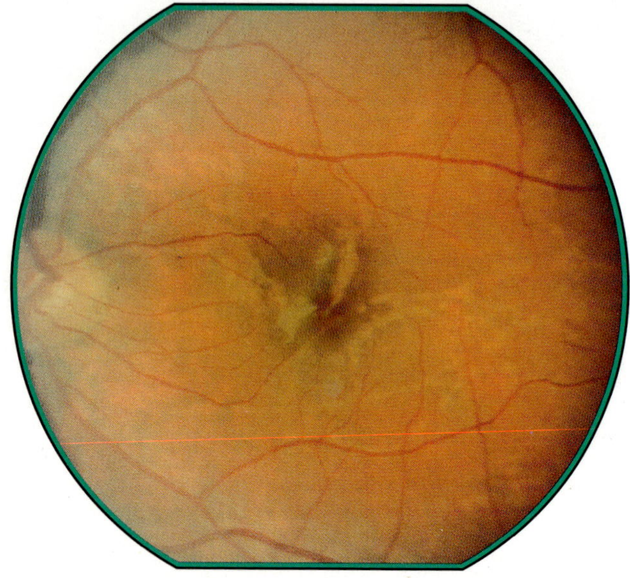

50–4

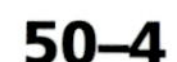

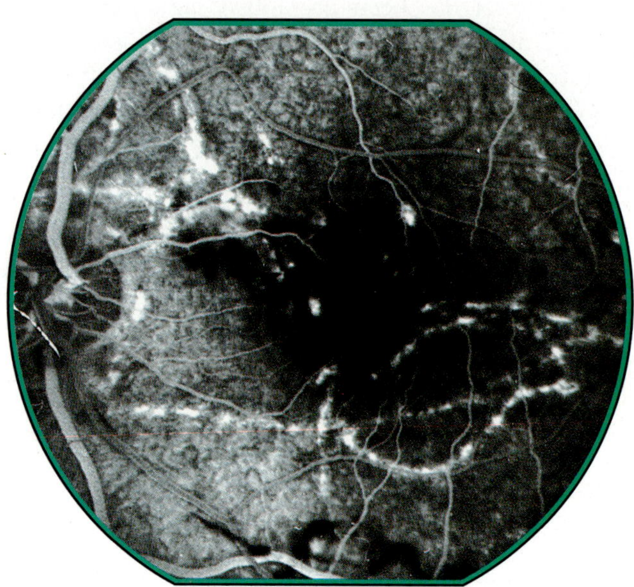

50–1 and 50–2 The following cases demonstrate examples of various worms that may invade the eye. A fly larva was noted in the vitreous cavity in this patient. One year later, the larva appeared stable.

50–3 and 50–4 This patient has atrophic tracks noted both clinically (50–3) and by fluorescein angiography (50–4).

50–1 *and* ***50–2,*** *Courtesy of Kenneth G. Julian, CRA, FOPS.* ***50–3*** *and* ***50–4,*** *From Fitzgerald, CR, and Rubin, ML: Intraocular parasite destroyed by photocoagulation: a case report, Arch Ophthalmol 91:162–164, 1974.Copyright 1974, American Medical Association.*

(Case continued on next page.)

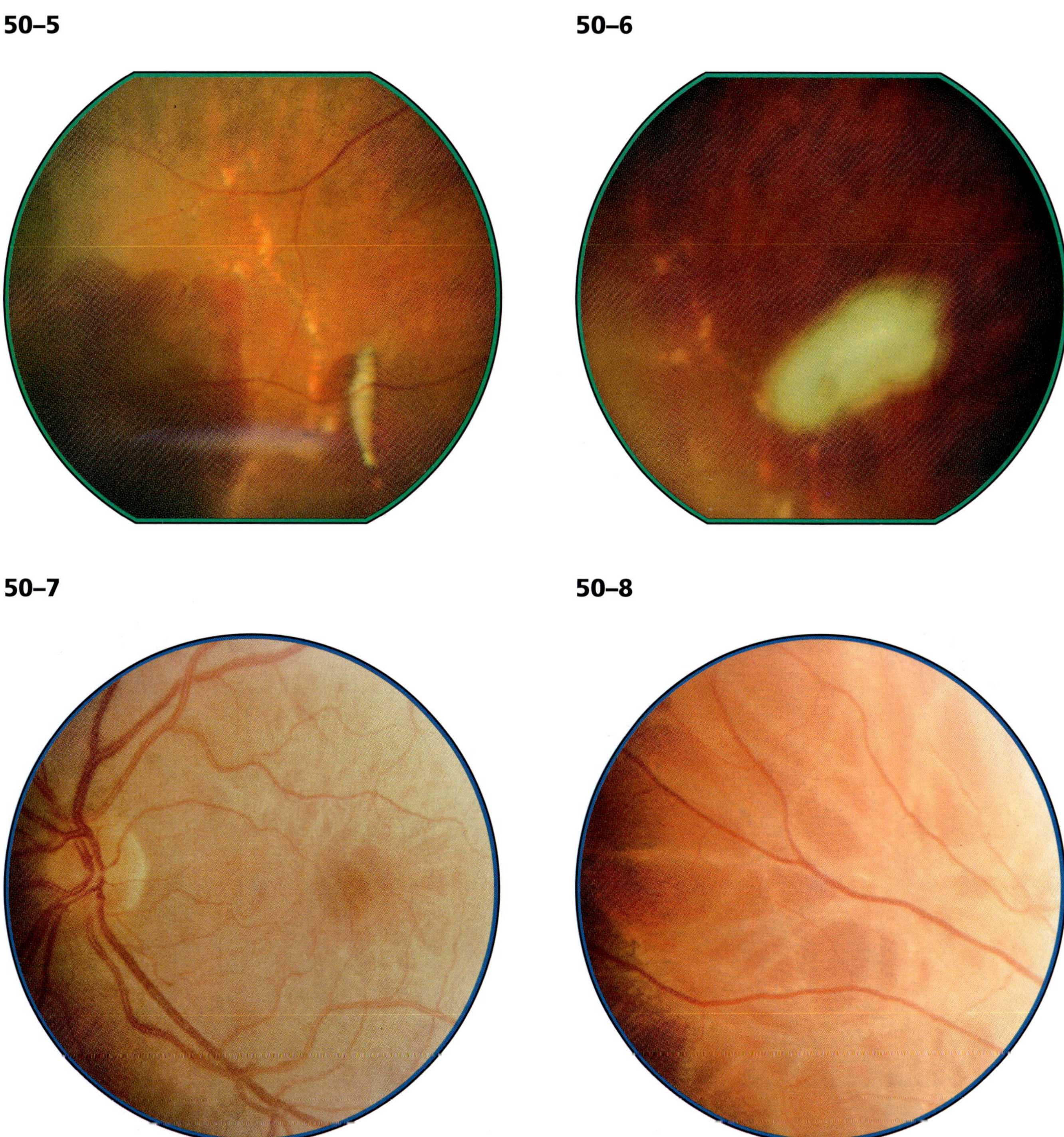

50–5 The worm was isolated near a patch of subretinal hemorrhage. Note the atrophic tract between the worm and hemorrhage.

50–6 Laser photocoagulation was applied to the worm with obliteration of the organism.

50–7 and 50–8 Atrophic tracts are also noted in this patient.

__50–5__ and __50–6,__ From Fitzgerald, CR, and Rubin, ML: Intraocular parasite destroyed by photocoagulation: a case report, Arch Ophthalmol 91:162–164, 1974. Copyright 1974, American Medical Association. __50–7__ and __50–8,__ Courtesy of Dr. Miriam Ridley.

(Case continued on next page.)

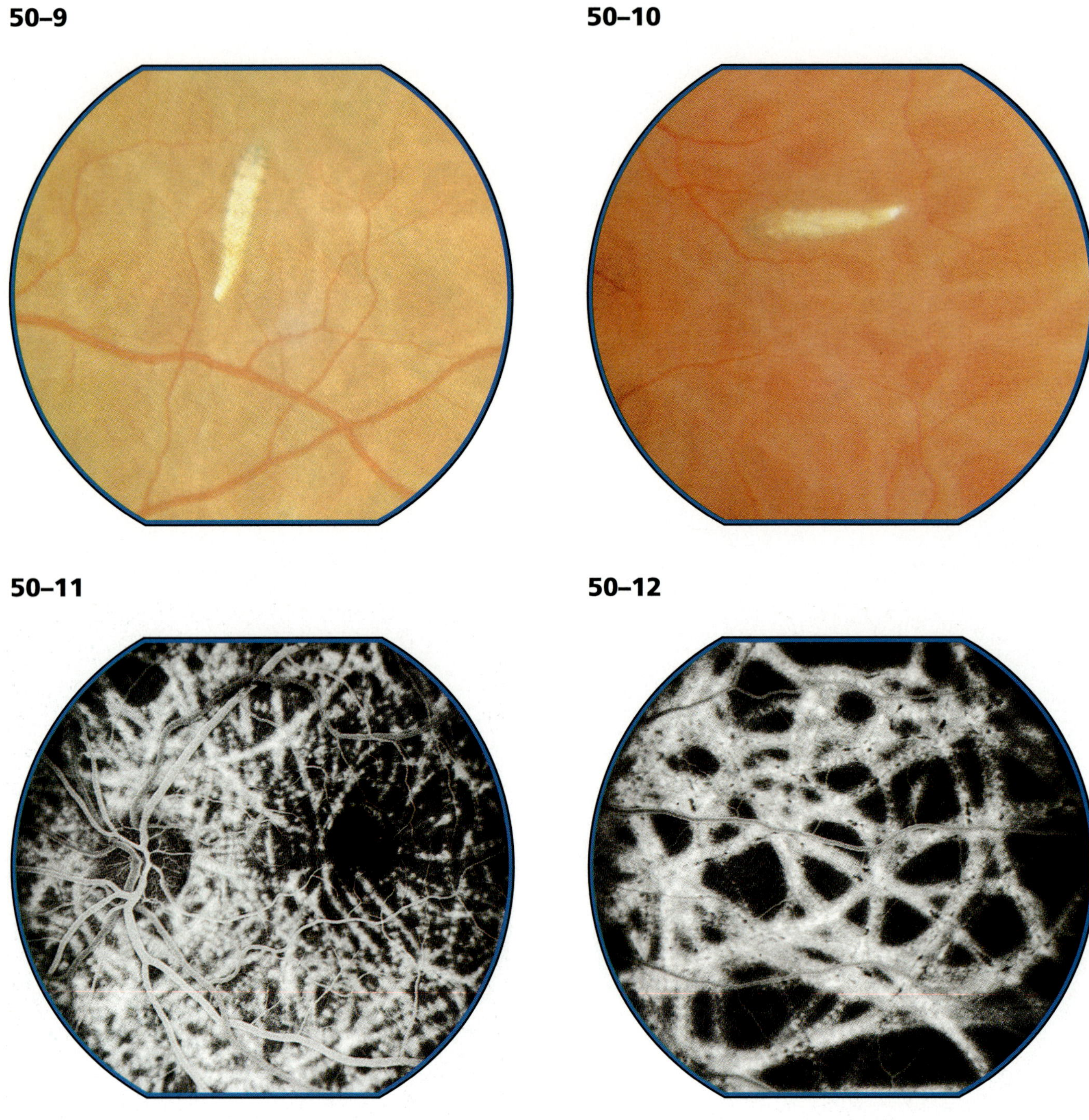

50–9 and 50–10 A motile maggot can be demonstrated in the midperiphery. Note the surrounding atrophic tracts.

50–11 and 50–12 The maggot is evident in the fovea (50–11). Fluorescein angiography illustrates the atrophic tracts.

50–9 *through* ***50–12,*** *Courtesy of Dr. Miriam Ridley.*

50–13 GNATHOSTOMIASIS

50–14

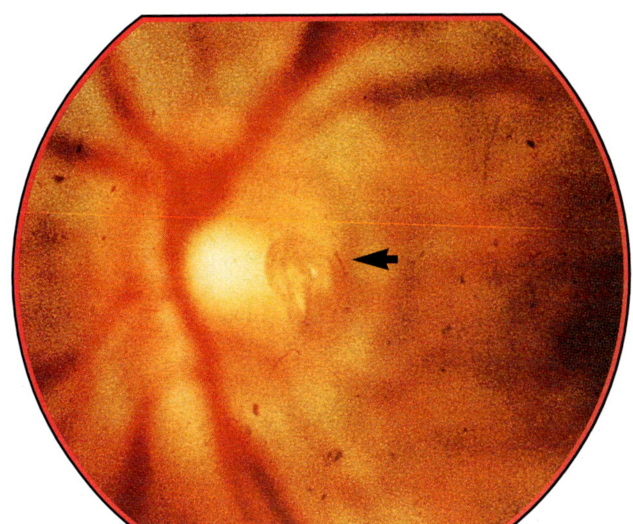

50–15

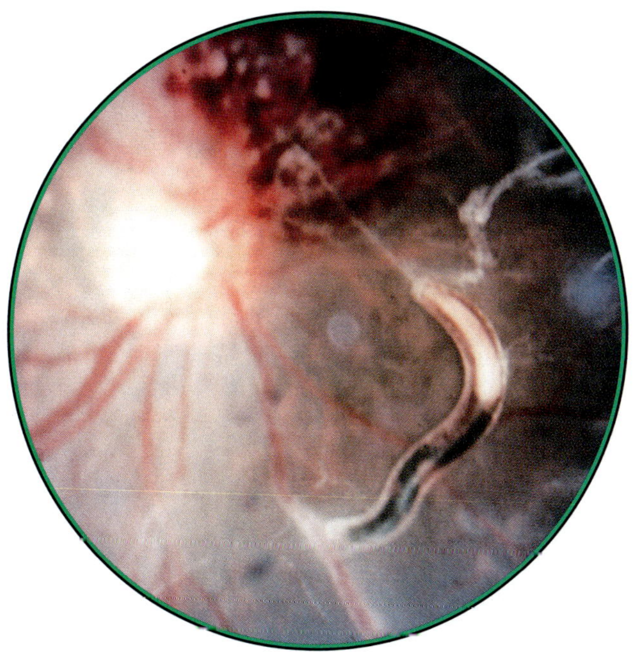

50–16

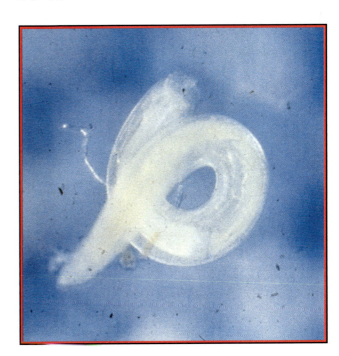

50–13 and 50–14 The next case illustrates gnathostomiasis, which is caused by the larva of the nematode *Gnathostoma spinigerum.* The living worm can be seen in the vitreous over the disc *(arrowheads).*

50–15 Another case of intraocular gnathostomiasis shows the worm, blood, and waste material.

50–16 The worm in 50–13 and 50–14 measures approximately 1.5 mm in length and has a knoblike structure at the cephalic end.

50–13, 50–14, *and* ***50–16,*** *From Funata, M, et al: Intraocular gnathostomiasis, Retina 13:240–244, 1993.* ***50–15,*** *Courtesy of Dr. Charles Mango.*

(Case continued on next page.)

50–17 GNATHOSTOMIASIS

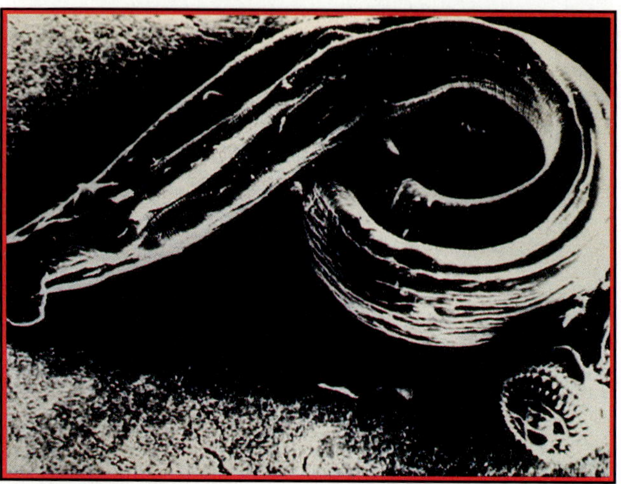

50–18

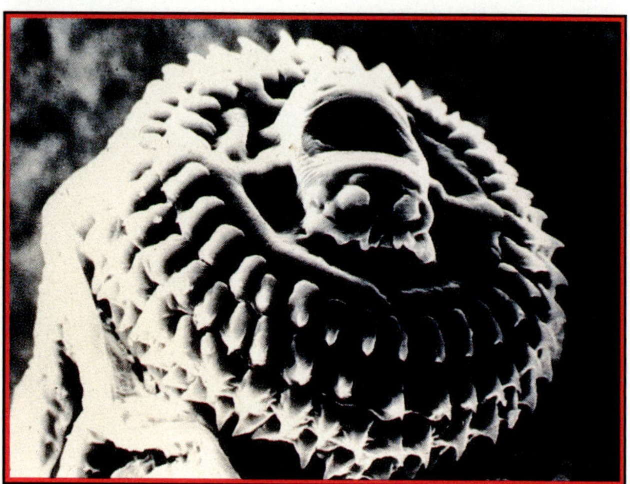

50–19

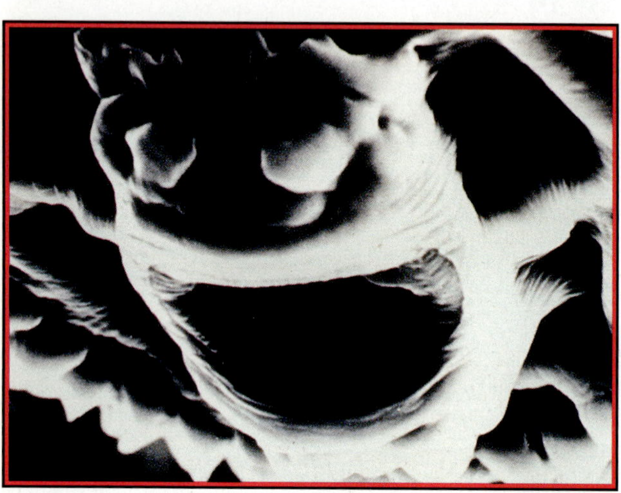

50–17 Scanning electron micrograph appearance of the parasite in 50–13 with a segmented head bulb *(bottom right).*

50–18 Higher-power view of the head bulb, with four rows of hooklets. The mouth is located at the center of the head bulb and has two lips with sensory papillae.

50–19 Higher view of the mouth and lips of the parasite. Each lip has a pair of sensory papillae.

50–17 *through* ***50–19,*** *From Funata, M, et al: Intraocular gnathostomiasis, Retina 13:240–244, 1993.*

50–20 ONCHOCERCIASIS

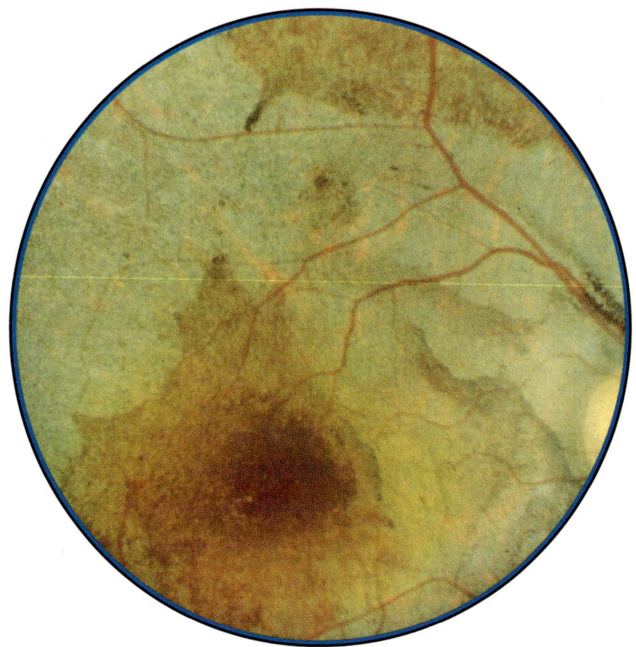

50–21

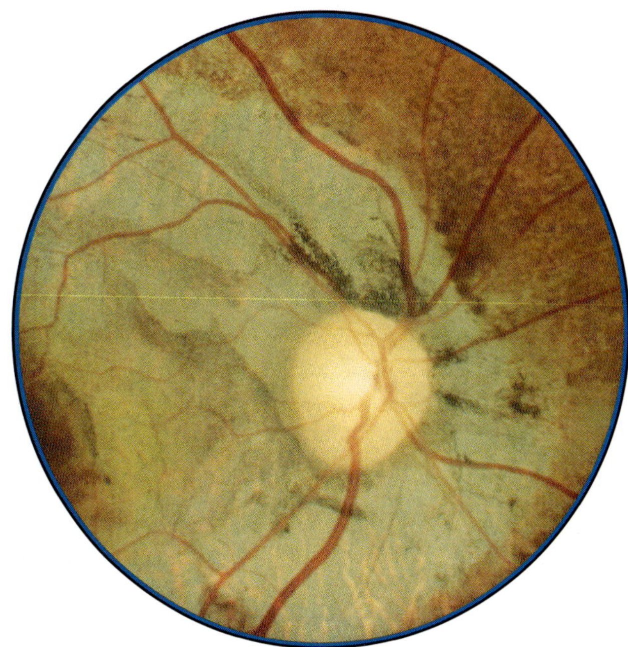

50–22

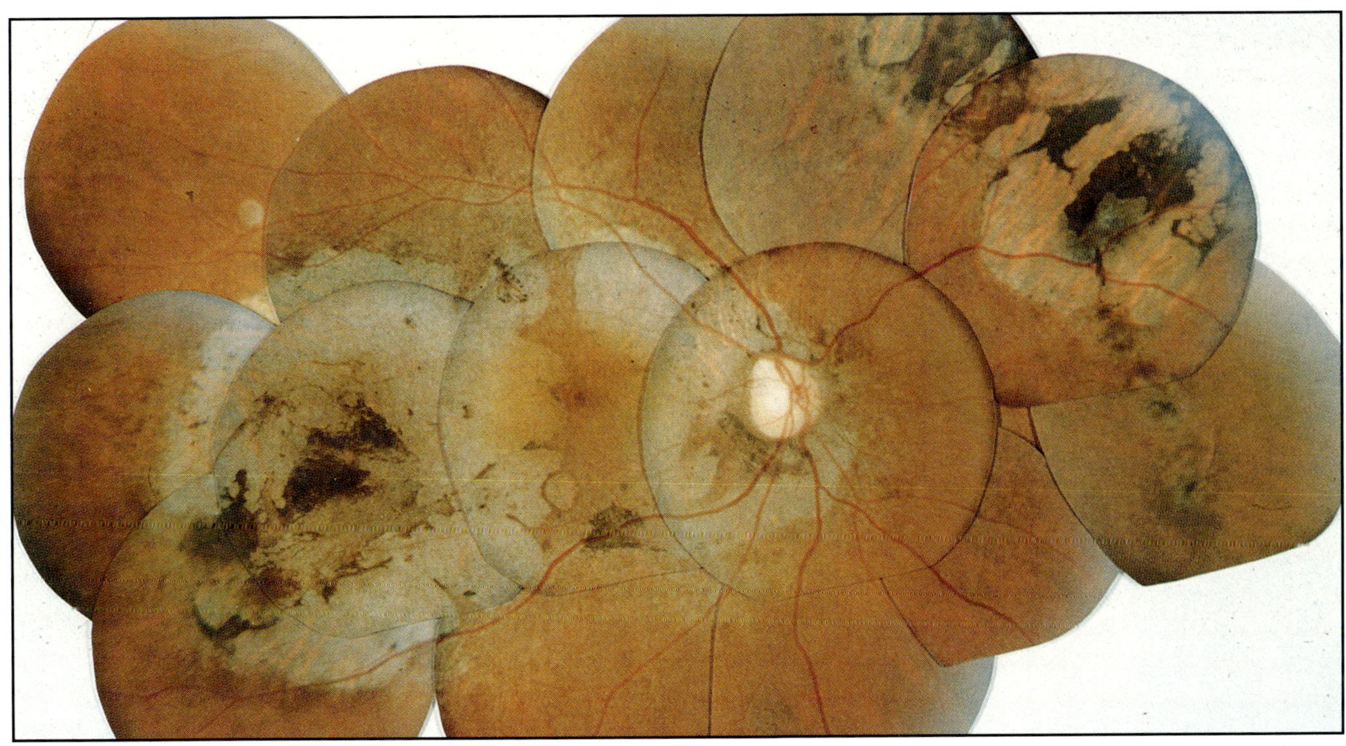

50–20 and 50–21 Extensive chorioretinal scarring can be seen secondary to onchocerciasis. Optic atrophy and vascular attenuation also may be noted (50–21).

50–22 The atrophy may be around the macula or disc or throughout the periphery. An irregular pigmentary response and atrophy are noted.

50–20 *through* ***50–22,*** *Courtesy of Dr. Robert Murphy.*

(Case continued on next page.)

50–23 ONCHOCERCIASIS

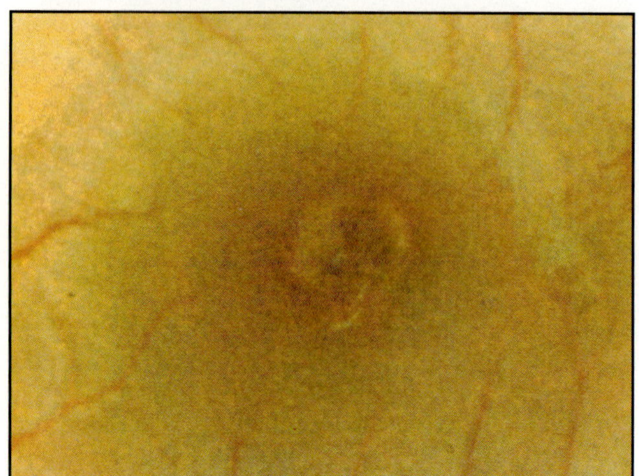

50–24

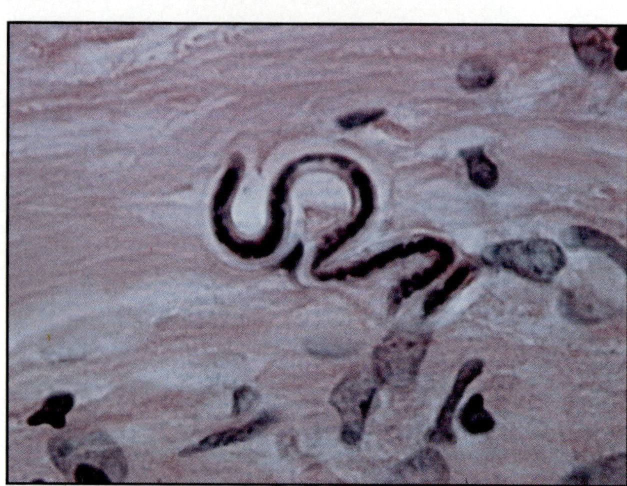

50–23 The macula may also be affected.

50–24 Histopathologic examination of another case reveals the microfilaria.

50–23 *and* ***50–24,*** *Courtesy of Dr. Robert Murphy.*

50–25 Diffuse Unilateral Subacute Neuroretinitis (DUSN)

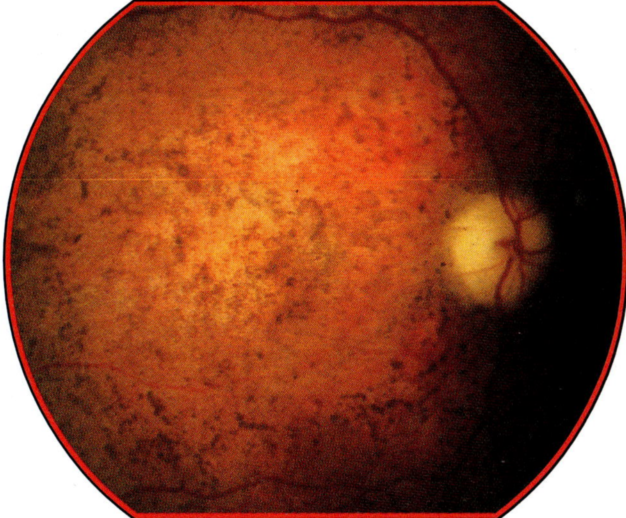

50–26

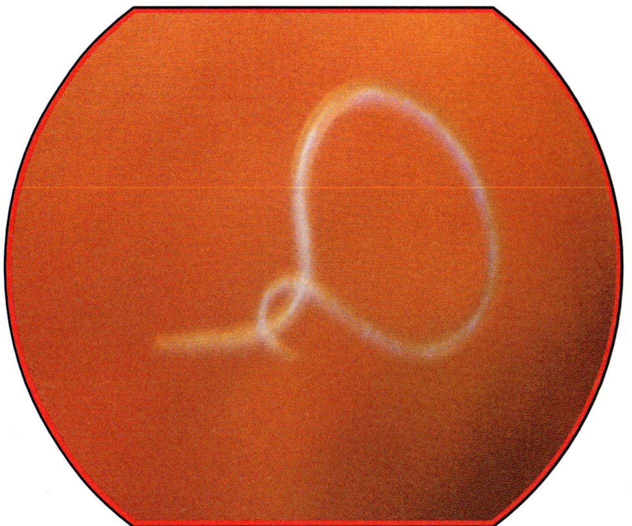

DUSN

Diffuse unilateral subacute neuroretinitis (DUSN), or the so-called unilateral wipeout syndrome, is a condition seen in healthy young patients, which consists of a unilateral severe loss of vision, vitritis, and a pigmentary retinopathy. Often there is optic disc atrophy and attenuation of the retinal vessels. The cause of the condition is a living nematode within the eye. The worm is usually found to lie beneath the retina, although it may rarely be seen in the vitreous. The worm's movement is accelerated by bright light and slowed by red-free illumination. Thus, red-free illumination is most useful to identify these organisms. Laser photocoagulation to the nematode may stop the progression of the disorder. Several types of nematodes may cause this condition, depending upon the geographic location. A smaller nematode (400–1000 μm) is noted in patients in the southeastern United States, whereas a larger nematode (1500–2000 μm) is noted in patients in the northern midwestern United States.

50–25 This patient has a unilateral pigmentary retinopathy with optic atrophy and attenuated vessels. The other eye was normal.

50–26 A coiled wormlike structure was seen in the vitreous cavity. Vitrectomy was performed by Dr. Mark Blumenkranz.

50–27 Scanning electron microscopic appearance of the worm.

***50–25** and **50–26**, Courtesy of Dr. Mark Blumenkranz. **50–27**, Courtesy of Drs. Mark Blumenkranz and W. Richard Green.*

50–27

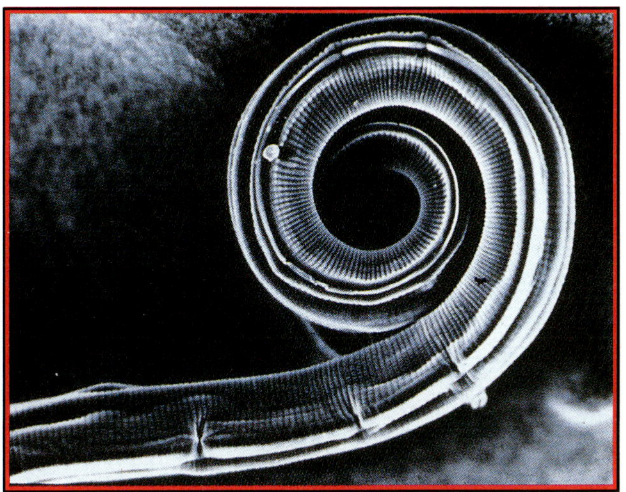

50–28 DUSN

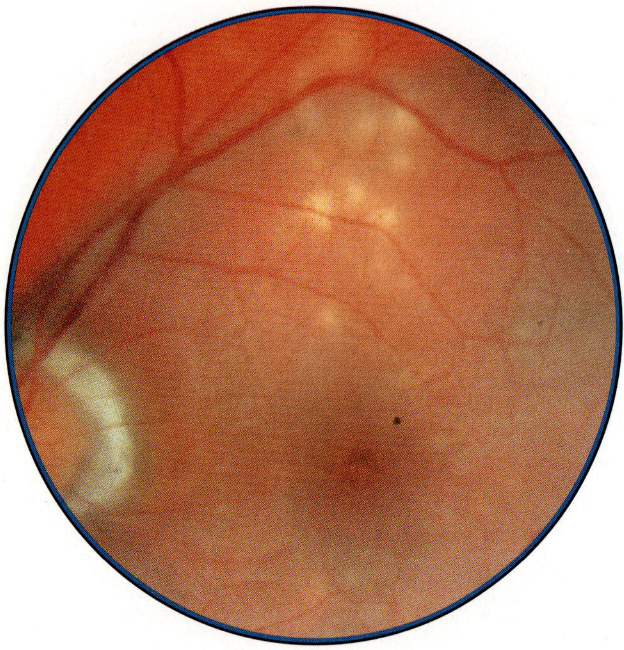

50–29

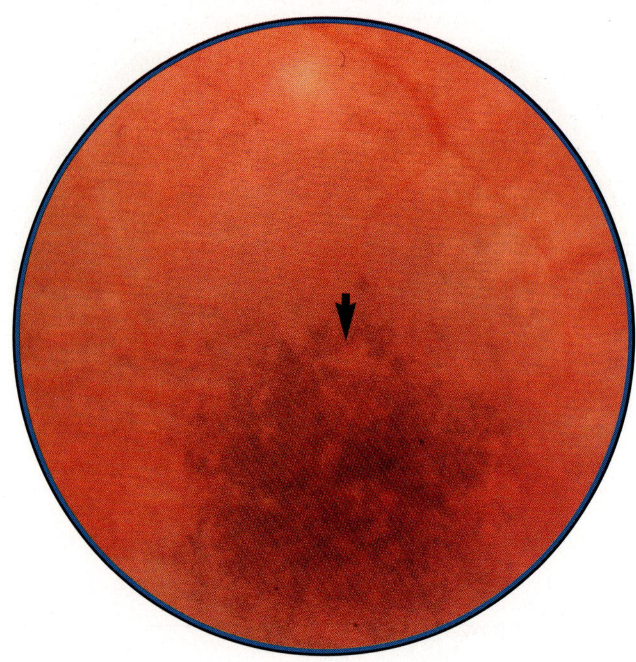

50–30

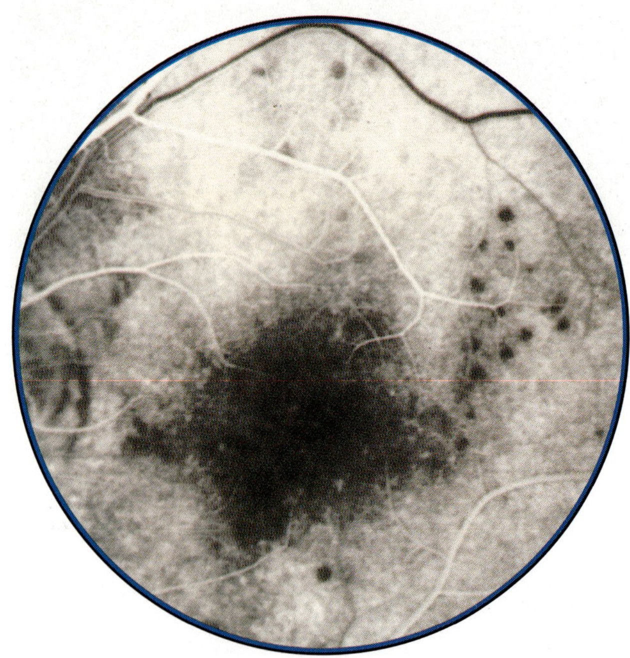

50–28 This 8-year-old boy with DUSN has widespread pigment epithelial atrophy and narrowing of the retinal vasculature. Peripapillary fibrous proliferation is also present, and there are multiple white subretinal spots. The small, 500-µm worm is in the superior juxtafoveal area, barely visible because of the glistening sheen and high reflectivity of the vitreoretinal interface.

50–29 The worm *(arrowhead)* can be identified with magnification in the superior juxtafoveal area overlying an atrophic and granular pigment epithelium. A singular white subretinal spot is demonstrated in the superior macula. Note the sheen to the inner retina.

50–30 The fluorescein angiogram in this case shows hypofluorescent spots, which are a reliable finding in identifying this inflammatory disease.

50–31

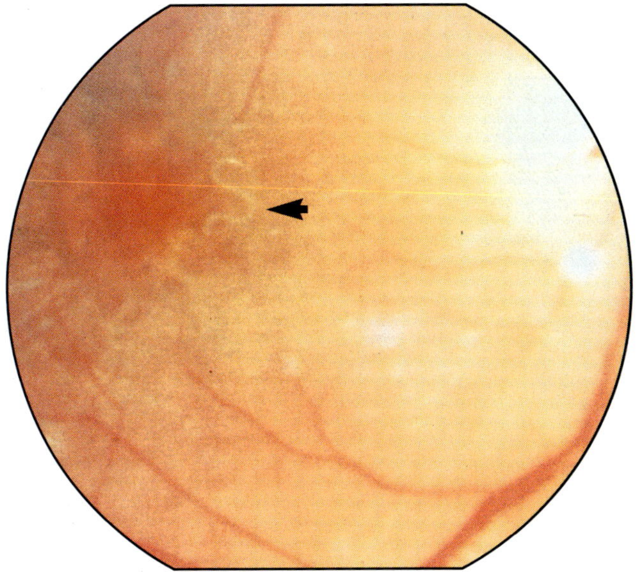

50–32

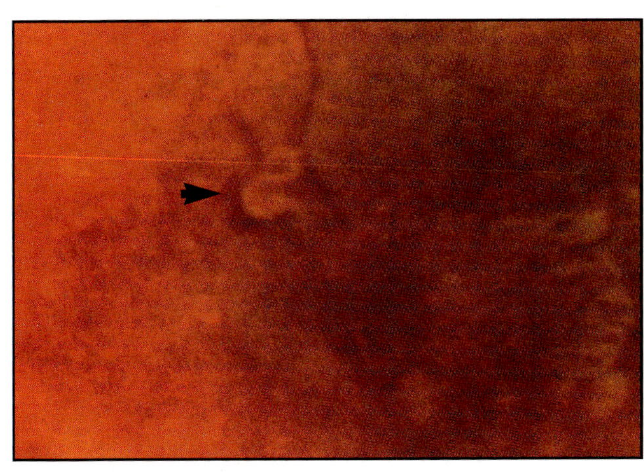

50–33

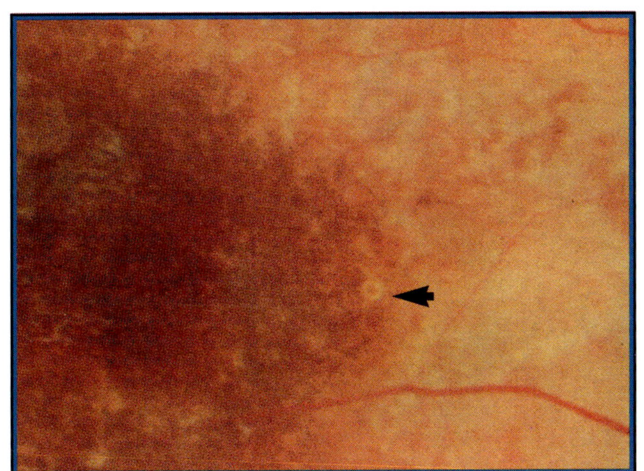

50–34

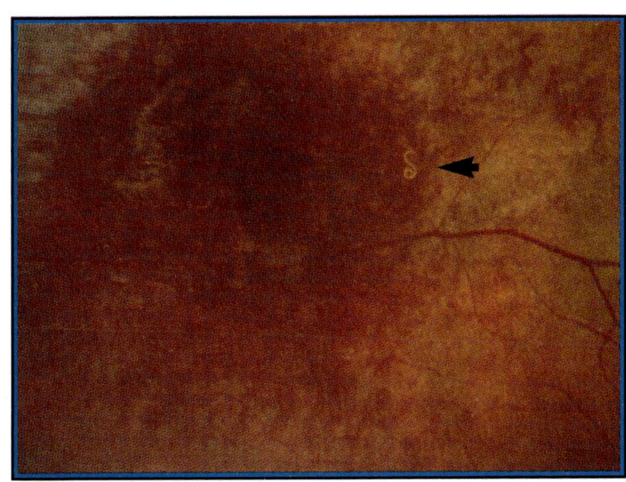

50–31 through 50–34 These photographs show various worms *(arrowheads)* that are responsible for the DUSN syndrome. The first patient has the large worm variant (50–31); the second patient shows the smaller worm (50–32), the third and fourth photographs show the same patient with the worm in a coiled position (50–33) and an uncoiled position (50–34).

50–31 *through* ***50–34,*** *Courtesy of Dr. J. Donald Gass.*

50–35 ANGIOSTRONGYLIASIS

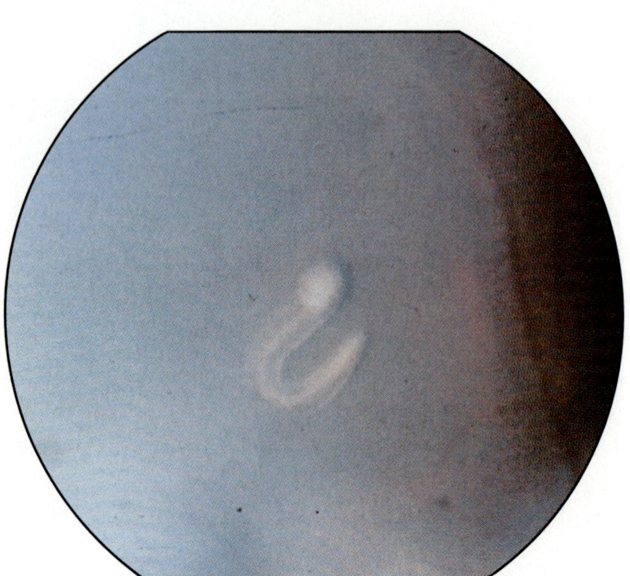

50–36

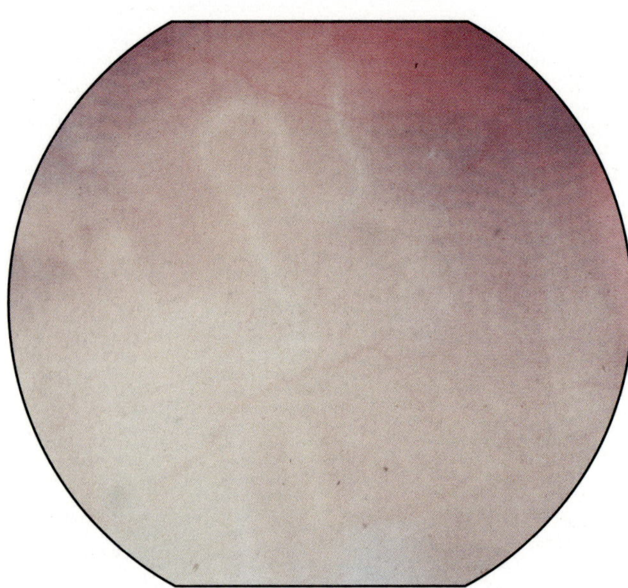

50–35 Gnathostomiasis intravitreal.

50–36 Angiostrongyliasis subretinal invasion. This is the most common nematode causing eosinophilic meningitis in Southeast Asia.

50–35 *and* ***50–36,*** *Courtesy of Dr. Prut Hanutsaha.*

50–37 *ALARIA MESOCERCARIAE*

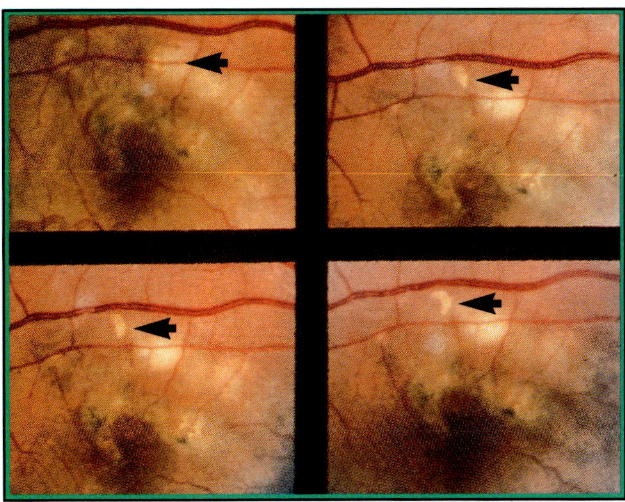

50–38

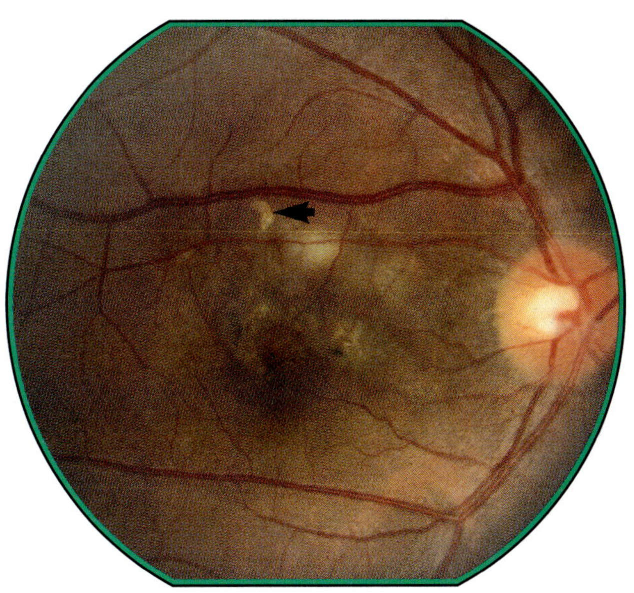

50–39

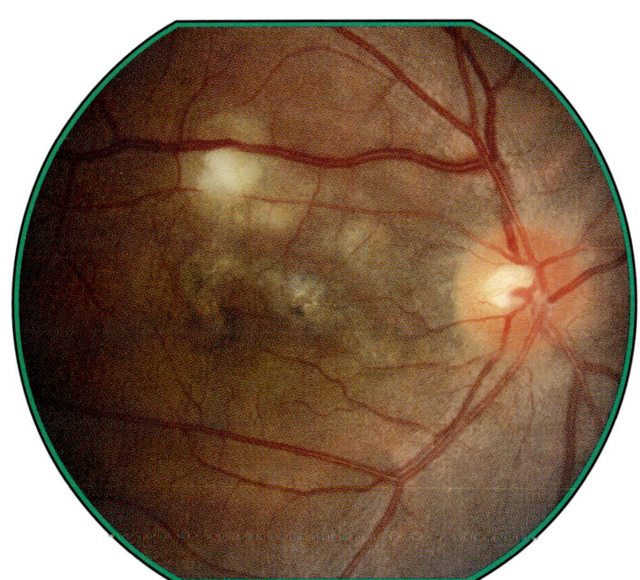

50–37 This patient has a subretinal worm, which can be seen moving in various positions *(arrowheads)*.

50–38 The higher magnification in the next photograph shows the worm *(arrowhead)*, a yellowish subretinal lesion and atrophy in the macular region.

50–39 The worm was successfully photocoagulated. This worm was believed to be the trematode *Alaria*. The worm was identified from analysis of projected fundus photographs and diagnosed based on its shape, size, and movement. Another worm had been identified as *Alaria* in a similar patient after being removed surgically. The most probable source of infection of these patients is ingestion of undercooked frogs' legs, which contain *Alaria*. Thus, DUSN may be caused by an organism other than an intraocular nematode larva. The most common types of larvae or nematodes that may cause DUSN include *Toxocara canis* of dogs and *Baylisascaris procyonis* of raccoons. In addition, the dog hookworm *Ancylostoma canium* has also been suggested as a cause of DUSN. *Alaria* thus represents another organism that may cause DUSN.

***50–37** through **50–39,** Courtesy of Dr. H. Richard McDonald. From McDonald, HR, et al: Two cases of intraocular infection with* Alaria mesocercariae *trematodes, Am J Ophthalmol 117:447, 1994. Published with permission of the American Journal of Ophthalmology. Copyright by the Ophthalmic Publishing Company.*

Suggested Readings

Fox, AS, Kazacos, KR, Gould, NS, Heyedemann, PT, Thomsa, C, and Boyer, KM: Fatal eosinophilic meningoencephalitis and visceral larva migrans caused by the raccoon ascarid *Baylisascaris procyonis*, N Engl J Med 312:1619–1623, 1985

Gass, JDM, and Braunstein, RA: Further observations concerning the diffuse unilateral subacute neuroretinitis syndrome, Arch Ophthalmol 101:1689–1697, 1983

Gass, JDM, Gilbert, WR, Jr, Guerry, RK, and Scelfo, R: Diffuse unilateral subacute neuroretinitis, Ophthalmology 85:521–545, 1978

Huff, DS, Neafie, RC, Binder, MJ, De Leon, GA, Brown, LW, and Kazacos, KR: The first fatal *Baylisascaris* infection in humans: an infant with eosinophilic meningoencephalitis, Pediatr Pathol 2:345–352, 1984

Kazacos, KR, Wirtz, WL, Burger, PP, and Christmas, CS: Raccoon ascarid larvae as a cause of fatal nervous system disease in subhuman primates, J Am Vet Med Assoc 179:1089–1094, 1981

Rubin, ML, Kaufman, HE, Tierney, JP, and Lucas, HC: An intraretinal nematode (a case report), Trans Acad Ophthalmol Otolaryngol 72:855–866, 1968

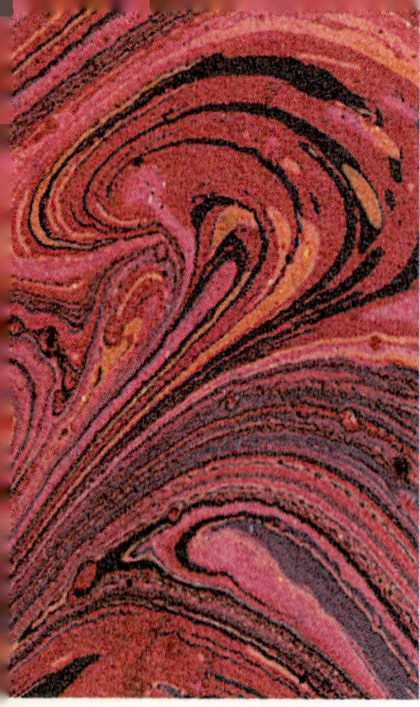

Chapter 51

Scleritis

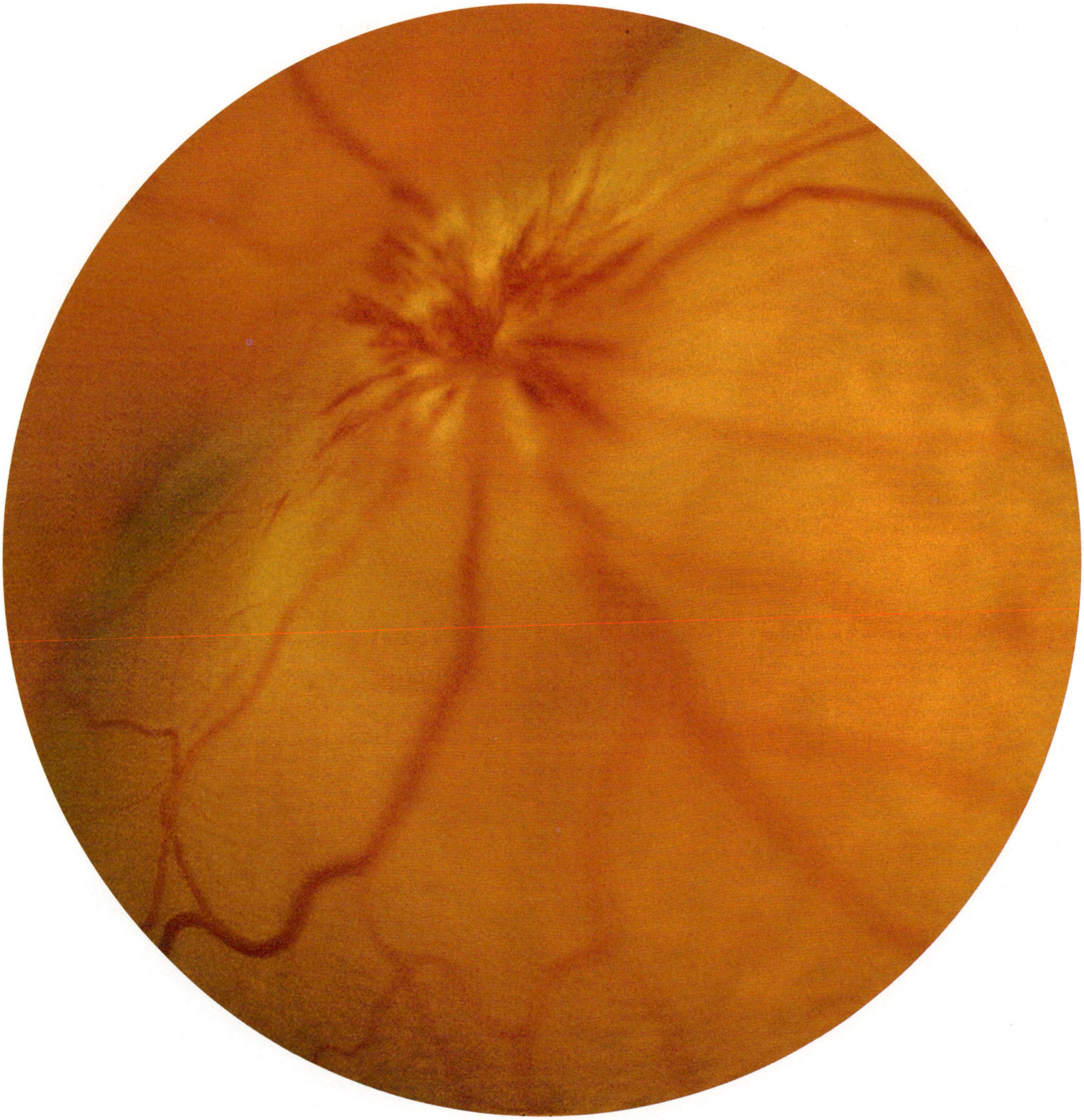

Posterior scleritis is an uncommon form of scleritis and usually affects women. It is unilateral and usually has an accompanying anterior scleritis and uveitis. Severe pain and limitations in extraocular movements may occur. Optic disc edema, exudative retinal detachment, proptosis, and chorioretinal folds may occur.

51–1

A

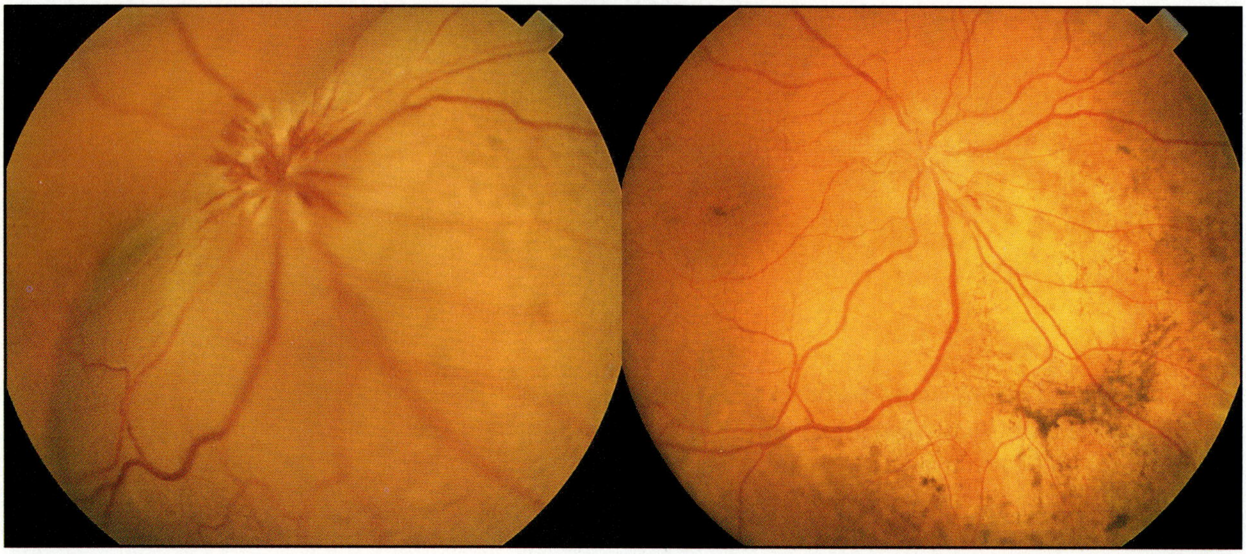

B

51–2

51–3

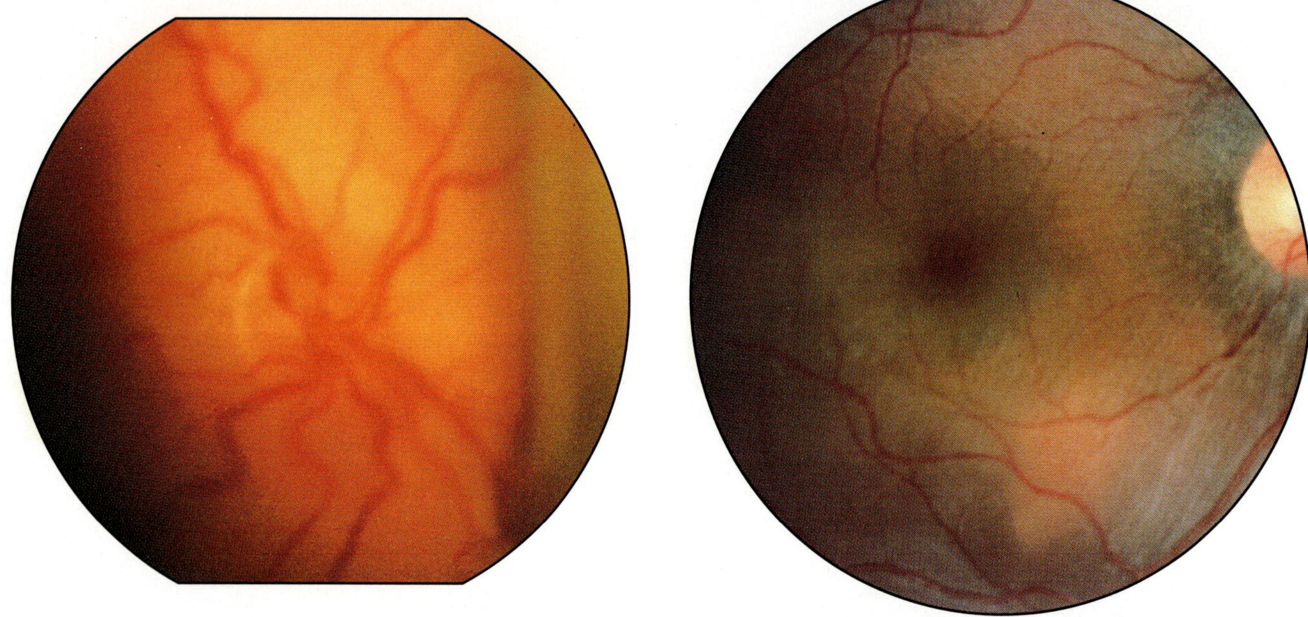

51–1 **A,** This is a case of posterior scleritis presenting as a solid juxtapopillary mass simulating an amelanotic melanoma. Note the hemorrhage and swelling of the disc. **B,** One month later there has been nearly complete and spontaneous flattening of the mass and resolution of the exudative change.

51–2 This patient has a choroidal effusion secondary to posterior scleritis.

51–3 Chorioretinal folds are demonstrated in this patient with posterior scleritis.

***51–1 A** and **B,** Courtesy of Dr. David Abramson, Dr. Mary Mendelsohn, and Dr. Jerry Shields.*

51–4

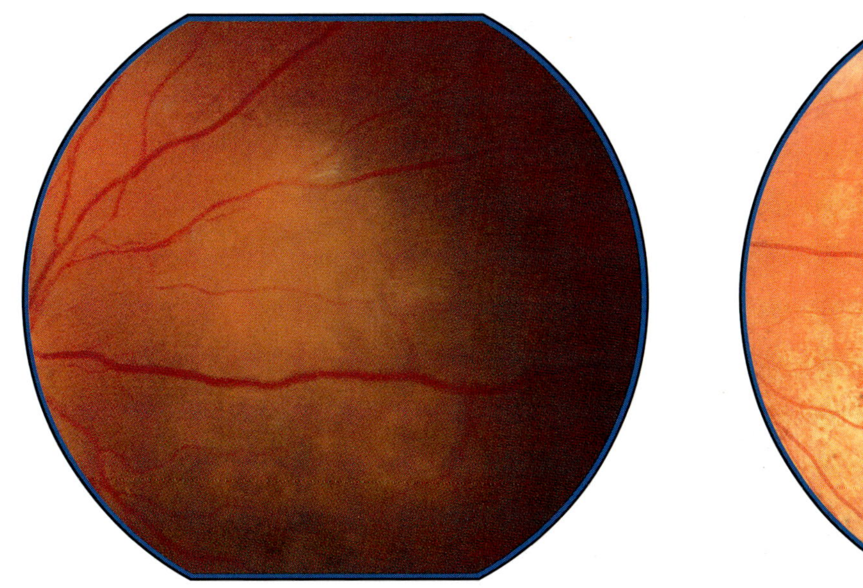

51–5

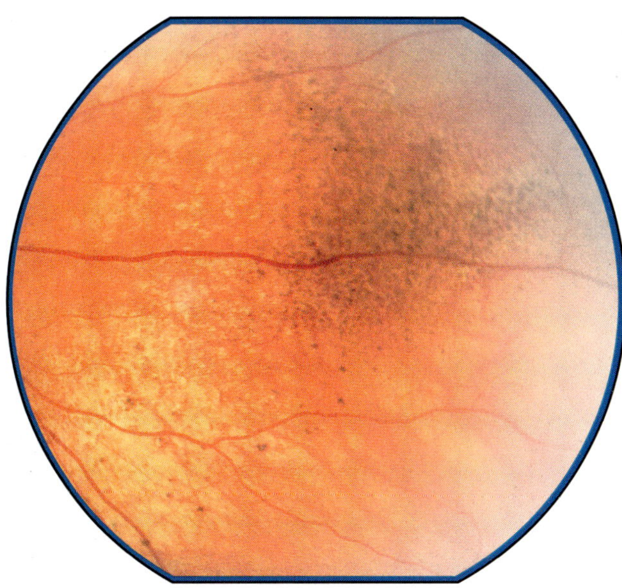

51–4 and 51–5 This 10-year-old boy presented with an elevated pigmented choroidal mass in the peripapillary region. The patient was referred for a possible choroidal melanoma. The mass resolved after steroid treatment, suggesting the diagnosis of posterior scleritis.

Suggested Readings

Benson, WE, Shields, JA, Tasman, W, and Crandall, AS: Posterior scleritis: a cause of diagnostic confusion, Arch Ophthalmol 97:1482–1486, 1979

Fong, LP, Maza, MS, Rice, BA, Kupferman, AE, and Foster, CS: Immunopathogy of scleritis, Opthalmology 98:472–479, 1991

Jampol, LM, West, C, and Goldberg, MF: Therapy of scleritis with cytotoxic agents, Am J Ophthalmol 86:266–271, 1978

Singh G, Guthoff, R, and Foster, CS: Observations on long-term follow-up of posterior scleritis, Am J Ophthalmol 101:570–575, 1986

Watson, PG, and Hazleman, BL: The sclera and systemic disorders, London, 1976, WB Saunders

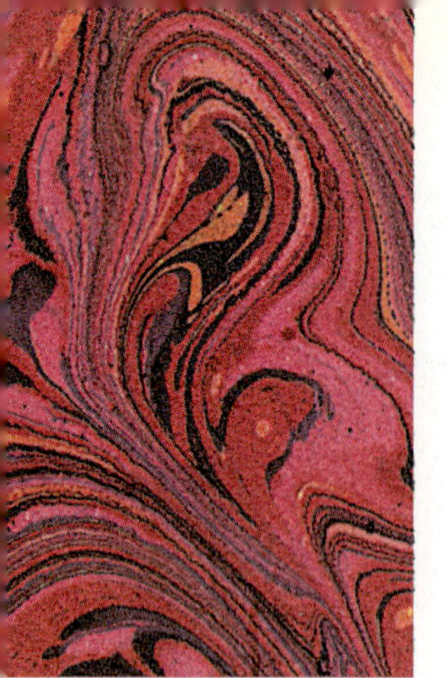

Chapter 52

Ocular Histoplasmosis

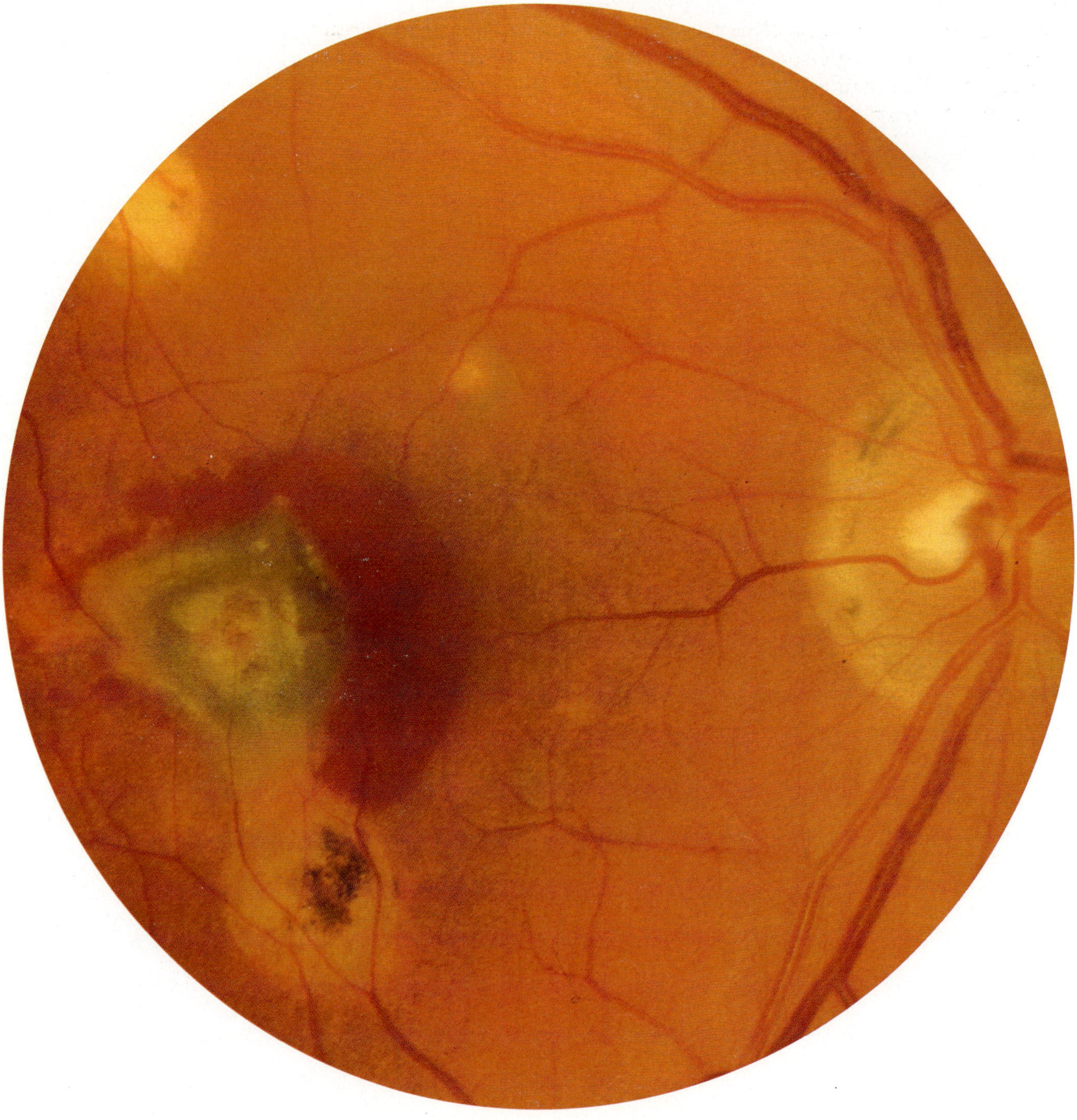

The presumed ocular histoplasmosis syndrome consists of chorioretinal whitish-yellow lesions (histospots), peripapillary atrophy, and an exudative maculopathy. This condition is a major cause of choroidal neovascularization in the Ohio Mississippi River Valley belt.

52–1

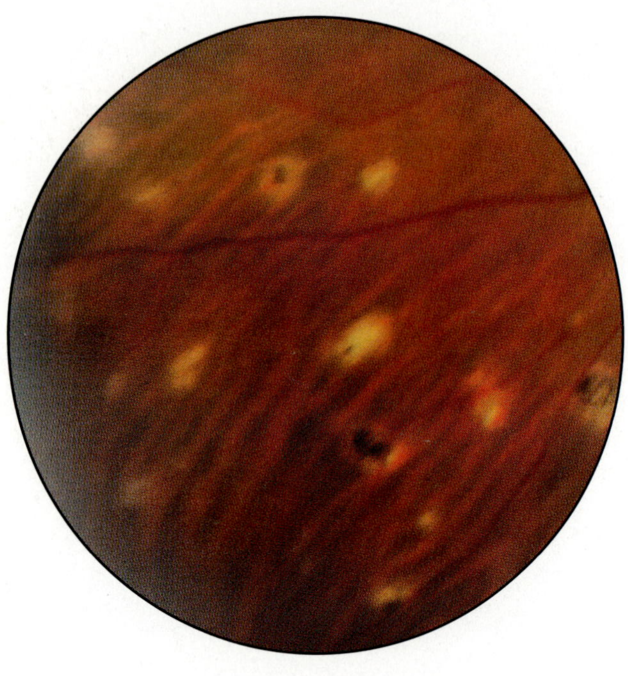

52–2 52–2A

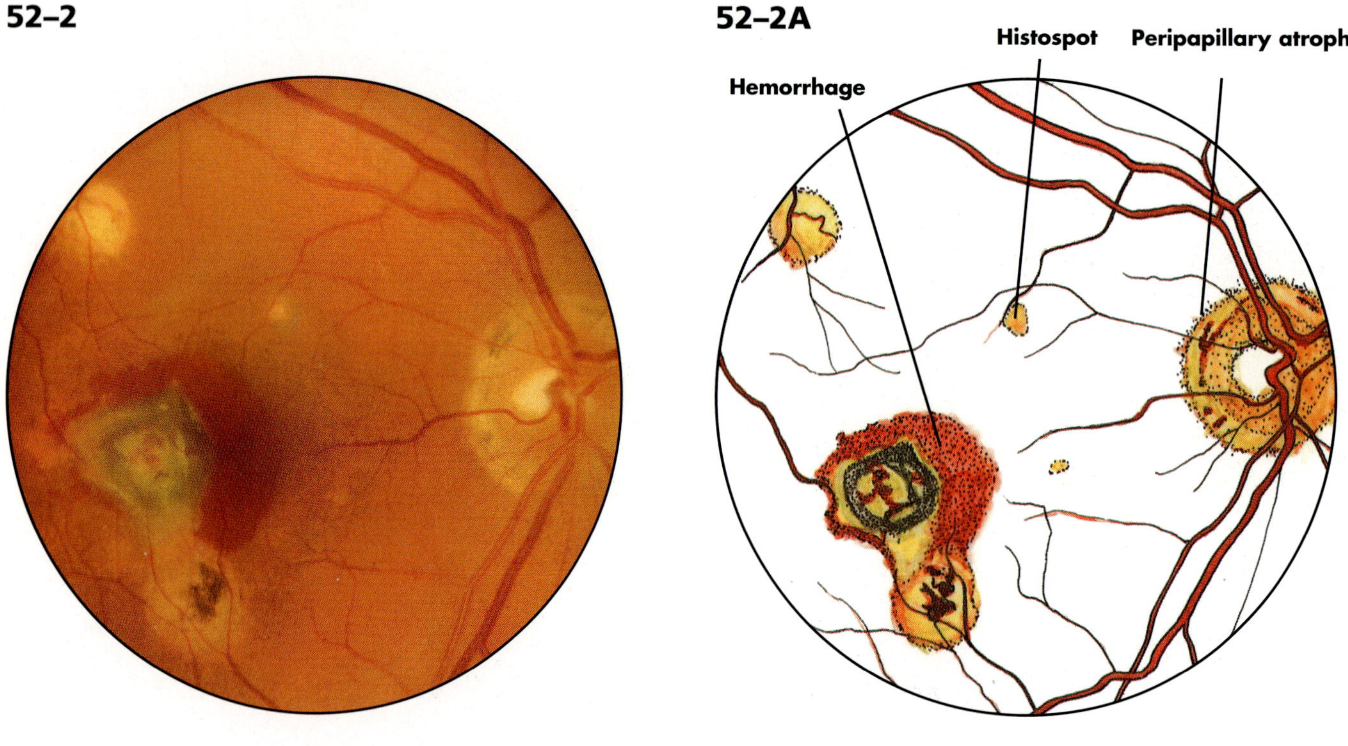

52–1 This photograph shows the peripheral chorioretinal scars secondary to ocular histoplasmosis, which are termed "histospots."

52–2 and 52–2A This patient illustrates the classic triad seen in ocular histoplasmosis, which includes peripapillary atrophy, atrophic chorioretinal "histospots," and subretinal hemorrhage with scarring from choroidal neovascularization.

52–2, *Courtesy of Bruce Morris, CRA.*

52–3

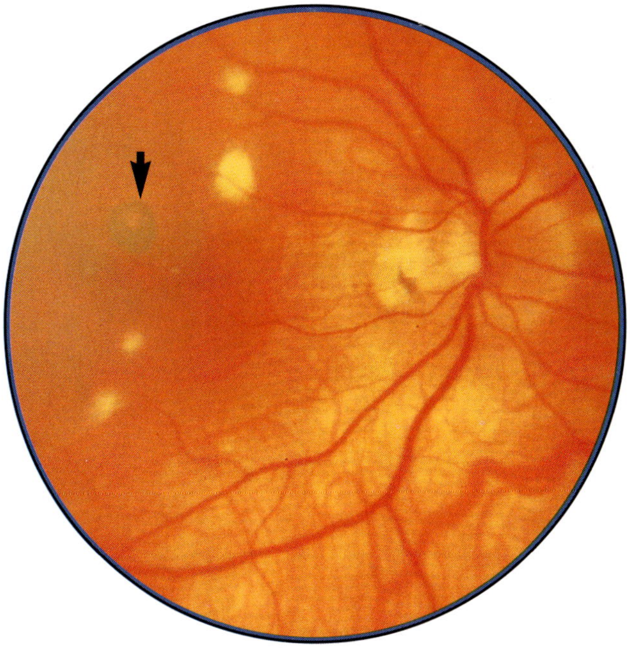

52–4

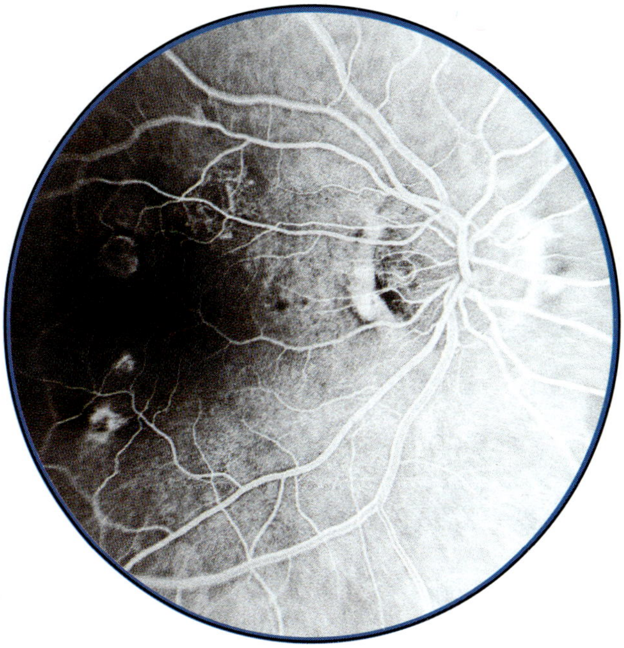

52–5

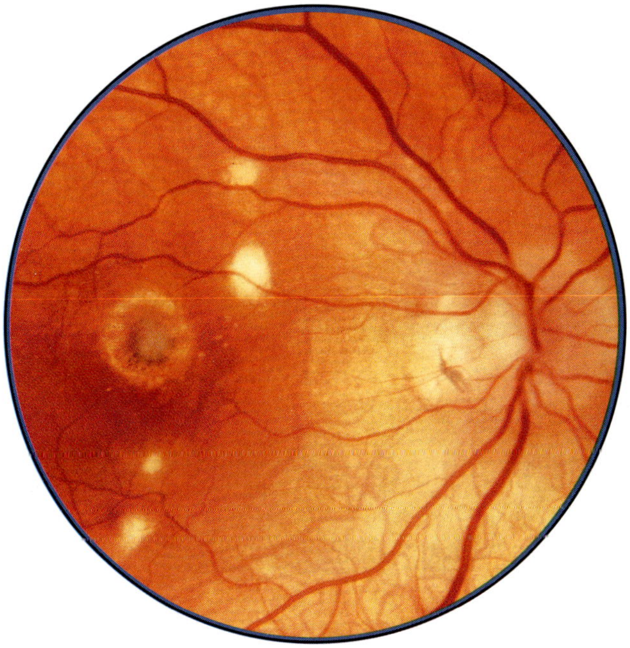

52–6

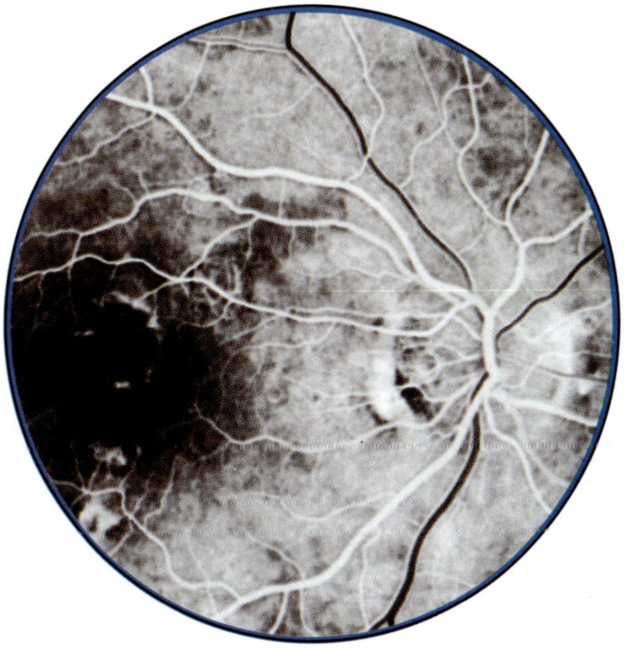

52–3 This patient has the presumed ocular histoplasmosis syndrome. Note the peripapillary atrophy, "histospots," and choroidal neovascularization *(arrowhead)*. The choroidal neovascularization emanates from an orange colored "histospot" with differential growth which is faster towards the fovea.

52–4 The fluorescein angiogram confirms the presence of choroidal neovascularization superotemporal to the fovea.

52–5 and 52–6 This area of neovascularization (52–5) was treated with laser photocoagulation. Note the atrophy surrounding the regressed vessel (52–6).

52–7

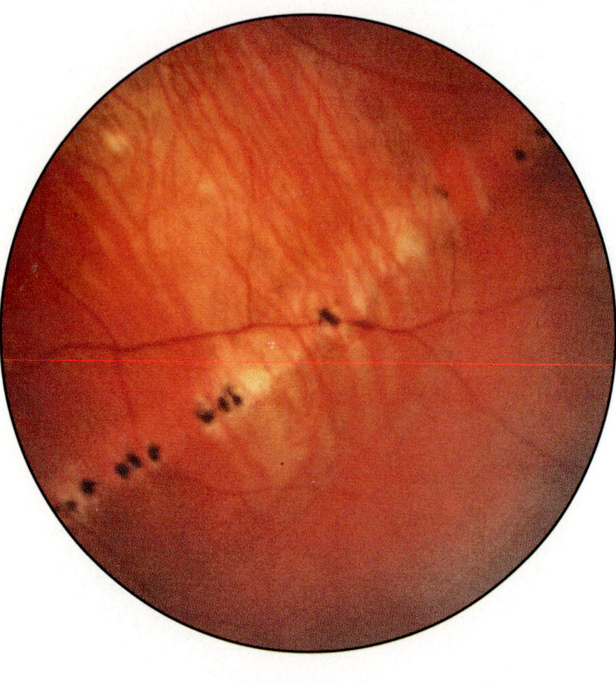

52–8

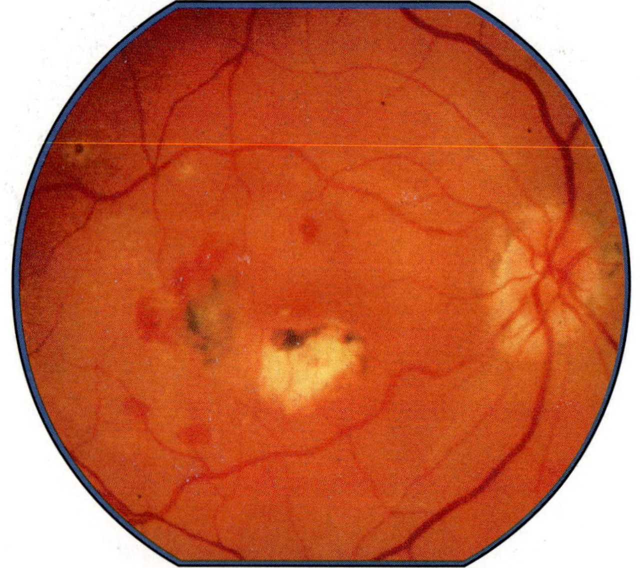

52–9

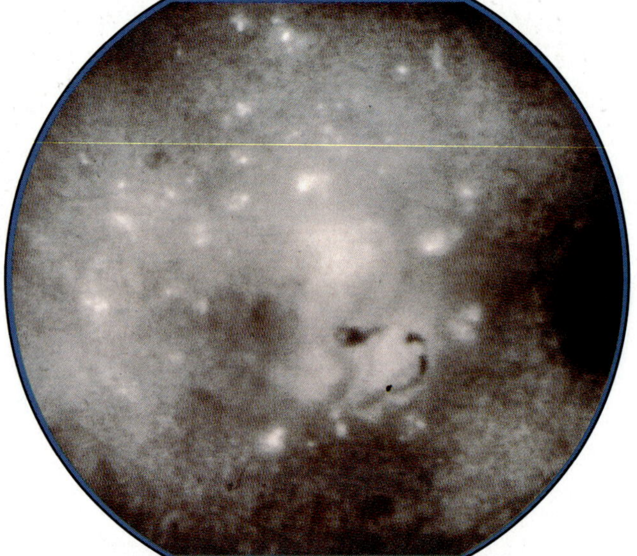

52–7 Another finding seen in ocular histoplasmosis is curvilinear streaks, as demonstrated in this patient.

52–8 and 52–9 The right eye of this patient with the presumed ocular histoplasmosis syndrome shows peripapillary atrophy, atrophic spots, and recurrent choroidal neovascularization. The indocyanine-green (ICG) angiogram of this eye shows multiple hyperfluorescent spots.

(Case continued on next page.)

52–10

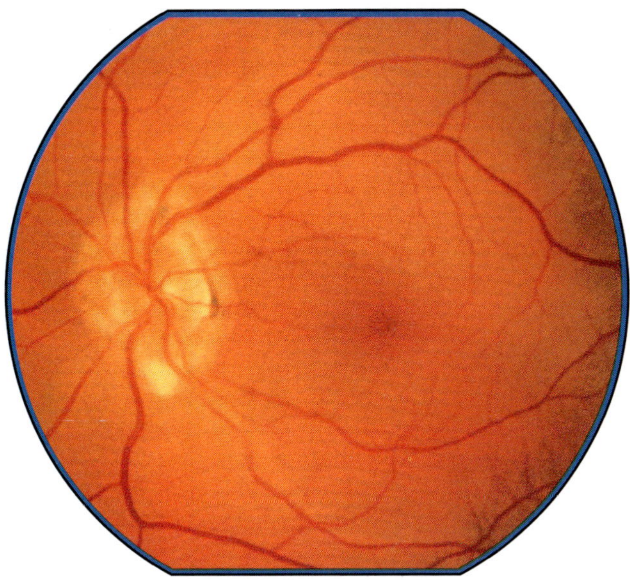

52–11

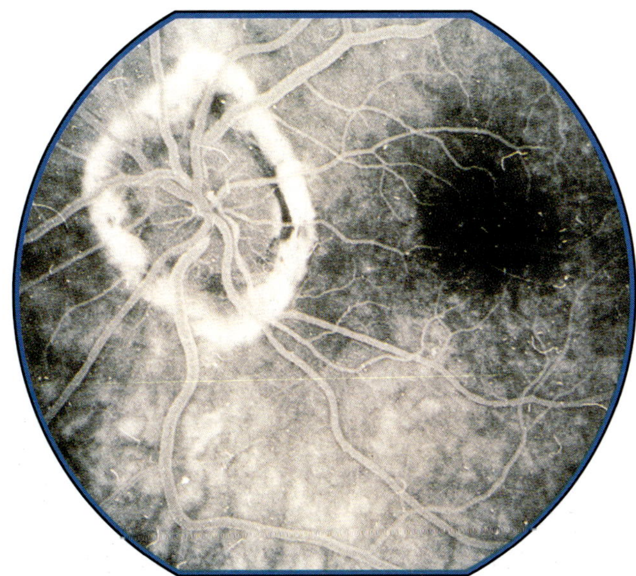

52–12

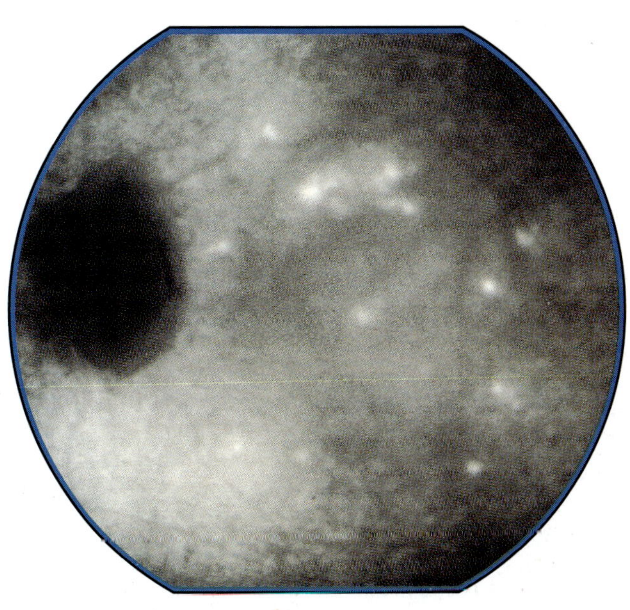

52–10 through 52–12 The color photograph of the fellow eye reveals atrophy surrounding regressed peripapillary choroidal neovascularization, but the macular region appears normal. Fluorescein angiography of this eye reveals staining secondary to the peripapillary atrophy. However, the macula appears normal. ICG angiography, however, reveals multiple hyperfluorescent spots throughout the macular region in this asymptomatic and, clinically and fluorescein angiographically unaffected eye. This case demonstrates that ICG angiography may be useful in identifying abnormalities in patients in whom the clinical examination and fluorescein angiogram fail to reveal any pathology. This finding is very preliminary, and further research is indicated in the use of ICG angiography in patients with this condition.

52–13

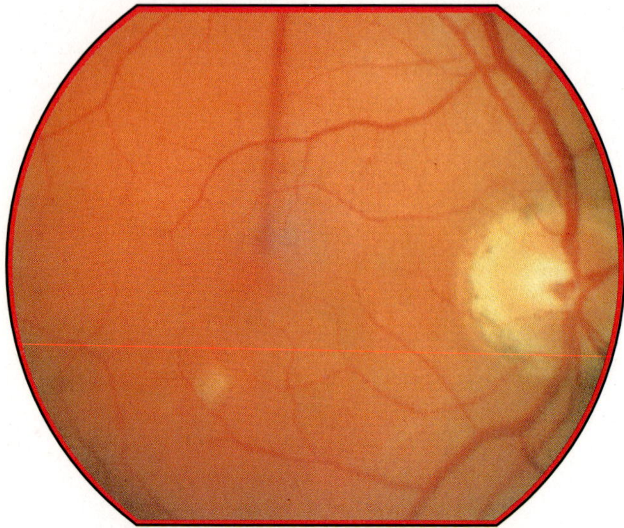

52–14

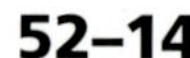

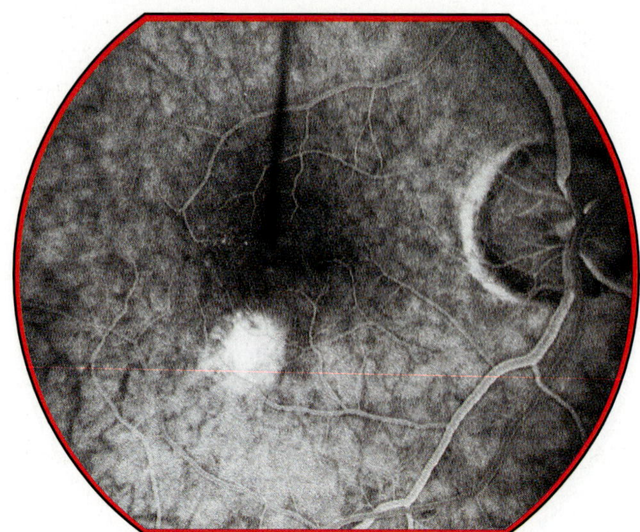

52–15

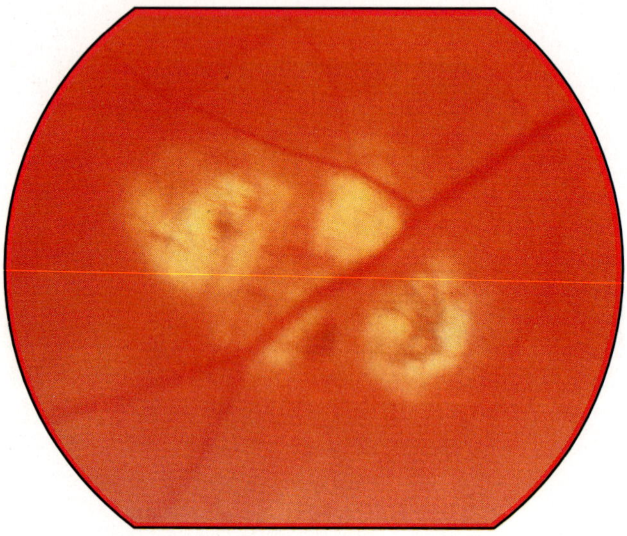

52–13 through 52–15 This clinicopathologic correlation of a patient with the ocular histoplasmosis syndrome illustrates peripapillary atrophy, peripheral chorioretinal "punched-out" lesions, and choroidal neovascularization. The clinical photographs illustrate an area of choroidal neovascularization inferotemporal to the macula, peripapillary scarring, and midperipheral chorioretinal scars. The fluorescein angiogram reveals choroidal neovascularization.

52–13 *through* ***52–15,*** *From Sheffer, A, Green, WR, Fine, SL, and Kincaid, M: Presumed ocular histoplasmosis syndrome: a clinicopathologic correlation of a treated case, Arch Ophthalmol 95:335–340, 1980. Copyright 1980, American Medical Association.*

(Case continued on next page.)

52–16

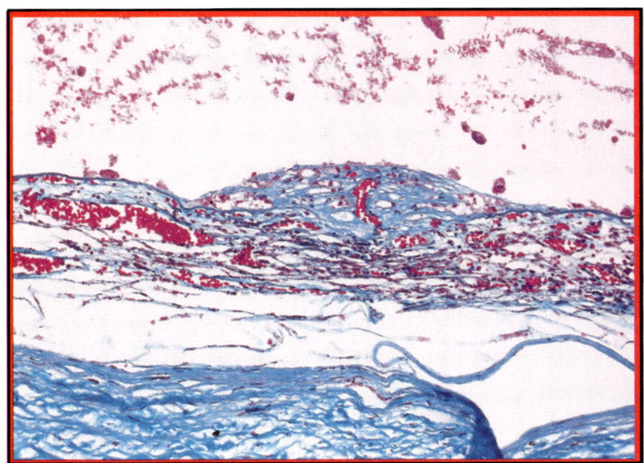

52–17

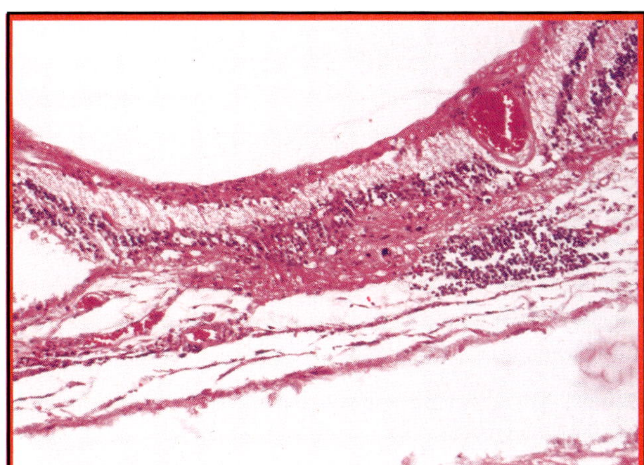

52–18

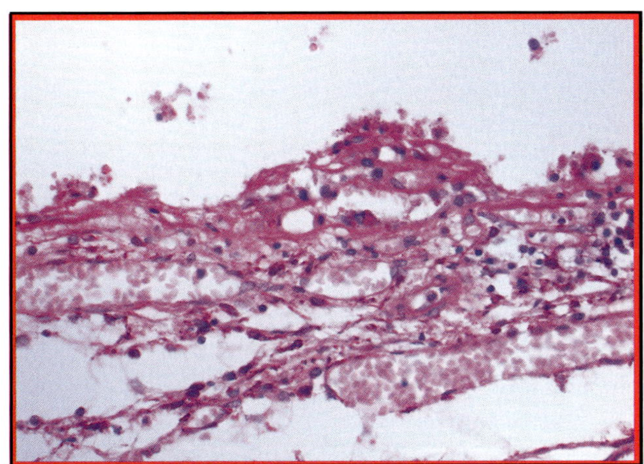

52–19

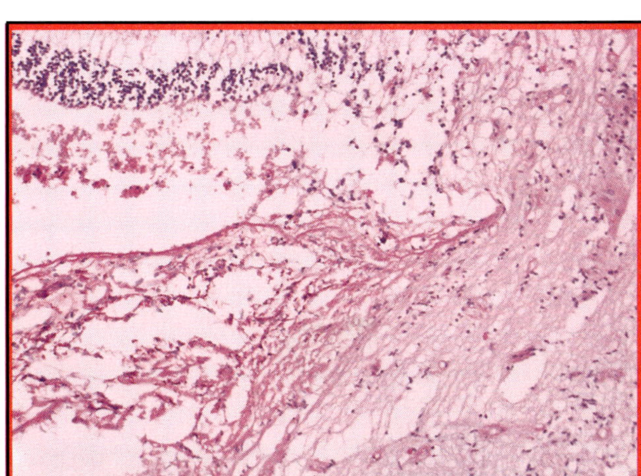

52–16 Histopathologic examination of the macular region reveals a scar composed of laminated hyperplastic retinal pigment epithelium and a disruption of Bruch's membrane with choroidal neovascularization.

52–17 The midperipheral chorioretinal lesion demonstrates an area of chorioretinal scarring with photoreceptor atrophy, a defect in Bruch's membrane, and gliosis extending into the choroid.

52–18 A lesion just superonasal to the disc shows two breaks in Bruch's membrane with early choroidal neovascularization.

52–19 Peripapillary scarring without neovascularization was also observed.

52–16 *through* ***52–19,*** *From Sheffer, A, Green, WR, Fine, SL, and Kincaid, M: Presumed ocular histoplasmosis syndrome: a clinicopathologic correlation of a treated case, Arch Ophthalmol 95:335–340, 1980. Copyright 1980, American Medical Association.*

Suggested Readings

Baskin, MA, Jampol, LM, Huamonte, FU, Rabb, MF, Vygantas, CM, and Wyhinny, G: Macular lesions in blacks with the presumed ocular histoplasmosis syndrome, Am J Ophthalmol 89:77–83, 1980

Bottoni, FG, Deutman, AF, and Aandekerk, AL: Presumed ocular histoplasmosis syndrome and linear streak lesions, Br J Ophthalmol 73:528–535, 1989

Craig, EL, and Suie, T: *Histoplasma capsulatum* in human ocular tissue, Arch Ophthalmol 91:285–289, 1974

Davidorf, FH: The role of T-lymphocytes in the reactivation of presumed ocular histoplasmosis scars, Int Ophthalmol Clin 15:111–124, 1975

Ganley, JP: Epidemiologic characteristics of presumed ocular histoplasmosis, Acta Ophthalmologica Suppl (Copenh) 119:1–63, 1973

Goldstein, BG, and Buettner, H: Histoplasmic endophthalmitis: a clinicopathologic correlation, Arch Ophthalmol 101:774–777, 1983

Kaplan, HJ, and Waldrep, JC: Immunological basis of presumed ocular histoplasmosis, Int Ophthalmol Clin 23:19–31, 1983

Lewis, ML, and Schiffman, JC: Long-term follow-up of the second eye in ocular histoplasmosis, Int Ophthalmol Clin 23:125–135, 1983

Macular Photocoagulation Study Group: Krypton laser photocoagulation for neovascular lesions of ocular histoplasmosis: results of a randomized clinical trial, Arch Ophthalmol 105:1499–1507, 1987

Macular Photocoagulation Study Group: Argon laser photocoagulation for neovascular maculopathy: five-year results from randomized clinical trials, Arch Ophthalmol 109:1109–1114, 1991

Meredith, TA, Smith, RE, Braley, RE, Witkowski, JA, and Koethe, SM: The prevalence of HLA-B7 in presumed ocular histoplasmosis in patients with peripheral atrophic scars, Am J Ophthalmol 86:325–328, 1978

Schlaegel, TF: Ocular histoplasmosis, New York, 1977, Grune & Stratton, pp 209–259

Scholz, R, Green, WR, Kutys, R, Sutherland, J, and Richards, RD: *Histoplasma capsulatum* in the eye, Ophthalmology 91:1100–1104, 1984

Sheffer, A, Green, WR, Fine, SL, and Kincaid, M: Presumed ocular histoplasmosis syndrome: a clinicopathologic correlation of a treated case, Arch Ophthalmol 98:335–345, 1980

Thomas, MA, and Kaplan, HJ: Surgical removal of subfoveal neovascularization in the presumed ocular histoplasmosis syndrome, Am J Ophthalmol 111:1–7, 1991

Weingeist, GA, and Watzke, RC: Ocular involvement by *Histoplasma capsulatum,* Int Ophthalmol Clin 23:33–47, 1983

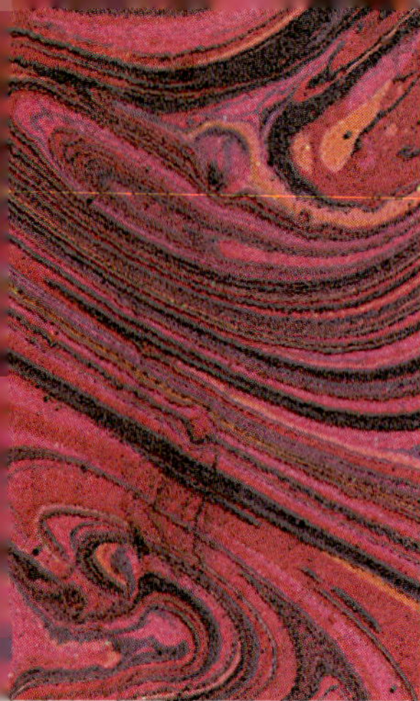

Chapter 53
Birdshot Chorioretinopathy

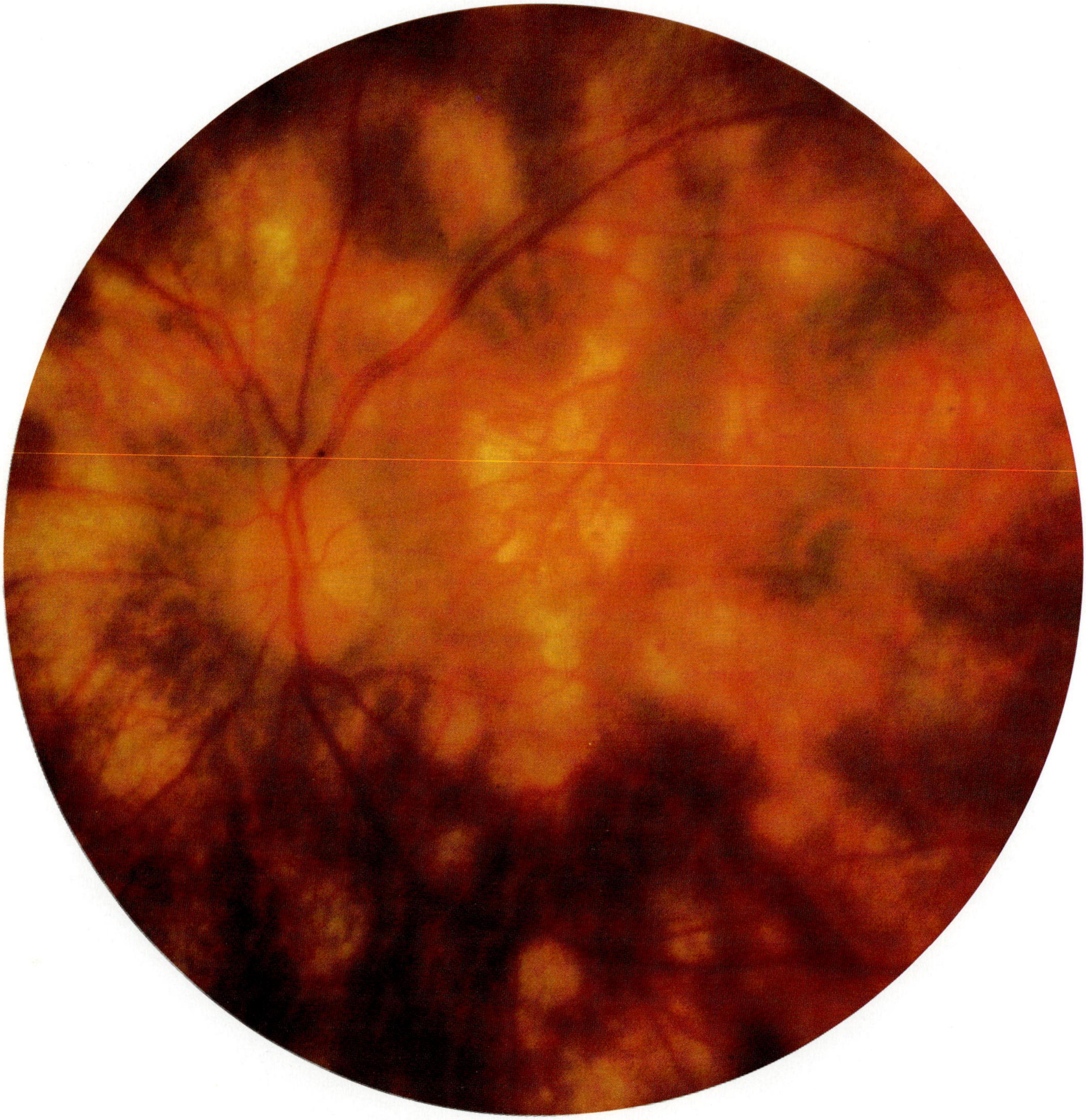

Birdshot chorioretinopathy is a rare acquired, bilateral inflammatory disorder first described by Ryan and Maumenee. Multiple cream-colored lesions are noted throughout the deep retina and choroid. These lesions appear to have a vascular predilection. Exacerbations or remissions are common. Vitreous debris and cystoid macular edema also may be noted.

The characteristic cream-colored spots are often oval. Patients with birdshot chorioretinopathy often have positive HLA A-29 antigen typing. Choroidal neovascularization as well as vitreous hemorrhage may occur in this condition. Cystoid macular edema commonly is responsible for the vision loss in this disease. Papilledema and chronic vitritis may also be noted.

53–1

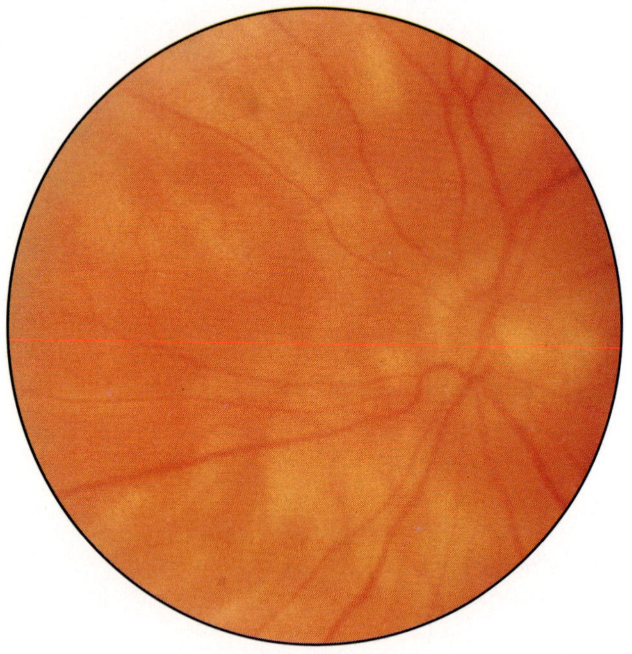

53–2

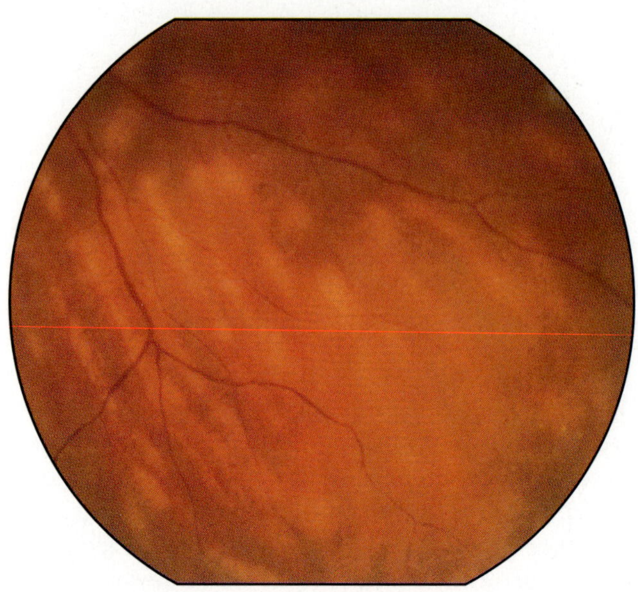

53–3

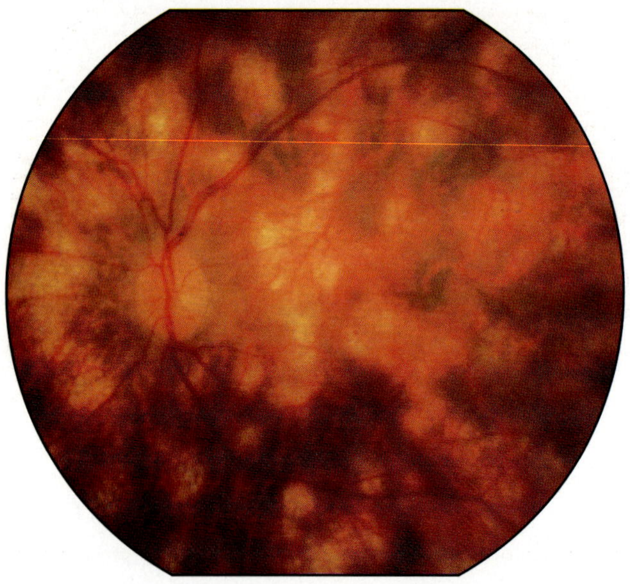

53–1 and 53–2 The classic appearance of birdshot chorioretinopathy is represented by these oval whitish-yellow chorioretinal lesions.

53–3 A more severe rarer form of birdshot chorioretinopathy with hyperpigmented and confluent hypopigmentary areas are noted in this patient.

53–4

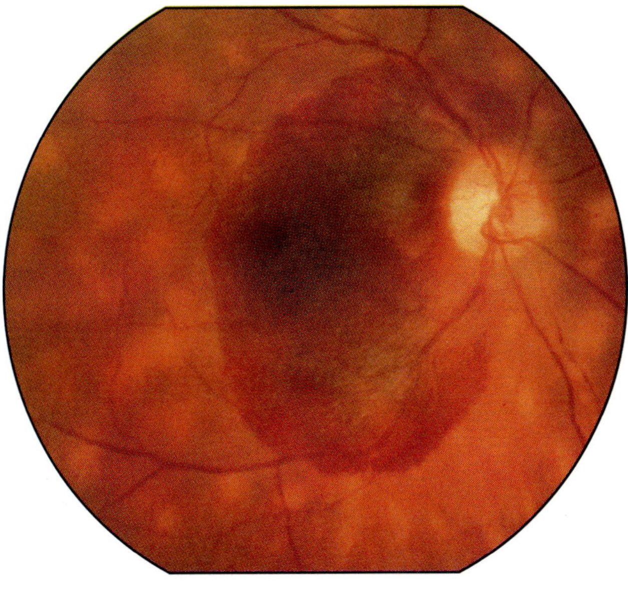

53–5 **53–6**

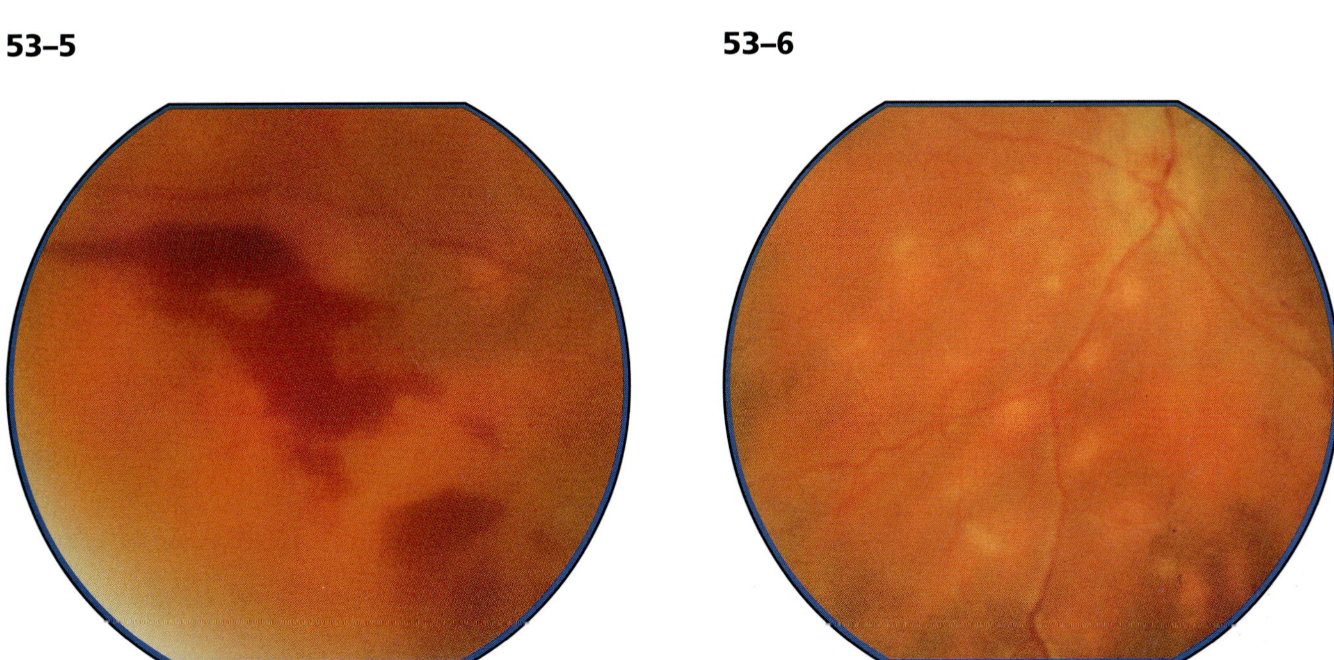

53–4 Choroidal neovascularization with subretinal hemorrhage may occur in some patients with birdshot chorioretinopathy.

53–5 and 53–6 Another complication of birdshot chorioretinopathy is vitreous hemorrhage, as demonstrated in this patient. Note also the periphlebitis and optic disc edema (53–6).

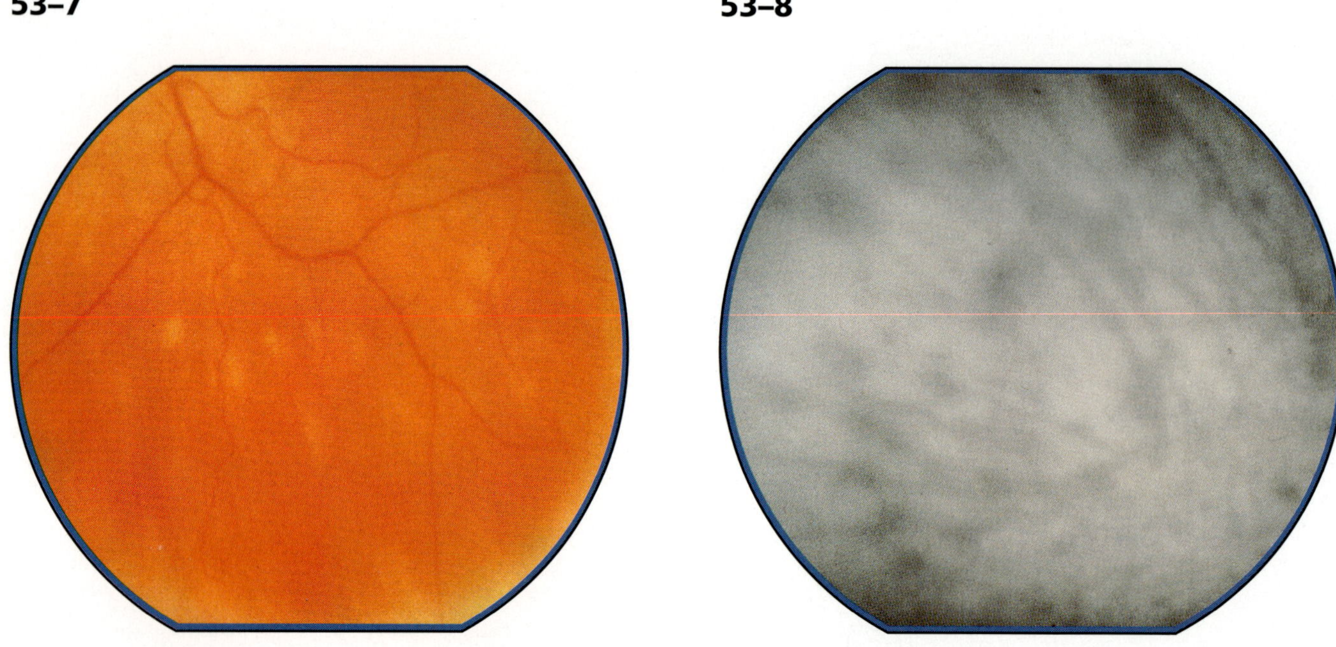

53–7 and 53–8 This patient with birdshot chorioretinopathy (53–7) illustrates the indocyanine-green (ICG) angiographic findings in this condition. Note the hypofluorescent lesions that appear in a vascular pattern in the peripapillary region (53–8).

Suggested Readings

Aaberg, TM: Diffuse inflammatory salmon patch choroidopathy syndrome, International Fluorescein Macula Symposium, Carmel, CA, October, 1979

Brucker, AJ, Deglin, EA, Bene, C, and Hoffman, ME: Subretinal choroidal neovascularization in birdshot retinochoroidopathy, Am J Ophthalmol 99:40–44, 1985

Feltkamp, TEW: Ophthalmological significance of HLA associated uveitis, Eye 4:839–844, 1990

Gass, JDM: Vitiliginous chorioretinitis, Arch Ophthalmol 99:1778–1787, 1981

Kaplan, HJ. and Aaberg, TM: Birdshot retinochoroidopathy, Am J Ophthalmol 90:773–782, 1980

Ohno, S: Immunogenetic studies on ocular diseases. In Blodi, F, Brancato, R, Cristini, G, d'Ermo, F, Esente, I, Musini, A, Philipson, B, Pintucci, F, Ponte, F, and Scuderi, G, eds: Acta XXV Concilium Ophthalmologicum, Berkely, CA, 1987, Kugler and Ghedini, 1:144–154

Oosterhuis, JA, Baarsma, GS, and Polak, BCP: Birdshot chorioretinopathy—vitiliginous chorioretinitis, Int Ophthalmol 5:137–144, 1982

Priem, HA, De Rouck, A, DeLaey, JJ, and Bird, AC: Electrophysiologic studies in birdshot chorioretinopathy, Am J Ophthalmol 106:430–436, 1988

Ryan, SJ, and Maumenee, AE: Birdshot retinochoroidopathy, Am J Ophthalmol 89:31–45, 1980

Soubrane, G, Bokobza, R, and Coscas, G: Late developing lesions in birdshot retinochoroidopathy, Am J Ophthalmol 109:204–210, 1990

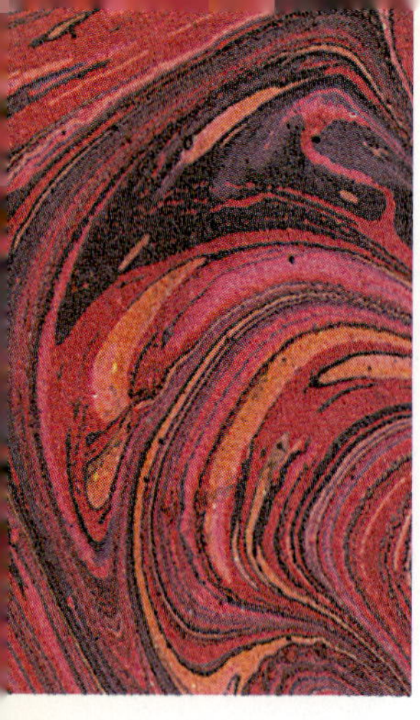

Chapter 54

Punctate Inner Choroidopathy, Multifocal Choroiditis, and Subretinal Fibrosis and Uveitis Syndrome

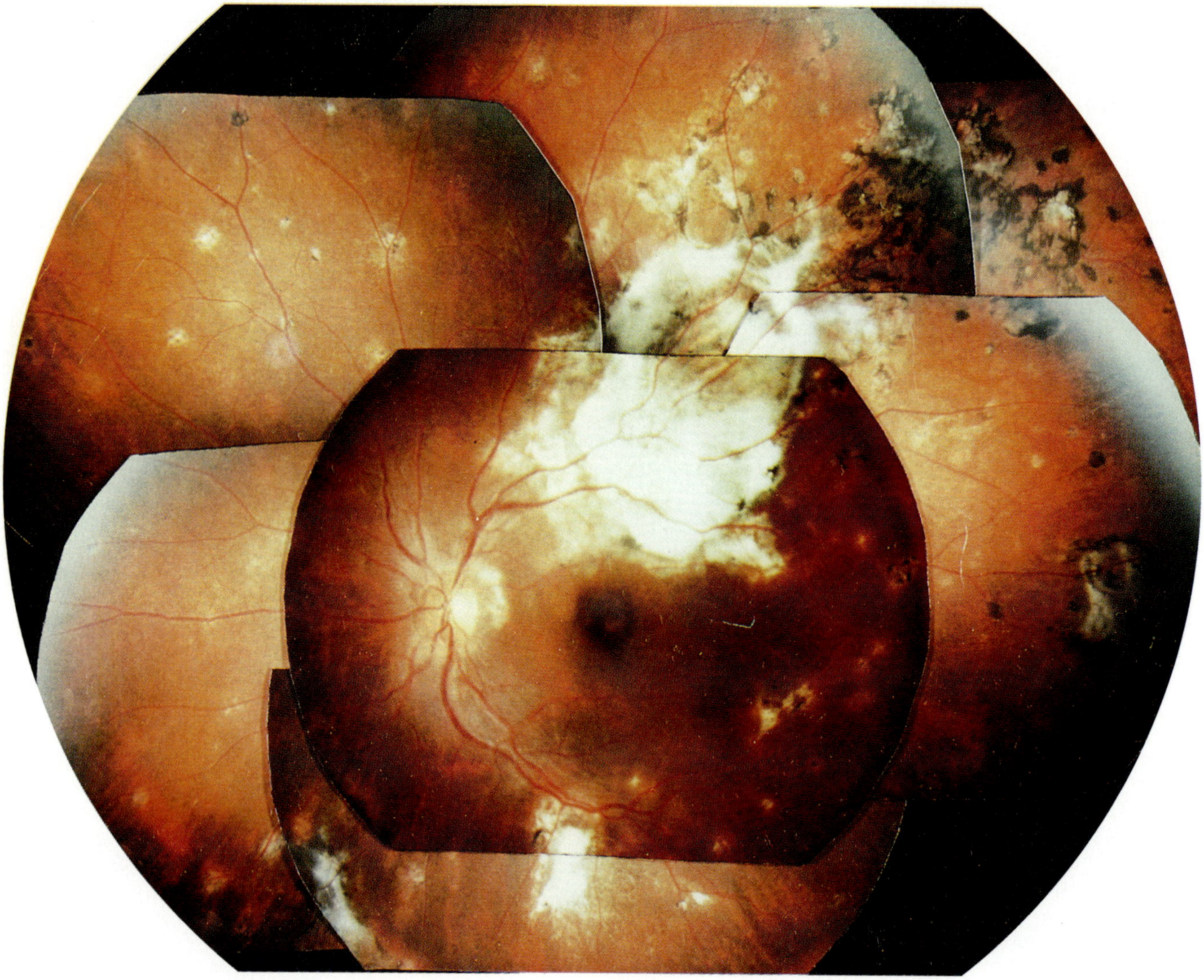

Punctate inner choroidopathy is seen in myopic females. Small yellow lesions in the inner choroid and retinal pigment epithelium are noted. Rarely, serous detachments may occur. These acute yellow infiltrates eventually evolve into chorioretinal scars. Choroidal neovascularization may occur. There is controversy as to whether this disease is different from multifocal choroiditis, in which whitish-yellow chorioretinal lesions are demonstrated, often with an accompanying vitritis and/or choroidal neovascularization. In addition, some investigators believe that both acute conditions may eventually evolve, in some cases, into the subretinal fibrosis and uveitis syndrome.

54–1 PUNCTATE INNER CHOROIDOPATHY

54–2

54–3

54–4

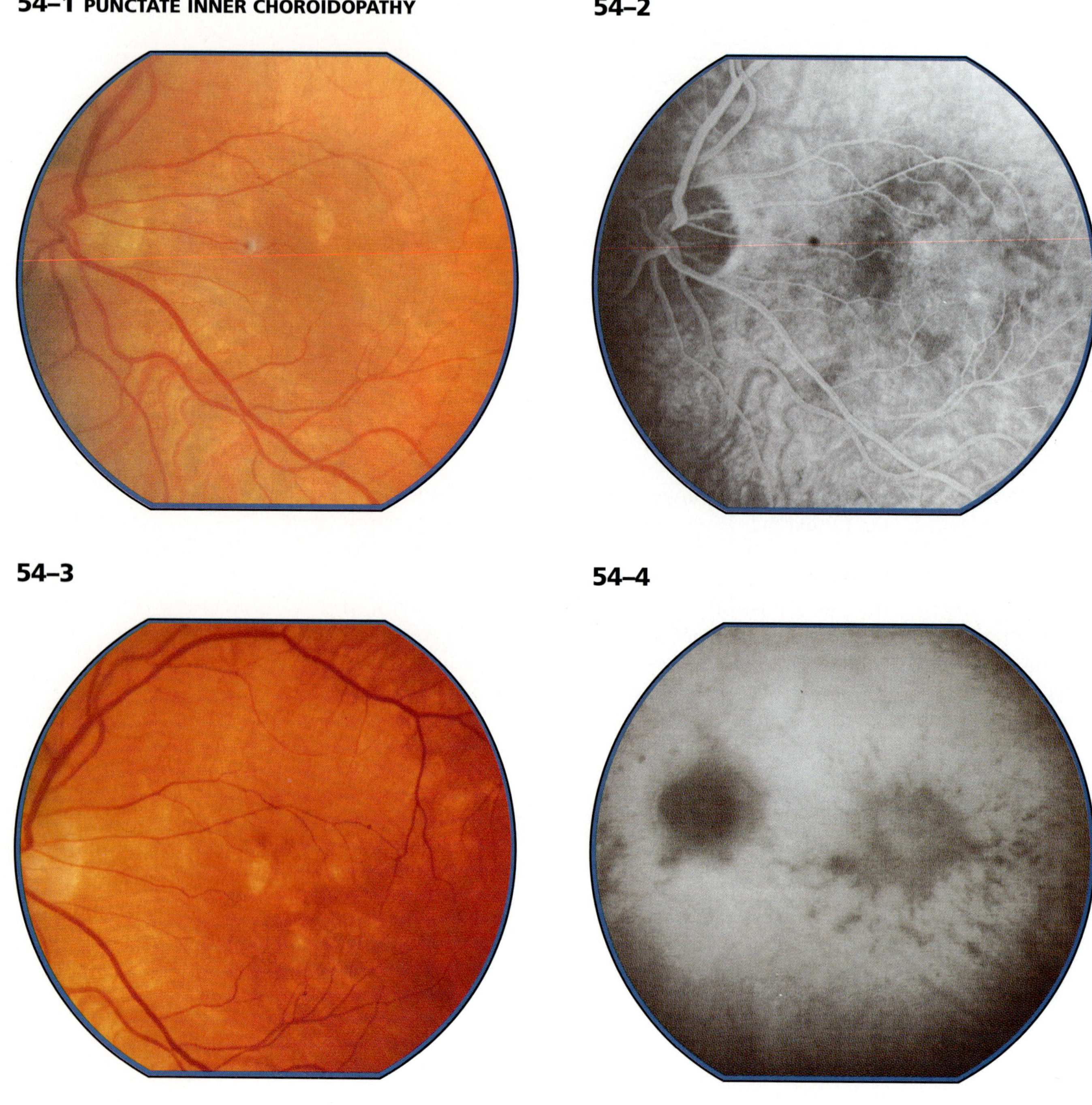

54–1 through 54–4 This 41-year-old myopic female noted a central scotoma in her left eye. She had a history of a recent upper respiratory infection. Visual acuity is 20/50 in the left eye; focal yellow spots are demonstrated in the macular region (54–1). An associated neurosensory detachment is noted. The fluorescein angiogram shows hypoflurescence of the lesions early with leakage late (54–2). There was a mild vitritis. Approximately 1 week later, she noted a decrease in her scotoma, and vision improved to 20/40 in the left eye. The lesions had become discrete, punctate atrophic spots (54–3). An indocyanine-green (ICG) angiogram revealed hypofluorescent spots in the macula and peripapillary area (54–4).

54–5

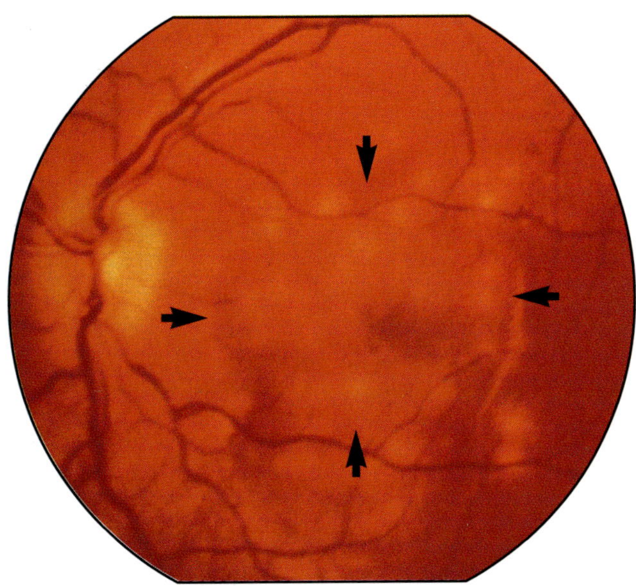

54–6 MULTIFOCAL CHOROIDITIS

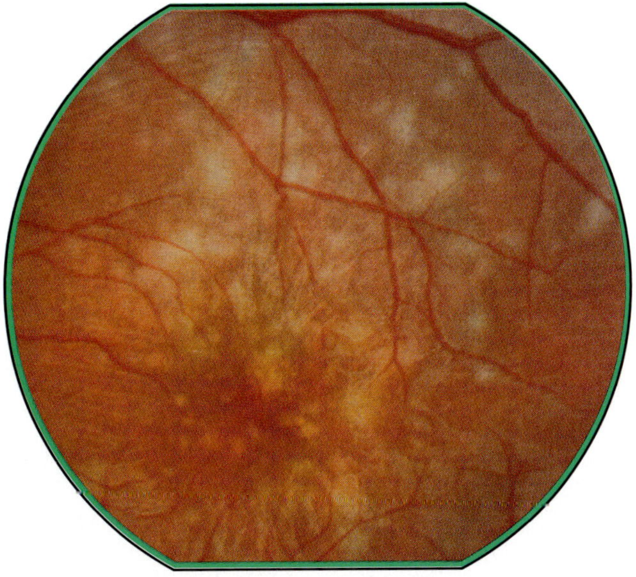

54–7

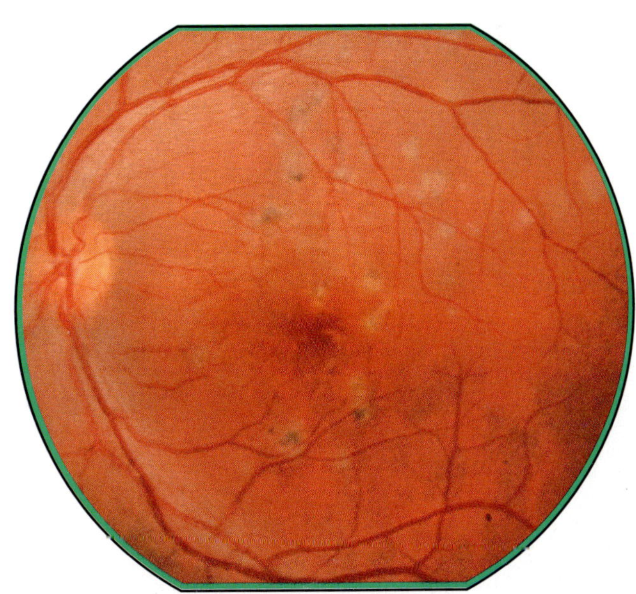

54–5 Punctate inner choroidopathy may occasionally cause a serous detachment *(arrowheads)*.

54–6 and 54–7 This case demonstrates the acute and resolved forms of multifocal choroiditis in the same patient. Note the whitish lesions in the acute phases (54–6) and the more hyperpigmented, more well-defined lesions in the chronic stage (54–7).

***54–5,** Courtesy of Dr. James Folk.*

54–8 MULTIFOCAL CHOROIDITIS

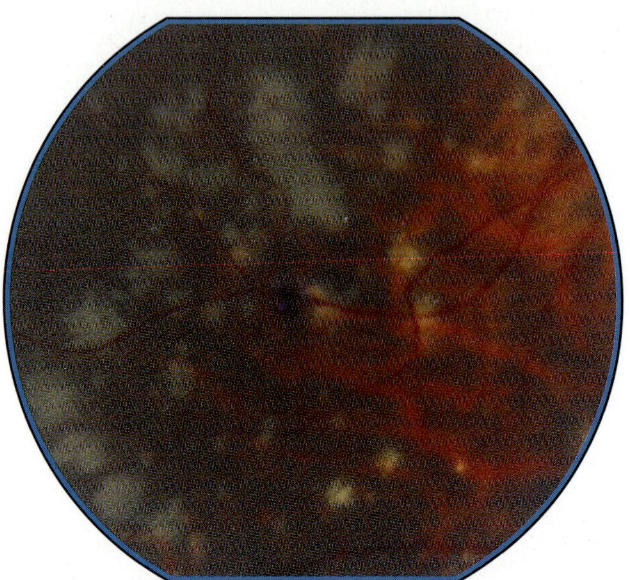

54–9

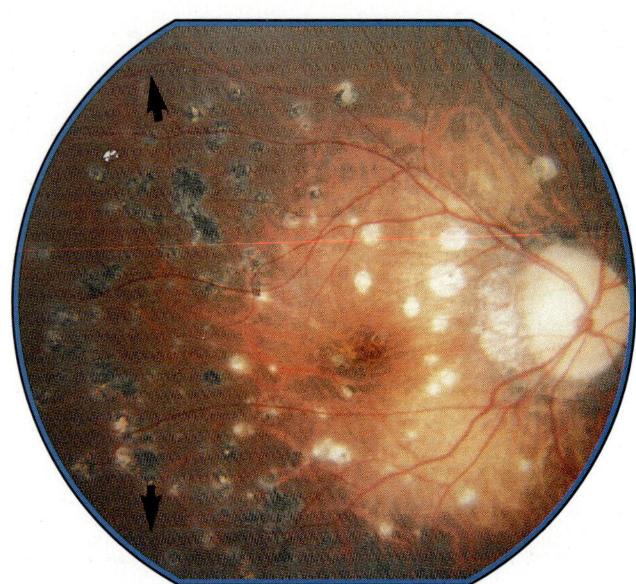

54–10

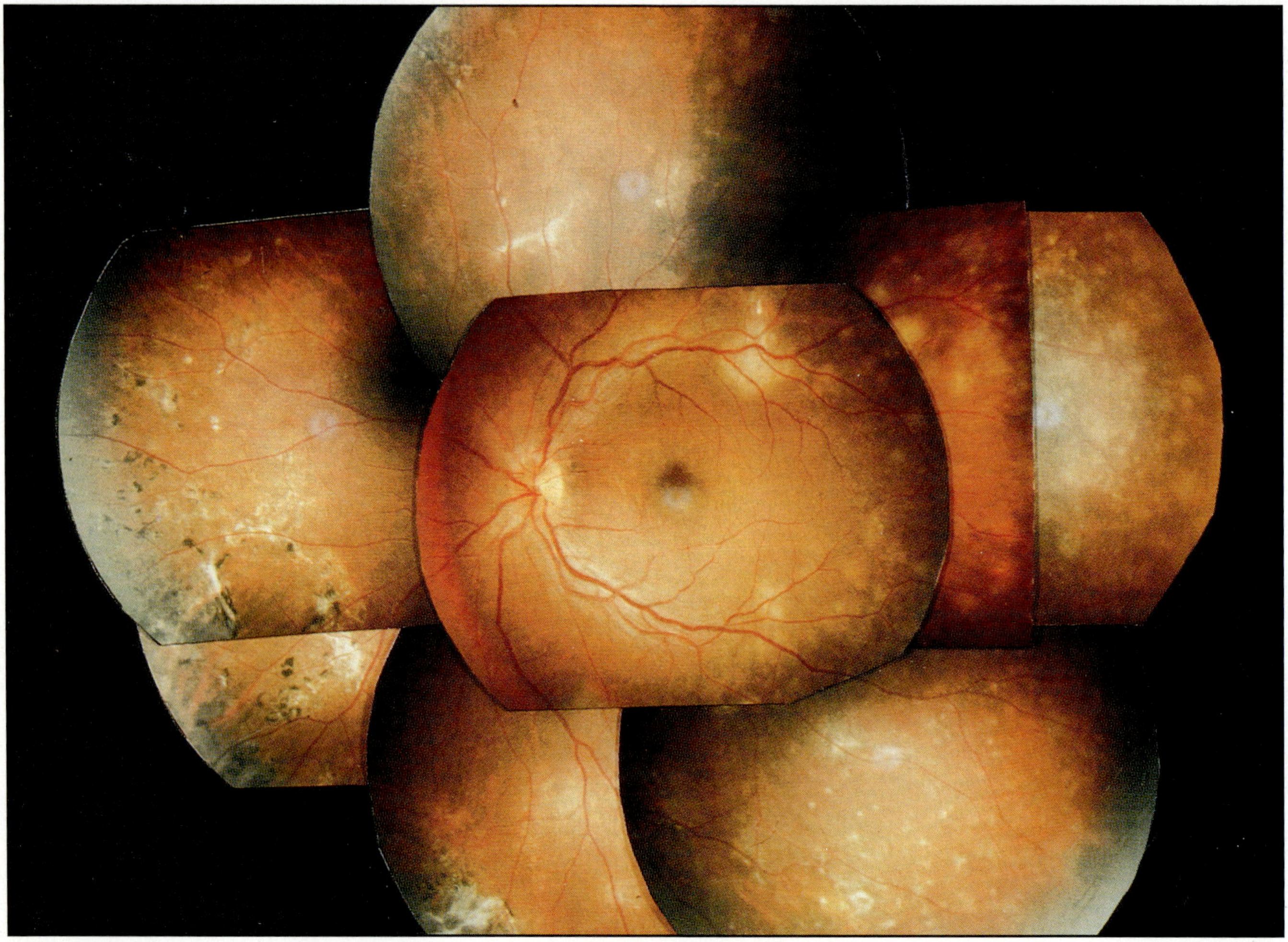

54–11

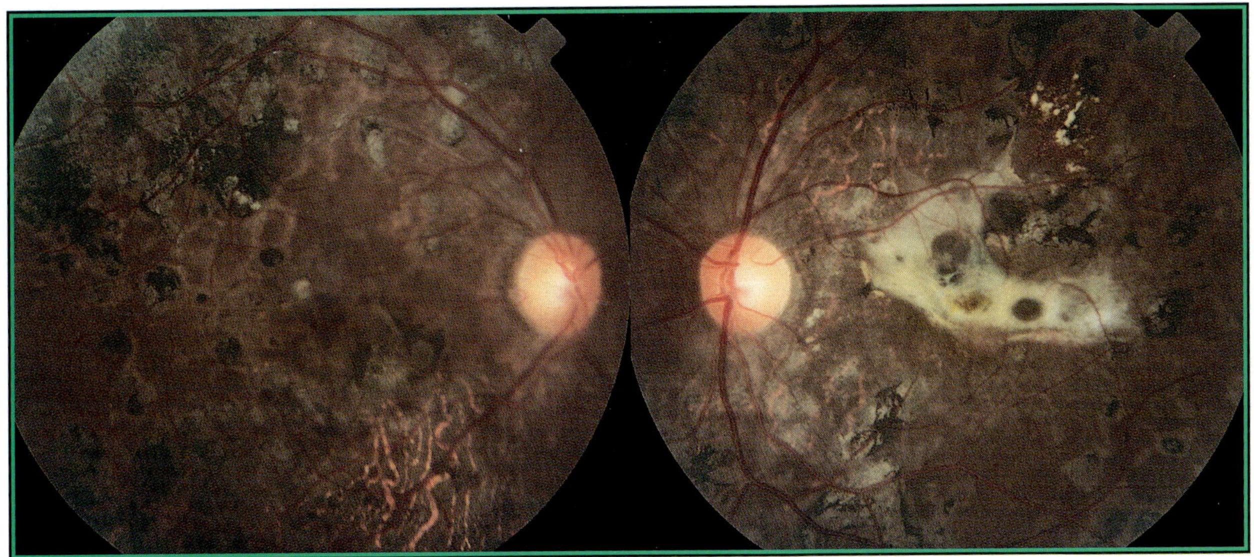

54–8 and 54–9 This patient shows the acute lesions of multifocal choroiditis (54–8). Chorioretinal scars are noted when the multifocal choroiditis resolved (54–9). Also note faint areas of phlebitis superiorly and inferiorly in this black myopic female *(arrowheads)*. The lesions in the posterior pole are atrophic, while in the periphery they are hyperpigmented. This finding may be due to minimal pigmentation within the thinned retina in a staphyloma.

54–10 This montage of a patient with multifocal choroiditis demonstrates both acute yellowish-white lesions in the periphery, as well as resolved hyperpigmented areas, noted especially in the nasal periphery.

54–11 This patient with multifocal choroiditis also shows extensive scarring.

54–12 MULTIFOCAL CHOROIDITIS

54–13

54–14

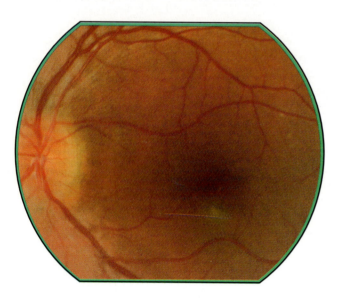

54–15

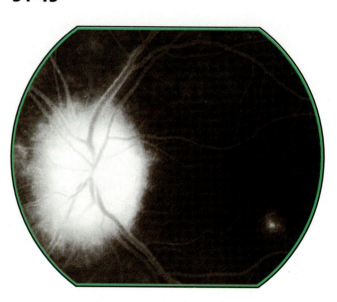

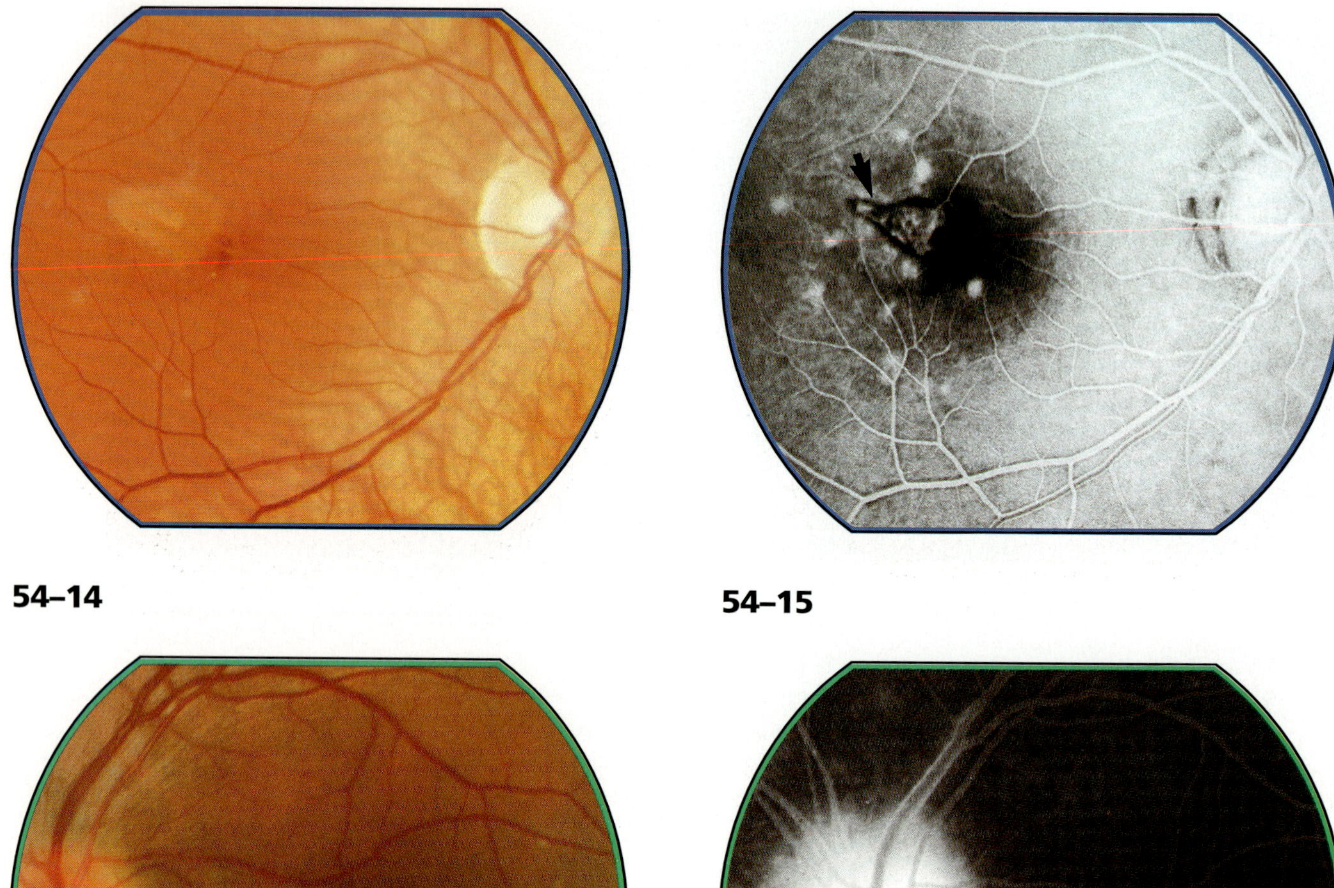

54–12 and 54–13 This patient has multifocal choroiditis with choroidal neovascularization (54–12). Fluorescein angiography confirms the diagnosis (54–13). Note the hyperfluorescent spots and choroidal neovascularization just temporal to the fovea *(arrowhead)*.

54–14 and 54–15 This patient has multifocal choroiditis and secondary choroidal neovascularization. Note the area of choroidal neovascularization and small atrophic spots near the macula in the color photograph (54–14). The fluorescein angiogram shows hyperfluorescence in the area of choroidal neovascularization near the macula and hyperfluorescence of the optic disc (54–15). Optic disc swelling is an important feature of multifocal choroiditis, which distinguishes it from cases of the presumed ocular histoplasmosis syndrome.

54–16

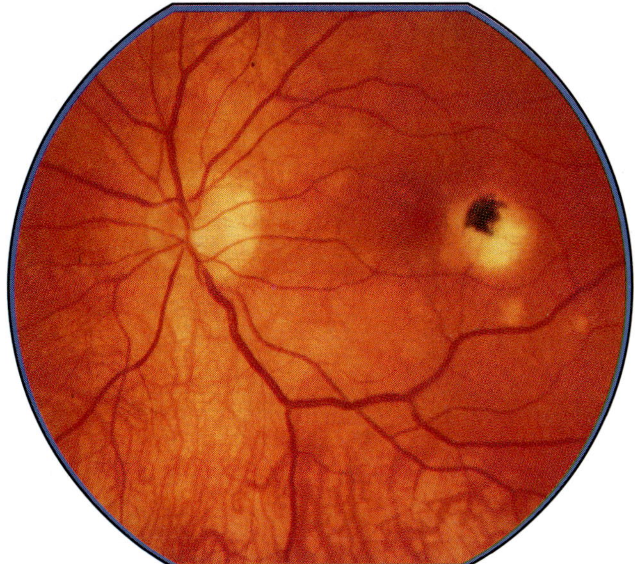

54–17

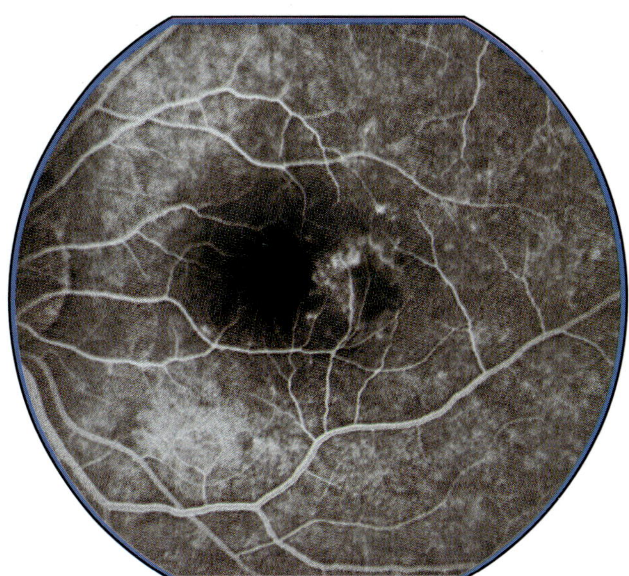

54–18

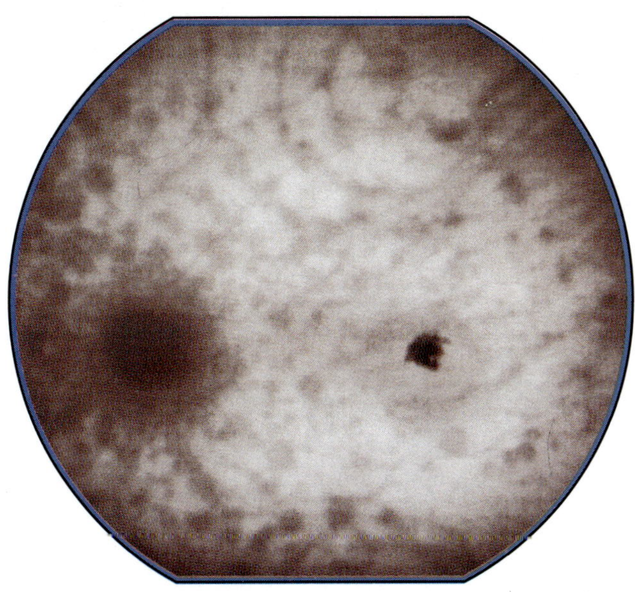

54–16 through 54–18 This patient also has chorioretinal scars from resolved multifocal choroiditis, as well as a disciform scar from choroidal neovascularization. The fluorescein angiogram illustrates choroidal neovascularization and a few hyperfluorescent areas, which represent old sites of choroiditis. Digital indocyanine-green angiography of the same case, however, reveals multiple hypofluorescent spots in areas that appeared normal by clinical examination and fluorescein angiography.

54–19

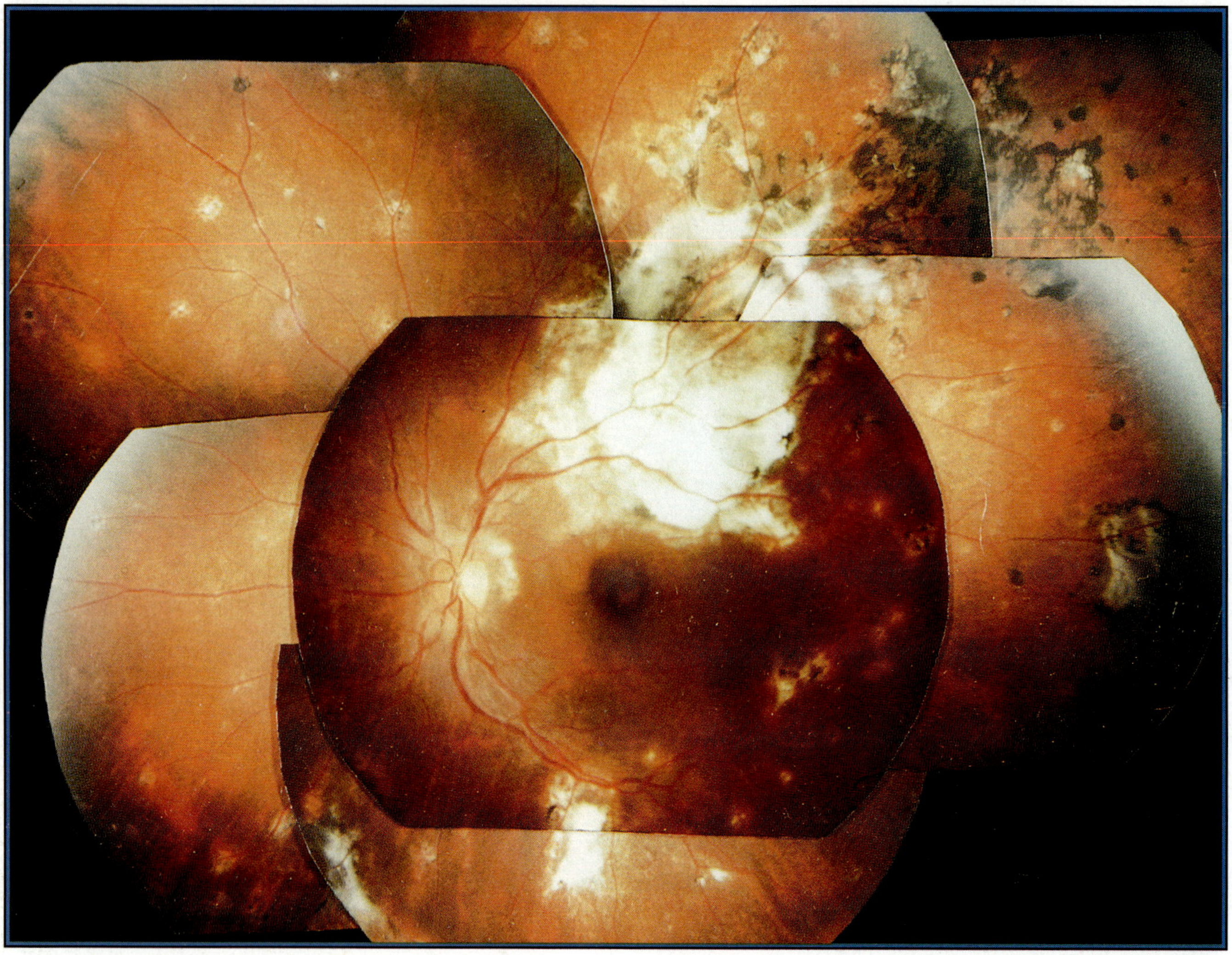

54–20

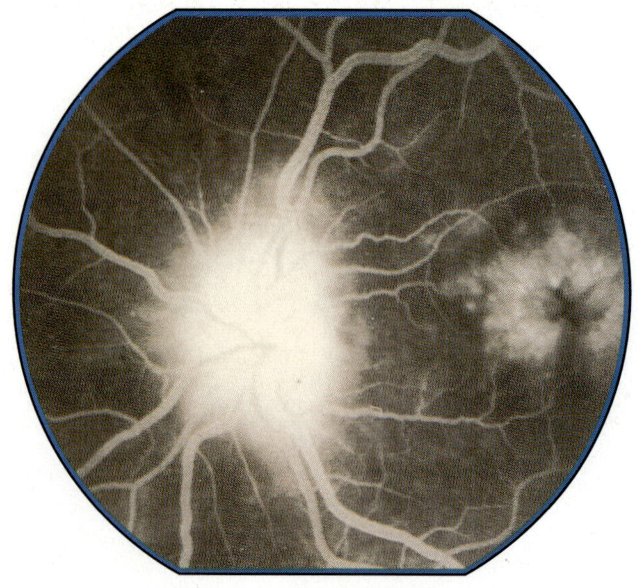

54–19 This montage demonstrates the extensive changes of a patient with multifocal choroiditis. Note the extensive atrophy in this case that extends far into the periphery. Also note the hyperpigmented spots that can be seen in the peripheral quandrants.

54–20 This fluorescein angiogram of a patient with multifocal choroiditis reveals optic disc staining and cystoid macular edema. Intraocular inflammation such as vitritis, phlebitis, and optic disc staining is helpful in distinguishing multifocal choroiditis from the presumed ocular histoplasmosis syndrome.

54–21 SUBRETINAL FIBROSIS AND UVEITIS SYNDROME

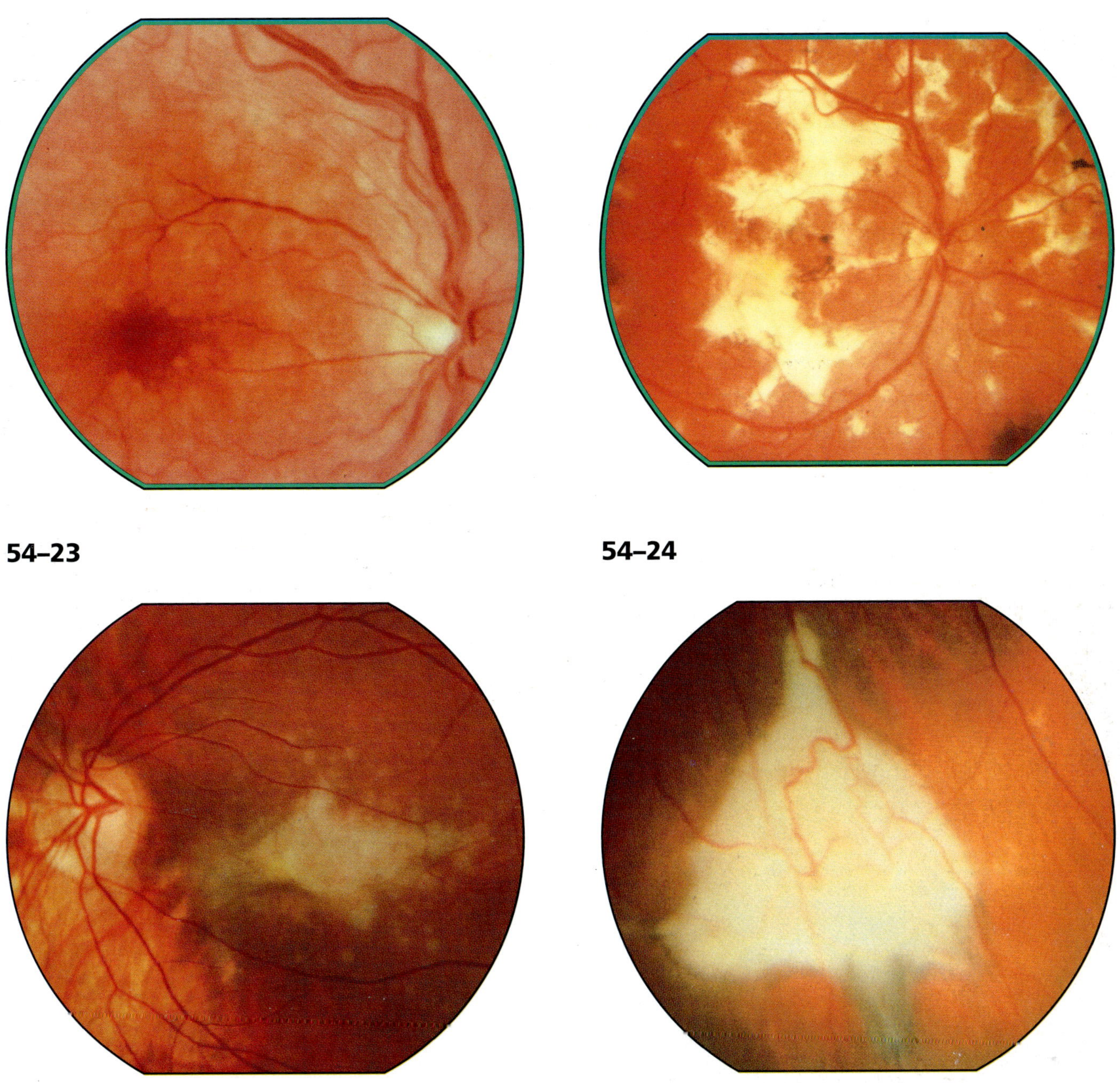

54–21 through 54–24 The subretinal fibrosis and uveitis syndrome shows extensive subretinal fibrosis with uveitis, as demonstrated in these cases (54–21 through 54–24). Note the acute lesions of multifocal choroiditis (54–21) and the resolved stage with subretinal fibrosis (54–22). Note the multifocal lesions surrounding the area of subretinal fibrosis in the macular region (54–23).

54–21 *and* ***54–22,*** *Courtesy of Dr. Herbert Cantrill. From Cantrill, HL, Folk, JC: Multifocal choroiditis associated with progressive subretinal fibrosis, Am J Ophthalmol 101:170–180, 1986.*
54–24, *Courtesy of Dr. Robert Nussenblatt.*

Suggested Readings

Cantrill, HL, and Folk, JC: Multifocal choroiditis associated with progressive subretinal fibrosis, Am J Ophthalmol 101:170–180, 1986

Dreyer, RF, and Gass, JDM: Multifocal choroiditis and panuveitis: a syndrome that mimics ocular histoplasmosis, Arch Ophthalmol 102:1776–1784, 1984

Folk, JC: Punctate inner choroidopathy. In Ryan, SJ, ed: Retina, vol 2, Schachat, AP, Murphy, RP, and Patz, A, eds: Medical retina, St Louis, 1989, Mosby–Year Book, pp 679–686

Morgan, CM, and Schatz, H: Recurrent multifocal choroiditis, Ophthalmology 93:1138–1147, 1986

Nozik, RA, and Dorsch, W: A new chorioretinopathy associated with anterior uveitis, Am J Ophthalmol 76:758–762, 1973

Nussenblatt, RB, and Palestine, AG: White dot syndromes. In Uveitis: fundamentals and clinical practice, St Louis, 1989, Mosby–Year Book

Palestine, AG, et al: Progressive subretinal fibrosis and uveitis, Br J Ophthalmol 68:667–673, 1984

Spaide, RF, et al: Lack of HLA-DR2 specificity in multifocal choroiditis and panuveitis, Br J Ophthalmol 74:536–537, 1990

Spaide, RF, et al: Epstein-Barr virus antibodies in multifocal choroiditis and panuveitis, Am J Ophthalmol 112:410–413, 1991

Spaide, RF, Yannuzzi, LA, and Freund, KB: Linear streaks in multifocal choroiditis and panuveitis, Retina 11:229–231, 1991

Tiedman, JS: Epstein-Barr viral antibodies in multifocal choroiditis and panuveitis, Am J Ophthalmol 103:659–663, 1987

Watzke, RC, et al: Punctate inner choroidopathy, Am J Ophthalmol 98:572–584, 1984

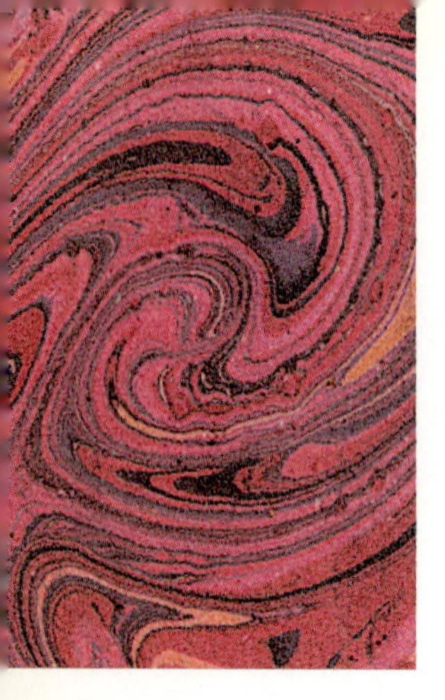

Chapter 55

Multiple Evanescent White Dot Syndrome, Acute Macular Neuroretinopathy, Acute Retinal Pigment Epitheliitis, and Unilateral Acute Idiopathic Maculopathy

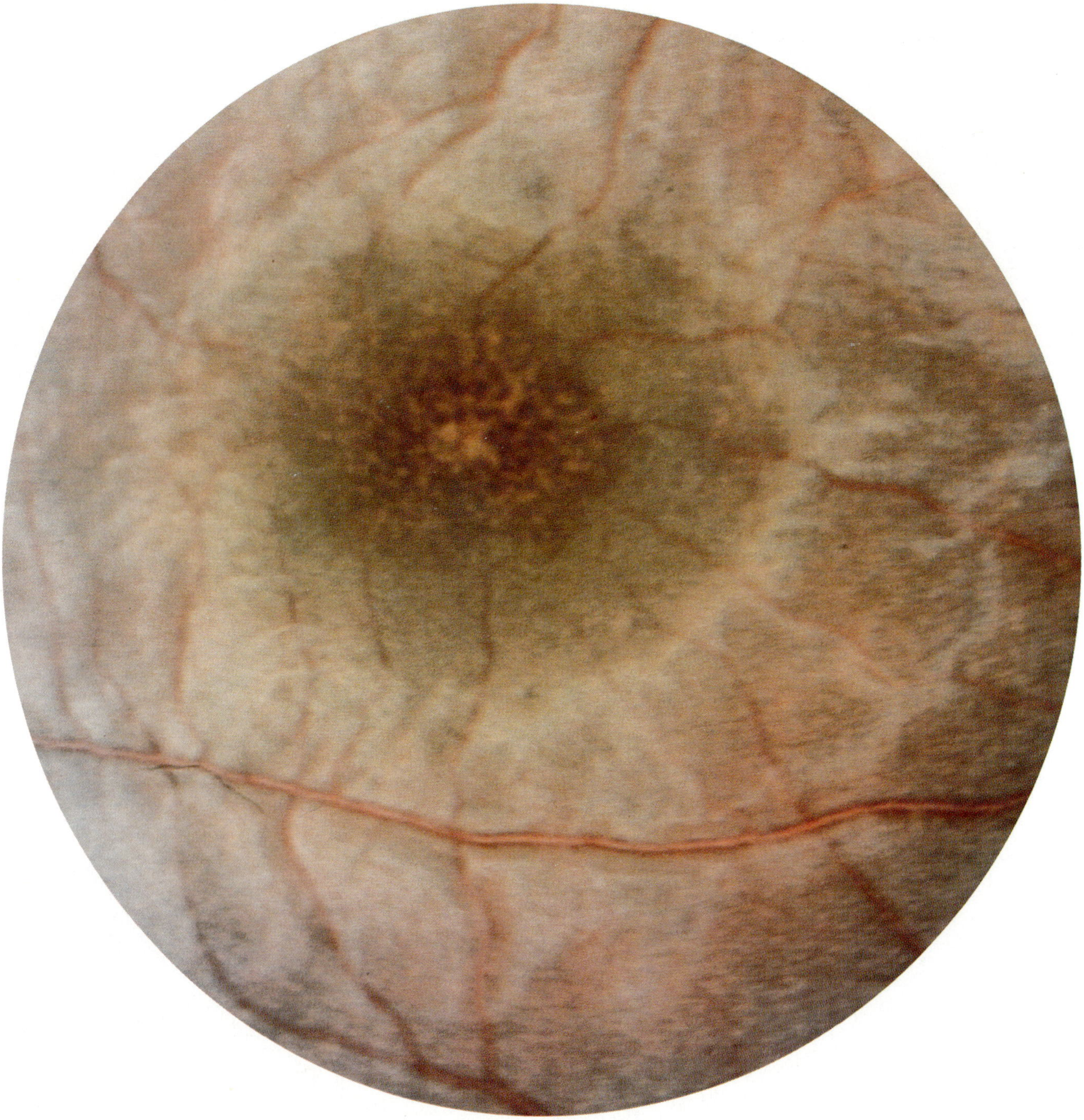

This chapter illustrates manifestations of various rare chorioretinal disorders.

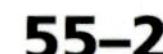

55–1 MEWDS

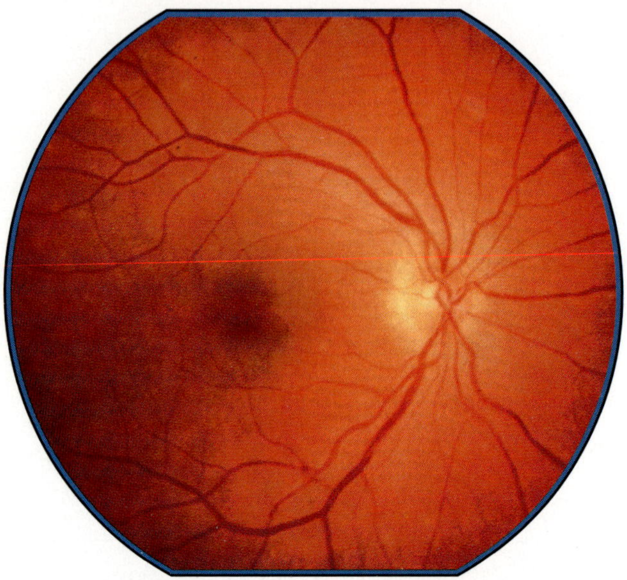

55–2

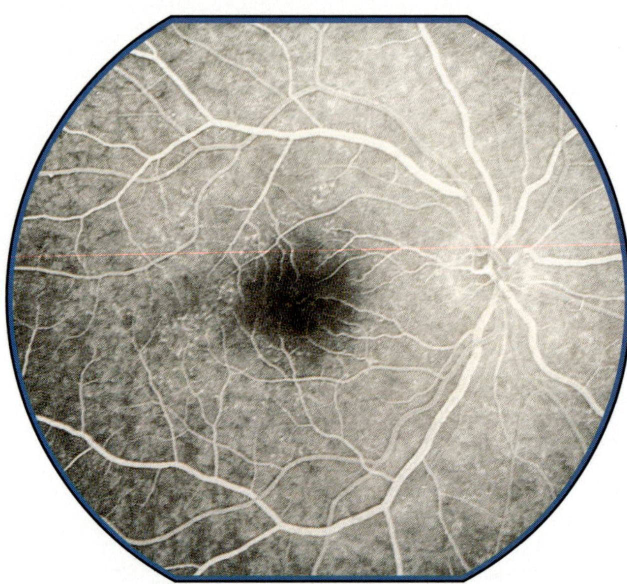

55–1 The multiple evanescent white dot syndrome (MEWDS) is a rare disorder often associated with a viral prodrome. An enlarged blind spot may be noted by visual field testing. This patient has a history of unilateral photopsia and reduction in central acuity. The fundus photograph reveals very faintly evident white spots—at the level of the outer retina and the retinal pigment epithelium—scattered throughout the posterior fundus. There is a mild erythematous change at the disc and a granular appearance to the fovea.

55–2 The fluorescein study reveals punctate hyperfluorescent spots, which do not stain extensively in the late study.

55–3

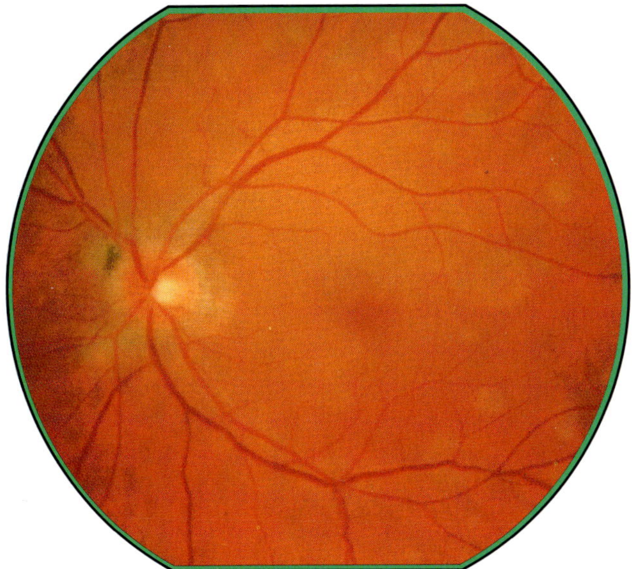

55–4

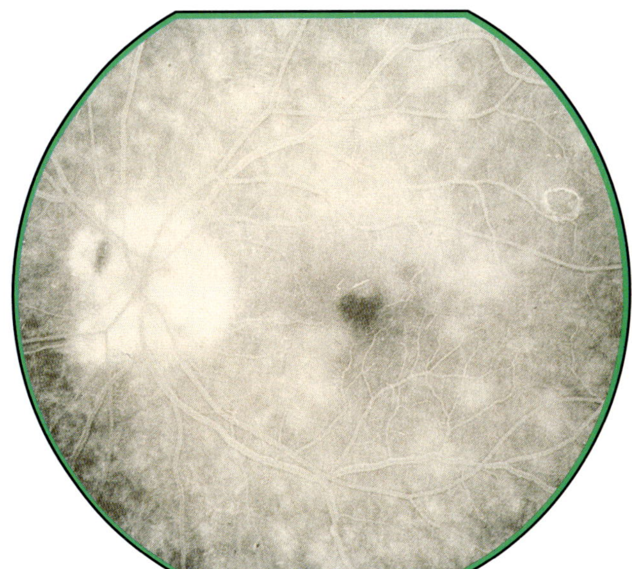

55–5

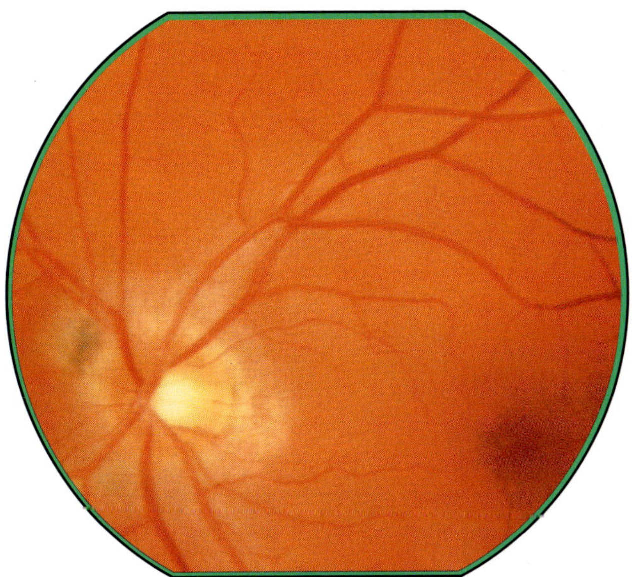

55–3 and 55–4 In this patient with MEWDS (55–3), the widespread spots are larger and possibly deeper in the fundus, causing an alteration in the posterior blood barrier evident as leakage on the late-stage fluorescein angiogram. There is disc staining in this patient as there is in most patients with this condition. Some peripapillary atrophy and pigmentary disturbance is demonstrated in some patients, which may or may not be associated with the overlying syndrome.

55–5 Three weeks later, there is disappearance of the spots and improvement of the vision.

55–6 MEWDS

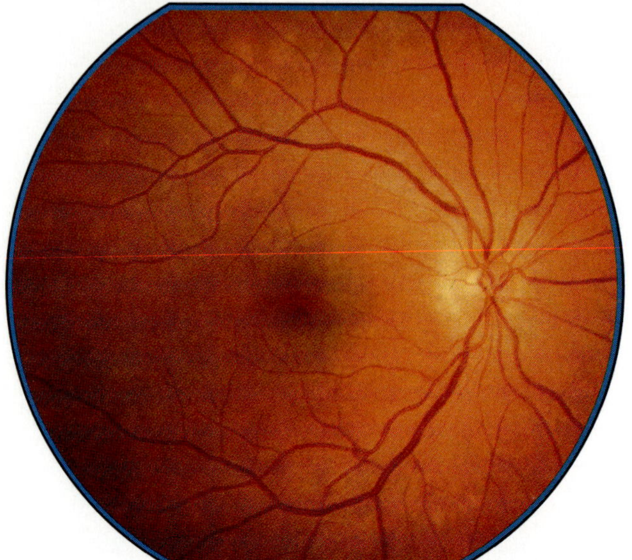

55–7

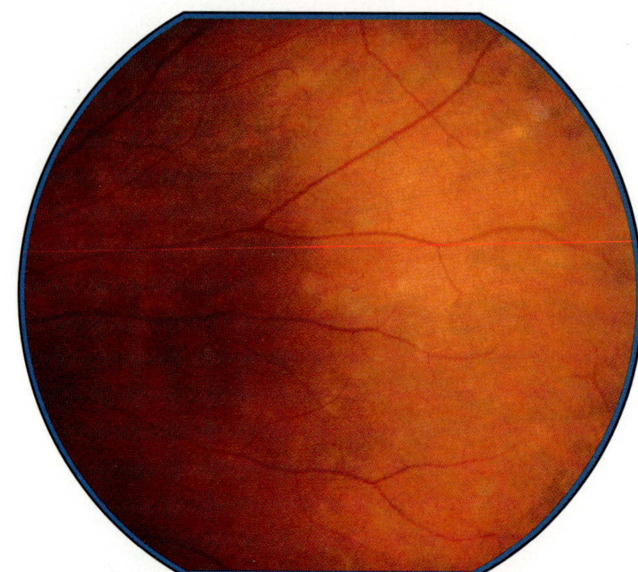

55–8

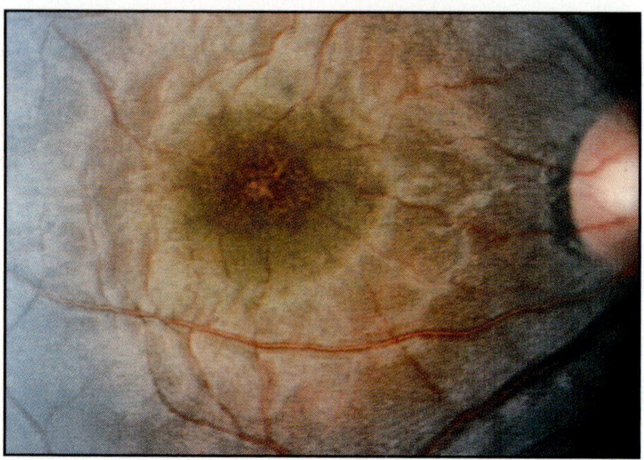

55–6 and 55–7 This patient also has MEWDS. The faint, small whitish lesions in this patient are more characteristic of the white spots noted in this condition.

55–8 Punctate neuroretinitis that appears as macular granularity in patients with MEWDS can be appreciated in this photograph.

55–8, *From Albert, DM, and Jakobiec, FA: Principles and practice of ophthalmology, Philadelphia, 1994, WB Saunders.*

55–9

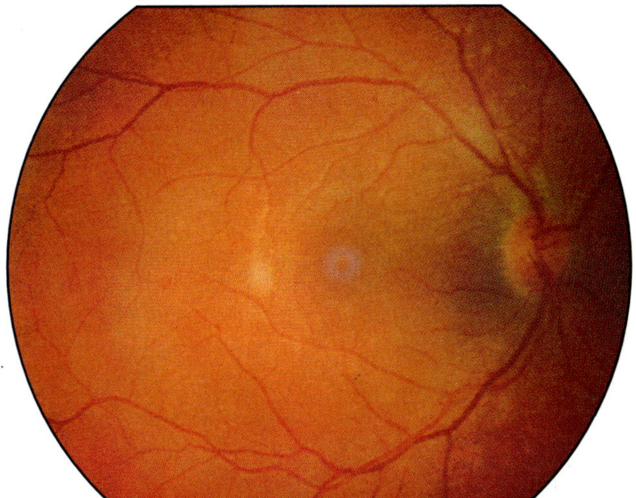

55–10

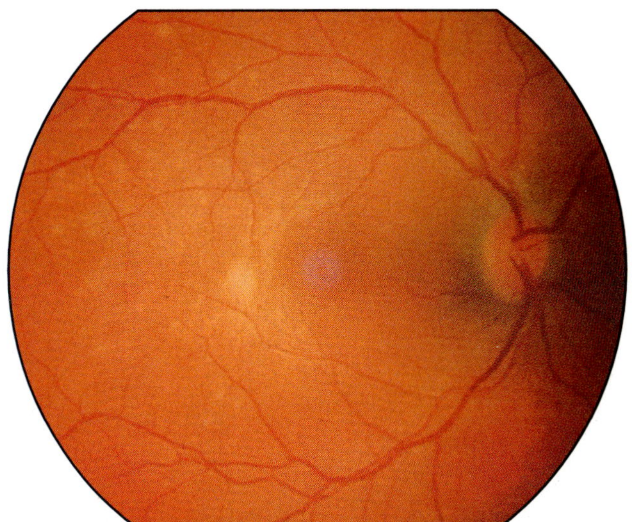

55–11

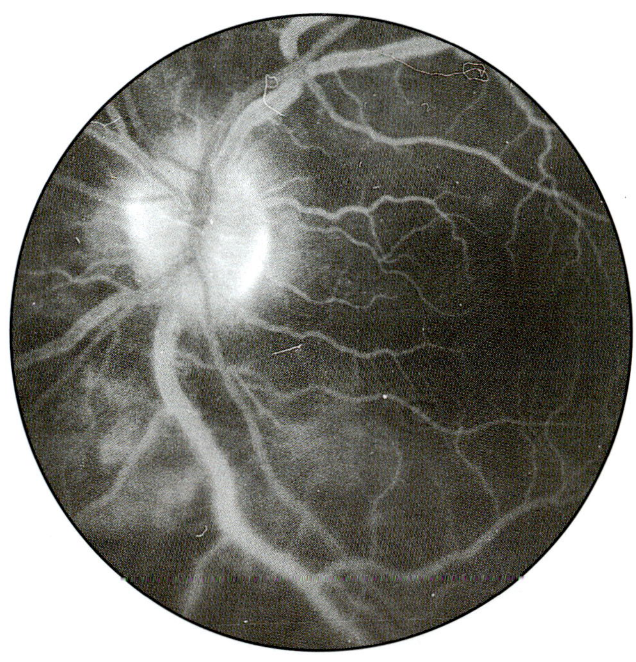

55–9 and 55–10 The evanescent nature of MEWDS is illustrated in this patient. Note that most of the white dots are initially seen inferior to the disc (55–9). Within a few days, this area resolved and more white spots can be seen superotemporal to the macula (55–10). There was a mild vitritis that cleared in this same time interval.

55–11 Fluorescein angiography of another patient with MEWDS shows hyperfluorescence of the optic disc and an inflamed dilated vessel inferiorly. Optic disc swelling is usually seen with this condition, and phlebitis may occasionally be noted. MEWDS has been associated with several other conditions including the idiopathic blind spot syndrome and acute macular neuroretinitis (AMN).

55–12 MEWDS AND AMN **55–13**

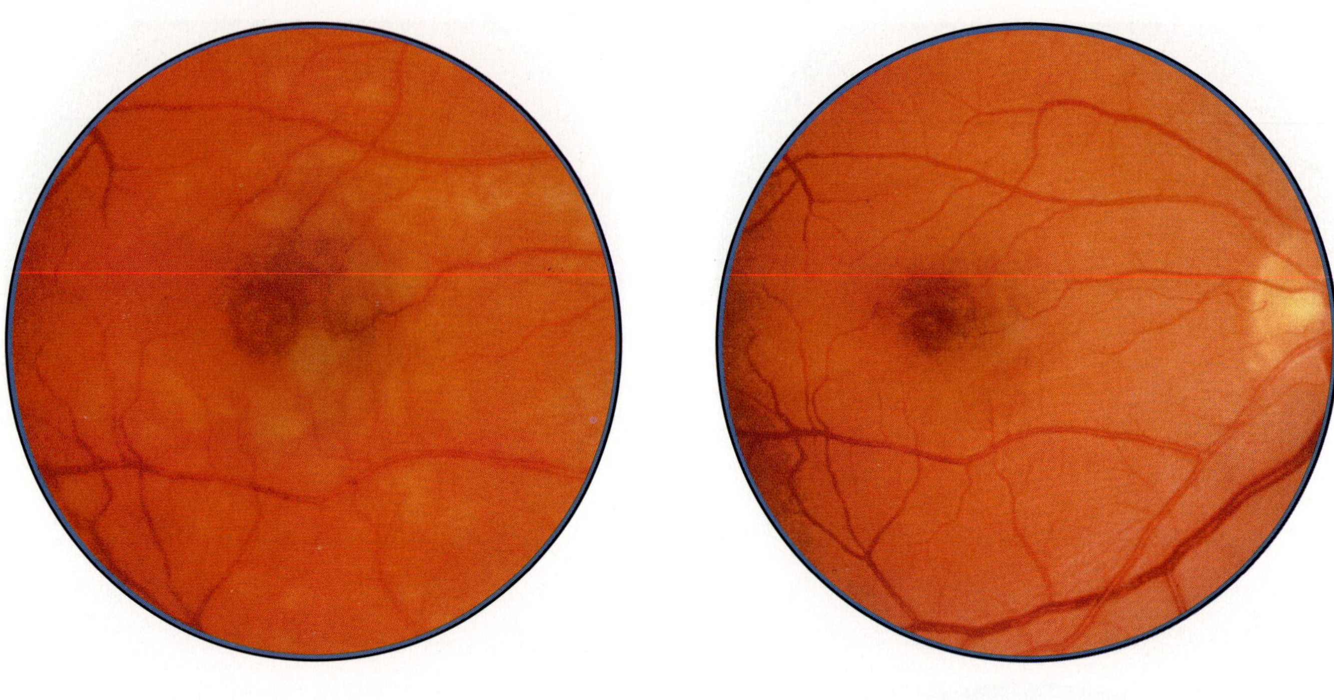

55–12 This patient initially had the characteristic findings of MEWDS with whitish spots and macular granularity.

55–13 The MEWDS resolved, and the patient was later found to have a wedge-shaped reddish macular lesion consistent with acute macular neuroretinopathy (AMN) in the same eye. A prominence in the tortuosity of the retinal veins suggests a mild phlebitis that accompanies the papillitis (papillophlebitis).

55–14 ACUTE MACULAR NEURORETINOPATHY (AMN) **55–15**

55–16 **55–17**

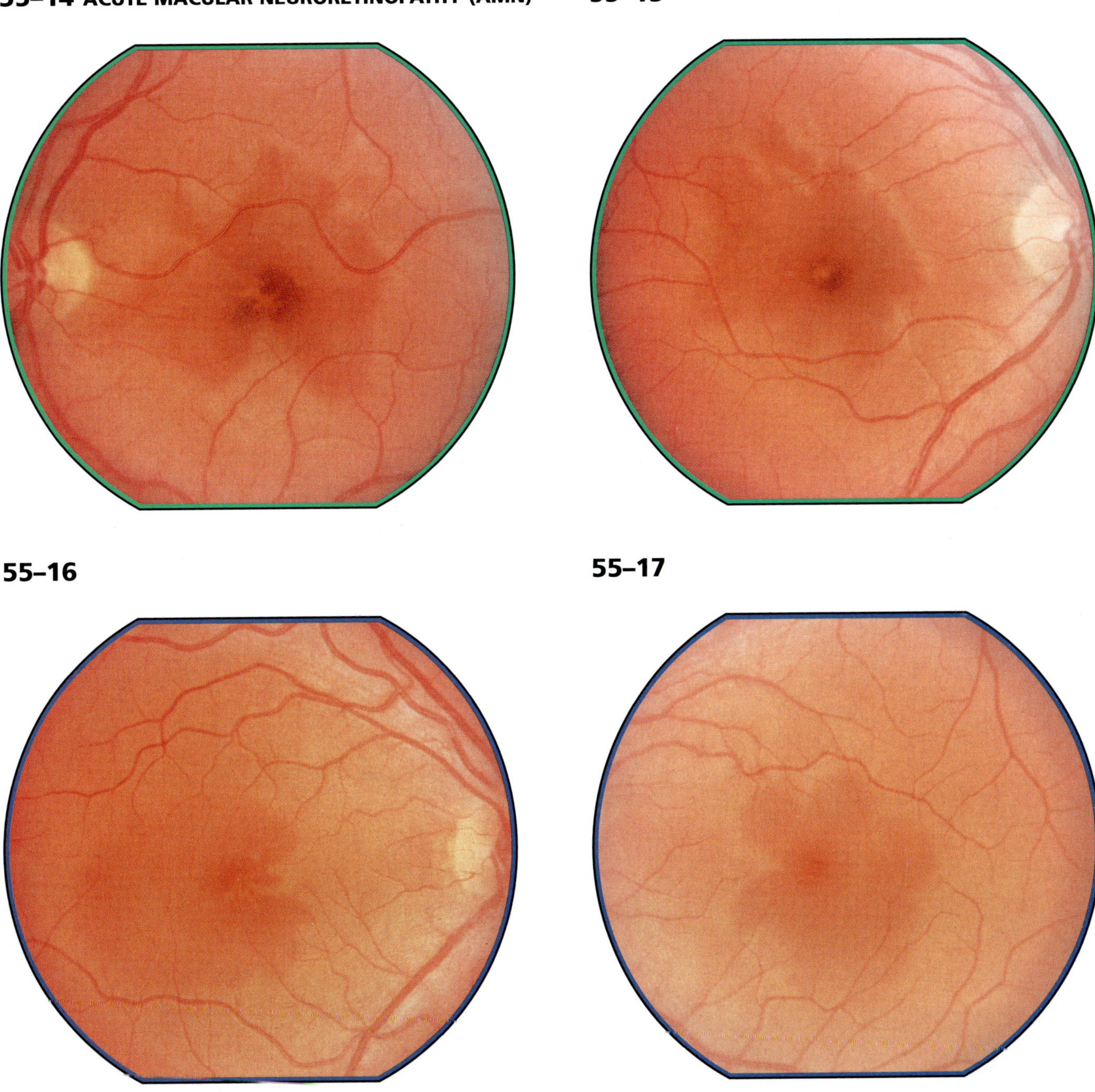

55–14 through 55–17 Acute vision loss is noted in the rare condition acute macular neuroretinopathy (AMN). The fundus shows a darkish, brownish-red often wedged-shaped lesion in the macula. These patients demonstrate the classic findings of AMN. One patient had AMN following an adverse reaction to intravenous contrast media and the other following a hypertensive episode. Note the darkish-red macular lesions that appear to be located in the outer retina. The lesions have a geographic pattern and wedgelike configuration.

55–14 *through* ***55–17,*** *Courtesy of Dr. Robert Kalina.*

55–18 ACUTE MACULAR NEURORETINOPATHY

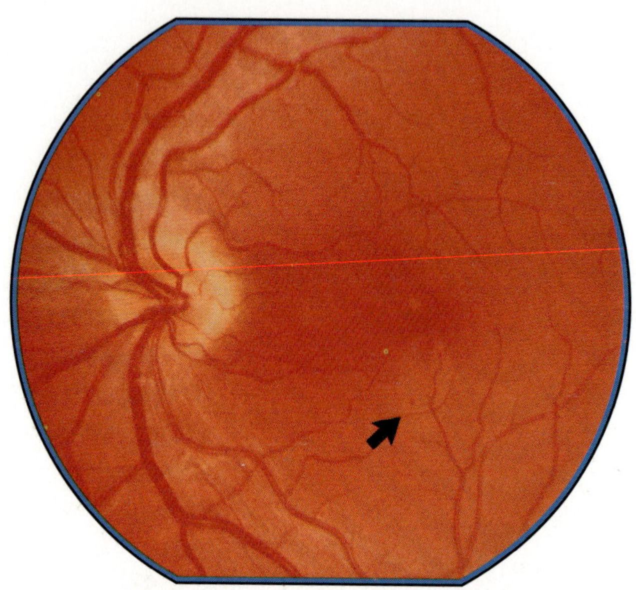

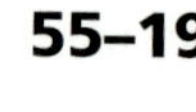

55–19

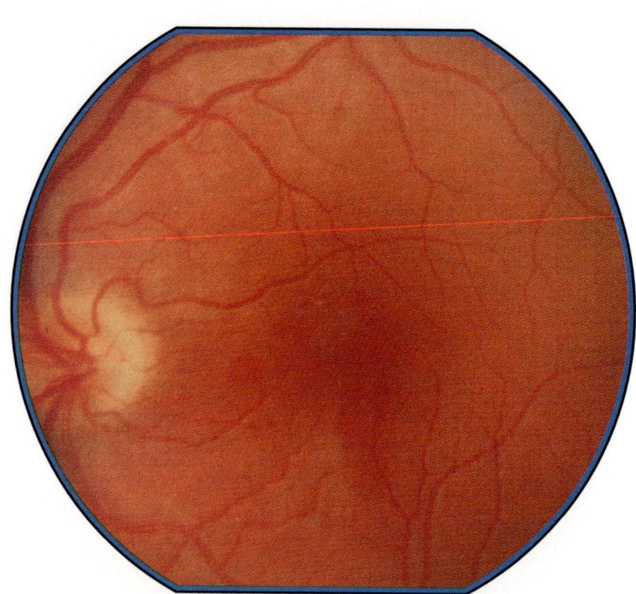

55–20

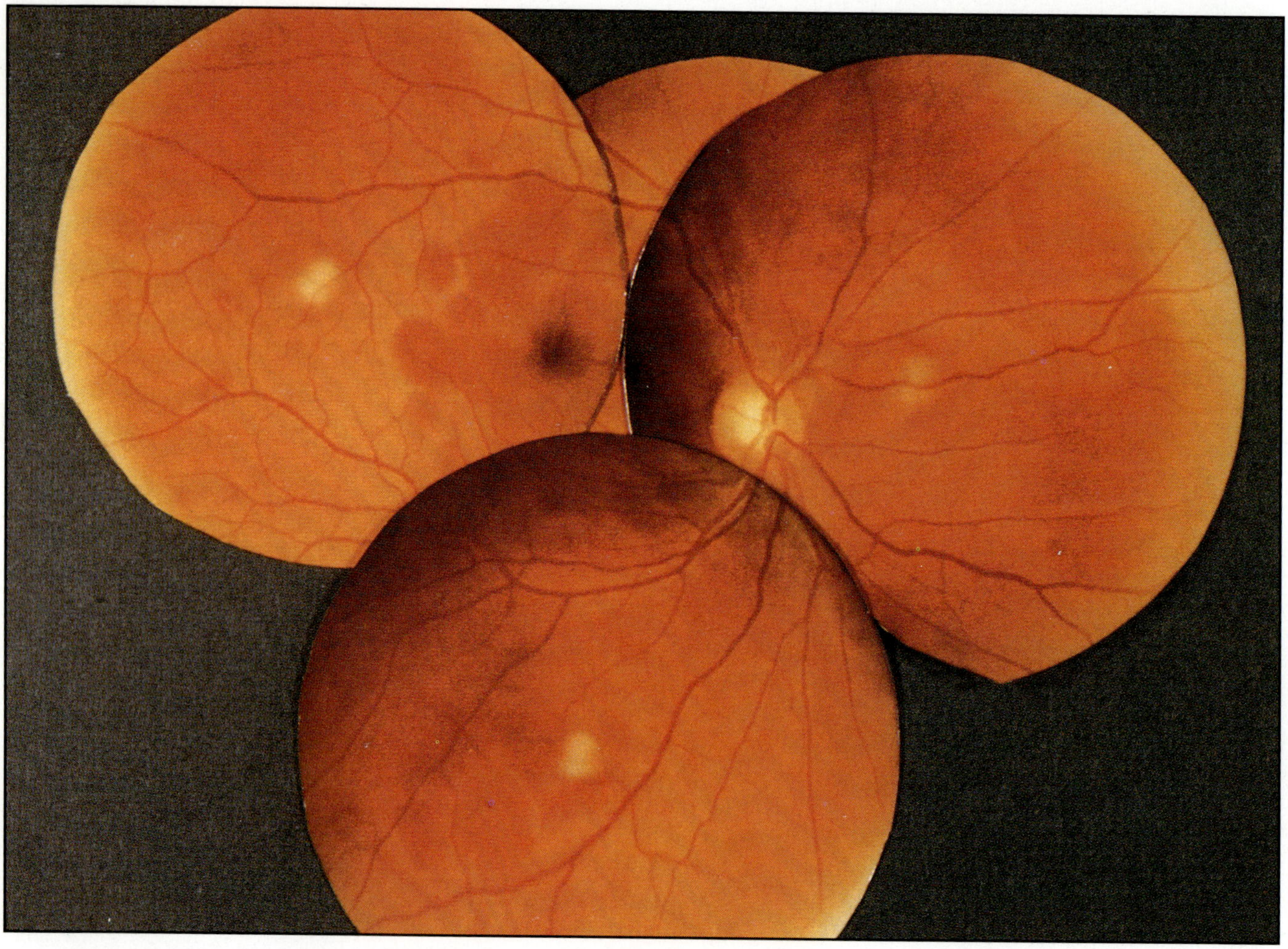

55–21 **ACUTE RETINAL PIGMENT EPITHELIITIS**

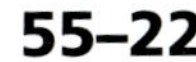

55–22

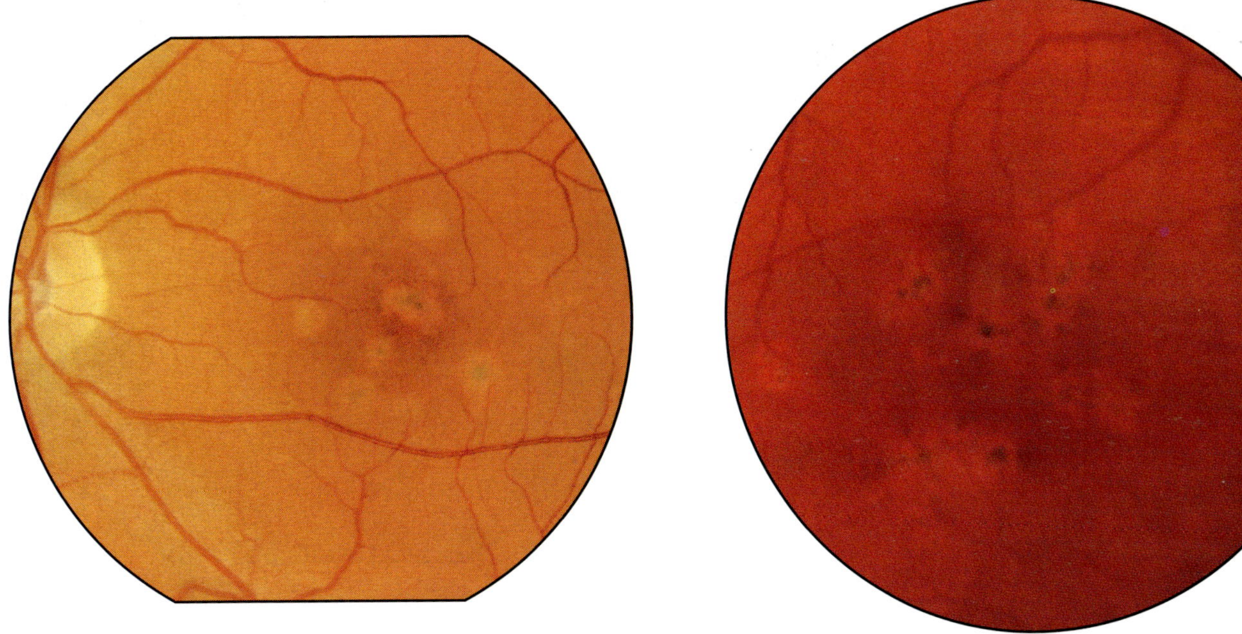

Acute Macular Neuroretinopathy

55–18 and 55–19 This 17-year-old patient had a flu-like illness and developed a central scotoma one week later. Initially, a small retinal hemorrhage in an area of retinal discoloration was noted *(arrow)*. A few days later, the classical petaloid changes of AMN had developed.

55–20 In this patient with AMN, there are huge areas of geographic involvement. Note the reddening of the outer retina in the central macula as well as superonasal to the vascular arcades. The three white spots seen on the photograph are artifacts.

Acute Retinal Pigment Epitheliitis

55–21 and 55–22 The rare condition acute pigment epitheliitis causes acute unilateral loss of vision. One or more clusters of dark areas is noted. These dark spots are surrounded by a small halo and/or atrophic areas. Some of the lesions resemble Elschnig's spots. This condition occurs in young adults and usually disappears within several months. Visual acuity often returns to normal. However, pigmentary changes may be permanent. This condition is probably due to a viral disorder.

55–18 *and* ***55–19,*** *Courtesy of Dr. Helmut Buettner.* ***55–20,*** *Courtesy of Dr. Sergio Cunha.*

55–23 UNILATERAL ACUTE IDIOPATHIC MACULOPATHY 55–24

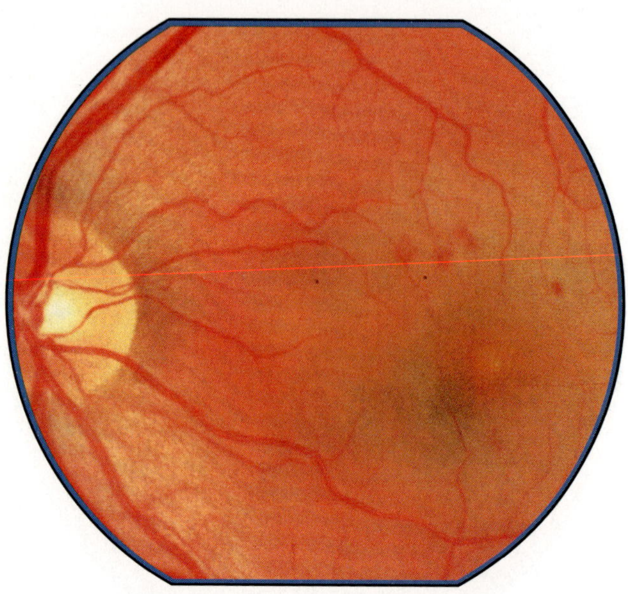

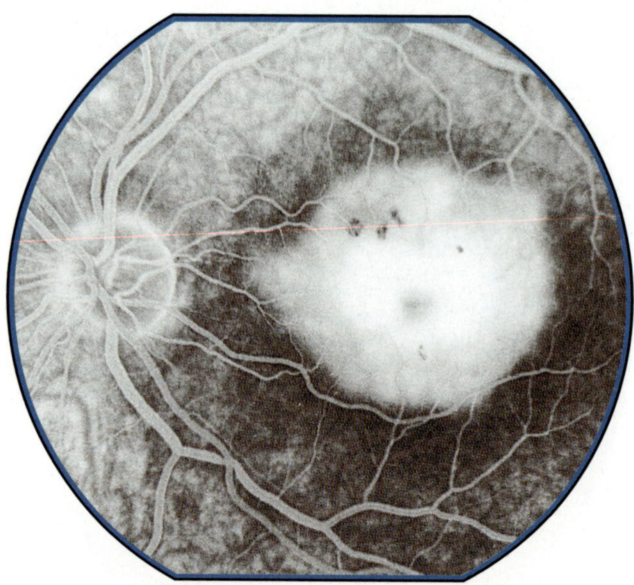

55–23 The unilateral acute idiopathic maculopathy syndrome (UAIM) is noted in patients who develop sudden severe unilateral loss of central vision following a flu-like illness. Acutely, these patients have exudative detachments of the macula. Spontaneous resolution of the clinical findings occurs with a near complete recovery of vision. A characteristic bull's eye appearance persists in the macula. This condition may be caused by inflammatory disease of the retinal pigment epithelium. A specific causative agent has not been identified. This 45-year-old man had a 3 day history of vision loss. He has an irregular exudative detachment of the neurosensory retina. There is an area of intraretinal hemorrhage superior to the macula. Perifoveal thickening at the level of the retinal pigment epithelium is also noted. Visual acuity was 20/200.

55–24 Late frames of the fluorescein angiogram reveal complete filling of the neurosensory retinal detachment. There are at least two irregular wedged-shaped margins. More intense hyperfluorescence is noted in the perifoveal region corresponding to the combined subretinal staining external to the retinal pigment epithelium and pooling within the subneurosensory retinal space. The detachment resolved.

(Case continued on next page.)

55–25

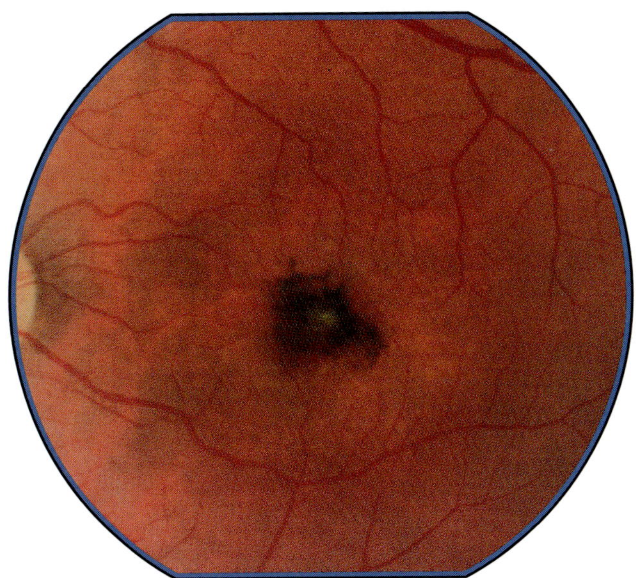

55–26

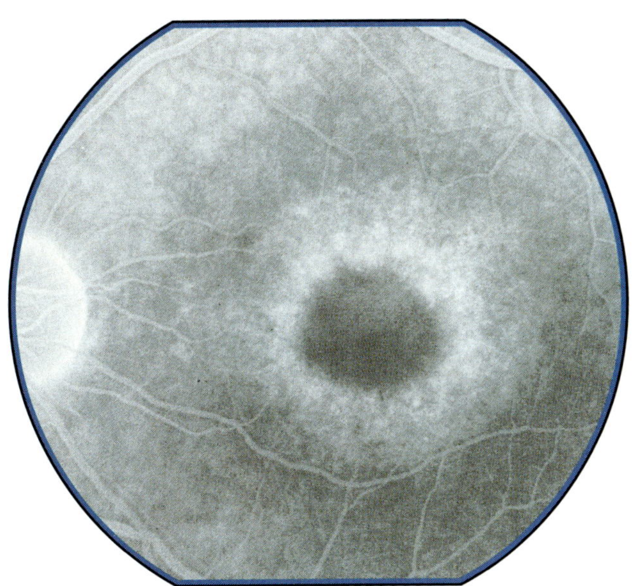

55–25 One year later, an irregular pigment epithelium hyperpigmentation surrounds a central area of presumed subretinal fibrous and metaplasia in the foveal region.

55–26 A broader area of pigment epithelial hypopigmentation is noted in a bull's eye appearance. Visual acuity improved to 20/25.

55–23 *through* ***55–26,*** *From Yannuzzi, LA, et al: Unilateral acute idiopathic maculopathy, Arch Ophthalmol 109:1411–1416, 1991.*

55–27 UAIM

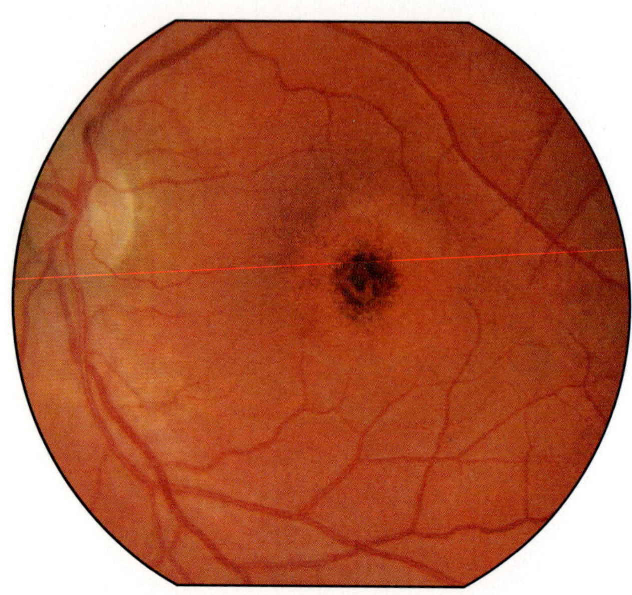

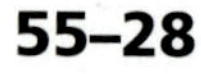

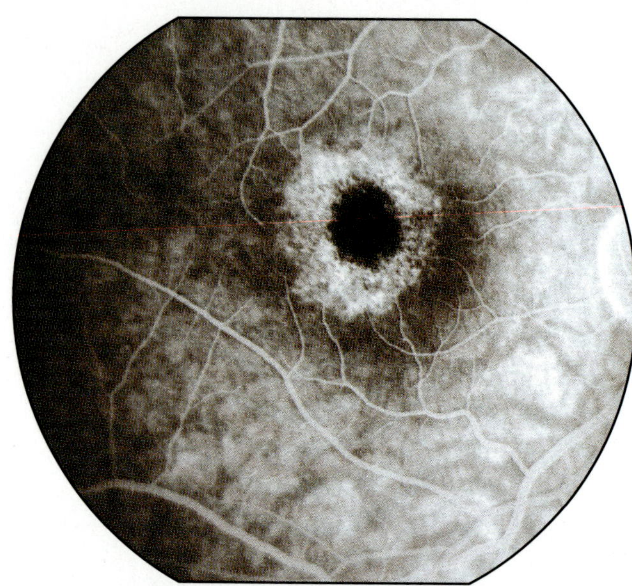

55–27 This patient with resolved UAIM demonstrates a macular lesion with central hyperpigmentation and surrounding atrophy.

55–28 This bull's eye lesion is noted in another resolved case of UAIM and is due to blockage by the pigmentation.

Suggested Readings

Aaberg, TM: Multiple evanescent white dot syndrome, Arch Ophthalmol 106:1162–1163, 1988

Aaberg, TM, Campo, RV, and Joffe, L: Recurrences and bilaterality in multiple evanescent white dot syndrome, Am J Ophthalmol 100:29–37, 1985

Gass, JDM, and Hamed, LM: Acute macular neuroretinopathy and multiple evanescent white dot syndrome occurring in the same patients, Arch Ophthalmol 107:189–193, 1989

Guzak, SV, Kalina, RE, and Chenoweth, RG: Acute macular neuroretinopathy following adverse reaction to intravenous contrast media, Retina 3:312–317, 1983

Hamed, LA, Schatz, NJ, Glaser, JS, and Gass, JDM: Acute idiopathic blind spot enlargement without optic disc edema, Arch Ophthalmol 106:1030–1031, 1988

Jampol, LM, Sieving, PA, Pugh, D, Fishman, GA, and Gilbert, H: Multiple evanescent white dot syndrome. I. Clinical findings, Arch Ophthalmol 102:671–674, 1984

Jost, BF, Olk, RJ, and McGaughy, A: Bilateral symptomatic multiple evanescent white dot syndrome, Am J Ophthalmol 101:489–490, 1986

Kimmel, AS, Folk, JC, Thompson, HS, and Strnad, LS: The multiple evanescent white dot syndrome with acute blind spot enlargement, Am J Ophthalmol 107:425–426, 1989

Leys, A, Leys, M, Jonckheere, P, and DeLaey, JJ: Multiple evanescent white dot syndrome (MEWDS), Bull Soc Belge Ophthalmol 236:97–108, 1990

Sieving, PA, Fishman, GA, Jampol, LM, and Pugh, D: Multiple evanescent white dot syndrome. II. Electrophysiology of the photoreceptors during retinal pigment epithelial disease, Arch Ophthalmol 102:675–679, 1984

Slusher, MM, and Weaver, RG: Multiple evanescent white dot syndrome, Retina 8:132–135, 1988

Wyhinny, GJ, Jackson, JL, Jampol, LM, and Caro, NC: Subretinal neovascularization following multiple evanescent white dot syndrome, Arch Ophthalmol 108:1384–1385, 1990

Yannuzzi, LA, et al: Unilateral acute idiopathic maculopathy, Arch Opthalmol 109:1411–1416, 1991

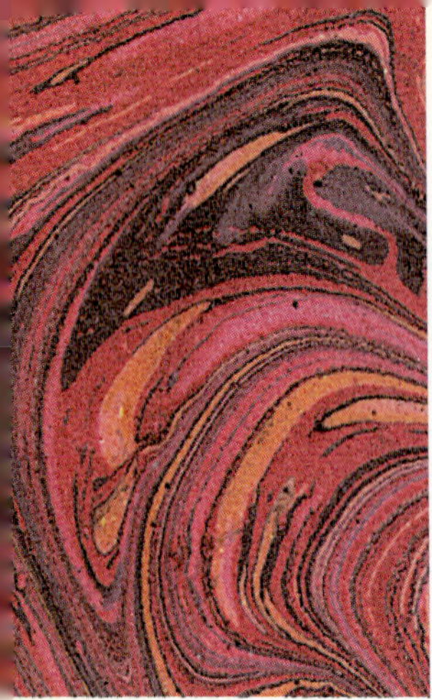

Chapter 56

Sarcoidosis

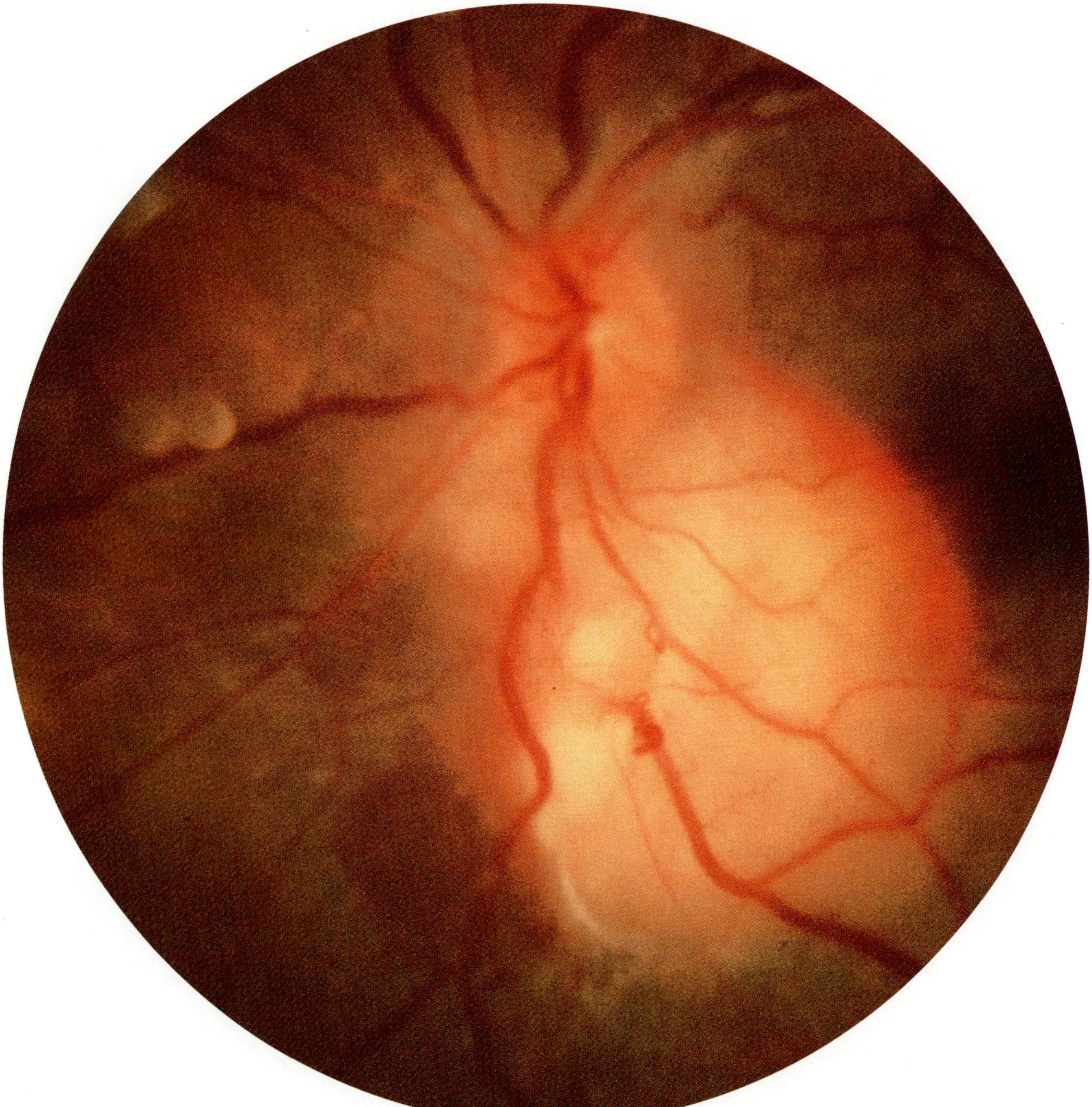

Sarcoidosis is a granulomatous disease of unknown etiology. It can affect various organ systems. Approximately 20% of patients with sarcoidosis have ophthalmic involvement including anterior uveitis, iris nodules, band keratopathy, interstitial keratitis, vitritis, periphlebitis, cystoid macular edema, chorioretinitis, choroidal nodules, retinal neovascularization, orbital disease, lacrimal gland disorder with keratoconjunctivitis sicca, and optic nerve granulomas. Posterior segment disease is noted in approximately 14% to 28% of patients with ocular sarcoid. Vitreous findings are the most common posterior segment finding. Vitreous clumping may occur with either snowballs or a string of pearls. The second most common posterior segment finding is perivascular sheathing. Severe forms of periphlebitis are termed "candle-wax drippings." Choroidal nodules or granulomas may also rarely occur.

56–1

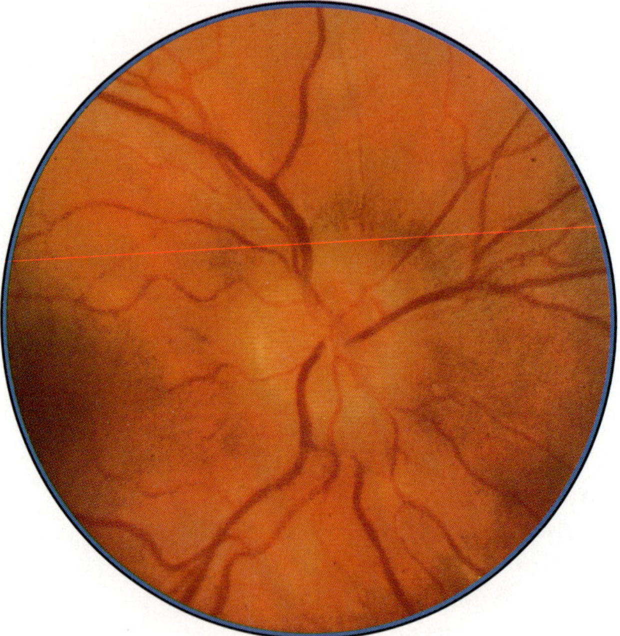

56–2

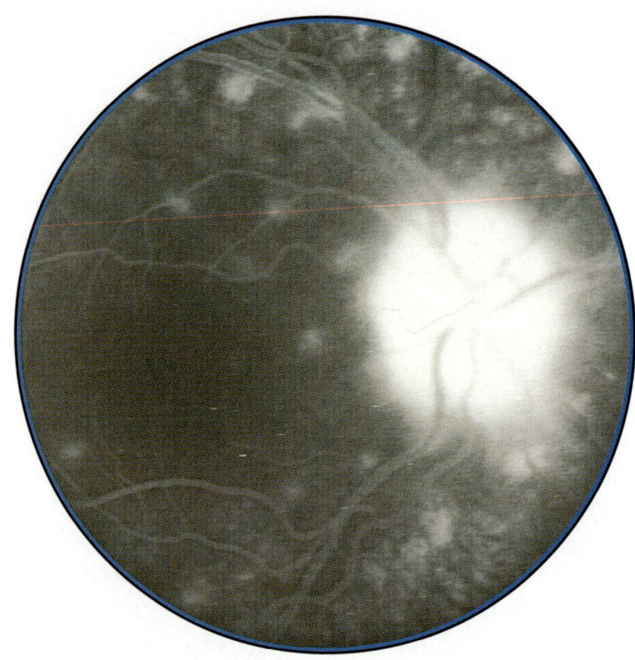

56–3

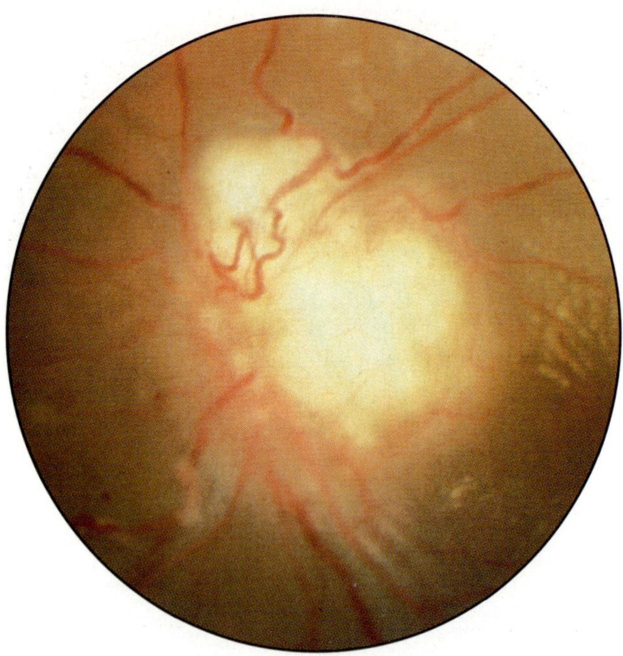

56–1 and 56–2 In this patient with sarcoidosis, which was diagnosed by mediastinal biospy, there is a shallow but clinically detectable elevation or swelling of the optic nerve. There are also faintly evident spots at the level of the retinal pigment epithelium and inner choroid in the peripapillary region. The fluorescein study shows late staining of the optic nerve, as well as the peripapillary spots.

56–3 This case shows an optic nerve mass in a patient with sarcoidosis. Retinal vessels communicate with the granulomatous lesion. Note the candle-wax drippings, which are inflammatory plaques along the venules, most prominently inferonasally in this case. Exudation in a starlike configuration is demonstrated in the macula.

56–3, *Courtesy of Drs. Robert Nussenblatt and Douglas A. Jabs. From Ryan, SJ: Retina, ed 2, St Louis, 1994, Mosby–Year Book.*

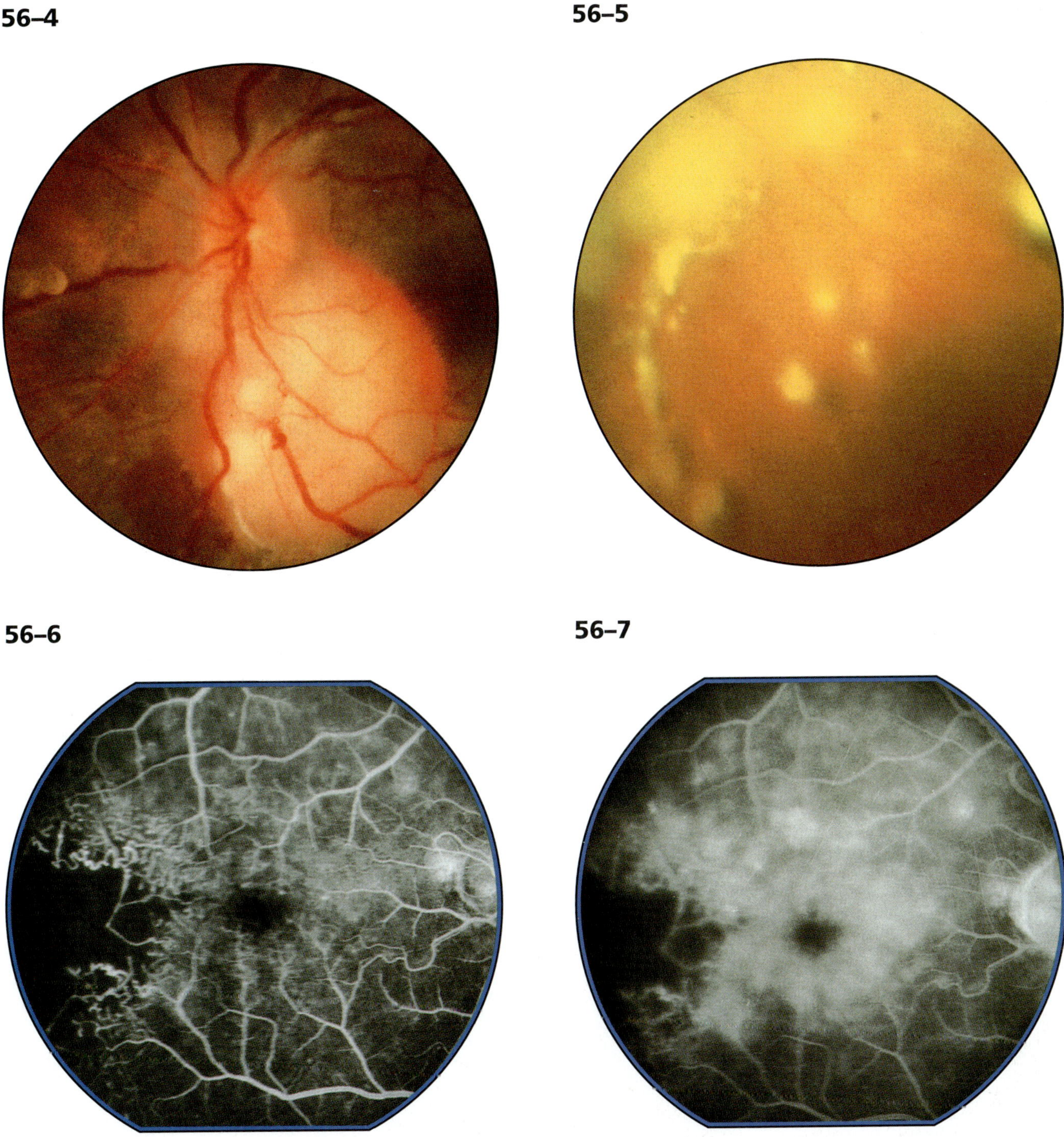

56–4 This patient also has a choroidal granuloma secondary to sarcoidosis. Note the subretinal hemorrhage and serous detachment; vision was 6/200. A retinal vascular anastomosis is noted within the scar, and there are a few plaques of inflammatory debris along the inferior vessel. This nodule shrunk after steroid treatment.

56–5 Vitreous inflammation is noted in this patient with sarcoidosis.

56–6 and 56–7 Fluorescein studies may reveal a microangiopathy, including telangiectatic vascular changes, ischemia, and leakage.

56–4, *Courtesy of Dr. Rollins Tindell, Jr.* ***56–5,*** *Courtesy of Dr. Douglas A. Jabs. From Ryan, SJ: Retina, ed 2, St Louis, 1994, Mosby–Year Book.*

56–8

56–9

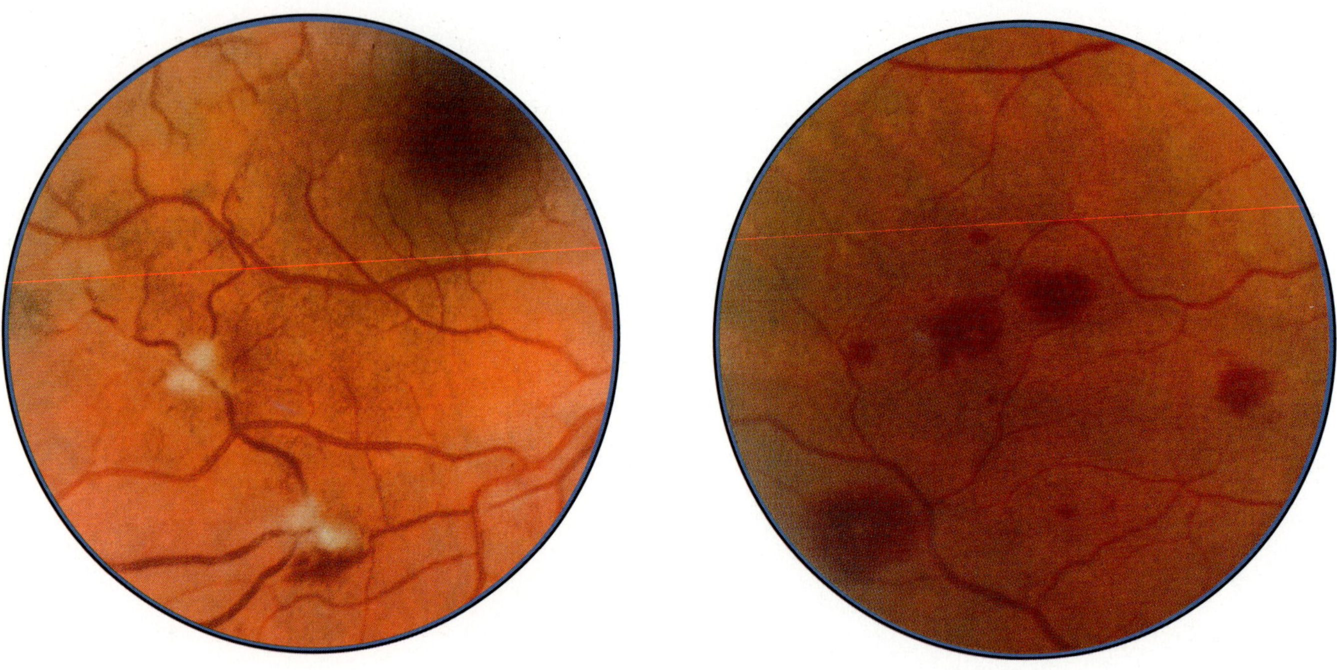

56–10

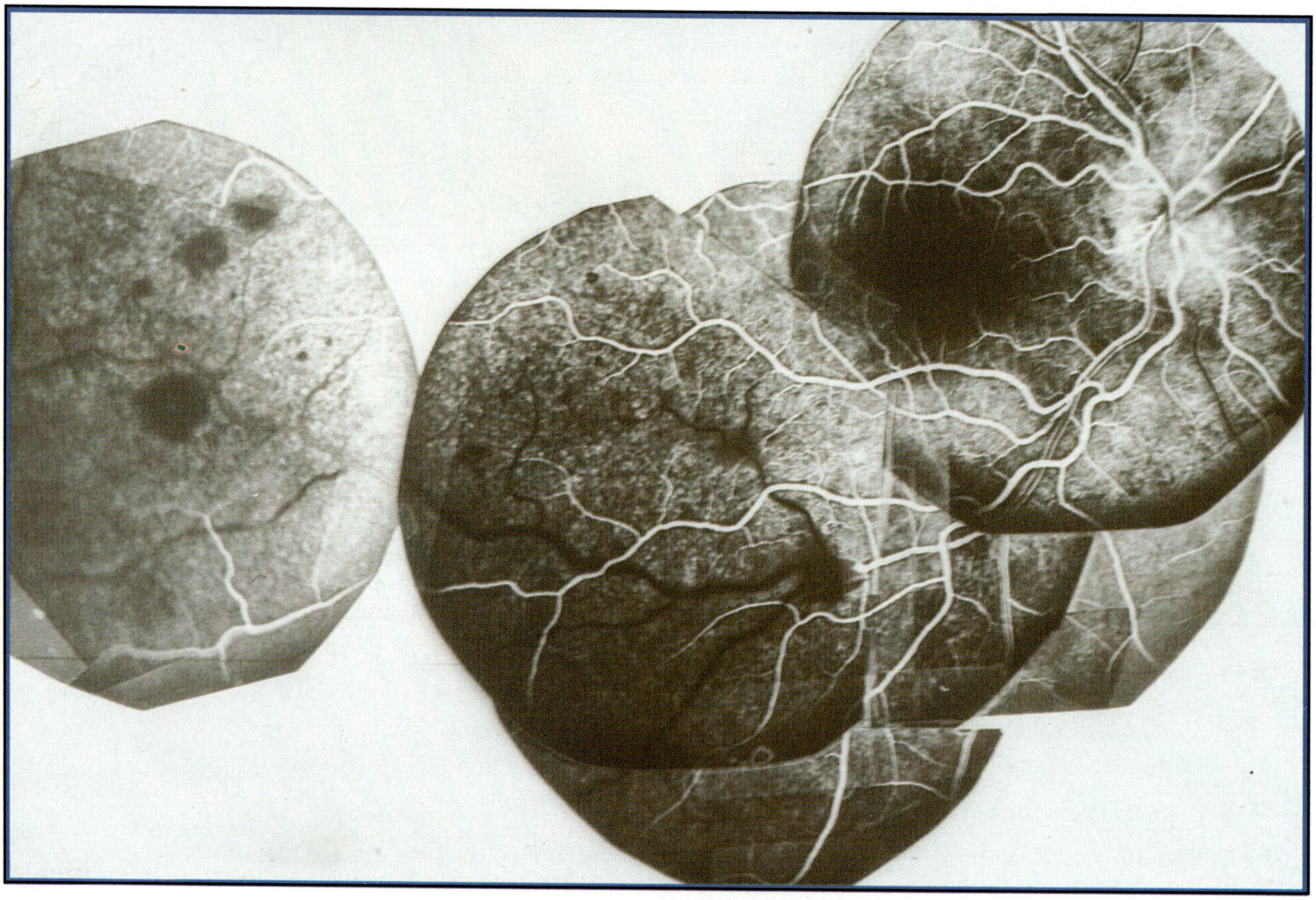

56–11

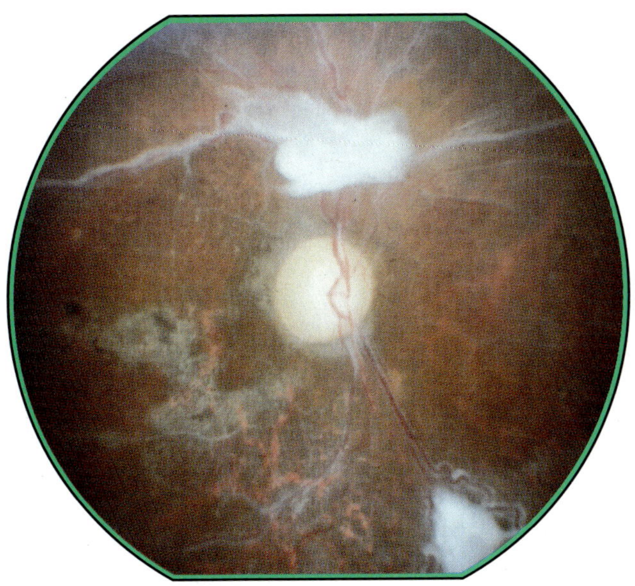

56–12

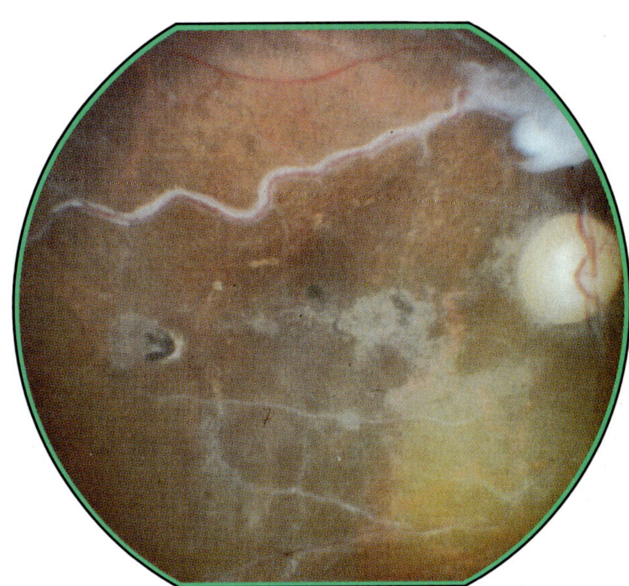

56–8 and 56–9 Intraretinal hemorrhages (56–8 and 56–9), cotton-wool spots (56–8), and Roth's spots (56–9) may also be demonstrated in patients with sarcoidosis.

56–10 This patient with sarcoidosis reveals retinal vascular changes including a branch retinal vein occlusion, arterial occlusion, and scattered hemorrhages—including a few with white centers (Roth's spots). Note that the vein occlusion occurs at the site of localized phlebitis rather than at an arteriovenous crossing. The arteriole occlusion is best demonstrated on the fluorescein angiogram.

56–11 and 56–12 Extensive sheathing of the vessels with fibrosis may occur in the end stage of ocular sarcoidosis. Note the extensive nonperfusion in these cases with optic disc atrophy, fibrous material at the vascular arcades, and pigment epithelium atrophy.

56–13

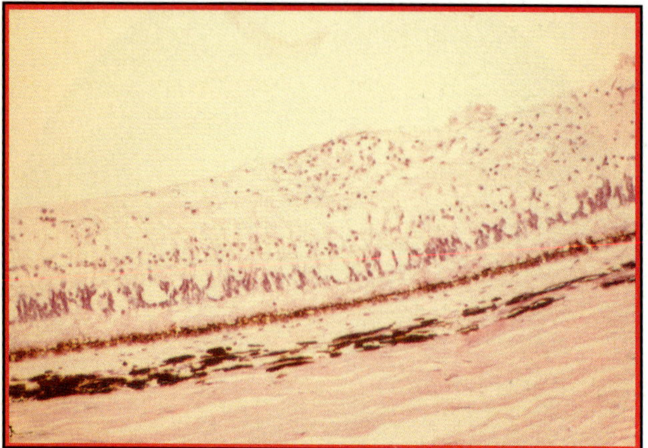

56–14

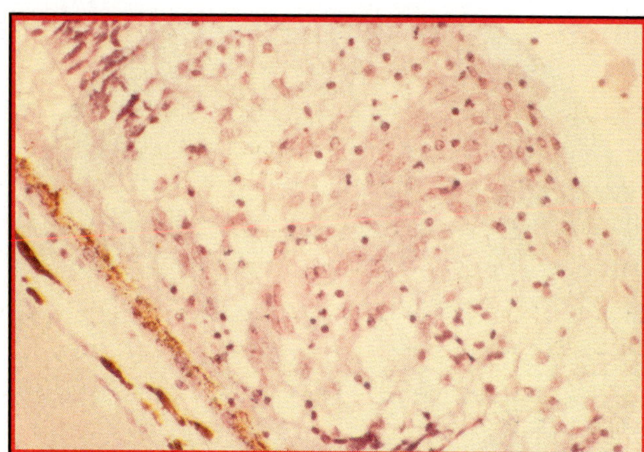

56–15

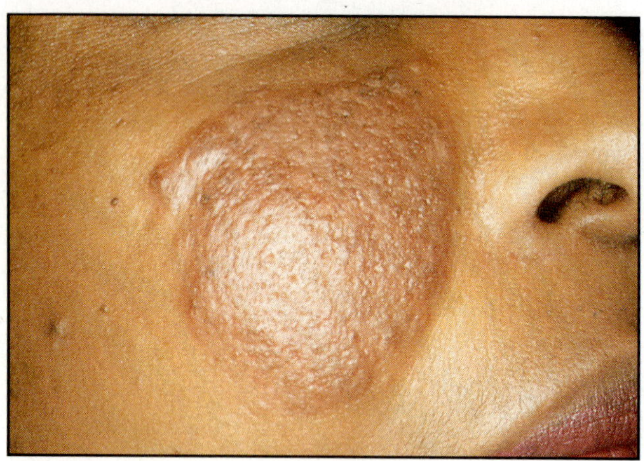

56–13 and 56–14 This patient with sarcoidosis has sarcoid granulomas in and on the inner surface of the retina. Higher-power view shows the sarcoid granuloma of the retina.

56–15 This patient has a sarcoid nodule on the cheek.

56–13 *and* ***56–14,*** *From Green, WR: Retina. In Spencer, WH, ed: Ophthalmic pathology. An atlas and textbook, vol 2, Philadelphia, 1985, WB Saunders, p 780.* ***56–15,*** *Courtesy of and copyright Dr. Mark Lebwohl.*

Suggested Readings

Asdourian, GK, Goldberg, MF, and Busse, BJ: Peripheral retinal neovascularization in sarcoidosis, Arch Ophthalmol 93:787–791, 1975

Baarsma, GS, La Hey, EL, Glasius, E, de Vries, J, and Kijlstra, A: The predictive value of serum angiotensin converting enzyme and lysozyme levels in the diagnosis of ocular sarcoidosis, Am J Ophthalmol 104:211–217, 1987

Beardsley, TL, Brown, SVL, Sydnor, CF, Grimson, BS, and Klintworth, GK: Eleven cases of sarcoidosis of the optic nerve, Am J Ophthalmol 97:62–77, 1984

Blain, JG, Riley, W, and Logothetis, J: Optic nerve manifestations of sarcoidosis, Arch Neurol 13:307–309, 1965

Campo, RV, and Aaberg, TM: Choroidal granuloma in sarcoidosis, Am J Ophthalmol 97:419–427, 1984

Chumbley, LC and Kearns, TP: Retinopathy of sarcoidosis, Am J Ophthalmol 73:123–131, 1972

Gass, JDM, and Olson, CL: Sarcoidosis with optic nerve and retinal involvement, Arch Ophthalmol 94:945–950, 1976

Green, WR: Inflammatory diseases and conditions of the eye. In Spencer, WH, ed: Ophthalmic pathology, an atlas and textbook, Philadelphia, 1986, WB Saunders

Jabs, DA, and Johns, CJ: Ocular involvement in chronic sarcoidosis, Am J Ophthalmol 102:297–301, 1986

James, DG, Neville, E, and Siltzbach, LE: A worldwide review of sarcoidosis, Ann NY Acad Sci 278:321–334, 1976

Karcioglu, ZA, and Brear, R: Conjunctival biopsy in sarcoidosis, Am J Ophthalmol 99:68–73, 1985

Letocha, CE, Shields, JA, and Goldberg, RE: Retinal changes in sarcoidosis, Can J Ophthalmol 10:184–192, 1975

Marcus, DF, Bovino, JA, and Burton, TC: Sarcoid granuloma of the choroid, Ophthalmology 89:1326–1330, 1982

Spalton, DJ, and Sanders, MD: Fundus changes in histologically confirmed sarcoidosis, Br J Ophthalmol 65:348–358, 1981

Weinreb, RN, and Tessler, H: Laboratory diagnosis of ophthalmic sarcoidosis, Surv Ophthalmol 28:653–664, 1984

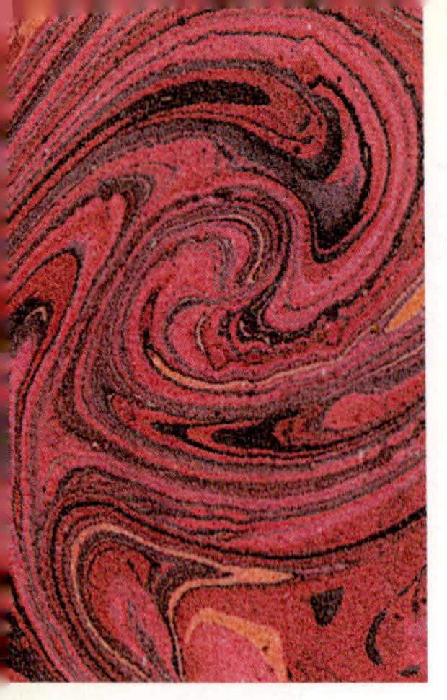

Chapter 57

Acute Multifocal Posterior Placoid Pigment Epitheliopathy

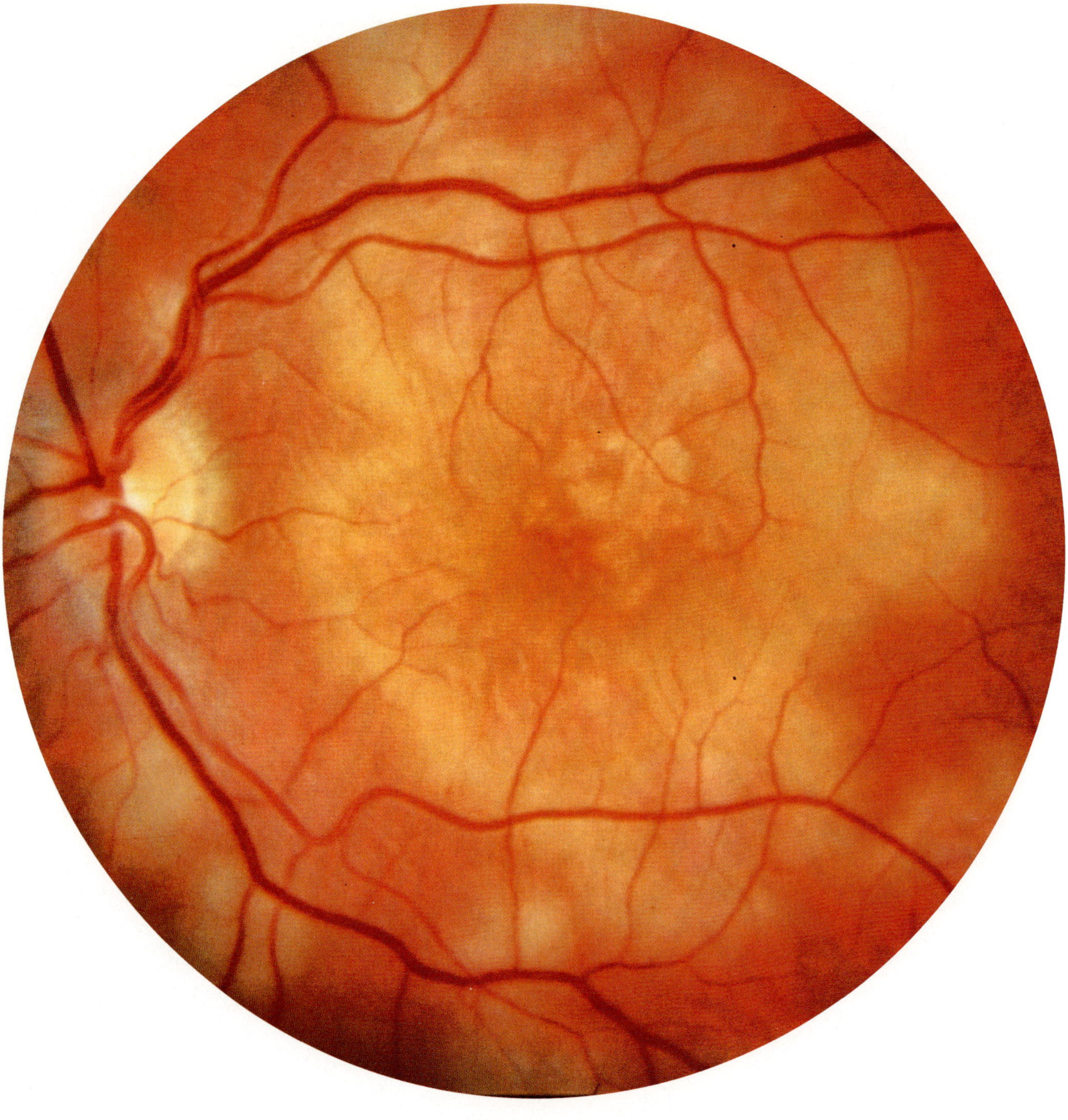

Acute multifocal posterior placoid pigment epitheliopathy (AMPPPE) is a condition characterized by an acute loss of vision with multiple yellow-whitish lesions at the level of the choroid and retinal pigment epithelium. The condition usually resolves within several weeks with a good prognosis. Rarely, hyperpigmentation may occur and cause permanent vision loss. AMPPPE has a rather characteristic fluorescein angiographic appearance. Early in the study, the lesions are hypofluorescent. Later in the study, they become hyperfluorescent. Rarely, an accompanying cerebral vasculitis may occur. There is great controversy over the pathogenesis of this disorder. However, a viral prodrome is common.

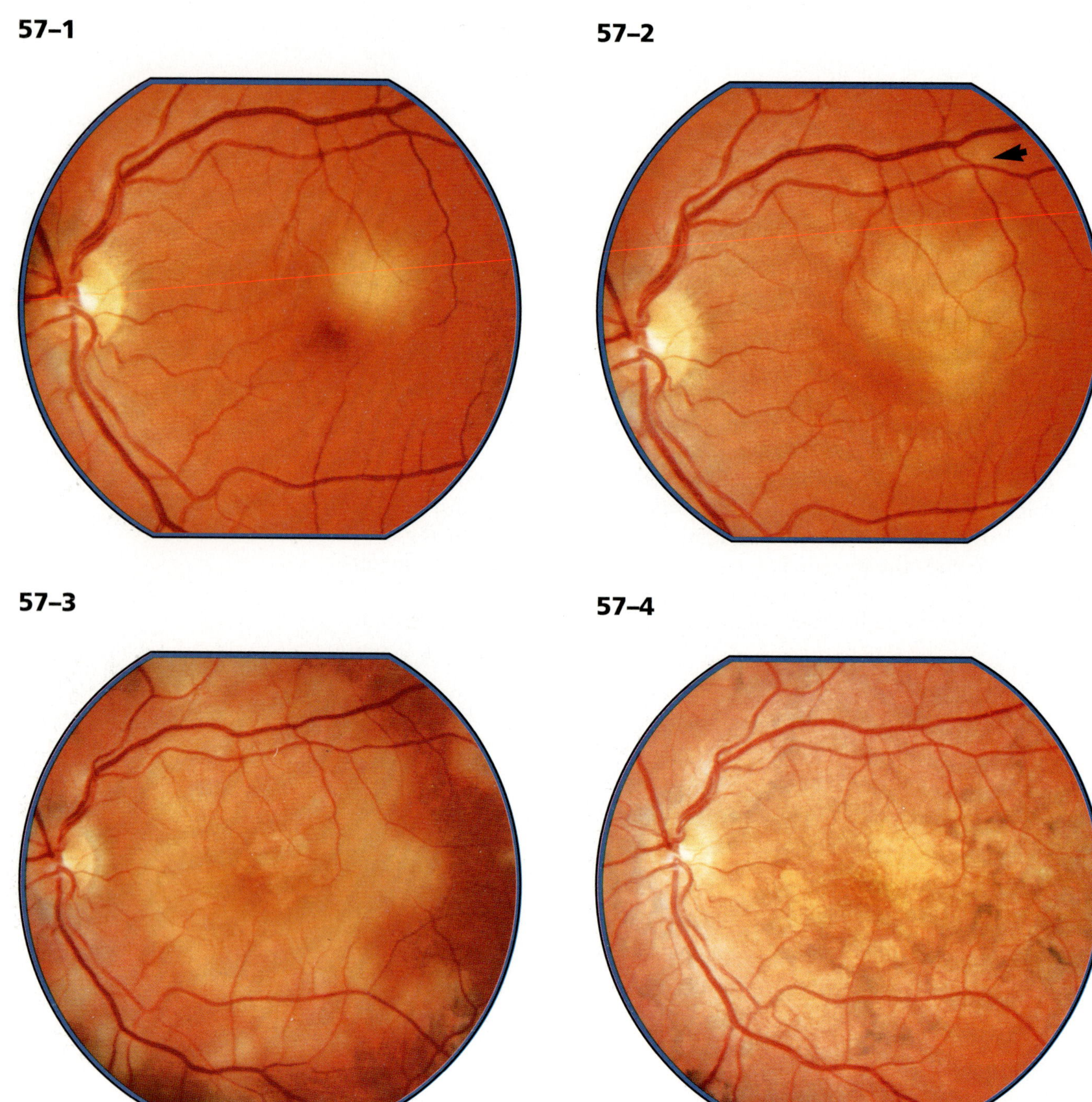

57–1 This patient with AMPPPE presented with a solitary deep whitish-yellow lesion near the macula.

57–2 Four days later, the lesion enlarged and a satellite lesion was also present *(arrowhead)*.

57–3 Two weeks after presentation, multiple acute and resolving lesions are noted.

57–4 Three months after presentation, the resolved lesions appeared atrophic and hyperpigmented.

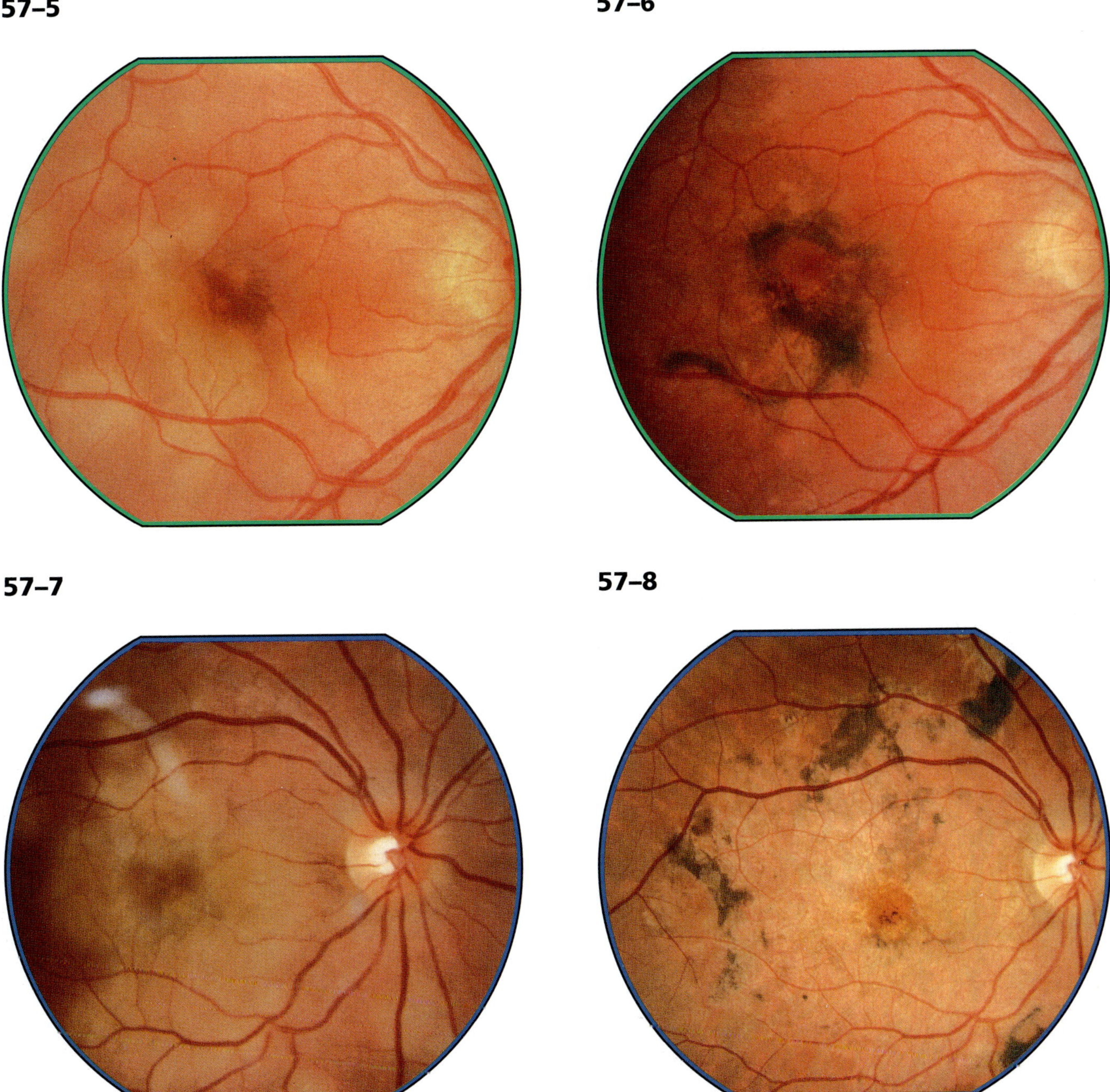

57–5 and 57–6 Note the creamy white lesions at the level of the choroid and retinal pigment epithelium in this patient with AMPPPE. Although most cases of AMPPPE resolve with a good prognosis, some patients may develop hyperpigmentation and have a poor prognosis, as occurred in this case.

57–7 and 57–8 This patient also had AMPPPE (57–7), which resulted in pigmentary changes and a poor visual outcome (57–8).

57–9

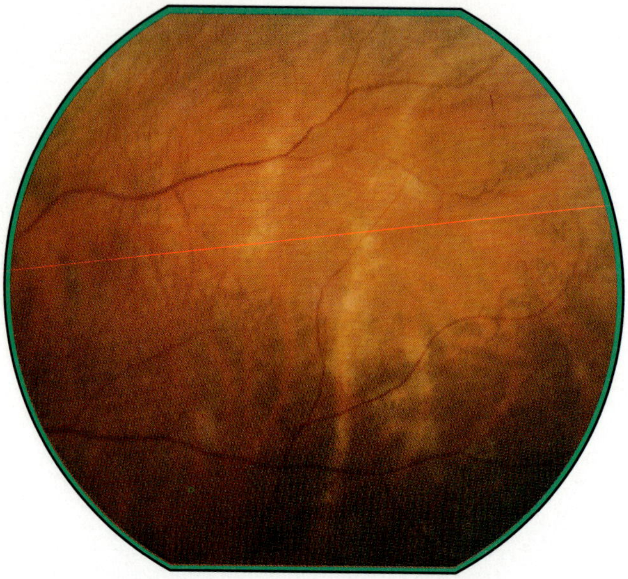

57–10

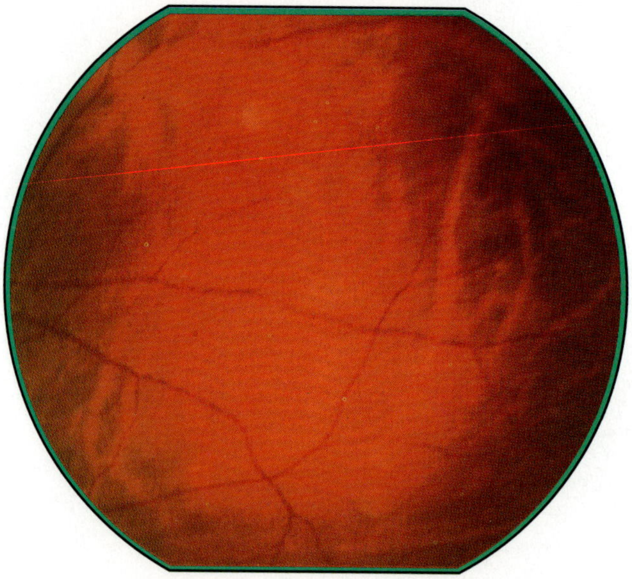

57–9 This patient demonstrates perivascular choroidal inflammation in the peripheral fundus during the acute stages of AMPPPE. The choroidal vasculitis seen in this patient may not necessarily reflect the primary mechanism of the disease but instead just a diffuse vasculitis.

57–10 The perivascular choroiditis resolved.

Suggested Readings

Bird, AC, and Hamilton, AM: Placoid pigment epitheliopathy presenting with bilateral serous retinal detachment, Br J Ophthalmol 56:881–886, 1972

Deutman, AF, and Lion, F: Choriocapillaris nonperfusion in acute multifocal placoid pigment epitheliopathy, Am J Ophthalmol 84:652–658, 1977

Fishman, GA, Rabb, MF, and Kaplan, J: Acute posterior multifocal placoid pigment epitheliopathy, Arch Ophthalmol 92:173–177, 1974

Gass, JDM: Acute posterior multifocal placoid pigment epitheliopathy, Arch Ophthalmol 80:177–184, 1968

Gass, JDM: Acute posterior multifocal placoid pigment epitheliopathy: a long-term follow-up. In Fine, SL, and Owen, SL, eds: Management of retinal vascular and macular disorders, Baltimore, 1983, Williams & Wilkins, pp 176–181

Kirkham, TH, Ffytche, TJ, and Sanders, MD: Placoid pigment epitheliopathy with retinal vasculitis and papillitis, Br J Ophthalmol 56:875–880, 1972

Ryan, SJ, and Maumenee, AE: Acute posterior multifocal placoid pigment epitheliopathy, Am J Ophthalmol 74:1066–1074, 1972

Spaide, RF, Yannuzzi, LA, and Slakter, JS: Choroidal vasculitis in acute posterior multifocal placoid pigment epitheliopathy, Br J Ophthalmol 75:685–687, 1991

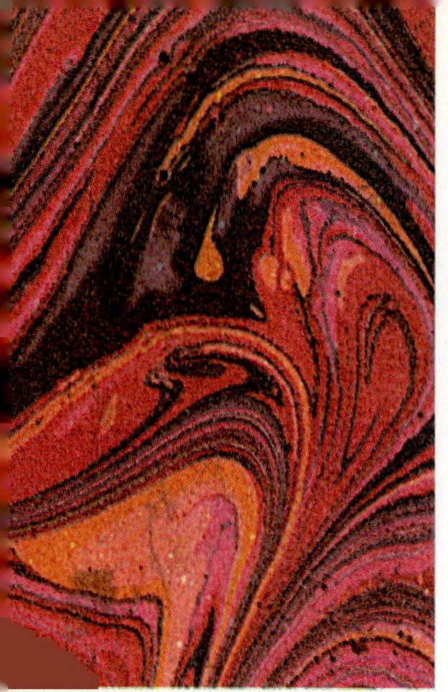

Chapter 58
Serpiginous Choroiditis

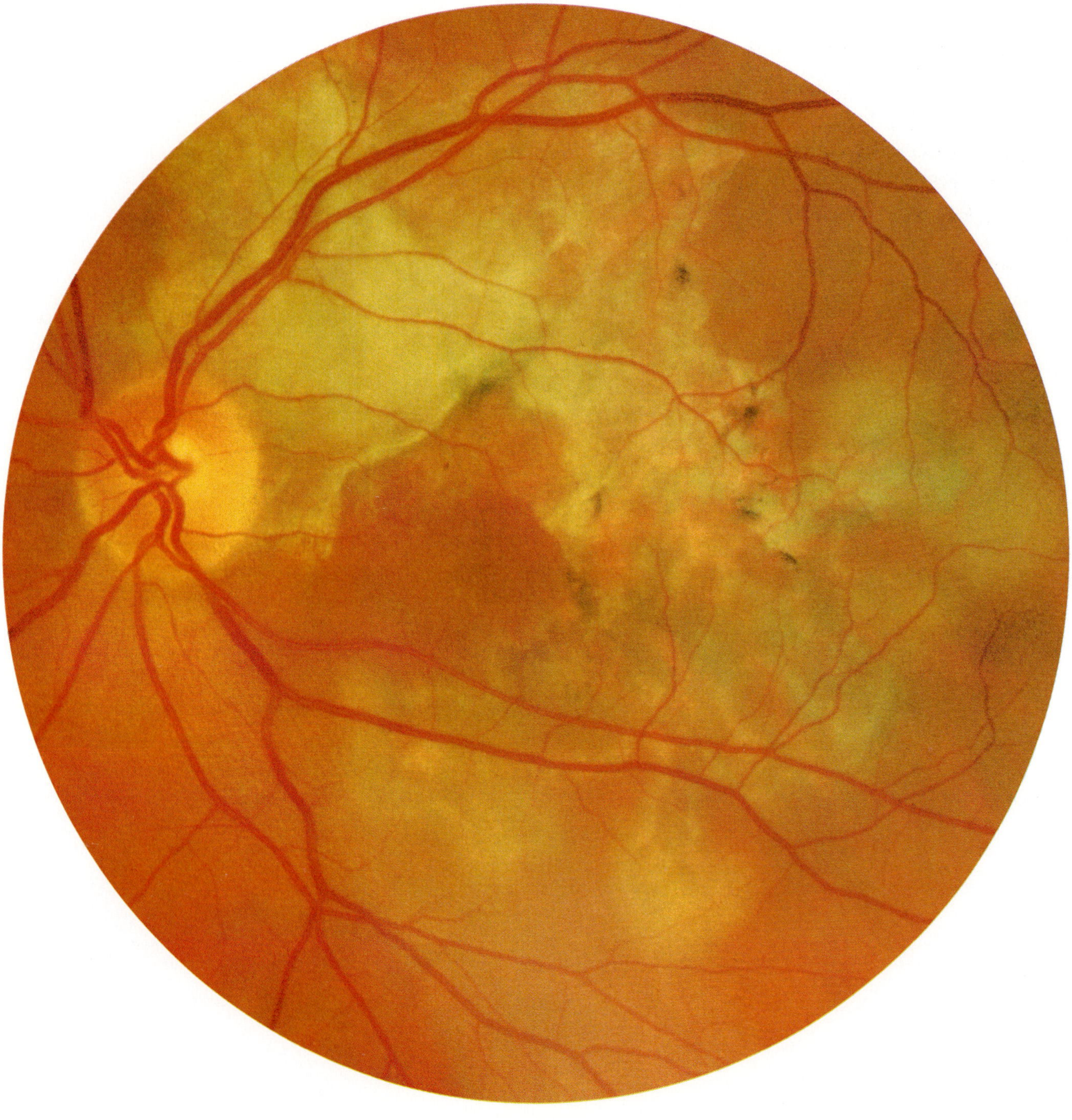

Serpiginous choroiditis is a rare bilateral inflammatory disorder. Recurrences are common with this condition, which usually occurs in the peripapillary region and progresses in a helicoid or serpiginous manner toward the macula. Acute lesions are grayish-white and occur at the retinal pigment epithelium or choroidal level. The fluorescein angiogram shows early blockage and late staining similar to acute multifocal posterior placoid pigment epitheliopathy (AMPPPE). Chronic lesions show pigmentary changes. Acute lesions occur at the edge of the chronic lesion. Choroidal neovascularization may occur in these patients.

58–1

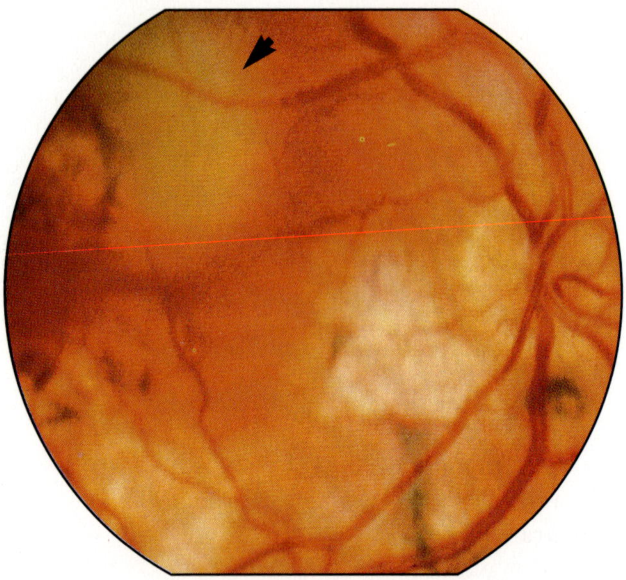

58–2 58–2A

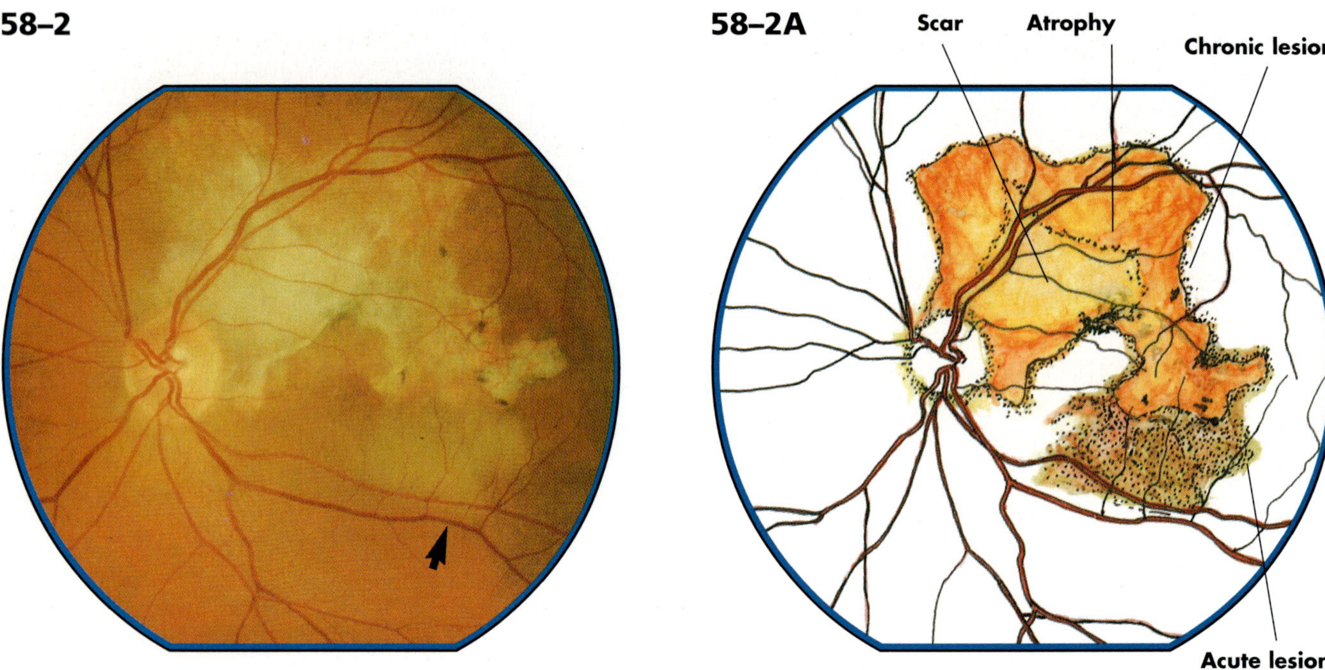

58–1 This patient has serpiginous choroidopathy. Note the pigmentary changes consistent with chronic serpiginous disease. Also note the fluffy whitish-yellow lesion superiorly that represents an active area of choroiditis *(arrowhead)*.

58–2 and 58–2A This patient has atrophy originating from the peripapillary area in a serpiginous-like pattern. Note the acute fluffy white lesion at the inferior most aspect of the lesion *(arrowhead),* which represents a recurrence. The chronic lesion shows atrophic and cicatricial scarring. There is atrophy, fibrous metaplasia, and retinal pigment epithelial hyperplasia.

58–2, *Courtesy of Dr. Stuart L. Fine.*

(Case continued on next page.)

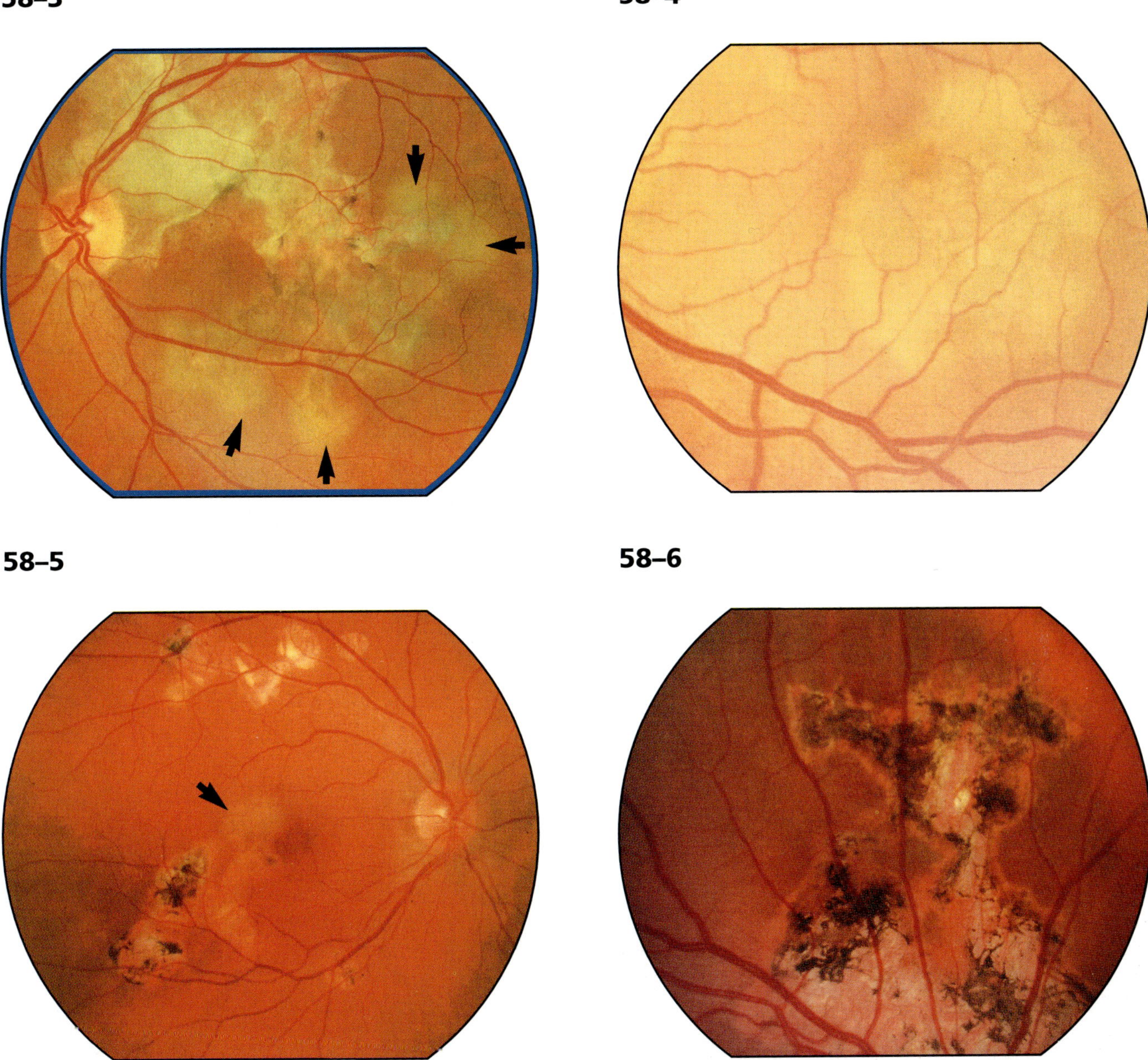

58–3 Approximately 2 months later, the acute lesion has resolved with atrophy and scarring, and there are now four additional acute lesions *(arrowheads).*

58–4 Serpiginous choroidopathy may begin anywhere. This patient has solitary serpiginous choroiditis that started in the macular region.

58–5 This patient with serpiginous choroidopathy demonstrates an acute lesion *(arrowhead)* near the macula, as well as areas of scarring. Also note the satellite or "skip" lesions, which are common in this disorder.

58–6 The chronic stage of serpiginous choroidopathy with atrophic areas can be demonstrated in this patient. Note that the choroidal vasculature can be observed because of the overlying atrophy.

58–3, *Courtesy of Dr. Stuart L. Fine.* ***58–4,*** *Courtesy of Dr. Maurice Rabb.*

58–7

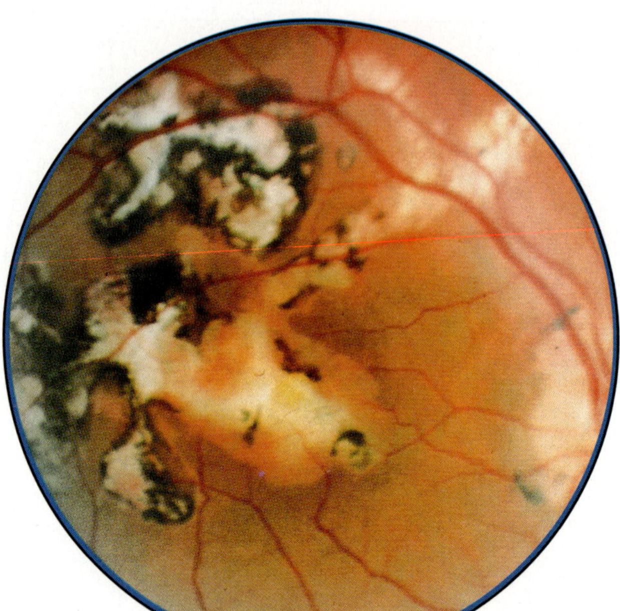

58–8

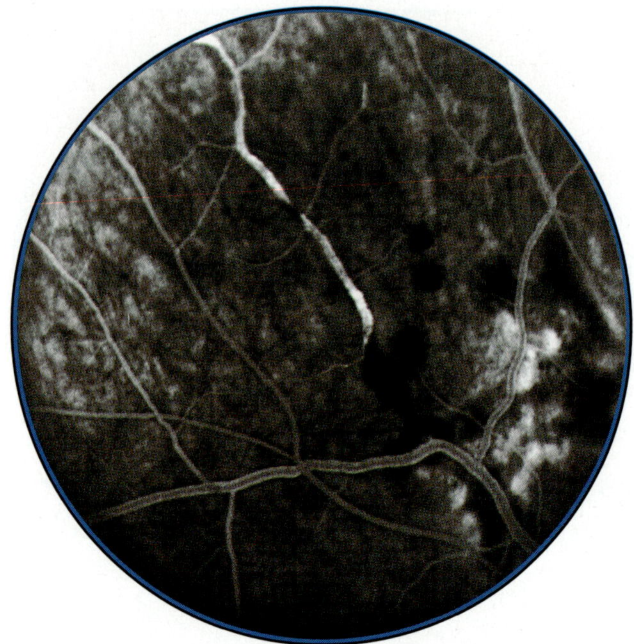

58–9

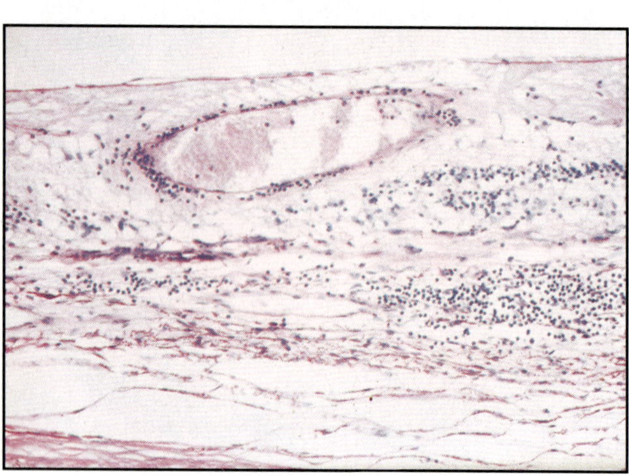

58–7 and 58–8 Serpiginous choroidopathy in this patient led to a retinal vein occlusion. In some patients, choroidal inflammation may extend to cause retinal inflammation, and the secondary inflammation may cause closure of a retinal vein. Note the occluded vessel as seen by fluorescein angiography.

58–9 This histopathologic photograph of a patient with serpiginous choroidopathy reveals retinal phlebitis and choroiditis.

Suggested Readings

Blumenkranz, MS, Gass, JDM, and Clarkson, JG: Atypical serpiginous choroiditis, Arch Ophthalmol 100:1773–1775, 1982

Hamilton, AM, and Bird, AC: Geographical choroidopathy, Br J Ophthalmol 58:784–797, 1974

Hardy, RA, and Schatz, H: Macular geographic helicoid choroidopathy, Arch Ophthalmol 105:1237–1242, 1987

Jampol, LM, Orth, D, Daily, MJ, and Rabb, MF: Subretinal neovascularization with geographic (serpiginous) choroiditis, Am J Ophthalmol 88:683–689, 1979

Laatikainen, L, and Erkkilä, H: Serpiginous choroiditis, Br J Ophthalmol 58:777–783, 1974

Mansour, AM, Jampol, LM, Packo, KH, and Hrisomalos, NF: Macular serpiginous choroiditis, Retina 8:125–131, 1988

Schatz, N, Maumenee, AE, and Patz, A: Geographic helicoid peripapillary choroidopathy: clinical presentation and fluorescein angiographic findings, Trans Am Acad Ophthalmol Otolaryngol 78:747–761, 1974

Wu, JS, Lewis, H, Fine, SL, Grover, DA, and Green, WR: Clinicopathologic findings in a patient with serpiginous choroiditis and treated choroidal neovascularization, Retina 9:292–301, 1989

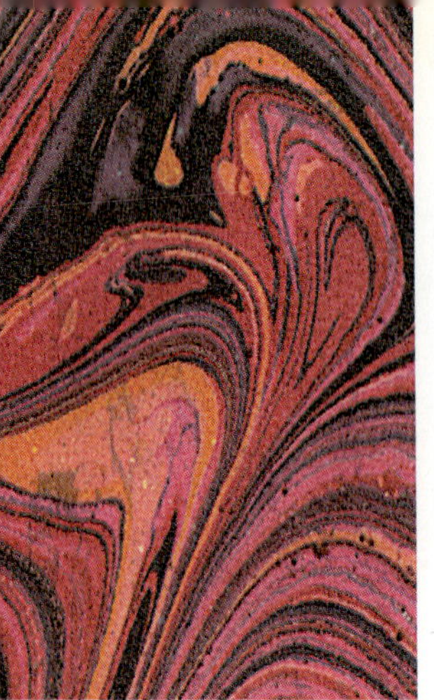

Chapter 59

Sympathetic Ophthalmia

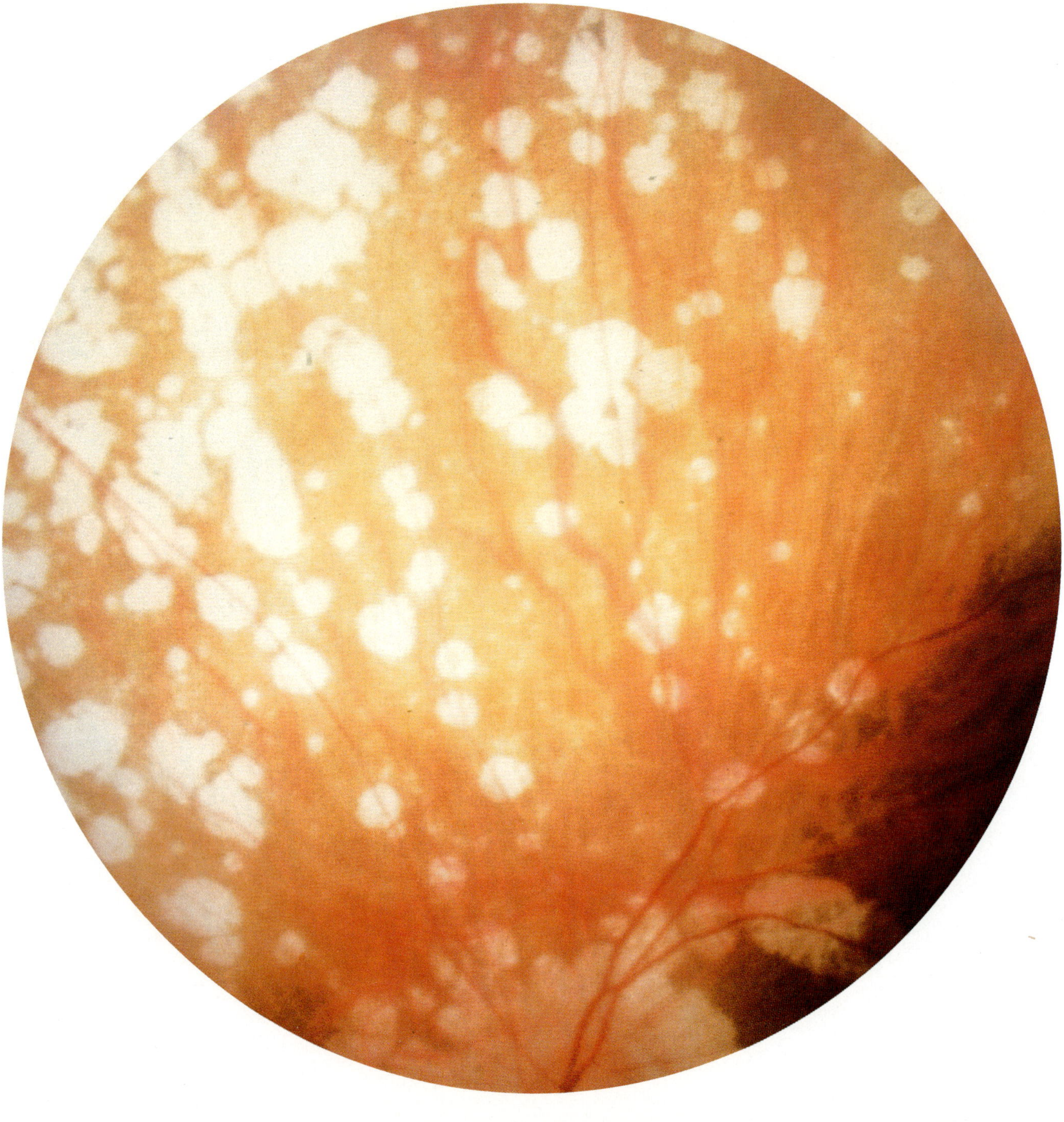

Sympathetic ophthalmia is a rare diffuse granulomatous uveitis that occurs days to decades after trauma. Ocular inflammation is common. Keratic precipitates on the endothelium of the cornea occur. Chorioretinal findings include edema, perivasculitis, yellow-white choroidal lesions, and yellowish-white exudates beneath the retinal pigment epithelium, which are termed Dalen-Fuchs nodules. Papillitis may also be noted. Exudative retinal detachments may rarely be seen. The condition often occurs approximately 6 weeks after trauma but may occur at any time. It rarely occurs earlier than 2 weeks after trauma. Corticosteroid and immunosuppressive therapy can be used to treat this condition.

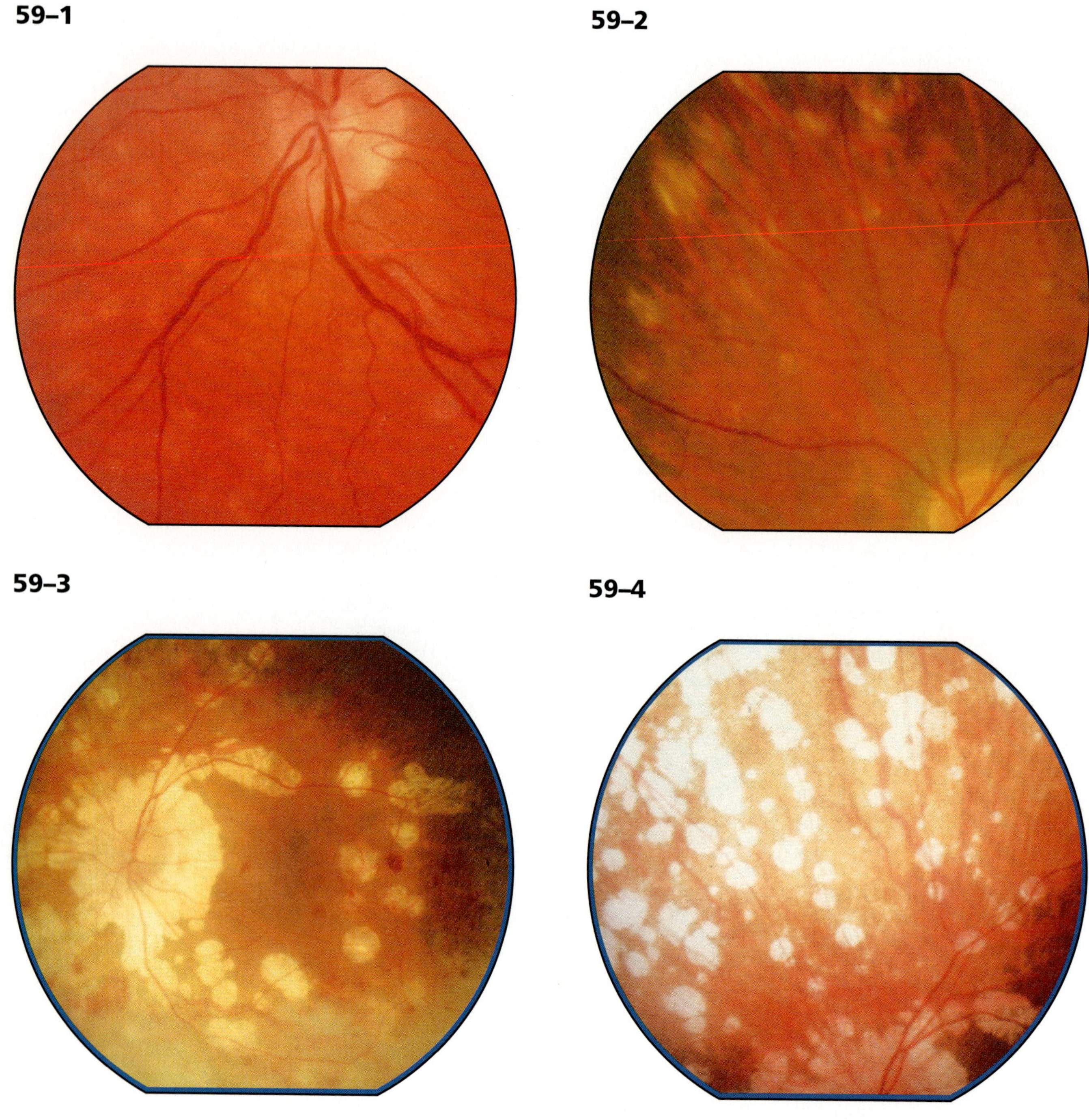

59–1 and 59–2 These small whitish-yellow choroidal lesions are noted acutely in patients with sympathetic ophthalmia.

59–3 and 59–4 In this patient with chronic sympathetic ophthalmia, widespread lesions at the level of the choroid have led to atrophy of the retinal pigment epithelium. There is papillotrophic involvement as well. Vitreous haze from inflammatory cells as well as blood and scattered intraretinal hemorrhages are also noted in this subacute stage. Many months later, the same patient demonstrates resolution of the acute inflammation and hemorrhage with residual widespread peripheral and posterior fundus atrophic lesions.

***59–3** and **59–4**, Courtesy of Dr. George Williams.*

59–5

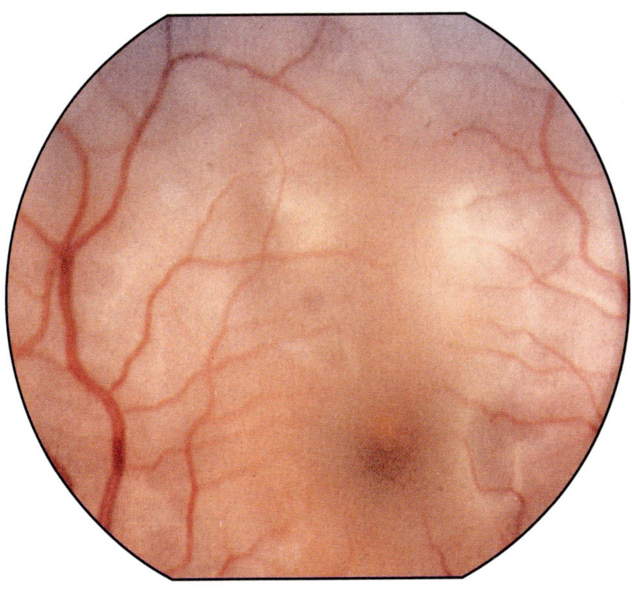

59–6

59–7

59–5 In this case of sympathetic ophthalmia, the manifestations resemble those seen in Harada's disease with multiple neurosensory retinal detachments forming bullous elevations in some areas. The retinal pigment epithelial whitish spots are associated with early hypofluorescence and late staining on fluorescein angiography. Multiple pinpoint leaks from the level of the pigment epithelium may also account for the overlying exudative detachment. The presumed whitish spots are Dalen-Fuchs nodules.

59–6 and 59–7 This patient appeared to have Harada's disease. Note the bullous neurosensory retinal detachments. The patient's condition improved after steroid treatment. Later histopathologic study suggested that the patient actually had sympathetic ophthalmia.

59–5, *From Dreyer, et al: Am J Ophthalmol 92:816–823, 1981. Published with permission of the American Journal of Ophthalmology. Copyright by the Ophthalmic Publishing Company.* ***59–6*** *and* ***59–7,*** *Courtesy of Dr. Thomas Aaberg.*

59–8

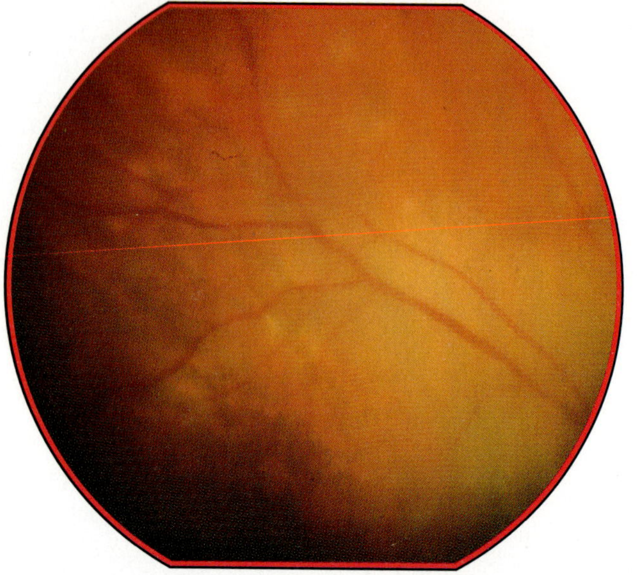

59–9

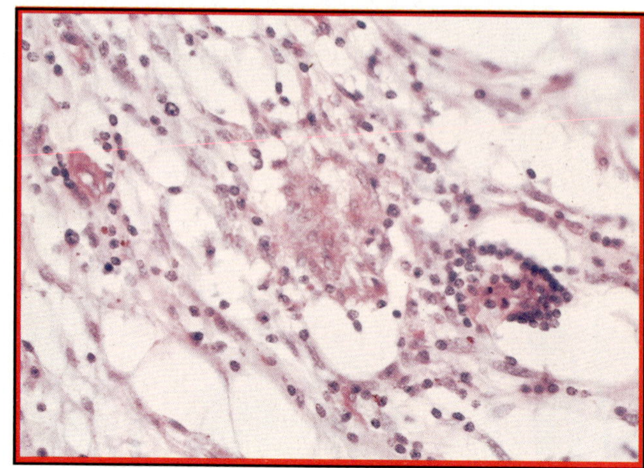

59–10

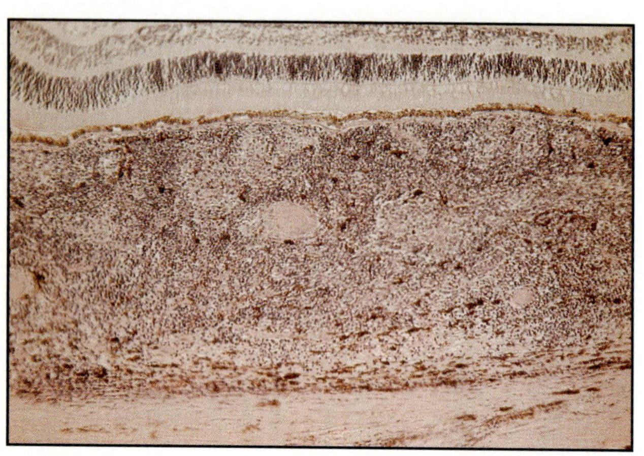

59–8 and 59–9 This patient developed vitritis and whitish-yellow lesions at the level of the choroid. Histopathologic examination reveals a diffuse infiltration of lymphocytes with foci of epithelioid cells.

59–10 Another histopathologic case of sympathetic ophthalmia reveals an extensive choroidal inflammatory reaction.

59–11 and 59–11A A characteristic Dalen-Fuchs nodule is noted with a cluster of epithelioid cells under the retinal pigment epithelium.

59–11

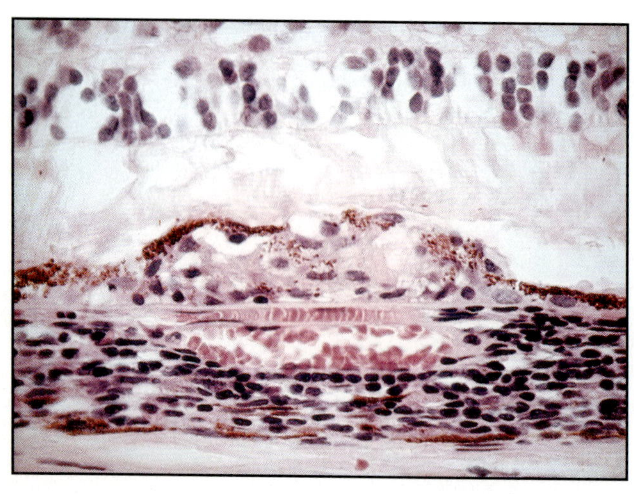

59–11A

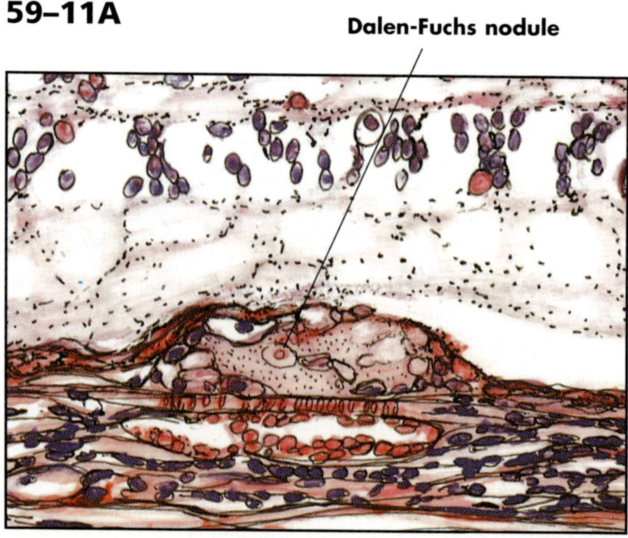

Suggested Readings

Albert, DM, and Diaz-Rohena, R: A historical review of sympathetic ophthalmia and its epidemiology, Surv Ophthalmol 34:1–14, 1989

Blodi, FC: Sympathetic uveitis. In Freeman, HM, ed: Ocular trauma, New York 1979, Appleton-Century-Crofts

Gass, JDM: Sympathetic ophthalmia following vitrectomy, Am J Ophthalmol 93:552–558, 1982

Goto, H, and Rao, NA: Sympathetic ophthalmia and Vogt-Koyanagi-Harada syndrome, Int Ophthalmol Clin 30:279–285, 1990

Hammer, H: Cellular hypersensitivity to uveal pigment confirmed by leucocyte migration tests in sympathetic ophthalmitis and the Vogt-Koyanagi-Harada syndrome, Br J Ophthalmol 58:773–776, 1974

Kraus-Mackiw, E: Sympathetic ophthalmia, a genuine autoimmune disease, Curr Eye Res 9(Suppl):1–5, 1990

Lubin, JR, Albert, DM, and Weinstein, M: Sixty-five years of sympathetic ophthalmia: a clinicopathologic review of 105 cases (1913–1978), Ophthalmology 87:109–121, 1980

Makley, TA, Jr, and Azar, A: Sympathetic ophthalmia: a long-term follow-up, Arch Ophthalmol 96:257–262, 1978

Rao, NA, and Marak, GE: Sympathetic ophthalmia simulating Vogt-Koyanagi-Harada's disease: A clinicopathologic study of four cases, Jpn J Ophthalmol 27:506–511, 1983

Tesseler, HH, and Jennings, T: High-dose short-term chlorambucil for intractable sympathetic ophthalmia and Behçet's disease, Br J Ophthalmol 74:353 357, 1990

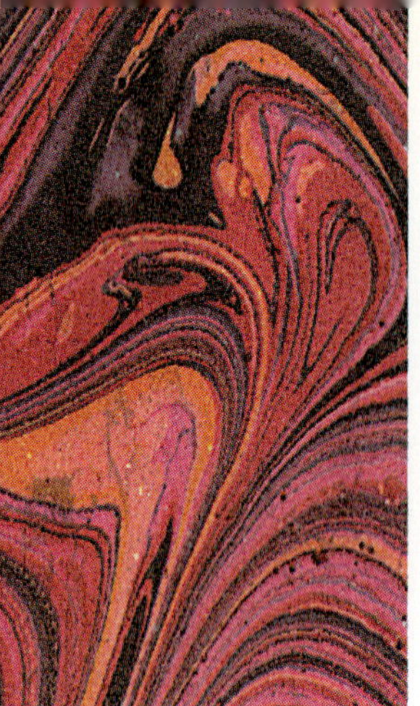

Chapter 60

Vogt-Koyanagi-Harada Syndrome

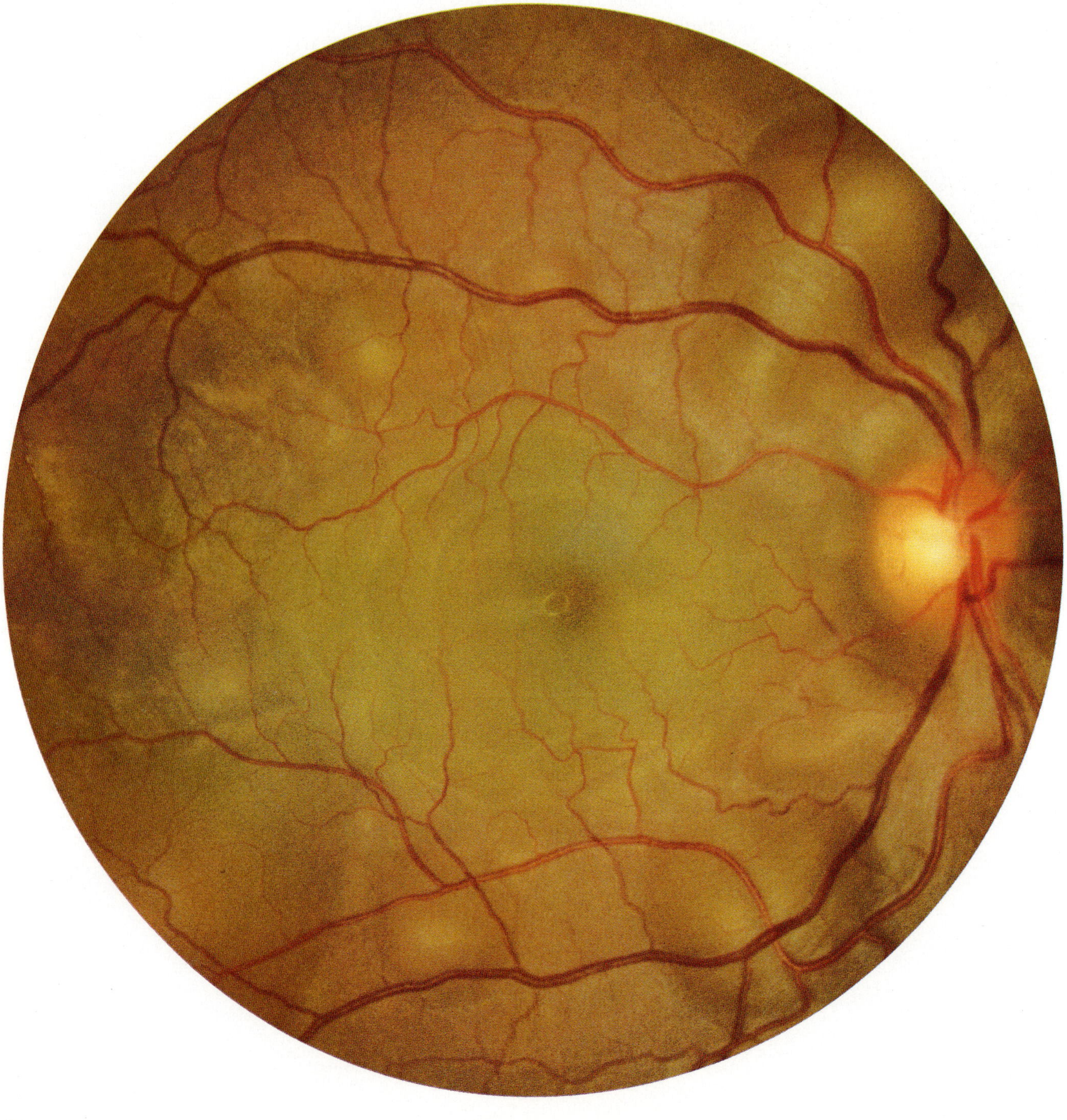

Vogt-Koyanagi-Harada syndrome, or the uveal meningitic syndrome, involves the ear, skin, and meninges, as well as the eye. Granulomatous keratic precipitates are noted. Iritis and vitritis may occur. This inflammation may be quite severe at times. Optic disc edema may be present. Exudative retinal detachment occurs, and yellowish-white lesions may appear in the retinal periphery. Retinal neovascularization with or without vitreous hemorrhage, choroidal neovascularization, and rhegmatogenous retinal detachments may also occur. Systemic findings in these patients include hair and skin changes, headaches, stiff neck, auditory problems, and fever. Vitiligo and poliosis are noted in the majority of patients. The condition is often highly sensitive to corticosteroid therapy.

60–1

60–2

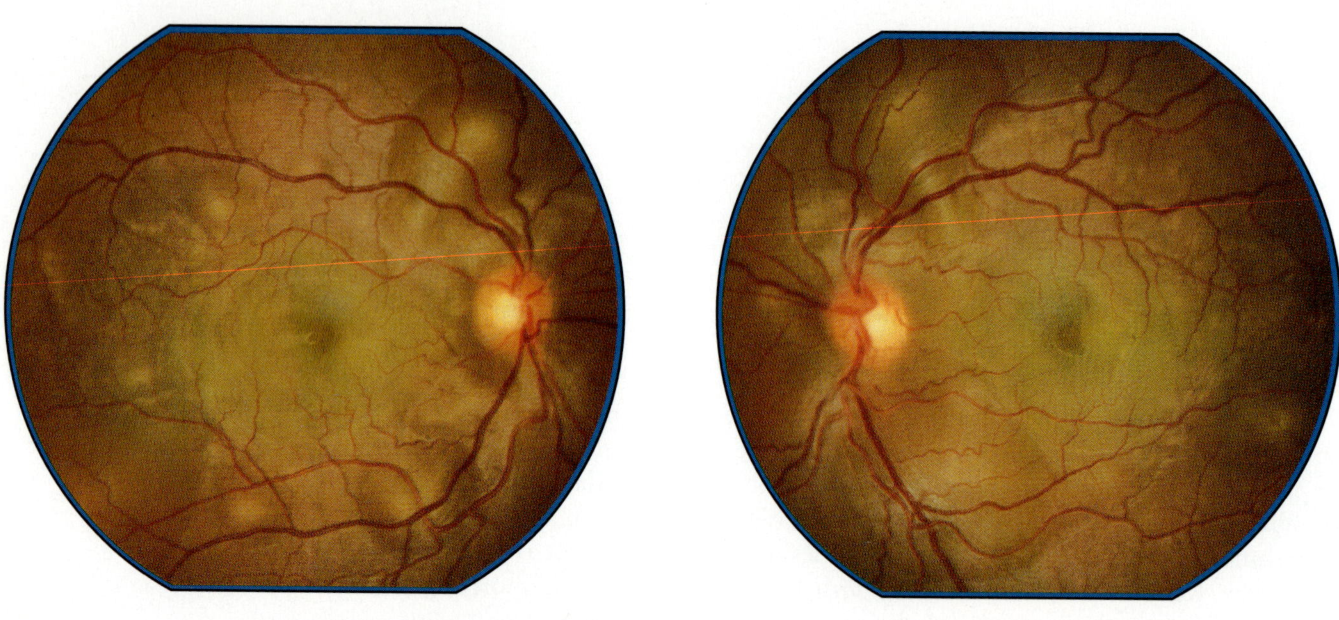

60–1 and 60–2 This patient illustrates the classic findings in Harada's disease. Note the multiple serous detachments of the neurosensory retina and retinal pigment epithelium. There is an inferior gravitating detachment. Also note the whitish spots resembling the Dalen-Fuchs nodules seen in sympathetic ophthalmia. Mild vitritis, a prominent vitreoretinal interface, and an erythematous optic disc also are noted. These changes may also be demonstrated in any infiltrative or inflammatory uveal process in the posterior fundus such as posterior scleritis, leukemia, sympathetic ophthalmia, disseminated intravascular coagulopathy, tumors—including diffuse melanocytic hyperplasia and eosinophilic granuloma, choroidal osteoma, toxemia of pregnancy, and malignant hypertension.

60–3

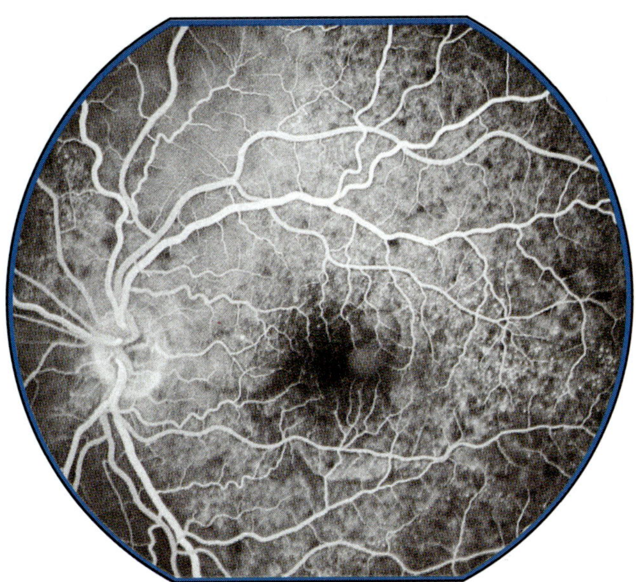

60–4

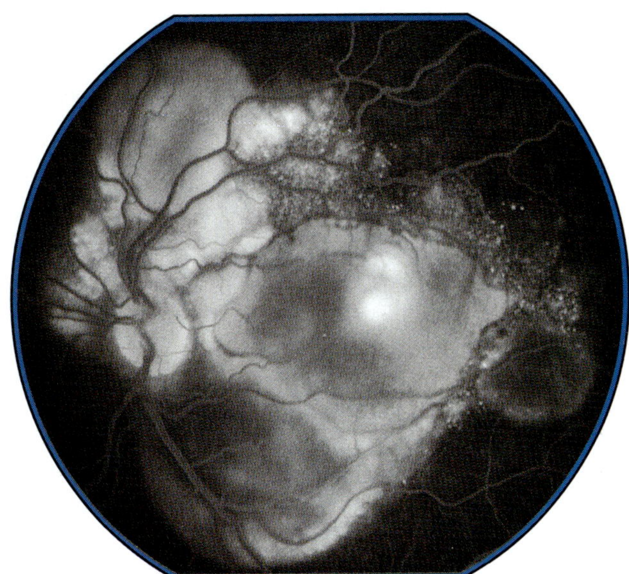

60–3 and 60–4 The fluorescein angiogram shows pinpoint areas of hyperfluorescence initially and later shows large sharply demarcated areas, which represent the detachments. Note that in the later angiogram the pinpoint hyperfluorescent lesions are still apparent. The dye may actually fill the subneurosensory retinal space, giving a fluorescein angiographic picture of a serous pigment epithelial detachment. This pattern is also characteristic of choroidal neovascularization or any inflammatory process, but not central serous chorioretinopathy—which may, in its most severe variant, delineate the outline of the detachment.

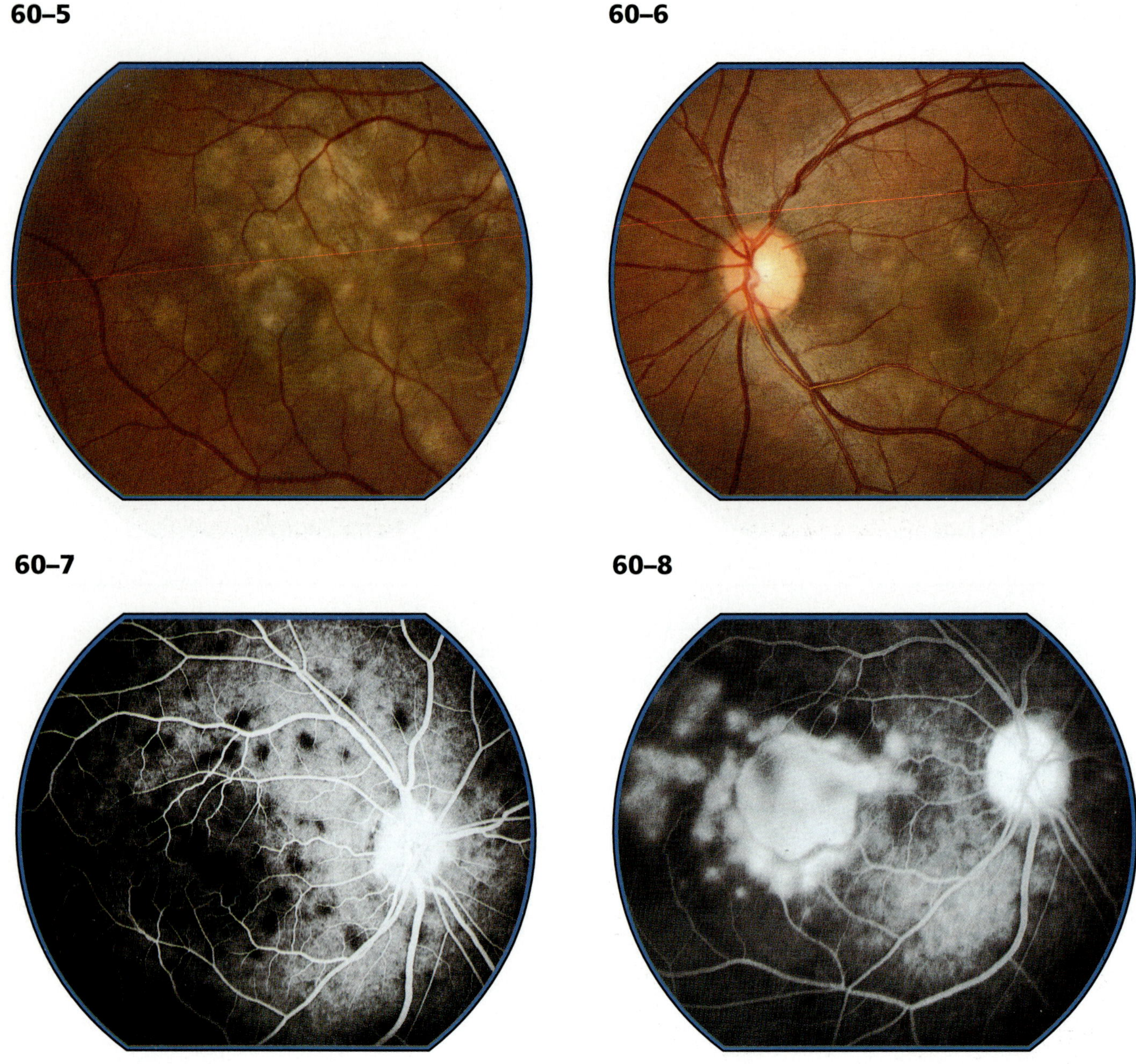

60–5 and 60–6 Another patient demonstrates multiple neurosensory detachments secondary to Harada's disease. In some patients, multiple yellowish-white spots beneath the detachments are the most conspicuous clinical feature.

60–7 and 60–8 Fluorescein findings in this patient demonstrate hypofluorescence at the site of the yellowish-orange spots and eventual filling of the neurosensory detachments with dye. Late staining of the optic nerve is also characteristic of this syndrome.

(Case continued on next page.)

60–9

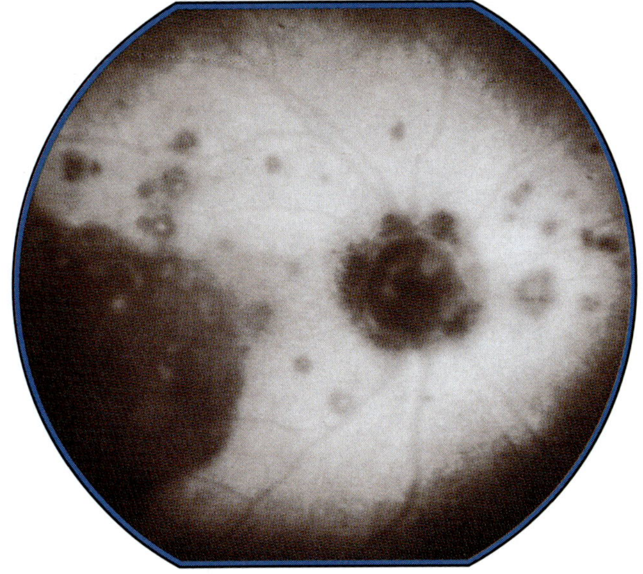

60–10

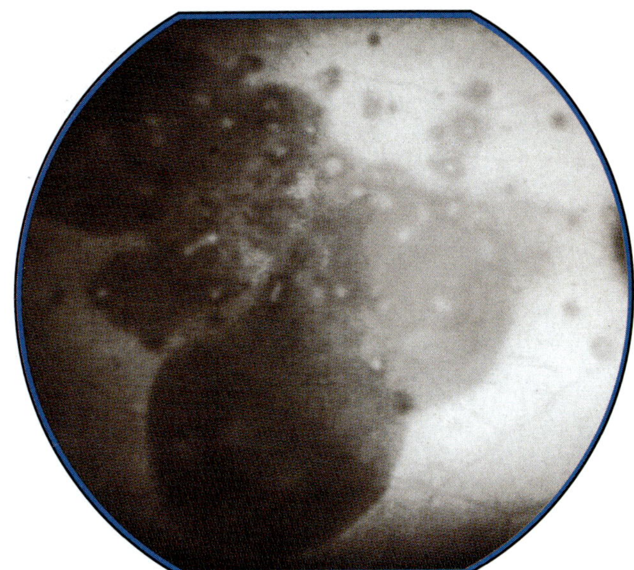

60–11

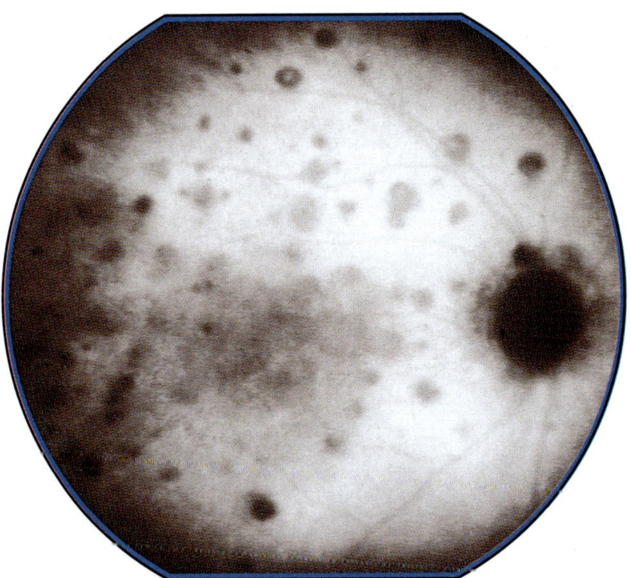

60–9 Digital indocyanine-green (ICG) angiography shows a plethora of hypofluorescent spots. More spots are noted on the ICG angiogram than the fluorescein study.

60–10 Later in the ICG study, there is masking of the background choroidal fluorescence by the neurosensory detachment. The masking effect covers a larger area than the clinically evident detachment. Also note the inferior gravitating extensions of the blockage. Hyperfluorescent foci are also present, which may represent sites of active leakage.

60–11 After 1 week of steroid therapy, there is marked clinical improvement. The ICG angiogram at this time shows that the masking effect is almost completely resolved and many of the hyperfluorescent spots have become dark spots. In addition, new dark spots are noted in previously uninvolved areas. The ICG angiogram may be allowing us to view an ongoing inflammatory process, which is resolving and evolving simultaneously.

60–12

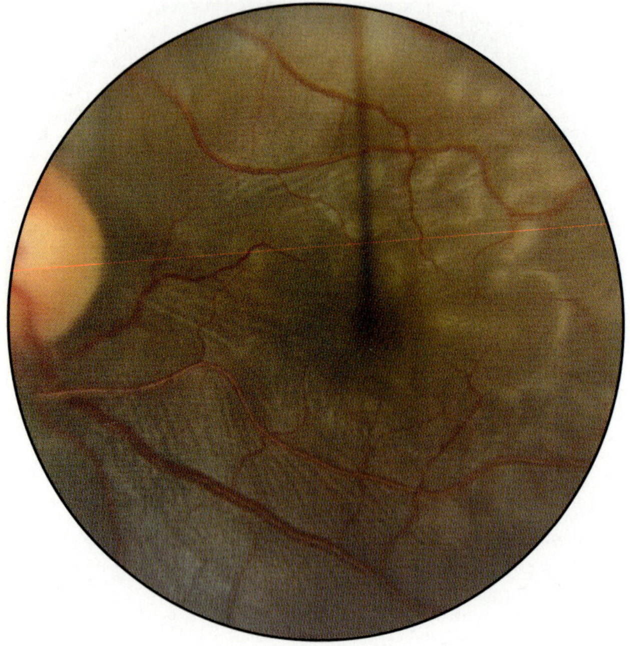

60–13

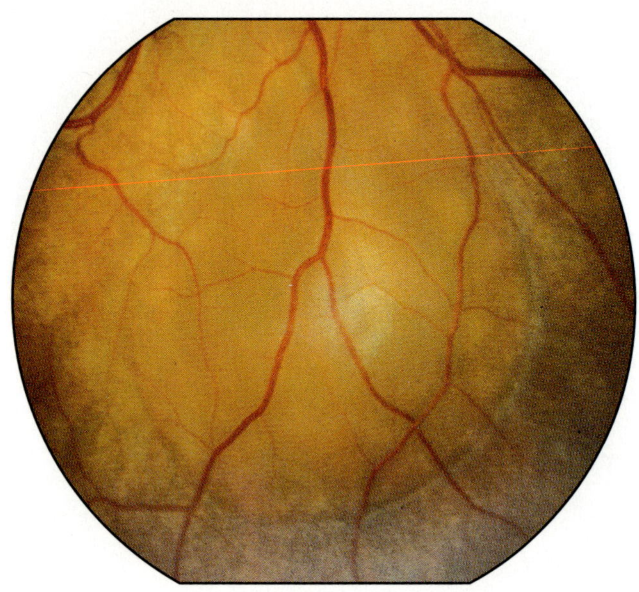

60–14

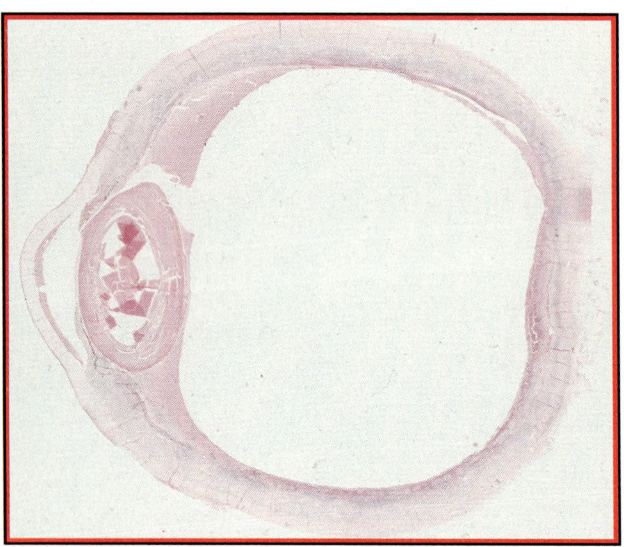

60–15

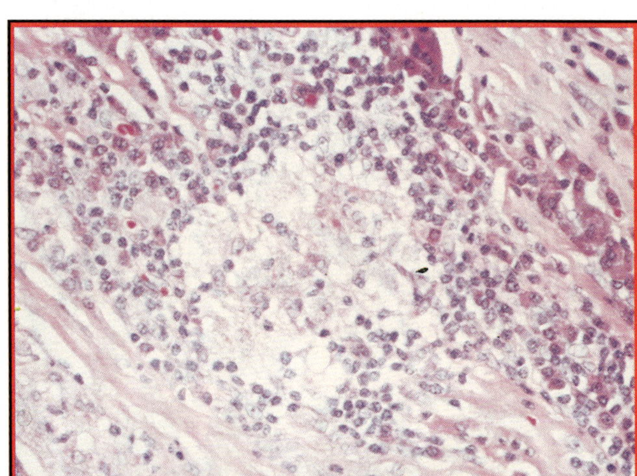

60–12 This patient also has Harada's disease. Note that extensive exudation has led to chorioretinal folds. There is a more proteinaceous exudate at the margins of some of the detachments, which is also characteristic of the disease.

60–13 Large detachments may also occur secondary to Harada's disease and gravitate inferiorly, as in this teardrop detachment.

60–14 and 60–15 This cross section of an eye with Harada's disease shows extensive choroidal thickening (60–14) by a granulomatous inflammatory cell infiltration (60–15).

Suggested Readings

Chan, CC, Palestine, AG, Nussenblatt, RB, Roberge, FG, and Ben-Ezra, D: Anti-retinal auto-antibodies in Vogt-Koyanagi-Harada syndrome, Behçet's disease, and sympathetic ophthalmia, Ophthalmology 92:1025–1028, 1985

Davis, JL, Mittal, KK, Freidlin, V, Mellow, S, Optican, DC, Palestine, AG, and Nussenblatt, RB: HLA associations and ancestry in Vogt-Koyanagi-Harada disease and sympathetic ophthalmia, Ophthalmology 97:1137–1142, 1990

Forster, DJ, Cano, MR, Green, RL, and Rao, NA: Echographic features of the Vogt-Koyanagi-Harada syndrome, Arch Ophthalmol 108:1421–1426, 1990

Koyanagi, Y: Dysakusis, Alopecia und Poliosis bei schwerer Uveitis nichttraumatischen Ursprungs, Klin Monatsbi Augenheilkd 82:194–211, 1929

Lindley, DM, Boosinger, TR, and Cox, NR: Ocular histopathology of Vogt-Koyanagi-Harada-like syndrome in an Akita dog, Vet Pathol 27:294–296, 1990

Nussenblatt, RB, Gery, I, Ballintine, EJ, and Wacker, WB: Cellular immune responsiveness of uveitis patients to retinal S-antigen, Am J Ophthalmol 89:173–179, 1980

Nussenblatt, RB, Palestine, AG, and Chan, CC: Cyclosporin A therapy in the treatment of intraocular inflammatory disease resistant to systemic corticosteroids and cytotoxic agents, Am J Ophthalmol 96:275–282, 1983

Rao, NA, and Marak, GE: Sympathetic ophthalmia simulating Vogt-Koyanagi-Harada's disease: a clinicopathologic study of four cases, Jpn J Ophthalmol 27:506–511, 1983

Sassamoto, Y, Ohno, S, and Matsuda, H: Studies on corticosteroid therapy in Vogt-Koyanagi-Harada disease, Ophthalmologica 201:162–167, 1990

To, KW, Nadel, AJ, and Brockhurst, RJ: Optic disc neovascularization in association with Vogt-Koyanagi-Harada syndrome, Arch Ophthalmol 108:918–919, 1990

Vogt, A: Frühzeitiges Ergrauen der Zilien und Bemerkungen über den sogenannten plötzlichen Eintritt dieser Veränderung, Klin Monatsbl Augenheilkd 44:228–242, 1906

Chapter 61
Uveal Effusion

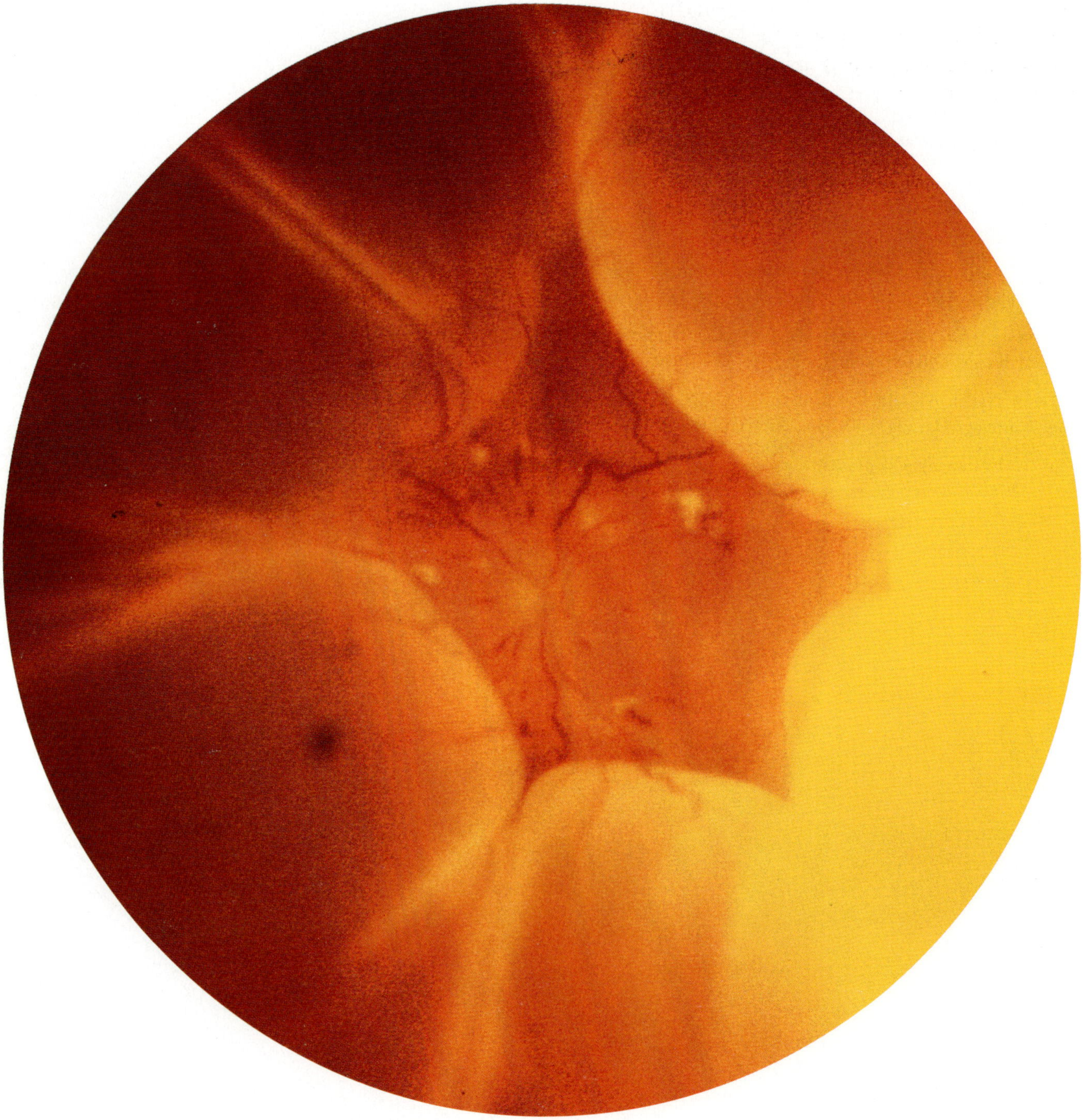

The uveal effusion syndrome consists of a choroidal detachment in which the retinal elevation is smooth and convex. Ciliochoroidal effusion may be idiopathic, inflammatory, or due to nanophthalmos.

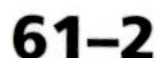

61–1

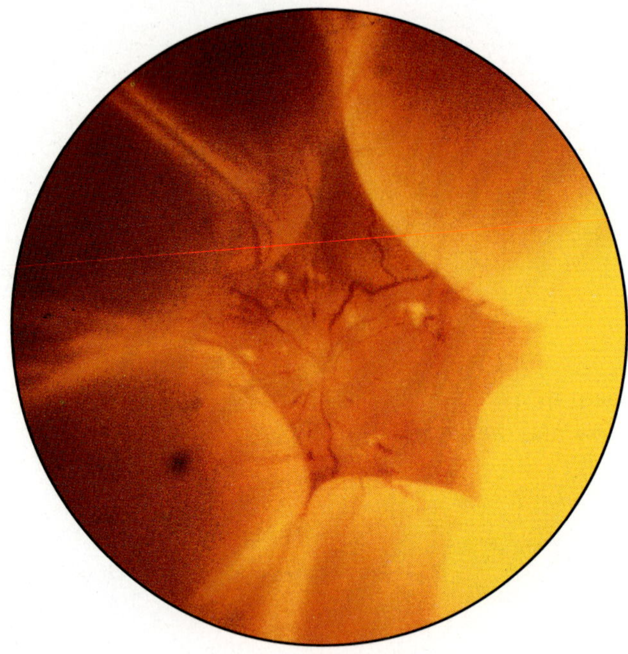

61–2

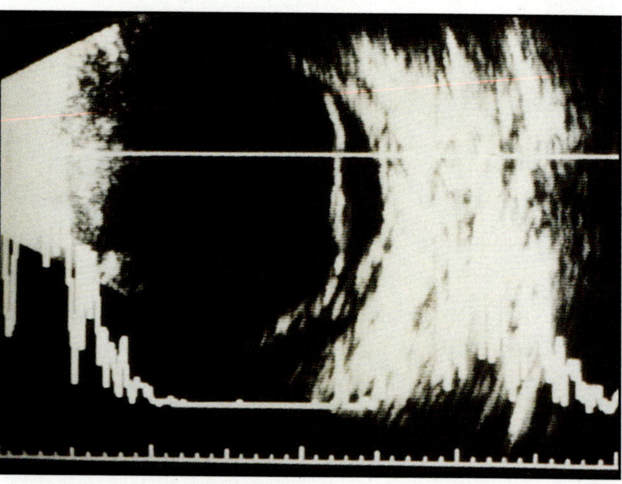

61–1 This photograph demonstrates extensive choroidal detachment in a case of ciliochoroidal effusion. Venous stasis changes are noted in the retinal vasculature. Note the smooth convex surface of the detached retina without fixed retinal folds.

61–2 Ultrasonography confirms the diagnosis.

61–1 *and* ***61–2,*** *Courtesy of Dr. Robert Brockhurst.*

61–3

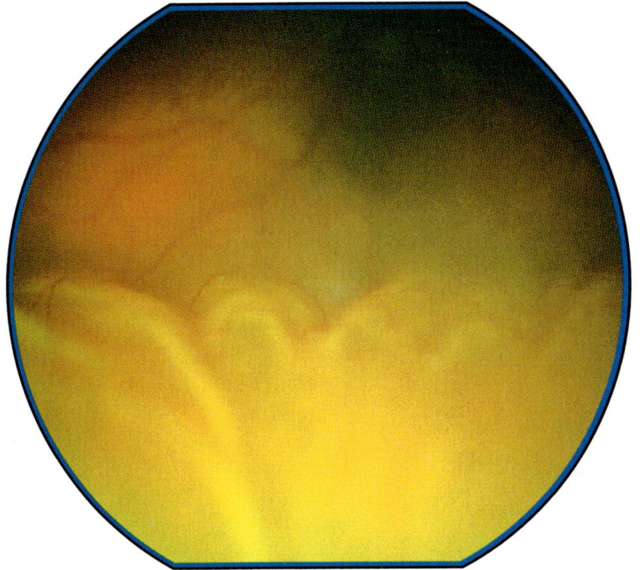

61–4

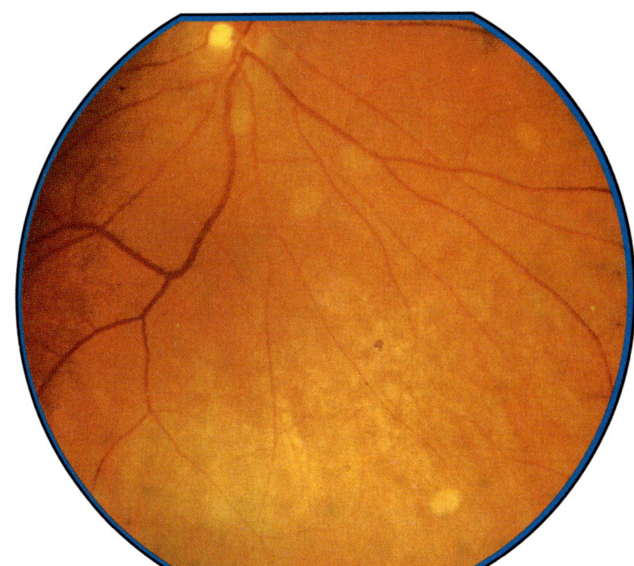

61–5

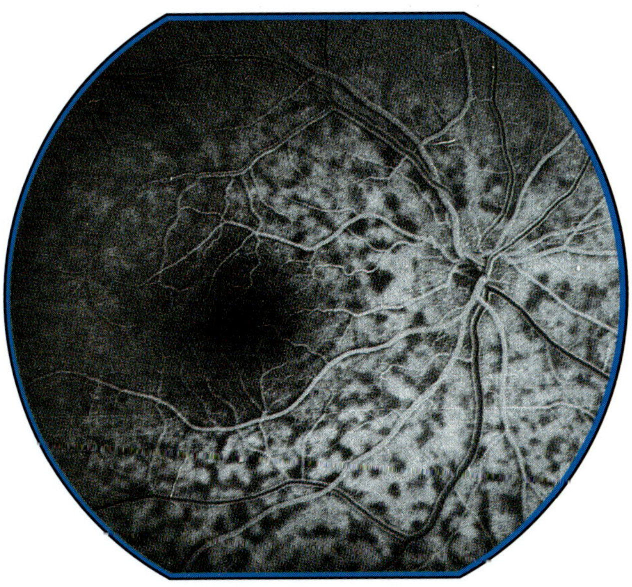

61–3 This patient also has the uveal effusion syndrome with massive detachment.

61–4 and 61–5 Note the leopard spots (diffuse spotty areas of pigmentation that occur after chronic detachment), which can be seen clinically (61–4) and by fluorescein angiography (61–5) in this condition. Fluorescein angiography reveals no leakage under the detachment.

Suggested Readings

Allen, KM, Meyers, SM, and Zegarra, H: Nanophthalmic uveal effusion, Retina 8:145–147, 1988

Brockhurst, RJ: Nanophthalmos with uveal effusion: a new clinical entity, Arch Ophthalmol 93:1289–1299, 1975

Brockhurst, RJ: Vortex vein decompression for nanophthalmic uveal effusion, Arch Ophthalmol 98:1987–1990, 1980

Gass, JDM: Uveal effusion syndrome: a new hypothesis concerning pathogenesis and technique of surgical treatment, Retina 3:159–163, 1983

Johnson, MW, and Gass, JDM: Surgical management of the idiopathic uveal effusion syndrome, Ophthalmology 97:998, 1990

Schepens, CL, and Brockhurst, RJ: Uveal effusion: clinical picture, Arch Ophthalmol 70:189–201, 1963

Vine, AK: Uveal effusion in Hunter's syndrome: evidence that abnormal sclera is responsible for the uveal effusion syndrome, Retina 6:57–60, 1986

Weiter, JJ, Brockhurst, RJ, and Tolentino, FI: Uveal effusion following pan-retinal photocoagulation, Ann Ophthalmol 11:1723–1727, 1979

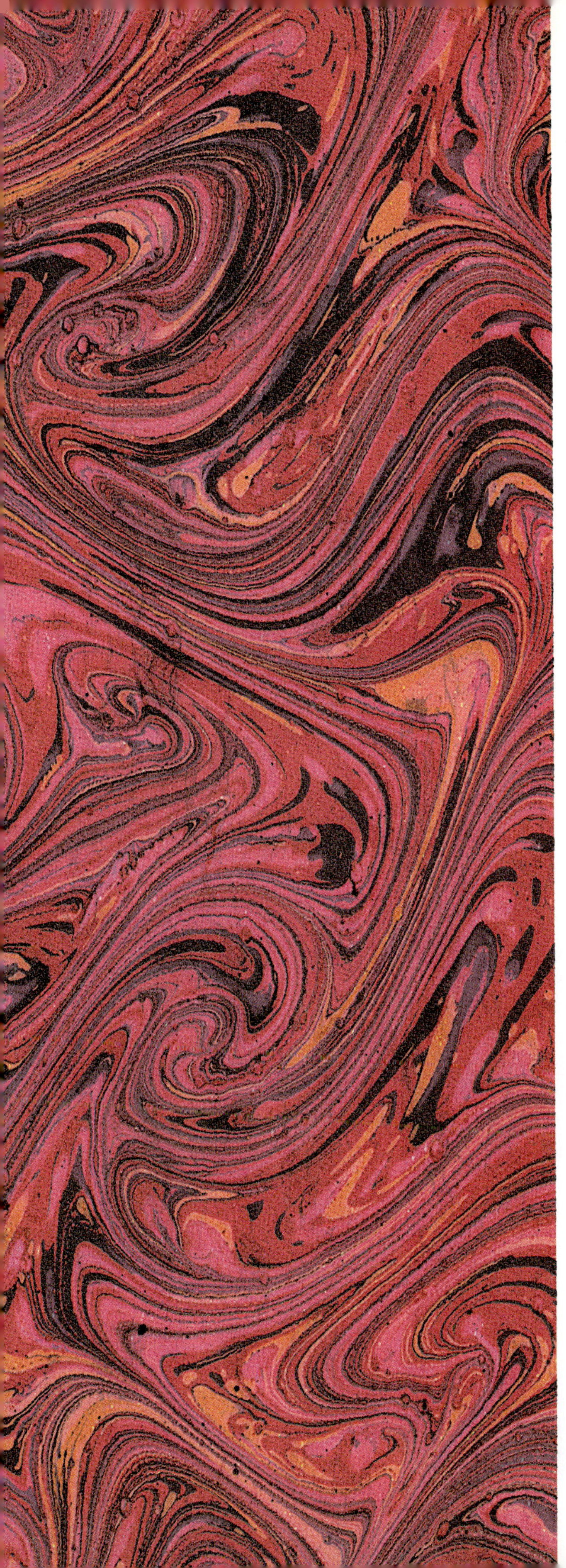

Part IX

Other Diseases

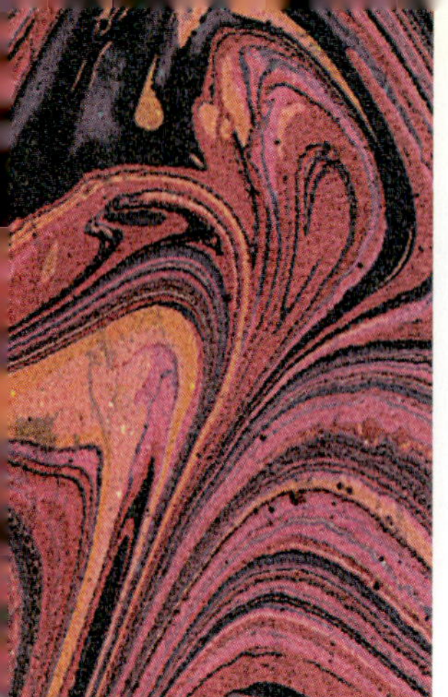

Chapter 62

Drug Toxicities

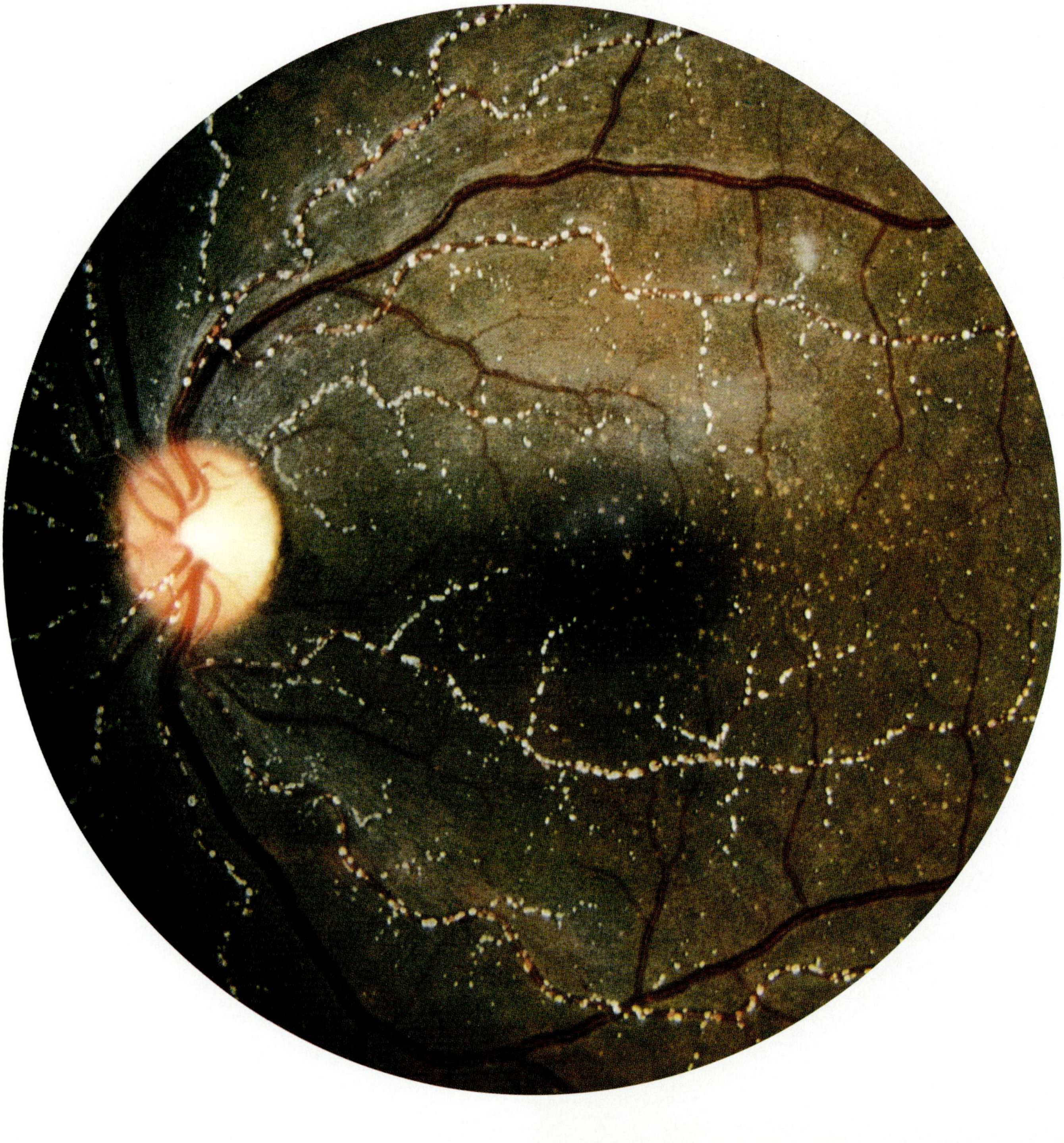

Various drug toxicities may affect the retina. (We are indebted to Dr. William Mieler in the preparation of this chapter.)

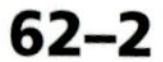

62–1 CHLOROQUINE

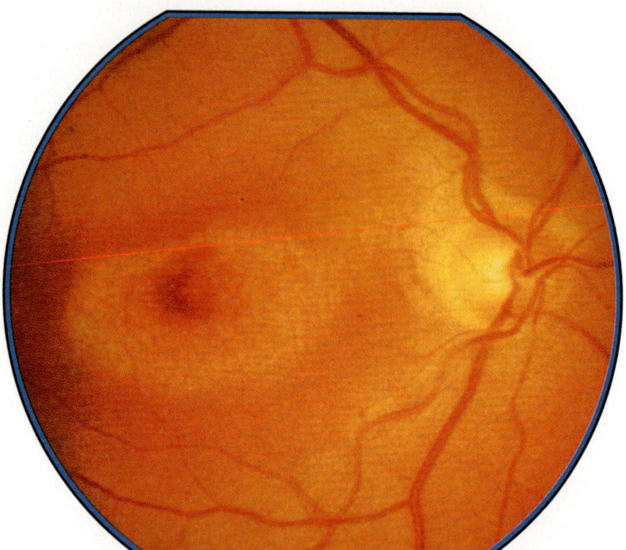

62–2

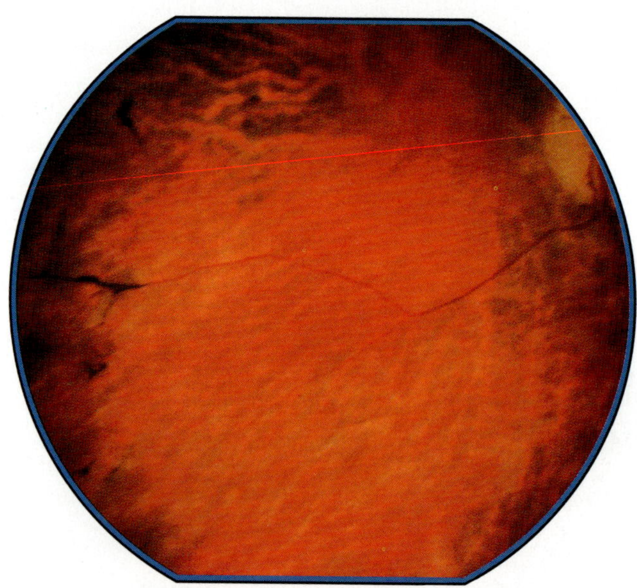

Chloroquine

Chloroquine (Aralen) is a four-aminoquinoline derivative, which was initially used in World War II as an antimalarial agent. It has since been used in the treatment of amebiasis, rheumatoid arthritis, and systemic lupus erythematosus. A retinal toxicity was first described in 1957 and initially involves asymptomatic perifoveal granularity at the level of the retinal pigment epithelium with loss of the foveal reflex. These findings are followed by a bull's eye pattern of atrophy of the retinal pigment epithelium, which is nonreversible. The retinal periphery may show nonspecific granularity and in later stages may progress into a marked pigmentary disturbance resembling an advanced tapetoretinal degeneration. Narrowing of the retinal arterioles may also occur late in the condition. Affected patients usually complain of decreased visual acuity, which may be accompanied by a scotoma or decrease in the peripheral visual field. Retinopathy rarely occurs with a total dose of less than 300 g or a daily dose of 250 mg/day.

62–1 and 62–2 This case demonstrates the classic bull's eye maculopathy (62–1) with a pigmentary disturbance in the periphery (62–2). Note that the bull's eye is asymmetric, with more atrophy inferiorly, which is a characteristic and poorly understood finding.

62–1 *and* ***62–2,*** *Courtesy of Dr. William Mieler.*

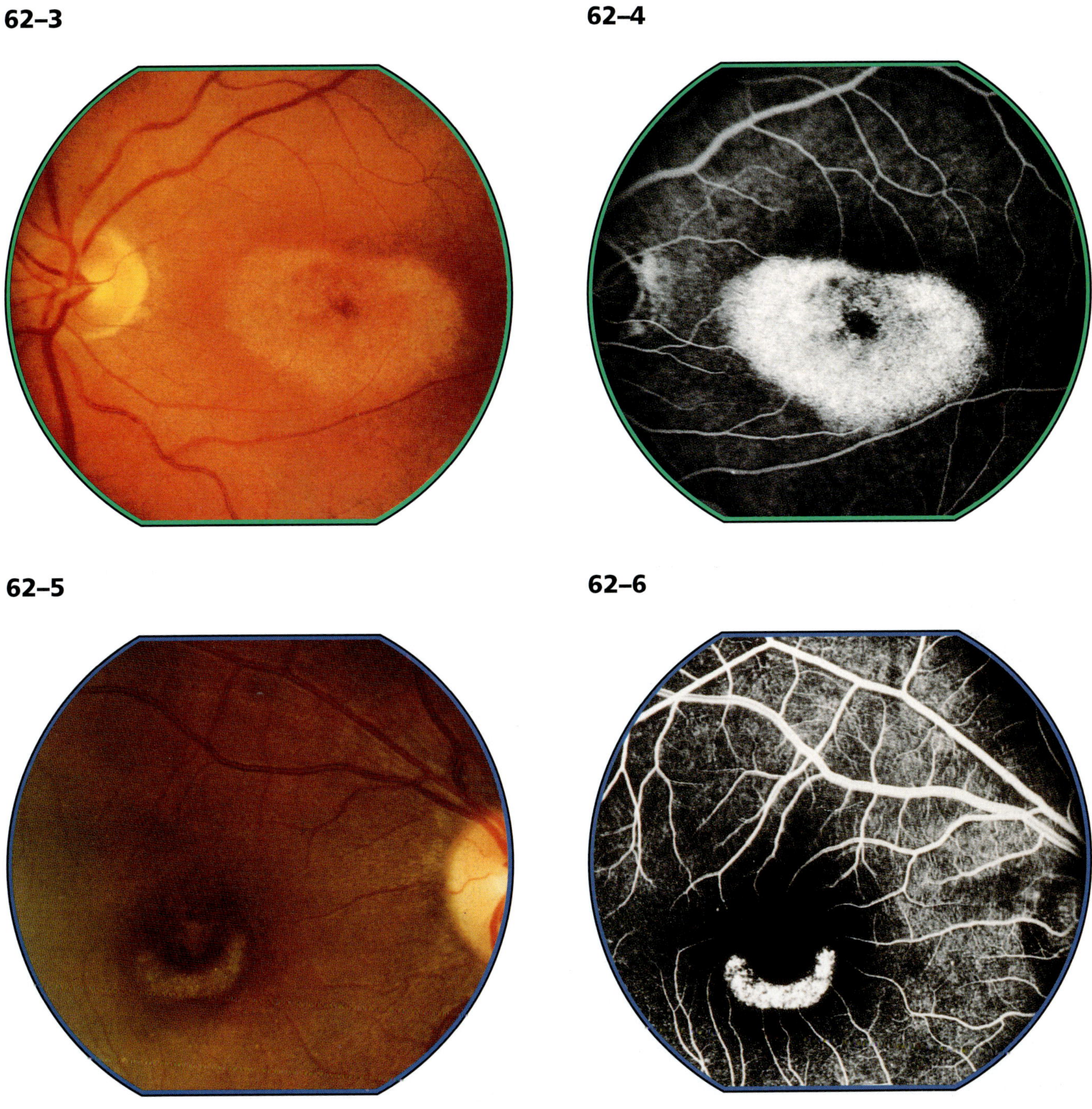

62–3 through 62–6 Bull's eye maculopathies secondary to chloroquine can also be demonstrated in the next two patients. Note the complete bull's eye pattern in the first case (62–3 and 62–4) and the inferior half-moon pattern of toxicity in the second case (62–5 and 62–6).

62–3 *through* ***62–6,*** *Courtesy of Dr. William Mieler.*

62–7 CHLOROQUINE

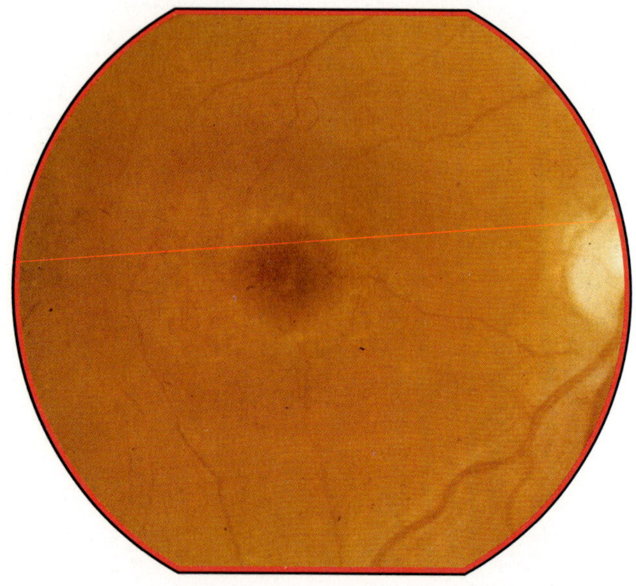

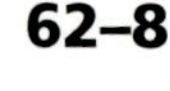

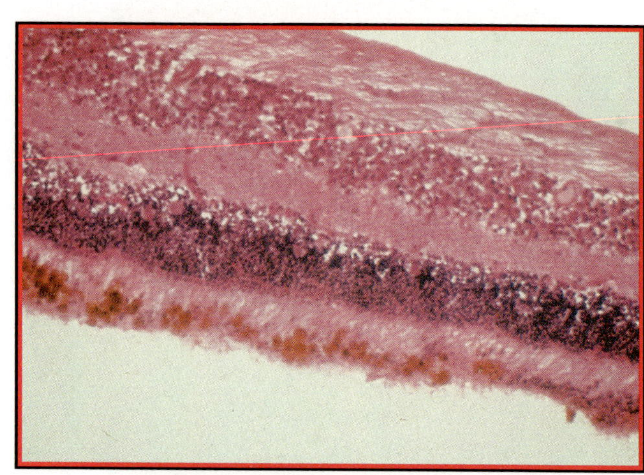

62–9

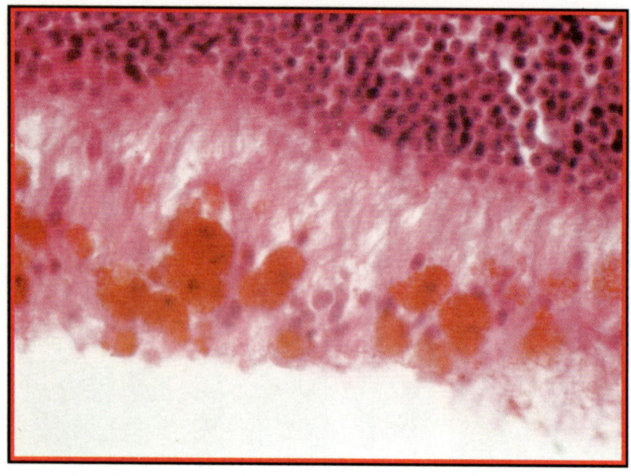

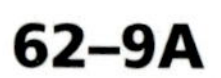

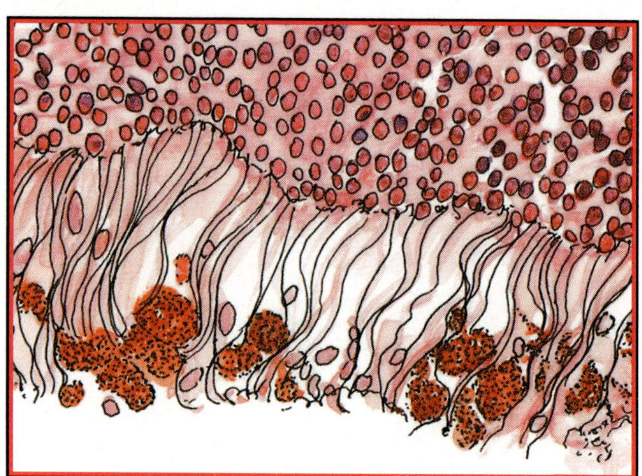

62–7 This patient has the characteristic bull's eye maculopathy of chloroquine retinopathy.

62–8 through 62–9A Light microscopy reveals that the ring corresponds to an area of loss of the photoreceptor cell layer and an aggregate of pigmented cells.

62–10 HYDROXYCHLOROQUINE (PLAQUENIL)

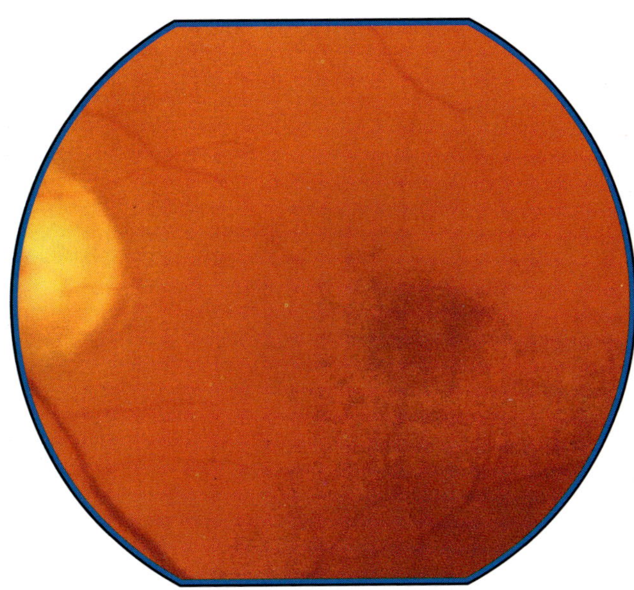

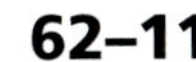
62–11

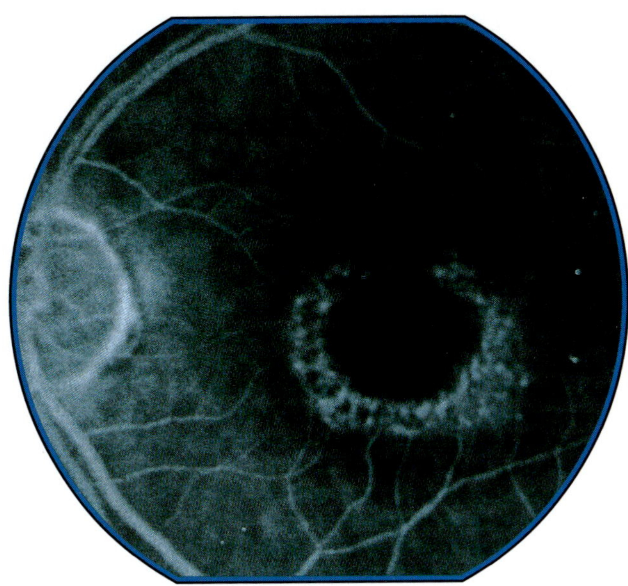

Hydroxychloroquine

62–10 and 62–11 Hydroxychloroquine (Plaquenil) is a derivative of chloroquine and causes an indistinguishable retinopathy. Plaquenil may be safer than chloroquine. Dosages up to 400 mg/day or 5–7 mg/kg/day are generally safe. This case demonstrates the characteristic bull's eye appearance with its corresponding fluorescein angiographic pattern.

62–12 **THIORIDAZINE (MELLARIL)**

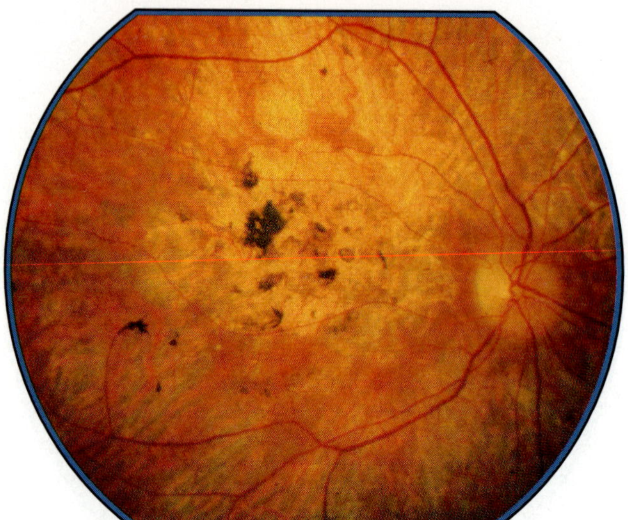

62–13

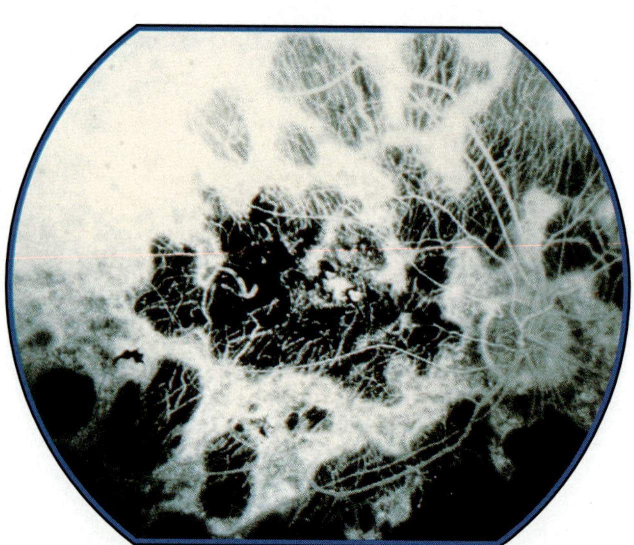

Thioridazine

Thioridazine (Mellaril) is used in the treatment of the psychoses. A pigmentary retinopathy was reported in 1960. The fundus changes initially have a salt-and-pepper appearance and are followed by pigment clumping in a plaquelike fashion. These changes usually occur at the level of the retinal pigment epithelium (RPE) between the optic disc and the equator. In advanced stages, atrophy of the RPE and choriocapillaris may occur. Retinal toxicity is usually seen in dosages in excess of 1000 mg/day with a total accumulation of 85 to 100 g over 30 to 50 days. The toxicity may progress even if the medication is discontinued.

62–12 and 62–13 Note the pigment clumping in a plaquelike fashion demonstrated with this toxicity (62–12), as well as atrophy of the RPE and choriocapillaris, which follows a lobular confluent pattern on the corresponding fluorescein angiogram (62–13).

62–12 *and* ***62–13,*** *Courtesy of Dr. William Mieler.*

62–14

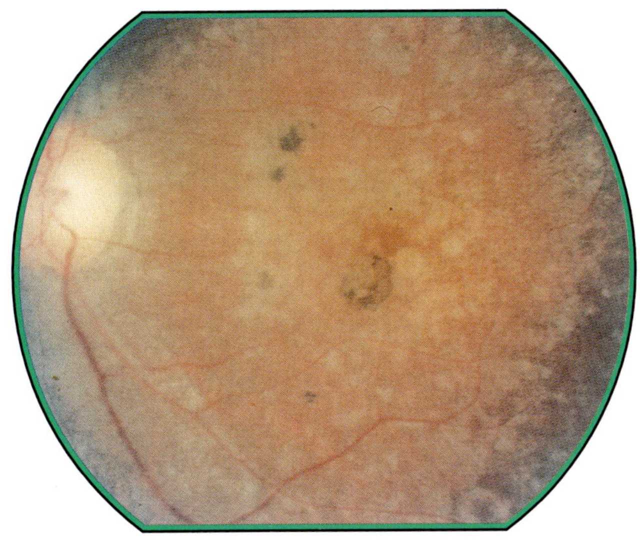

62–15

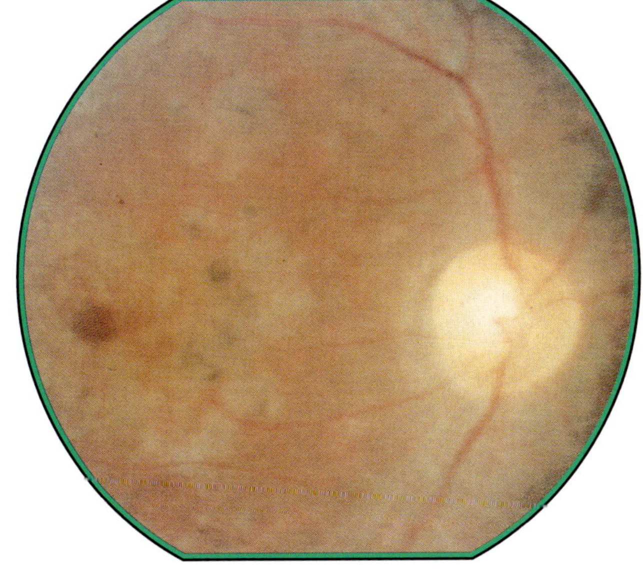

62–16

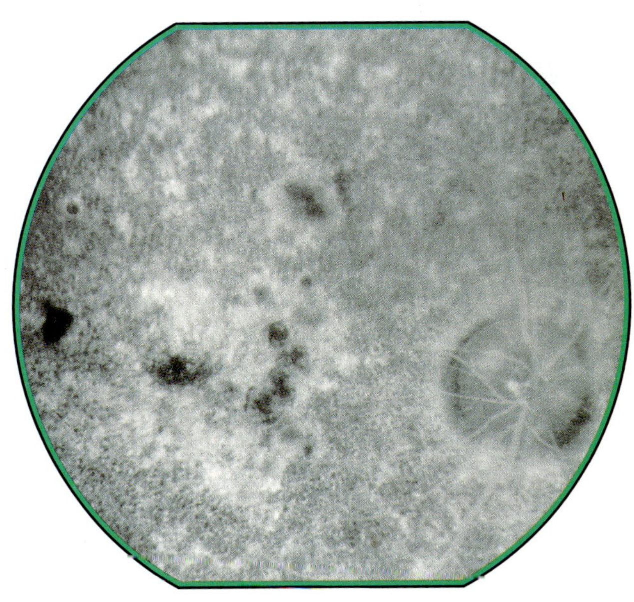

62–14 through 62–16 These eyes also illustrate thioridazine toxicity with pigment clumping.

62–14 *through* ***62–16,*** *Courtesy of Dr. William Mieler.*

62–17 THIORIDAZINE (MELLARIL)

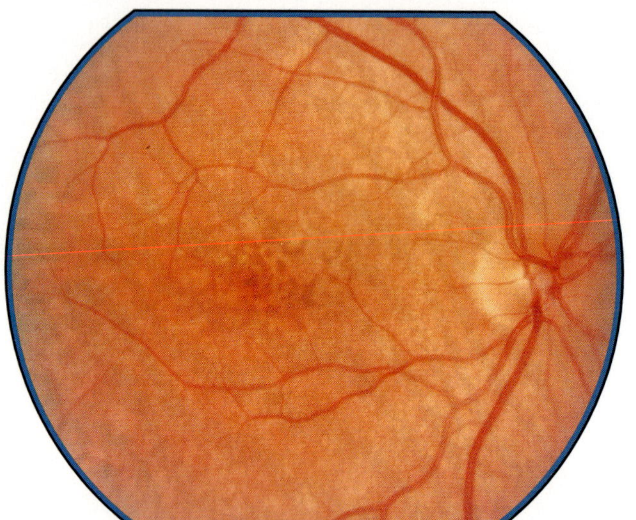

62–18

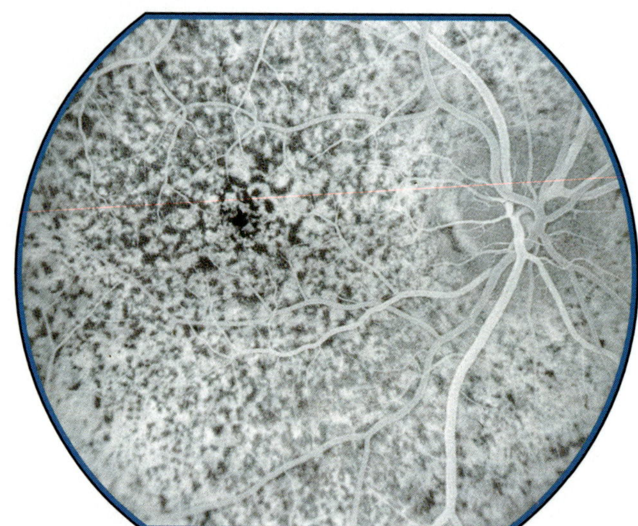

62–19

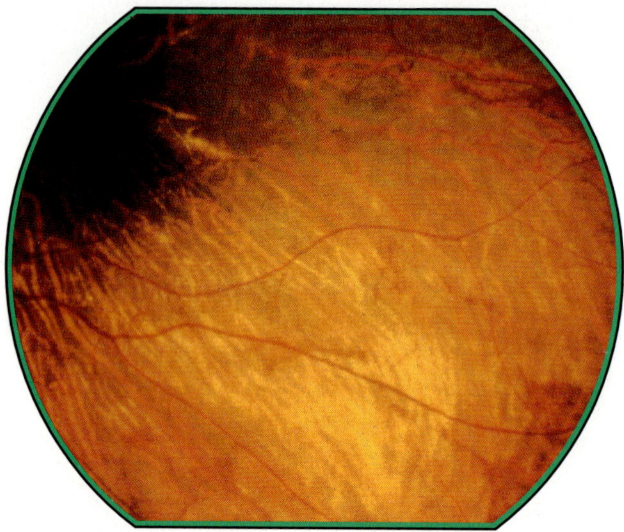

62–20

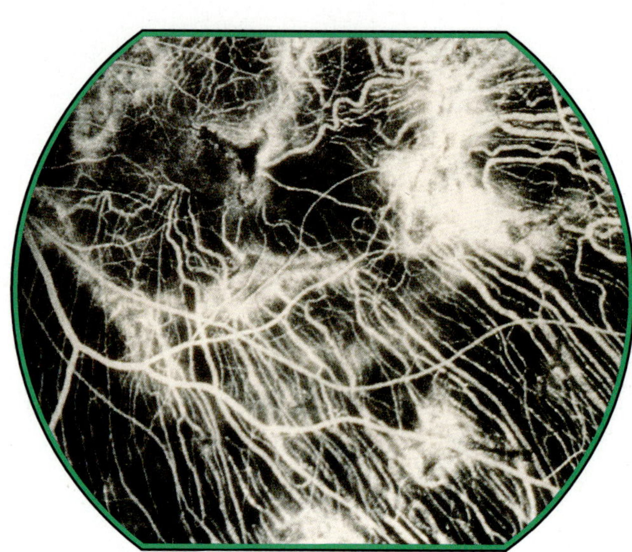

62–17 and 62–18 The early salt-and-pepper–like changes in the macular region are demonstrated in this patient.

62–19 and 62–20 This case shows more pigment clumping with hypopigmented areas and vessel attenuation.

62–17 *through* ***62–20,*** *Courtesy of Dr. William Mieler.*

62–21

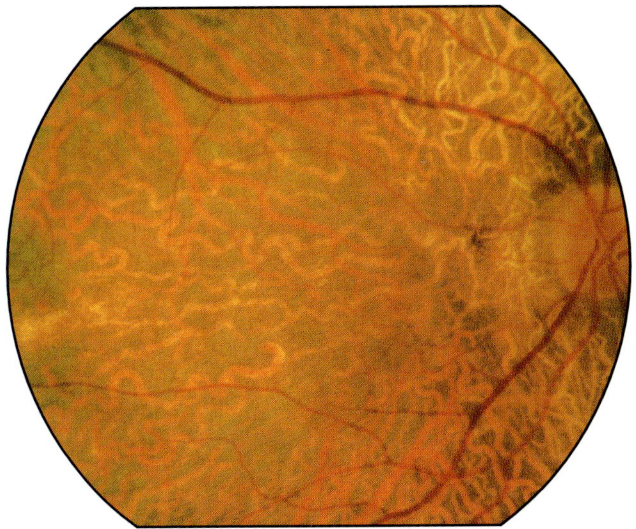

62–22

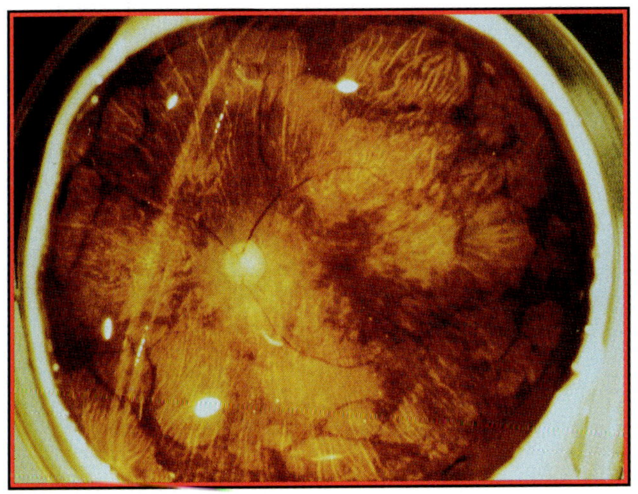

62–23

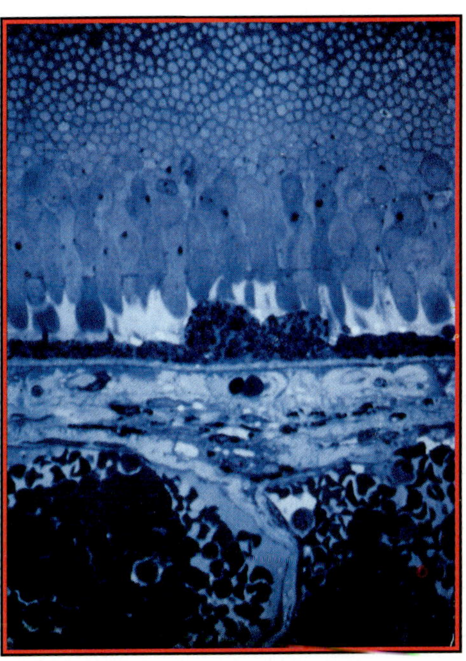

62–21 This 59-year-old schizophrenic male was treated with thioridazine at a dosage of 200 mg at bedtime. Visual acuity was 20/70; an atrophic retinopathy is noted.

62–22 and 62–23 Gross appearance of thioridazine retinopathy reveals widespread atrophy of the retinal pigment epithelium. An area near the macula demonstrates that the RPE is intact and that there is partial atrophy of the photoreceptors.

62–21, *Courtesy of Tina Dominquez.* ***62–22*** *and* ***62–23,*** *From Miller, et al: Clinical-ultrastructural study of thioridazine retinopathy, Ophthalmology 89:1478–1488, 1982.*

62–24 CHLORPROMAZINE (THORAZINE)

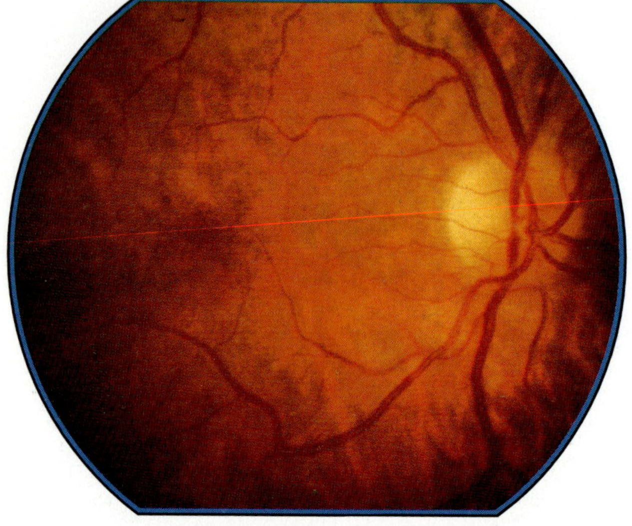

62–25

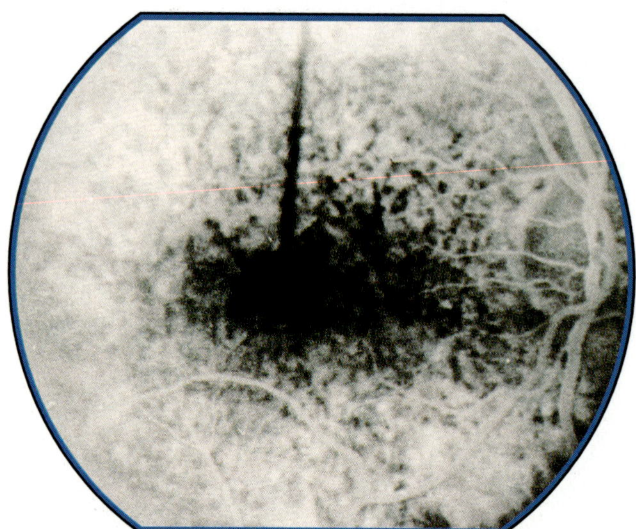

62–26 QUININE SULFATE

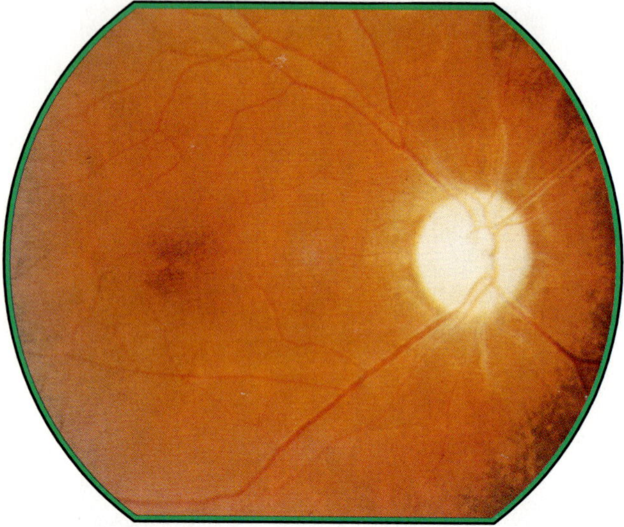

62–27

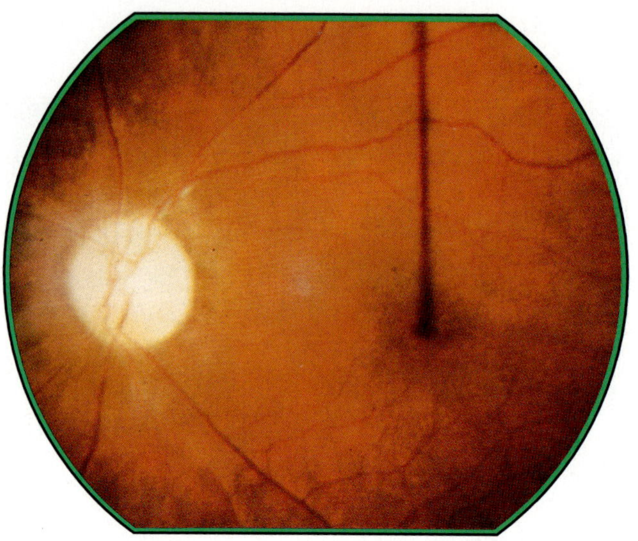

Chlorpromazine

Chlorpromazine (Thorazine) is used in the treatment of schizophrenia, anxiety, tension, nausea, vomiting, and porphyria. Infrequently, a retinal toxicity is noted in which a nonspecific retinal granularity with fine pigment clumping can be seen. This is usually noted when 800 mg/day is used for 20 months or more.

62–24 and 62–25 Nonspecific granularity in the macular region with fine pigment clumping can be noted in this patient who was taking chlorpromazine.

Quinine Sulfate

Quinine sulfate has been used as an antimalarial agent and as a muscle relaxant. Toxicity has been noted in dosages greater than 4 g. Initial ocular toxicity findings are subtle. However, optic disc pallor and retinal vessel attenuation may eventually occur.

62–26 and 62–27 This patient has quinine toxicity. Note the optic disc pallor and retinal vessel attenuation.

62–24 *through* **62–27,** *Courtesy of Dr. William Mieler.*

62–28 NICOTINIC ACID

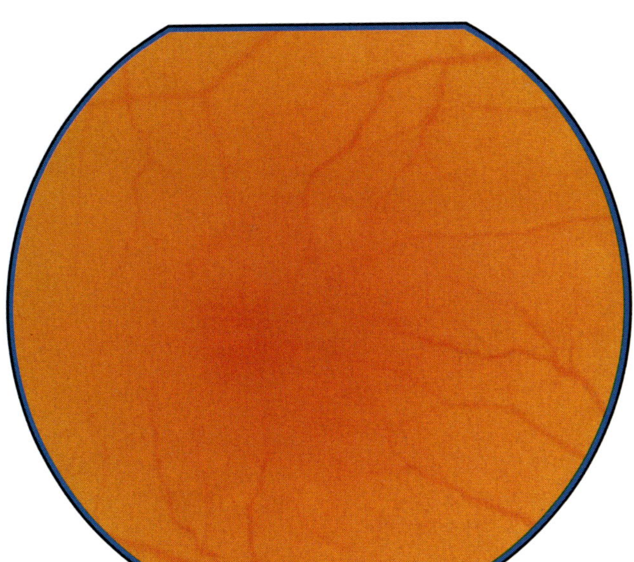

62–29

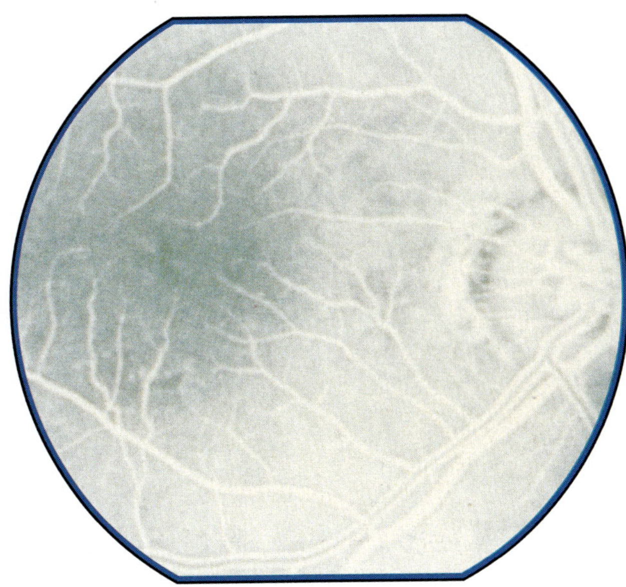

Nicotinic Acid

Nicotinic acid (niacin) has been used to treat hypercholesterolemia. An atypical form of macular edema has been reported in which there is no capillary permeability alteration on the fluorescein angiogram. Toxicity has been noted with dosages greater than 3 g/day. Visual acuity returns to normal if the drug is discontinued.

62–28 and 62–29 In this case, a nonleaking cystoid macular edema can be seen. Permeability changes of the capillaries in the macula region are not noted in this type of cystoid macular edema on fluorescein angiography.

62–28 *and* ***62–69,*** *Courtesy of Drs. William Mieler and J. Donald Gass.*

62–30 METHOXYFLURANE

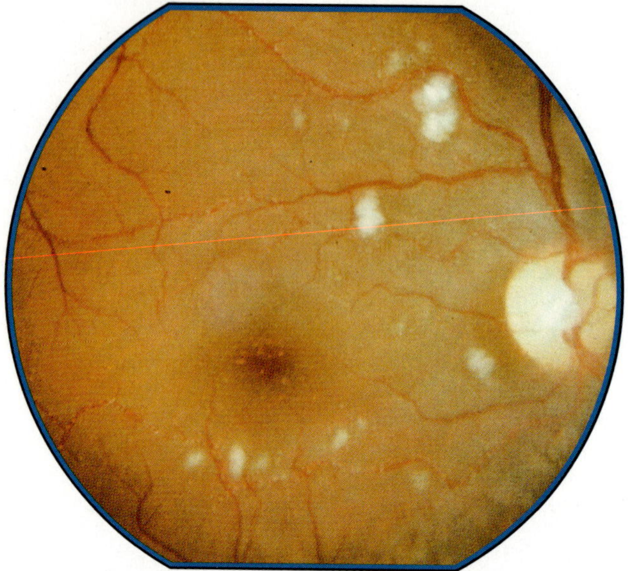

62–31

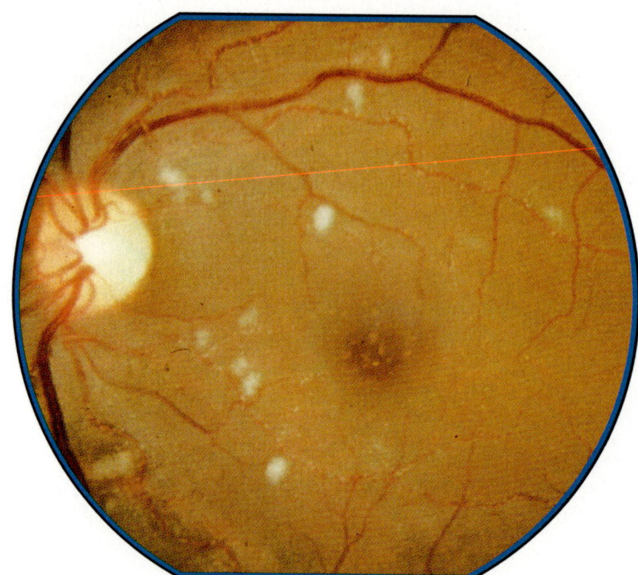

62–32

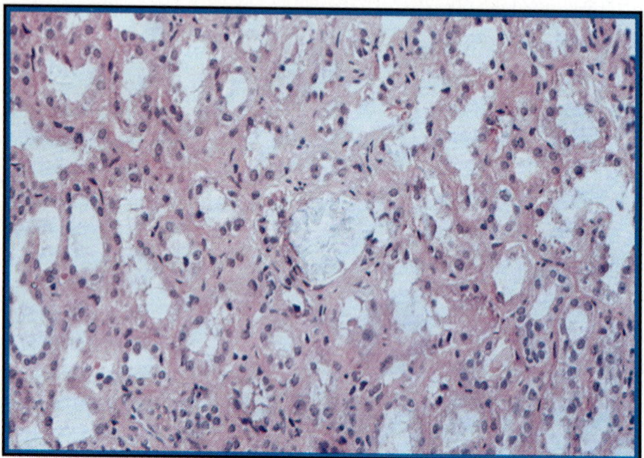

Methoxyflurane

Methoxyflurane (Penthrane) is a nonflammable anesthetic agent that may cause secondary hyperoxalosis. Deposition of calcium oxalate crystals at the level of the retinal pigment epithelium and retina may occur. This disorder may resemble a flecked retinal syndrome and may have diffuse retinal involvement.

62–30 and 62–31 This patient had a crystalline deposition secondary to methoxyflurane ingestion. Initially, multiple cotton-wool spots and highly refractile yellow-white crystals were noted.

62–32 Renal biopsy revealed calcium oxalate crystals in the renal tubular lumens, epithelial cells, and interstitium.

62–30 *through* ***62–32,*** *Courtesy of Dr. Michael Novak. From Novak, MA, et al: Calcium oxalate retinopathy associated with methoxyflurane abuse, Retina 8:230–236, 1988.*

(Case continued on next page.)

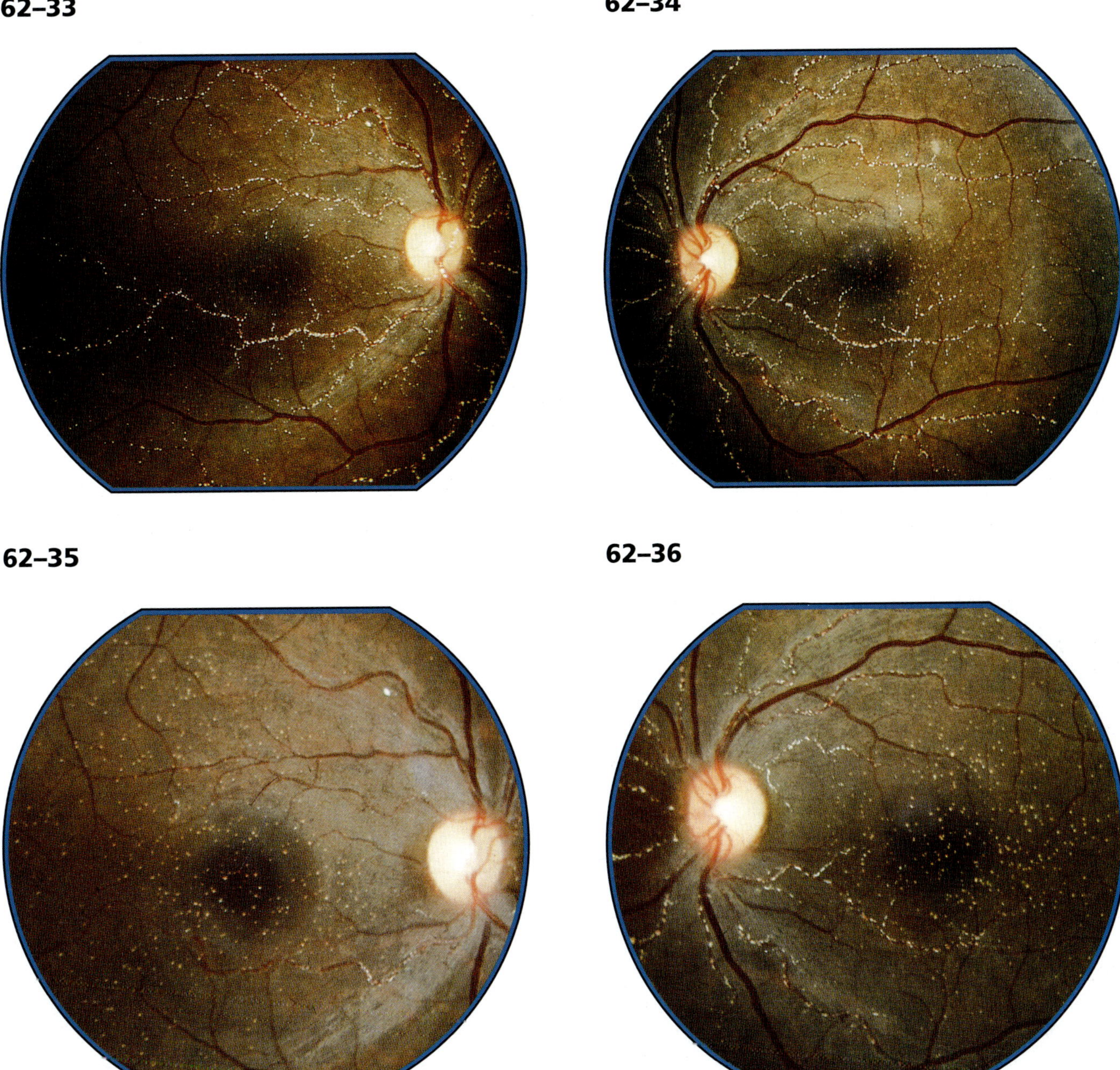

62–33 and 62–34 The crystals then became much more abundant and the cotton-wool spots disappeared. Note that the crystal-like deposition follows the vasculature pattern. There are also scattered lesions in the choroid, which are modified in their appearance by the RPE. In the retinal vessels, the deposits are predominantly crystalline or glistening, although there are a few orange-colored deposits as well.

62–35 and 62–36 Six months later the crystals have partially resolved.

62–33 *through* ***62–36,*** *Courtesy of Dr. Michael Novak. From Novak, MA, et al: Calcium oxalate retinopathy associated with methoxyflurane abuse, Retina 8:230–236, 1988.*

62–37 METHOXYFLURANE

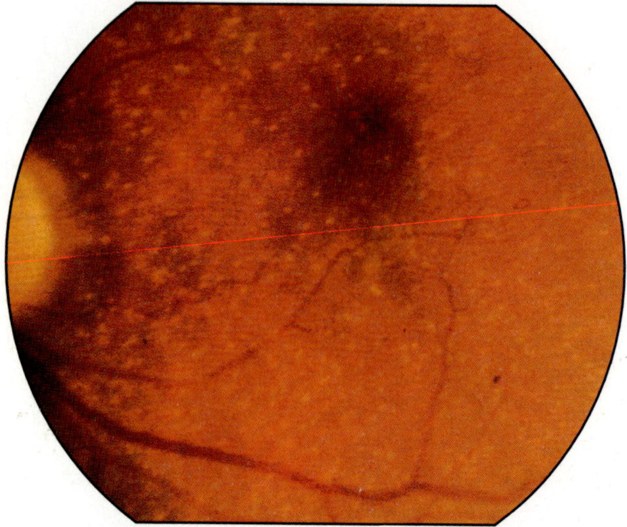

62–38 PRIMARY HYPEROXALURIA

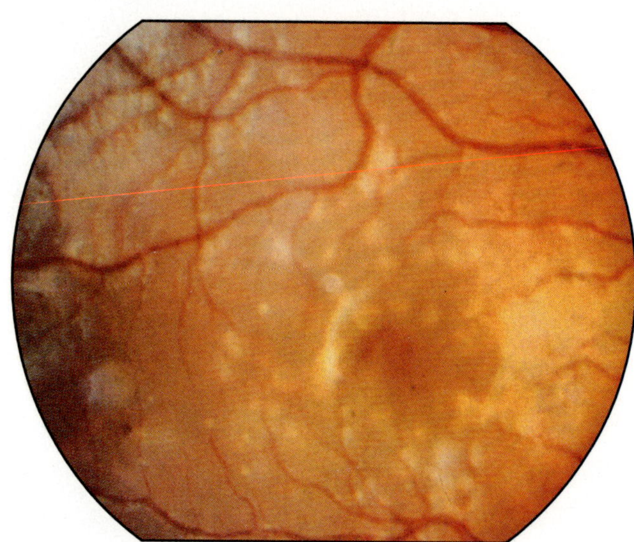

62–39 PRIMARY HYPEROXALURIA

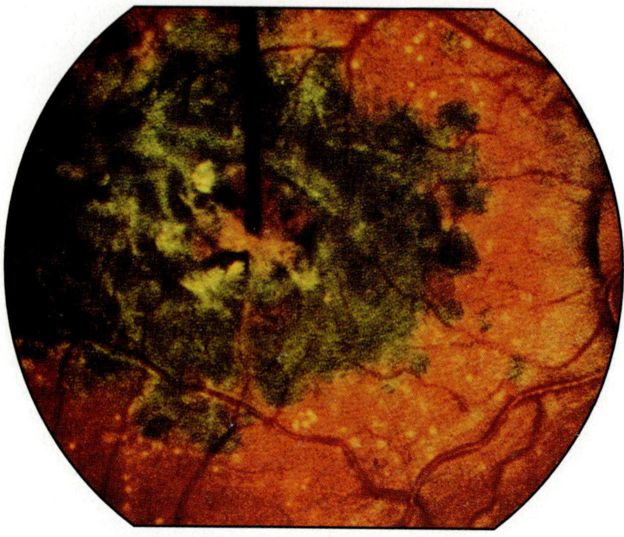

62–40

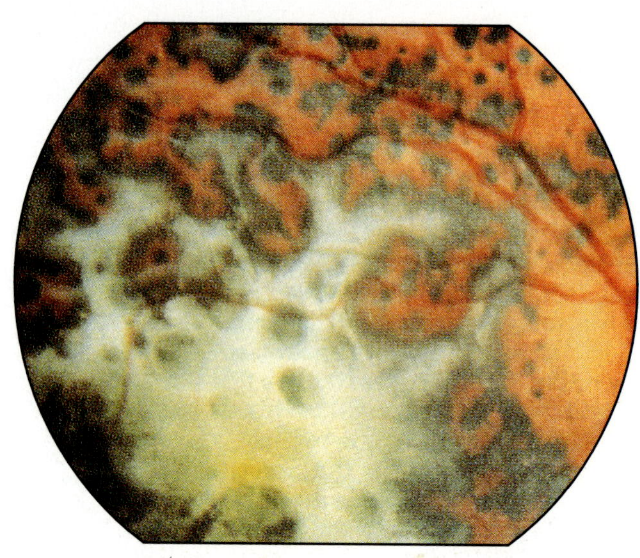

Methoxyflurane

62–37 This patient also has methoxyflurane toxicity with a whitish-yellow fleck-like deposition, which is not evident in the larger retinal vessels, as in the last case.

Primary Hyperoxaluria

62–38 through 62–40 Primary hyperoxaluria is a rare autosomal recessive condition. Ocular findings include crystalline or flecked-shaped lesions (62–38) with or without pigmentation, fibrosis, and scarring (62–39 and 62–40).

62–37, *Courtesy of Dr. William Mieler.* ***62–38,*** *Courtesy of Dr. Elias Traboulsi.* ***62–39*** *and* ***62–40,*** *From Smale, et al: Ocular findings in primary oxalosis, Arch Ophthalmol 108:89–93, 1990.*

62–41 PRIMARY HYPEROXALURIA

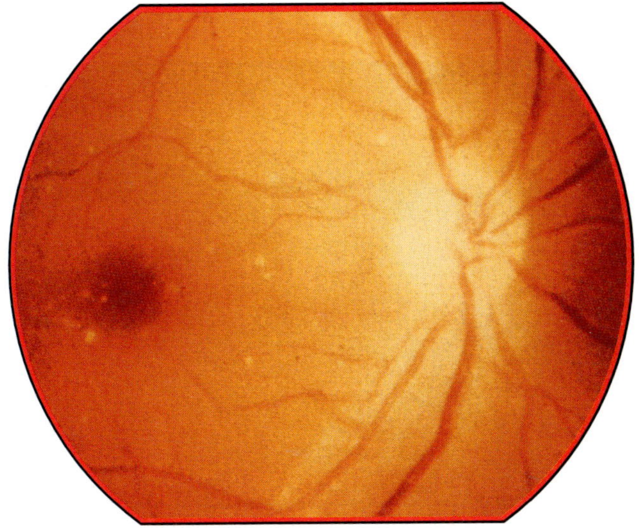

62–42

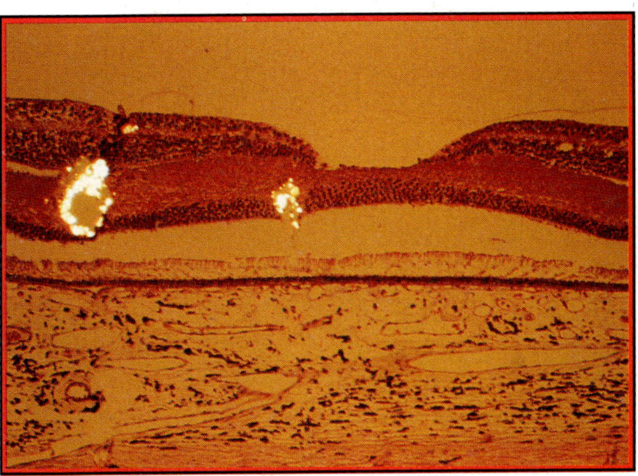

62–43 TAMOXIFEN

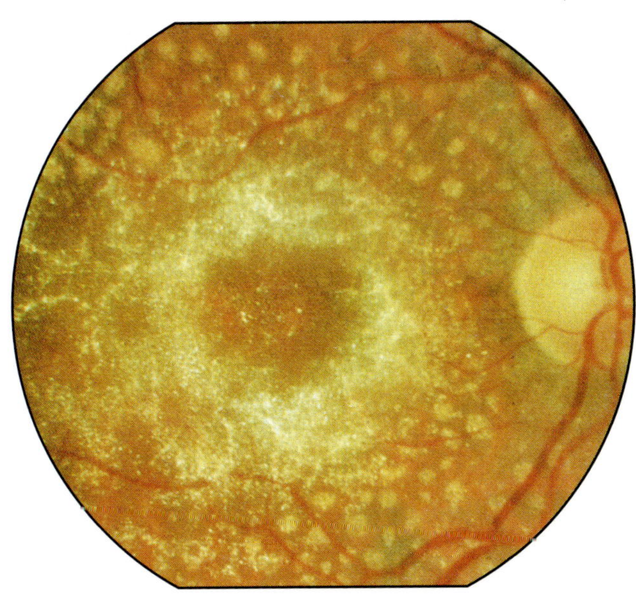

Primary Hyperoxaluria

62–41 and 62–42 Clinicopathologic correlation of a patient with primary hyperoxaluria demonstrates crystals in the fundus. With polarized light, the crystals are birefringent.

Tamoxifen

Tamoxifen (Nolvadex) is a nonsteroidal antiestrogen agent used in the treatment of metastatic breast carcinoma. Bilateral refractile opacities may be seen with tamoxifen toxicity. These changes are usually limited to the perifoveal region. Macular edema has also been noted. The abnormalities appear to be permanent.

62–43 This patient demonstrates tamoxifen toxicity. Note the refractive opacities in the perifoveal region. Note the scattered areas of atrophy and an irregular encircling area of preretinal fibrosis.

62–41 *and* **62–42,** *Reprinted from Sakamoto, I, et al: Arch Ophthalmol 109:384, 1991.* **62–43,** *Courtesy of Dr. William Mieler.*

62–44 CANTHAXANTHIN

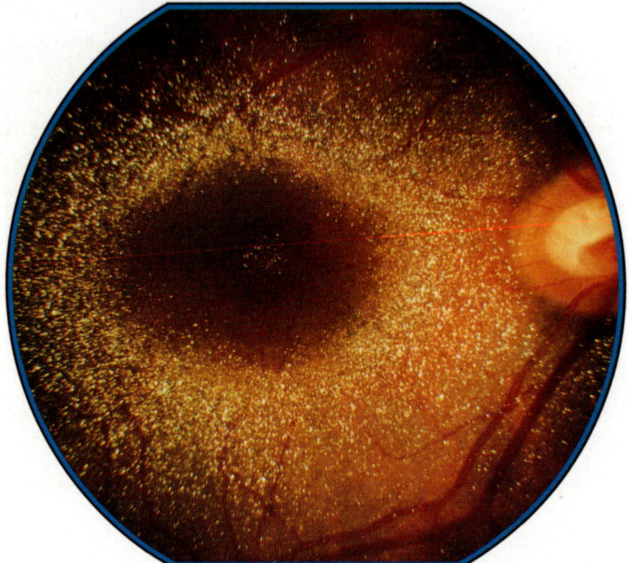

62–45

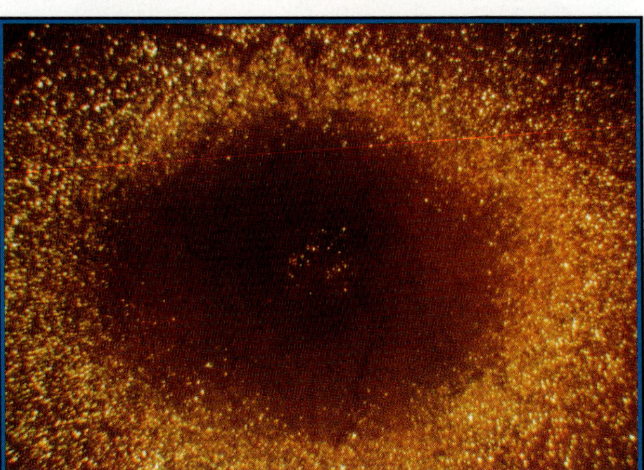

62–46

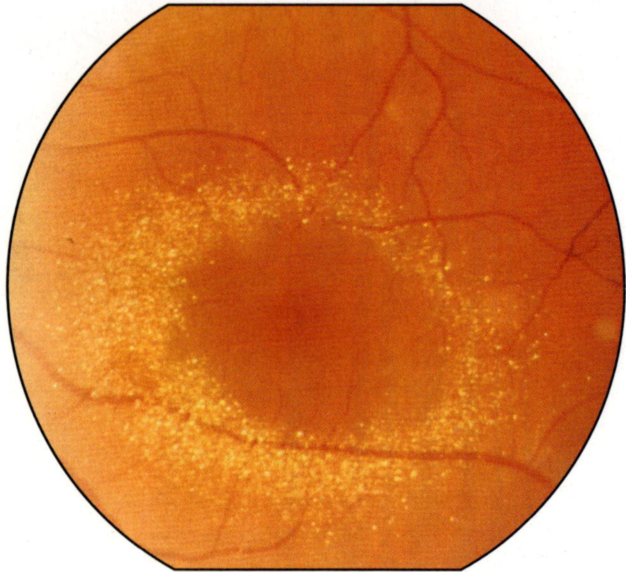

Canthaxanthin

Canthaxanthin is a carotinoid used as a food-coloring agent. It has also been used as a suntanning agent, although it has not been approved in the USA. It has been marketed for that purpose in Canada and Europe. The retinopathy consists of yellow glistening dots in a donut-shaped pattern around the macula. Toxicity is usually demonstrated after ingestion of 3.6 to 66 g of the drug over 24 months. Patients are generally asymptomatic.

62–44 and 62–45 This patient shows the characteristic yellow glistening crystalline deposits of canthaxanthin. Note the donut-shaped pattern around the macula.

62–46 This patient also exhibits the characteristic donut-shaped pattern of canthaxanthin deposition.

62–46, *Courtesy of Dr. Dean Eliott.*

62–47 CANTHAXANTHIN

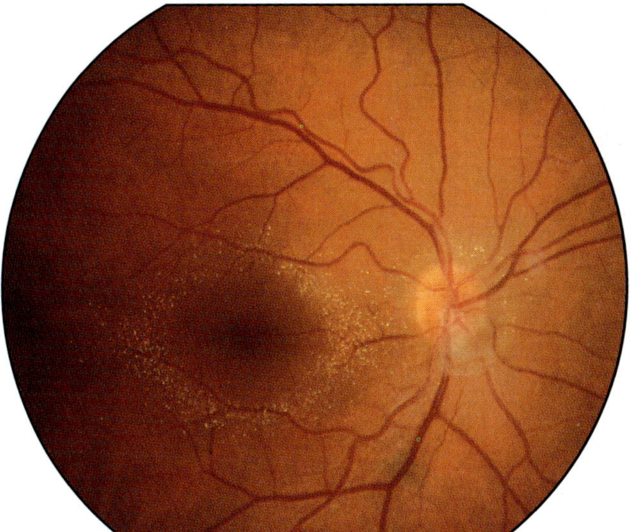

62–48

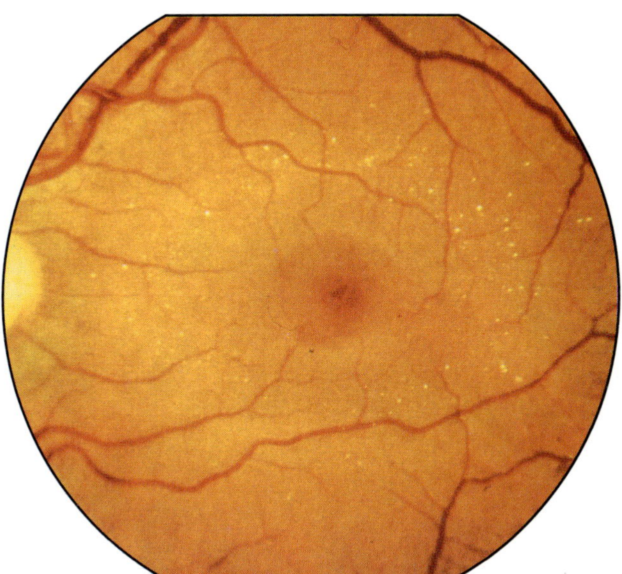

62–49 NITROFURANTOIN

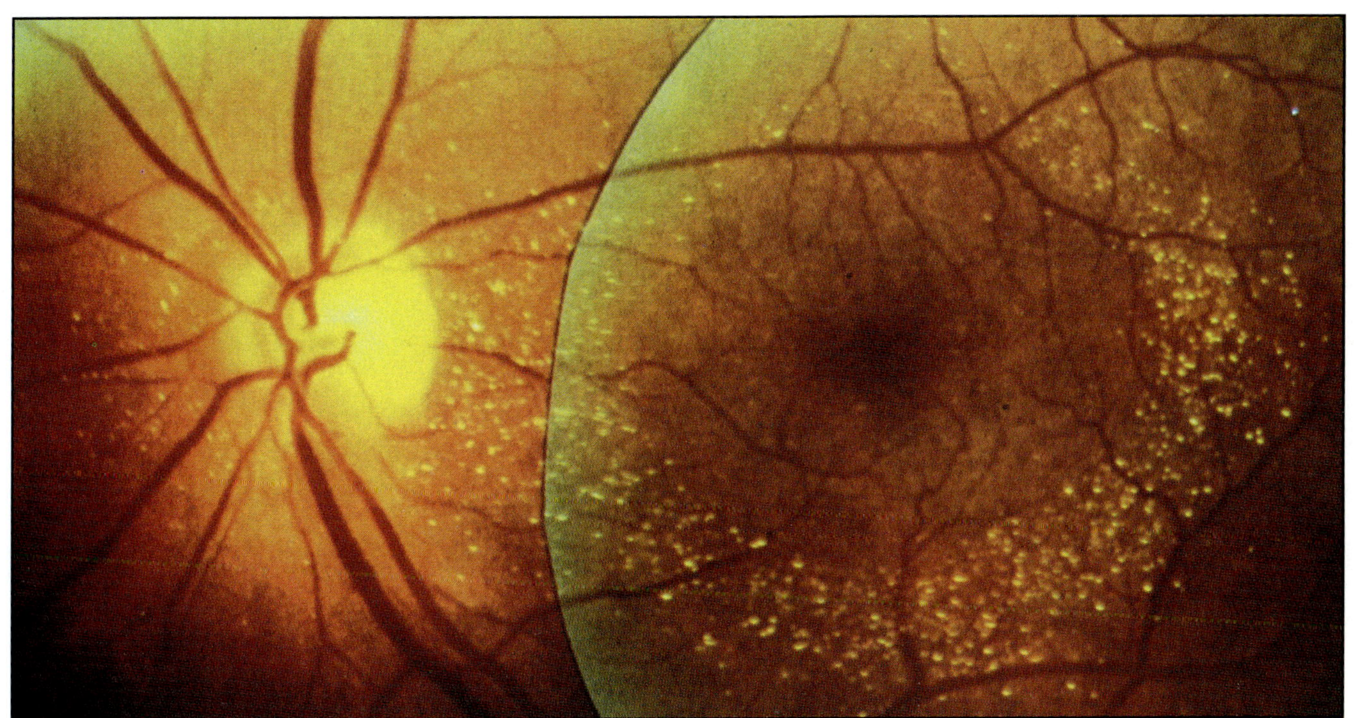

62–47 and 62–48 The next two patients show more subtle forms of canthaxanthin toxicity. Note that these eyes have fewer crystals. The characteristic glistening crystals in a donut-shaped pattern are consistent with this toxicity.

62–49 This patient has a crystalline retinopathy in the macular and peripapillary areas due to long-term nitrofurantoin therapy, which resembles canthaxanthin toxicity.

62–48, *Courtesy of Dr. William Mieler.* **62–49,** *Courtesy of Dr. David Williams.*

62–50 TALC

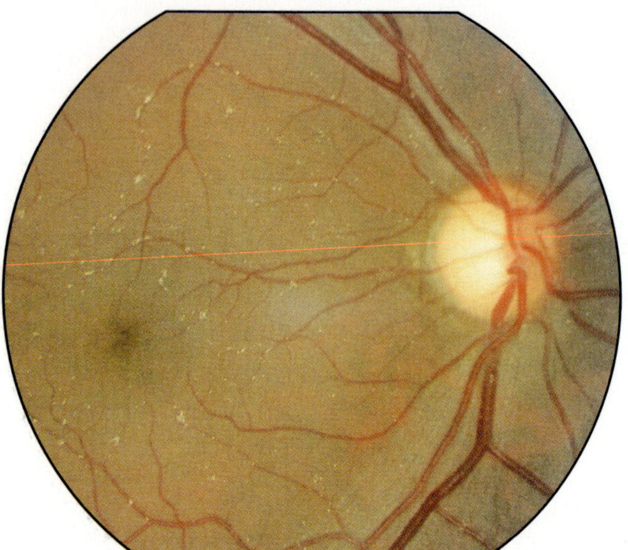

62–51

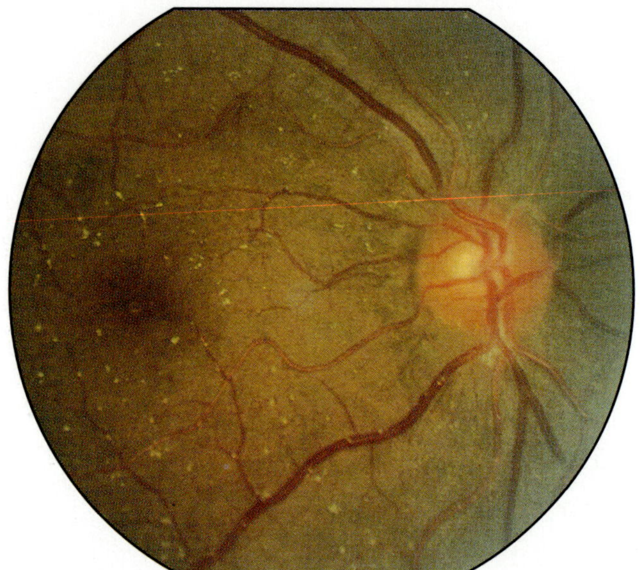

62–52

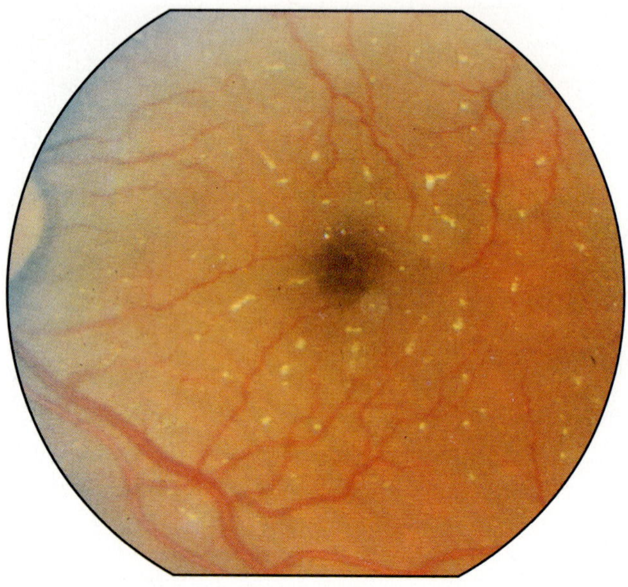

Talc

62–50 through 62–52 These patients with talc retinopathy demonstrate whitish lesions in the retina, which often follow a vascular distribution.

***62–50** and **62–51**, Courtesy of Dr. Alexander Brucker.*

62–53 PROCAINAMIDE

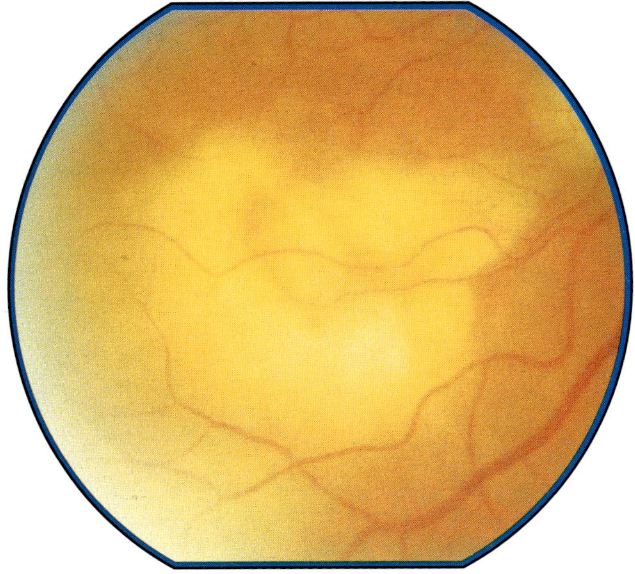

62–54

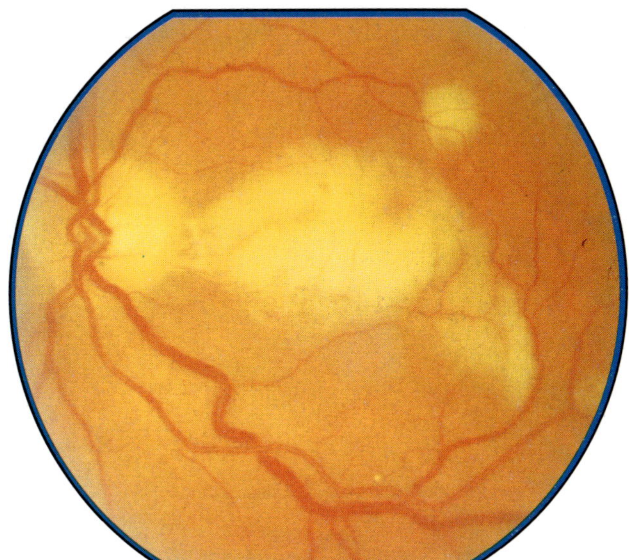

62–55

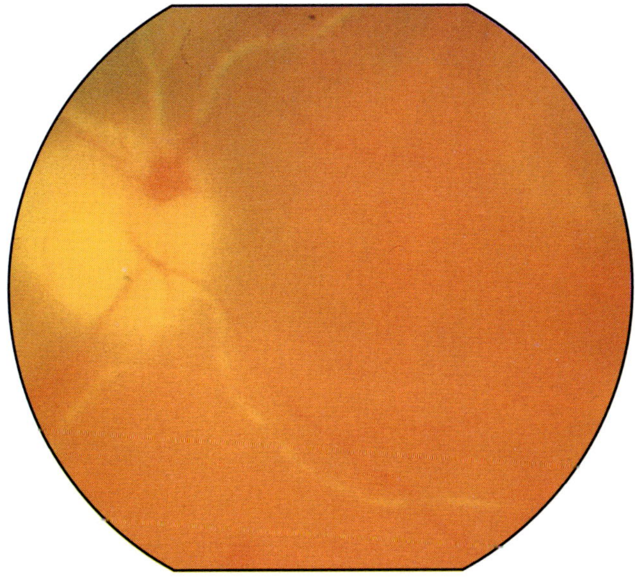

Procainamide

62–53 through 62–55 Procainamide can produce zones of retinal whitening secondary to vascular ischemic disease, as demonstrated in these patients. A variable yellowish-white deposition can be seen at the level of the choroid and retinal pigment epithelium. This whitening resembles an ischemic retinopathy. Vascular occulsion with nonperfusion and optic atrophy can be extensive (62–55).

***62–53** through **62–55,** Courtesy of Dr. William Mieler.*

62–56 GENTAMYCIN

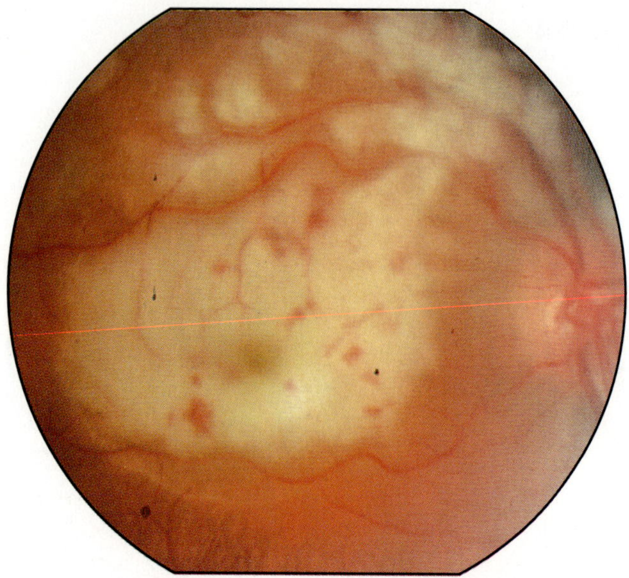

62–57

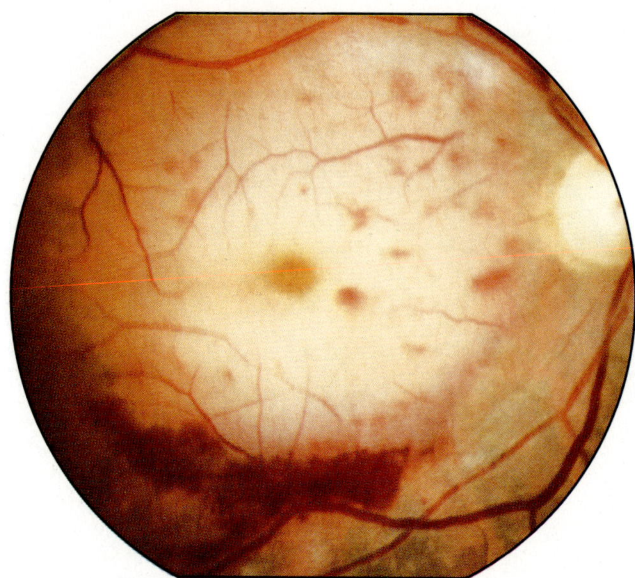

62–58 VANCOMYCIN

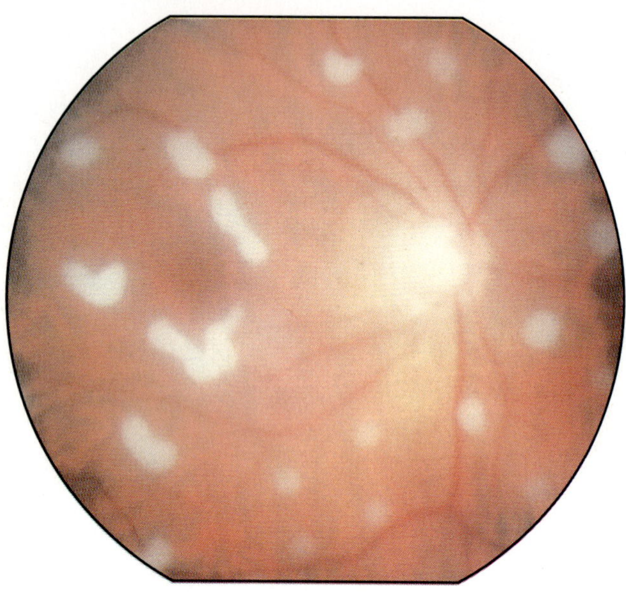

Gentamycin

62–56 and 62–57 Gentamycin toxicity can lead to massive destruction of the posterior pole, as observed in these two patients. Intense inflammation, hemorrhage, sheathed vessels, and optic atrophy can occur. Whitish areas of infarction caused by a necrotizing obliterative hemorrhagic retinopathy in the macular region are characteristically noted in this condition; in this case there is also a cherry-red spot, which is not characteristically seen.

Vancomycin

62–58 This patient has whitish particles in the vitreous and on the surface of the retina that were believed to be due to particulate matter from vancomycin after intraocular injection of a preparation of the drug after vitrectomy for endophthalmitis.

62–58, *Courtesy of Dr. Jeffrey Shakin.*

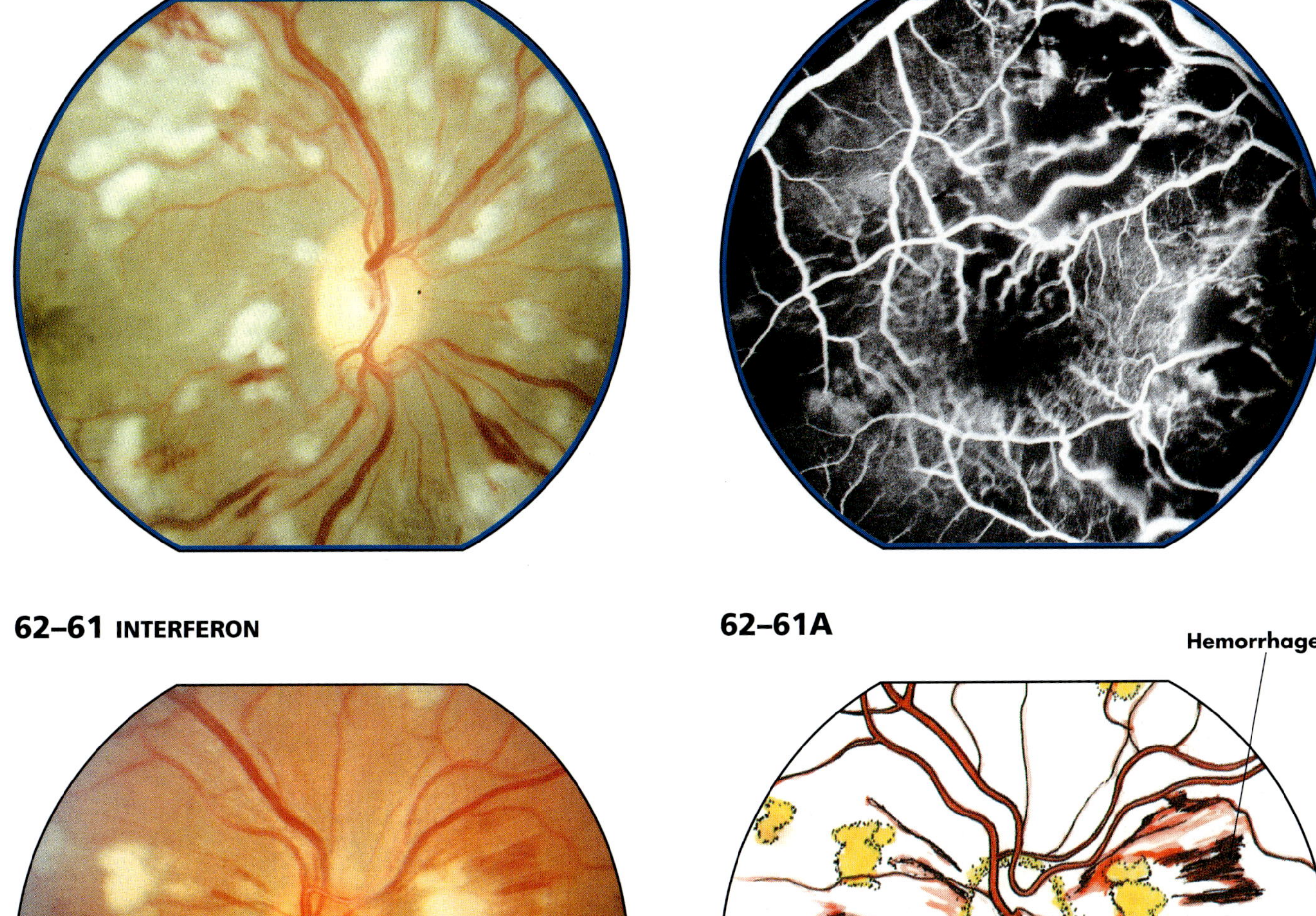

Cocaine

62–59 Cocaine toxicity can result in multiple cotton-wool spots and intraretinal hemorrhages.

62–60 Fluorescein angiography reveals telangiectatic vessels and areas of capillary non-perfusion.

Interferon

62–61 and 62–61A Interferon is another drug that can result in multiple cotton-wool spots with intraretinal hemorrhages, as demonstrated in this patient with interferon-associated retinopathy. The condition may be due to an immune complex deposition in the retinal vessels.

62–61, *From Guyer, DR, et al: Interferon-associated retinopathy, Arch Ophthalmol 111:350–356, 1992. Copyright 1992, American Medical Association.*

62–62 CARBON MONOXIDE

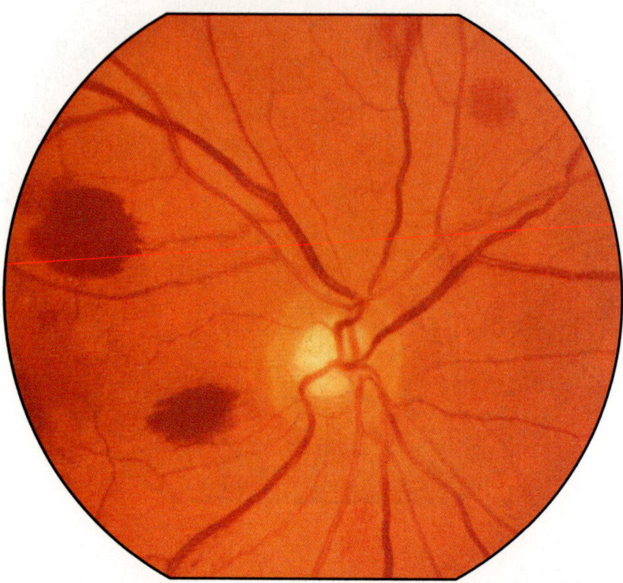

62–63 HEPARIN

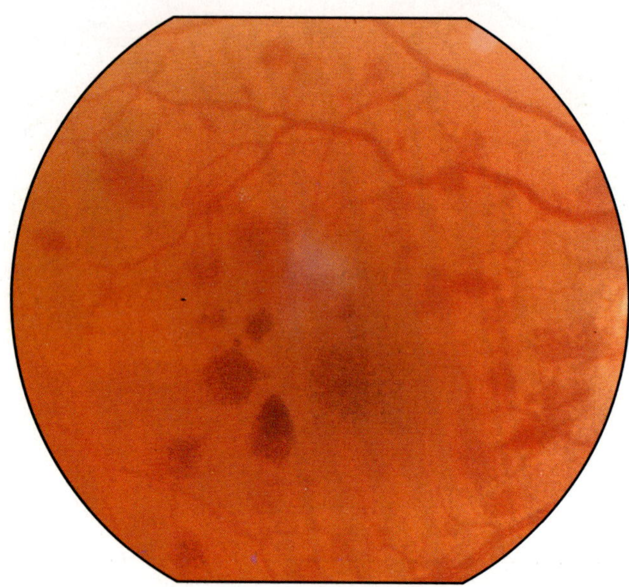

Carbon Monoxide

62–62 This patient has intraretinal hemorrhages secondary to carbon monoxide poisoning.

Heparin

62–63 Multiple intraretinal hemorrhages secondary to heparin toxicity are demonstrated in this patient.

62–62, *Courtesy of Terry George.* **62–63,** *Courtesy of Dr. Kurt Gitter.*

62–64 CORTICOSTEROIDS

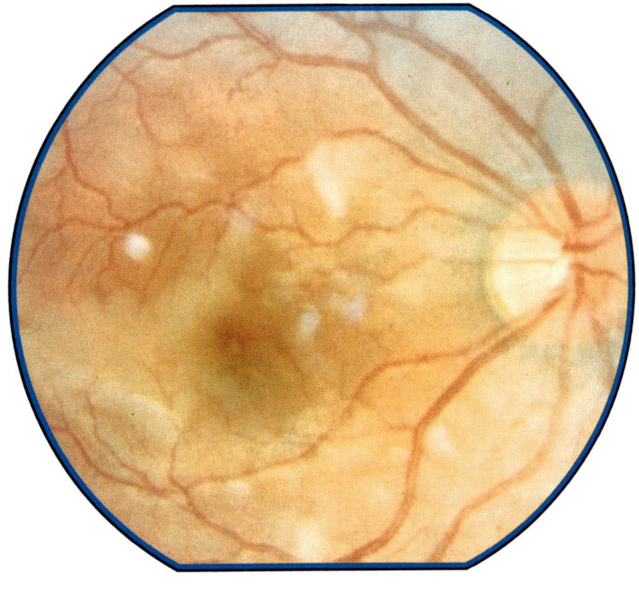

62–65

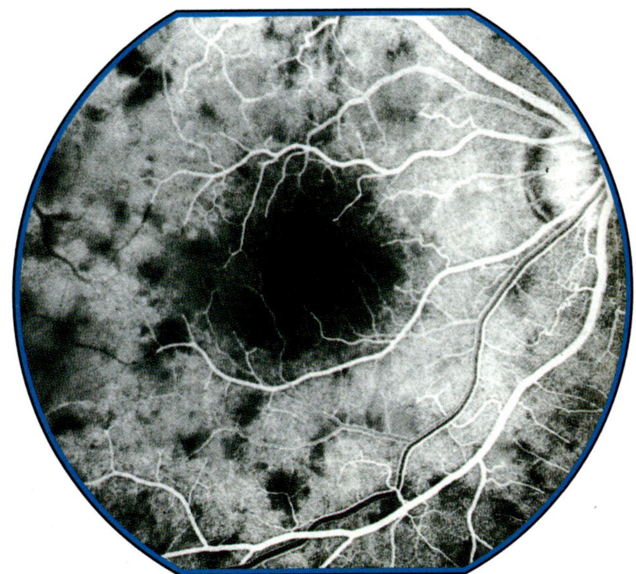

62–66

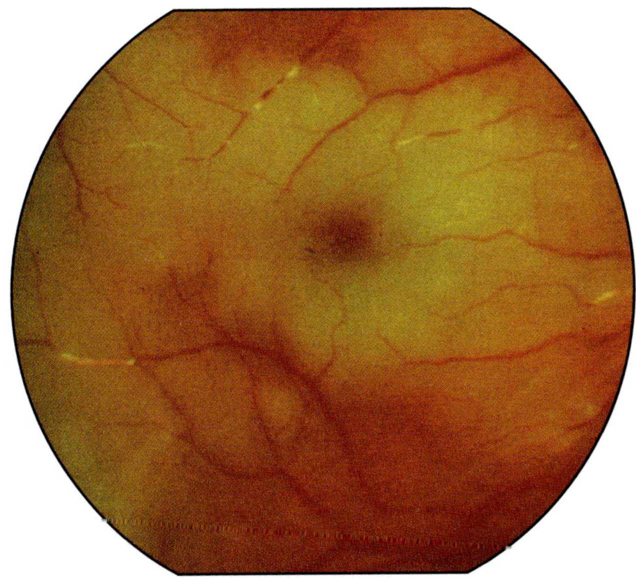

62–67

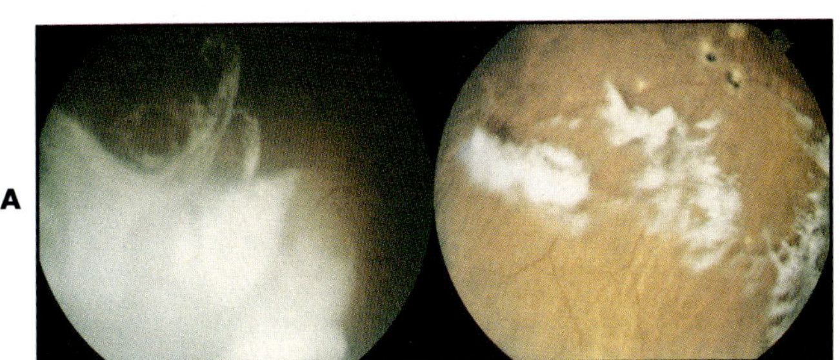

Corticosteroids

62–64 and 62–65 This patient had retinal and choroidal occlusions secondary to multiple emboli from corticosteroid injection into the nasal cavity. Note the multiple retinal as well as choroidal occlusions with inner and outer retinal whitening.

62–66 This patient also had emboli from a nasal injection of corticosteroids. Note the cherry-red spot, retinal whitening, particulate matter in the vessels, and vasculature sheathing.

62–67 This patient had a sub-tenon steroid injection with inadvertent globe perforation. Part of the steroid solution is seen within the vitreous five minutes after injection **(A).** Seven days later much of the material had resorbed and the remaining material had a cottage-cheese-like appearance **(B).** Complete resolution was noted by one month.

62–64 *and* ***62–65,*** *Courtesy of Dr. Kurt Gitter.* ***62–67,*** *Courtesy of Dr. Fransisco Gomez-Ulla. From Gomez-Ulla, et al: Unintentional intraocular injection of corticosteroids, Acta Ophthalmologica 71:419–421, 1993.*

Suggested Readings

Albert, DM, Bullock, JD, Lahav, M, and Caine, R: Flecked retinal secondary to oxalate crystals from methoxyflurane anesthesia: clinical and experimental studies, Trans Am Acad Ophthalmol Otolaryngol 79:817–826, 1975

Arden, GB, and Kolb, HE: Screening test for chloroquine retinopathy, Lancet 2:41, 1964

Bluth, LL, and Hanscom, TA: Retinal detachment and vitreous hemorrhage due to talc emboli, JAMA 246:980–981, 1981

Connell, MM, Poley, BJ, and McFarlane, JR: Chorioretinopathy associated with thioridazine therapy, Arch Ophthalmol 71:816–821, 1964

Conway, BP, and Campochiaro, PA: Macular infarction after endophthalmitis treated with vitrectomy and intravitreal gentamycin, Arch Ophthalmol 104:367–371, 1986

Cortin, P, Corriveau, LA, Rousseau, A, Boudreault, G, Malenfant, M, and Angers, Y: Canthaxanthine retinopathy, J Ophthalmic Photogr 6:68, 1983

Finbloom, DS, Silver, K, Newsome, DA, and Gunkel, R: Comparison of hydroxychloroquine and chloroquine use and the development of retinal toxicity, J Rheumatol 12:692–694, 1985

Gass, JDM: Nicotinic acid maculopathy, Am J Ophthalmol 76:500–510, 1973

Guyer, DR, et al: Interferon-associated retinopathy, Arch Ophthalmol 111:350–356, 1992

Hart, WM, Jr, Burde, RM, Johnston, GP, and Drews, RC: Static perimetry in chloroquine retinopathy. Perifoveal patterns of visual field depression, Arch Ophthalmol 102:377–380, 1984

Kaiser-Kupfer, MI, Kupfer, C, and Rodrigues, MM: Tamoxifen retinopathy: a clinicopathologic report, Ophthalmology 88:89–93, 1981

Kaiser-Kupfer, MI, and Lippman, ME: Tamoxifen retinopathy, Cancer Treat Rep 62:315–320, 1978

Leopold, IH: Ocular complications of drugs: visual changes, JAMA 205:631–633, 1968

McDonald, HR, Schatz, H, Allen, AW, Chenoveth, RG, Cohen, HB, Crawford, JB, Klein, R, May, DR, and Snider, JD, III: Retinal toxicity secondary to intraocular gentamycin injection, Ophthalmology 93:871–877, 1986

McKeown, CA, Swartz, M, Blom, J, and Maggiano, JM: Tamoxifen retinopathy, Br J Ophthalmol 65:177–179, 1981

Meredith, TA, Aaberg, TM, and Willerson, WD: Progressive chorioretinopathy after receiving thioridazine, Arch Ophthalmol 96:1172–1176, 1978

Meredith, TA, Wright, JD, Gammon, JA, Fellner, SK, Warshaw, BL, and Maio, M: Ocular involvement in primary hyperoxaluria, Arch Ophthalmol 102:584–587, 1984

Mieler, WF, Williams, DF, Sneed, SR, and Williams, GA: Systemic therapeutic agents and retinal toxicity, Semin Ophthalmol 6:45–64, 1991

Miller, FS, III, Bunt-Milam, AH, and Kalina, RE: Clinical-ultrastructural study of thioridazine retinopathy, Ophthalmology 89:1478–1488, 1982

Novak, MA, et al: Calcium oxalate retinopathy associated with methoxyflurane abuse, Retina 8:230–236, 1988

Rosenthal, AR, Kolb, H, Bergsma, D, Huxsoll, D, and Hopkins, JL: Chloroquine retinopathy in the rhesus monkey, Invest Ophthalmol Vis Sci 17:1158–1175, 1978

Sakamoto, T, Maeda, K, Sueishi, K, Inomata, H, and Onoyama, K: Ocular histopathologic findings in a 46-year-old man with primary hyperoxaluria, Arch Ophthalmol 109:384–387, 1991

Siddall, JR: The ocular toxic findings with prolonged and high dosage chlorpromazine intake, Arch Ophthalmol 74:460–464, 1965

Small, KW, Letson, R, and Scheinman, J: Ocular findings in primary hyperoxaluria, Arch Ophthalmol 108:89–93, 1990

Weiner, A, Sandberg, MA, Gaudio, AR, Kini, MM, and Berson, EL: Hydroxychloroquine retinopathy, Am J Ophthalmol 112:528–534, 1991

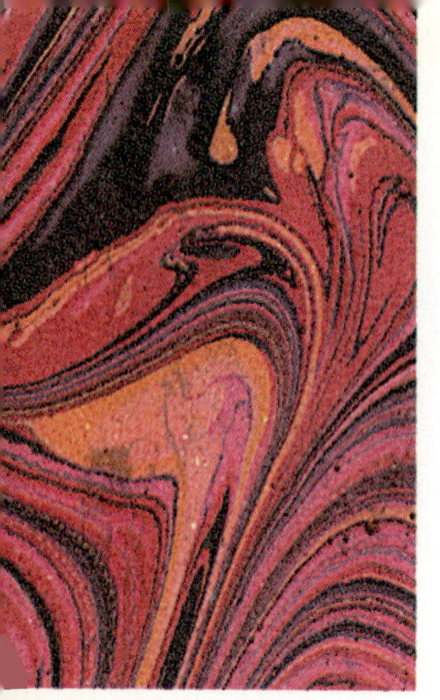

Chapter 63

Photic Retinal Injury

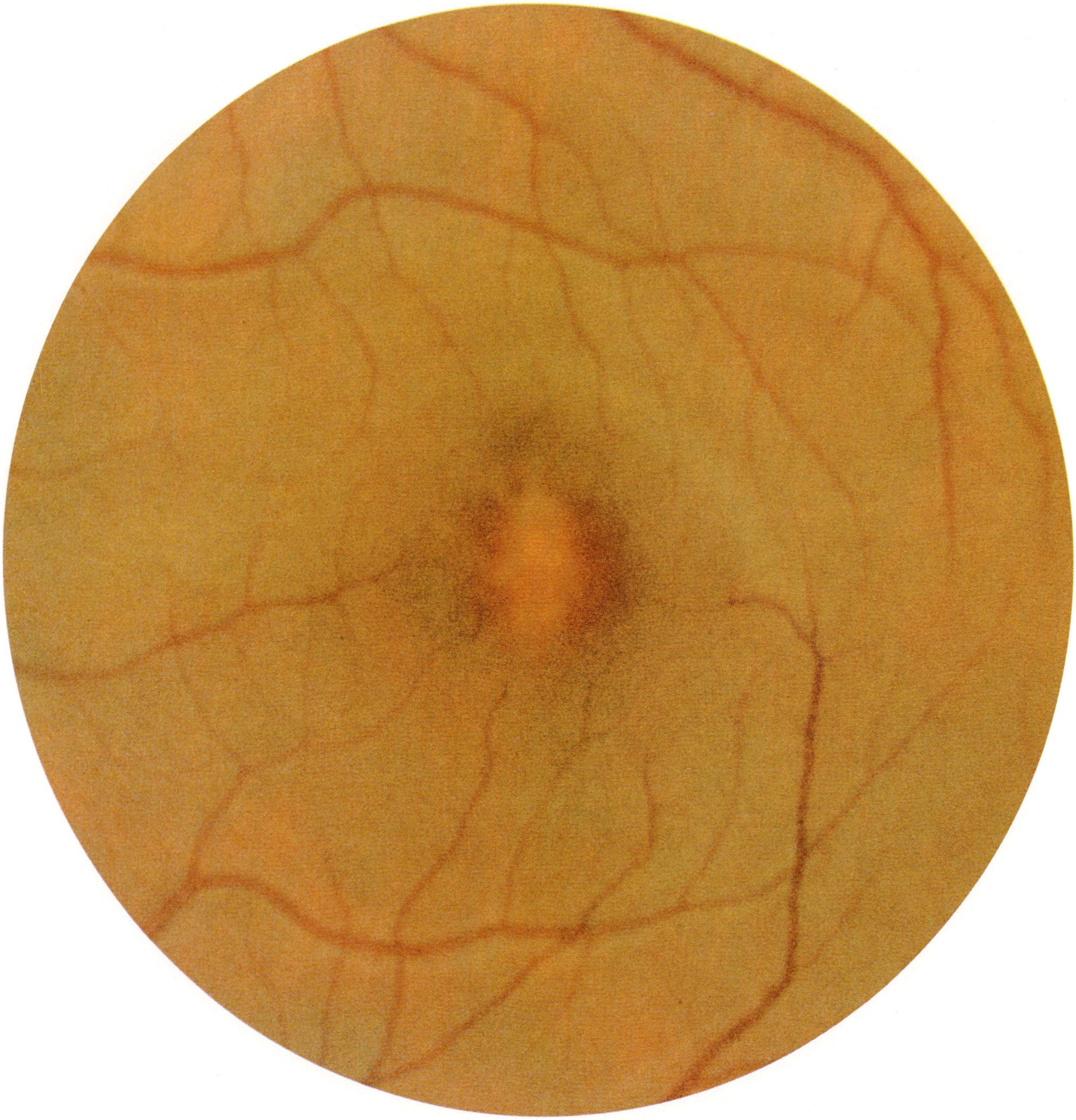

Solar retinopathy appears as a small yellow-whitish foveolar lesion. However, in approximately 1 to 2 weeks, the lesion fades and a reddish or lamellar holelike lesion is noted. Visual acuity is usually minimally disturbed and often returns to normal after many months.

63–1

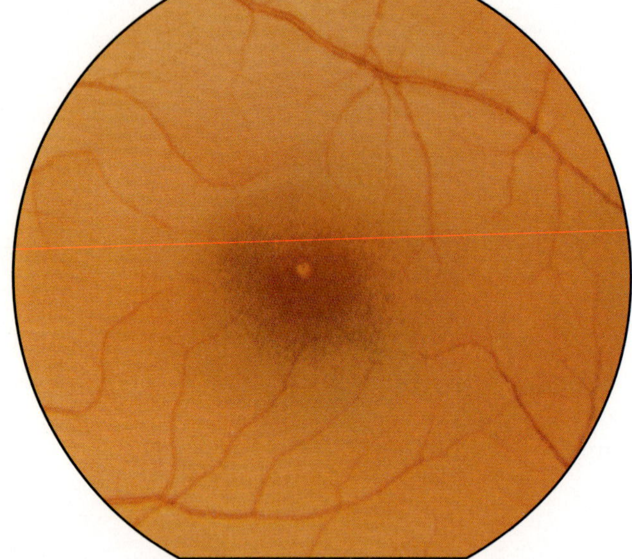

63–2

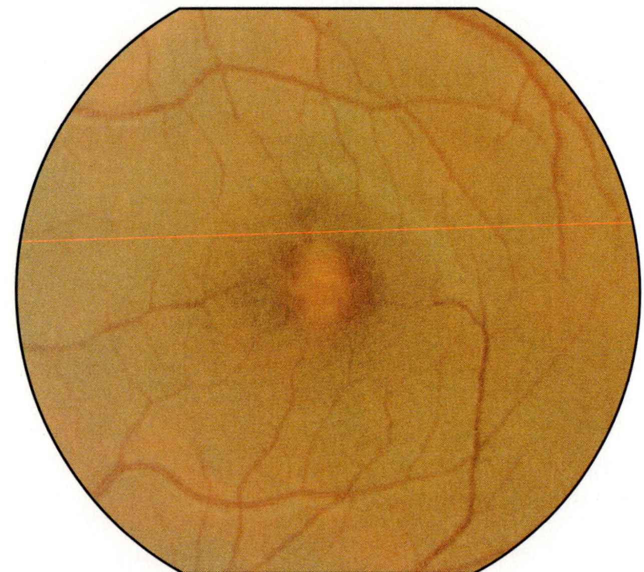

63–3

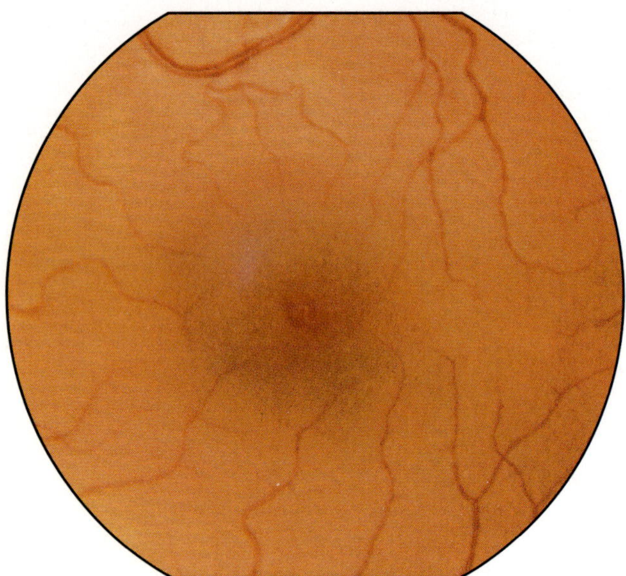

63–1 Note the yellowish ovoid reaction at the level of the outer retina and pigment epithelium in this patient who experienced inadvertent sun gazing.

63–2 Sun exposure was more intentional and the reaction is more pronounced in this patient.

63–3 In this patient with inadvertent sun gazing, an outer retinal, juxtafoveal ovoid reddish excavation corresponds to the healed state of solar retinopathy. Although visual acuity in this patient returned to 20/20, there was a persistent juxtafoveal scotoma. Although this lesion is typical of the healed solar retinopathy response, some patients have minimal evidence of previous phototoxicity with only a barely detectable pigment epithelial granular response.

63–4

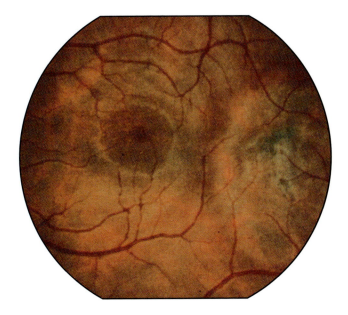

63–5

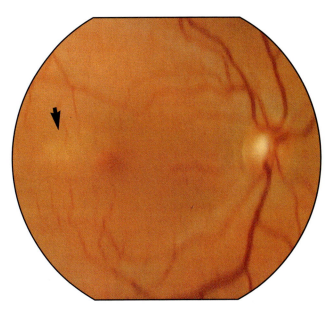

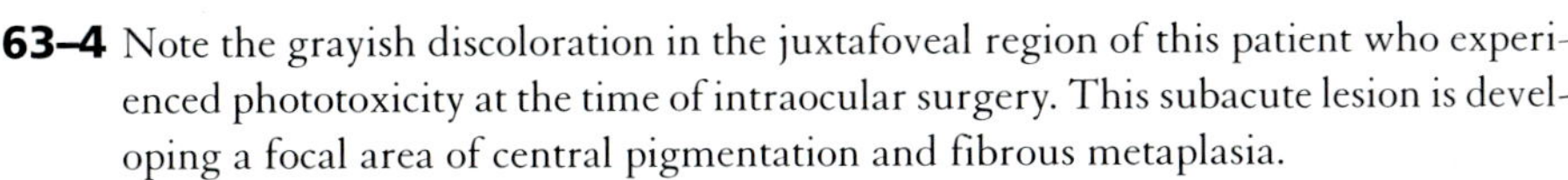

63–4 Note the grayish discoloration in the juxtafoveal region of this patient who experienced phototoxicity at the time of intraocular surgery. This subacute lesion is developing a focal area of central pigmentation and fibrous metaplasia.

63–5 This patient demonstrates an early whitish retinal change secondary to light exposure during cataract extraction *(arrowhead)*.

63–6

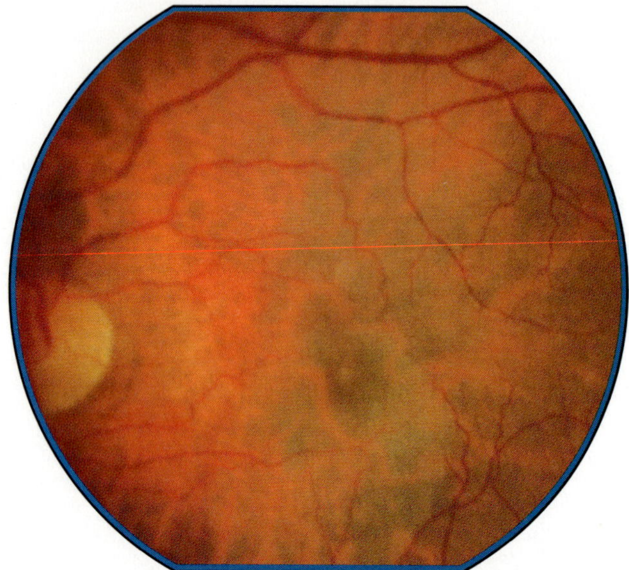

63–7

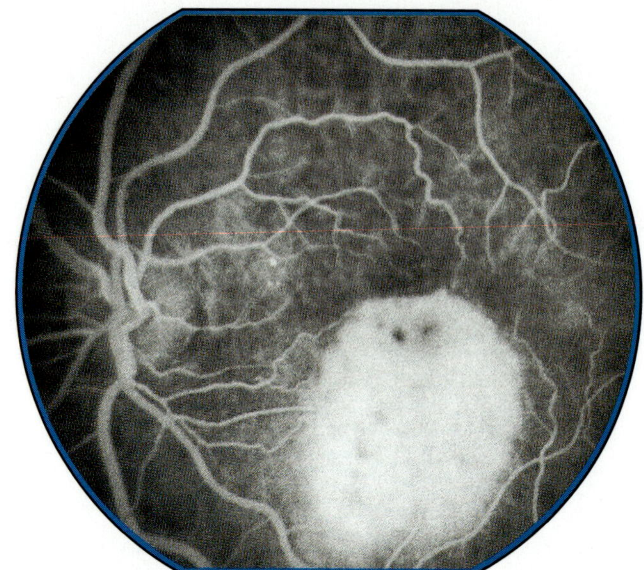

63–8

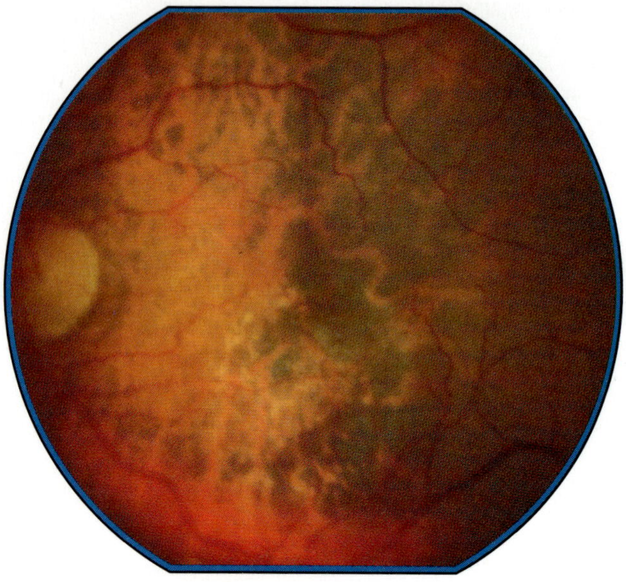

63–6 In this patient, the acute phototoxic lesion is barely evident a few days after cataract surgery as a faintly grayish discoloration in the inferior macula with some foveal involvement and noticeable visual dysfunction.

63–7 The fluorescein angiogram reveals an area of hyperfluorescence from disturbance of the outer blood-retinal barrier. Note that there is no cystoid edema pattern.

63–8 Later in the course of this patient, there is an atrophic and pigmentary disturbance corresponding to the light toxicity.

63–6 *through* ***63–8,*** *Courtesy of Dr. Richard McDonald.*

63–9

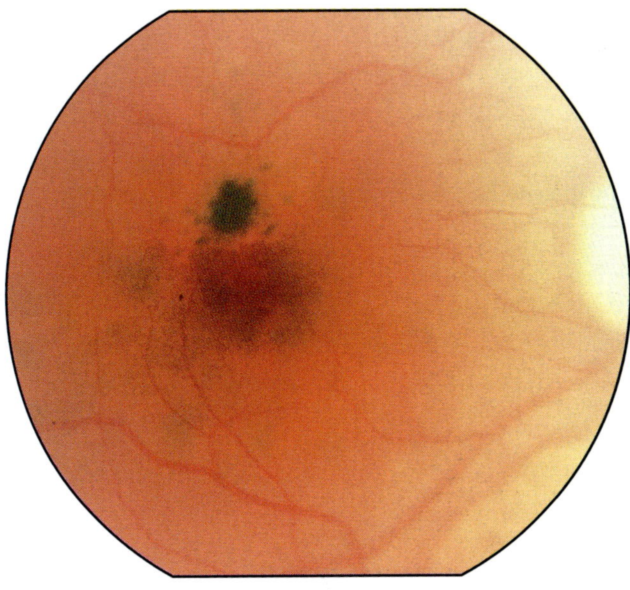

63–10

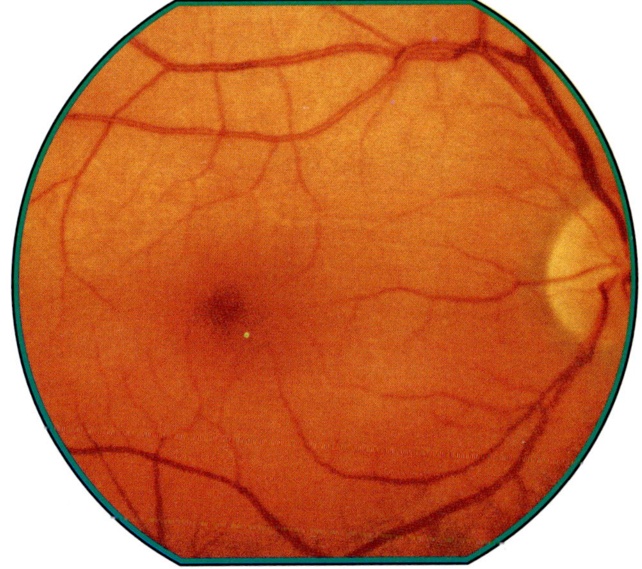

63–11

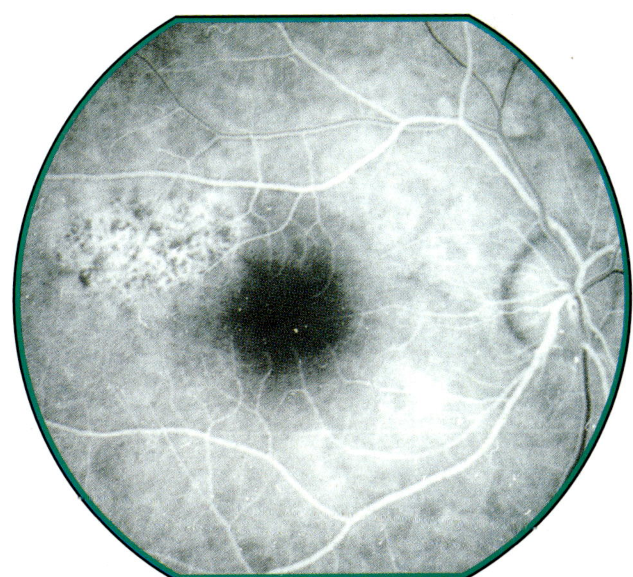

63–9 Pigment scarring is more intense in some patients. There may also be a more prominent pigment epithelial hyperplastic response, fibrous metaplasia, choroidal folds, or even disciform scarring.

63–10 and 63–11 Phototoxicity associated with vitreous surgery using a mobile intraocular light pipe has a different appearance. Note the irregular atrophic and pigmentary change in this patient following vitreous surgery for membrane peeling.

Suggested Readings

Boldrey, EE, Ho, BT, and Griffith, RD: Retinal burns occurring at cataract extraction, Ophthalmology 91:1297–1302, 1984

Fuller, D, Machemer, R, and Knighton, RW: Retinal damage produced by intraocular fiber optic light, Am J Ophthalmol 85:519–537, 1978

Ham, WT, Jr: Action spectrum for retinal injury from near ultraviolet radiation in the aphakic monkey, Am J Ophthalmol 93:299–396, 1982

Jampol, LM, Kraff, MC, Sanders, DR, Alexander, K, and Lieberman, H: Near-UV radiation from the operating microscope and pseudophakic cystoid macular edema, Arch Ophthalmol 103:28–30, 1985

Lawwill, T: Three major pathologic processes caused by light in the primate retina: a search for mechanisms, Trans Am Ophthalmol Soc 80:517–579, 1982

Mainster, MA: Destructive light adaptation, Ann Ophthalmol 2:44–48, 1970

Mainster, MA: Wavelength selection in macular photocoagulation tissue optics, thermal effects and laser systems, Ophthalmology 93:952–958, 1986

Mainster, MA, White, TJ, Tips, JH, and Wilson, PW: Retinal temperature increases produced by intense light sources, J Opt Soc Am (A) 60:264–270, 1970

McDonald, HR, and Irvine, AR: Light-induced maculopathy from the operating microscope in extracapsular cataract extraction and intraocular lens implantation, Ophthalmology 90:945–951, 1983

Noell, WK: Possible mechanisms of photoreceptor damage by light in mammalian eyes, Vision Res 20:1163–1171, 1980

Robertson, DM, and Feldman, RB: Photic retinopathy from the operating room microscope, Am J Ophthalmol 101:561–569, 1986

Tso, MOM, and LaPiana, FG: The human fovea after sungazing, Trans Am Acad Ophthalmol Otolaryngol 79:788–795, 1975

Yannuzzi, LA, Fisher, YL, Krueger, A, and Slakter, J: Solar retinopathy: a photobiological and geophysical analysis, Trans Am Ophthalmol Soc 85:120–158, 1987

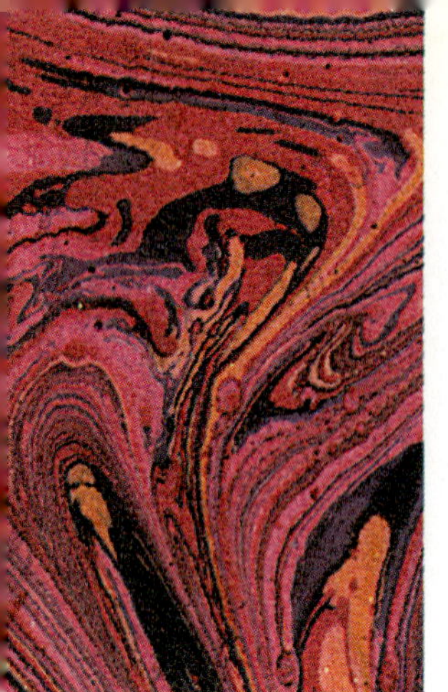

Chapter 64

Traumatic Chorioretinopathies

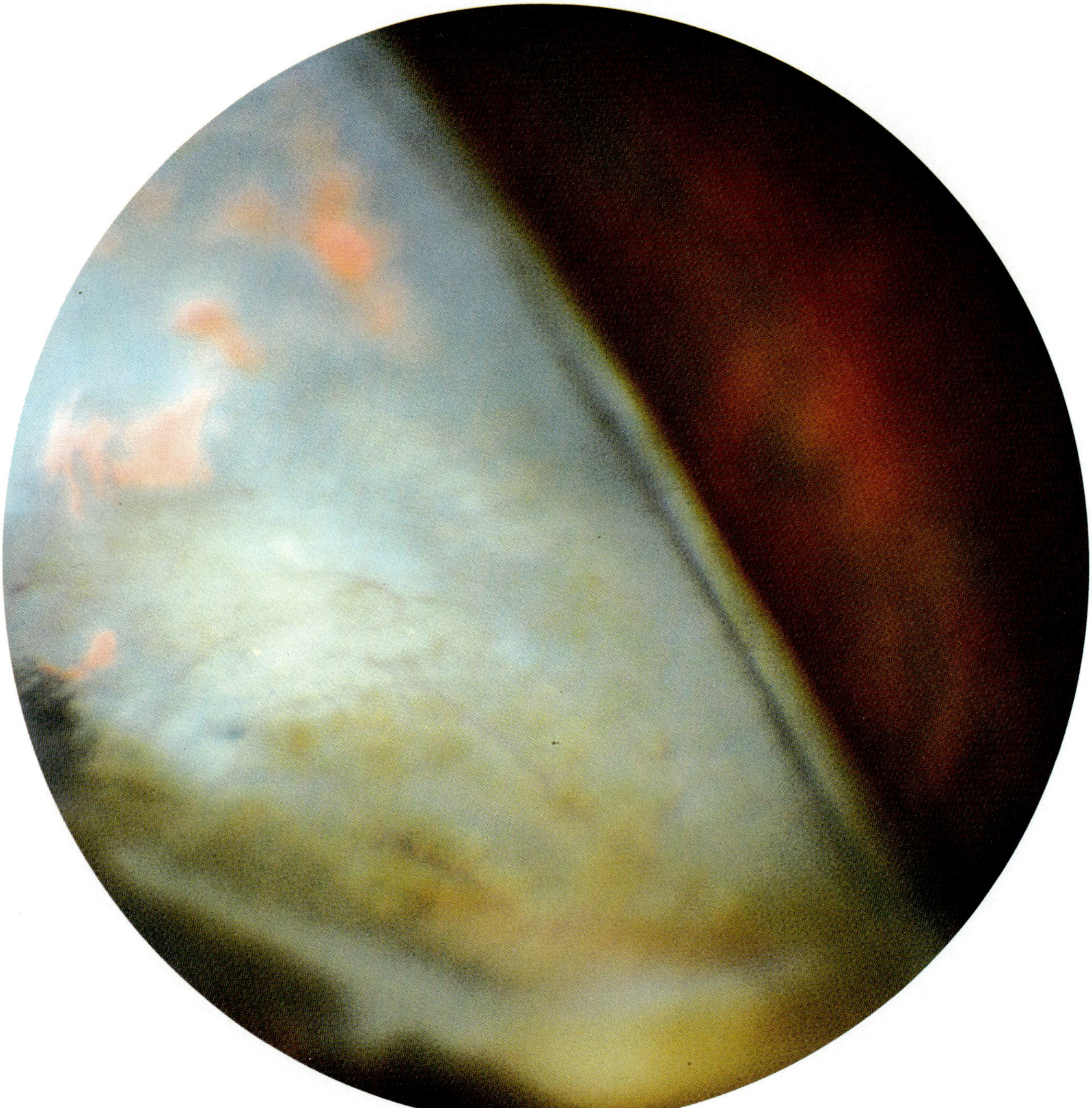

Trauma can cause various injuries to the choroid and/or retina. These traumatic chorioretinopathies include commotio retinae, traumatic macular holes, choroidal ruptures, Purtscher's retinopathy, the shaken baby syndrome secondary to child abuse, intraocular foreign bodies, and traumatic retinal tears and retinal detachments.

64–1 VALSALVA RETINOPATHY

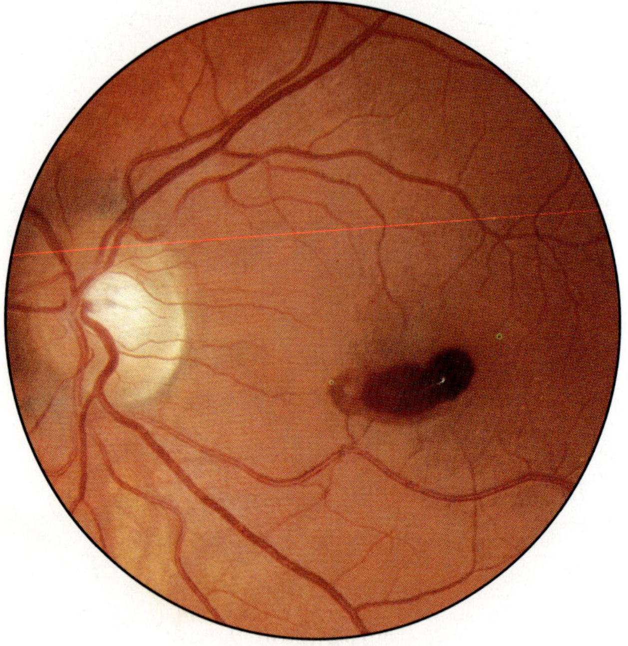

64–2

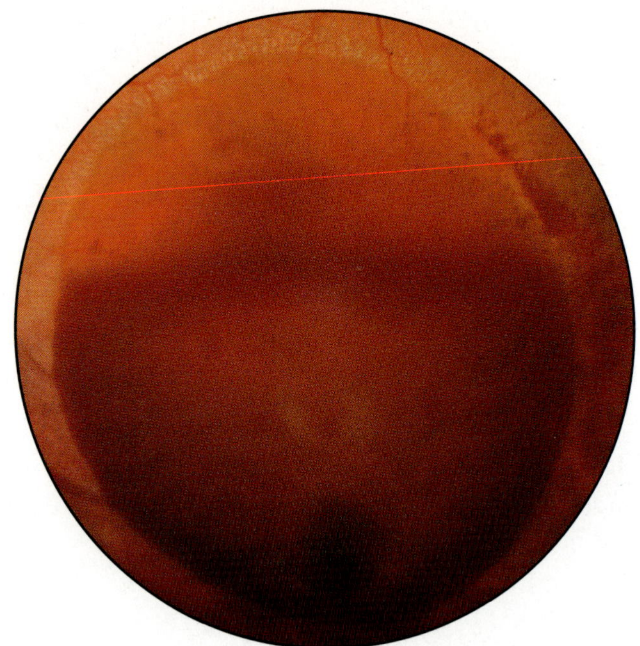

64–3

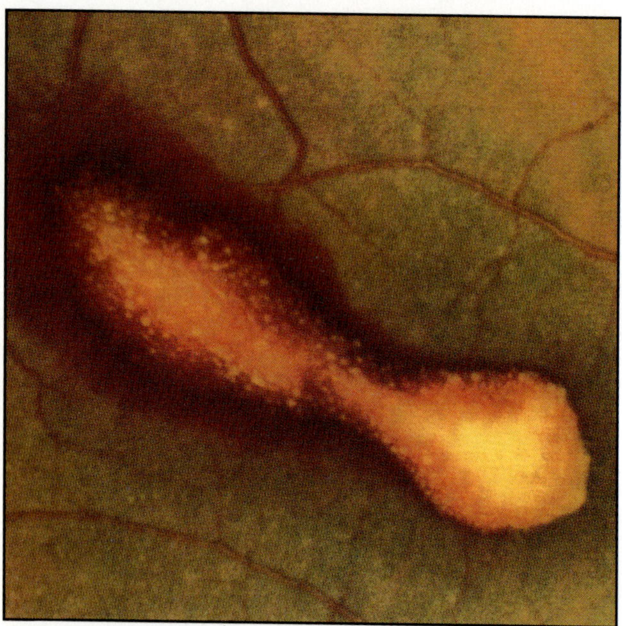

64–1 Subhyaloid hemorrhage may be noted in patients with Valsalva retinopathy.

64–2 The size of the hemorrhage can vary. This second case shows an extremely large hemorrhage secondary to Valsalva retinopathy with layering of the various components.

64–3 A case of resolving Valsalva retinopathy illustrates the yellowish discoloration of the dehemoglobinized blood.

64–4 PERFORATIONS

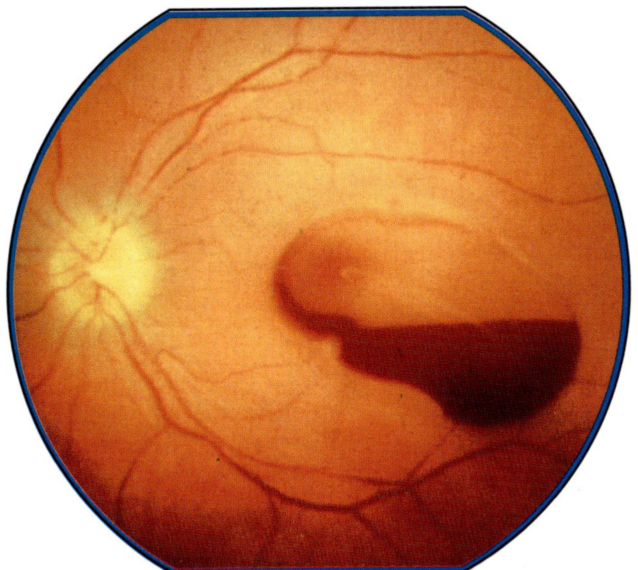

64–5

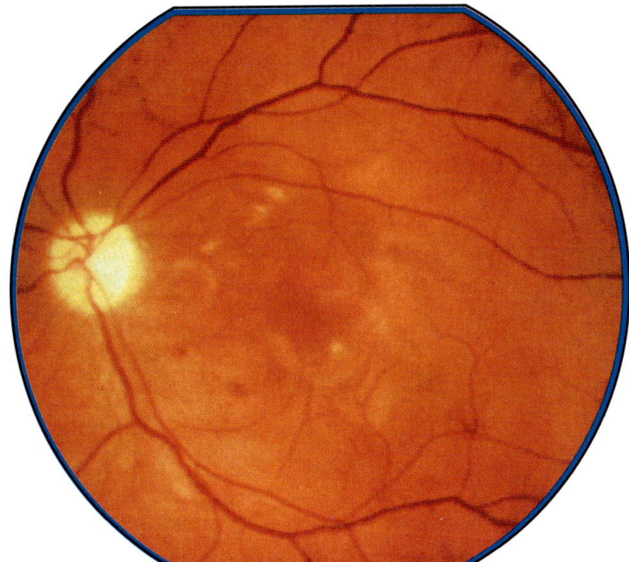

64–6

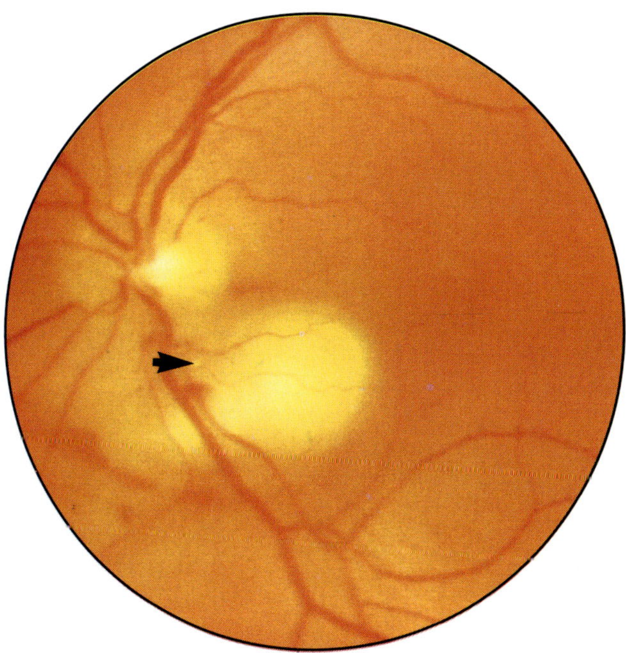

64–4 and 64–5 Perforation of the globe during retrobulbar injection may also lead to hemorrhage, which can be confused with Valsalva retinopathy. This patient has hemorrhage secondary to an intrasheath-injection with an arterial obstruction and a Terson's like effect. Note the optic nerve swelling, irregular vascular caliber, and Terson's like syndrome. Resolution of most of the blood is noted with retinal pigment epithelial changes and optic atrophy.

64–6 This patient also had a perforation after retrobulbar injection. The yellowish material represents the anesthetic. Note the hemorrhage surrounding this area. A piece of particulate material from the injection is also present *(arrowhead)*.

***64–4** and **64–5,** Courtesy of Dr. Gary Brown. **64–6,** Courtesy of Dr. Kurt Gitter.*

64–7 PURTSCHER'S RETINOPATHY

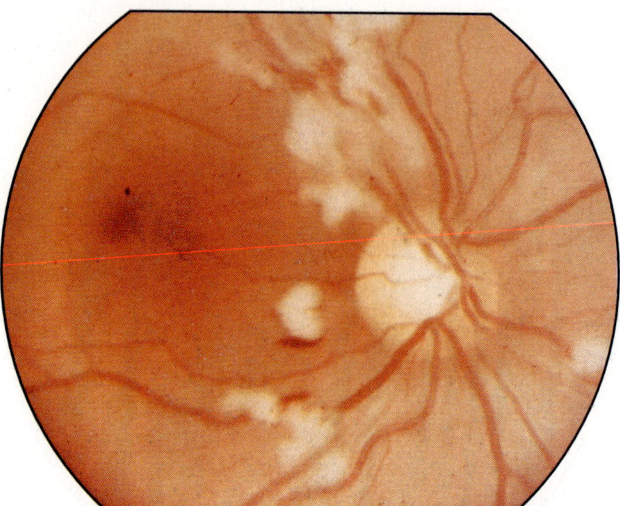

64–8

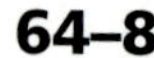

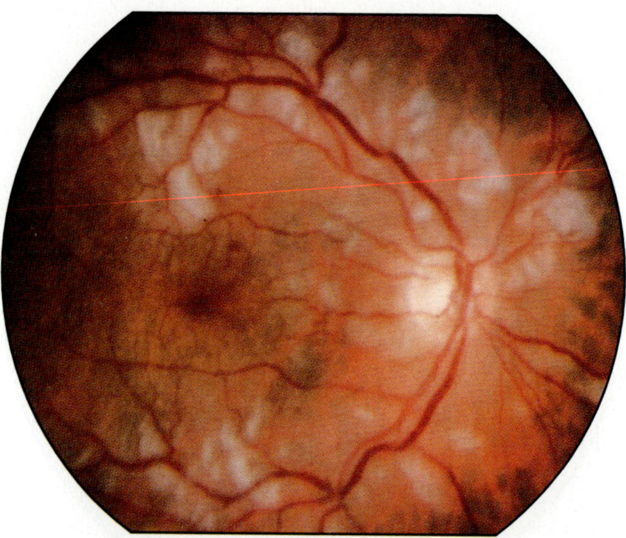

64–7 Purtscher's retinopathy secondary to trauma produces cotton-wool spots and intraretinal hemorrhages as demonstrated in this patient. Note the inner retinal hemorrhages and axoplasmic debris accumulation. Purtscher's retinopathy secondary to trauma is believed to be due to leukoembolization.

64–8 A Purtscher's-like retinopathy picture can also be seen in several other conditions. For example, this patient has retinal and choroidal ischemia secondary to a perforation after a retrobulbar injection. Note the inner retinal axoplasmic debris (retinal ischemia) and the outer retinal debris (choroidal ischemia or outer retinal infarction).

64–9

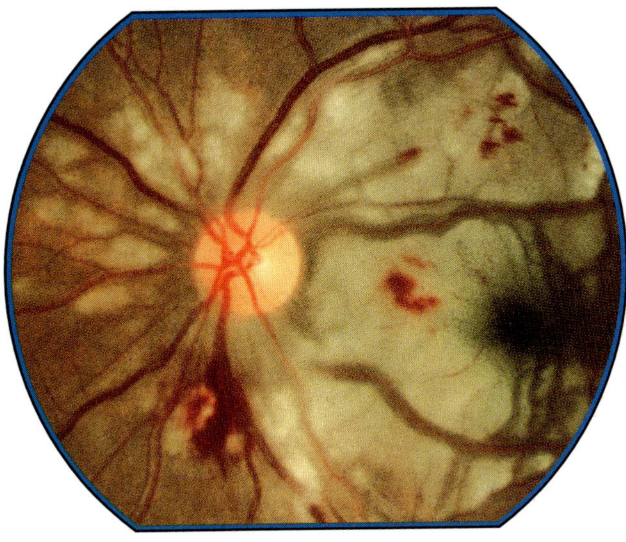

64–10

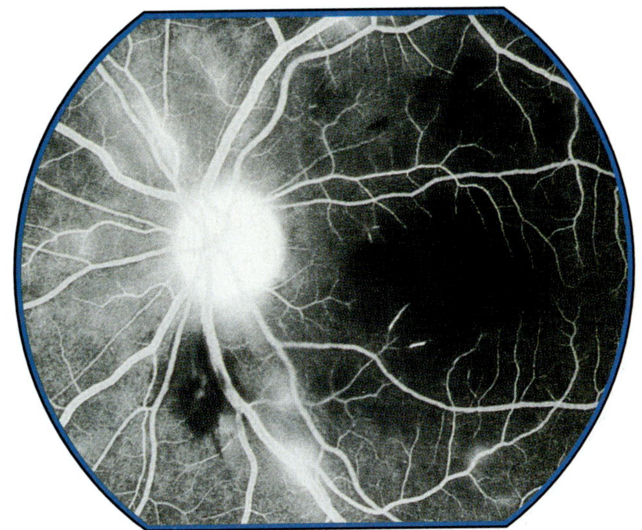

64–9 This patient also has a Purtscher's-like retinopathy picture with retinal whitening and hemorrhage. Note the sparing around the arterioles.

64–10 The fluorescein angiogram in this case shows blunting of the perifoveal capillaries. There is also closure of small vessels in the central macula and optic disc staining. This Purtscher's-like retinopathy was secondary to acute pancreatitis. Collagen vascular disorders may also demonstrate such Purtscher's-like changes; one such example can be seen in the Rheumatic Disease section in this atlas.

64–11 COMMOTIO RETINAE

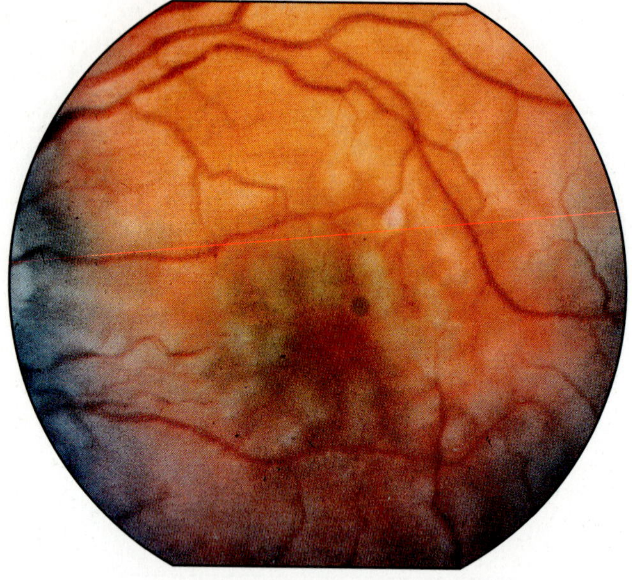

64–12

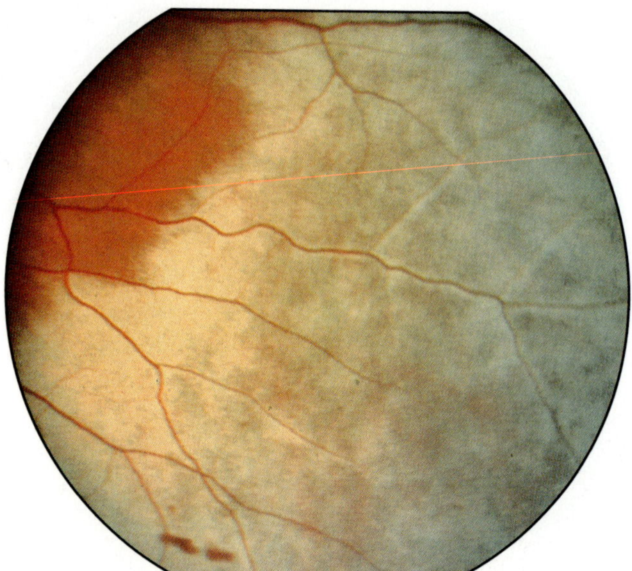

64–13

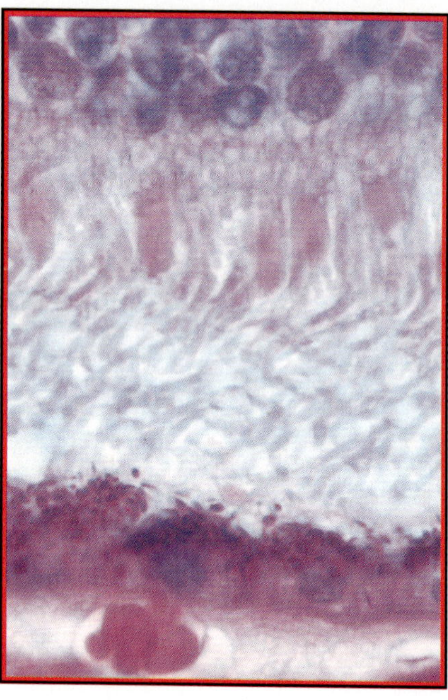

64–14

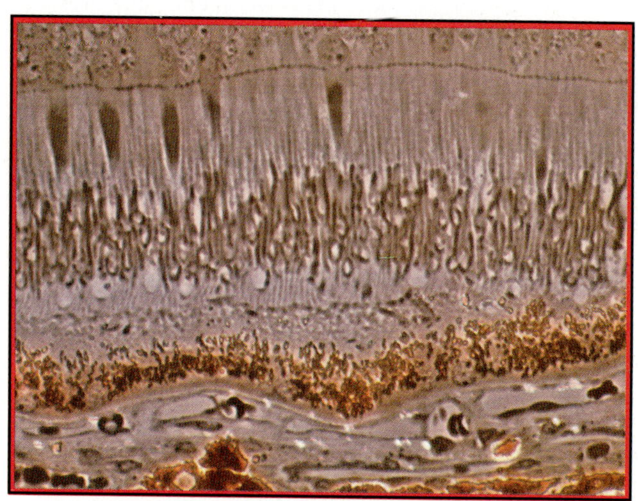

64–11 Berlin's edema or commotio retinae consists of a deep retinal whitening secondary to trauma. This case shows multiple whitish lesions at the level of the deep retina secondary to Berlin's edema.

64–12 Deep retinal whitening due to commotio retinae may be more extensive. Note the hemorrhage inferiorly.

64–15

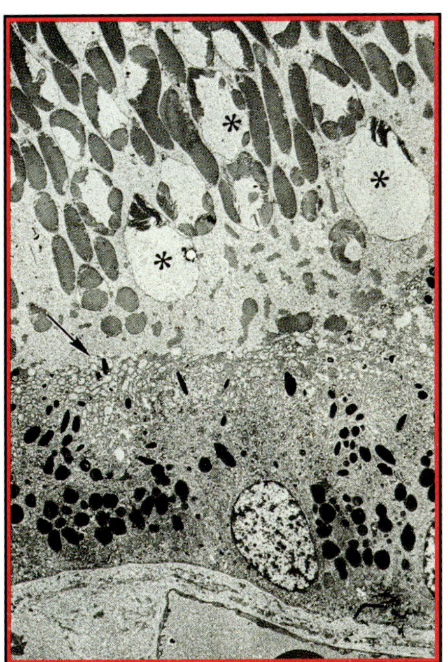

64–16

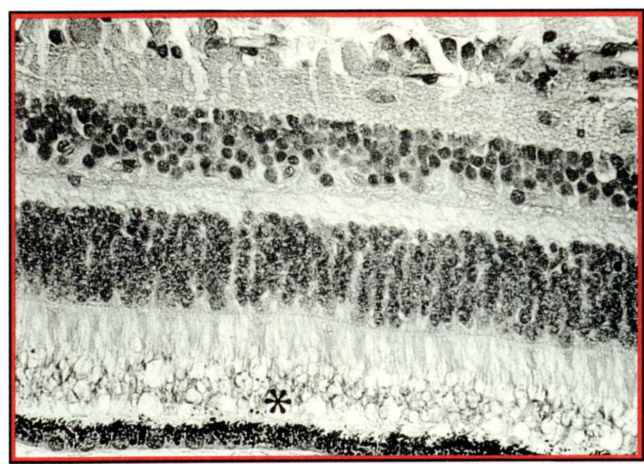

64–17

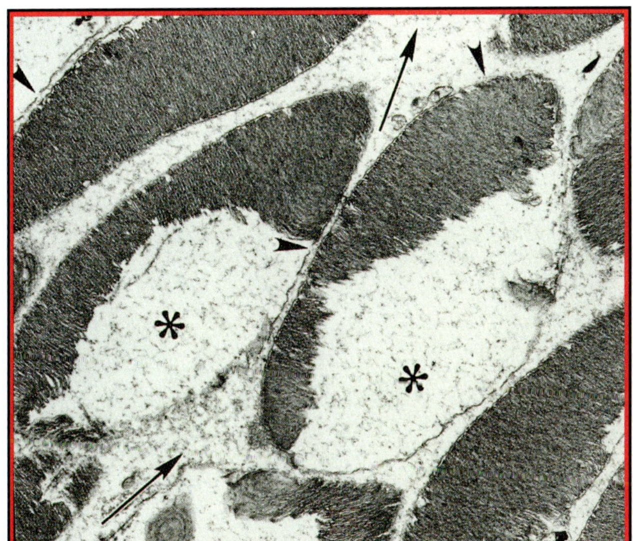

64–13 through 64–17 Commotio retinae (Berlin's edema) microscopically shows disruption of the outer segments of the photoreceptors, as demonstrated in this acute case. Later, fluid may collect in the outer layers of the retina. When the edema subsides, there may be retinal pigment epithelial degeneration and cystoid edema. Coalescence of cystoid areas may produce a large cyst and a macular hole.

64–13 *through* ***64–17,*** *From Mansour, AM, Green, WR, and Hogge, C: Histopathology of commotio retinae, Retina 12:24–28, 1992.*

64–18 SHAKEN BABY SYNDROME

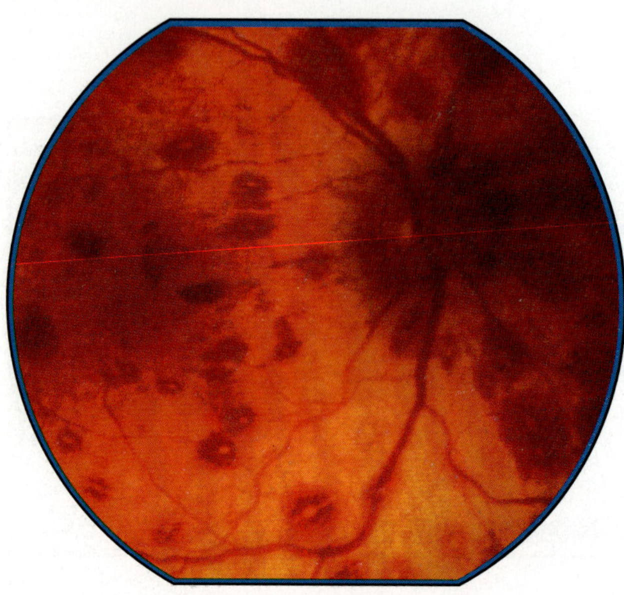

64–19

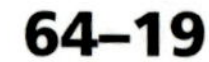

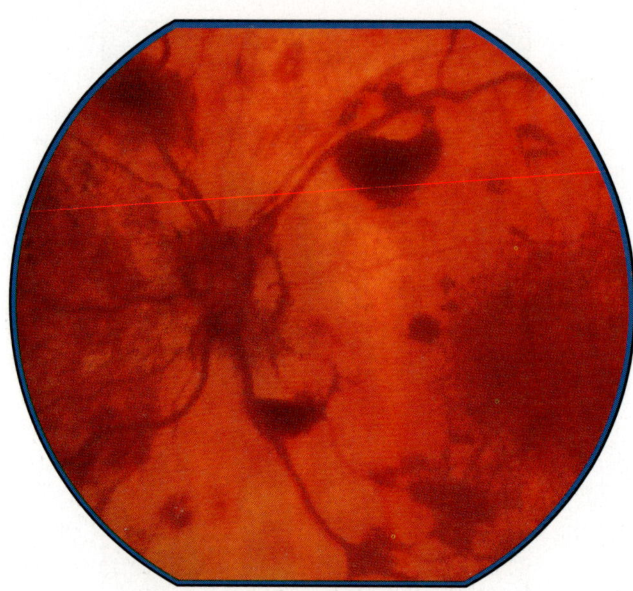

64–18 and 64–19 Child abuse or the shaken baby syndrome may result in retinal hemorrhages, white-centered retinal hemorrhages, and/or cotton-wool spots. Neurologic damage and skin bruises are commonly seen in these cases.

64–18 *and* ***64–19,*** *Courtesy of Dr. Richard Spaide.*

64–20 CHOROIDAL RUPTURES

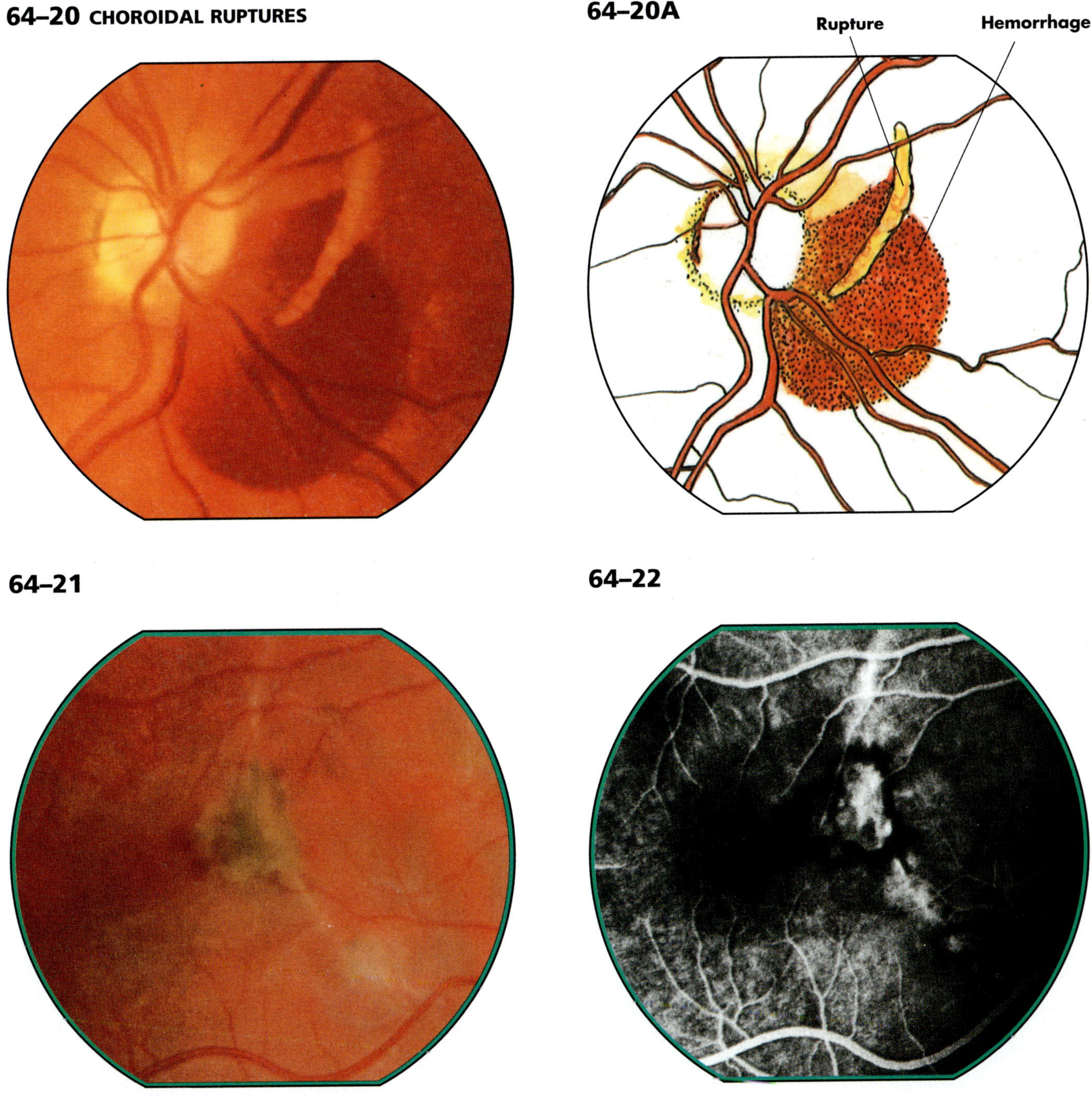

64–20 and 64–20A Choroidal ruptures may occur secondary to trauma. Note the vertical linear hypopigmented choroidal rupture with secondary choroidal neovascularization and subretinal hemorrhage.

64–21 This patient also has a choroidal rupture with choroidal neovascularization. Note the subretinal hemorrhage.

64–22 The vertical hyperfluorescent area on the fluorescein angiogram shows the area of choroidal rupture. In the middle of the choroidal rupture, areas of neovascularization and blockage secondary to hemorrhage can be demonstrated.

64–23 TRAUMATIC RETINAL DETACHMENT

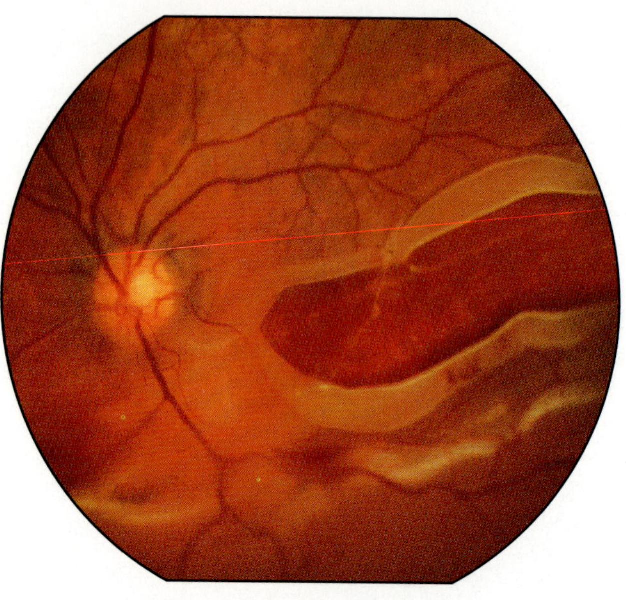

64–24 INTRAOCULAR FOREIGN BODY

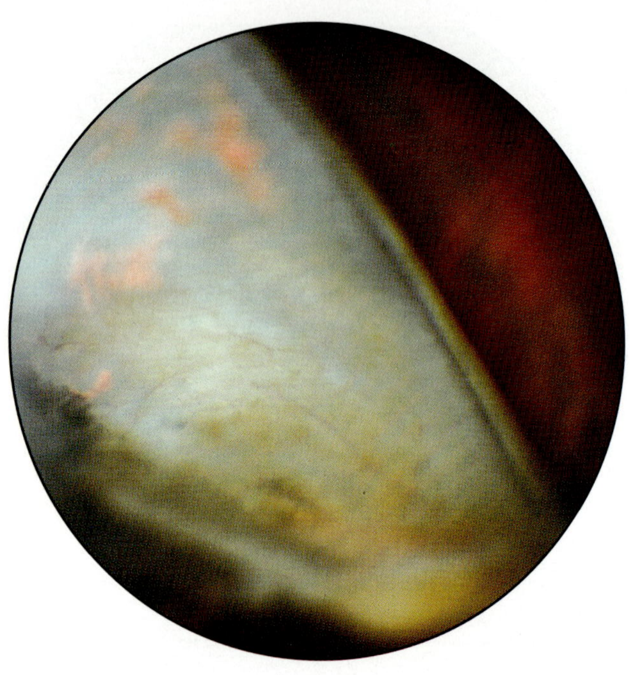

64–25

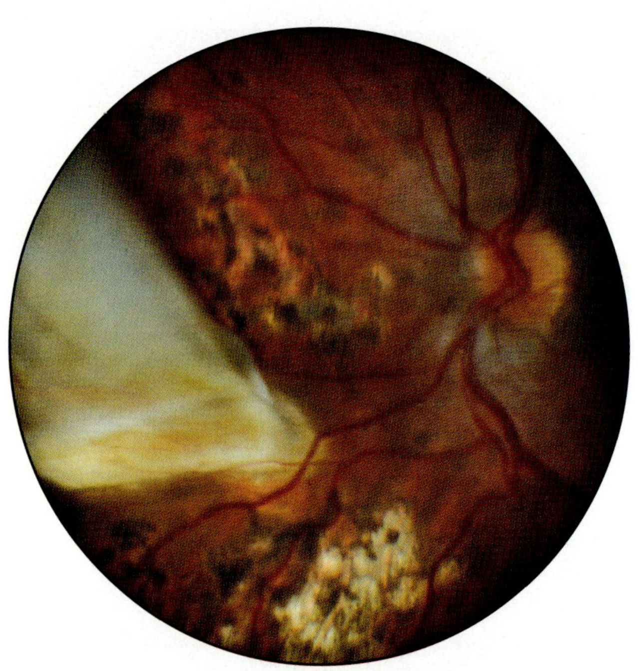

64–23 This patient has a traumatic retinal detachment with a large hole in the macular region. Note the elevated edges of the hole and detachment that extends inferiorly.

64–24 and 64–25 Intraocular foreign bodies can also occur following trauma. This patient had a piece of glass enter the eye. Postoperatively, the retina was stable. Note the laser photocoagulation scars.

64–23, *Courtesy of Chris Barry.* **64–24** *and* **64–25,** *Courtesy of Yale Fisher.*

Suggested Readings

Archer, DB, and Canavan, YM: Contusional eye injuries: retinal and choroidal lesions, Aust J Ophthalmol 11:251–264, 1983

Blodi, B, Johnson, MW, Gass, JDM, Fine, SL, and Joffe, LM: Purtscher's-like retinopathy after childbirth, Ophthalmology 97:1654–1659, 1990

Burton, TC: Unilateral Purtscher's retinopathy, Ophthalmology 87:1096–1105, 1980

Fischbein, F, and Safir, A: Monocular Purtscher's retinopathy: a fluorescein angiographic study, Arch Ophthalmol 85:480–484, 1971

Friberg, TR: Traumatic retinal pigment epithelial edema, Am J Ophthamol 88:18–21, 1979

Fuller, B, and Gitter, KA: Traumatic choroidal rupture with late serous detachment of macula: report of successful argon laser treatment, Arch Ophthalmol 89:354–355, 1973

Giovinazzo, V, Yannuzzi, L, Sorenson, J, Delrowe, D, and Campbell, E: The ocular complications of boxing, Ophthalmol 6:587–595, 1987

Hilton, GF: Late serosanguinous detachment of the macula after traumatic choroidal rupture, Am J Ophthalmol 79:997–1000, 1975

Kelley, JS: Purtscher's retinopathy related to chest compression by safety belts: fluorescein angiographic findings, Am J Ophthalmol 74:278–283, 1972

LaRoche, GR, McIntyre, L, and Schertzer, RM: Epidemiology of severe eye injuries in childhood, Ophthalmology 95:1603–1607, 1988

Liggett, PE, Pince, KJ, Barlow, W, Ragen, M, and Ryan, SJ: Ocular trauma in an urban population: review of 1132 cases, Ophthalmology 97:581–584, 1990

Pulido, JS, and Blair, NP: The blood-retinal barrier in Berlin's edema, Retina 7:233–236, 1987

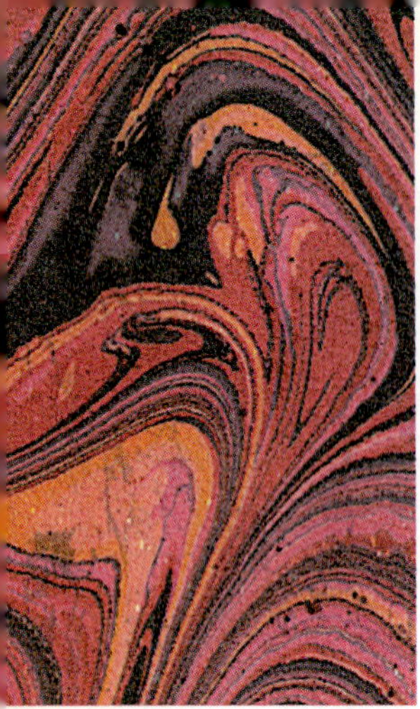

Chapter 65

Cystoid Macular Edema

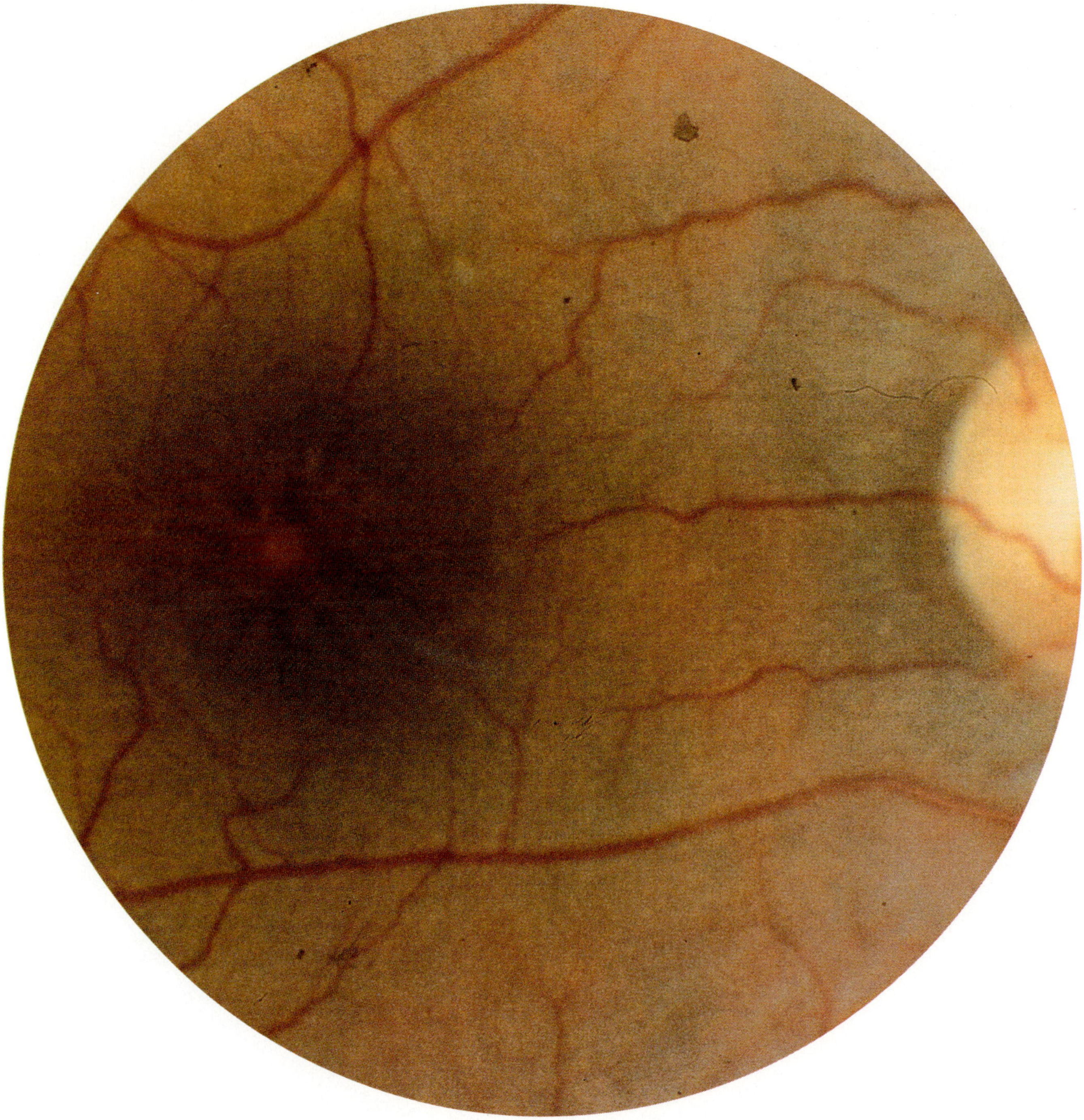

Cystoid macular edema may commonly occur following cataract extraction. A petaloid pattern of macular edema is noted. Topical anti-inflammatory agents are useful to treat this condition. Cystoid macular edema is a nonspecific manifestation that may be due to pseudophakia, aphakia, inflammatory diseases, vein occlusions, and hereditary conditions. Edema is best demonstrated with fluorescein angiography rather than color photography.

65–1

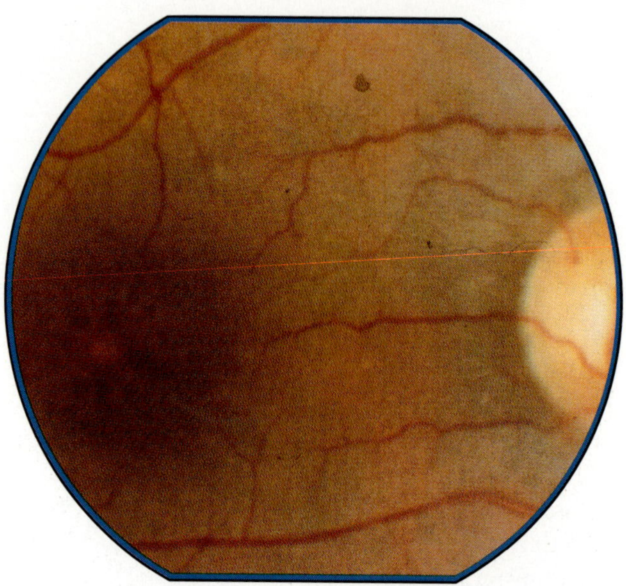

65–2

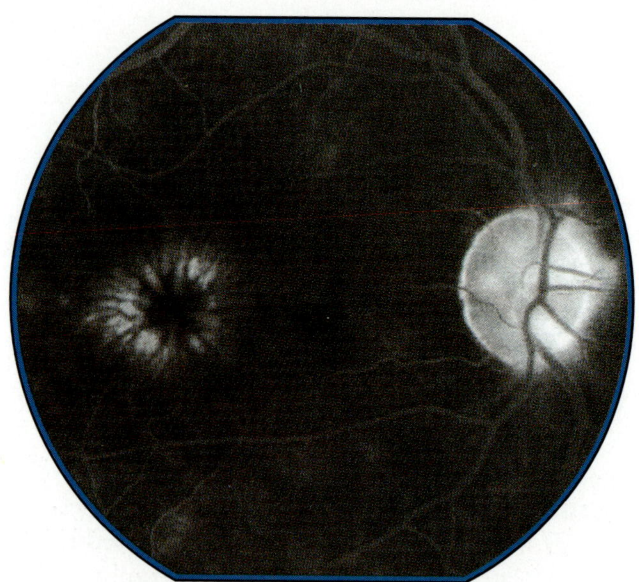

65–1 This pseudophakic patient had cystic changes in the macular region with accompanying fluid, which is seen in patients with pseudophakic cystoid macular edema.

65–2 The characteristic fluorescein angiographic pattern of cystoid macular edema can be demonstrated in this same patient. Accumulation of fluorescein dye in the cystoid spaces of Henle's layer is noted. Pseudophakic cystoid macular edema often is accompanied by optic disc leakage, unlike macular edema secondary to diabetic retinopathy in which the optic disc usually demonstrates no leakage.

65–3 65–4

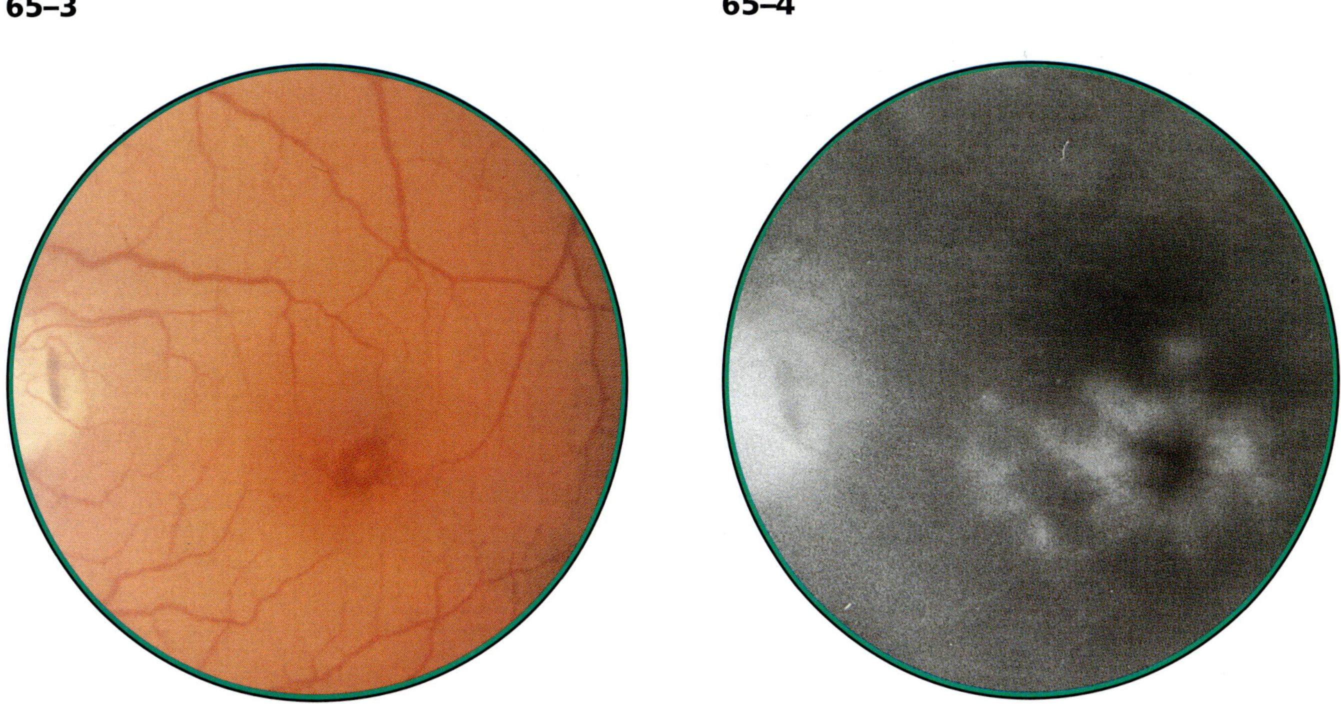

65–3 Patient with aphakic cystoid macular edema with cysts in the outer plexiform and inner nuclear layers.

65–4 The fluorescein angiogram confirms the cystoid pattern of leakage.

65–5

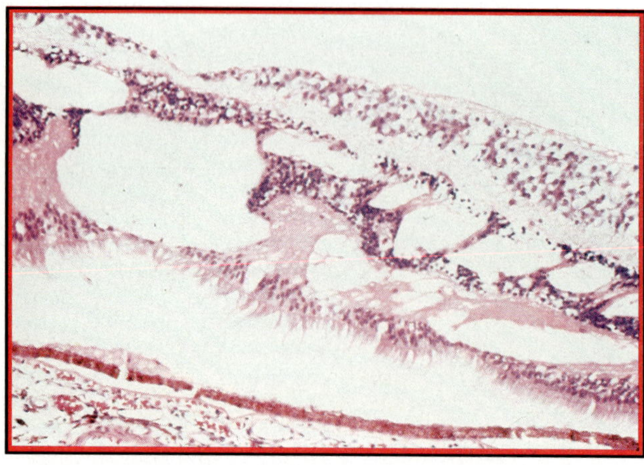

65–6

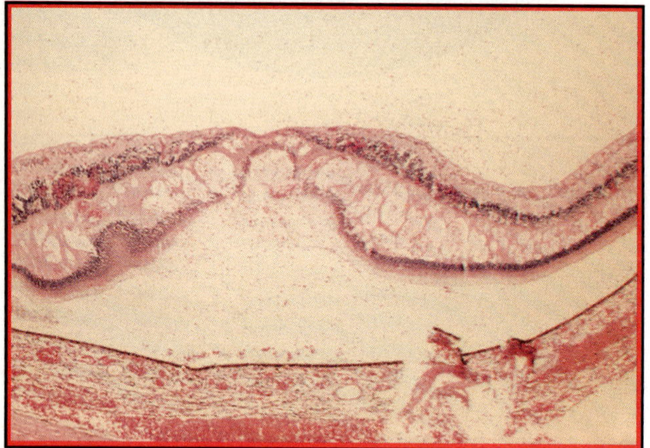

65–7

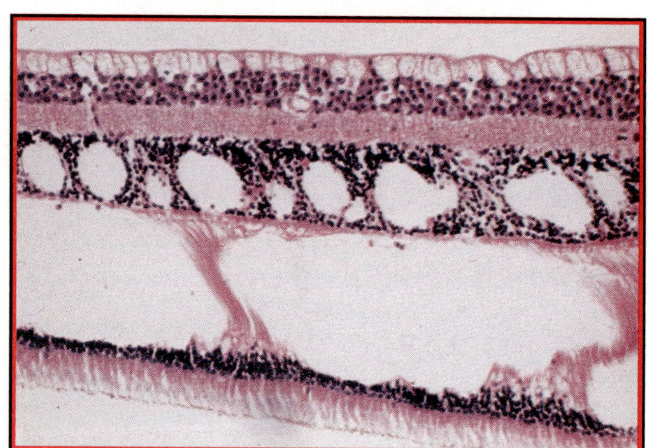

65–5 This histopathologic photograph demonstrates a pseudophakic eye with cystoid macular edema. Note the large cystic cavities.

65–6 This histopathologic correlate also demonstrates cystoid macular edema in a pseudophakic patient.

65–7 Extensive cystoid macular edema with large cystic cavities is noted in this patient.

Suggested Readings

Coscas, G, and Gaudrice, A: Natural course of nonaphakic cystoid macular edema, Surv Ophthalmol 28:471–484, 1984

Fine, BS, and Brucker, AJ: Macular edema and cystoid macular edema, Am J Ophthalmol 92:466–481, 1981

Gass, JDM, Anderson, DR, and Davis, EB: A clinical, fluorescein angiographic and electron microscopic correlation of cystoid macular edema, Am J Ophthalmol 100:82–86, 1985

Kramer, SG: Cystoid macular edema after aphakic penetrating keratoplasty, Ophthalmology 88:782–787, 1981

Meredith, TA, Reeser, FH, Topping, TM, and Aaberg, TM: Cystoid macular edema after retinal detachment surgery, Ophthalmology 87:1090–1095, 1980

Yanoff, M, Fine, BS, Brucker, AJ, and Eagle, RC, Jr: Pathology of human cystoid macular edema, Surv Ophthalmol 28:505–511, 1984

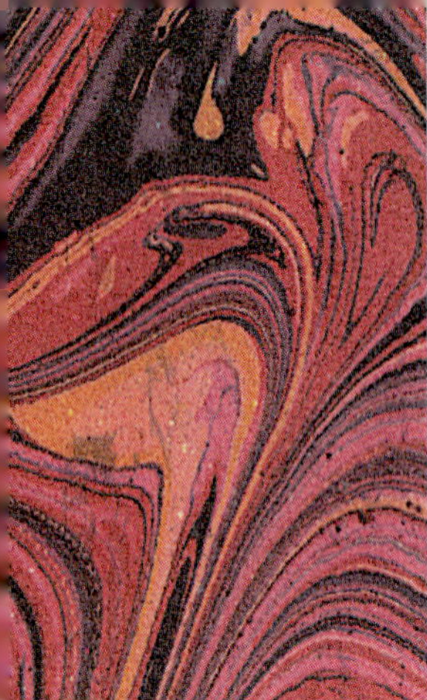

Chapter 66

Epiretinal Membranes

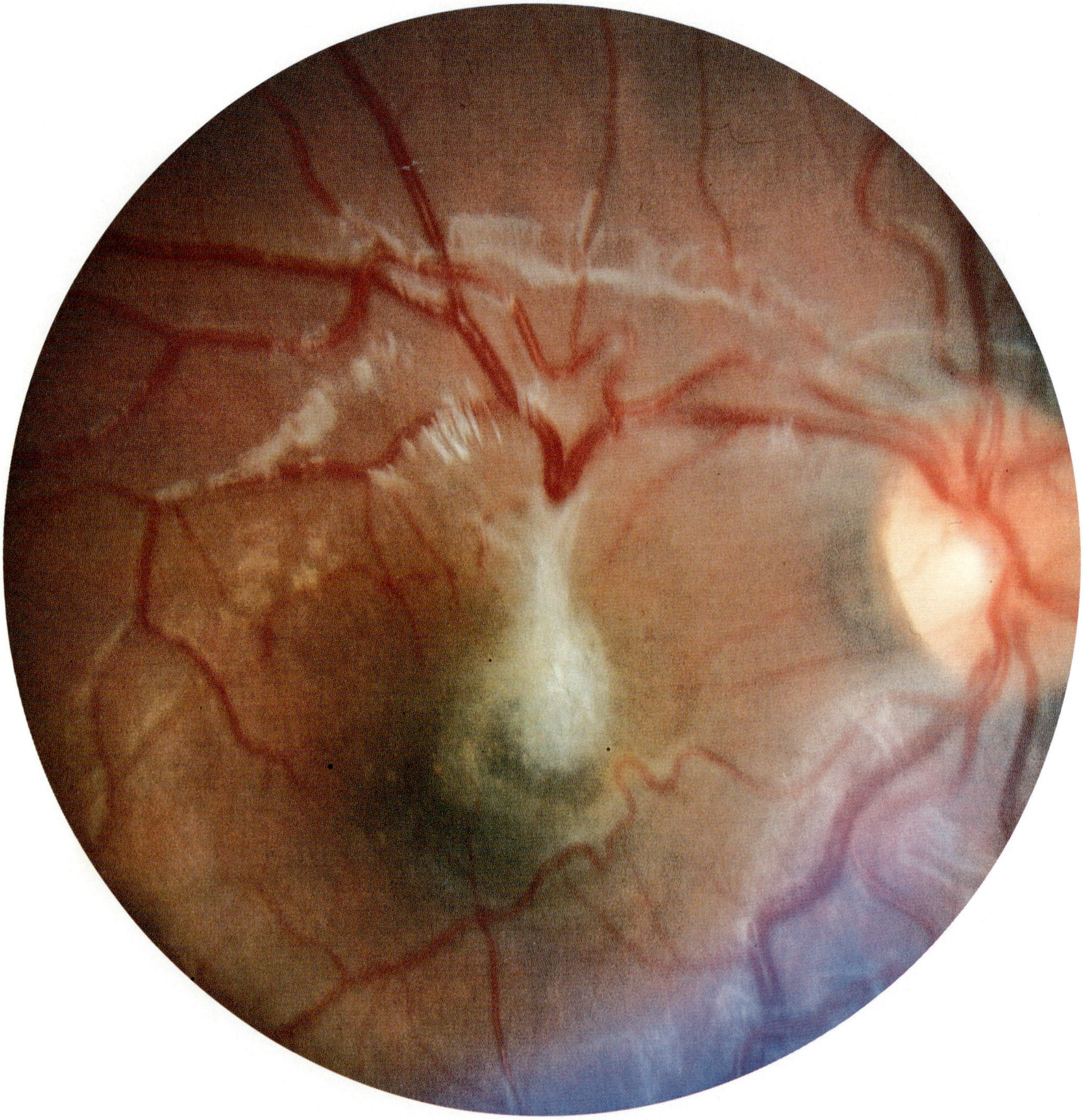

Idiopathic epiretinal membranes or macular puckers are usually seen in patients over 50 years of age. A glistening irregular light reflex may be noted early in this condition. Wrinkling of the internal limiting membrane, retinal striae, retinal tortuosity, cystoid macular edema, and fibrosis may also be noted. Foveal ectopia, punctate hemorrhages, and cotton-wool spots may also occur. Rarely, microaneurysm formation and dilation of the retinal capillaries are present. A pseudohole is an epiretinal membrane that gives the impression of a full-thickness macular hole. Epiretinal membranes can be removed via pars plana vitrectomy.

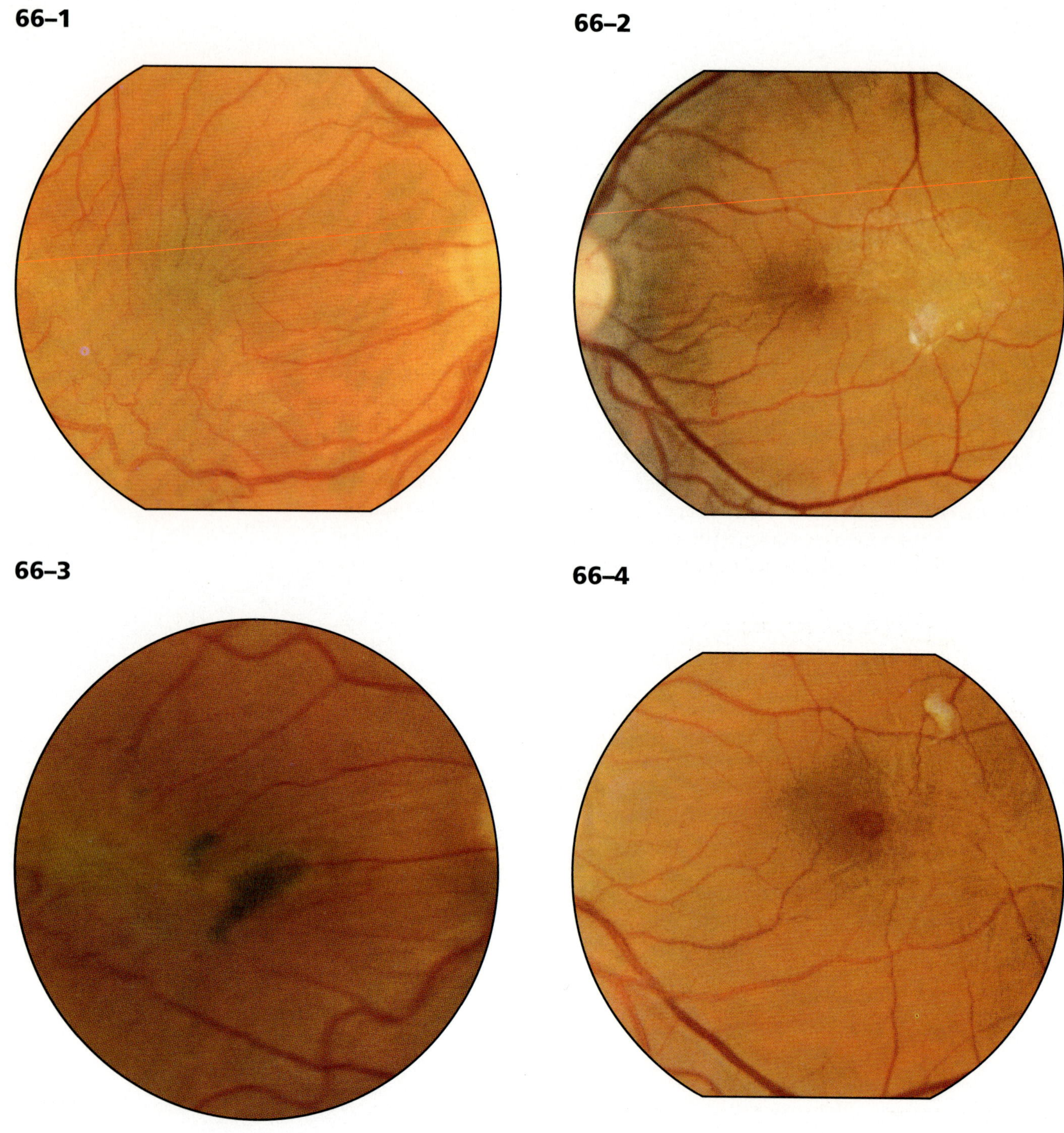

66–1 and 66–2 Idiopathic epiretinal membranes or macular puckers are demonstrated in these patients. Glial tissue is noted in front of the retina with tortuosity of the retinal vessels. Secondary folds may also develop. Note the cystic foveal changes due to traction (66–2).

66–3 Epiretinal membranes may be hyperpigmented, as demonstrated in this case.

66–4 This patient has an idiopathic epiretinal membrane, which is noted especially temporally. Ectopia of the fovea occurred secondary to traction from the epiretinal membrane. A pseudohole is evident.

66–5

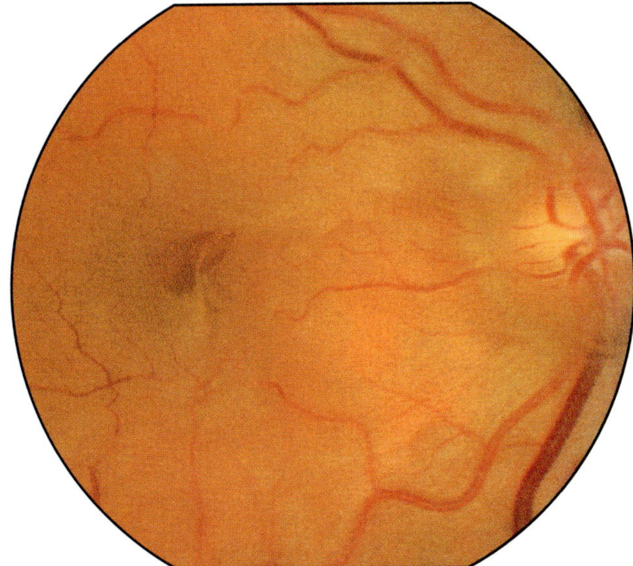

66–6

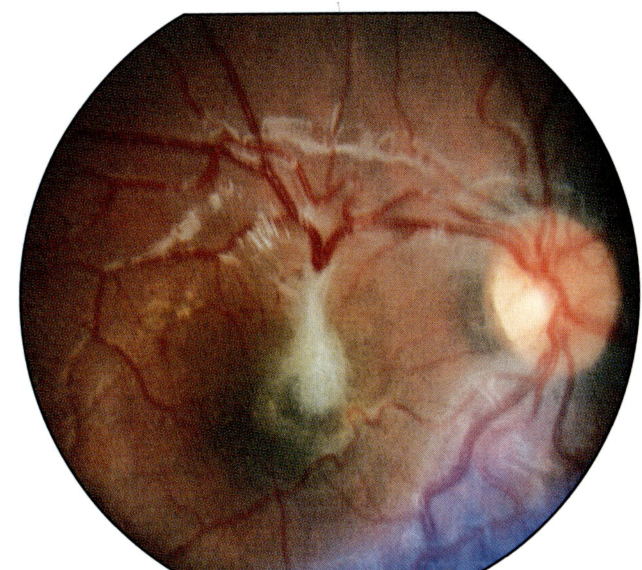

66–7

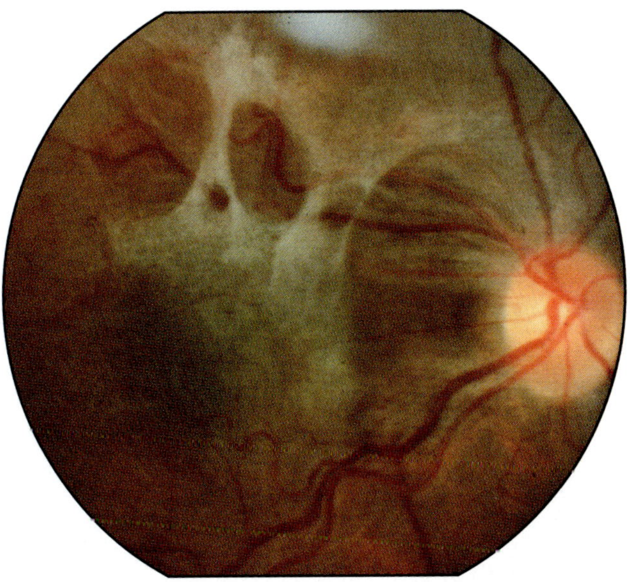

66–5 In the differential diagnosis of an epiretinal membrane is the vitreomacular traction syndrome. This patient has incomplete detachment of the posterior hyaloid. Note the early Vossius ring formation overlying and obscuring the optic nerve. This eye illustrates a maculopapillary tractional effect.

66–6 This case is an example of a congenital epiretinal membrane. Note the extensive glial tissue and tortuosity of the vessels induced by fibrous tractional bands.

66–7 Epiretinal membranes may vary from very minimally evident translucent tissue layers to semitranslucent membranes, and in some cases to extensive fibrous proliferation, as demonstrated in this patient.

66–5, *Courtesy of Mark Croswell.*

66–8

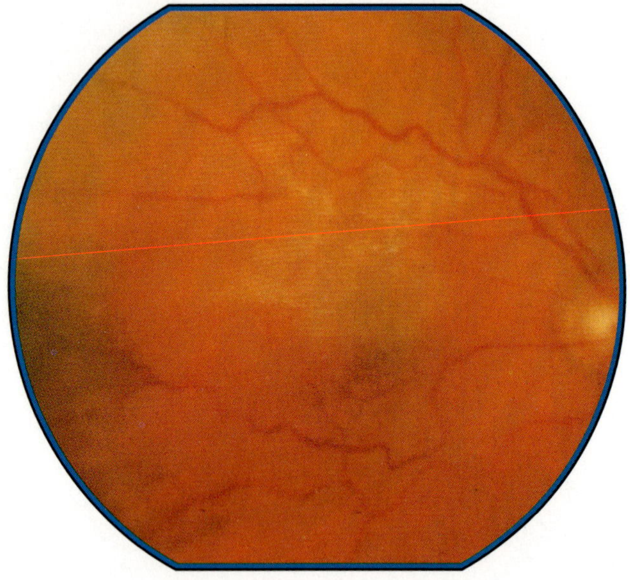

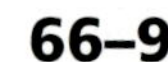

66–9

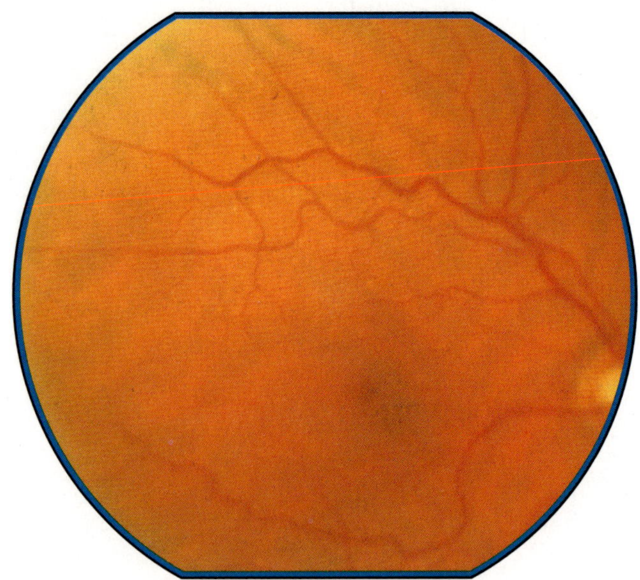

66–10

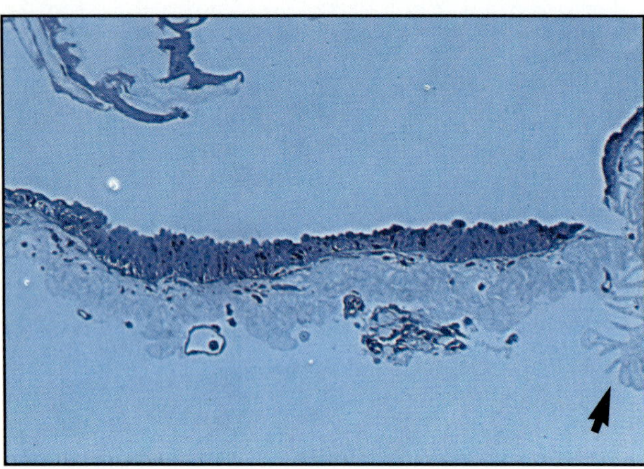

66–8 and 66–9 Epiretinal membranes can be removed by pars plana vitrectomy. Often there is a residual vitreoretinal interface disturbance, which will still be detectable postoperatively, as demonstrated in this patient (66–9).

66–10 This specimen from a pars plana vitrectomy for idiopathic macular pucker is composed of fibrovascular tissue, a fragment of internal limiting membrane at one end *(arrowhead),* and is lined internally by a single layer of tall retinal pigment epithelium.

66–8 *and* ***66–9,*** *Courtesy of Yale Fisher.*

Suggested Readings

Clarkson, JG, Green, WR, and Massof, D: A histopathologic review of 168 cases of preretinal membrane, Am J Ophthalmol 84:1–17, 1977

Fine, SL: Idiopathic preretinal macular fibrosis, Int Ophthalmol Clin 17:183–189, 1977

Green, WR, Kenyon, KR, Michels, RG, Gilbert, HD, and de la Cruz, Z: Ultrastructure of epiretinal membranes causing macular pucker after retinal re-attachment surgery, Trans Ophthalmol Soc UK 99:63–77, 1979

Green, WR: Periretinal proliferation. In Franklin, RM, ed: Proceedings of the symposium on retina and vitreous, New Orleans Academy of Ophthalmology, New Orleans, LA, 1993, New York, Kugler Publications, pp 195–222

Hagler, WS, and Aturaliya, U: Macular puckers after retinal detachment surgery, Br J Ophthalmol 55:451–457, 1971

Kampik, A, Kenyon, KR, Michels, RG, Green, WR, and de la Cruz, Z: Epiretinal and vitreous membranes: comparative study of 56 cases, Arch Ophthalmol 99:1445–1454, 1981

Kimmel, AS, Weingeist, TA, Blodi, CF, and Wells, KK: Idiopathic premacular gliosis in children and adolescents, Am J Ophthalmol 108:578–581, 1989

Lobes, LA, Jr, and Burton, TC: The incidence of macular pucker after retinal detachment surgery, Am J Ophthalmol 85:72–77, 1978

Margherio, RR, Cox, JS, Jr, Trese, MT, Murphy, PL, Johnson, J, and Minor, LA: Removal of epimacular membranes, Ophthalmology 92:1075–1083, 1985

McDonald, HR, and Aaberg, TM: Idiopathic epiretinal membranes, Semin Ophthalmol 1:189–195, 1986

McDonald, HR, Verre, WP, and Aaberg, TM: Surgical management of idiopathic epiretinal membranes, Ophthalmology 93:978–983, 1986

Michels, RG: Vitrectomy for macular pucker, Ophthalmology 91:1384–1388, 1984

Noble, KG, and Carr, RE: Idiopathic preretinal gliosis, Ophthalmology 89:521–523, 1982

Schatz, H: Essential fluorescein angiography: a conpendium of 100 classic cases, San Francisco, 1982, Pacific Medical Press

Smiddy, WE, Maguire, AM, Green, WR, Michels, RG, de la Cruz, Z, Enger, C, Jaeger, M, and Rice, TA: Idiopathic epiretinal membranes: ultrastructural characteristics and clinicopathologic correlation, Ophthalmology 96:811–821, 1989

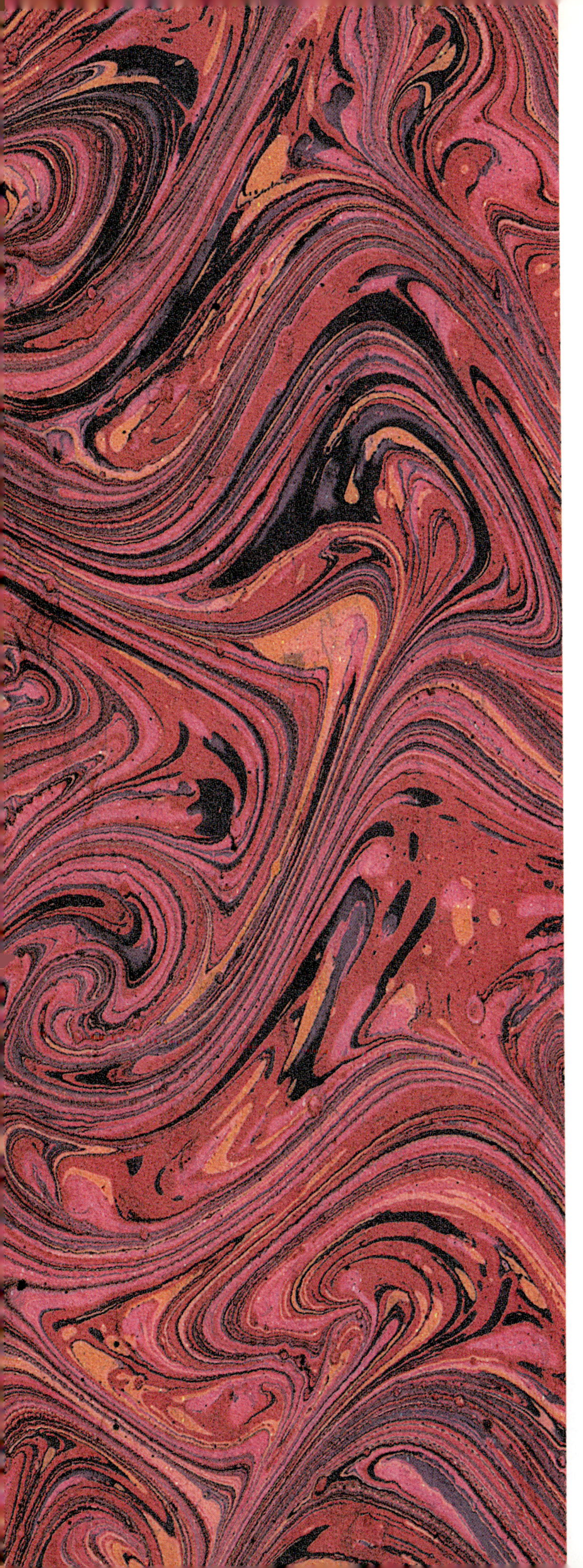

Part X

Optic Nerve Diseases

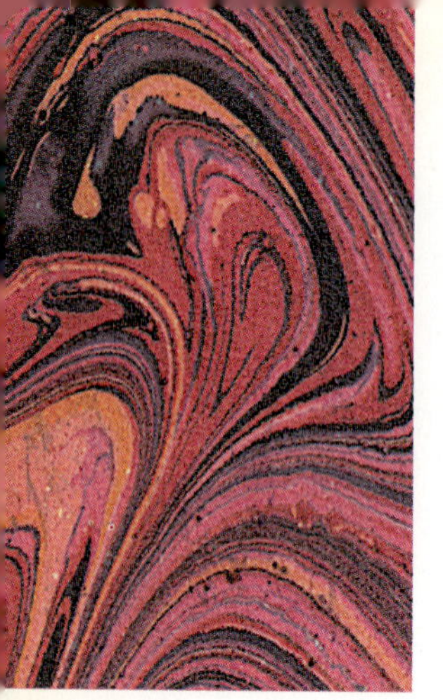

Chapter 67

Optic Disc Pits and Associated Serous Macular Detachments

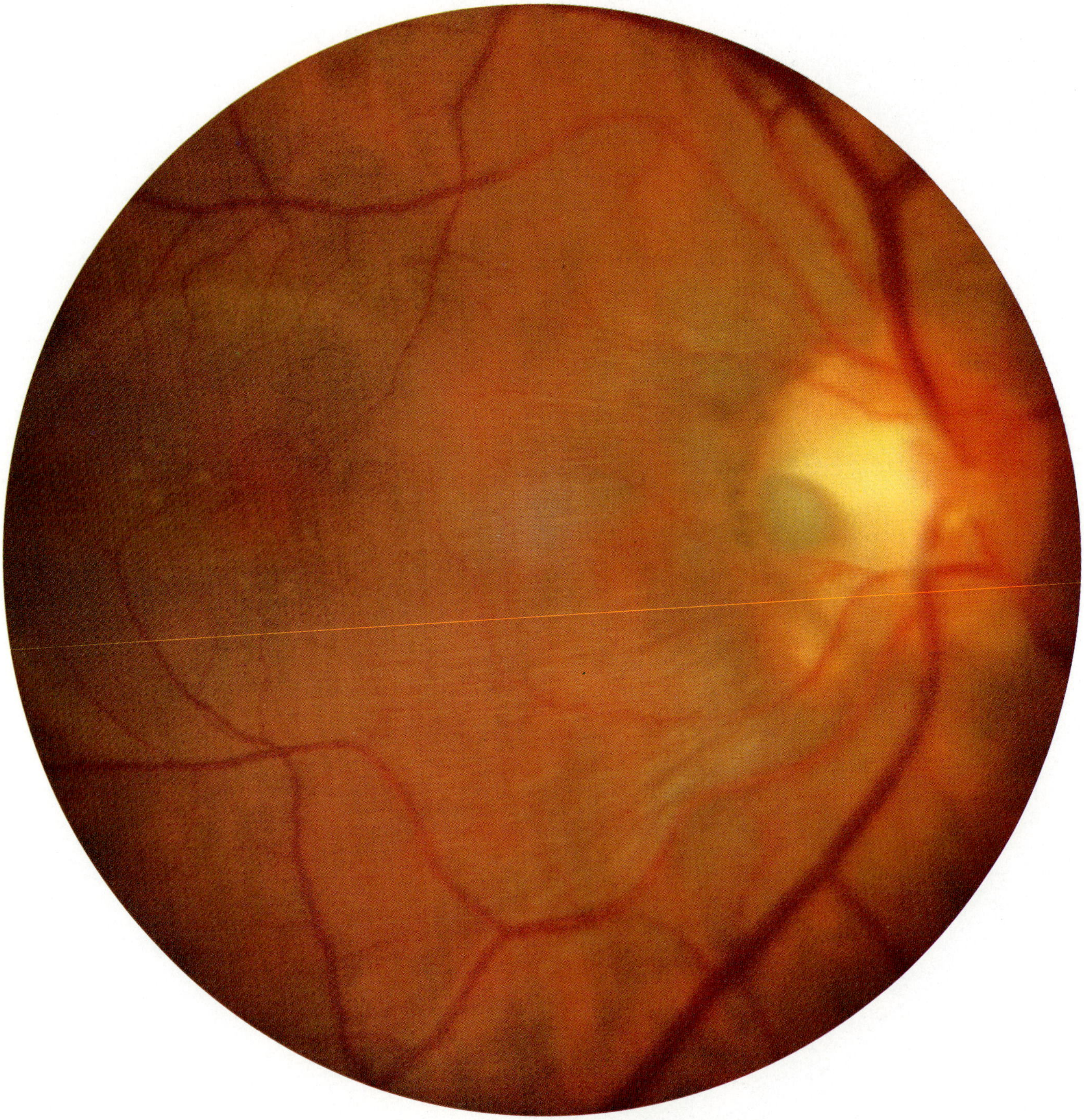

Optic disc pits may be associated with serous macular detachments. Subretinal fluid may occur from liquefied vitreous that travels through the optic pit. Optic disc pits are bilateral in approximately 10% to 15% of cases. Approximately 50% of patients with optic nerve pits have an associated serous retinal detachment or retinal pigment epithelial changes suggestive of a previous detachment. Rarely, a macular hole may be seen associated with an optic pit.

67–1 **67–1A**

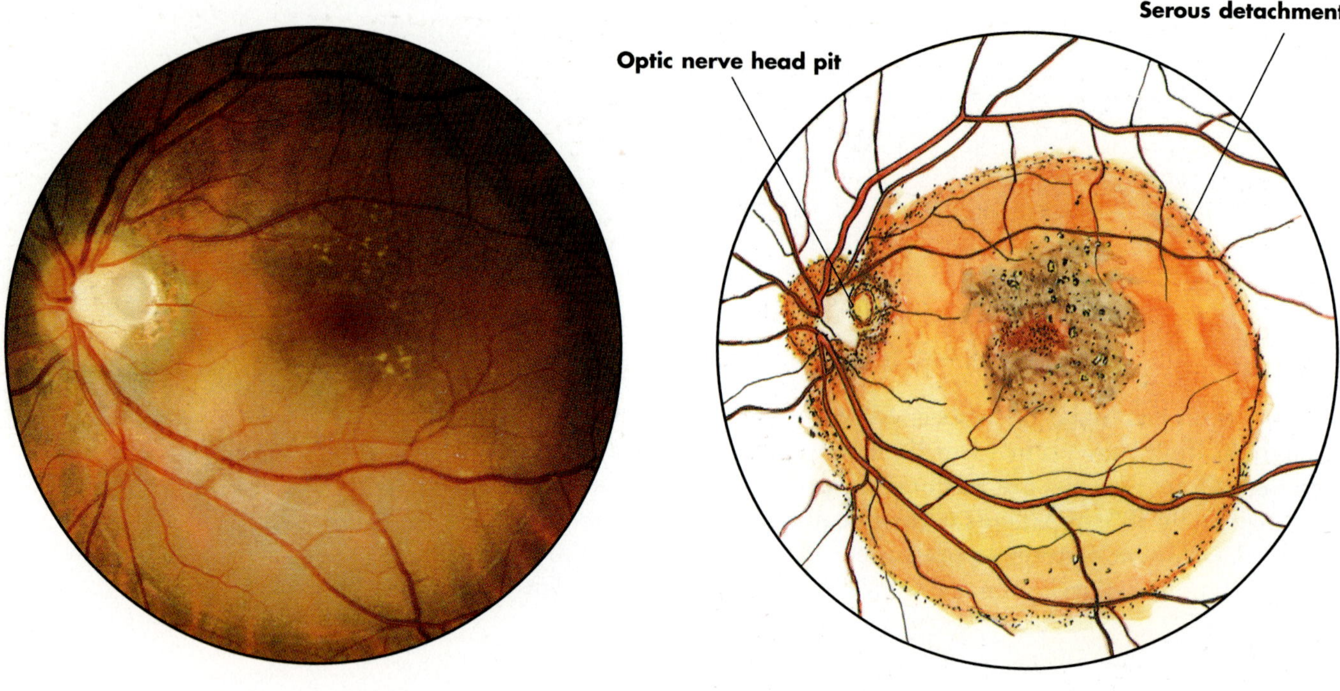

67–2

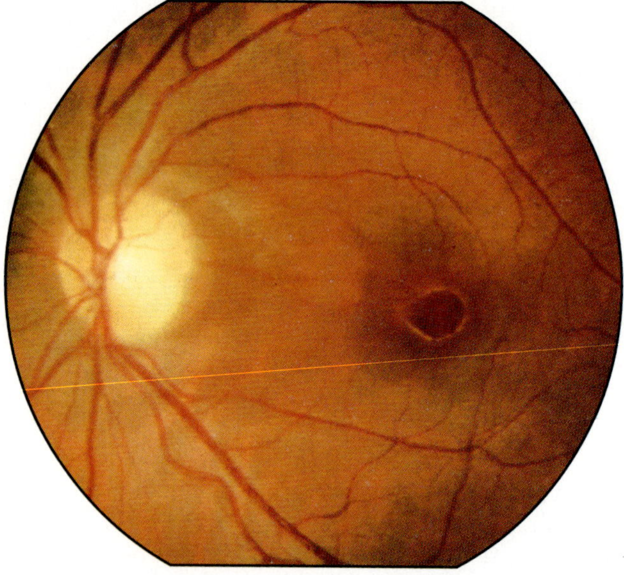

67–1 and 67–1A An optic disc pit with an associated serous detachment of the macula is demonstrated in this patient. An optic pit with secondary macular manifestations is believed to be due to a splitting of the retina or retinoschisis emanating from the optic disc margin toward the central macula. Subsequently, an outer retinal cyst may form in the schisis cavity. This leads to the commonly appreciated full retinal detachment or, in some instances, a dual elevation, consisting of the schisis cavity and the neurosensory retinal detachment as well.

67–2 This patient has an optic disc pit with a secondary macular hole.

67–3

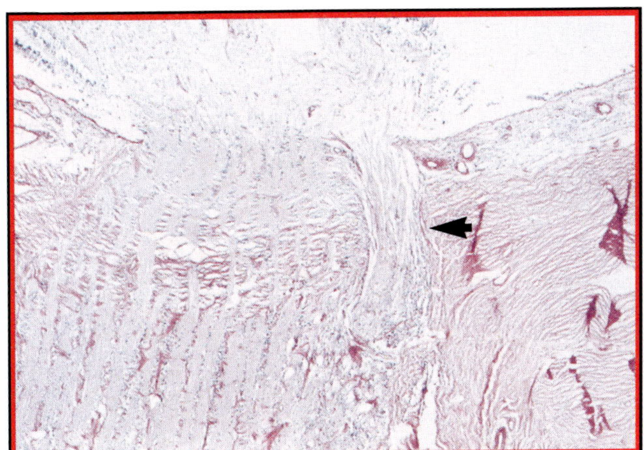

67–3A

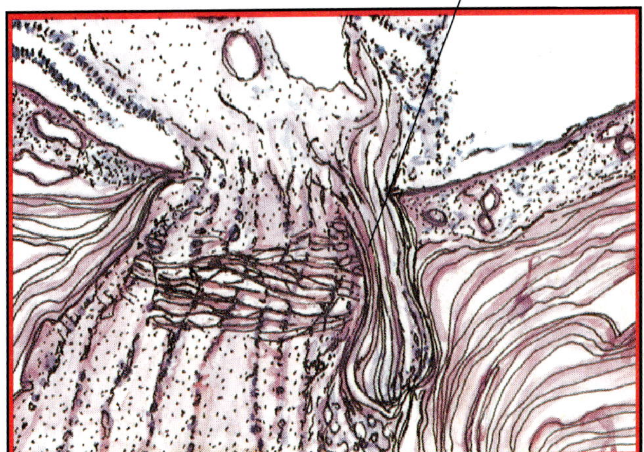

67–4

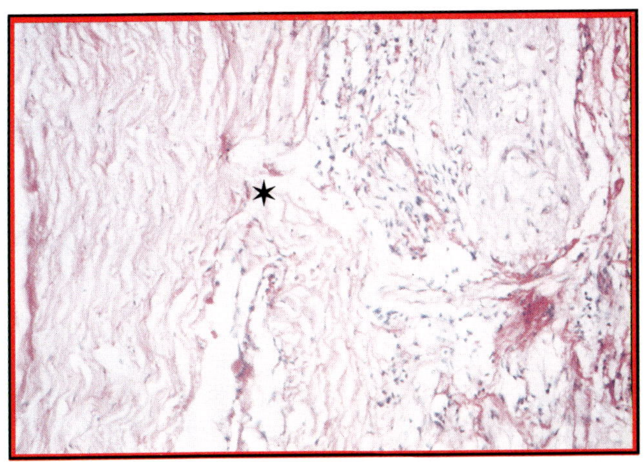

67–3 and 67–3A Light microscopy of an optic nerve head pit *(arrowhead)* in the temporal aspect of the optic nerve head.

67–4 Only a thin diaphanous tissue *(asterisk)* separates the optic pit from the subarachnoid space.

67–5

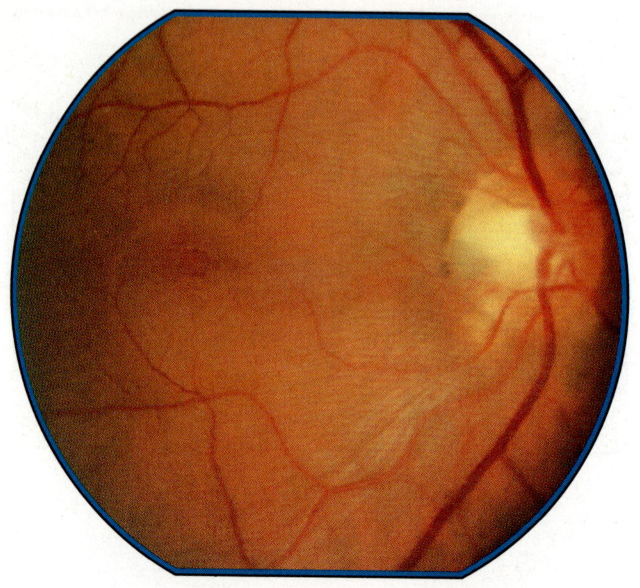

67–6

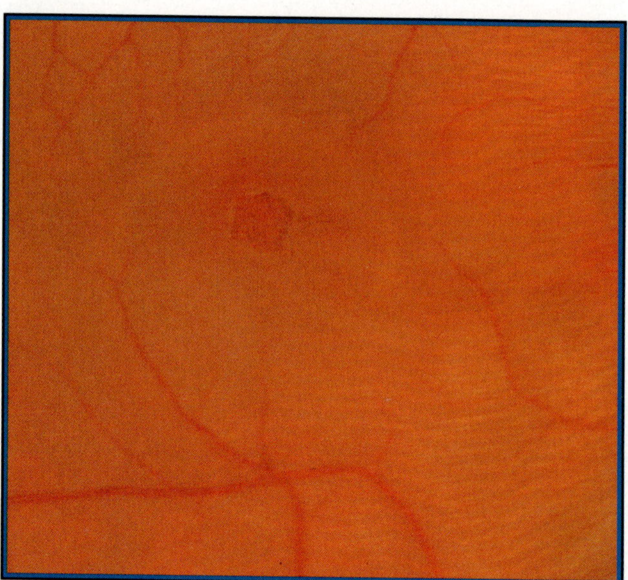

67–7 **67–8**

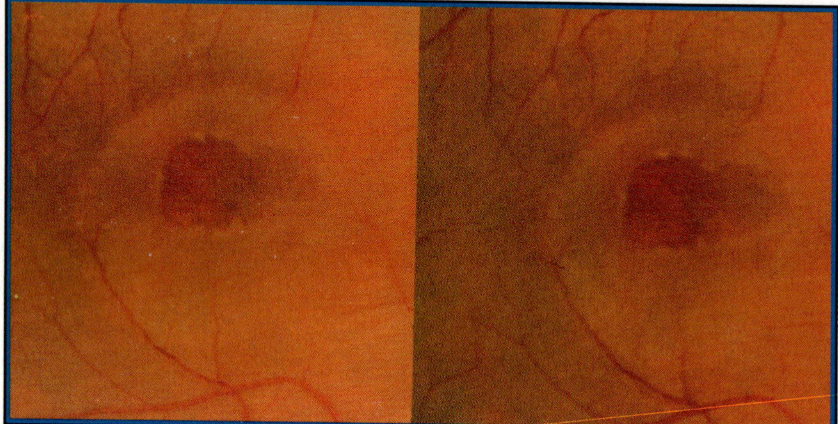

67–5 and 67–6 This patient has a schisis-like separation of the inner layers of the retina that connects to an optic pit and a hole in an outer layer separation.

67–7 and 67–8 With time, the macular hole in the outer layers enlarged (stereo view).

67–5 *through* ***67–8,*** *Courtesy of Dr. Harvey Lincoff. From Lincoff, H, Lopez, R, Kreissig, I, Yannuzzi, L, Cox, M, and Burton, T: Retinoschisis associated with optic nerve pits, Arch Ophthalmol 106:61–67, 1988.*

(Case continued on next page.)

67–9

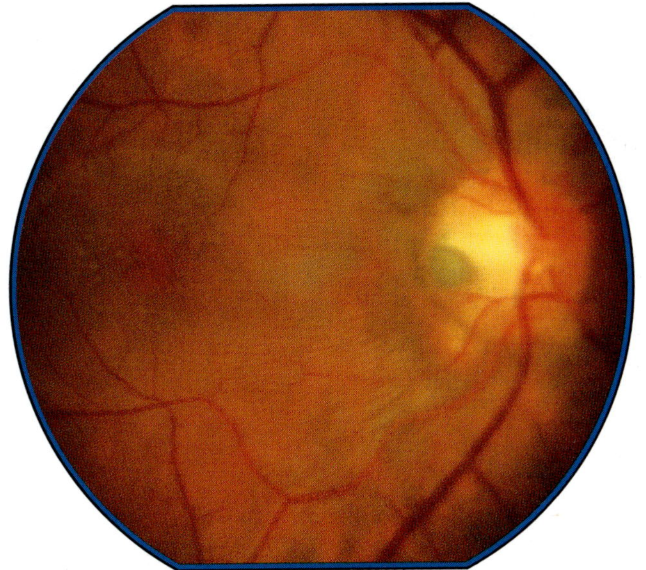

67–10

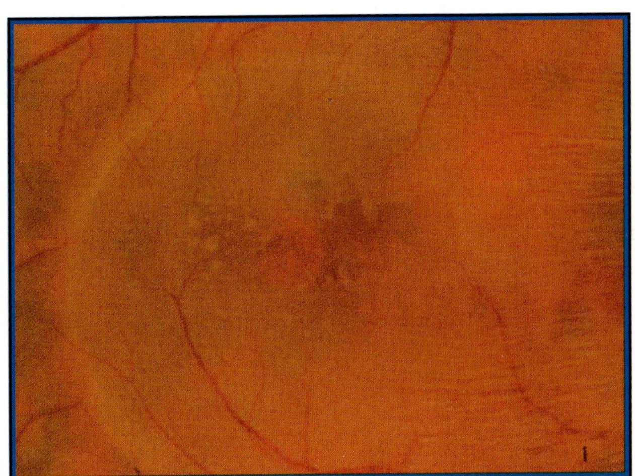

67–11

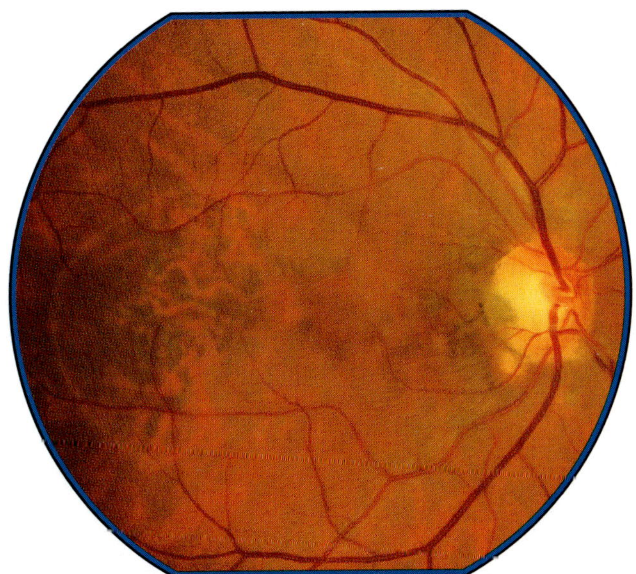

67–9 and 67–10 Further separation occurred.

67–11 Postoperatively, the lesion flattened.

67–9 *through* ***67–11,*** *Courtesy of Dr. Harvey Lincoff. From Lincoff, H, Lopez, R, Kreissig, I, Yannuzzi, L, Cox, M, and Burton, T: Retinoschisis associated with optic nerve pits, Arch Ophthalmol 106:61–67, 1988.*

Suggested Readings

Bonnet, M: Serous macular detachment associated with optic nerve pits, Graefe's Arch Clin Exp Ophthalmol 229:526–532, 1991

Brown, GC, Shields, JA, Patty, BE, and Goldberg, RE: Congenital pits of the optic nerve head. I. Experimental studies in collie dogs, Arch Ophthalmol 97:1341–1344, 1979

Brown, GC, and Tasman, WC: Congenital anomalies of the optic disk, New York, 1983, Grune & Stratton, Inc, pp 97–126

Cox, MS, Witherspoon, CD, Morris, RE, and Flynn, HW: Evolving techniques in the treatment of macular detachment caused by optic nerve pits, Ophthalmology 95:889–896, 1988

Ferry, AP: Macular detachment associated with congenital pit of the optic nerve head: pathologic findings in two cases simulating malignant melanoma of the choroid, Arch Ophthalmol 70:346–357, 1963

Gass, JDM: Steroscopic atlas of macular diseases, St Louis, 1977, Mosby–Year Book, pp 368–371

Kalina, RE, and Conrad, WC: Intrathecal fluorescein for serous macular detachment, Arch Ophthalmol 94:1421, 1976

Lincoff, H, Lopez, R, Kreissig, I, Yannuzzi, L, Cox, M, and Burton, T: Retinoschisis associated with optic nerve pits, Arch Ophthalmol 106:61–67, 1988

Pahwa, V: Optic pit and central serous detachment, Indian J Ophthalmol 33:175–176, 1985

Schatz, H, and McDonald, HR: Treatment of sensory retinal detachment associated optic nerve pit or coloboma, Ophthalmology 95:178–186, 1988

Slusher, MM, Weaver, RG, Greven, CM, Mundorf, TK, and Cashwell, LF: The spectrum of cavitary optic disc anomalies in a family, Ophthalmology 96:342–347, 1989

Sugar, HS: An explanation for the acquired macular pathology associated with congenital pits of the optic disc, Am J Ophthalmol 57:833–835, 1964

Theodossiadis, G: Evolution of congenital pit of the optic disk with macular detachment in photocoagulated and nonphotocoagulated eyes, Am J Ophthalmol 84:620–631, 1977

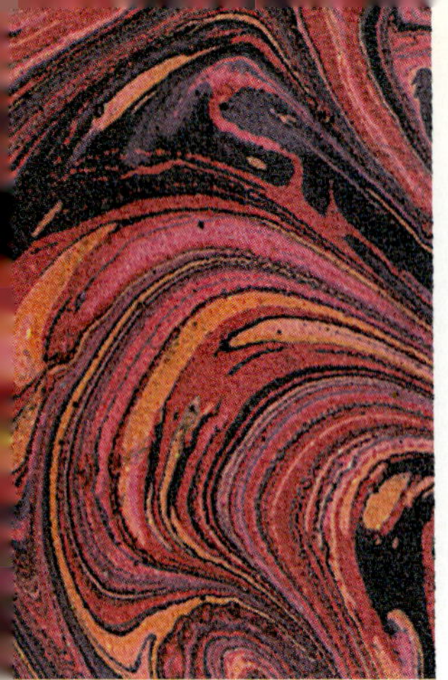

Chapter 68

Optic Disc Drusen

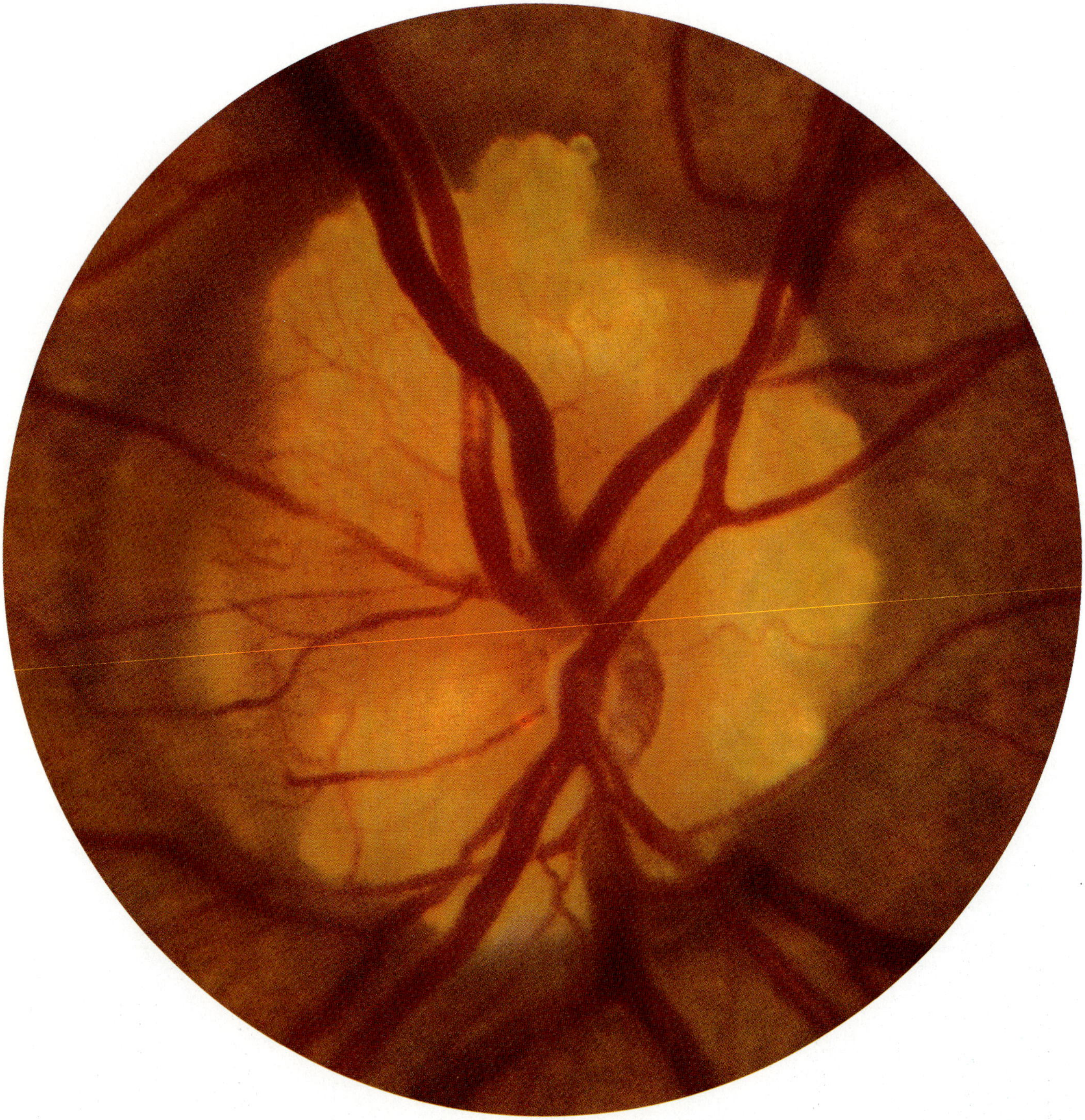

Optic disc drusen are bilateral in approximately two-thirds of cases. Usually, visual acuity is not affected. Visual field abnormalities, however, may be noted. Tumors should always be suspected in cases with optic disc drusen in which the visual acuity is abnormal.

68–1

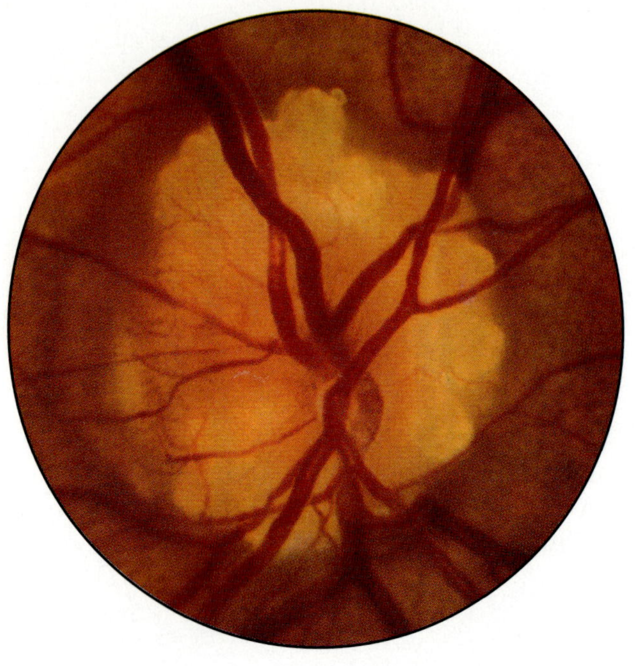

68–2

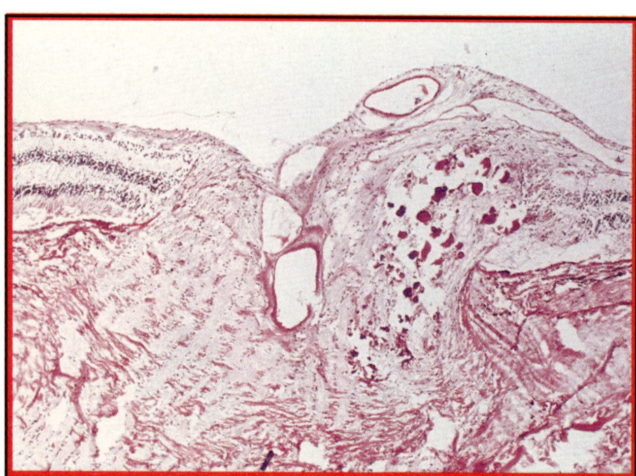

68–3

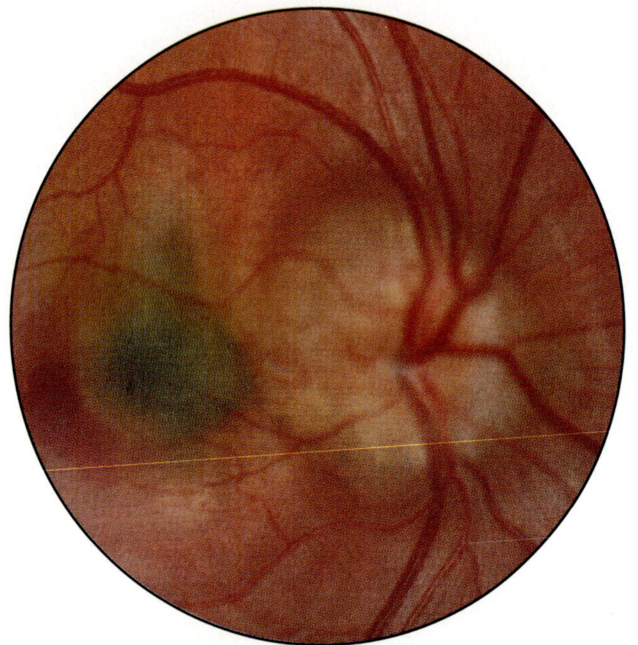

68–4

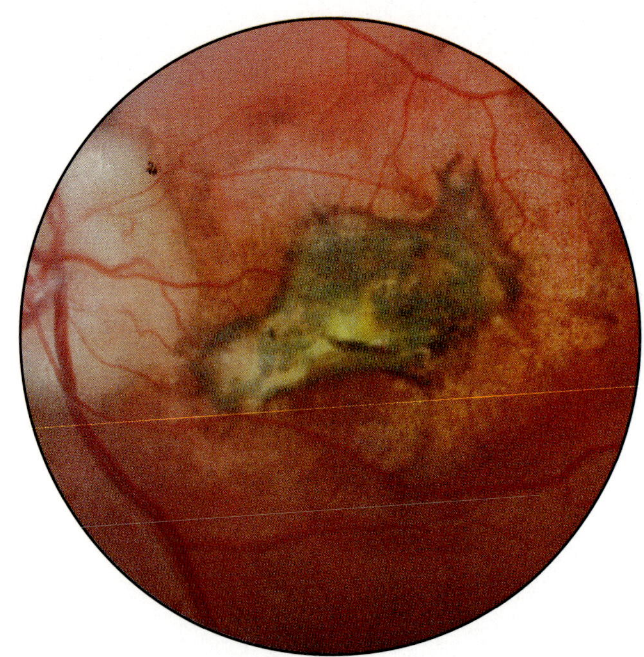

68–1 Optic disc drusen may appear as yellowish glistening globular masses at the optic disc. More commonly, optic nerve drusen are more subtle, with just one or two drusen noted on the optic disc.

68–2 Histopathologically, optic disc drusen consist of multiple globular calcified deposits in the nasal aspect of the optic disc.

68–3 Choroidal neovascularization may be associated with optic disc drusen.

68–4 This patient has disciform scarring secondary to choroidal neovascularization secondary to optic disc drusen.

68–1, *Courtesy of Mark Croswell.*

Suggested Readings

Arnold, AC: Improvement of visual field defects associated with optic disc drusen, North American Neuro-Ophthalmology Society Meeting, Steamboat Springs, Co, February 4–8, 1990

Bishara, S, and Feinsod, M: Visual evoked response as an aid in diagnosing optic nerve head drusen: Case report, J Pediatr Ophthalmol Strabismus 17:396–398, 1980

Friedman, DH, Gartner, S, and Modi, SS: Drusen of the optic disc: a retrospective study in cadaver eyes, Br J Ophthalmol 59:413–421, 1975

Gartner, S: Drusen of the optic disk in retinitis pigmentosa, Am J Ophthalmol 103:845, 1987

Hoyt, WF, and Beeston, D: The ocular fundus in neurologic disease, St Louis, 1966, Mosby–Year Book

Novack, RL, and Foos, RY: Drusen of the optic disk in retinitis pigmentosa, Am J Ophthalmol 103:44–47, 1987

Purcell, JJ, Jr, and Goldberg, RE: Hyaline bodies of the optic papilla and bilateral acute vascular occlusions, Ann Ophthalmol 6:1069–1076, 1974

Spencer, WH: In discussion of Tso, MOM: Pathology and pathogenesis of drusen of the optic nervehead, Ophthalmology 88:1079–1080, 1981

Ten Doesschate, MJL, and Manshot, WA: Optic disc drusen and central vein occlusion, Doc Ophthalmol 59:27–31, 1985

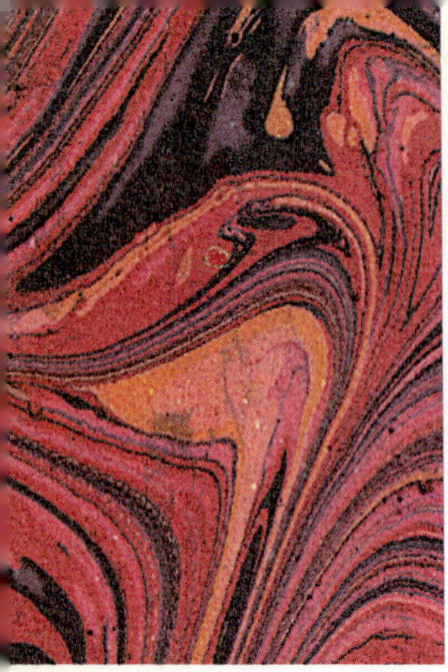

Chapter 69

Other Optic Nerve Diseases

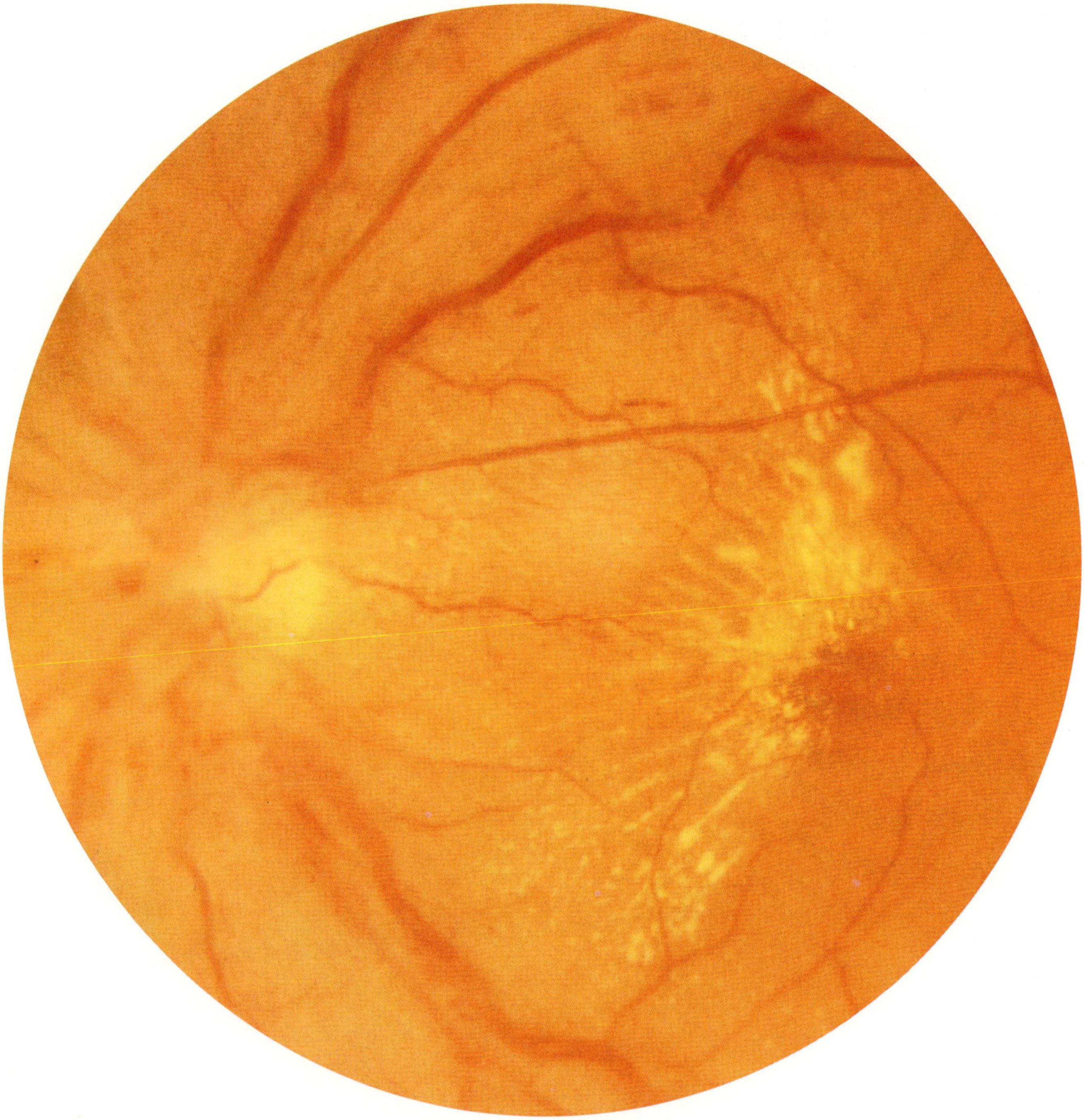

Various other optic nerve diseases may affect the retina. These conditions include Leber's stellate neuroretinitis, and optic disc abnormalities from tumors with secondary retinal changes.

69–1 MENINGIOMAS

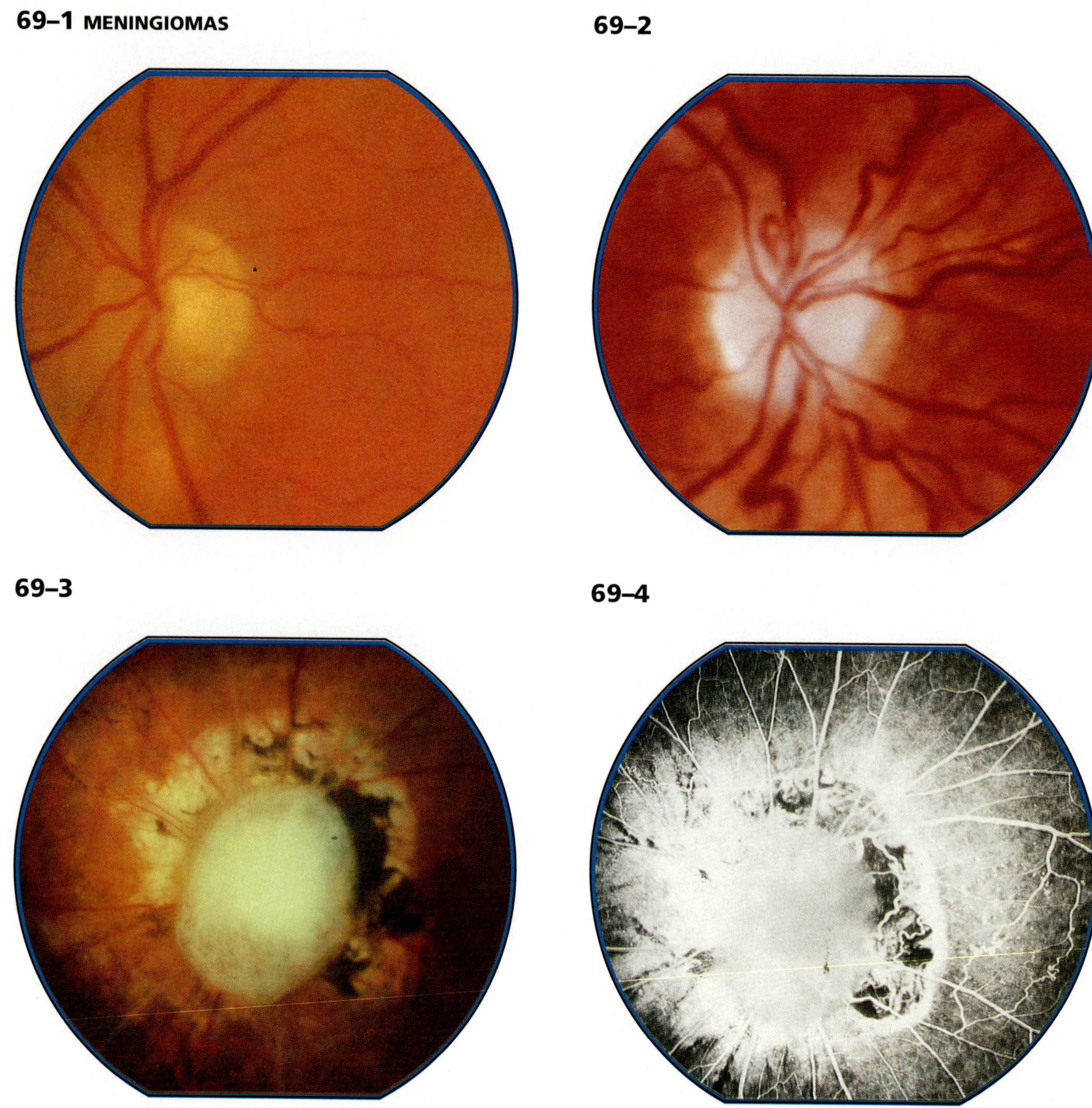

69–1 through 69–4 An optic nerve sheath meningioma may present as optic atrophy (69–1), optic atrophy with cilioretinal shunt vessels (69–2), or rarely with ill-defined optic nerve pathology and intraretinal anastomoses or shunts (69–3). Each of these patients had an optic nerve sheath meningioma. Note that optic nerve atrophy in combination with cilioretinal shunts is reflective of this disease; whereas cilioretinal shunts without optic neuropathy is indicative of an antecedent central retinal vein occlusion. Note also that in 69–3, the shunting is between the venous vessels within the retina, as is evident on the fluorescein angiogram (69–4).

69–2, *Courtesy of Dr. Jim Bollings.*

69–5

69–6 LEBER'S STELLATE NEURORETINITIS

69–7

69–8

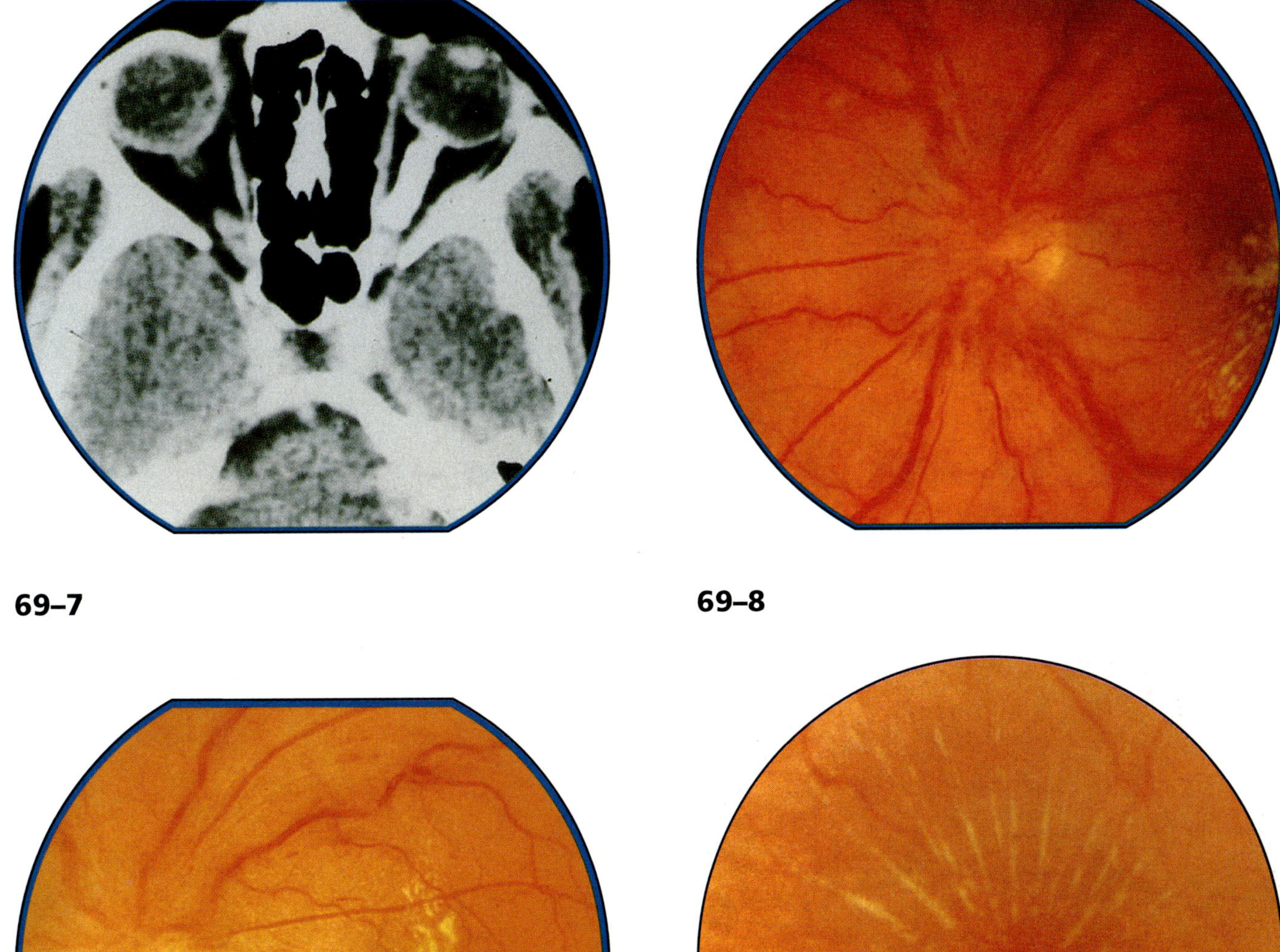

69–5 The optic nerve meningioma is imaged with computed axial tomography.

69–6 and 69–7 Leber's stellate neuroretinitis is a rare disorder in which there is hyperpermeability of the optic nerve vessels. Optic disc edema and a secondary macular star may be noted. Paramacular vessels do not show permeability abnormalities in this condition, which suggests that this disease is of optic nerve origin with secondary macular exudation.

69–8 This patient also has Leber's stellate neuroretinitis. Note the macular star.

***69–6** and **69–7,** Courtesy of Dr. Donald D'Amico. From Guyer, et al: Leber's idiopathic stellate neuroretinitis. In Albert and Jakobiec, eds: Principles and practice of ophthalmology, vol 2, Philadelphia, 1994, WB Saunders, pp 809–813.*

69–9 MULTIPLE SCLEROSIS

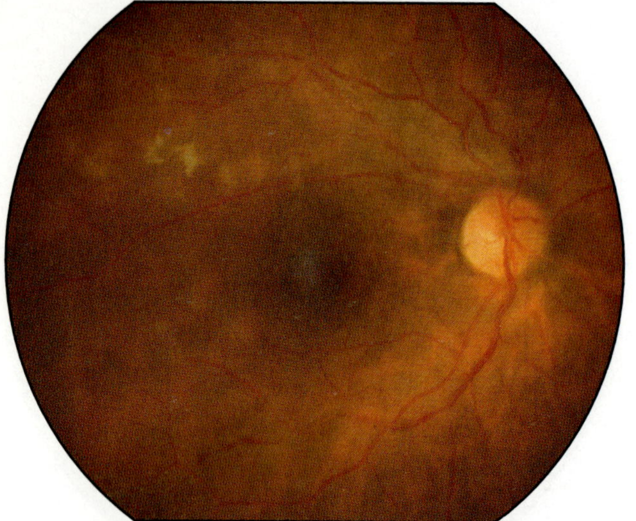

69–10

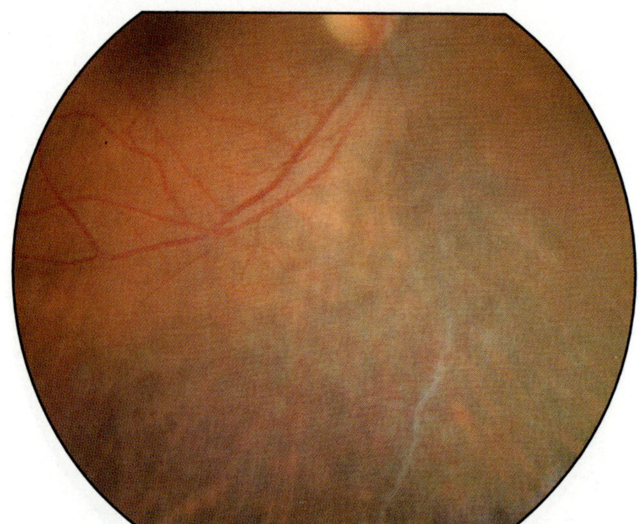

69–11

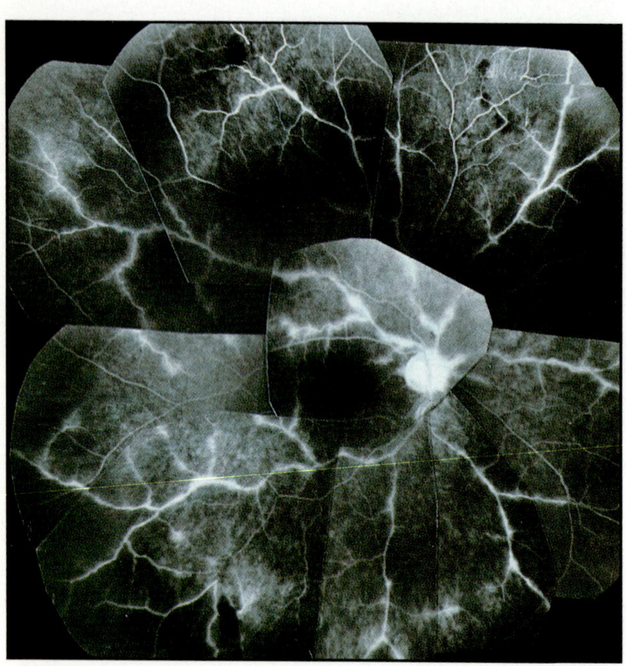

69–9 through 69–11 In addition to optic nerve pallor, patients with multiple sclerosis may show retinal vessel tortuosity, sheathing, and whitish-yellow deposition (69–9). Note the sheathing and capillary non-perfusion in this case (69–10). Fluorescein angiography shows vessel staining, non-perfusion, and blockage secondary to blood.

69–9 *through* ***69–11,*** *Courtesy of Dr. Anita Leys.*

Suggested Readings

Albert, DM, Searl, SS, and Craft, JL: Histologic and ultrastructural characteristics of temporal arteritis: the value of the temporal artery biopsy, Ophthalmology 89:1111, 1982

Francois, J, Verriest, G, and DeLaey, JJ: Leber's idiopathic stellate retinopathy, Am J Ophthalmol 68:340, 1969

Hayreh, SS: Anterior ischemic optic neuropathy. IV. Occurrence after cataract extraction, Arch Ophthalmol 98:1410, 1980

Kindler, P: Morning glory syndrome: unusual congenital optic disk anomaly, Am J Ophthalmol 69:376, 1970

Morse, PH, Leveille, AS, Antel, JP, and Burch, JV: Bilateral juxtapapillary subretinal neovascularization associated with pseudotumor cerebri, Am J Ophthalmol 91:312, 1981

Mosier, MA, Lieberman, MF, Green, WR, and Knox, DL: Hypoplasia of the optic nerve, Arch Ophthalmol 96:1437, 1978

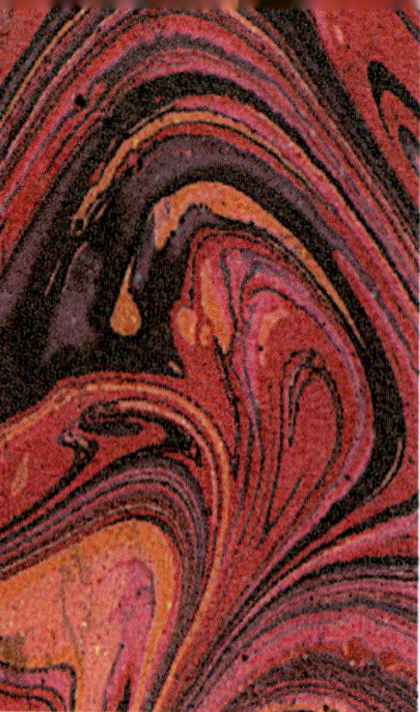

Chapter 70

Peripheral Retinal Diseases

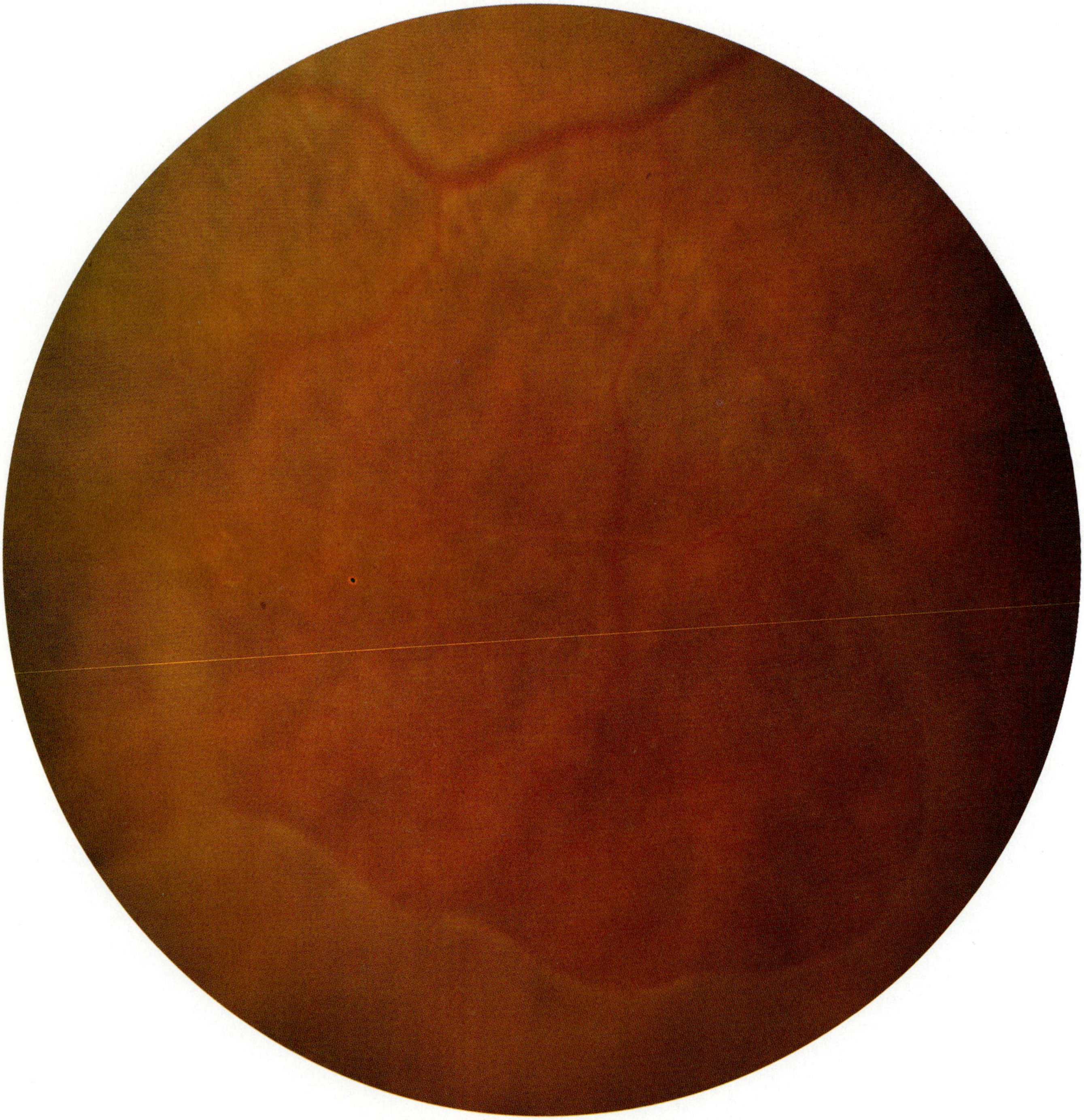

Various peripheral retinal conditions may predispose to retinal detachment. Other peripheral retinal lesions have little risk of progression to retinal detachment. In this chapter we survey various types of peripheral retinal pathology thanks to the contribution of Dr. Norman Byer.

70–1 MERIDIONAL FOLDS

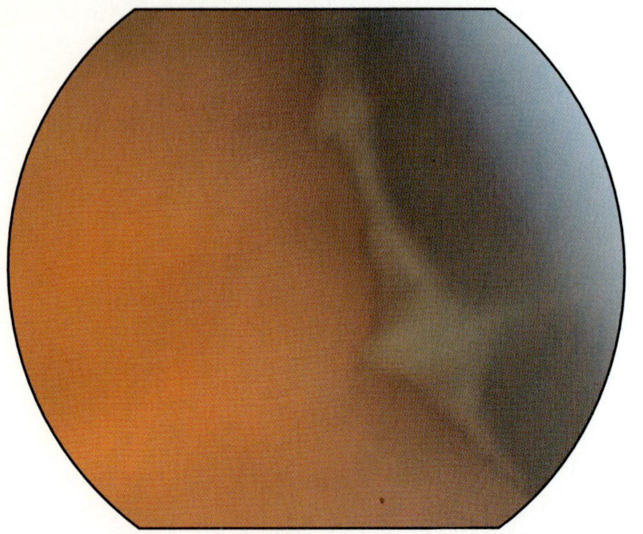

70–2 ENCLOSED ORA BAY

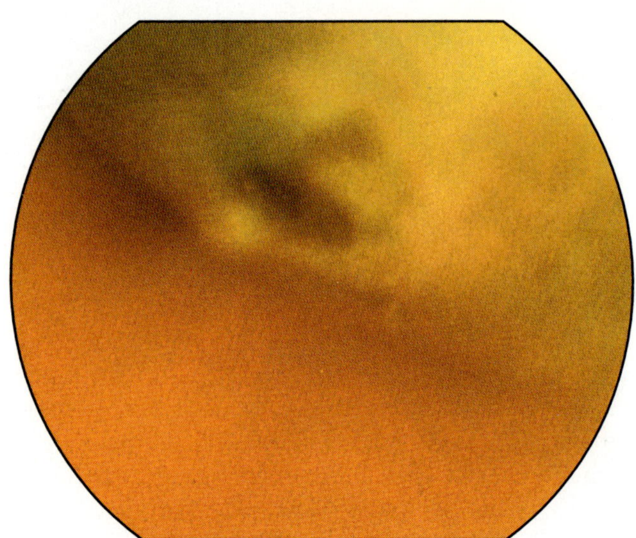

70–3 ORA PEARL

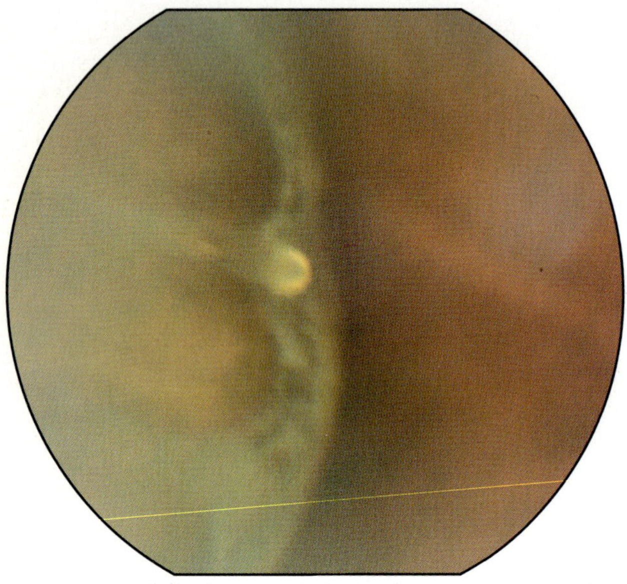

70–4 PARS PLANA CYST

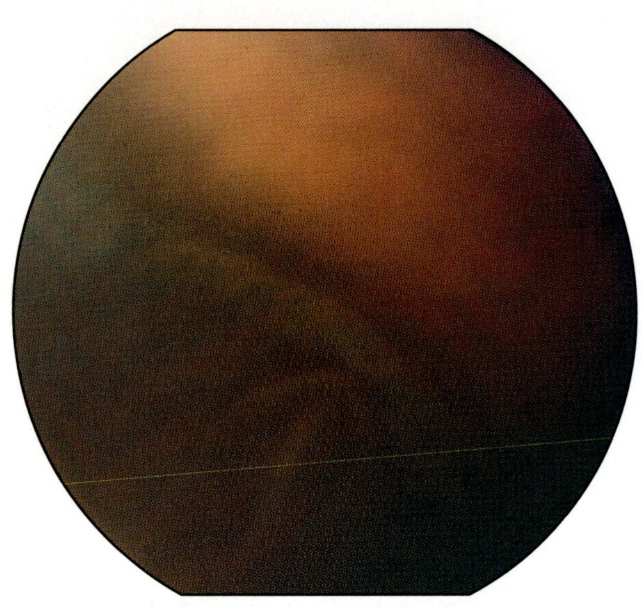

70–1 This patient has a meridional fold in the nasal ora serrata. Approximately 26% of the population have such meridional folds, which are elevated folds of retina. They are generally not of clinical significance.

70–2 An enclosed ora bay is demonstrated in this patient. This yellowish area represents an abortive dentate process. Enclosed ora bays are normal areas of the pars plana epithelium that have become enclosed as the developing teeth of the ora joins together. Enclosed ora bays are seen in approximately 6% of the population. They also are not of any clinical importance. However, they may be mistaken as retinal tears.

70–3 A pearl of the ora serrata is demonstrated in this patient. Note the whitish-yellow pearl at the ora.

70–4 This patient has a pars plana cyst.

***70-1** through **70-4,** Courtesy of Dr. Norman E. Byer. Reprinted from Byer, NE: The peripheral retina in profile: a stereoscopic atlas, Criterion Press.*

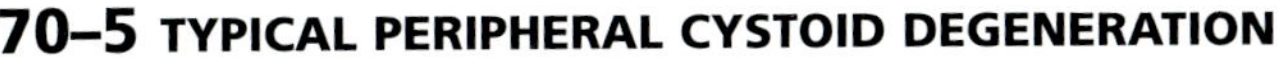

70–5 TYPICAL PERIPHERAL CYSTOID DEGENERATION

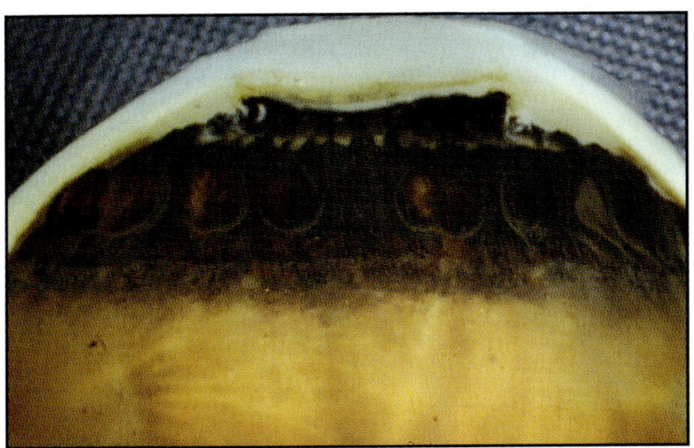

70–6 WHITE WITHOUT PRESSURE

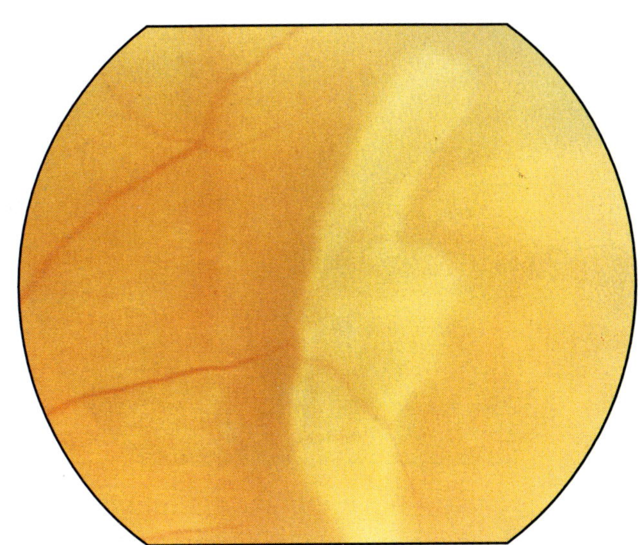

70–7 PAVING STONE DEGENERATION

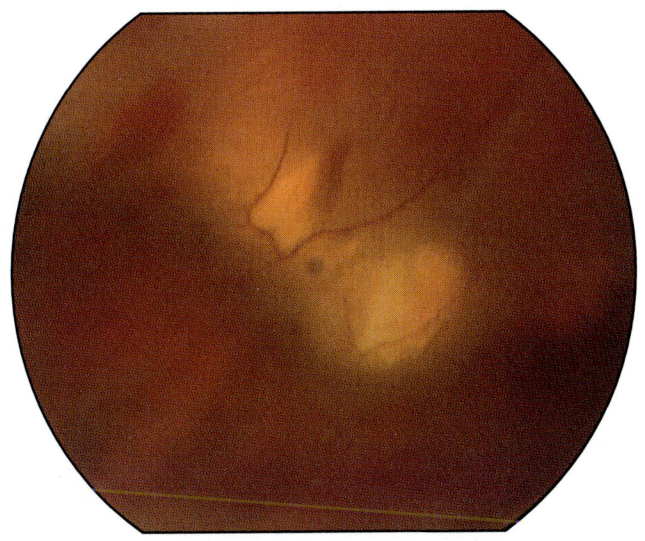

70–8 CYSTIC RETINAL TUFT

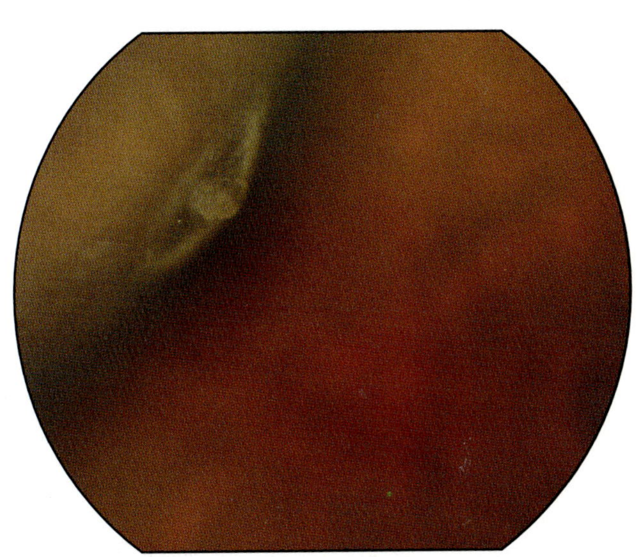

70–5 Gross appearance of typical peripheral cystoid degeneration.

70–6 This patient has white without pressure. This lesion is also not of clinical importance.

70–7 Paving stone or cobblestone degeneration is demonstrated in this patient. Note the yellow areas as well as the reddish areas of paving stone, which appear as pseudobreaks.

70–8 This 27-year-old white female has a cystic retinal tuft with subretinal fluid. Cystic retinal tufts are congenital lesions of the peripheral retina. They are noted in 5% of the population in autopsy studies and are a clinically significant lesion in that they are responsible for approximately 10% of primary retinal detachments. Approximately 0.28% of patients with these lesions will have retinal detachments secondary to the tuft. Cystic tufts are usually chalky white and elevated. Due to the high prevalence of these tufts in the general population, and the low risk of retinal detachment, cystic retinal tufts usually are not considered for prophylactic laser photocoagulation treatment.

***70-6** through **70-8**, Courtesy of Dr. Norman E. Byer. Reprinted from Byer, NE: The peripheral retina in profile: a stereoscopic atlas, Criterion Press.*

70–9 **LATTICE DEGENERATION**

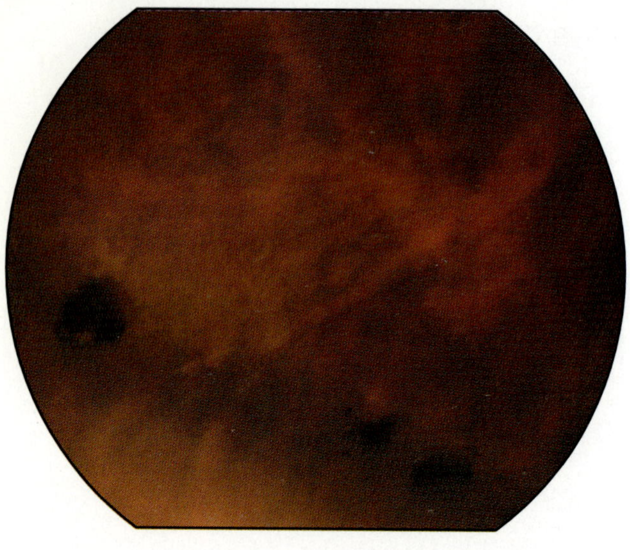

70–10

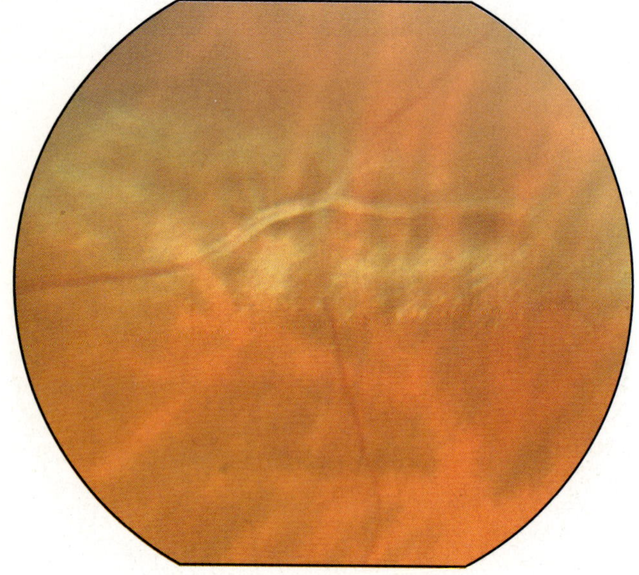

70–11

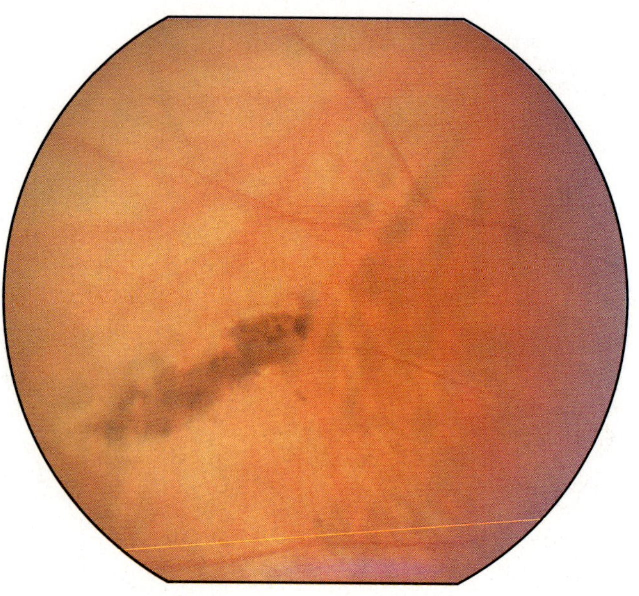

70–9 through 70–11 These patients have lattice degeneration, which is a common vitreoretinal degenerative disorder. It is a significant lesion in that it is associated with approximately 30% of clinical retinal detachments. However, only approximately 1% of eyes with lattice degeneration develop a retinal detachment. The first patient has lattice degeneration with a reddish crater, pigmentation, and whitish lines (70–9). The next two cases illustrate craters of lattice degeneration. These craters may be between horizontal whitish lines or be reddish and/or associated with pigmentary changes. On histopathologic examination, lattice degeneration consists of localized thinning of the inner retinal layers, a pocket of liquefied vitreous adjacent to the lesion, and abnormal attachments of the vitreous at the edge of the lesion. Most retinal detachments in lattice degeneration occur secondary to retinal tears that are not within the area of lattice degeneration.

70-9 *through* **70-11,** *Courtesy of Dr. Norman E. Byer. Reprinted from Byer, NE: The peripheral retina in profile: a stereoscopic atlas, Criterion Press.*

70–12 ATROPHIC RETINAL HOLES

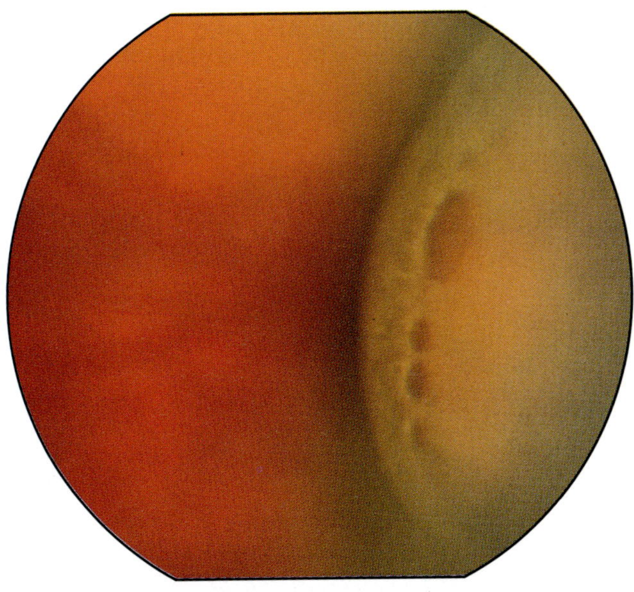

70–13 SYMPTOMATIC RETINAL TEAR WITH CYSTIC RETINAL TUFT

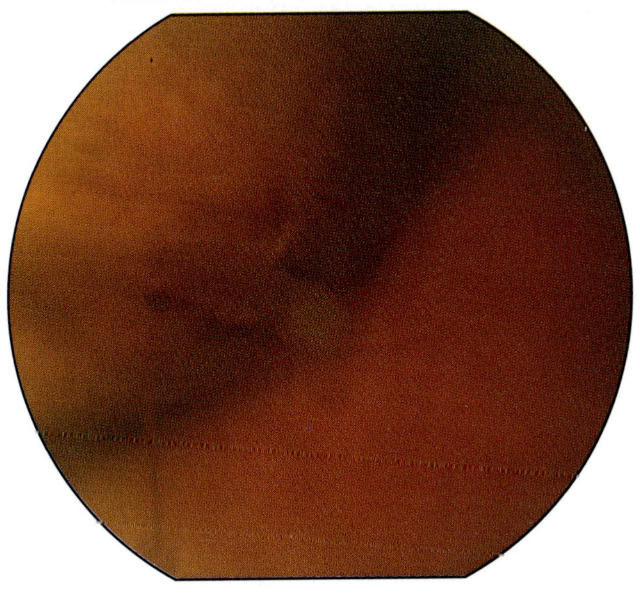

70–14 HORSESHOE RETINAL TEAR

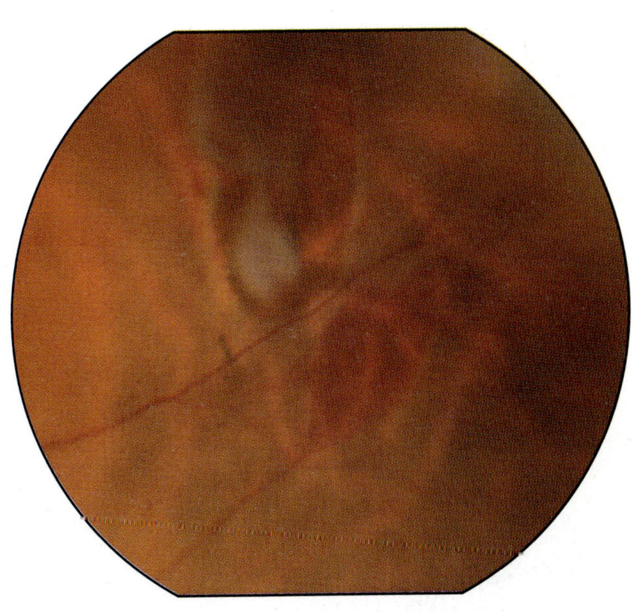

70–12 This patient has four asymptomatic round atrophic holes with a sizable subclinical retinal detachment. This eye has been stable for 21 years.

70–13 A symptomatic tear with a cystic retinal tuft is noted in this patient. Also note the hemorrhage around the tear.

70–14 This patient has an acute horseshoe-shaped retinal tear. The tear occurred secondary to a posterior vitreous detachment. Note the vitreous hemorrhage and the operculum. There are some mild pigmentary changes under the flap. In this case, the retina is torn in two places. Symptomatic retinal tears with associated vitreous traction have a high risk of developing a retinal detachment.

***70-12** through **70-14,** Courtesy of Dr. Norman E. Byer. Reprinted from Byer, NE: The peripheral retina in profile: a stereoscopic atlas, Criterion Press.*

70–15 RETINOSCHISIS

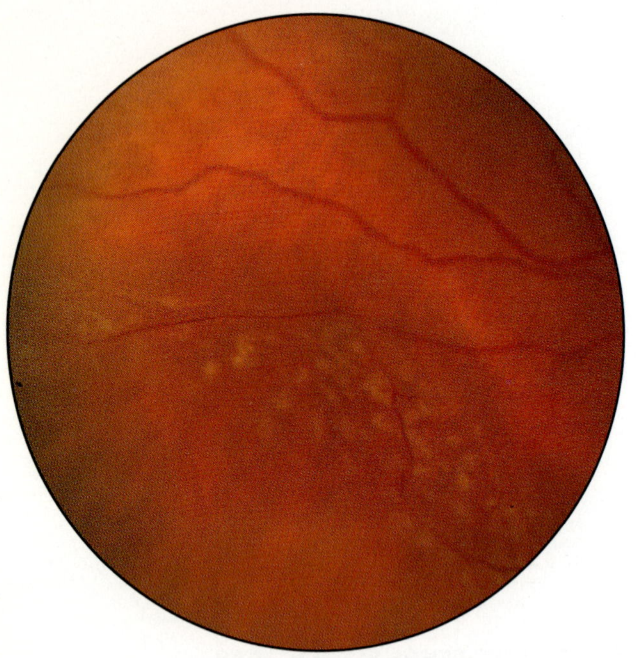

70–16

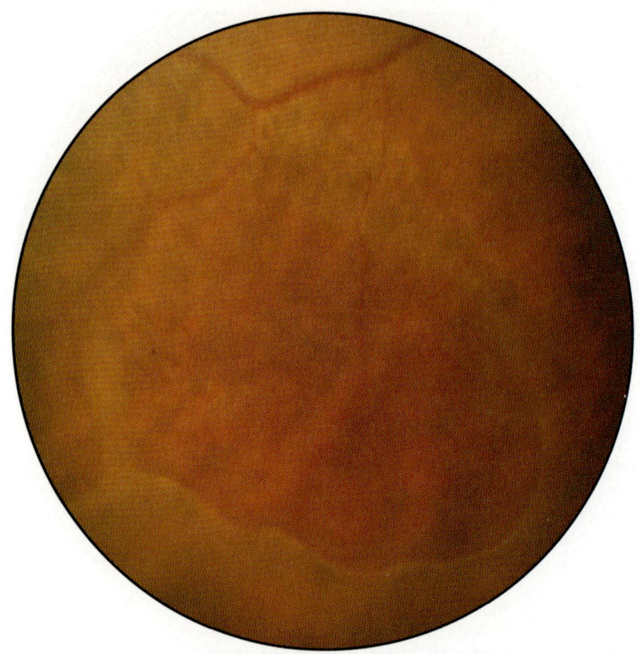

70–17 RHEGMATOGENOUS RETINAL DETACHMENT

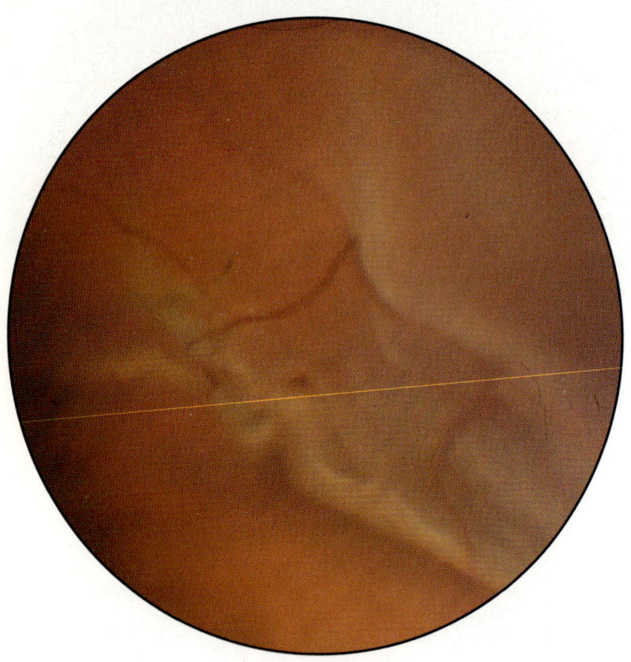

70–15 Senile retinoschisis or degenerative retinoschisis is an intraretinal degenerative disorder in the peripheral retina. It is noted in approximately 7% of the population over age 40. A separation of the retina into two separate layers occurs. A dome-shaped elevation in the peripheral retina is noted. This patient demonstrates retinoschisis. Note the small yellow-white flecks on the retinal surface. These spots are in the inner layer.

70–16 This patient also has retinoschisis with an outer layer hole. The lesion has been stable for 8 years. Note the yellow dots on the inner layer. Retinoschisis may be confused with a rhegmatogenous retinal detachment. Retinoschisis may develop true breaks in the outer layer in about 6% of cases and rarely in the inner layer (3% of cases). The risk of clinical retinal detachment in a patient with retinoschisis is probably 0.05%. The lesion should probably be treated only if there is a complicating associated clinical retinal detachment, which is extremely rare.

70–17 This patient has a rhegmatogenous retinal detachment with a tear in the lower retinal fold.

***70-15** and **70-16,** Courtesy of Dr. Norman E. Byer. Reprinted from Byer, NE: The peripheral retina in profile: a stereoscopic atlas, Criterion Press. **70-17,** Courtesy of Dr. Norman E. Byer.*

70–18 PROLIFERATIVE VITREORETINOPATHY (PVR)

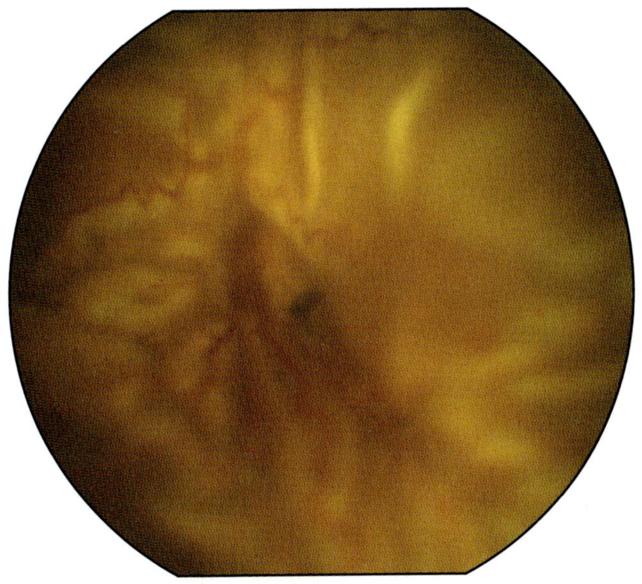

70–19

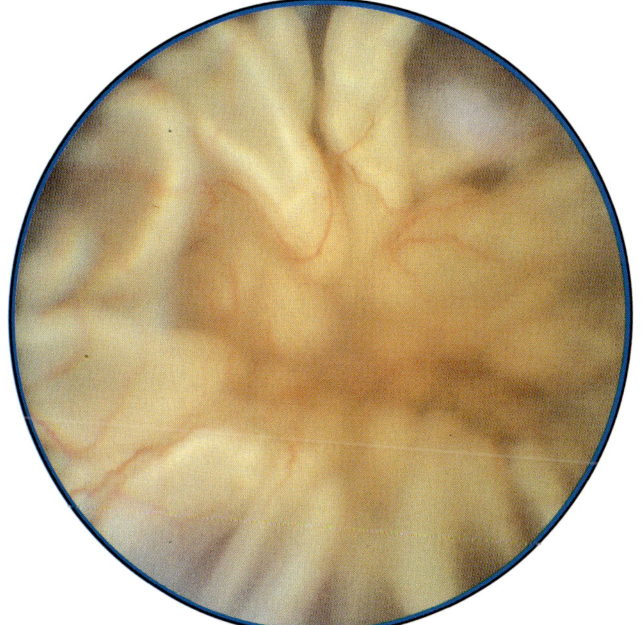

70–20

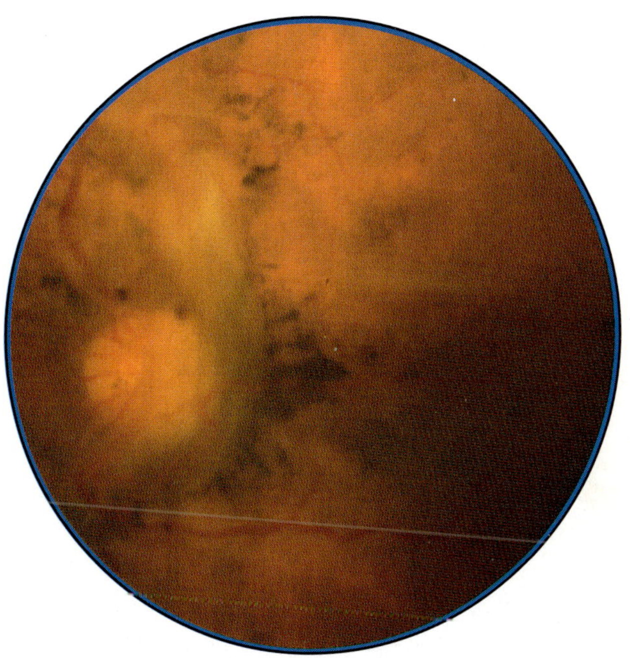

70–18 through 70–20 Proliferative vitreoretinopathy (PVR) is the leading cause of failure of retinal reattachment surgery. Note the fixed folds and PVR preoperatively (70–19); the retina was reattached following vitrectomy (70–20).

70-18 *through* ***70-20,*** *Courtesy of Dr. Yale Fisher.*

70–21 GIANT RETINAL TEARS

70–22

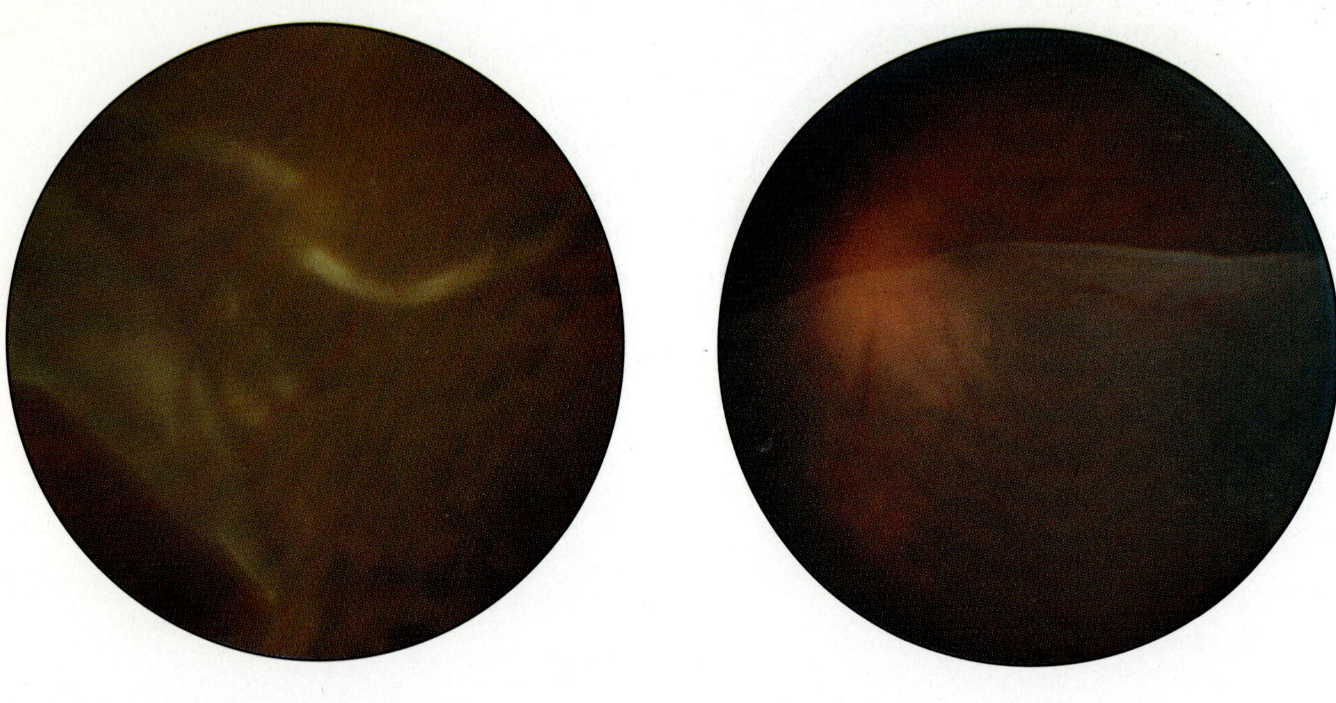

70–21 and 70–22 Giant retinal tears may also lead to retinal detachments.

70-21 *and* ***70-22,*** *Courtesy of Dr. Yale Fisher.*

Suggested Readings

Bell, F, and Stenstrom, W: Atlas of the peripheral retina, Philadelphia, 1983, WB Saunders

Byer, N: The peripheral retina in profile, Torrance, 1982, Criterion Press

Lewis, H, and Ryan, S: Medical and surgical retina, St Louis, 1994, Mosby–Year Book

Michels, RG, Wilkinson, CP, and Rice, TA: Retinal detachment, St Louis, 1990, Mosby–Year Book

Peyman, GA, and Schulman, JA: Intravitreal surgery, principles and practice, Connecticut, 1994, Appleton & Lange

Zinn, K: Clinical atlas of peripheral retina disorders, New York, 1988, Springer-Verlag

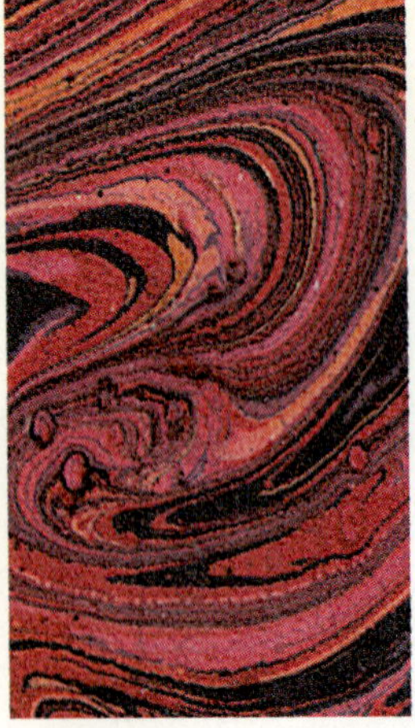

Credits

The Publisher wishes to acknowledge the following credits for figures found in *The Retina Atlas* by Lawrence A. Yannuzzi, David R. Guyer, and W. Richard Green

2-25 Courtesy of Dr. Albert Aandekerk. Spencer W: Ophthalmic pathology: an atlas and a textbook, ed 3, Philadelphia, 1985, WB Saunders.

2-66 Courtesy of Drs. Ron Carr and Ken Noble. Noble K: Hereditary chorioretinal dystrohies. In Freenean WA, ed: Practical atlas of retinal diseases and therapy, New York, 1993, Raven Press.

2-78 Courtesy of Dr. Jeffrey Shakin. Mietz H, Green WR, Wolff SM, Abundo GP: Foveal hypoplasia in complete oculocutaneous albinism. A histopathological study, Retina 12:254-260, 1992.

4-1, 4-2 Courtesy of Dr. Jerry Shields. Augsburger JJ: Fluorescein angiography of retinal and choroidal tumors. In Tasman W, Jaegar EA, eds: Duane's foundation of clinical ophthalmology, Philadelphia, 1991, JB Lippincott.

4-4, 4-5 Courtesy of Dr. Jerry Shields. Shields JA, Sanborn GE, Augsburger JJ, et al: Fluorescein angiography of retinoblastoma, Trans Am Ophthalmol Soc 80:98, 1982.

11-2 Courtesy of Dr. Edward B. McLean. McLean EB: Hamartoma of the retinal pigment epithelium, Am J Ophthalmol 82:227-231, 1976.

13-5 Courtesy of Dr. Evangelos Gragoudas. Augsburger JJ: Fluorescein angiography of retinal and choroidal tumors. In Tasman W, Jaegar EA, eds: Duane's foundation of clinical ophthalmology, Philadelphia, 1991, JB Lippincott.

13-6 Courtesy of Dr. Jerry Shields. Augsburger JJ, Golden MI, Shields JA: Fluorescein angiography of choroidal malignant melanomas with retinal invasion, Retina 4: 232-241, 1984.

13-7 Augsburger JJ: Fluorescein angiography of retinal and choroidal tumors. In Tasman W, Jaegar EA, eds: Duane's foundation of clinical ophthalmology, Philadelphia, 1991, JB Lippincott.

14-14 Courtesy of Dr. Evangelos Gragoudas. Guyer DG, et al: Indocyanine-green angiography of intraocular tumors, Semin Ophthalmol (Dec) 1993.

15-1 Courtesy of Dr. Jerry Shields. Augsburger JJ, Shields JA, Rafe CJ: Bilateral choroidal osteoma after nine years, Can J Ophthalmol 14:281-284, 1979.

15-3 Courtesy of Dr. Jerry Shields. Joffe L, Shields JA, Fitzgerald JR: Osseous choristoma of the choroid, Arch Ophthalmol 96: 1809-1812, 1978. Copyright 1978, American Medical Association.

15-6 Guyer DG, et al: Indocyanine-green angiography of intraocular tumors, Semin Ophthalmol (Dec) 1993.

17-5 Courtesy of WH Spencer. Green WR, McLean IW: In Spencer WH, ed: Ophthalmic pathology, ed 4, Philadelphia, 1995, WB Saunders.

18-22, 18-23
Sarks JP, Sarks SH, Killingsworth AI: Evolution of geographic atrophy of the retinal pigment epithelium, Eye 2: 552-577, 1988.

18-39 Macular Photocoagulation Study Group: Argon laser photocoagulation for senile macular degeneration: results of a randomized clinical trial, Arch Ophthalmol 100: 912-918, 1992.

22-8, 22-25, 22-104
Courtesy of Drs. Ron Carr and Ken Noble. Noble K: Hereditary chorioretinal dystrophies. In Freenean WA, ed: Practical atlas of retinal diseases and therapy, New York, 1993, Raven Press.

22-102, 22-103
Courtesy of Drs. Ron Carr and Ken Noble. From O'Donnell FE, Welch RB: Fenestrated sheen macular dystrophy, Arch Ophthalmol 97:1292-1296, 1979. Copyright 1979, American Medical Association.

24-17 Courtesy of Dr. Mark Lebwohl. Lebwohl M: Atlas of the skin and systemic disease, New York, 1995, Churchill Livingstone.

28-24, 28-25, 28-26
From Vaghefi HA, Green WR, Kelly JS, Sloan LL, Hoover RE, Patz A: Correlation of clinicopathologic findings in a patient: congenital night blindness, branch retinal vein occlusion, drusen of the optic nerve head, intraretinal pigmented lesion, Arch Ophthalmol 96: 2097-2104, 1978. Copyright 1978, American Medical Association.

31-15 Courtesy of Dr. Mark Lebwohl. Lebwohl M: Atlas of the skin and systemic disease, New York, 1995, Churchill Livingstone.

40-10 Courtesy of Dr. Jim Bollings. Buettner H, Bollings JP: Retinal arteriovenous communication in carotid occlusive disease, Amsterdam, 1992, Elsevier.

50-16 Funata M, et al: Intraocular gnathostomiasis, Retina 13:240-244, 1993.

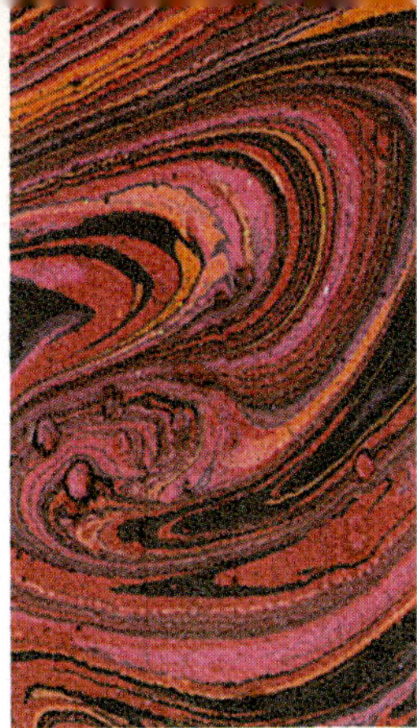

Index

D

E

V

W

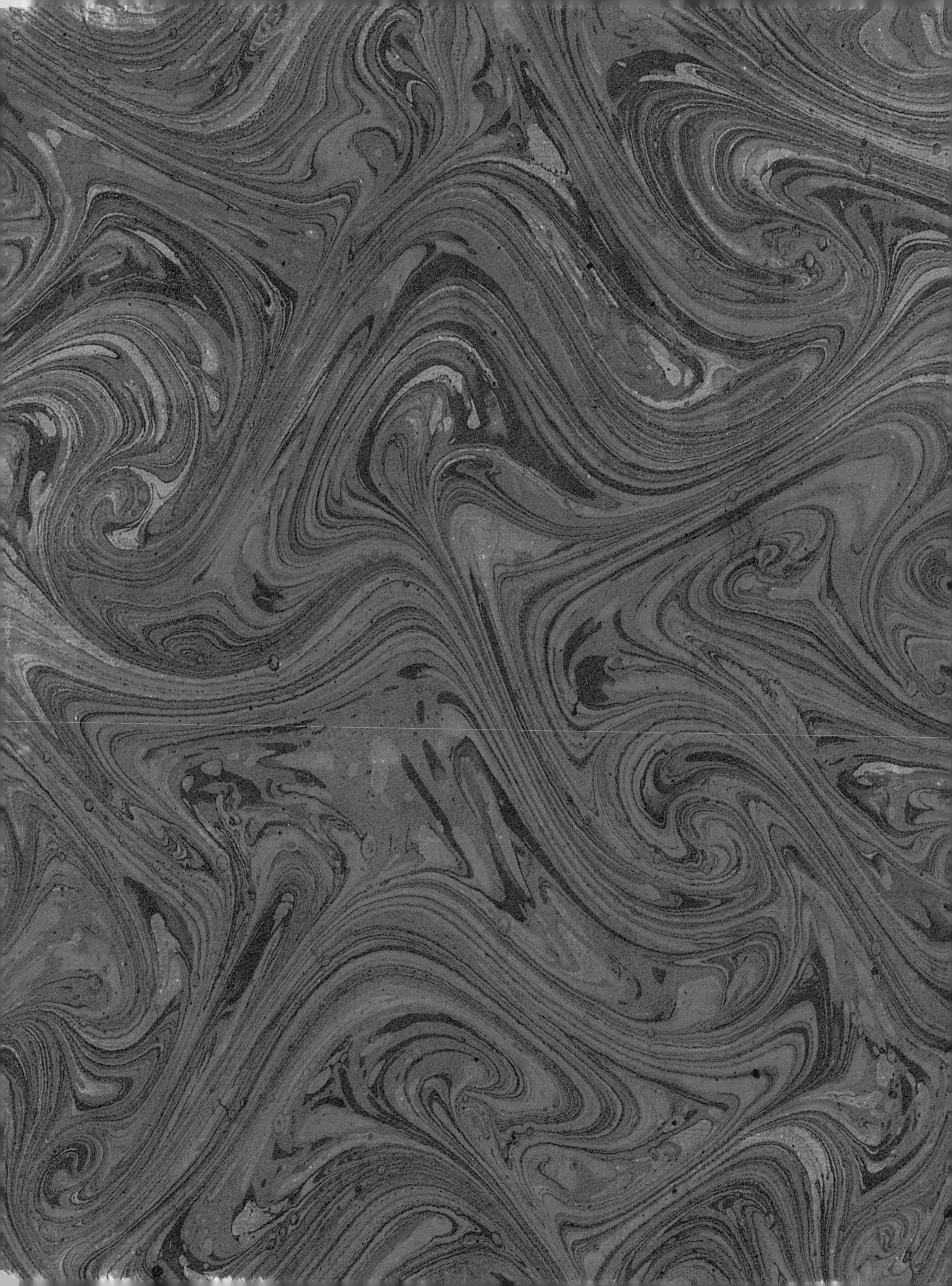